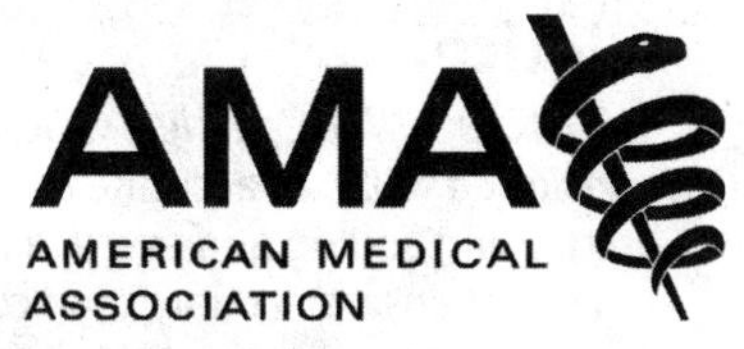

ICD-10-PCS
The Complete Official Draft Codebook

2015

Notice

ICD-10-PCS: The Complete Official Draft Codebook is designed to be an accurate and authoritative source regarding coding and every reasonable effort has been made to ensure accuracy and completeness of the content. However, the AMA makes no guarantee, warranty, or representation that this publication is accurate, complete, or without errors. It is understood that the AMA is not rendering any legal or other professional services or advice in this publication and that the AMA bears no liability for any results or consequences that may arise from the use of this book.

Our Commitment to Accuracy

The AMA is committed to producing accurate and reliable materials. To report corrections, please call the AMA Unified Service Center at (800) 621-8335.

Copyright

Made in the USA
ISBN 978-1-62202-012-6
OP201115
BQ45:09/14:13-0577

Acknowledgments

Anita Schmidt, BS, RHIT, *Clinical Technical Editor*
Karen Schmidt, BSN, *Technical Director*
Peggy Willard, CCS, ICD-10-CM/PCS Trainer, *Clinical Technical Editor*
Stacy Perry, *Manager, Desktop Publishing*
Tracy Betzler, *Senior Desktop Publishing Specialist*
Hope M. Dunn, *Senior Desktop Publishing Specialist*
Katie Russell, *Desktop Publishing Specialist*
Kate Holden, *Editor*

Anita Schmidt, BS, RHIT

Ms. Schmidt has expertise in Level I Adult and Pediatric Trauma hospital coding, specializing in ICD-9-CM, DRG, and CPT coding. Her experience includes analysis of medical record documentation and assignment of ICD-9-CM codes and DRGs, and CPT code assignments for same-day surgery cases. She has conducted coding training and auditing inclusive of DRG validation, conducted electronic health record training, and worked with clinical documentation specialists to identify documentation needs and potential areas for physician education. Ms. Schmidt is an active member of the American Health Information Management Association (AHIMA) and the Minnesota Health Information Management Association (MHIMA).

Karen Schmidt, BSN

Ms. Schmidt has more than 25 years of health care experience beginning with a strong clinical background in critical care nursing and later functioning as director of case management, including the components of quality assurance, utilization management, concurrent coding, case-mix analysis, and discharge planning. Her areas of expertise include ICD-9-CM/DRG coding, outpatient observation, billing compliance, implementation of concurrent coding methodology, and physician documentation education. She is an active member of the American Health Information Management Association (AHIMA).

Peggy Willard, CCS, AHIMA ICD1Ø-CM/PCS Trainer

Ms. Willard has several years of experience in Level I Adult and Pediatric Trauma hospital coding, specializing in ICD-9-CM, DRG, and CPT coding. She has been extensively trained in ICD-10-CM and PCS. Her recent experience includes in-depth analysis of medical record documentation, ICD-10-CM code assignment, and DRG shifts based on ICD-10-CM code assignment. Ms. Willard's expertise includes conducting coding audits, conducting coding training for coding staff and clinical documentation specialists, and creating internal ICD-10-CM coding guidelines/tips. Ms. Willard is an active member of the American Health Information Management Association (AHIMA) and the Minnesota Health Information Management Association (MHIMA).

Contents

Preface ... iii

What's New for 2015 ... v

Introduction ... 1
- History of ICD-10-PCS ... 1
- Number of Codes in ICD-10-PCS ... 2
- ICD-10-PCS Manual ... 2
- Medical and Surgical Section (0) ... 4
- Obstetrics Section ... 8
- Placement Section ... 8
- Administration Section ... 9
- Measurement and Monitoring Section ... 10
- Extracorporeal Assistance and Performance Section ... 10
- Extracorporeal Therapies Section ... 11
- Osteopathic Section ... 11
- Other Procedures Section ... 12
- Chiropractic Section ... 12
- Imaging Section ... 12
- Nuclear Medicine Section ... 13
- Radiation Therapy Section ... 14
- Physical Rehabilitation and Diagnostic Audiology Section ... 14
- Mental Health Section ... 15
- Substance Abuse Treatment Section ... 16
- Comparison of ICD-10-PCS and ICD-9-CM ... 17
- Conclusion ... 17

ICD-10-PCS Official Conventions ... 19
- Index ... 19
- Code Tables ... 19

ICD-10-PCS Additional Conventions ... 21

ICD-10-PCS Coding Guidelines ... 23
- Conventions ... 23
- Medical and Surgical Section Guidelines ... 24
- Obstetric Section Guidelines ... 27
- Selection of Principal Procedure ... 27

Coding Exercises ... 29
- Medical Surgical Section ... 29
- Obstetrics ... 33
- Placement ... 33
- Administration ... 33
- Measurement and Monitoring ... 33
- Extracorporeal Assistance and Performance ... 33
- Extracorporeal Therapies ... 34
- Osteopathic ... 34
- Other Procedures ... 34
- Chiropractic ... 34
- Imaging ... 34
- Nuclear Medicine ... 34
- Radiation Therapy ... 35
- Physical Rehabilitation and Diagnostic Audiology ... 35
- Mental Health ... 35
- Substance Abuse Treatment ... 35

ICD-10-PCS Index ... 37

ICD-10-PCS Tables ... 131
- Central Nervous System ... 131
- Peripheral Nervous System ... 139
- Heart and Great Vessels ... 145
- Upper Arteries ... 154
- Lower Arteries ... 165
- Upper Veins ... 175
- Lower Veins ... 185
- Lymphatic and Hemic Systems ... 195
- Eye ... 203
- Ear, Nose, Sinus ... 213
- Respiratory System ... 223
- Mouth and Throat ... 233
- Gastrointestinal System ... 242
- Hepatobiliary System and Pancreas ... 258
- Endocrine System ... 266
- Skin and Breast ... 272
- Subcutaneous Tissue and Fascia ... 283
- Muscles ... 294
- Tendons ... 303
- Bursae and Ligaments ... 312
- Head and Facial Bones ... 321
- Upper Bones ... 331
- Lower Bones ... 341
- Upper Joints ... 351
- Lower Joints ... 362
- Urinary System ... 373
- Female Reproductive System ... 382
- Male Reproductive System ... 392
- Anatomical Regions, General ... 400
- Anatomical Regions, Upper Extremities ... 408
- Anatomical Regions, Lower Extremities ... 414
- Obstetrics ... 420
- Placement—Anatomical Regions ... 423
- Placement—Anatomical Orifices ... 428
- Administration ... 429
- Measurement and Monitoring ... 436
- Extracorporeal Assistance and Performance ... 440
- Extracorporeal Therapies ... 441
- Osteopathic ... 443
- Other Procedures ... 444
- Chiropractic ... 445
- Imaging ... 446
- Nuclear Medicine ... 475
- Radiation Therapy ... 484
- Physical Rehabilitation and Diagnostic Audiology ... 497
- Mental Health ... 509
- Substance Abuse Treatment ... 511

Appendix A: Root Operations Definitions ... 513

Appendix B: Comparison of Medical and Surgical Root Operations ... 519

Appendix C: Body Part Key ... 523

Appendix D: Device Key and Aggregation Table ... 541

Appendix E: Type and Type Qualifier Definitions Sections B–H ... 551

Appendix F: Components of the Medical and Surgical Approach Definitions ... 561

Appendix G: Character Meanings ... 563

Appendix H: Answers to Coding Exercises ... 623

Appendix I: Procedure Combination Tables ... 633

Appendix J: Administration/Substance Key ... 645

Appendix K: Illustrations ... 647

Preface

This draft of the International Classification of Diseases, 10th Revision, Procedure Coding System (ICD-10-PCS) has been developed as a replacement for volume 3 of the International Classification of Diseases, Ninth Revision (ICD-9-CM). The development of ICD-10-PCS was funded by the U.S. Centers for Medicare and Medicaid Services under contract nos. 90-138, 91-22300 500-95-0005 and HHSM-550-2004-00011C to 3M Health Information Systems. ICD-10-PCS has a multi-axial, seven-character, alphanumeric code structure that provides a unique code for all substantially different procedures and allows new procedures to be easily incorporated as new codes. The initial draft was formally tested and evaluated by an independent contractor; the final version was released in 1998, with annual updates since the final release.

What's New for 2015

The Centers for Medicare and Medicaid Services is the agency charged with maintaining and updating ICD-10-PCS. CMS released the most current revisions, a summary of which may be found on the CMS website at: http://www.cms.gov/Medicare/Coding/ICD10/2015-ICD-10-PCS-and-GEMs.html.

Due to the unique structure of ICD-10-PCS, a change in a character value may affect individual codes and several code tables.

Change Summary Table

2013 Total	New Codes	Revised Titles	Deleted Codes	2015Total
71,924	0	0	0	71,924

ICD-10-PCS Code 2014 Totals, by Section

Medical and Surgical	61,898
Obstetrics	300
Placement	861
Administration	1,388
Measurement and Monitoring	339
Extracorporeal Assistance and Performance	41
Extracorporeal Therapies	42
Osteopathic	100
Other Procedures	60
Chiropractic	90
Imaging	2,934
Nuclear Medicine	463
Radiation Oncology	1,939
Rehabilitation and Diagnostic Audiology	1,380
Mental Health	30
Substance Abuse Treatment	59
Total	**71,924**

ICD-10-PCS Code Changes

- No new codes were added or deleted for fiscal 2015.
- No codes were deleted for fiscal 2015.
- No code titles were revised for fiscal 2015.

New Index Entries

Addenda

The 2015 ICD-10-PCS index addenda reflected new, revised, and deleted index entries in response to public comment.

New Definitions Addenda

Body Part Key

Term	Includes	
Costotransverse joint	Delete	thoracic vertebral joints, 8 or more
	Delete	thoracic vertebral joints, 2 to 7
Costovertebral joint	Delete	thoracic vertebral joints, 8 or more
	Delete	thoracic vertebral joints, 2 to 7
Thoracic facet joint	Delete	thoracic vertebral joints, 8 or more
	Delete	thoracic vertebral joints, 2 to 7
Lumbar facet joint	Delete	lumbar vertebral joints, 2 or more

Device Key

PCS Description	Device Term	
Cardiac Resynchronization Pacemaker Pulse Generator for Insertion in Subcutaneous Tissue and Fascia	Add	Viva (XT) (S)
(Delete) Cardiac Rhythm Related Device in Subcutaneous Tissue and Fascia	Delete	Baroreflex Activation Therapy® (BAT®)
	Delete	Rheos® System device
Defibrillator Generator for Insertion in Subcutaneous Tissue and Fascia	Add	Evera (XT)(S)(DR/VR)
External Heart Assist System in Heart and Great Vessels	Add	Centrimag® Blood Pump
Infusion Device	Add	Ascenda Intrathecal Catheter
Infusion Device, Pump in Subcutaneous Tissue and Fascia	Add	SynchroMed pump
Intraluminal Device	Delete	Centrimag® Blood Pump
	Delete	Impella (2.5)(5.0)(LD) cardiac assist device
	Delete	Stent (angioplasty)(embolization)
	Add	Absolute Pro Vascular (OTW) Self-Expanding Stent System
	Add	Acculink (RX) Carotid Stent System
	Add	Herculink (RX) Elite Renal Stent System
	Add	MULTI-LINK (VISION)(MINI-VISION)(ULTRA) Coronary Stent System
	Add	Omnilink Elite Vascular Balloon Expandable Stent System
	Add	Stent, intraluminal (cardiovascular) (gastrointestinal) (hepatobiliary) (urinary)
	Add	Xact Carotid Stent System
Intraluminal Device, Drug-eluting in Heart and Great Vessels	Delete	XIENCE V Everolimus Eluting Coronary Stent System
	Add	XIENCE Everolimus Eluting Coronary Stent System
Pacemaker, Dual Chamber for Insertion in Subcutaneous Tissue and Fascia	Add	Advisa (MRI)

PCS Description	Device Term	
Stimulator Generator in Subcutaneous Tissue and Fascia	Add	Baroreflex Activation Therapy® (BAT®)
	Add	Rheos® System device
Stimulator Generator, Multiple Array for Insertion in Subcutaneous Tissue and Fascia	Delete	Kinetra® neurostimulator
	Delete	PrimeAdvanced neurostimulator
	Add	PrimeAdvanced neurostimulator (SureScan)(MRI Safe)
Stimulator Generator, Multiple Array Rechargeable for Insertion in Subcutaneous Tissue and Fascia	Delete	RestoreAdvanced neurostimulator
	Delete	RestoreSensor neurostimulator
	Delete	RestoreUltra neurostimulator
	Add	RestoreAdvanced neurostimulator (SureScan)(MRI Safe)
	Add	RestoreSensor neurostimulator (SureScan)(MRI Safe)
	Add	RestoreUltra neurostimulator (SureScan)(MRI Safe)
Stimulator Generator, Single Array for Insertion in Subcutaneous Tissue and Fascia	Delete	Soletra® neurostimulator
Synthetic Substitute	Add	Open Pivot (mechanical) valve
	Add	Open Pivot Aortic Valve Graft (AVG)
Zooplastic Tissue in Heart and Great Vessels	Add	Mosaic Bioprosthesis (aortic) (mitral) valve

Administration/Substance Key

Trade Name or Synonym		PCS Substance Category	
Add	AIGISRx Antibacterial Envelope	Add	Anti-Infective Envelope
Add	Antimicrobial envelope	Add	Anti-Infective Envelope
Add	Bone morphogenetic protein 2 (BMP 2)	Add	Recombinant Bone Morphogenetic Protein
Add	Clolar	Add	Clofarabine
Add	Kcentra	Add	4-Factor Prothrombin Complex Concentrate
Add	Nesiritide	Add	Human B-type Natriutretic Peptide
Add	rhBMP-2	Add	Recombinant Bone Morphogenetic Protein
Add	Seprafilm	Add	Adhesion Barrier
Add	Tissue Plasminogen Activator (tPA)(r-tPA)	Add	Other Thrombolytic
Add	Voraxaze	Add	Glucarpidase
Add	Zyvox	Add	Oxazolidinones

List of Updated Files

2Ø15 Official ICD-1Ø-PCS Coding Guidelines

- Downloadable PDF file
- No guideline changes for fiscal 2Ø15

2Ø15 ICD-1Ø-PCS Code Tables and Index (Zip file)

- No code table changes for fiscal 2Ø15, minor index changes only
- Downloadable PDF, file name PCS_2Ø15.pdf
- Downloadable xml files for developers, file names icd1Øpcs_tabular_2Ø15.xml, icd1Øpcs_index_2Ø15.xml, icd1Øpcs_definitions_2Ø15.xml
- Accompanying schema for developers, file names icd1Øpcs_tabular_2Ø15.xsd, icd1Øpcs_index_2Ø15.xsd, icd1Øpcs_definitions_2Ø15.xsd

2Ø15 ICD-1Ø-PCS Code Titles, Long and Abbreviated (Zip file)

- No tabular order file changes for fiscal 2Ø15
- Tabular order file defines an unambiguous order for all ICD-1Ø-CM/PCS codes
- Text file format, file name icd1Øpcs_order_2Ø15.txt
- Provides a unique five-digit "order number" for each ICD-1Ø-PCS table and code, as well as a long and abbreviated code title
- Accompanying documentation, file name ICD1ØOrderFiles.pdf

2Ø15 ICD-1Ø-PCS Final Addenda (Zip file)

- Index addenda in downloadable PDF, file name index_addenda_2Ø15.pdf
- PCS Definitions addenda in downloadable PDF, file name definitions_addenda_2Ø15.pdf
- Index and Definitions addenda in machine readable text format for developers, file names index_addenda_2Ø15.txt, definitions_addenda_2Ø15.txt

2Ø15 ICD-1Ø-PCS Reference Manual (Zip file)

- Downloadable PDF, file name ICD-1Ø-PCS Reference Manual.pdf
- Addenda to 2Ø15 version of reference manual specifies the changes, file name pcs_ref_addenda_2Ø15.pdf

2Ø15 ICD-1Ø-PCS and ICD-9-CM General Equivalence Mappings (Zip file)

- Downloadable text format, file names gem_i9pcs.txt, gem_pcsi9.txt
- Summary of mapping entries revised in response to public comment and internal review, file name Gems2Ø15UpdateSummary.pdf
- Documentation for general and technical users, file names pcs_gemguide_2Ø15.pdf, GemsTechDoc.pdf

2Ø15 ICD-1Ø Reimbursement Mappings (Zip file)

- Downloadable text format, file names reimb_map_dx_2Ø15.txt, reimb_map_pr_2Ø15.txt
- Fiscal 2Ø15 version uses the fiscal 2Ø15 GEM files
- Accompanying documentation, file name reimb_map_guide_2Ø15.pdf

Introduction

Volume 3 of the International Classification of Diseases Ninth Revision Clinical Modification (ICD-9-CM) has been used in the United States for reporting inpatient procedures since 1979. The structure of volume 3 of ICD-9-CM has not allowed new procedures associated with rapidly changing technology to be effectively incorporated as new codes. As a result, in 1992 the U.S. Centers for Medicare and Medicaid Services funded a project to design a replacement for volume 3 of ICD-9-CM. In 1995 CMS awarded 3M Health Information Systems a three-year contract to complete development of the replacement system. The new system is the ICD-1Ø Procedure Coding System (ICD-1Ø-PCS).

History of ICD-1Ø-PCS

The World Health Organization has maintained the International Classification of Diseases (ICD) for recording cause of death since 1893. It has updated the ICD periodically to reflect new discoveries in epidemiology and changes in medical understanding of disease.

The International Classification of Diseases Tenth Revision (ICD-1Ø), published in 1992, is the latest revision of the ICD. The WHO authorized the National Center for Health Statistics (NCHS) to develop a clinical modification of ICD-1Ø for use in the United States. This version, called ICD-1Ø-CM, is intended to replace the previous U.S. clinical modification, ICD-9-CM, that has been in use since 1979. ICD-9-CM contains a procedure classification; ICD-1Ø-CM does not.

CMS, the agency responsible for maintaining the inpatient procedure code set in the United States, contracted with 3M Health Information Systems in 1993 to design and then develop a procedure classification system to replace volume 3 of ICD-9-CM.

The result, ICD-1Ø-PCS, was initially completed in 1998. The code set has been updated annually since that time to ensure that ICD-1Ø-PCS includes classifications for new procedures, devices, and technologies.

The development of ICD-1Ø-PCS had as its goal the incorporation of the following major attributes:

- **Completeness:** There should be a unique code for all substantially different procedures. In volume 3 of ICD-9-CM, procedures on different body parts, with different approaches, or of different types are sometimes assigned to the same code.
- **Unique definitions:** Because ICD-1Ø-PCS codes are constructed of individual values rather than lists of fixed codes and text descriptions, the unique, stable definition of a code in the system is retained. New values may be added to the system to represent a specific new approach or device or qualifier, but whole codes by design cannot be given new meanings and reused.
- **Expandability:** As new procedures are developed, the structure of ICD-1Ø-PCS should allow them to be easily incorporated as unique codes.
- **Multi-axial codes:** ICD-1Ø-PCS codes should consist of independent characters, with each individual component retaining its meaning across broad ranges of codes to the extent possible.
- **Standardized terminology:** ICD-1Ø-PCS should include definitions of the terminology used. While the meaning of specific words varies in common usage, ICD-1Ø-PCS should not include multiple meanings for the same term, and each term must be assigned a specific meaning. There are no eponyms or common procedure terms in ICD-1Ø-PCS.
- **Structural integrity:** ICD-1Ø-PCS can be easily expanded without disrupting the structure of the system. ICD-1Ø-PCS allows unique new codes to be added to the system because values for the seven characters that make up a code can be combined as needed. The system can evolve as medical technology and clinical practice evolve, without disrupting the ICD-1Ø-PCS structure.

In the development of ICD-1Ø-PCS, several additional general characteristics were added:

- **Diagnostic information is not included in procedure description:** When procedures are performed for specific diseases or disorders, the disease or disorder is not contained in the procedure code. The diagnosis codes, not the procedure codes, specify the disease or disorder.
- **Explicit not otherwise specified (NOS) options are restricted:** Explicit "not otherwise specified," (NOS) options are restricted in ICD-1Ø-PCS. A minimal level of specificity is required for each component of the procedure.
- **Limited use of not elsewhere classified (NEC) option:** Because all significant components of a procedure are specified in ICD-1Ø-PCS, there is generally no need for a "not elsewhere classified" (NEC) code option. However, limited NEC options are incorporated into ICD-1Ø-PCS where necessary. For example, new devices are frequently developed, and therefore it is necessary to provide an "other device" option for use until the new device can be explicitly added to the coding system.
- **Level of specificity:** All procedures currently performed can be specified in ICD-1Ø-PCS. The frequency with which a procedure is performed was not a consideration in the development of the system. A unique code is available for variations of a procedure that can be performed.

ICD-1Ø-PCS code structure results in qualities that optimize the performance of the system in electronic applications, and maximize the usefulness of the coded healthcare data. These qualities include:

- **Optimal search capability:** ICD-1Ø-PCS is designed for maximum versatility in the ability to aggregate coded data. Values belonging to the same character as defined in a section or sections can be easily compared, since they occupy the same position in a code. This provides a high degree of flexibility and functionality for data mining.
- **Consistent characters and values:** Stability of characters and values across vast ranges of codes provides the maximum degree of functionality and flexibility for the collection and analysis of data. Because the character definition is consistent, and only the individual values assigned to that character differ as needed, meaningful comparisons of data over time can be conducted across a virtually infinite range of procedures.
- **Code readability:** ICD-1Ø-PCS resembles a language in the sense that it is made up of semi-independent values combined by following the rules of the system, much the way a sentence is formed by combining words and following the rules of grammar and syntax. As with words in their context, the meaning of any

single value is a combination of its position in the code and any preceding values on which it may be dependent.

ICD-10-PCS Code Structure

ICD-10-PCS has a seven-character alphanumeric code structure. Each character contains up to 34 possible values. Each value represents a specific option for the general character definition. The 10 digits 0–9 and the 24 letters A–H, J–N, and P–Z may be used in each character. The letters O and I are not used so as to avoid confusion with the digits 0 and 1. An ICD-10-PCS code is the result of a process rather than as a single fixed set of digits or alphabetic characters. The process consists of combining semi-independent values from among a selection of values, according to the rules governing the construction of codes.

	Section	Body System	Root Operation	Body Part	Approach	Device	Qualifier
Characters:	1	2	3	4	5	6	7

A code is derived by choosing a specific value for each of the seven characters. Based on details about the procedure performed, values for each character specifying the section, body system, root operation, body part, approach, device, and qualifier are assigned. Because the definition of each character is also a function of its physical position in the code, the same letter or number placed in a different position in the code has different meaning.

The seven characters that make up a complete code have specific meanings that vary for each of the 16 sections of the manual. (The resource section of this manual lists character meanings for each section along with body part definitions.)

Procedures are then divided into sections that identify the general type of procedure (e.g., Medical and Surgical, Obstetrics, Imaging). The first character of the procedure code always specifies the section. The second through seventh characters have the same meaning within each section, but may mean different things in other sections. In all sections, the third character specifies the general type of procedure performed (e.g., Resection, Transfusion, Fluoroscopy), while the other characters give additional information such as the body part and approach.

In ICD-10-PCS, the term *procedure* refers to the complete specification of the seven characters.

Number of Codes in ICD-10-PCS

The table structure of ICD-10-PCS permits the specification of a large number of codes on a single page. At the time of this publication, there are 71,924 codes in the 2015 ICD-10-PCS. This is a substantial increase over the number of ICD-9-CM procedure codes. However, many codes have been eliminated from ICD-10-PCS from the Medical and Surgical section as part of a planned streamlining and refinement initiated in 2006. This code reduction has also included the deletion of certain body system values specified as "other" in order to facilitate more selective body part and system values.

The ICD-9-CM Coordination and Maintenance Committee are suspending regular updates to the ICD code sets to ease the ICD-10 transition process. These limited updates are required by section 503(a) of the Medicare Prescription Drug, Improvement, and Modernization Act of 2003.

ICD-10-PCS Manual

Index

Codes may be found in the index based on the general type of procedure (e.g., resection, transfusion, fluoroscopy), or a more commonly used term (e.g., appendectomy). For example, the code for percutaneous intraluminal dilation of the coronary arteries with an intraluminal device can be found in the Index under *Dilation*, or a synonym of *Dilation* (e.g., angioplasty). The Index then specifies the first three or four values of the code or directs the user to see another term.

Example:

Dilation
Artery
Coronary
One Site 0270

Based on the first three values of the code provided in the Index, the corresponding table can be located. In the example above, the first three values indicate table 027 is to be referenced for code completion.

The tables and characters are arranged first by number and then by letter for each character (tables for 00-, 01-, 02-, etc., are followed by those for 0B-, 0C-, 0D-, etc., followed by 0B1, 0B2, etc., followed by 0BB, 0BC, 0BD, etc.).

Note: The Tables section must be used to construct a complete and valid code by specifying the last three or four values.

Tables

The Tables section is organized differently from ICD-9-CM. Each page in the section is composed of rows that specify the valid combinations of code values. In most sections of the system, the upper portion of each table contains a description of the first three characters of the procedure code. In the Medical and Surgical section, for example, the first three characters contain the name of the section, the body system, and the root operation performed.

For instance, the values *027* specify the section *Medical and Surgical* (0), the body system *Heart and Great Vessels* (2) and the root operation *Dilation* (7). As shown in table 027, the root operation (*Dilation*) is accompanied by its definition.

The lower portion of the table specifies all the valid combinations of characters 4 through 7. The four columns in the table specify the last four characters. In the Medical and Surgical section they are labeled body part, approach, device and qualifier, respectively. Each row in the table specifies the valid combination of values for characters 4 through 7.

Ø Medical and Surgical
2 Heart and Great Vessels
7 Dilation Expanding an orifice or the lumen of a tubular body part

Body Part Character 4	Approach Character 5	Device Character 6	Qualifier Character 7
Ø Coronary Artery, One Site **1** Coronary Artery, Two Sites **2** Coronary Artery, Three Sites **3** Coronary Artery, Four or More Sites	**Ø** Open **3** Percutaneous **4** Percutaneous Endoscopic	**4** Intraluminal Device, Drug-eluting **D** Intraluminal Device **T** Intraluminal Device, Radioactive **Z** No Device	**6** Bifurcation **Z** No Qualifier
F Aortic Valve **G** Mitral Valve **H** Pulmonary Valve **J** Tricuspid Valve **K** Ventricle, Right **P** Pulmonary Trunk **Q** Pulmonary Artery, Right **S** Pulmonary Vein, Right **T** Pulmonary Vein, Left **V** Superior Vena Cava **W** Thoracic Aorta	**Ø** Open **3** Percutaneous **4** Percutaneous Endoscopic	**4** Intraluminal Device, Drug-eluting **D** Intraluminal Device **Z** No Device	**Z** No Qualifier
R Pulmonary Artery, Left	**Ø** Open **3** Percutaneous **4** Percutaneous Endoscopic	**4** Intraluminal Device, Drug-eluting **D** Intraluminal Device **Z** No Device	**T** Ductus Arteriosus **Z** No Qualifier

The rows of this table can be used to construct 213 unique procedure codes. For example, code Ø27Ø3DZ specifies the procedure for dilation of one coronary artery using an intraluminal device via percutaneous approach (i.e., percutaneous transluminal coronary angioplasty with stent).

Following are the 24 valid combinations of characters 5 through 7 for the Medical and Surgical procedure dilation of the heart and great vessels coronary artery, one site (Ø27Ø):

Ø27ØØ46	Dilation of Coronary Artery, One Site, Bifurcation, with Drug-eluting Intraluminal Device, Open Approach
Ø27ØØ4Z	Dilation of Coronary Artery, One Site with Drug-eluting Intraluminal Device, Open Approach
Ø27ØØD6	Dilation of Coronary Artery, One Site, Bifurcation, with Intraluminal Device, Open Approach
Ø27ØØDZ	Dilation of Coronary Artery, One Site with Intraluminal Device, Open Approach
Ø27ØØT6	Dilation of Coronary Artery, One Site, Bifurcation, with Radioactive Intraluminal Device, Open Approach
Ø27ØØTZ	Dilation of Coronary Artery, One Site with Radioactive Intraluminal Device, Open Approach
Ø27ØØZ6	Dilation of Coronary Artery, One Site, Bifurcation, Open Approach
Ø27ØØZZ	Dilation of Coronary Artery, One Site, Open Approach
Ø27Ø346	Dilation of Coronary Artery, One Site, Bifurcation, with Drug-eluting Intraluminal Device, Percutaneous Approach
Ø27Ø34Z	Dilation of Coronary Artery, One Site with Drug-eluting Intraluminal Device, Percutaneous Approach
Ø27Ø3D6	Dilation of Coronary Artery, One Site, Bifurcation, with Intraluminal Device, Percutaneous Approach
Ø27Ø3DZ	Dilation of Coronary Artery, One Site with Intraluminal Device, Percutaneous Approach
Ø27Ø3T6	Dilation of Coronary Artery, One Site, Bifurcation, with Radioactive Intraluminal Device, Percutaneous Approach
Ø27Ø3TZ	Dilation of Coronary Artery, One Site with Radioactive Intraluminal Device, Percutaneous Approach
Ø27Ø3Z6	Dilation of Coronary Artery, One Site, Bifurcation, Percutaneous Approach
Ø27Ø3ZZ	Dilation of Coronary Artery, One Site, Percutaneous Approach
Ø27Ø446	Dilation of Coronary Artery, One Site, Bifurcation, with Drug-eluting Intraluminal Device, Percutaneous Endoscopic Approach
Ø27Ø44Z	Dilation of Coronary Artery, One Site with Drug-eluting Intraluminal Device, Percutaneous Endoscopic Approach
Ø27Ø4D6	Dilation of Coronary Artery, One Site, Bifurcation, with Intraluminal Device, Percutaneous Endoscopic Approach
Ø27Ø4DZ	Dilation of Coronary Artery, One Site with Intraluminal Device, Percutaneous Endoscopic Approach
Ø27Ø4T6	Dilation of Coronary Artery, One Site, Bifurcation, with Radioactive Intraluminal Device, Percutaneous Endoscopic Approach
Ø27Ø4TZ	Dilation of Coronary Artery, One Site with Radioactive Intraluminal Device, Percutaneous Endoscopic Approach
Ø27Ø4Z6	Dilation of Coronary Artery, One Site, Bifurcation, Percutaneous Endoscopic Approach
Ø27Ø4ZZ	Dilation of Coronary Artery, One Site, Percutaneous Endoscopic Approach

Each table contains only those combinations of values that make up a valid procedure code. In some instances, the tables are split, indicating that there is a restriction in the combination of character choices. In table Ø27 above, character 7, qualifier 6 Bifurcation can be used only with coronary artery body part characters Ø–3. Character 7, qualifier T Ductus Arteriosus can be used only with body part character R Pulmonary Artery, Left.

The lower portion of table ØØ1, shown below, is split into two sections; values of characters must be selected from within the same section (row) of the table.

Ø Medical and Surgical
Ø Central Nervous System
1 Bypass Altering the route of passage of the contents of a tubular body part

Body Part Character 4	Approach Character 5	Device Character 6	Qualifier Character 7
6 Cerebral Ventricle	**Ø** Open **3** Percutaneous	**7** Autologous Tissue Substitute **J** Synthetic Substitute **K** Nonautologous Tissue Substitute	**Ø** Nasopharynx **1** Mastoid Sinus **2** Atrium **3** Blood Vessel **4** Pleural Cavity **5** Intestine **6** Peritoneal Cavity **7** Urinary Tract **8** Bone Marrow **B** Cerebral Cisterns
U Spinal Canal	**Ø** Open **3** Percutaneous	**7** Autologous Tissue Substitute **J** Synthetic Substitute **K** Nonautologous Tissue Substitute	**4** Pleural Cavity **6** Peritoneal Cavity **7** Urinary Tract **9** Fallopian Tube

Body part value *6* may be in combination with device values *7, J,* or *K.* Body part (character 4) value *U* may be used only in combination with qualifier (character 7) values of 4, 6, 7, and 9. In other words, code ØØ1UØ73 is invalid since the qualifier character appears above the line separating the two sections of the table.

Note: In this manual, there are instances in which some tables due to length must be continued on the next page. Each section must be used separately and value selection must be made within the same section (row) of the table.

Character Meanings

In each section each character has a specific meaning. Within a section all character meanings remain constant. The resource section of this manual lists character meanings for each section.

Sections

Procedures are divided into sections that identify the general type of procedure (e.g., Medical and Surgical, Obstetrics, Imaging). The first character of the procedure code always specifies the section.

The sections are listed below:

Medical and Surgical-related sections

- Ø Medical and Surgical
- 1 Obstetrics
- 2 Placement
- 3 Administration
- 4 Measurement and Monitoring
- 5 Extracorporeal Assistance and Performance
- 6 Extracorporeal Therapies
- 7 Osteopathic
- 8 Other Procedures
- 9 Chiropractic

Ancillary Sections

- B Imaging
- C Nuclear Medicine
- D Radiation Therapy
- F Physical Rehabilitation and Diagnostic Audiology
- G Mental Health
- H Substance Abuse Treatment

Medical and Surgical Section (Ø)

Character Meaning

The seven characters for Medical and Surgical procedures have the following meaning:

Character	Meaning
1	Section
2	Body System
3	Root Operation
4	Body Part
5	Approach
6	Device
7	Qualifier

The Medical and Surgical section constitutes the vast majority of procedures reported in an inpatient setting. Medical and Surgical procedure codes all have a first-character value of *Ø*. The second character indicates the general body system (e.g., Mouth and Throat, Gastrointestinal). The third character indicates the root operation, or specific objective, of the procedure (e.g., Excision). The fourth character indicates the specific body part on which the procedure was performed (e.g., Tonsils, Duodenum). The fifth character indicates the approach used to reach the procedure site (e.g., Open). The sixth character indicates whether a device was left in place during in the procedure (e.g., Synthetic Substitute). The seventh character is qualifier, which has a specific meaning for each root operation. For example, the qualifier can be used to identify the destination site of a *Bypass*. The first through fifth characters are always assigned a specific value, but the device (sixth character) and the qualifier (seventh character) are not applicable to all procedures. The value *Z* is used for the sixth and seventh characters to indicate that a specific device or qualifier does not apply to the procedure.

Section (Character 1)

Medical and Surgical procedure codes all have a first-character value of *Ø*.

Body Systems (Character 2)

Body systems for Medical and Surgical section codes are specified in the second character.

Body Systems

Ø Central Nervous System

1 Peripheral Nervous System

2 Heart and Great Vessels

3 Upper Arteries

4 Lower Arteries

5 Upper Veins

6 Lower Veins

7 Lymphatic and Hemic Systems

8 Eye

9 Ear, Nose, Sinus

B Respiratory System

C Mouth and Throat

D Gastrointestinal System

F Hepatobiliary System and Pancreas

G Endocrine System

H Skin and Breast

J Subcutaneous Tissue and Fascia

K Muscles

L Tendons

M Bursae and Ligaments

N Head and Facial Bones

P Upper Bones

Q Lower Bones

R Upper Joints

S Lower Joints

T Urinary System

U Female Reproductive System

V Male Reproductive System

W Anatomical Regions, General

X Anatomical Regions, Upper Extremities

Y Anatomical Regions, Lower Extremities

Root Operations (Character 3)

The root operation is specified in the third character. In the Medical and Surgical section there are 31 different root operations. The root operation identifies the objective of the procedure. Each root operation has a precise definition.

- *Alteration:* Modifying the natural anatomic structure of a body part without affecting the function of the body part
- *Bypass:* Altering the route of passage of the contents of a tubular body part
- *Change:* Taking out or off a device from a body part and putting back an identical or similar device in or on the same body part without cutting or puncturing the skin or a mucous membrane
- *Control:* Stopping, or attempting to stop, postprocedural bleeding
- *Creation:* Making a new genital structure that does not take over the function of a body part
- *Destruction:* Physical eradication of all or a portion of a body part by the direct use of energy, force, or a destructive agent
- *Detachment:* Cutting off all or a portion of the upper or lower extremities
- *Dilation:* Expanding an orifice or the lumen of a tubular body part
- *Division:* Cutting into a body part without draining fluids and/or gases from the body part in order to separate or transect a body part
- *Drainage:* Taking or letting out fluids and/or gases from a body part
- *Excision:* Cutting out or off, without replacement, a portion of a body part
- *Extirpation:* Taking or cutting out solid matter from a body part
- *Extraction:* Pulling or stripping out or off all or a portion of a body part by the use of force
- *Fragmentation:* Breaking solid matter in a body part into pieces
- *Fusion:* Joining together portions of an articular body part rendering the articular body part immobile
- *Insertion:* Putting in a nonbiological appliance that monitors, assists, performs, or prevents a physiological function but does not physically take the place of a body part
- *Inspection:* Visually and/or manually exploring a body part
- *Map:* Locating the route of passage of electrical impulses and/or locating functional areas in a body part
- *Occlusion:* Completely closing an orifice or lumen of a tubular body part
- *Reattachment:* Putting back in or on all or a portion of a separated body part to its normal location or other suitable location
- *Release:* Freeing a body part from an abnormal physical constraint by cutting or by use of force
- *Removal:* Taking out or off a device from a body part
- *Repair:* Restoring, to the extent possible, a body part to its normal anatomic structure and function
- *Replacement:* Putting in or on biological or synthetic material that physically takes the place and/or function of all or a portion of a body part
- *Reposition:* Moving to its normal location or other suitable location all or a portion of a body part
- *Resection:* Cutting out or off, without replacement, all of a body part
- *Restriction:* Partially closing an orifice or lumen of a tubular body part
- *Revision:* Correcting, to the extent possible, a portion of a malfunctioning device or the position of a displaced device
- *Supplement:* Putting in or on biological or synthetic material that physically reinforces and/or augments the function of a portion of a body part
- *Transfer:* Moving, without taking out, all or a portion of a body part to another location to take over the function of all or a portion of a body part

- *Transplantation:* Putting in or on all or a portion of a living body part taken from another individual or animal to physically take the place and/or function of all or a portion of a similar body part

The above definitions of root operation illustrate the precision of code values defined in the system. There is a clear distinction between each root operation.

A root operation specifies the objective of the procedure. The term *anastomosis* is not a root operation, because it is a means of joining and is always an integral part of another procedure (e.g., Bypass, Resection) with a specific objective. Similarly, *incision* is not a root operation, since it is always part of the objective of another procedure (e.g., Division, Drainage). The root operation *Repair* in the Medical and Surgical section functions as a "not elsewhere classified" option. *Repair* is used when the procedure performed is not one of the other specific root operations.

Appendix A provides additional explanation and representative examples of the Medical and Surgical root operations. Appendix B groups all root operations in the Medical and Surgical section into subcategories and provides an example of each root operation.

Body Part (Character 4)

The body part is specified in the fourth character. The body part indicates the specific anatomical site of the body system on which the procedure was performed (e.g., Duodenum). Tubular body parts are defined in ICD-10-PCS as those hollow body parts that provide a route of passage for solids, liquids, or gases. They include the cardiovascular system and body parts such as those contained in the gastrointestinal tract, genitourinary tract, biliary tract, and respiratory tract.

Approach (Character 5)

The technique used to reach the site of the procedure is specified in the fifth character. There are seven different approaches:

- *Open*: Cutting through the skin or mucous membrane and any other body layers necessary to expose the site of the procedure
- *Percutaneous*: Entry, by puncture or minor incision, of instrumentation through the skin or mucous membrane and any other body layers necessary to reach the site of the procedure
- *Percutaneous Endoscopic*: Entry, by puncture or minor incision, of instrumentation through the skin or mucous membrane and any other body layers necessary to reach and visualize the site of the procedure
- *Via Natural or Artificial Opening*: Entry of instrumentation through a natural or artificial external opening to reach the site of the procedure
- *Via Natural or Artificial Opening Endoscopic*: Entry of instrumentation through a natural or artificial external opening to reach and visualize the site of the procedure
- *Via Natural or Artificial Opening with Percutaneous Endoscopic Assistance:* Entry of instrumentation through a natural or artificial external opening and entry, by puncture or minor incision, of instrumentation through the skin or mucous membrane and any other body layers necessary to aid in the performance of the procedure
- *External*: Procedures performed directly on the skin or mucous membrane and procedures performed indirectly by the application of external force through the skin or mucous membrane

The approach comprises three components: the access location, method, and type of instrumentation.

Access location: For procedures performed on an internal body part, the access location specifies the external site through which the site of the procedure is reached. There are two general types of access locations: skin or mucous membranes, and external orifices. Every approach value except external includes one of these two access locations. The skin or mucous membrane can be cut or punctured to reach the procedure site. All open and percutaneous approach values use this access location. The site of a procedure can also be reached through an external opening. External openings can be natural (e.g., mouth) or artificial (e.g., colostomy stoma).

Method: For procedures performed on an internal body part, the method specifies how the external access location is entered. An open method specifies cutting through the skin or mucous membrane and any other intervening body layers necessary to expose the site of the procedure. An instrumentation method specifies the entry of instrumentation through the access location to the internal procedure site. Instrumentation can be introduced by puncture or minor incision, or through an external opening. The puncture or minor incision does not constitute an open approach because it does not expose the site of the procedure. An approach can define multiple methods. For example, *Via Natural or Artificial Opening with Percutaneous Endoscopic Assistance* includes both the initial entry of instrumentation to reach the site of the procedure, and the placement of additional percutaneous instrumentation into the body part to visualize and assist in the performance of the procedure.

Type of instrumentation: For procedures performed on an internal body part, instrumentation means that specialized equipment is used to perform the procedure. Instrumentation is used in all internal approaches other than the basic open approach. Instrumentation may or may not include the capacity to visualize the procedure site. For example, the instrumentation used to perform a sigmoidoscopy permits the internal site of the procedure to be visualized, while the instrumentation used to perform a needle biopsy of the liver does not. The term "endoscopic" as used in approach values refers to instrumentation that permits a site to be visualized.

Procedures performed directly on the skin or mucous membrane are identified by the external approach (e.g., skin excision). Procedures performed indirectly by the application of external force are also identified by the external approach (e.g., closed reduction of fracture).

Appendix B compares the components (access location, method, and type of instrumentation) of each approach and provides an example of each approach.

Device (Character 6)

The device is specified in the sixth character and is used only to specify devices that remain after the procedure is completed. There are four general types of devices:

- Grafts and Prostheses
- Implants
- Simple or Mechanical Appliances
- Electronic Appliances

While all devices can be removed, some cannot be removed without putting in another nonbiological appliance or body-part substitute.

When a specific device value is used to identify the device for a root operation, such as *Insertion* and that same device value is not an option for a more broad range root operation such as *Removal*, select the general device value. For example, in the body system Heart and Great Vessels, the specific device character for Cardiac Lead, Pacemaker in root operation *Insertion* is J. For the root operation *Removal*, the general device character M Cardiac Lead would be selected for the pacemaker lead.

ICD-10-PCS contains a PCS Device Aggregation Table (see appendix D) that crosswalks the *specific* device character values that have been created for specific root operations and specific body part character values to the *general* device character value that would be used for root operations that represent a broad range of procedures and general body part character values, such as Removal and Revision.

Instruments used to visualize the procedure site are specified in the approach, not the device, value.

If the objective of the procedure is to put in the device, then the root operation is *Insertion*. If the device is put in to meet an objective other than *Insertion*, then the root operation defining the underlying objective of the procedure is used, with the device specified in the device character. For example, if a procedure to replace the hip joint is performed, the root operation *Replacement* is coded, and the prosthetic device is specified in the device character. Materials that are incidental to a procedure such as clips, ligatures, and sutures are not specified in the device character. Because new devices can be developed, the value *Other Device* is provided as a temporary option for use until a specific device value is added to the system.

Qualifier (Character 7)

The qualifier is specified in the seventh character. The qualifier contains unique values for individual procedures. For example, the qualifier can be used to identify the destination site in a *Bypass*.

Medical and Surgical Section Principles

In developing the Medical and Surgical procedure codes, several specific principles were followed.

Composite Terms Are Not Root Operations

Composite terms such as colonoscopy, sigmoidectomy, or appendectomy do not describe root operations, but they do specify multiple components of a specific root operation. In ICD-10-PCS, the components of a procedure are defined separately by the characters making up the complete code. And the only component of a procedure specified in the root operation is the objective of the procedure. With each complete code the underlying objective of the procedure is specified by the root operation (third character), the precise part is specified by the body part (fourth character), and the method used to reach and visualize the procedure site is specified by the approach (fifth character). While colonoscopy, sigmoidectomy, and appendectomy are included in the Index, they do not constitute root operations in the Tables section. The objective of colonoscopy is the visualization of the colon and the root operation (character 3) is *Inspection*. Character 4 specifies the body part, which in this case is part of the colon. These composite terms, like colonoscopy or appendectomy, are included as cross-reference only. The index provides the correct root operation reference. Examples of other types of composite terms not representative of root operations are *partial* sigmoidectomy, *total* hysterectomy, and *partial* hip replacement. Always refer to the correct root operation in the Index and Tables section.

Root Operation Based on Objective of Procedure

The root operation is based on the objective of the procedure, such as *Resection* of transverse colon or *Dilation* of an artery. The assignment of the root operation is based on the procedure actually performed, which may or may not have been the intended procedure. If the intended procedure is modified or discontinued (e.g., excision instead of resection is performed), the root operation is determined by the procedure actually performed. If the desired result is not attained after completing the procedure (i.e., the artery does not remain expanded after the dilation procedure), the root operation is still determined by the procedure actually performed.

Examples:

- Dilating the urethra is coded as *Dilation* since the objective of the procedure is to dilate the urethra. If dilation of the urethra includes putting in an intraluminal stent, the root operation remains *Dilation* and not *Insertion* of the intraluminal device because the underlying objective of the procedure is dilation of the urethra. The stent is identified by the intraluminal device value in the sixth character of the dilation procedure code.
- If the objective is solely to put a radioactive element in the urethra, then the procedure is coded to the root operation *Insertion*, with the radioactive element identified in the sixth character of the code.
- If the objective of the procedure is to correct a malfunctioning or displaced device, then the procedure is coded to the root operation *Revision*. In the root operation *Revision*, the original device being revised is identified in the device character. *Revision* is typically performed on mechanical appliances (e.g., pacemaker) or materials used in replacement procedures (e.g., synthetic substitute). Typical revision procedures include adjustment of pacemaker position and correction of malfunctioning knee prosthesis.

Combination Procedures Are Coded Separately

If multiple procedures as defined by distinct objectives are performed during an operative episode, then multiple codes are used. For example, obtaining the vein graft used for coronary bypass surgery is coded as a separate procedure from the bypass itself.

Redo of Procedures

The complete or partial redo of the original procedure is coded to the root operation that identifies the procedure performed rather than *Revision*.

Example:

A complete redo of a hip replacement procedure that requires putting in a new prosthesis is coded to the root operation *Replacement* rather than *Revision*.

The correction of complications arising from the original procedure, other than device complications, is coded to the procedure performed. Correction of a malfunctioning or displaced device would be coded to the root operation *Revision*.

Example:

A procedure to control hemorrhage arising from the original procedure is coded to *Control* rather than *Revision*.

Examples of Procedures Coded in the Medical Surgical Section

The following are examples of procedures from the Medical and Surgical section, coded in ICD-10-PCS.

- Suture of skin laceration, left lower arm: 0HQEXZZ

  Medical and Surgical section (0), body system *Skin and Breast* (H), root operation *Repair* (Q), body part *Skin, Left Lower Arm* (E), *External* Approach (X) *No device* (Z), and *No qualifier* (Z).

- Laparoscopic appendectomy: ØDTJ4ZZ

  Medical and Surgical section (Ø), body system *Gastrointestinal* (D), root operation *Resection* (T), body part *Appendix* (J), *Percutaneous Endoscopic* approach (4), No Device (Z), and No qualifier (Z).

- Sigmoidoscopy with biopsy: ØDBN8ZX

  Medical and Surgical section (Ø), body system *Gastrointestinal* (D), root operation *Excision* (B), body part *Sigmoid Colon* (N), *Via Natural or Artificial Opening Endoscopic* approach (8), *No Device* (Z), and with qualifier *Diagnostic* (X).

- Tracheostomy with tracheostomy tube: ØB11ØF4

  Medical and Surgical section (Ø), body system *Respiratory* (B), root operation *Bypass* (1), body part *Trachea* (1), *Open* approach (Ø), with *Tracheostomy Device* (F), and qualifier *Cutaneous* (4).

Obstetrics Section

Character Meanings

The seven characters in the Obstetrics section have the same meaning as in the Medical and Surgical section.

Character	Meaning
1	Section
2	Body System
3	Root Operation
4	Body Part
5	Approach
6	Device
7	Qualifier

The Obstetrics section includes procedures performed on the products of conception only. Procedures on the pregnant female are coded in the Medical and Surgical section (e.g., episiotomy). The term "products of conception" refers to all physical components of a pregnancy, including the fetus, amnion, umbilical cord, and placenta. There is no differentiation of the products of conception based on gestational age. Thus, the specification of the products of conception as a zygote, embryo or fetus, or the trimester of the pregnancy is not part of the procedure code but can be found in the diagnosis code.

Section (Character 1)

Obstetrics procedure codes have a first-character value of *1*.

Body System (Character 2)

The second-character value for body system is *Pregnancy*.

Root Operation (Character 3)

The root operations *Change, Drainage, Extraction, Insertion, Inspection, Removal, Repair, Reposition, Resection,* and *Transplantation* are used in the obstetrics section and have the same meaning as in the Medical and Surgical section.

The Obstetrics section also includes two additional root operations, *Abortion* and *Delivery*, defined below:

- *Abortion*: Artificially terminating a pregnancy
- *Delivery*: Assisting the passage of the products of conception from the genital canal

A cesarean section is not a separate root operation because the underlying objective is *Extraction* (i.e., pulling out all or a portion of a body part).

Body Part (Character 4)

The body-part values in the obstetrics section are:

- *Products of conception*
- *Products of conception, retained*
- *Products of conception, ectopic*

Approach (Character 5)

The fifth character specifies approaches and is defined as are those in the Medical and Surgical section. In the case of an abortion procedure that uses a laminaria or an abortifacient, the approach is *Via Natural or Artificial Opening.*

Device (Character 6)

The sixth character is used for devices such as fetal monitoring electrodes.

Qualifier (Character 7)

Qualifier values are specific to the root operation and are used to specify the type of extraction (e.g., low forceps, high forceps, etc.), the type of cesarean section (e.g., classical, low cervical, etc.), or the type of fluid taken out during a drainage procedure (e.g., amniotic fluid, fetal blood, etc.).

Placement Section

Character Meanings

The seven characters in the Placement section have the following meaning:

Character	Meaning
1	Section
2	Anatomical Region
3	Root Operation
4	Body Region/Orifice
5	Approach
6	Device
7	Qualifier

Placement section codes represent procedures for putting a device in or on a body region for the purpose of protection, immobilization, stretching, compression, or packing.

Section (Character 1)

Placement procedure codes have a first-character value of *2*.

Body System (Character 2)

The second character contains two values specifying either *Anatomical Regions* or *Anatomical Orifices*.

Root Operation (Character 3)

The root operations in the Placement section include only those procedures that are performed without making an incision or a puncture. The root operations *Change* and *Removal* are in the

Placement section and have the same meaning as in the Medical and Surgical section.

The Placement section also includes five additional root operations, defined as follows:

- *Compression*: Putting pressure on a body region
- *Dressing*: Putting material on a body region for protection
- *Immobilization*: Limiting or preventing motion of an external body region
- *Packing*: Putting material in a body region or orifice
- *Traction*: Exerting a pulling force on a body region in a distal direction

Body Region (Character 4)

The fourth-character values are either body regions (e.g., *Upper Leg*) or natural orifices (e.g., *Ear*).

Approach (Character 5)

Since all placement procedures are performed directly on the skin or mucous membrane, or performed indirectly by applying external force through the skin or mucous membrane, the approach value is always *External*.

Device (Character 6)

The device character is always specified (except in the case of manual traction) and indicates the device placed during the procedure (e.g., cast, splint, bandage, etc.). Except for casts for fractures and dislocations, devices in the Placement section are off the shelf and do not require any extensive design, fabrication, or fitting. Placement of devices that require extensive design, fabrication, or fitting are coded in the Rehabilitation section.

Qualifier (Character 7)

The qualifier character is not specified in the Placement section; the qualifier value is always *No Qualifier*.

Administration Section

Character Meanings

The seven characters in the Administration section have the following meaning:

Character	Meaning
1	Section
2	Physiological System and Anatomical Region
3	Root Operation
4	Body System/Region
5	Approach
6	Substance
7	Qualifier

Administration section codes represent procedures for putting in or on a therapeutic, prophylactic, protective, diagnostic, nutritional, or physiological substance. The section includes transfusions, infusions, and injections, along with other similar services such as irrigation and tattooing.

Section (Character 1)

Administration procedure codes have a first-character value of *3*.

Body System (Character 2)

The body-system character contains only three values: *Indwelling Device, Physiological Systems and Anatomical Regions,* or *Circulatory System*. The *Circulatory System* is used for transfusion procedures.

Root Operation (Character 3)

There are three root operations in the Administration section.

- *Introduction*: Putting in or on a therapeutic, diagnostic, nutritional, physiological, or prophylactic substance except blood or blood products
- *Irrigation*: Putting in or on a cleansing substance
- *Transfusion*: Putting in blood or blood products

Body/System Region (Character 4)

The fourth character specifies the body system/region. The fourth character identifies the site where the substance is administered, not the site where the substance administered takes effect. Sites include *Skin and Mucous Membrane, Subcutaneous Tissue* and *Muscle*. These differentiate intradermal, subcutaneous, and intramuscular injections, respectively. Other sites include *Eye, Respiratory Tract, Peritoneal Cavity,* and *Epidural Space*.

The body systems/regions for arteries and veins are *Peripheral Artery, Central Artery, Peripheral Vein,* and *Central Vein*. The *Peripheral Artery* or *Vein* is typically used when a substance is introduced locally into an artery or vein. For example, chemotherapy is the introduction of an antineoplastic substance into a peripheral artery or vein by a percutaneous approach. In general, the substance introduced into a peripheral artery or vein has a systemic effect.

The *Central Artery* or *Vein* is typically used when the site where the substance is introduced is distant from the point of entry into the artery or vein. For example, the introduction of a substance directly at the site of a clot within an artery or vein using a catheter is coded as an introduction of a thrombolytic substance into a central artery or vein by a percutaneous approach. In general, the substance introduced into a central artery or vein has a local effect.

Approach (Character 5)

The fifth character specifies approaches as defined in the Medical and Surgical section. The approach for intradermal, subcutaneous, and intramuscular introductions (i.e., injections) is *Percutaneous*. If a catheter is placed to introduce a substance into an internal site within the circulatory system, then the approach is also *Percutaneous*. For example, if a catheter is used to introduce contrast directly into the heart for angiography, then the procedure would be coded as a percutaneous introduction of contrast into the heart.

Substance (Character 6)

The sixth character specifies the substance being introduced. Broad categories of substances are defined, such as anesthetic, contrast, dialysate, and blood products such as platelets.

Qualifier (Character 7)

The seventh character is a qualifier and is used to indicate whether the substance is *Autologous* or *Nonautologous*, or to further specify the substance.

Measurement and Monitoring Section

Character Meanings

The seven characters in the Measurement and Monitoring section have the following meaning:

Character	Meaning
1	Section
2	Physiological System
3	Root Operation
4	Body System
5	Approach
6	Function/Device
7	Qualifier

Measurement and Monitoring section codes represent procedures for determining the level of a physiological or physical function.

Section (Character 1)

Measurement and Monitoring procedure codes have a first-character value of *4*.

Body System (Character 2)

The second-character values for body system are A, *Physiological Systems* or B, *Physiological Devices*.

Root Operation (Character 3)

There are two root operations in the Measurement and Monitoring section, as defined below:

- *Measurement*: Determining the level of a physiological or physical function at a point in time
- *Monitoring*: Determining the level of a physiological or physical function repetitively over a period of time

Body System (Character 4)

The fourth character specifies the specific body system measured or monitored.

Approach (Character 5)

The fifth character specifies approaches as defined in the Medical and Surgical section.

Function/Device (Character 6)

The sixth character specifies the physiological or physical function being measured or monitored. Examples of physiological or physical functions are *Conductivity, Metabolism, Pulse, Temperature,* and *Volume*. If a device used to perform the measurement or monitoring is inserted and left in, then insertion of the device is coded as a separate Medical and Surgical procedure.

Qualifier (Character 7)

The seventh-character qualifier contains specific values as needed to further specify the body part (e.g., central, portal, pulmonary) or a variation of the procedure performed (e.g., ambulatory, stress). Examples of typical procedures coded in this section are EKG, EEG, and cardiac catheterization. An EKG is the measurement of cardiac electrical activity, while an EEG is the measurement of electrical activity of the central nervous system. A cardiac catheterization performed to measure the pressure in the heart is coded as the measurement of cardiac pressure by percutaneous approach.

Extracorporeal Assistance and Performance Section

Character Meanings

The seven characters in the Extracorporeal Assistance and Performance section have the following meaning:

Character	Meaning
1	Section
2	Physiological System
3	Root Operation
4	Body System
5	Duration
6	Function
7	Qualifier

In Extracorporeal Assistance and Performance procedures, equipment outside the body is used to assist or perform a physiological function. The section includes procedures performed in a critical care setting, such as mechanical ventilation and cardioversion; it also includes other services such as hyperbaric oxygen treatment and hemodialysis.

Section (Character 1)

Extracorporeal Assistance and Performance procedure codes have a first-character value of *5*.

Body System (Character 2)

The second-character value for body system is A, *Physiological Systems*.

Root Operation (Character 3)

There are three root operations in the Extracorporeal Assistance and Performance section, as defined below.

- *Assistance*: Taking over a portion of a physiological function by extracorporeal means
- *Performance*: Completely taking over a physiological function by extracorporeal means
- *Restoration*: Returning, or attempting to return, a physiological function to its natural state by extracorporeal means

The root operation *Restoration* contains a single procedure code that identifies extracorporeal cardioversion.

Body System (Character 4)

The fourth character specifies the body system (e.g., cardiac, respiratory) to which extracorporeal assistance or performance is applied.

Duration (Character 5)

The fifth character specifies the duration of the procedure—*Single, Intermittent*, or *Continuous*. For respiratory ventilation assistance or performance, the duration is specified in hours— *< 24 Consecutive Hours*, *24–96 Consecutive Hours*, or *> 96 Consecutive Hours*. Value 6, *Multiple* identifies serial procedure treatment.

Function (Character 6)

The sixth character specifies the physiological function assisted or performed (e.g., oxygenation, ventilation) during the procedure.

Qualifier (Character 7)
The seventh-character qualifier specifies the type of equipment used, if any.

Extracorporeal Therapies Section

Character Meanings
The seven characters in the Extracorporeal Therapies section have the following meaning:

Character	Meaning
1	Section
2	Physiological Systems
3	Root Operation
4	Body System
5	Duration
6	Qualifier
7	Qualifier

In extracorporeal therapy, equipment outside the body is used for a therapeutic purpose that does not involve the assistance or performance of a physiological function.

Section (Character 1)
Extracorporeal Therapy procedure codes have a first-character value of 6.

Body System (Character 2)
The second-character value for body system is *Physiological Systems*.

Root Operation (Character 3)
There are 10 root operations in the Extracorporeal Therapy section, as defined below.

- *Atmospheric Control*: Extracorporeal control of atmospheric pressure and composition
- *Decompression*: Extracorporeal elimination of undissolved gas from body fluids

  Coding note: The root operation *Decompression* involves only one type of procedure: treatment for decompression sickness (the bends) in a hyperbaric chamber.
- *Electromagnetic Therapy*: Extracorporeal treatment by electromagnetic rays
- *Hyperthermia*: Extracorporeal raising of body temperature

  Coding note: The term hyperthermia is used to describe both a temperature imbalance treatment and also as an adjunct radiation treatment for cancer. When treating the temperature imbalance, it is coded to this section; for the cancer treatment, it is coded in section *D Radiation Therapy.*
- *Hypothermia*: Extracorporeal lowering of body temperature
- *Pheresis*: Extracorporeal separation of blood products

  Coding note: Pheresis may be used for two main purposes: to treat diseases when too much of a blood component is produced (e.g., leukemia) and to remove a blood product such as platelets from a donor, for transfusion into another patient.
- *Phototherapy*: Extracorporeal treatment by light rays

  Coding note: Phototherapy involves using a machine that exposes the blood to light rays outside the body, recirculates it, and then returns it to the body.
- *Shock Wave Therapy*: Extracorporeal treatment by shock waves
- *Ultrasound Therapy*: Extracorporeal treatment by ultrasound
- *Ultraviolet Light Therapy*: Extracorporeal treatment by ultraviolet light

Body System (Character 4)
The fourth character specifies the body system on which the extracorporeal therapy is performed (e.g., skin, circulatory).

Duration (Character 5)
The fifth character specifies the duration of the procedure (e.g., single or intermittent).

Qualifier (Character 6)
The sixth character is not specified for Extracorporeal Therapies and always has the value *No Qualifier*.

Qualifier (Character 7)
The seventh-character qualifier is used in the root operation *Pheresis* to specify the blood component on which pheresis is performed and in the root operation *Ultrasound Therapy* to specify site of treatment.

Osteopathic Section

Character Meanings
The seven characters in the Osteopathic section have the following meaning:

Character	Meaning
1	Section
2	Anatomical Region
3	Root Operation
4	Body Region
5	Approach
6	Method
7	Qualifier

Section (Character 1)
Osteopathic procedure codes have a first-character value of *7*.

Body System (Character 2)
The body-system character contains the value *Anatomical Regions*.

Root Operation (Character 3)
There is only one root operation in the Osteopathic section.

- *Treatment*: Manual treatment to eliminate or alleviate somatic dysfunction and related disorders

Body Region (Character 4)
The fourth character specifies the body region on which the osteopathic treatment is performed.

Approach (Character 5)
The approach for osteopathic treatment is always *External*.

Method (Character 6)

The sixth character specifies the method by which the treatment is accomplished.

Qualifier (Character 7)

The seventh character is not specified in the Osteopathic section and always has the value *None*.

Other Procedures Section

Character Meanings

The seven characters in the Other Procedures section have the following meaning:

Character	Meaning
1	Section
2	Body System
3	Root Operation
4	Body Region
5	Approach
6	Method
7	Qualifier

The Other Procedures section includes acupuncture, suture removal, and in vitro fertilization.

Section (Character 1)

Other Procedure section codes have a first-character value of *8*.

Body System (Character 2)

The second-character values for body systems are *Physiological Systems and Anatomical Regions* and *Indwelling Device*.

Root Operation (Character 3)

The Other Procedures section has only one root operation, defined as follows:

- *Other Procedures*: Methodologies that attempt to remediate or cure a disorder or disease.

Body Region (Character 4)

The fourth character contains specified body-region values, and also the body-region value *None* for Extracorporeal Procedures.

Approach (Character 5)

The fifth character specifies approaches as defined in the Medical and Surgical section.

Method (Character 6)

The sixth character specifies the method (e.g., *Acupuncture, Therapeutic Massage*).

Qualifier (Character 7)

The seventh character is a qualifier and contains specific values as needed.

Chiropractic Section

Character Meanings

The seven characters in the Chiropractic section have the following meaning:

Character	Meaning
1	Section
2	Anatomical Regions
3	Root Operation
4	Body Region
5	Approach
6	Method
7	Qualifier

Section (Character 1)

Chiropractic section procedure codes have a first-character value of *9*.

Body System (Character 2)

The second-character value for body system is *Anatomical Regions*.

Root Operation (Character 3)

There is only one root operation in the *Chiropractic* section.

- *Manipulation:* Manual procedure that involves a directed thrust to move a joint past the physiological range of motion, without exceeding the anatomical limit.

Body Region (Character 4)

The fourth character specifies the body region on which the chiropractic manipulation is performed.

Approach (Character 5)

The approach for chiropractic manipulation is always *External*.

Method (Character 6)

The sixth character is the method by which the manipulation is accomplished.

Qualifier (Character 7)

The seventh character is not specified in the Chiropractic section and always has the value *None*.

Imaging Section

Character Meanings

The seven characters in Imaging procedures have the following meaning:

Character	Meaning
1	Section
2	Body System
3	Root Type
4	Body Part
5	Contrast
6	Qualifier
7	Qualifier

Imaging procedures include plain radiography, fluoroscopy, CT, MRI, and ultrasound. Nuclear medicine procedures, including PET, uptakes, and scans, are in the nuclear medicine section. Therapeutic radiation procedure codes are in a separate radiation therapy section.

Section (Character 1)
Imaging procedure codes have a first-character value of *B*.

Body System (Character 2)
In the Imaging section, the second character defines the body system, such as *Heart* or *Gastrointestinal System*.

Root Type (Character 3)
The third character defines the type of imaging procedure (e.g., MRI, ultrasound). The following list includes all types in the *Imaging* section with a definition of each type:

- *Computerized Tomography (CT Scan)* : Computer-reformatted digital display of multiplanar images developed from the capture of multiple exposures of external ionizing radiation
- *Fluoroscopy*: Single plane or bi-plane real-time display of an image developed from the capture of external ionizing radiation on fluorescent screen. The image may also be stored by either digital or analog means
- *Magnetic Resonance Imaging (MRI)* : Computer reformatted digital display of multiplanar images developed from the capture of radiofrequency signals emitted by nuclei in a body site excited within a magnetic field
- *Plain Radiography*: Planar display of an image developed from the capture of external ionizing radiation on photographic or photoconductive plate
- *Ultrasonography*: Real-time display of images of anatomy or flow information developed from the capture of reflected and attenuated high-frequency sound waves

Body Part(Character 4)
The fourth character defines the body part with different values for each body system (character 2) value.

Contrast (Character 5)
The fifth character specifies whether the contrast material used in the imaging procedure is *High* or *Low Osmolar*, when applicable.

Qualifier (Character 6)
The sixth-character qualifier provides further detail regarding the nature of the substance or technologies used, such as *Unenhanced and Enhanced (contrast), Laser, or Intravascular Optical Coherence*.

Qualifier (Character 7)
The seventh character is a qualifier that may be used to specify certain procedural circumstances, the method by which the procedure was performed, or technologies utilized, such as *Intraoperative, Intravascular, or Transesophageal.*

Nuclear Medicine Section

Character Meanings
The seven characters in the Nuclear Medicine section have the following meaning:

Character	Meaning
1	Section
2	Body System
3	Root Type
4	Body Part
5	Radionuclide
6	Qualifier
7	Qualifier

Nuclear Medicine is the introduction of radioactive material into the body to create an image, to diagnose and treat pathologic conditions, or to assess metabolic functions. The Nuclear Medicine section does not include the introduction of encapsulated radioactive material for the treatment of cancer. These procedures are included in the Radiation Therapy section.

Section (Character 1)
Nuclear Medicine procedure codes have a first-character value of *C*.

Body System (Character 2)
The second character specifies the body system on which the nuclear medicine procedure is performed.

Root Type (Character 3)
The third character indicates the type of nuclear medicine procedure (e.g., planar imaging or nonimaging uptake). The following list includes the types of nuclear medicine procedures with a definition of each type.

- *Nonimaging Uptake:* Introduction of radioactive materials into the body for measurements of organ function, from the detection of radioactive emissions
- *Nonimaging Probe:* Introduction of radioactive materials into the body for the study of distribution and fate of certain substances by the detection of radioactive emissions; or alternatively, measurement of absorption of radioactive emissions from an external source
- *Nonimaging Assay:* Introduction of radioactive materials into the body for the study of body fluids and blood elements, by the detection of radioactive emissions
- *Planar Imaging*: Introduction of radioactive materials into the body for single-plane display of images developed from the capture of radioactive emissions
- *Positron Emission Tomography (PET):* Introduction of radioactive materials into the body for three-dimensional display of images developed from the simultaneous capture, 180 degrees apart, of radioactive emissions
- *Systemic Therapy:* Introduction of unsealed radioactive materials into the body for treatment
- *Tomographic (Tomo) Imaging*: Introduction of radioactive materials into the body for three dimensional display of images developed from the capture of radioactive emissions

Body Part (Character 4)

The fourth character indicates the body part or body region studied. *Regional* (e.g., lower extremity veins) and *Combination* (e.g., liver and spleen) body parts are commonly used in this section.

Radionuclide (Character 5)

The fifth character specifies the radionuclide, the radiation source. The option *Other Radionuclide* is provided in the nuclear medicine section for newly approved radionuclides until they can be added to the coding system. If more than one radiopharmaceutical is given to perform the procedure, then more than one code is used.

Qualifier (Character 6 and 7)

The sixth and seventh characters are qualifiers but are not specified in the *Nuclear Medicine* section; the value is always *None.*

Radiation Therapy Section

Character Meanings

The seven characters in the Radiation Therapy section have the following meaning:

Character	Meaning
1	Section
2	Body System
3	Root Type
4	Treatment Site
5	Modality Qualifier
6	Isotope
7	Qualifier

Section (Character 1)

Radiation therapy procedure codes have a first-character value of *D.*

Body System (Character 2)

The second character specifies the body system (e.g., central nervous system, musculoskeletal) irradiated.

Root Type (Character 3)

The third character specifies the general modality used (e.g., beam radiation).

Treatment Site (Character 4)

The fourth character specifies the body part that is the focus of the radiation therapy.

Modality Qualifier (Character 5)

The fifth character further specifies the radiation modality used (e.g., photons, electrons).

Isotope (Character 6)

The sixth character specifies the isotopes introduced into the body, if applicable.

Qualifier (Character 7)

The seventh character may specify whether the procedure was performed intraoperatively.

Physical Rehabilitation and Diagnostic Audiology Section

Character Meanings

The seven characters in the Physical Rehabilitation and Diagnostic Audiology section have the following meaning:

Character	Meaning
1	Section
2	Section Qualifier
3	Root Type
4	Body System & Region
5	Type Qualifier
6	Equipment
7	Qualifier

Physical rehabilitation procedures include physical therapy, occupational therapy, and speech-language pathology. Osteopathic procedures and chiropractic procedures are in separate sections.

Section (Character 1)

Physical Rehabilitation and Diagnostic Audiology procedure codes have a first-character value of *F.*

Section Qualifier (Character 2)

The section qualifier *Rehabilitation* or *Diagnostic Audiology* is specified in the second character.

Root Type (Character 3)

The third character specifies the root type. There are 14 different root type values, which can be classified into four basic types of rehabilitation and diagnostic audiology procedures, defined as follows:

Assessment: Includes a determination of the patient's diagnosis when appropriate, need for treatment, planning for treatment, periodic assessment, and documentation related to these activities

Assessments are further classified into more than 100 different tests or methods. The majority of these focus on the faculties of hearing and speech, but others focus on various aspects of body function, and on the patient's quality of life, such as muscle performance, neuromotor development, and reintegration skills.

- *Speech Assessment*: Measurement of speech and related functions
- *Motor and/or Nerve Function Assessment*: Measurement of motor, nerve, and related functions
- *Activities of Daily Living Assessment*: Measurement of functional level for activities of daily living
- *Hearing Assessment*: Measurement of hearing and related functions
- *Hearing Aid Assessment*: Measurement of the appropriateness and/or effectiveness of a hearing device
- *Vestibular Assessment*: Measurement of the vestibular system and related functions

Caregiver Training: Educating caregiver with the skills and knowledge used to interact with and assist the patient

Caregiver Training is divided into 18 different broad subjects taught to help a caregiver provide proper patient care.

- *Caregiver Training*: Training in activities to support patient's optimal level of function

Fitting(s): Design, fabrication, modification, selection, and/or application of splint, orthosis, prosthesis, hearing aids, and/or other rehabilitation device

The fifth character used in *Device Fitting* procedures describes the device being fitted rather than the method used to fit the device. Definitions of devices, when provided, are located in the definitions portion of the ICD-1Ø-PCS tables and index, under section F, character 5.

- *Device Fitting*: Fitting of a device designed to facilitate or support achievement of a higher level of function

Treatment: Use of specific activities or methods to develop, improve, and/or restore the performance of necessary functions, compensate for dysfunction and/or minimize debilitation

Treatment procedures include swallowing dysfunction exercises, bathing and showering techniques, wound management, gait training, and a host of activities typically associated with rehabilitation.

- *Speech Treatment*: Application of techniques to improve, augment, or compensate for speech and related functional impairment
- *Motor Treatment*: Exercise or activities to increase or facilitate motor function
- *Activities of Daily Living Treatment*: Exercise or activities to facilitate functional competence for activities of daily living
- *Hearing Treatment*: Application of techniques to improve, augment, or compensate for hearing and related functional impairment
- *Cochlear Implant Treatment*: Application of techniques to improve the communication abilities of individuals with cochlear implant
- *Vestibular Treatment*: Application of techniques to improve, augment, or compensate for vestibular and related functional impairment

The type of treatment includes training as well as activities that restore function.

Body System & Region (Character 4)

The fourth character specifies the body region and/or system on which the procedure is performed.

Type Qualifier (Character 5)

The fifth character is a type qualifier that further specifies the procedure performed. Examples include therapy to improve the range of motion and training for bathing techniques. Refer to appendix D for definitions of these types of procedures.

Equipment (Character 6)

The sixth character specifies the equipment used. Specific equipment is not defined in the equipment value. Instead, broad categories of equipment are specified (e.g., aerobic endurance and conditioning, assistive/adaptive/supportive, etc.)

Qualifier (Character 7)

The seventh character is not specified in the Physical Rehabilitation and Diagnostic Audiology section and always has the value *None*.

Mental Health Section

Character Meanings

The seven characters in the Mental Health section have the following meaning:

Character	Meaning
1	Section
2	Body System
3	Root Type
4	Type Qualifier
5	Qualifier
6	Qualifier
7	Qualifier

Section (Character 1)

Mental health procedure codes have a first-character value of *G*.

Body System (Character 2)

The second character is used to identify the body system elsewhere in ICD-1Ø-PCS. In this section it always has the value *None*.

Root Type (Character 3)

The third character specifies the procedure type, such as crisis intervention or counseling. There are 12 types of mental health procedures, some of which are defined below.

Psychological Tests:

- Developmental: Age-normed developmental status of cognitive, social, and adaptive behavior skills
- Intellectual and Psychoeducational: Intellectual abilities, academic achievement, and learning capabilities (including behavior and emotional factors affecting learning)
- Neurobehavioral and Cognitive Status: Includes neurobehavioral status exam, interview(s), and observation for the clinical assessment of thinking, reasoning, and judgment, acquired knowledge, attention, memory, visual spatial abilities, language functions, and planning
- Neuropsychological: Thinking, reasoning and judgment, acquired knowledge, attention, memory, visual spatial abilities, language functions, planning
- Personality and Behavioral: Mood, emotion, behavior, social functioning, psychopathological conditions, personality traits, and characteristics

Crisis intervention: Includes defusing, debriefing, counseling, psychotherapy, and/or coordination of care with other providers or agencies

Individual Psychotherapy:

- Behavior: Primarily to modify behavior. Includes modeling and role playing, positive reinforcement of target behaviors, response cost, and training of self-management skills

- Cognitive/behavioral: Combining cognitive and behavioral treatment strategies to improve functioning. Maladaptive responses are examined to determine how cognitions relate to behavior patterns in response to an event. Uses learning principles and information-processing models
- Cognitive: Primarily to correct cognitive distortions and errors
- Interactive: Uses primarily physical aids and other forms of nonoral interaction with a patient who is physically, psychologically, or developmentally unable to use ordinary language for communication (e.g., the use of toys in symbolic play)
- Interpersonal: Helps an individual make changes in interpersonal behaviors to reduce psychological dysfunction. Includes exploratory techniques, encouragement of affective expression, clarification of patient statements, analysis of communication patterns, use of therapy relationship, and behavior change techniques.
- Psychoanalysis: Methods of obtaining a detailed account of past and present mental and emotional experiences to determine the source and eliminate or diminish the undesirable effects of unconscious conflicts by making the individual aware of their existence, origin, and inappropriate expression in emotions and behavior.
- Psychodynamic: Exploration of past and present emotional experiences to understand motives and drives using insight-oriented techniques (e.g., empathetic listening, clarifying self-defeating behavior patterns, and exploring adaptive alternatives) to reduce the undesirable effects of internal conflicts on emotions and behavior
- Psychophysiological: Monitoring and alternation of physiological processes to help the individual associate physiological reactions combined with cognitive and behavioral strategies to gain improved control of these processes to help the individual cope more effectively
- Supportive: Formation of therapeutic relationship primarily for providing emotional support to prevent further deterioration in functioning during periods of particular stress. Often used in conjunction with other therapeutic approaches

Counseling:

- Vocational: Exploration of vocational interest, aptitudes, and required adaptive behavior skills to develop and carry out a plan for achieving a successful vocational placement, enhancing work-related adjustment, and/or pursuing viable options in training education or preparation

Family Psychotherapy:

- Remediation of emotional or behavioral problems presented by one or more family members when psychotherapy with more than one family member is indicated

Electroconvulsive Therapy:

- Includes appropriate sedation and other preparation of the individual

Biofeedback: Includes electroencephalogram (EEG), blood pressure, skin temperature or peripheral blood flow, electrocardiogram (ECG), electrooculogram, electromyogram (EMG), respirometry or capnometry, galvanic skin response (GSR) or electrodermal response (EDR), perineometry to monitor and regulate bowel or bladder activity, and electrogastrogram to monitor and regulate gastric motility

Other Mental Health procedures include *Hypnosis, Narcosynthesis, Group Psychotherapy,* and *Light Therapy*. There are no ICD-1Ø-PCS definitions of these procedures at this time.

Type Qualifier (Character 4)

The fourth character is a type qualifier (e.g., to indicate that counseling was educational or vocational).

Qualifier (Character 5, 6 and 7)

The fifth, sixth, and seventh characters are not specified and always have the value *None.*

Substance Abuse Treatment Section

Character Meanings

The seven characters in the Substance Abuse Treatment section have the following meaning:

Character	Meaning
1	Section
2	Body System
3	Root Type
4	Type Qualifier
5	Qualifier
6	Qualifier
7	Qualifier

Section (Character 1)

Substance Abuse Treatment codes have a first-character value of *H.*

Body System (Character 2)

The second character is used to identify the body system elsewhere in ICD-1Ø-PCS. In this section, it always has the value *None.*

Root Type (Character 3)

The third character specifies the procedure. There are seven root type values classified in this section, as listed below:

- *Detoxification Services:* Not a treatment modality but helps the patient stabilize physically and psychologically until the body becomes free of drugs and the effects of alcohol
- *Individual Counseling:* Comprising several techniques, which apply various strategies to address drug addiction
- *Group Counseling:* Provides structured group counseling sessions and healing power through the connection with others
- *Family Counseling:* Provides support and education for family members of addicted individuals. Family member participation seen as critical to substance abuse treatment
- Other root type values in this section include *Individual Psychotherapy, Medication Management,* and *Pharmacotherapy*; there are no ICD-1Ø-PCS definitions of these procedures at this time.

Type Qualifier (Character 4)

The fourth character further specifies the procedure type. Type Qualifier values vary dependent upon the Root Type procedure (Character 3). Root type 2, *Detoxification Services* contains only the value Z, *None* and Root type 6, *Family Counseling* contains only the value 3, *Other Family Counseling*, whereas the remainder Root Type procedures include nine to twelve total possible values.

Qualifier (Character 5, 6 and 7)

The fifth through seventh characters are designated as qualifiers but are never specified, so they always have the value *None*.

Comparison of ICD-10-PCS and ICD-9-CM

In 1993, the National Committee on Vital and Health Statistics (NCVHS) issued a report specifying recommendations for a new procedure classification system. NCVHS identified the essential characteristics that a procedure classification system should possess. Those characteristics include hierarchical structure, expandability, comprehensive, nonoverlapping, ease of use, setting and provider neutrality, multi-axial structure, and limited to classification of procedures.

ICD-10-PCS meets virtually all NCVHS characteristics, while ICD-9-CM fails to meet many NCVHS characteristics. In addition to the NCVHS characteristics, there are several other attributes of a procedure coding system that should be taken into consideration when comparing systems.

Completeness and Accuracy of Codes

The procedures coded in ICD-10-PCS provided a much more complete and accurate description of the procedure performed. The specification of the procedures performed not only affects payment, but is integral to internal management systems, external performance comparisons, and the assessment of quality of care. The detail and completeness of ICD-10-PCS is essential in today's health care environment.

General Equivalence Mappings

Due to the complexities of ICD-10-PCS and the drastic structural differences between the two coding systems, a direct code crosswalk is not possible. However, a general "mapping" of similar code choices has been developed. This network of relationships between the two code sets may be referred to as general equivalence mappings (GEMs). The purpose of these mappings, from ICD-9-CM to ICD-10-PCS, and vice versa, is to attempt to find corresponding procedure codes in lieu of a direct translation. For example:

- The ICD-9-CM to ICD-10-PCS GEM may help with analyzing or comparing data coded using the ICD-9-CM system to facilitate "forward mapping" to ICD-10-PCS.
- The ICD-10-PCS to ICD-9-CM GEM may help in comparing coded data using the ICD-10-PCS system to facilitate "backward mapping" to ICD-9-CM.

The 2015 update of the ICD-10 general equivalence mappings are posted for reference on the CMS website at the URL below: http://www.cms.gov/Medicare/Coding/ICD10/2015-ICD-10-PCS-and-GEMs.html.

Communications with Physicians

ICD-9-CM procedure codes often poorly describe the precise procedure performed. Physicians or others reviewing or analyzing data coded in ICD-9-CM may have difficulty developing clinical pathways, evaluating the coding for possible fraud and abuse, or conducting research. The ICD-10-PCS codes provide more clinically relevant procedure descriptions that can be more readily understood and used by physicians.

Independent evaluation of ICD-10-PCS demonstrated that there is a learning curve associated with ICD-10-PCS. Because of the additional specificity in ICD-10-PCS, it probably takes longer to attain a minimum level of coding proficiency for ICD-10-PCS than for ICD-9-CM. However, it should take less time to become *highly* proficient with ICD-10-PCS than with ICD-9-CM due to the consistency of character and value definitions. ICD-9-CM lacks clear definitions, and many substantially different procedures are coded with the same code. Therefore, identifying the correct code required extensive knowledge of the American Hospital Association's *Coding Clinic for ICD-9-CM* and other coding guidelines.

Conclusion

ICD-10-PCS has been developed as a replacement for volume 3 of ICD-9-CM. The system has evolved during its development based on extensive input from many segments of the health care industry. The multi-axial structure of the system, combined with its detailed definition of terminology, permits a precise specification of procedures for use in health services research, epidemiology, statistical analysis, and administrative areas. ICD-10-PCS will also allow health information coders to assign accurate procedure codes with minimal effort.

Sources

All material contained in this manual is derived from the ICD-10-PCS Coding System, Reference Manual and related files revised and distributed by the Centers for Medicare and Medicaid Services, FY 2015.

ICD-10-PCS Official Conventions

The *ICD-10-PCS: The Complete Official Draft Code Set* is based on the official draft version of the International Classification of Diseases, 10th Revision, Procedure Classification System, issued by the U.S. Department of Health and Human Services, Centers for Medicare and Medicaid Services. This book is consistent with the content of the government's version of ICD-10-PCS and follows the official conventions.

Index

The user can use the Alphabetic Index to locate the appropriate table containing all the information necessary to construct a procedure code. The PCS tables should always be consulted to find the most appropriate valid code. Users may choose a valid code directly from the tables—he or she need not consult the index before proceeding to the tables to complete the code.

Main Terms

The Alphabetic Index reflects the structure of the tables. Therefore, the index is organized as an alphabetic listing. The index:

- Is based on the value of the third character
- Contains common procedure terms
- Lists anatomic sites
- Uses device terms

The main terms in the Alphabetic Index are root operations, root procedure types, or common procedure names. In addition, anatomic sites from the Body Part Key and device terms from the Device Key have been added for ease of use.

Examples:

Resection (root operation)

Fluoroscopy (root type)

Prostatectomy (common procedure name)

Brachial artery (body part)

Bard® Dulex™ mesh (device)

The index provides at least the first three or four values of the code, and some entries may provide complete valid codes. However, the user should always consult the appropriate table to verify that the most appropriate valid code has been selected.

Root Operation and Procedure Type Main Terms

For the *Medical and Surgical* and related sections, the root operation values are used as main terms in the index. The subterms under the root operation main terms are body parts. For the Ancillary section of the tables, the main terms in the index are the general type of procedure performed.

Examples:

Destruction
Acetabulum
Left 0Q55
Right 0Q54
Adenoids 0C5Q
Ampulla of Vater 0F5C
Biofeedback GZC9ZZZ
Planar Nuclear Medicine Imaging CP1

See Reference

The second type of term in the index uses common procedure names, such as "appendectomy" or "fundoplication." These common terms are listed as main terms with a "see" reference noting the PCS root operations that are possible valid code tables based on the objective of the procedure.

Examples:

Tendonectomy
see Excision, Tendon 0LB
see Resection, Tendon 0LT

Use Reference

The index also lists anatomic sites from the Body Part Key and device terms from the Device Key. These terms are listed with a "use" reference. The purpose of these references is to act as an additional reference to the terms located in the Appendix Keys. The term provided is the Body Part value or Device value to be selected when constructing a procedure code using the code tables. This type of index reference is not intended to direct the user to another term in the index, but to provide guidance regarding character value selection. Therefore, "use" references generally do not refer to specific valid code tables.

Examples:

Epitrochlear lymph node
use Lymphatic, Upper Extremity, Left
use Lymphatic, Upper Extremity, Right
CoAxia NeuroFlo catheter
use Intraluminal Device
SynCardia Total Artificial Heart
use Synthetic Substitute

Code Tables

ICD-10-PCS contains 16 sections of Code Tables organized by general type of procedure. The first three characters of a procedure code define each table. The tables consist of columns providing the possible last four characters of codes and rows providing valid values for each character. Within a PCS table, valid codes include all combinations of choices in characters 4 through 7 contained in the same row of the table. All seven characters must be specified to form a valid code.

There are three main sections of tables:

- *Medical and Surgical* section:
  - *Medical and Surgical* (0)
- *Medical and Surgical*-related sections:

- *Obstetrics* (1)
- *Placement* (2)
- *Administration* (3)
- *Extracorporeal Assistance and Performance* (5)
- *Extracorporeal Therapies* (6)
- *Osteopathic* (7)
- *Other Procedures* (8)
- *Chiropractic* (9)

• Ancillary sections:

- *Imaging* (B)
- *Nuclear Medicine* (C)
- *Radiation Therapy* (D)
- *Physical Rehabilitation and Diagnostic Audiology* (F)
- *Mental Health* (G)
- *Substance Abuse Treatment* (H)

The first three character values define each table. The root operation or root type designated for each table is accompanied by its official definition.

Examples:

Table ØØF provides codes for procedures on the central nervous system that involve breaking up of solid matter into pieces:

Character 1, Section Ø: Medical and Surgical

Character 2, Body System Ø: Central Nervous System

Character 3, Root Operation F: Fragmentation: Breaking solid matter in a body part to pieces

Tables are arranged numerically, then alphabetically.

Examples:

Section order: Numerically ordered Ø through 9, then alphabetically ordered B through H

Table order: Tables under body system *Central Nervous System* are ordered ØØ1 through ØØ9, then ØØB though ØØX.

Character value order: As an example, table ØØF in the *Central Nervous* body system, the character values for body part are arranged as follows:

3 Epidural Space

4 Subdural Space

5 Subarachnoid Space

6 Cerebral Ventricle

U Spinal Canal

When reviewing tables, the user should keep in mind that:

- There are multiple tables for the first three characters.
- Some tables may cover multiple pages in the code book—to ensure maximum clarity about character choices, valid entries do not split rows between pages. For instance, the entire table of valid characters completing a code beginning with 4A1 is split between two pages, but the split is between, not within, rows. This means that all the valid sixth and seventh characters for, say, body system *Arterial* (3) and approach *External* (X) are contained on one page.
- Individual entries may be listed in several horizontal "selection" lines.

When a table is continued onto another page, a note to this effect has been added in red.

Examples:

Ø Medical and Surgical
Ø Central Nervous System
F Fragmentation Breaking solid matter in a body part into pieces

Body Part Character 4	Approach Character 5	Device Character 6	Qualifier Character 7
3 Epidural Space NC **4** Subdural Space NC **5** Subarachnoid Space NC **6** Cerebral Ventricle NC **U** Spinal Canal	**Ø** Open **3** Percutaneous **4** Percutaneous Endoscopic **X** External	**Z** No Device	**Z** No Qualifier

NC **ØØF[3,4,5,6]XZZ**
Non-OR **ØØF[3,4,5,6]XZZ**

ICD-10-PCS Additional Conventions

New and Revised Text

To highlight changes to the tables with each new edition, the new and revised text is in green font.

Color-Coding and Symbol Annotations

An annotation box has been appended to every table with color-coding or symbols identifying Medicare code edits or other reimbursement edits. The box provides critical information on how the edits are applied. For example, the box may list all valid codes to which the edit applies or conditional criteria that must be met to satisfy the edits. Each table that includes a Medicare code edit or a reimbursement edit will have an annotation box. For example, see Table 00F provided on the previous page. There are two annotations one for Noncovered Procedure edit and one for Non-operating room Procedure edit. The codes to which those edits apply are listed. In some cases there will be additional criteria to satisfy the edit application, such as procedures that are noncovered except when reported with specific diagnosis codes. Because of the inherent structure of ICD-10-PCS, the edits do not always apply to all valid codes in a horizontal row of a table. The edit color-coding and symbols have been placed to the right of the fourth character for consistency and should be viewed as alerts to refer to the annotation box. It is important to *always* refer to the annotation box when applying the edits.

Bracketed Code Notation

The use of bracketed codes is an efficient convention to provide all valid character value alternatives for a specific set of circumstances. The character values in the brackets correspond to the valid values for the character in the position the bracket appears.

Examples:

In the annotation box for Table 00F provided on the previous page the Noncovered Procedure edit (NC) applies to codes represented in the bracketed code 00F[3,4,5,6]XZZ.

00F[3,4,5,6]XZZ Fragmentation in (Central Nervous System), External Approach

The valid fourth character values, Body Part that may be selected for this specific circumstance are as follows:

3 Epidural Space

4 Subdural Space

5 Subarachnoid Space

6 Cerebral Space

The fragmentation of matter in the spinal canal, Body Part value U, is not considered as having the noncovered edit apply under the Medicare Code Editor v30.0.

AHA's *Coding Clinic for ICD-10-CM/ PCS* References

The four cooperating parties have designated the AHA's *Coding Clinic for ICD-10-CM/PCS* as the official publication for coding guidance. The previous *Coding Clinic for ICD-9-CM* will not be carried over into ICD-10-CM/PCS edition. AHA began publishing Coding Clinic's specific to ICD-10-CM/PCS beginning with the 4th quarter of 2012. The references in this book include Coding Clinics released though the 2nd quarter of 2014 and are identified by the notation AHA: followed by the year, quarter and page number.

Due to the table format of ICD-10-PCS, a coding clinic may pertain to several codes within a specific table. You will find the AHA *Coding Clinic for ICD-10-CM/PCS* reference beneath the three character table that most fits the scenario of the coding clinic. For example, AHA's Coding Clinic 3rd quarter, 2013, page 18, contains a discussion regarding the correct code assignment for the placement of a peripherally inserted central catheter (PICC line). Since this code falls into Section **0** - Medical/Surgical, Body System **2** - Heart and Great Vessel and Root Operation **H** -Insertion, the reference will appear in blue ink beneath the 02H Table.

Medicare Code Edits

Medicare administrative contractors and many payers use Medicare code edits to check the coding accuracy on claims under the inpatient prospective payment system (IPPS). The Medicare code edits that apply to procedures are listed below. The coding edit information in this manual is effective from October 1, 2014, to September 30, 2015. This ICD-10 version of the Medicare Code Editor (MCE) is version 31R. However, the MCE is not intended to be used to process claims since the ICD-10 code set will not be mandated for use until the implementation of ICD-10 beginning on October 1, 2015.

- Invalid procedure code (for a list of all valid ICD-10-PCS codes, see the International Classification of Diseases, Tenth Revision, Procedures Classification System)
- *Sex conflict
- *Noncovered procedure
- Nonspecific O.R. procedure (Discontinued. Effective only for claims processed using MCE version 2.0-23.0)
- *Limited coverage procedure
- Open biopsy check (Discontinued. Effective only for claims processed using MCE version 2.0-26.0)
- Bilateral procedure (Discontinued. Effective only for claims processed using MCE version 2.0-28.0)

Starred edits are identified by colors, symbols, or footnotes as described below. For a quick reference to the color codes and symbols, look at the legend/key located at the bottom of each page.

Sex Edit Symbols

The sex edit symbols below address MCE and are used to detect inconsistencies between the patient's sex and the procedure. These symbols appear in the tables to the right of the body part value (character 4):

♂ Male procedure only: this symbol appears to the right of the body part value (character 4).

♀ Female procedure only: this symbol appears to the right of the body part value (character 4).

Noncovered Procedure

Medicare does not cover all procedures. However, some noncovered procedures, due to the presence of certain diagnoses, are reimbursed. Noncovered procedures are designated by the NC symbol.

Limited Coverage

For certain procedures whose medical complexity and serious nature incur extraordinary associated costs, Medicare limits coverage to a portion of the cost. The limited coverage edit indicates the type of limited coverage. Limited procedures are designated by the LC symbol to the right of the body part value.

Other Notations in the Tabular

Under the Medicare severity diagnosis-related group (MS-DRG) system, in addition to the MCEs there are certain other circumstances that affect MS-DRG assignment. The following notations alert users to reimbursement issues related to procedure reporting.

Non-Operating Room Procedures Not Affecting MS-DRG Assignment

Some ICD-10-PCS procedure codes are valid but do not affect MS-DRG assignment when reported on a claim. These codes represent non-operating room (non-OR) procedures. A gray color bar over the body part value indicates a procedure code that does not affect MS-DRG assignment and appears **only** in the Medical/Surgical and Obstetrical tables (001-10Y).

Non-Operating Room Procedures Affecting MS- DRG Assignment

A blue color bar over a body part value indicates a non-operating room procedure that does affect MS-DRG assignment (DRG non-OR).

Hospital-Acquired Condition Related Procedures

Procedures associated with hospital-acquired conditions (HAC) are identified with the yellow color bar over the body part value.

Combination Only

Some ICD-10-PCS procedure codes are considered "noncovered procedures" except when reported in combination with certain other procedure codes. Such codes are designated by a red color bar over the body part value.

Combination Member

A combination member is an ICD-10-PCS procedure code that can influence MS-DRG assignment either on its own or in combination with other specific ICD-10-PCS procedure codes. Combination member codes are designated by a plus sign (+) to the right of the body part value.

See Appendix I for Procedure Combinations

Under certain circumstances, more than one procedure code is needed in order to group to a specific MS-DRG. When codes within a table have been identified as a Combination Only (red color bar) or Combination Member (+) code, there is also a footnote instructing the coder to *see Appendix I*. Appendix I contains tables that identify the other procedure codes needed in the combination and the title and number of the MS-DRG to which the combination will group.

No Procedure Combinations Specified

There are some codes, although identified as a Combination Only or Combination Member codes, that are not part of a procedure combination that would group to a different MS-DRG. Codes within a table that have been identified as Combination Only (red color bar) or Combination Member (+) codes but are not found as part of a combination are listed under the footnote titled *No Procedure Combinations Specified.*

Other Notation in the Index

▼ Subterms under main terms may continue to the next column or page. This warning statement is a reminder to always check for additional subterms and information that may continue onto the next page or column before making a final selection.

ICD-10-PCS Coding Guidelines

Conventions

A1. ICD-10-PCS codes are composed of seven characters. Each character is an axis of classification that specifies information about the procedure performed. Within a defined code range, a character specifies the same type of information in that axis of classification.

Example: The fifth axis of classification specifies the approach in sections Ø through 4 and 7 through 9 of the system.

A2. One of 34 possible values can be assigned to each axis of classification in the seven-character code: they are the numbers Ø through 9 and the alphabet (except I and O because they are easily confused with the numbers 1 and Ø). The number of unique values used in an axis of classification differs as needed.

Example: Where the fifth axis of classification specifies the approach, seven different approach values are currently used to specify the approach.

A3. The valid values for an axis of classification can be added to as needed.

Example: If a significantly distinct type of device is used in a new procedure, a new device value can be added to the system.

A4. As with words in their context, the meaning of any single value is a combination of its axis of classification and any preceding values on which it may be dependent.

Example: The meaning of a body part value in the Medical and Surgical section is always dependent on the body system value. The body part value Ø in the Central Nervous body system specifies Brain and the body part value Ø in the Peripheral Nervous body system specifies Cervical Plexus.

A5. As the system is expanded to become increasingly detailed, over time more values will depend on preceding values for their meaning.

Example: In the Lower Joints body system, the device value 3 in the root operation Insertion specifies Infusion Device and the device value 3 in the root operation Replacement specifies Ceramic Synthetic Substitute.

A6. The purpose of the alphabetic index is to locate the appropriate table that contains all information necessary to construct a procedure code. The PCS Tables should always be consulted to find the most appropriate valid code.

A7. It is not required to consult the index first before proceeding to the tables to complete the code. A valid code may be chosen directly from the tables.

A8. All seven characters must be specified to be a valid code. If the documentation is incomplete for coding purposes, the physician should be queried for the necessary information.

A9. Within a PCS table, valid codes include all combinations of choices in characters 4 through 7 contained in the same row of the table. In the example below, ØJHT3VZ is a valid code, and ØJHW3VZ is *not* a valid code.

A10. "And," when used in a code description, means "and/or."

Example: Lower Arm and Wrist Muscle means lower arm and/or wrist muscle.

A11. Many of the terms used to construct PCS codes are defined within the system. It is the coder's responsibility to determine what the documentation in the medical record equates to in the PCS definitions. The physician is not expected to use the terms used in PCS code descriptions, nor is the coder required to query the physician when the correlation between the documentation and the defined PCS terms is clear.

Example: When the physician documents "partial resection" the coder can independently correlate "partial resection" to the root operation Excision without querying the physician for clarification.

Sample ICD-10-PCS Table

Ø Medical and Surgical
J Subcutaneous Tissue and Fascia
H Insertion Putting in a nonbiological appliance that monitors, assists, performs, or prevents a physiological function but does not physically take the place of a body part

Body Part Character 4	Approach Character 5	Device Character 6	Qualifier Character 7
S Subcutaneous Tissue and Fascia, Head and Neck **V** Subcutaneous Tissue and Fascia, Upper Extremity **W** Subcutaneous Tissue and Fascia, Lower Extremity	**Ø** Open **3** Percutaneous	**1** Radioactive Element **3** Infusion Device	**Z** No Qualifier
T Subcutaneous Tissue and Fascia, Trunk	**Ø** Open **3** Percutaneous	**1** Radioactive Element **3** Infusion Device **V** Infusion Pump	**Z** No Qualifier

Medical and Surgical Section Guidelines

B2. Body System

General guidelines

B2.1a. The procedure codes in the general anatomical regions body systems should only be used when the procedure is performed on an anatomical region rather than a specific body part (e.g., root operations Control and Detachment, drainage of a body cavity) or on the rare occasion when no information is available to support assignment of a code to a specific body part.

Example: Control of postoperative hemorrhage is coded to the root operation Control found in the general anatomical regions body systems.

B2.1b. Where the general body part values "upper" and "lower" are provided as an option in the Upper Arteries, Lower Arteries, Upper Veins, Lower Veins, Muscles and Tendons body systems, "upper" or "lower "specifies body parts located above or below the diaphragm respectively.

Example: Vein body parts above the diaphragm are found in the Upper Veins body system; vein body parts below the diaphragm are found in the Lower Veins body system.

B3. Root Operation

General guidelines

B3.1a. In order to determine the appropriate root operation, the full definition of the root operation as contained in the PCS Tables must be applied.

B3.1b. Components of a procedure specified in the root operation definition and explanation are not coded separately. Procedural steps necessary to reach the operative site and close the operative site are also not coded separately.

Example: Resection of a joint as part of a joint replacement procedure is included in the root operation definition of Replacement and is not coded separately. Laparotomy performed to reach the site of an open liver biopsy is not coded separately. In a resection of sigmoid colon with anastomosis of descending colon to rectum, the anastomosis is not coded separately.

Multiple procedures

B3.2. During the same operative episode, multiple procedures are coded if:

a. The same root operation is performed on different body parts as defined by distinct values of the body part character.

   Example: Diagnostic excision of liver and pancreas are coded separately.

b. The same root operation is repeated at different body sites that are included in the same body part value.

   Example: Excision of the sartorius muscle and excision of the gracilis muscle are both included in the upper leg muscle body part value, and multiple procedures are coded.

c. Multiple root operations with distinct objectives are performed on the same body part.

   Example: Destruction of sigmoid lesion and bypass of sigmoid colon are coded separately.

d. The intended root operation is attempted using one approach, but is converted to a different approach.

   Example: Laparoscopic cholecystectomy converted to an open cholecystectomy is coded as percutaneous endoscopic Inspection and open Resection.

Discontinued procedures

B3.3. If the intended procedure is discontinued, code the procedure to the root operation performed. If a procedure is discontinued before any other root operation is performed, code the root operation Inspection of the body part or anatomical region inspected.

Example: A planned aortic valve replacement procedure is discontinued after the initial thoracotomy and before any incision is made in the heart muscle, when the patient becomes hemodynamically unstable. This procedure is coded as an open Inspection of the mediastinum.

Biopsy procedures

B3.4a. Biopsy procedures are coded using the root operations Excision, Extraction, or Drainage and the qualifier Diagnostic. The qualifier Diagnostic is used only for biopsies.

Examples: Fine needle aspiration biopsy of lung is coded to the root operation Drainage with the qualifier Diagnostic. Biopsy of bone marrow is coded to the root operation Extraction with the qualifier Diagnostic. Lymph node sampling for biopsy is coded to the root operation Excision with the qualifier Diagnostic.

Biopsy followed by more definitive treatment

B3.4b. If a diagnostic Excision, Extraction, or Drainage procedure (biopsy) is followed by a more definitive procedure, such as Destruction, Excision or Resection at the same procedure site, both the biopsy and the more definitive treatment are coded.

Example: Biopsy of breast followed by partial mastectomy at the same procedure site, both the biopsy and the partial mastectomy procedure are coded.

Overlapping body layers

B3.5. If the root operations Excision, Repair or Inspection are performed on overlapping layers of the musculoskeletal system, the body part specifying the deepest layer is coded.

Example: Excisional debridement that includes skin and subcutaneous tissue and muscle is coded to the muscle body part.

Bypass procedures

B3.6a. Bypass procedures are coded by identifying the body part bypassed "from" and the body part bypassed "to." The fourth character body part specifies the body part bypassed from, and the qualifier specifies the body part bypassed to.

Example: Bypass from stomach to jejunum, stomach is the body part and jejunum is the qualifier.

B3.6b. Coronary arteries are classified by number of distinct sites treated, rather than number of coronary arteries or anatomic name of a coronary artery (e.g., left anterior descending). Coronary artery bypass procedures are coded differently than other bypass procedures as described in the previous guideline. Rather than identifying the body part bypassed from, the body part identifies the number of coronary artery sites bypassed to, and the qualifier specifies the vessel bypassed from.

Example: Aortocoronary artery bypass of one site on the left anterior descending coronary artery and one site on the obtuse marginal coronary artery is classified in the body part axis of classification as two coronary artery sites and the qualifier specifies the aorta as the body part bypassed from.

B3.6c. If multiple coronary artery sites are bypassed, a separate procedure is coded for each coronary artery site that uses a different device and/or qualifier.

Example: Aortocoronary artery bypass and internal mammary coronary artery bypass are coded separately.

Control vs. more definitive root operations

B3.7. The root operation Control is defined as, "Stopping, or attempting to stop, postprocedural bleeding." If an attempt to stop postprocedural bleeding is initially unsuccessful, and to stop the bleeding requires performing any of the definitive root operations Bypass, Detachment, Excision, Extraction, Reposition, Replacement, or Resection, then that root operation is coded instead of Control.

Example: Resection of spleen to stop postprocedural bleeding is coded to Resection instead of Control.

Excision vs. Resection

B3.8. PCS contains specific body parts for anatomical subdivisions of a body part, such as lobes of the lungs or liver and regions of the intestine. Resection of the specific body part is coded whenever all of the body part is cut out or off, rather than coding Excision of a less specific body part.

Example: Left upper lung lobectomy is coded to Resection of Upper Lung Lobe, Left rather than Excision of Lung, Left.

Excision for graft

B3.9. If an autograft is obtained from a different body part in order to complete the objective of the procedure, a separate procedure is coded.

Example: Coronary bypass with excision of saphenous vein graft, excision of saphenous vein is coded separately.

Fusion procedures of the spine

B3.10a. The body part coded for a spinal vertebral joint(s) rendered immobile by a spinal fusion procedure is classified by the level of the spine (e.g. thoracic). There are distinct body part values for a single vertebral joint and for multiple vertebral joints at each spinal level.

Example: Body part values specify Lumbar Vertebral Joint, Lumbar Vertebral Joints, 2 or More and Lumbosacral Vertebral Joint.

B3.10b. If multiple vertebral joints are fused, a separate procedure is coded for each vertebral joint that uses a different device and/or qualifier.

Example: Fusion of lumbar vertebral joint, posterior approach, anterior column and fusion of lumbar vertebral joint, posterior approach, posterior column are coded separately.

B3.10c. Combinations of devices and materials are often used on a vertebral joint to render the joint immobile. When combinations of devices are used on the same vertebral joint, the device value coded for the procedure is as follows:

- If an interbody fusion device is used to render the joint immobile (alone or containing other material like bone graft), the procedure is coded with the device value Interbody Fusion Device
- If bone graft is the *only* device used to render the joint immobile, the procedure is coded with the device value Nonautologous Tissue Substitute or Autologous Tissue Substitute
- If a mixture of autologous and nonautologous bone graft (with or without biological or synthetic extenders or binders) is used to render the joint immobile, code the procedure with the device value Autologous Tissue Substitute

Examples: Fusion of a vertebral joint using a cage style interbody fusion device containing morsellized bone graft is coded to the device Interbody Fusion Device.

Fusion of a vertebral joint using a bone dowel interbody fusion device made of cadaver bone and packed with a mixture of local morsellized bone and demineralized bone matrix is coded to the device Interbody Fusion Device.

Fusion of a vertebral joint using both autologous bone graft and bone bank bone graft is coded to the device Autologous Tissue Substitute.

Inspection procedures

B3.11a. Inspection of a body part(s) performed in order to achieve the objective of a procedure is not coded separately.

Example: Fiberoptic bronchoscopy performed for irrigation of bronchus, only the irrigation procedure is coded.

B3.11b. If multiple tubular body parts are inspected, the most distal body part inspected is coded. If multiple non-tubular body parts in a region are inspected, the body part that specifies the entire area inspected is coded.

Examples: Cystoureteroscopy with inspection of bladder and ureters is coded to the ureter body part value.

Exploratory laparotomy with general inspection of abdominal contents is coded to the peritoneal cavity body part value.

B3.11c. When both an Inspection procedure and another procedure are performed on the same body part during the same episode, if the Inspection procedure is performed using a different approach than the other procedure, the Inspection procedure is coded separately.

Example: Endoscopic Inspection of the duodenum is coded separately when open Excision of the duodenum is performed during the same procedural episode.

Occlusion vs. Restriction for vessel embolization procedures

B3.12. If the objective of an embolization procedure is to completely close a vessel, the root operation Occlusion is coded. If the objective of an embolization procedure is to narrow the lumen of a vessel, the root operation Restriction is coded.

Examples: Tumor embolization is coded to the root operation Occlusion, because the objective of the procedure is to cut off the blood supply to the vessel.

Embolization of a cerebral aneurysm is coded to the root operation Restriction, because the objective of the procedure is not to close off the vessel entirely, but to narrow the lumen of the vessel at the site of the aneurysm where it is abnormally wide.

Release procedures

B3.13. In the root operation Release, the body part value coded is the body part being freed and not the tissue being manipulated or cut to free the body part.

Example: Lysis of intestinal adhesions is coded to the specific intestine body part value.

Release vs. Division

B3.14. If the sole objective of the procedure is freeing a body part without cutting the body part, the root operation is Release. If the sole objective of the procedure is separating or transecting a body part, the root operation is Division.

Examples: Freeing a nerve root from surrounding scar tissue to relieve pain is coded to the root operation Release. Severing a nerve root to relieve pain is coded to the root operation Division.

Reposition for fracture treatment

B3.15. Reduction of a displaced fracture is coded to the root operation Reposition and the application of a cast or splint in conjunction with the Reposition procedure is not coded separately. Treatment of a nondisplaced fracture is coded to the procedure performed.

Examples: Casting of a nondisplaced fracture is coded to the root operation Immobilization in the Placement section.

Putting a pin in a nondisplaced fracture is coded to the root operation Insertion.

Transplantation vs. Administration

B3.16. Putting in a mature and functioning living body part taken from another individual or animal is coded to the root operation Transplantation. Putting in autologous or nonautologous cells is coded to the Administration section.

Example: Putting in autologous or nonautologous bone marrow, pancreatic islet cells or stem cells is coded to the Administration section.

B4. Body Part

General guidelines

B4.1a. If a procedure is performed on a portion of a body part that does not have a separate body part value, code the body part value corresponding to the whole body part.

Example: A procedure performed on the alveolar process of the mandible is coded to the mandible body part.

B4.1b. If the prefix "peri" is combined with a body part to identify the site of the procedure, the procedure is coded to the body part named.

Example: A procedure site identified as perirenal is coded to the kidney body part.

Branches of body parts

B4.2. Where a specific branch of a body part does not have its own body part value in PCS, the body part is coded to the closest proximal branch that has a specific body part value.

Example: A procedure performed on the mandibular branch of the trigeminal nerve is coded to the trigeminal nerve body part value

Bilateral body part values

B4.3. Bilateral body part values are available for a limited number of body parts. If the identical procedure is performed on contralateral body parts, and a bilateral body part value exists for that body part, a single procedure is coded using the bilateral body part value. If no bilateral body part value exists, each procedure is coded separately using the appropriate body part value.

Example: The identical procedure performed on both fallopian tubes is coded once using the body part value Fallopian Tube, Bilateral. The identical procedure performed on both knee joints is coded twice using the body part values Knee Joint, Right and Knee Joint, Left.

Coronary arteries

B4.4. The coronary arteries are classified as a single body part that is further specified by number of sites treated and not by name or number of arteries. Separate body part values are used to specify the number of sites treated when the same procedure is performed on multiple sites in the coronary arteries.

Examples: Angioplasty of two distinct sites in the left anterior descending coronary artery with placement of two stents is coded as Dilation of Coronary Arteries, Two Sites, with Intraluminal Device.

Angioplasty of two distinct sites in the left anterior descending coronary artery, one with stent placed and one without, is coded separately as Dilation of Coronary Artery, One Site with Intraluminal Device, and Dilation of Coronary Artery, One Site with no device.

Tendons, ligaments, bursae and fascia near a joint

B4.5. Procedures performed on tendons, ligaments, bursae and fascia supporting a joint are coded to the body part in the respective body system that is the focus of the procedure. Procedures performed on joint structures themselves are coded to the body part in the joint body systems.

Example: Repair of the anterior cruciate ligament of the knee is coded to the knee bursae and ligament body part in the bursae and ligaments body system. Knee arthroscopy with shaving of articular cartilage is coded to the knee joint body part in the Lower Joints body system.

Skin, subcutaneous tissue and fascia overlying a joint

B4.6. If a procedure is performed on the skin, subcutaneous tissue or fascia overlying a joint, the procedure is coded to the following body part:

- Shoulder is coded to Upper Arm
- Elbow is coded to Lower Arm
- Wrist is coded to Lower Arm
- Hip is coded to Upper Leg
- Knee is coded to Lower Leg
- Ankle is coded to Foot

Fingers and toes

B4.7. If a body system does not contain a separate body part value for fingers, procedures performed on the fingers are coded to the body part value for the hand. If a body system does not contain a separate body part value for toes, procedures performed on the toes are coded to the body part value for the foot.

Example: Excision of finger muscle is coded to one of the hand muscle body part values in the Muscles body system.

Upper and lower intestinal tract

B4.8 In the Gastrointestinal body system, the general body part values Upper Intestinal Tract and Lower Intestinal Tract are provided as an option for the root operations Change, Inspection, Removal and Revision. Upper Intestinal Tract includes the portion of the gastrointestinal tract from the esophagus down to and including the duodenum, and Lower Intestinal Tract includes the portion of the gastrointestinal tract from the jejunum down to and including the rectum and anus.

Example: In the root operation Change table, change of a device in the jejunum is coded using the body part Lower Intestinal Tract.

B5. Approach

Open approach with percutaneous endoscopic assistance

B5.2 Procedures performed using the open approach with percutaneous endoscopic assistance are coded to the approach Open.

Example: Laparoscopic-assisted sigmoidectomy is coded to the approach Open.

External approach

B5.3a Procedures performed within an orifice on structures that are visible without the aid of any instrumentation are coded to the approach External.

Example: Resection of tonsils is coded to the approach External.

B5.3b Procedures performed indirectly by the application of external force through the intervening body layers are coded to the approach External.

Example: Closed reduction of fracture is coded to the approach External.

Percutaneous procedure via device

B5.4 Procedures performed percutaneously via a device placed for the procedure are coded to the approach Percutaneous.

Example: Fragmentation of kidney stone performed via percutaneous nephrostomy is coded to the approach Percutaneous.

B6. Device

General guidelines

B6.1a. A device is coded only if a device remains after the procedure is completed. If no device remains, the device value No Device is coded.

B6.1b. Materials such as sutures, ligatures, radiological markers and temporary post-operative wound drains are considered integral to the performance of a procedure and are not coded as devices.

B6.1c. Procedures performed on a device only and not on a body part are specified in the root operations Change, Irrigation, Removal and Revision, and are coded to the procedure performed.

Example: Irrigation of percutaneous nephrostomy tube is coded to the root operation Irrigation of indwelling device in the Administration section.

Drainage device

B6.2. A separate procedure to put in a drainage device is coded to the root operation Drainage with the device value Drainage Device.

Obstetric Section Guidelines

C. Obstetrics Section

Products of conception

C1. Procedures performed on the products of conception are coded to the Obstetrics section. Procedures performed on the pregnant female other than the products of conception are coded to the appropriate root operation in the Medical and Surgical section.

Example: Amniocentesis is coded to the products of conception body part in the Obstetrics section. Repair of obstetric urethral laceration is coded to the urethra body part in the Medical and Surgical section.

Procedures following delivery or abortion

C2. Procedures performed following a delivery or abortion for curettage of the endometrium or evacuation of retained products of conception are all coded in the Obstetrics section, to the root operation Extraction and the body part Products of Conception, Retained. Diagnostic or therapeutic dilation and curettage performed during times other than the postpartum or post-abortion period are all coded in the Medical and Surgical section, to the root operation Extraction and the body part Endometrium.

Selection of Principal Procedure

D. Selection of Principal Procedure

The following instructions should be applied in the selection of principal procedure and clarification on the importance of the relation to the principal diagnosis when more than one procedure is performed:

1. Procedure performed for definitive treatment of both principal diagnosis and secondary diagnosis
    a. Sequence procedure performed for definitive treatment most related to principal diagnosis as principal procedure.
2. Procedure performed for definitive treatment and diagnostic procedures performed for both principal diagnosis and secondary diagnosis
    a. Sequence procedure performed for definitive treatment most related to principal diagnosis as principal procedure
3. A diagnostic procedure was performed for the principal diagnosis and a procedure is performed for definitive treatment of a secondary diagnosis.
    a. Sequence diagnostic procedure as principal procedure, since the procedure most related to the principal diagnosis takes precedence.
4. No procedures performed that are related to principal diagnosis; procedures performed for definitive treatment and diagnostic procedures were performed for secondary diagnosis
    a. Sequence procedure performed for definitive treatment of secondary diagnosis as principal procedure, since there are no procedures (definitive or nondefinitive treatment) related to principal diagnosis.

Coding Exercises

Using the ICD-10-PCS tables construct the code that accurately represents the procedure performed. Answers to these coding exercises may be found in appendix H.

Medical Surgical Section

Procedure	Code
Excision of malignant melanoma from skin of right ear	
Laparoscopy with excision of endometrial implant from left ovary	
Percutaneous needle core biopsy of right kidney	
EGD with gastric biopsy	
Open endarterectomy of left common carotid artery	
Excision of basal cell carcinoma of lower lip	
Open excision of tail of pancreas	
Percutaneous biopsy of right gastrocnemius muscle	
Sigmoidoscopy with sigmoid polypectomy	
Open excision of lesion from right Achilles tendon	
Open resection of cecum	
Total excision of pituitary gland, open	
Explantation of left failed kidney, open	
Open left axillary total lymphadenectomy	
Laparoscopic-assisted total vaginal hysterectomy	
Right total mastectomy, open	
Open resection of papillary muscle	
Radical retropubic prostatectomy, open	
Laparoscopic cholecystectomy	
Endoscopic bilateral total maxillary sinusectomy	
Amputation at right elbow level	
Right below-knee amputation, proximal tibia/fibula	
Fifth ray carpometacarpal joint amputation, left hand	
Right leg and hip amputation through ischium	
DIP joint amputation of right thumb	
Right wrist joint amputation	
Trans-metatarsal amputation of foot at left big toe	
Mid-shaft amputation, right humerus	
Left fourth toe amputation, mid-proximal phalanx	
Right above-knee amputation, distal femur	
Cryotherapy of wart on left hand	
Percutaneous radiofrequency ablation of right vocal cord lesion	

Medical Surgical Section (Continued)

Procedure	Code
Left heart catheterization with laser destruction of arrhythmogenic focus, A-V node	
Cautery of nosebleed	
Transurethral endoscopic laser ablation of prostate	
Cautery of oozing varicose vein, left calf	
Laparoscopy with destruction of endometriosis, bilateral ovaries	
Laser coagulation of right retinal vessel hemorrhage, percutaneous	
Thoracoscopic pleurodesis, left side	
Percutaneous insertion of Greenfield IVC filter	
Forceps total mouth extraction, upper and lower teeth	
Removal of left thumbnail	
Extraction of right intraocular lens without replacement, percutaneous	
Laparoscopy with needle aspiration of ova for in vitro fertilization	
Nonexcisional debridement of skin ulcer, right foot	
Open stripping of abdominal fascia, right side	
Hysteroscopy with D&C, diagnostic	
Liposuction for medical purposes, left upper arm	
Removal of tattered right ear drum fragments with tweezers	
Microincisional phlebectomy of spider veins, right lower leg	
Routine Foley catheter placement	
Incision and drainage of external perianal abscess	
Percutaneous drainage of ascites	
Laparoscopy with left ovarian cystotomy and drainage	
Laparotomy and drain placement for liver abscess, right lobe	
Right knee arthrotomy with drain placement	
Thoracentesis of left pleural effusion	
Phlebotomy of left median cubital vein for polycythemia vera	
Percutaneous chest tube placement for right pneumothorax	
Endoscopic drainage of left ethmoid sinus	
External ventricular CSF drainage catheter placement via burr hole	
Removal of foreign body, right cornea	
Percutaneous mechanical thrombectomy, left brachial artery	

Medical Surgical Section (Continued)

Procedure	Code
Esophagogastroscopy with removal of bezoar from stomach	
Foreign body removal, skin of left thumb	
Transurethral cystoscopy with removal of bladder stone	
Forceps removal of foreign body in right nostril	
Laparoscopy with excision of old suture from mesentery	
Incision and removal of right lacrimal duct stone	
Nonincisional removal of intraluminal foreign body from vagina	
Right common carotid endarterectomy, open	
Open excision of retained sliver, subcutaneous tissue of left foot	
Extracorporeal shock-wave lithotripsy (ESWL), bilateral ureters	
Endoscopic retrograde cholangiopancreatography (ERCP) with lithotripsy of common bile duct stone	
Thoracotomy with crushing of pericardial calcifications	
Transurethral cystoscopy with fragmentation of bladder calculus	
Hysteroscopy with intraluminal lithotripsy of left fallopian tube calcification	
Division of right foot tendon, percutaneous	
Left heart catheterization with division of bundle of HIS	
Open osteotomy of capitate, left hand	
EGD with esophagotomy of esophagogastric junction	
Sacral rhizotomy for pain control, percutaneous	
Laparotomy with exploration and adhesiolysis of right ureter	
Incision of scar contracture, right elbow	
Frenulotomy for treatment of tongue-tie syndrome	
Right shoulder arthroscopy with coracoacromial ligament release	
Mitral valvulotomy for release of fused leaflets, open approach	
Percutaneous left Achilles tendon release	
Laparoscopy with lysis of peritoneal adhesions	
Manual rupture of right shoulder joint adhesions under general anesthesia	
Open posterior tarsal tunnel release	
Laparoscopy with freeing of left ovary and fallopian tube	
Liver transplant with donor matched liver	
Orthotopic heart transplant using porcine heart	
Right lung transplant, open, using organ donor match	
Transplant of large intestine, organ donor match	
Left kidney/pancreas organ bank transplant	

Medical Surgical Section (Continued)

Procedure	Code
Replantation of avulsed scalp	
Reattachment of severed right ear	
Reattachment of traumatic left gastrocnemius avulsion, open	
Closed replantation of three avulsed teeth, lower jaw	
Reattachment of severed left hand	
Right open palmaris longus tendon transfer	
Endoscopic radial to median nerve transfer	
Fasciocutaneous flap closure of left thigh, open	
Transfer left index finger to left thumb position, open	
Percutaneous fascia transfer to fill defect, anterior neck	
Trigeminal to facial nerve transfer, percutaneous endoscopic	
Endoscopic left leg flexor hallucis longus tendon transfer	
Right scalp advancement flap to right temple	
Bilateral TRAM pedicle flap reconstruction status post mastectomy, muscle only, open	
Skin transfer flap closure of complex open wound, left lower back	
Open fracture reduction, right tibia	
Laparoscopy with gastropexy for malrotation	
Left knee arthroscopy with reposition of anterior cruciate ligament	
Open transposition of ulnar nerve	
Closed reduction with percutaneous internal fixation of right femoral neck fracture	
Trans-vaginal intraluminal cervical cerclage	
Cervical cerclage using Shirodkar technique	
Thoracotomy with banding of left pulmonary artery using extraluminal device	
Restriction of thoracic duct with intraluminal stent, percutaneous	
Craniotomy with clipping of cerebral aneurysm	
Nonincisional, transnasal placement of restrictive stent in right lacrimal duct	
Catheter-based temporary restriction of blood flow in abdominal aorta for treatment of cerebral ischemia	
Percutaneous ligation of esophageal vein	
Percutaneous embolization of left internal carotid-cavernous fistula	
Laparoscopy with bilateral occlusion of fallopian tubes using Hulka extraluminal clips	
Open suture ligation of failed A-V graft, left brachial artery	
Percutaneous embolization of vascular supply, intracranial meningioma	
Percutaneous embolization of right uterine artery, using coils	

Medical Surgical Section (Continued)

Procedure	Code
Open occlusion of left atrial appendage, using extraluminal pressure clips	
Percutaneous suture exclusion of left atrial appendage, via femoral artery access	
ERCP with balloon dilation of common bile duct	
PTCA of two coronary arteries, LAD with stent placement, RCA with no stent	
Cystoscopy with intraluminal dilation of bladder neck stricture	
Open dilation of old anastomosis, left femoral artery	
Dilation of upper esophageal stricture, direct visualization, with Bougie sound	
PTA of right brachial artery stenosis	
Transnasal dilation and stent placement in right lacrimal duct	
Hysteroscopy with balloon dilation of bilateral fallopian tubes	
Tracheoscopy with intraluminal dilation of tracheal stenosis	
Cystoscopy with dilation of left ureteral stricture, with stent placement	
Open gastric bypass with Roux-en-Y limb to jejunum	
Right temporal artery to intracranial artery bypass using Gore-Tex graft, open	
Tracheostomy formation with tracheostomy tube placement, percutaneous	
PICVA (percutaneous in situ coronary venous arterialization) of single coronary artery	
Open left femoral-popliteal artery bypass using cadaver vein graft	
Shunting of intrathecal cerebrospinal fluid to peritoneal cavity using synthetic shunt	
Colostomy formation, open, transverse colon to abdominal wall	
Open urinary diversion, left ureter, using ileal conduit to skin	
CABG of LAD using left internal mammary artery, open off-bypass	
Open pleuroperitoneal shunt, right pleural cavity, using synthetic device	
Percutaneous placement of ventriculoperitoneal shunt for treatment of hydrocephalus	
End-of-life replacement of spinal neurostimulator generator, multiple array, in lower abdomen	
Percutaneous insertion of spinal neurostimulator lead, lumbar spinal cord	
Percutaneous placement of pacemaker lead in left atrium	
Open placement of dual chamber pacemaker generator in chest wall	
Percutaneous placement of venous central line in right internal jugular	

Medical Surgical Section (Continued)

Procedure	Code
Open insertion of multiple channel cochlear implant, left ear	
Percutaneous placement of Swan-Ganz catheter in superior vena cava	
Bronchoscopy with insertion of brachytherapy seeds, right main bronchus	
Placement of intrathecal infusion pump for pain management, percutaneous	
Open insertion of interspinous process device into lumbar vertebral joint	
Open placement of bone growth stimulator, left femoral shaft	
Cystoscopy with placement of brachytherapy seeds in prostate gland	
Percutaneous insertion of Greenfield IVC filter	
Full-thickness skin graft to right lower arm, autograft (do not code graft harvest for this exercise)	
Excision of necrosed left femoral head with bone bank bone graft to fill the defect, open	
Penetrating keratoplasty of right cornea with donor matched cornea, percutaneous approach	
Bilateral mastectomy with concomitant saline breast implants, open	
Excision of abdominal aorta with Gore-Tex graft replacement, open	
Total right knee arthroplasty with insertion of total knee prosthesis	
Bilateral mastectomy with free TRAM flap reconstruction	
Tenonectomy with graft to right ankle using cadaver graft, open	
Mitral valve replacement using porcine valve, open	
Percutaneous phacoemulsification of right eye cataract with prosthetic lens insertion	
Transcatheter replacement of pulmonary valve using of bovine jugular vein valve	
Total left hip replacement using ceramic on ceramic prosthesis, without bone cement	
Aortic valve annuloplasty using ring, open	
Laparoscopic repair of left inguinal hernia with marlex plug	
Autograft nerve graft to right median nerve, percutaneous endoscopic (do not code graft harvest for this exercise)	
Exchange of liner in femoral component of previous left hip replacement, open approach	
Anterior colporrhaphy with polypropylene mesh reinforcement, open approach	
Implantation of CorCap cardiac support device, open approach	
Abdominal wall herniorrhaphy, open, using synthetic mesh	

Medical Surgical Section (Continued)

Procedure	Code
Tendon graft to strengthen injured left shoulder using autograft, open (do not code graft harvest for this exercise)	
Onlay lamellar keratoplasty of left cornea using autograft, external approach	
Resurfacing procedure on right femoral head, open approach	
Exchange of drainage tube from right hip joint	
Tracheostomy tube exchange	
Change chest tube for left pneumothorax	
Exchange of cerebral ventriculostomy drainage tube	
Foley urinary catheter exchange	
Open removal of lumbar sympathetic neurostimulator lead	
Nonincisional removal of Swan-Ganz catheter from right pulmonary artery	
Laparotomy with removal of pancreatic drain	
Extubation, endotracheal tube	
Nonincisional PEG tube removal	
Transvaginal removal of brachytherapy seeds	
Transvaginal removal of extraluminal cervical cerclage	
Incision with removal of K-wire fixation, right first metatarsal	
Cystoscopy with retrieval of left ureteral stent	
Removal of nasogastric drainage tube for decompression	
Removal of external fixator, left radial fracture	
Reposition of Swan-Ganz catheter insertion to superior vena cava	
Open revision of right hip replacement, with readjustment of prosthesis	
Adjustment of position, pacemaker lead in left ventricle, percutaneous	
External repositioning of Foley catheter to bladder	
Taking out loose screw and putting larger screw in fracture repair plate, left tibia	
Revision of VAD reservoir placement in chest wall, causing patient discomfort, open	
Thoracotomy with exploration of right pleural cavity	
Diagnostic laryngoscopy	
Exploratory arthrotomy of left knee	
Colposcopy with diagnostic hysteroscopy	
Digital rectal exam	
Diagnostic arthroscopy of right shoulder	
Endoscopy of bilateral maxillary sinus	
Laparotomy with palpation of liver	
Transurethral diagnostic cystoscopy	

Medical Surgical Section (Continued)

Procedure	Code
Colonoscopy, abandoned at sigmoid colon	
Percutaneous mapping of basal ganglia	
Heart catheterization with cardiac mapping	
Intraoperative whole brain mapping via craniotomy	
Mapping of left cerebral hemisphere, percutaneous endoscopic	
Intraoperative cardiac mapping during open heart surgery	
Hysteroscopy with cautery of post-hysterectomy oozing and evacuation of clot	
Open exploration and ligation of post-op arterial bleeder, left forearm	
Control of postoperative retroperitoneal bleeding via laparotomy	
Reopening of thoracotomy site with drainage and control of post-op hemopericardium	
Arthroscopy with drainage of hemarthrosis at previous operative site, right knee	
Radiocarpal fusion of left hand with internal fixation, open	
Posterior spinal fusion at L1–L3 level with BAK cage interbody fusion device, open	
Intercarpal fusion of right hand with bone bank bone graft, open	
Sacrococcygeal fusion with bone graft from same operative site, open	
Interphalangeal fusion of left great toe, percutaneous pin fixation	
Suture repair of left radial nerve laceration	
Laparotomy with suture repair of blunt force duodenal laceration	
Cosmetic face lift, open, no other information available	
Bilateral breast augmentation with silicone implants, open	
Cosmetic rhinoplasty with septal reduction and tip elevation using local tissue graft, open	
Abdominoplasty (tummy tuck), open	
Liposuction of bilateral thighs	
Creation of penis in female patient using tissue bank donor graft	
Creation of vagina in male patient using synthetic material	
Laparoscopic vertical sleeve gastrectomy	
Left uterine artery embolization, intraluminal biosphere injection	

Obstetrics

Procedure	Code
Abortion by dilation and evacuation following laminaria insertion	
Manually assisted spontaneous abortion	
Abortion by abortifacient insertion	
Bimanual pregnancy examination	
Extraperitoneal C-section, low transverse incision	
Fetal spinal tap, percutaneous	
Fetal kidney transplant, laparoscopic	
Open in utero repair of congenital diaphragmatic hernia	
Laparoscopy with total excision of tubal pregnancy	
Transvaginal removal of fetal monitoring electrode	

Placement

Procedure	Code
Placement of packing material, right ear	
Mechanical traction of entire left leg	
Removal of splint, right shoulder	
Placement of neck brace	
Change of vaginal packing	
Packing of wound, chest wall	
Sterile dressing placement to left groin region	
Removal of packing material from pharynx	
Placement of intermittent pneumatic compression device, covering entire right arm	
Exchange of pressure dressing to left thigh	

Administration

Procedure	Code
Peritoneal dialysis via indwelling catheter	
Transvaginal artificial insemination	
Infusion of total parenteral nutrition via central venous catheter	
Esophagogastroscopy with Botox injection into esophageal sphincter	
Percutaneous irrigation of knee joint	
Epidural injection of mixed steroid and local anesthetic for pain control	
Transfusion of antihemophilic factor, (nonautologous) via arterial central line	
Transabdominal in vitro fertilization, implantation of donor ovum	

Administration (Continued)

Procedure	Code
Autologous bone marrow transplant via central venous line	
Implantation of anti-microbial envelope with cardiac defibrillator placement, open	
Sclerotherapy of brachial plexus lesion, alcohol injection	
Percutaneous peripheral vein injection, glucarpidase	
Introduction of anti-infective envelope into subcutaneous tissue, open	

Measurement and Monitoring

Procedure	Code
Cardiac stress test, single measurement	
EGD with biliary flow measurement	
Right and left heart cardiac catheterization with bilateral sampling and pressure measurements	
Temperature monitoring, rectal	
Peripheral venous pulse, external, single measurement	
Holter monitoring	
Respiratory rate, external, single measurement	
Fetal heart rate monitoring, transvaginal	
Visual mobility test, single measurement	
Left ventricular cardiac output monitoring from pulmonary artery wedge (Swan-Ganz) catheter	
Olfactory acuity test, single measurement	

Extracorporeal Assistance and Performance

Procedure	Code
Intermittent mechanical ventilation, 16 hours	
Liver dialysis, single encounter	
Cardiac countershock with successful conversion to sinus rhythm	
IPPB (intermittent positive pressure breathing) for mobilization of secretions, 22 hours	
Renal dialysis, series of encounters	
IABP (intra-aortic balloon pump) continuous	
Intra-operative cardiac pacing, continuous	
ECMO (extracorporeal membrane oxygenation), continuous	
Controlled mechanical ventilation (CMV), 45 hours	
Pulsatile compression boot with intermittent inflation	

Extracorporeal Therapies

Procedure	Code
Donor thrombocytapheresis, single encounter	
Bili-lite phototherapy, series treatment	
Whole body hypothermia, single treatment	
Circulatory phototherapy, single encounter	
Shock wave therapy of plantar fascia, single treatment	
Antigen-free air conditioning, series treatment	
TMS (transcranial magnetic stimulation), series treatment	
Therapeutic ultrasound of peripheral vessels, single treatment	
Plasmapheresis, series treatment	
Extracorporeal electromagnetic stimulation (EMS) for urinary incontinence, single treatment	

Osteopathic

Procedures	Code
Isotonic muscle energy treatment of right leg	
Low velocity-high amplitude osteopathic treatment of head	
Lymphatic pump osteopathic treatment of left axilla	
Indirect osteopathic treatment of sacrum	
Articulatory osteopathic treatment of cervical region	

Other Procedures

Procedure	Code
Near infrared spectroscopy of leg vessels	
CT computer assisted sinus surgery	
Suture removal, abdominal wall	
Isolation after infectious disease exposure	
Robotic assisted open prostatectomy	
In vitro fertilization	

Chiropractic

Procedure	Code
Chiropractic treatment of lumbar region using long lever specific contact	
Chiropractic manipulation of abdominal region, indirect visceral	
Chiropractic extra-articular treatment of hip region	
Chiropractic treatment of sacrum using long and short lever specific contact	
Mechanically-assisted chiropractic manipulation of head	

Imaging

Procedure	Code
Noncontrast CT of abdomen and pelvis	
Ultrasound guidance for catheter placement, left subclavian artery	
Intravascular ultrasound, left subclavian artery	
Fluoroscopic guidance for insertion of central venous catheter in SVC, low osmolar contrast	
Chest x-ray, AP/PA and lateral views	
Endoluminal ultrasound of gallbladder and bile ducts	
MRI of thyroid gland, contrast unspecified	
Esophageal videofluoroscopy study with oral barium contrast	
Portable x-ray study of right radius/ulna shaft, standard series	
Routine fetal ultrasound, second trimester twin gestation	
CT scan of bilateral lungs, high osmolar contrast with densitometry	
Fluoroscopic guidance for percutaneous transluminal angioplasty (PTA) of left common femoral artery, low osmolar contrast	

Nuclear Medicine

Procedure	Code
Tomo scan of right and left heart, unspecified radiopharmaceutical, qualitative gated rest	
Technetium pentetate assay of kidneys, ureters, and bladder	
Uniplanar scan of spine using technetium oxidronate, with first-pass study	
Thallous chloride tomographic scan of bilateral breasts	
PET scan of myocardium using rubidium	
Gallium citrate scan of head and neck, single plane imaging	

Nuclear Medicine (Continued)

Procedure	Code
Xenon gas nonimaging probe of brain	
Upper GI scan, radiopharmaceutical unspecified, for gastric emptying	
Carbon 11 PET scan of brain with quantification	
Iodinated albumin nuclear medicine assay, blood plasma volume study	

Radiation Therapy

Procedure	Code
Plaque radiation of left eye, single port	
8 MeV photon beam radiation to brain	
IORT of colon, 3 ports	
HDR brachytherapy of prostate using palladium-103	
Electron radiation treatment of right breast, with custom device	
Hyperthermia oncology treatment of pelvic region	
Contact radiation of tongue	
Heavy particle radiation treatment of pancreas, four risk sites	
LDR brachytherapy to spinal cord using iodine	
Whole body phosphorus-32 administration with risk to hematopoetic system	

Physical Rehabilitation and Diagnostic Audiology

Procedure	Code
Bekesy assessment using audiometer	
Individual fitting of left eye prosthesis	
Physical therapy for range of motion and mobility, patient right hip, no special equipment	
Bedside swallow assessment using assessment kit	
Caregiver training in airway clearance techniques	
Application of short arm cast in rehabilitation setting	
Verbal assessment of patient's pain level	
Caregiver training in communication skills using manual communication board	
Group musculoskeletal balance training exercises, whole body, no special equipment	
Individual therapy for auditory processing using tape recorder	

Mental Health

Procedure	Code
Cognitive-behavioral psychotherapy, individual	
Narcosynthesis	
Light therapy	
ECT (electroconvulsive therapy), unilateral, multiple seizure	
Crisis intervention	
Neuropsychological testing	
Hypnosis	
Developmental testing	
Vocational counseling	
Family psychotherapy	

Substance Abuse Treatment

Procedure	Code
Naltrexone treatment for drug dependency	
Substance abuse treatment family counseling	
Medication monitoring of patient on methadone maintenance	
Individual interpersonal psychotherapy for drug abuse	
Patient in for alcohol detoxification treatment	
Group motivational counseling	
Individual 12-step psychotherapy for substance abuse	
Post-test infectious disease counseling for IV drug abuser	
Psychodynamic psychotherapy for drug-dependent patient	
Group cognitive-behavioral counseling for substance abuse	

3f (Aortic) Bioprosthesis valve *use* Zooplastic Tissue in Heart and Great Vessels

Abdominal aortic plexus *use* Nerve, Abdominal Sympathetic
Abdominal esophagus *use* Esophagus, Lower
Abdominohysterectomy
see Excision, Uterus ØUB9
see Resection, Uterus ØUT9
Abdominoplasty
see Alteration, Abdominal Wall ØWØF
see Repair, Abdominal Wall ØWQF
see Supplement, Abdominal Wall ØWUF
Abductor hallucis muscle
use Muscle, Foot, Left
use Muscle, Foot, Right
AbioCor® Total Replacement Heart *use* Synthetic Substitute
Ablation *see* Destruction
Abortion
Abortifacient 1ØAØ7ZX
Laminaria 1ØAØ7ZW
Products of Conception 1ØAØ
Vacuum 1ØAØ7Z6
Abrasion *see* Extraction
Absolute Pro Vascular (OTW) Self-Expanding Stent System *use* Intraluminal Device
Accessory cephalic vein
use Vein, Cephalic, Left
use Vein, Cephalic, Right
Accessory obturator nerve *use* Nerve, Lumbar Plexus
Accessory phrenic nerve *use* Nerve, Phrenic
Accessory spleen *use* Spleen
Acculink (RX) Carotid Stent System *use* Intraluminal Device
Acellular Hydrated Dermis *use* Nonautologous Tissue Substitute
Acetabulectomy
see Excision, Lower Bones ØQB
see Resection, Lower Bones ØQT
Acetabulofemoral joint
use Joint, Hip, Left
use Joint, Hip, Right
Acetabuloplasty
see Repair, Lower Bones ØQQ
see Replacement, Lower Bones ØQR
see Supplement, Lower Bones ØQU
Achilles tendon
use Tendon, Lower Leg, Left
use Tendon, Lower Leg, Right
Achillorrhaphy *see* Repair, Tendons ØLQ
Achillotenotomy, achillotomy
see Division, Tendons ØL8
see Drainage, Tendons ØL9
Acromioclavicular ligament
use Bursa and Ligament, Shoulder, Left
use Bursa and Ligament, Shoulder, Right
Acromion (process)
use Scapula, Left
use Scapula, Right
Acromionectomy
see Excision, Upper Joints ØRB
see Resection, Upper Joints ØRT
Acromioplasty
see Repair, Upper Joints ØRQ
see Replacement, Upper Joints ØRR
see Supplement, Upper Joints ØRU
Activa PC neurostimulator *use* Stimulator Generator, Multiple Array in ØJH
Activa RC neurostimulator *use* Stimulator Generator, Multiple Array Rechargeable in ØJH
Activa SC neurostimulator *use* Stimulator Generator, Single Array in ØJH
Activities of Daily Living Assessment FØ2
Activities of Daily Living Treatment FØ8
ACUITY™ Steerable Lead
use Cardiac Lead, Defibrillator in Ø2H
use Cardiac Lead, Pacemaker in Ø2H
Acupuncture
Breast
Anesthesia 8EØH3ØØ
No Qualifier 8EØH3ØZ
Integumentary System
Anesthesia 8EØH3ØØ
No Qualifier 8EØH3ØZ
Adductor brevis muscle
use Muscle, Upper Leg, Left
use Muscle, Upper Leg, Right
Adductor hallucis muscle
use Muscle, Foot, Left
use Muscle, Foot, Right
Adductor longus muscle
use Muscle, Upper Leg, Left
use Muscle, Upper Leg, Right
Adductor magnus muscle
use Muscle, Upper Leg, Left
use Muscle, Upper Leg, Right
Adenohypophysis *use* Gland, Pituitary
Adenoidectomy
see Excision, Adenoids ØCBQ
see Resection, Adenoids ØCTQ
Adenoidotomy *see* Drainage, Adenoids ØC9Q
Adhesiolysis *see* Release
Administration
Blood products *see* Transfusion
Other substance *see* Introduction of substance in or on
Adrenalectomy
see Excision, Endocrine System ØGB
see Resection, Endocrine System ØGT
Adrenalorrhaphy *see* Repair, Endocrine System ØGQ
Adrenalotomy *see* Drainage, Endocrine System ØG9
Advancement
see Reposition
see Transfer
Advisa (MRI) *use* Pacemaker, Dual Chamber in ØJH
AIGISRx Antibacterial Envelope *use* Anti-Infective Envelope
Alar ligament of axis *use* Bursa and Ligament, Head and Neck
Alimentation *see* Introduction of substance in or on
Alteration
Abdominal Wall ØWØF
Ankle Region
Left ØYØL
Right ØYØK
Arm
Lower
Left ØXØF
Right ØXØD
Upper
Left ØXØ9
Right ØXØ8
Axilla
Left ØXØ5
Right ØXØ4
Back
Lower ØWØL
Upper ØWØK
Breast
Bilateral ØHØV
Left ØHØU
Right ØHØT
Buttock
Left ØYØ1
Right ØYØØ
Chest Wall ØWØ8
Ear
Bilateral Ø9Ø2
Left Ø9Ø1
Right Ø9ØØ
Elbow Region
Left ØXØC
Right ØXØB
Extremity
Lower
Left ØYØB
Right ØYØ9
Upper
Left ØXØ7
Right ØXØ6
Eyelid
Lower
Alteration — continued
Eyelid — continued
Lower — continued
Left Ø8ØR
Right Ø8ØQ
Upper
Left Ø8ØP
Right Ø8ØN
Face ØWØ2
Head ØWØØ
Jaw
Lower ØWØ5
Upper ØWØ4
Knee Region
Left ØYØG
Right ØYØF
Leg
Lower
Left ØYØJ
Right ØYØH
Upper
Left ØYØD
Right ØYØC
Lip
Lower ØCØ1X
Upper ØCØØX
Neck ØWØ6
Nose Ø9ØK
Perineum
Female ØWØN
Male ØWØM
Shoulder Region
Left ØXØ3
Right ØXØ2
Subcutaneous Tissue and Fascia
Abdomen ØJØ8
Back ØJØ7
Buttock ØJØ9
Chest ØJØ6
Face ØJØ1
Lower Arm
Left ØJØH
Right ØJØG
Lower Leg
Left ØJØP
Right ØJØN
Neck
Anterior ØJØ4
Posterior ØJØ5
Upper Arm
Left ØJØF
Right ØJØD
Upper Leg
Left ØJØM
Right ØJØL
Wrist Region
Left ØXØH
Right ØXØG
Alveolar process of mandible
use Mandible, Left
use Mandible, Right
Alveolar process of maxilla
use Maxilla, Left
use Maxilla, Right
Alveolectomy
see Excision, Head and Facial Bones ØNB
see Resection, Head and Facial Bones ØNT
Alveoloplasty
see Repair, Head and Facial Bones ØNQ
see Replacement, Head and Facial Bones ØNR
see Supplement, Head and Facial Bones ØNU
Alveolotomy
see Division, Head and Facial Bones ØN8
see Drainage, Head and Facial Bones ØN9
Ambulatory cardiac monitoring 4A12X45
Amniocentesis *see* Drainage, Products of Conception 1Ø9Ø
Amnioinfusion *see* Introduction of substance in or on, Products of Conception 3EØE
Amnioscopy 1ØJØ8ZZ
Amniotomy *see* Drainage, Products of Conception 1Ø9Ø
AMPLATZER® Muscular VSD Occluder *use* Synthetic Substitute
Amputation *see* Detachment
AMS 800® Urinary Control System *use* Artificial Sphincter in Urinary System

Anal orifice *use* Anus
Analog radiography *see* Plain Radiography
Analog radiology *see* Plain Radiography
Anastomosis *see* Bypass
Anatomical snuffbox
use Muscle, Lower Arm and Wrist, Left
use Muscle, Lower Arm and Wrist, Right
AneuRx® AAA Advantage® *use* Intraluminal Device
Angiectomy
see Excision, Heart and Great Vessels Ø2B
see Excision, Lower Arteries Ø4B
see Excision, Lower Veins Ø6B
see Excision, Upper Arteries Ø3B
see Excision, Upper Veins Ø5B
Angiocardiography
Combined right and left heart *see* Fluoroscopy, Heart, Right and Left B216
Left Heart *see* Fluoroscopy, Heart, Left B215
Right Heart *see* Fluoroscopy, Heart, Right B214
SPY *see* Fluoroscopy, Heart B21
Angiography
see Fluoroscopy, Heart B21
see Plain Radiography, Heart B2Ø
Angioplasty
see Dilation, Heart and Great Vessels Ø27
see Dilation, Lower Arteries Ø47
see Dilation, Upper Arteries Ø37
see Repair, Heart and Great Vessels Ø2Q
see Repair, Lower Arteries Ø4Q
see Repair, Upper Arteries Ø3Q
see Replacement, Heart and Great Vessels Ø2R
see Replacement, Lower Arteries Ø4R
see Replacement, Upper Arteries Ø3R
see Supplement, Heart and Great Vessels Ø2U
see Supplement, Lower Arteries Ø4U
see Supplement, Upper Arteries Ø3U
Angiorrhaphy
see Repair, Heart and Great Vessels Ø2Q
see Repair, Lower Arteries Ø4Q
see Repair, Upper Arteries Ø3Q
Angioscopy Ø4JY4ZZ
Angiotripsy
see Occlusion, Lower Arteries Ø4L
see Occlusion, Upper Arteries Ø3L
Angular artery *use* Artery, Face
Angular vein
use Vein, Face, Left
use Vein, Face, Right
Annular ligament
use Bursa and Ligament, Elbow, Left
use Bursa and Ligament, Elbow, Right
Annuloplasty
see Repair, Heart and Great Vessels Ø2Q
see Supplement, Heart and Great Vessels Ø2U
Annuloplasty ring *use* Synthetic Substitute
Anoplasty
see Repair, Anus ØDQQ
see Supplement, Anus ØDUQ
Anorectal junction *use* Rectum
Anoscopy ØDJD8ZZ
Ansa cervicalis *use* Nerve, Cervical Plexus
Antabuse therapy HZ93ZZZ
Antebrachial fascia
use Subcutaneous Tissue and Fascia, Lower Arm, Left
use Subcutaneous Tissue and Fascia, Lower Arm, Right
Anterior cerebral artery *use* Artery, Intracranial
Anterior cerebral vein *use* Vein, Intracranial
Anterior choroidal artery *use* Artery, Intracranial
Anterior circumflex humeral artery
use Artery, Axillary, Left
use Artery, Axillary, Right
Anterior communicating artery *use* Artery, Intracranial
Anterior cruciate ligament (ACL)
use Bursa and Ligament, Knee, Left
use Bursa and Ligament, Knee, Right
Anterior crural nerve *use* Nerve, Femoral
Anterior facial vein
use Vein, Face, Left
use Vein, Face, Right
Anterior intercostal artery
use Artery, Internal Mammary, Left
use Artery, Internal Mammary, Right
Anterior interosseous nerve *use* Nerve, Median
Anterior lateral malleolar artery
use Artery, Anterior Tibial, Left
use Artery, Anterior Tibial, Right
Anterior lingual gland *use* Gland, Minor Salivary
Anterior (pectoral) lymph node
use Lymphatic, Axillary, Left
use Lymphatic, Axillary, Right
Anterior medial malleolar artery
use Artery, Anterior Tibial, Left
use Artery, Anterior Tibial, Right
Anterior spinal artery
use Artery, Vertebral, Left
use Artery, Vertebral, Right
Anterior tibial recurrent artery
use Artery, Anterior Tibial, Left
use Artery, Anterior Tibial, Right
Anterior ulnar recurrent artery
use Artery, Ulnar, Left
use Artery, Ulnar, Right
Anterior vagal trunk *use* Nerve, Vagus
Anterior vertebral muscle
use Muscle, Neck, Left
use Muscle, Neck, Right
Antihelix
use Ear, External, Bilateral
use Ear, External, Left
use Ear, External, Right
Antimicrobial envelope *use* Anti-Infective Envelope
Antitragus
use Ear, External, Bilateral
use Ear, External, Left
use Ear, External, Right
Antrostomy *see* Drainage, Ear, Nose, Sinus Ø99
Antrotomy *see* Drainage, Ear, Nose, Sinus Ø99
Antrum of Highmore
use Sinus, Maxillary, Left
use Sinus, Maxillary, Right
Aortic annulus *use* Valve, Aortic
Aortic arch *use* Aorta, Thoracic
Aortic intercostal artery *use* Aorta, Thoracic
Aortography
see Fluoroscopy, Lower Arteries B41
see Fluoroscopy, Upper Arteries B31
see Plain Radiography, Lower Arteries B4Ø
see Plain Radiography, Upper Arteries B3Ø
Aortoplasty
see Repair, Aorta, Abdominal Ø4QØ
see Repair, Aorta, Thoracic Ø2QW
see Replacement, Aorta, Abdominal Ø4RØ
see Replacement, Aorta, Thoracic Ø2RW
see Supplement, Aorta, Abdominal Ø4UØ
see Supplement, Aorta, Thoracic Ø2UW
Apical (subclavicular) lymph node
use Lymphatic, Axillary, Left
use Lymphatic, Axillary, Right
Apneustic center *use* Pons
Appendectomy
see Excision, Appendix ØDBJ
see Resection, Appendix ØDTJ
Appendicolysis *see* Release, Appendix ØDNJ
Appendicotomy *see* Drainage, Appendix ØD9J
Application *see* Introduction of substance in or on
Aquapheresis 6A55ØZ3
Aqueduct of Sylvius *use* Cerebral Ventricle
Aqueous humour
use Anterior Chamber, Left
use Anterior Chamber, Right
Arachnoid mater
use Cerebral Meninges
use Spinal Meninges
Arcuate artery
use Artery, Foot, Left
use Artery, Foot, Right
Areola
use Nipple, Left
use Nipple, Right
AROM (artificial rupture of membranes) 1Ø9Ø7ZC
Arterial canal (duct) *use* Artery, Pulmonary, Left
Arterial pulse tracing *see* Measurement, Arterial 4AØ3
Arteriectomy
see Excision, Heart and Great Vessels Ø2B
see Excision, Lower Arteries Ø4B
see Excision, Upper Arteries Ø3B
Arteriography
see Fluoroscopy, Heart B21
see Fluoroscopy, Lower Arteries B41
see Fluoroscopy, Upper Arteries B31
see Plain Radiography, Heart B2Ø
see Plain Radiography, Lower Arteries B4Ø
see Plain Radiography, Upper Arteries B3Ø
Arterioplasty
see Repair, Heart and Great Vessels Ø2Q
see Repair, Lower Arteries Ø4Q
see Repair, Upper Arteries Ø3Q
see Replacement, Heart and Great Vessels Ø2R
see Replacement, Lower Arteries Ø4R
see Replacement, Upper Arteries Ø3R
see Supplement, Heart and Great Vessels Ø2U
see Supplement, Lower Arteries Ø4U
see Supplement, Upper Arteries Ø3U
Arteriorrhaphy
see Repair, Heart and Great Vessels Ø2Q
see Repair, Lower Arteries Ø4Q
see Repair, Upper Arteries Ø3Q
Arterioscopy Ø4JY4ZZ
Arthrectomy
see Excision, Lower Joints ØSB
see Excision, Upper Joints ØRB
see Resection, Lower Joints ØST
see Resection, Upper Joints ØRT
Arthrocentesis
see Drainage, Lower Joints ØS9
see Drainage, Upper Joints ØR9
Arthrodesis
see Fusion, Lower Joints ØSG
see Fusion, Upper Joints ØRG
Arthrography
see Plain Radiography, Non-Axial Lower Bones BQØ
see Plain Radiography, Non-Axial Upper Bones BPØ
see Plain Radiography, Skull and Facial Bones BNØ
Arthrolysis
see Release, Lower Joints ØSN
see Release, Upper Joints ØRN
Arthropexy
see Repair, Lower Joints ØSQ
see Repair, Upper Joints ØRQ
see Reposition, Lower Joints ØSS
see Reposition, Upper Joints ØRS
Arthroplasty
see Repair, Lower Joints ØSQ
see Repair, Upper Joints ØRQ
see Replacement, Lower Joints ØSR
see Replacement, Upper Joints ØRR
see Supplement, Lower Joints ØSU
see Supplement, Upper Joints ØRU
Arthroscopy
see Inspection, Lower Joints ØSJ
see Inspection, Upper Joints ØRJ
Arthrotomy
see Drainage, Lower Joints ØS9
see Drainage, Upper Joints ØR9
Artificial anal sphincter (AAS) *use* Artificial Sphincter in Gastrointestinal System
Artificial bowel sphincter (neosphincter) *use* Artificial Sphincter in Gastrointestinal System
Artificial Sphincter
Insertion of device in
Anus ØDHQ
Bladder ØTHB
Bladder Neck ØTHC
Urethra ØTHD
Removal of device from
Anus ØDPQ
Bladder ØTPB
Urethra ØTPD
Revision of device in
Anus ØDWQ
Bladder ØTWB
Urethra ØTWD
Artificial urinary sphincter (AUS) *use* Artificial Sphincter in Urinary System
Aryepiglottic fold *use* Larynx
Arytenoid cartilage *use* Larynx
Arytenoid muscle
use Muscle, Neck, Left
use Muscle, Neck, Right
Arytenoidectomy *see* Excision, Larynx ØCBS

Arytenoidopexy *see* Repair, Larynx ØCQS
Ascenda Intrathecal Catheter *use* Infusion Device
Ascending aorta *use* Aorta, Thoracic
Ascending palatine artery *use* Artery, Face
Ascending pharyngeal artery
  use Artery, External Carotid, Left
  use Artery, External Carotid, Right
Aspiration *see* Drainage
Assessment
  Activities of daily living *see* Activities of Daily Living Assessment, Rehabilitation FØ2
  Hearing *see* Hearing Assessment, Diagnostic Audiology F13
  Hearing aid *see* Hearing Aid Assessment, Diagnostic Audiology F14
  Motor function *see* Motor Function Assessment, Rehabilitation FØ1
  Nerve function *see* Motor Function Assessment, Rehabilitation FØ1
  Speech *see* Speech Assessment, Rehabilitation FØØ
  Vestibular *see* Vestibular Assessment, Diagnostic Audiology F15
  Vocational *see* Activities of Daily Living Treatment, Rehabilitation FØ8
Assistance
  Cardiac
    Continuous
      Balloon Pump 5AØ221Ø
      Impeller Pump 5AØ221D
      Other Pump 5AØ2216
      Pulsatile Compression 5AØ2215
    Intermittent
      Balloon Pump 5AØ211Ø
      Impeller Pump 5AØ211D
      Other Pump 5AØ2116
      Pulsatile Compression 5AØ2115
  Circulatory
    Continuous
      Hyperbaric 5AØ5221
      Supersaturated 5AØ522C
    Intermittent
      Hyperbaric 5AØ5121
      Supersaturated 5AØ512C
  Respiratory
    24-96 Consecutive Hours
      Continuous Negative Airway Pressure 5AØ9459
      Continuous Positive Airway Pressure 5AØ9457
      Intermittent Negative Airway Pressure 5AØ945B
      Intermittent Positive Airway Pressure 5AØ9458
      No Qualifier 5AØ945Z
    Greater than 96 Consecutive Hours
      Continuous Negative Airway Pressure 5AØ9559
      Continuous Positive Airway Pressure 5AØ9557
      Intermittent Negative Airway Pressure 5AØ955B
      Intermittent Positive Airway Pressure 5AØ9558
      No Qualifier 5AØ955Z
    Less than 24 Consecutive Hours
      Continuous Negative Airway Pressure 5AØ9359
      Continuous Positive Airway Pressure 5AØ9357
      Intermittent Negative Airway Pressure 5AØ935B
      Intermittent Positive Airway Pressure 5AØ9358
      No Qualifier 5AØ935Z
Assurant (Cobalt) stent *use* Intraluminal Device
Atherectomy
  see Extirpation, Heart and Great Vessels Ø2C
  see Extirpation, Lower Arteries Ø4C
  see Extirpation, Upper Arteries Ø3C
Atlantoaxial joint *use* Joint, Cervical Vertebral
Atmospheric Control 6AØZ
Atrioseptoplasty
  see Repair, Heart and Great Vessels Ø2Q
  see Replacement, Heart and Great Vessels Ø2R
  see Supplement, Heart and Great Vessels Ø2U
Atrioventricular node *use* Conduction Mechanism
Atrium dextrum cordis *use* Atrium, Right
Atrium pulmonale *use* Atrium, Left
Attain Ability® lead Ø2H
  use Cardiac Lead, Defibrillator in Ø2H
  use Cardiac Lead, Pacemaker in Ø2H
Attain Starfix® (OTW) lead
  use Cardiac Lead, Defibrillator in Ø2H
  use Cardiac Lead, Pacemaker in Ø2H
Audiology, diagnostic
  see Hearing Aid Assessment, Diagnostic Audiology F14
  see Hearing Assessment, Diagnostic Audiology F13
  see Vestibular Assessment, Diagnostic Audiology F15
Audiometry *see* Hearing Assessment, Diagnostic Audiology F13
Auditory tube
  use Eustachian Tube, Left
  use Eustachian Tube, Right
Auerbach's (myenteric) plexus *use* Nerve, Abdominal Sympathetic
Auricle
  use Ear, External, Bilateral
  use Ear, External, Left
  use Ear, External, Right
Auricularis muscle *use* Muscle, Head
Autograft *use* Autologous Tissue Substitute
Autologous artery graft
  use Autologous Arterial Tissue in Heart and Great Vessels
  use Autologous Arterial Tissue in Lower Arteries
  use Autologous Arterial Tissue in Lower Veins
  use Autologous Arterial Tissue in Upper Arteries
  use Autologous Arterial Tissue in Upper Veins
Autologous vein graft
  use Autologous Venous Tissue in Heart and Great Vessels
  use Autologous Venous Tissue in Lower Arteries
  use Autologous Venous Tissue in Lower Veins
  use Autologous Venous Tissue in Upper Arteries
  use Autologous Venous Tissue in Upper Veins
Autotransfusion *see* Transfusion
Autotransplant
  Adrenal tissue *see* Reposition, Endocrine System ØGS
  Kidney *see* Reposition, Urinary System ØTS
  Pancreatic tissue *see* Reposition, Pancreas ØFSG
  Parathyroid tissue *see* Reposition, Endocrine System ØGS
  Thyroid tissue *see* Reposition, Endocrine System ØGS
  Tooth *see* Reattachment, Mouth and Throat ØCM
Avulsion *see* Extraction
Axial Lumbar Interbody Fusion System *use* Interbody Fusion Device in Lower Joints
AxiaLIF® System *use* Interbody Fusion Device in Lower Joints
Axillary fascia
  use Subcutaneous Tissue and Fascia, Upper Arm, Left
  use Subcutaneous Tissue and Fascia, Upper Arm, Right
Axillary nerve *use* Nerve, Brachial Plexus

B

BAK/C® Interbody Cervical Fusion System *use* Interbody Fusion Device in Upper Joints
BAL (bronchial alveolar lavage), diagnostic *see* Drainage, Respiratory System ØB9
Balanoplasty
  see Repair, Penis ØVQS
  see Supplement, Penis ØVUS
Balloon Pump
  Continuous, Output 5AØ221Ø
  Intermittent, Output 5AØ211Ø
Bandage, Elastic *see* Compression
Banding
  see Occlusion
  see Restriction
Bard® Composix® Kugel® patch *use* Synthetic Substitute
Bard® Composix® (E/X) (LP) mesh *use* Synthetic Substitute
Bard® Dulex™ mesh *use* Synthetic Substitute
Bard® Ventralex™ Hernia Patch *use* Synthetic Substitute
Barium swallow *see* Fluoroscopy, Gastrointestinal System BD1
Baroreflex Activation Therapy® (BAT®)
  use Stimulator Generator in Subcutaneous Tissue and Fascia
  use Stimulator Lead in Upper Arteries
Bartholin's (greater vestibular) gland *use* Gland, Vestibular
Basal (internal) cerebral vein *use* Vein, Intracranial
Basal metabolic rate (BMR) *see* Measurement, Physiological Systems 4AØZ
Basal nuclei *use* Basal Ganglia
Basilar artery *use* Artery, Intracranial
Basis pontis *use* Pons
Beam Radiation
  Abdomen DWØ3
    Intraoperative DWØ33ZØ
  Adrenal Gland DGØ2
    Intraoperative DGØ23ZØ
  Bile Ducts DFØ2
    Intraoperative DFØ23ZØ
  Bladder DTØ2
    Intraoperative DTØ23ZØ
  Bone
    Intraoperative DPØC3ZØ
    Other DPØC
  Bone Marrow D7ØØ
    Intraoperative D7ØØ3ZØ
  Brain DØØØ
    Intraoperative DØØØ3ZØ
  Brain Stem DØØ1
    Intraoperative DØØ13ZØ
  Breast
    Left DMØØ
      Intraoperative DMØØ3ZØ
    Right DMØ1
      Intraoperative DMØ13ZØ
  Bronchus DBØ1
    Intraoperative DBØ13ZØ
  Cervix DUØ1
    Intraoperative DUØ13ZØ
  Chest DWØ2
    Intraoperative DWØ23ZØ
  Chest Wall DBØ7
    Intraoperative DBØ73ZØ
  Colon DDØ5
    Intraoperative DDØ53ZØ
  Diaphragm DBØ8
    Intraoperative DBØ83ZØ
  Duodenum DDØ2
    Intraoperative DDØ23ZØ
  Ear D9ØØ
    Intraoperative D9ØØ3ZØ
  Esophagus DDØØ
    Intraoperative DDØØ3ZØ
  Eye D8ØØ
    Intraoperative D8ØØ3ZØ
  Femur DPØ9
    Intraoperative DPØ93ZØ
  Fibula DPØB
    Intraoperative DPØB3ZØ
  Gallbladder DFØ1
    Intraoperative DFØ13ZØ
  Gland
    Adrenal DGØ2
      Intraoperative DGØ23ZØ
    Parathyroid DGØ4
      Intraoperative DGØ43ZØ
    Pituitary DGØØ
      Intraoperative DGØØ3ZØ
    Thyroid DGØ5
      Intraoperative DGØ53ZØ
  Glands
    Intraoperative D9Ø63ZØ
    Salivary D9Ø6
  Head and Neck DWØ1
    Intraoperative DWØ13ZØ
  Hemibody DWØ4
    Intraoperative DWØ43ZØ
  Humerus DPØ6
    Intraoperative DPØ63ZØ
  Hypopharynx D9Ø3
    Intraoperative D9Ø33ZØ
  Ileum DDØ4
    Intraoperative DDØ43ZØ
  Jejunum DDØ3
    Intraoperative DDØ33ZØ
  Kidney DTØØ
    Intraoperative DTØØ3ZØ
  Larynx D9ØB
    Intraoperative D9ØB3ZØ
  Liver DFØØ
    Intraoperative DFØØ3ZØ
  Lung DBØ2
    Intraoperative DBØ23ZØ

Beam Radiation — continued
Lymphatics
Abdomen D7Ø6
Intraoperative D7Ø63ZØ
Axillary D7Ø4
Intraoperative D7Ø43ZØ
Inguinal D7Ø8
Intraoperative D7Ø83ZØ
Neck D7Ø3
Intraoperative D7Ø33ZØ
Pelvis D7Ø7
Intraoperative D7Ø73ZØ
Thorax D7Ø5
Intraoperative D7Ø53ZØ
Mandible DPØ3
Intraoperative DPØ33ZØ
Maxilla DPØ2
Intraoperative DPØ23ZØ
Mediastinum DBØ6
Intraoperative DBØ63ZØ
Mouth D9Ø4
Intraoperative D9Ø43ZØ
Nasopharynx D9ØD
Intraoperative D9ØD3ZØ
Neck and Head DWØ1
Intraoperative DWØ13ZØ
Nerve
Intraoperative DØØ73ZØ
Peripheral DØØ7
Nose D9Ø1
Intraoperative D9Ø13ZØ
Oropharynx D9ØF
Intraoperative D9ØF3ZØ
Ovary DUØØ
Intraoperative DUØØ3ZØ
Palate
Hard D9Ø8
Intraoperative D9Ø83ZØ
Soft D9Ø9
Intraoperative D9Ø93ZØ
Pancreas DFØ3
Intraoperative DFØ33ZØ
Parathyroid Gland DGØ4
Intraoperative DGØ43ZØ
Pelvic Bones DPØ8
Intraoperative DPØ83ZØ
Pelvic Region DWØ6
Intraoperative DWØ63ZØ
Pineal Body DGØ1
Intraoperative DGØ13ZØ
Pituitary Gland DGØØ
Intraoperative DGØØ3ZØ
Pleura DBØ5
Intraoperative DBØ53ZØ
Prostate DVØØ
Intraoperative DVØØ3ZØ
Radius DPØ7
Intraoperative DPØ73ZØ
Rectum DDØ7
Intraoperative DDØ73ZØ
Rib DPØ5
Intraoperative DPØ53ZØ
Sinuses D9Ø7
Intraoperative D9Ø73ZØ
Skin
Abdomen DHØ8
Intraoperative DHØ83ZØ
Arm DHØ4
Intraoperative DHØ43ZØ
Back DHØ7
Intraoperative DHØ73ZØ
Buttock DHØ9
Intraoperative DHØ93ZØ
Chest DHØ6
Intraoperative DHØ63ZØ
Face DHØ2
Intraoperative DHØ23ZØ
Leg DHØB
Intraoperative DHØB3ZØ
Neck DHØ3
Intraoperative DHØ33ZØ
Skull DPØØ
Intraoperative DPØØ3ZØ
Spinal Cord DØØ6
Intraoperative DØØ63ZØ
Spleen D7Ø2

Beam Radiation — continued
Spleen — continued
Intraoperative D7Ø23ZØ
Sternum DPØ4
Intraoperative DPØ43ZØ
Stomach DDØ1
Intraoperative DDØ13ZØ
Testis DVØ1
Intraoperative DVØ13ZØ
Thymus D7Ø1
Intraoperative D7Ø13ZØ
Thyroid Gland DGØ5
Intraoperative DGØ53ZØ
Tibia DPØB
Intraoperative DPØB3ZØ
Tongue D9Ø5
Intraoperative D9Ø53ZØ
Trachea DBØØ
Intraoperative DBØØ3ZØ
Ulna DPØ7
Intraoperative DPØ73ZØ
Ureter DTØ1
Intraoperative DTØ13ZØ
Urethra DTØ3
Intraoperative DTØ33ZØ
Uterus DUØ2
Intraoperative DUØ23ZØ
Whole Body DWØ5
Intraoperative DWØ53ZØ
Bedside swallow FØØZJWZ
Berlin Heart Ventricular Assist Device *use* Implantable Heart Assist System in Heart and Great Vessels
Biceps brachii muscle
use Muscle, Upper Arm, Left
use Muscle, Upper Arm, Right
Biceps femoris muscle
use Muscle, Upper Leg, Left
use Muscle, Upper Leg, Right
Bicipital aponeurosis
use Subcutaneous Tissue and Fascia, Lower Arm, Left
use Subcutaneous Tissue and Fascia, Lower Arm, Right
Bicuspid valve *use* Valve, Mitral
Bililite therapy *see* Ultraviolet Light Therapy, Skin 6A8Ø
Bioactive embolization coil(s) *use* Intraluminal Device, Bioactive in Upper Arteries
Biofeedback GZC9ZZZ
Biopsy
see Drainage with qualifier Diagnostic
see Excision with qualifier Diagnostic
Bone Marrow *see* Extraction with qualifier Diagnostic
BiPAP *see* Assistance, Respiratory 5AØ9
Bisection *see* Division
Biventricular external heart assist system *use* External Heart Assist System in Heart and Great Vessels
Blepharectomy
see Excision, Eye Ø8B
see Resection, Eye Ø8T
Blepharoplasty
see Repair, Eye Ø8Q
see Replacement, Eye Ø8R
see Reposition, Eye Ø8S
see Supplement, Eye Ø8U
Blepharorrhaphy *see* Repair, Eye Ø8Q
Blepharotomy *see* Drainage, Eye Ø89
Block, Nerve, anesthetic injection 3EØT3CZ
Blood glucose monitoring system *use* Monitoring Device
Blood pressure *see* Measurement, Arterial 4AØ3
BMR (basal metabolic rate) *see* Measurement, Physiological Systems 4AØZ
Body of femur
use Femoral Shaft, Left
use Femoral Shaft, Right
Body of fibula
use Fibula, Left
use Fibula, Right
Bone anchored hearing device
use Hearing Device, Bone Conduction in Ø9H
use Hearing Device in Head and Facial Bones
Bone bank bone graft *use* Nonautologous Tissue Substitute

Bone Growth Stimulator
Insertion of device in
Bone
Facial ØNHW
Lower ØQHY
Nasal ØNHB
Upper ØPHY
Skull ØNHØ
Removal of device from
Bone
Facial ØNPW
Lower ØQPY
Nasal ØNPB
Upper ØPPY
Skull ØNPØ
Revision of device in
Bone
Facial ØNWW
Lower ØQWY
Nasal ØNWB
Upper ØPWY
Skull ØNWØ
Bone marrow transplant *see* Transfusion
Bone morphogenetic protein 2 (BMP 2) *use* Recombinant Bone Morphogenetic Protein
Bone screw (interlocking) (lag) (pedicle) (recessed)
use Internal Fixation Device in Head and Facial Bones
use Internal Fixation Device in Lower Bones
use Internal Fixation Device in Upper Bones
Bony labyrinth
use Ear, Inner, Left
use Ear, Inner, Right
Bony orbit
use Orbit, Left
use Orbit, Right
Bony vestibule
use Ear, Inner, Left
use Ear, inner, Right
Botallo's duct *use* Artery, Pulmonary, Left
Bovine pericardial valve *use* Zooplastic Tissue in Heart and Great Vessels
Bovine pericardium graft *use* Zooplastic Tissue in Heart and Great Vessels
BP (blood pressure) *see* Measurement, Arterial 4AØ3
Brachial (lateral) lymph node
use Lymphatic, Axillary, Left
use Lymphatic, Axillary, Right
Brachialis muscle
use Muscle, Upper Arm, Left
use Muscle, Upper Arm, Right
Brachiocephalic artery *use* Artery, Innominate
Brachiocephalic trunk *use* Artery, Innominate
Brachiocephalic vein
use Vein, Innominate, Left
use Vein, Innominate, Right
Brachioradialis muscle
use Muscle, Lower Arm and Wrist, Left
use Muscle, Lower Arm and Wrist, Right
Brachytherapy
Abdomen DW13
Adrenal Gland DG12
Bile Ducts DF12
Bladder DT12
Bone Marrow D71Ø
Brain DØ1Ø
Brain Stem DØ11
Breast
Left DM1Ø
Right DM11
Bronchus DB11
Cervix DU11
Chest DW12
Chest Wall DB17
Colon DD15
Diaphragm DB18
Duodenum DD12
Ear D91Ø
Esophagus DD1Ø
Eye D81Ø
Gallbladder DF11
Gland
Adrenal DG12
Parathyroid DG14
Pituitary DG1Ø
Thyroid DG15

Subterms under main terms may continue to next column or page

- **Brachytherapy** — continued
  - Glands, Salivary D916
  - Head and Neck DW11
  - Hypopharynx D913
  - Ileum DD14
  - Jejunum DD13
  - Kidney DT1Ø
  - Larynx D91B
  - Liver DF1Ø
  - Lung DB12
  - Lymphatics
    - Abdomen D716
    - Axillary D714
    - Inguinal D718
    - Neck D713
    - Pelvis D717
    - Thorax D715
  - Mediastinum DB16
  - Mouth D914
  - Nasopharynx D91D
  - Neck and Head DW11
  - Nerve, Peripheral DØ17
  - Nose D911
  - Oropharynx D91F
  - Ovary DU1Ø
  - Palate
    - Hard D918
    - Soft D919
  - Pancreas DF13
  - Parathyroid Gland DG14
  - Pelvic Region DW16
  - Pineal Body DG11
  - Pituitary Gland DG1Ø
  - Pleura DB15
  - Prostate DV1Ø
  - Rectum DD17
  - Sinuses D917
  - Spinal Cord DØ16
  - Spleen D712
  - Stomach DD11
  - Testis DV11
  - Thymus D711
  - Thyroid Gland DG15
  - Tongue D915
  - Trachea DB1Ø
  - Ureter DT11
  - Urethra DT13
  - Uterus DU12
- **Brachytherapy seeds** *use* Radioactive Element
- **Broad ligament** *use* Uterine Supporting Structure
- **Bronchial artery** *use* Aorta, Thoracic
- **Bronchography**
  - *see* Fluoroscopy, Respiratory System BB1
  - *see* Plain Radiography, Respiratory System BBØ
- **Bronchoplasty**
  - *see* Repair, Respiratory System ØBQ
  - *see* Supplement, Respiratory System ØBU
- **Bronchorrhaphy** *see* Repair, Respiratory System ØBQ
- **Bronchoscopy** ØBJØ8ZZ
- **Bronchotomy** *see* Drainage, Respiratory System ØB9
- **BRYAN® Cervical Disc System** *use* Synthetic Substitute
- **Buccal gland** *use* Buccal Mucosa
- **Buccinator lymph node** *use* Lymphatic, Head
- **Buccinator muscle** *use* Muscle, Facial
- **Buckling, scleral with implant** *see* Supplement, Eye Ø8U
- **Bulbospongiosus muscle** *use* Muscle, Perineum
- **Bulbourethral (Cowper's) gland** *use* Urethra
- **Bundle of His** *use* Conduction Mechanism
- **Bundle of Kent** *use* Conduction Mechanism
- **Bunionectomy** *see* Excision, Lower Bones ØQB
- **Bursectomy**
  - *see* Excision, Bursae and Ligaments ØMB
  - *see* Resection, Bursae and Ligaments ØMT
- **Bursocentesis** *see* Drainage, Bursae and Ligaments ØM9
- **Bursography**
  - *see* Plain Radiography, Non-Axial Lower Bones BQØ
  - *see* Plain Radiography, Non-Axial Upper Bones BPØ
- **Bursotomy**
  - *see* Division, Bursae and Ligaments ØM8
  - *see* Drainage, Bursae and Ligaments ØM9
- **BVS 5ØØØ Ventricular Assist Device** *use* External Heart Assist System in Heart and Great Vessels
- **Bypass**
  - Anterior Chamber
    - Left Ø8133
    - Right Ø8123
  - Aorta
    - Abdominal Ø41Ø
    - Thoracic Ø21W
  - Artery
    - Axillary
      - Left Ø316Ø
      - Right Ø315Ø
    - Brachial
      - Left Ø318Ø
      - Right Ø317Ø
    - Common Carotid
      - Left Ø31JØ
      - Right Ø31HØ
    - Common Iliac
      - Left Ø41D
      - Right Ø41C
    - Coronary
      - Four or More Sites Ø213
      - One Site Ø21Ø
      - Three Sites Ø212
      - Two Sites Ø211
    - External Carotid
      - Left Ø31NØ
      - Right Ø31MØ
    - External Iliac
      - Left Ø41J
      - Right Ø41H
    - Femoral
      - Left Ø41L
      - Right Ø41K
    - Innominate Ø312Ø
    - Internal Carotid
      - Left Ø31LØ
      - Right Ø31KØ
    - Internal Iliac
      - Left Ø41F
      - Right Ø41E
    - Intracranial Ø31GØ
    - Popliteal
      - Left Ø41N
      - Right Ø41M
    - Radial
      - Left Ø31CØ
      - Right Ø31BØ
    - Splenic Ø414
    - Subclavian
      - Left Ø314Ø
      - Right Ø313Ø
    - Temporal
      - Left Ø31TØ
      - Right Ø31SØ
    - Ulnar
      - Left Ø31AØ
      - Right Ø319Ø
  - Atrium
    - Left Ø217
    - Right Ø216
  - Bladder ØT1B
  - Cavity, Cranial ØW11ØJ
  - Cecum ØD1H
  - Cerebral Ventricle ØØ16
  - Colon
    - Ascending ØD1K
    - Descending ØD1M
    - Sigmoid ØD1N
    - Transverse ØD1L
  - Duct
    - Common Bile ØF19
    - Cystic ØF18
    - Hepatic
      - Left ØF16
      - Right ØF15
    - Lacrimal
      - Left Ø81Y
      - Right Ø81X
    - Pancreatic ØF1D
      - Accessory ØF1F
  - Duodenum ØD19
  - Ear
    - Left Ø91EØ
    - Right Ø91DØ
  - Esophagus ØD15
- **Bypass** — continued
  - Esophagus — continued
    - Lower ØD13
    - Middle ØD12
    - Upper ØD11
  - Fallopian Tube
    - Left ØU16
    - Right ØU15
  - Gallbladder ØF14
  - Ileum ØD1B
  - Jejunum ØD1A
  - Kidney Pelvis
    - Left ØT14
    - Right ØT13
  - Pancreas ØF1G
  - Pelvic Cavity ØW1J
  - Peritoneal Cavity ØW1G
  - Pleural Cavity
    - Left ØW1B
    - Right ØW19
  - Spinal Canal ØØ1U
  - Stomach ØD16
  - Trachea ØB11
  - Ureter
    - Left ØT17
    - Right ØT16
  - Ureters, Bilateral ØT18
  - Vas Deferens
    - Bilateral ØV1Q
    - Left ØV1P
    - Right ØV1N
  - Vein
    - Axillary
      - Left Ø518
      - Right Ø517
    - Azygos Ø51Ø
    - Basilic
      - Left Ø51C
      - Right Ø51B
    - Brachial
      - Left Ø51A
      - Right Ø519
    - Cephalic
      - Left Ø51F
      - Right Ø51D
    - Colic Ø617
    - Common Iliac
      - Left Ø61D
      - Right Ø61C
    - Esophageal Ø613
    - External Iliac
      - Left Ø61G
      - Right Ø61F
    - External Jugular
      - Left Ø51Q
      - Right Ø51P
    - Face
      - Left Ø51V
      - Right Ø51T
    - Femoral
      - Left Ø61N
      - Right Ø61M
    - Foot
      - Left Ø61V
      - Right Ø61T
    - Gastric Ø612
    - Greater Saphenous
      - Left Ø61Q
      - Right Ø61P
    - Hand
      - Left Ø51H
      - Right Ø51G
    - Hemiazygos Ø511
    - Hepatic Ø614
    - Hypogastric
      - Left Ø61J
      - Right Ø61H
    - Inferior Mesenteric Ø616
    - Innominate
      - Left Ø514
      - Right Ø513
    - Internal Jugular
      - Left Ø51N
      - Right Ø51M
    - Intracranial Ø51L

Bypass — continued
Vein — continued
Lesser Saphenous
Left Ø61S
Right Ø61R
Portal Ø618
Renal
Left Ø61B
Right Ø619
Splenic Ø611
Subclavian
Left Ø516
Right Ø515
Superior Mesenteric Ø615
Vertebral
Left Ø51S
Right Ø51R
Vena Cava
Inferior Ø61Ø
Superior Ø21V
Ventricle
Left Ø21L
Right Ø21K
Bypass, cardiopulmonary 5A1221Z

C

Caesarean section *see* Extraction, Products of Conception 1ØDØ
Calcaneocuboid joint
use Joint, Tarsal, Left
use Joint, Tarsal, Right
Calcaneocuboid ligament
use Bursa and Ligament, Foot, Left
use Bursa and Ligament, Foot, Right
Calcaneofibular ligament
use Bursa and Ligament, Ankle, Left
use Bursa and Ligament, Ankle, Right
Calcaneus
use Tarsal, Left
use Tarsal, Right
Cannulation
see Bypass
see Dilation
see Drainage
see Irrigation
Canthorrhaphy *see* Repair, Eye Ø8Q
Canthotomy *see* Release, Eye Ø8N
Capitate bone
use Carpal, Left
use Carpal, Right
Capsulectomy, lens *see* Excision, Eye Ø8B
Capsulorrhaphy, joint
see Repair, Lower Joints ØSQ
see Repair, Upper Joints ØRQ
Cardia *use* Esophagogastric Junction
Cardiac contractility modulation lead *use* Cardiac Lead in Heart and Great Vessels
Cardiac event recorder *use* Monitoring Device
Cardiac Lead
Defibrillator
Atrium
Left Ø2H7
Right Ø2H6
Pericardium Ø2HN
Vein, Coronary Ø2H4
Ventricle
Left Ø2HL
Right Ø2HK
Insertion of device in
Atrium
Left Ø2H7
Right Ø2H6
Pericardium Ø2HN
Vein, Coronary Ø2H4
Ventricle
Left Ø2HL
Right Ø2HK
Pacemaker
Atrium
Left Ø2H7
Right Ø2H6
Pericardium Ø2HN
Vein, Coronary Ø2H4

Cardiac Lead — continued
Pacemaker — continued
Ventricle
Left Ø2HL
Right Ø2HK
Removal of device from, Heart Ø2PA
Revision of device in, Heart Ø2WA
Cardiac plexus *use* Nerve, Thoracic Sympathetic
Cardiac Resynchronization Defibrillator Pulse Generator
Abdomen ØJH8
Chest ØJH6
Cardiac Resynchronization Pacemaker Pulse Generator
Abdomen ØJH8
Chest ØJH6
Cardiac resynchronization therapy (CRT) lead
use Cardiac Lead, Defibrillator in Ø2H
use Cardiac Lead, Pacemaker in Ø2H
Cardiac Rhythm Related Device
Insertion of device in
Abdomen ØJH8
Chest ØJH6
Removal of device from, Subcutaneous Tissue and Fascia, Trunk ØJPT
Revision of device in, Subcutaneous Tissue and Fascia, Trunk ØJWT
Cardiocentesis *see* Drainage, Pericardial Cavity ØW9D
Cardioesophageal junction *use* Esophagogastric Junction
Cardiolysis *see* Release, Heart and Great Vessels Ø2N
CardioMEMS® pressure sensor *use* Monitoring Device, Pressure Sensor in Ø2H
Cardiomyotomy *see* Division, Esophagogastric Junction ØD84
Cardioplegia *see* Introduction of substance in or on, Heart 3EØ8
Cardiorrhaphy *see* Repair, Heart and Great Vessels Ø2Q
Cardioversion 5A22Ø4Z
Caregiver Training FØFZ
Caroticotympanic artery
use Artery, Internal Carotid, Left
use Artery, Internal Carotid, Right
Carotid glomus
use Carotid Bodies, Bilateral
use Carotid Body, Left
use Carotid Body, Right
Carotid sinus
use Artery, Internal Carotid, Left
use Artery, Internal Carotid, Right
Carotid (artery) sinus (baroreceptor) lead *use* Stimulator Lead in Upper Arteries
Carotid sinus nerve *use* Nerve, Glossopharyngeal
Carotid WALLSTENT® Monorail® Endoprosthesis *use* Intraluminal Device
Carpectomy
see Excision, Upper Bones ØPB
see Resection, Upper Bones ØPT
Carpometacarpal (CMC) joint
use Joint, Metacarpocarpal, Left
use Joint, Metacarpocarpal, Right
Carpometacarpal ligament
use Bursa and Ligament, Hand, Left
use Bursa and Ligament, Hand, Right
Casting *see* Immobilization
CAT scan *see* Computerized Tomography (CT Scan)
Catheterization
see Dilation
see Drainage
see Insertion of device in
see Irrigation
Heart *see* Measurement, Cardiac 4AØ2
Umbilical vein, for infusion Ø6HØ33T
Cauda equina *use* Spinal Cord, Lumbar
Cauterization
see Destruction
see Repair
Cavernous plexus *use* Nerve, Head and Neck Sympathetic
Cecectomy
see Excision, Cecum ØDBH
see Resection, Cecum ØDTH
Cecocolostomy
see Bypass, Gastrointestinal System ØD1
see Drainage, Gastrointestinal System ØD9

Cecopexy
see Repair, Cecum ØDQH
see Reposition, Cecum ØDSH
Cecoplication *see* Restriction, Cecum ØDVH
Cecorrhaphy *see* Repair, Cecum ØDQH
Cecostomy
see Bypass, Cecum ØD1H
see Drainage, Cecum ØD9H
Cecotomy *see* Drainage, Cecum ØD9H
Celiac ganglion *use* Nerve, Abdominal Sympathetic
Celiac lymph node *use* Lymphatic, Aortic
Celiac (solar) plexus *use* Nerve, Abdominal Sympathetic
Celiac trunk *use* Artery, Celiac
Central axillary lymph node
use Lymphatic, Axillary, Left
use Lymphatic, Axillary, Right
Central venous pressure *see* Measurement, Venous 4AØ4
Centrimag® Blood Pump *use* External Heart Assist System in Heart and Great Vessels
Cephalogram BNØØZZZ
Cerclage *see* Restriction
Cerebral aqueduct (Sylvius) *use* Cerebral Ventricle
Cerebrum *use* Brain
Cervical esophagus *use* Esophagus, Upper
Cervical facet joint
use Joint, Cervical Vertebral
use Joint, Cervical Vertebral, 2 or more
Cervical ganglion *use* Nerve, Head and Neck Sympathetic
Cervical interspinous ligament *use* Bursa and Ligament, Head and Neck
Cervical intertransverse ligament *use* Bursa and Ligament, Head and Neck
Cervical ligamentum flavum *use* Bursa and Ligament, Head and Neck
Cervical lymph node
use Lymphatic, Neck, Left
use Lymphatic, Neck, Right
Cervicectomy
see Excision, Cervix ØUBC
see Resection, Cervix ØUTC
Cervicothoracic facet joint *use* Joint, Cervicothoracic Vertebral
Cesarean section *see* Extraction, Products of Conception 1ØDØ
Change device in
Abdominal Wall ØW2FX
Back
Lower ØW2LX
Upper ØW2KX
Bladder ØT2BX
Bone
Facial ØN2WX
Lower ØQ2YX
Nasal ØN2BX
Upper ØP2YX
Bone Marrow Ø72TX
Brain ØØ2ØX
Breast
Left ØH2UX
Right ØH2TX
Bursa and Ligament
Lower ØM2YX
Upper ØM2XX
Cavity, Cranial ØW21X
Chest Wall ØW28X
Cisterna Chyli Ø72LX
Diaphragm ØB2TX
Duct
Hepatobiliary ØF2BX
Pancreatic ØF2DX
Ear
Left Ø92JX
Right Ø92HX
Epididymis and Spermatic Cord ØV2MX
Extremity
Lower
Left ØY2BX
Right ØY29X
Upper
Left ØX27X
Right ØX26X
Eye
Left Ø821X

Change device in — continued
Eye — continued
Right Ø82ØX
Face ØW22X
Fallopian Tube ØU28X
Gallbladder ØF24X
Gland
Adrenal ØG25X
Endocrine ØG2SX
Pituitary ØG2ØX
Salivary ØC2AX
Head ØW2ØX
Intestinal Tract
Lower ØD2DXUZ
Upper ØD2ØXUZ
Jaw
Lower ØW25X
Upper ØW24X
Joint
Lower ØS2YX
Upper ØR2YX
Kidney ØT25X
Larynx ØC2SX
Liver ØF2ØX
Lung
Left ØB2LX
Right ØB2KX
Lymphatic Ø72NX
Thoracic Duct Ø72KX
Mediastinum ØW2CX
Mesentery ØD2VX
Mouth and Throat ØC2YX
Muscle
Lower ØK2YX
Upper ØK2XX
Neck ØW26X
Nerve
Cranial ØØ2EX
Peripheral Ø12YX
Nose Ø92KX
Omentum ØD2UX
Ovary ØU23X
Pancreas ØF2GX
Parathyroid Gland ØG2RX
Pelvic Cavity ØW2JX
Penis ØV2SX
Pericardial Cavity ØW2DX
Perineum
Female ØW2NX
Male ØW2MX
Peritoneal Cavity ØW2GX
Peritoneum ØD2WX
Pineal Body ØG21X
Pleura ØB2QX
Pleural Cavity
Left ØW2BX
Right ØW29X
Products of Conception 1Ø2Ø7
Prostate and Seminal Vesicles ØV24X
Retroperitoneum ØW2HX
Scrotum and Tunica Vaginalis ØV28X
Sinus Ø92YX
Skin ØH2PX
Skull ØN2ØX
Spinal Canal ØØ2UX
Spleen Ø72PX
Subcutaneous Tissue and Fascia
Head and Neck ØJ2SX
Lower Extremity ØJ2WX
Trunk ØJ2TX
Upper Extremity ØJ2VX
Tendon
Lower ØL2YX
Upper ØL2XX
Testis ØV2DX
Thymus Ø72MX
Thyroid Gland ØG2KX
Trachea ØB21
Tracheobronchial Tree ØB2ØX
Ureter ØT29X
Urethra ØT2DX
Uterus and Cervix ØU2DXHZ
Vagina and Cul-de-sac ØU2HXGZ
Vas Deferens ØV2RX
Vulva ØU2MX

Change device in or on
Abdominal Wall 2WØ3X
Anorectal 2YØ3X5Z
Arm
Lower
Left 2WØDX
Right 2WØCX
Upper
Left 2WØBX
Right 2WØAX
Back 2WØ5X
Chest Wall 2WØ4X
Ear 2YØ2X5Z
Extremity
Lower
Left 2WØMX
Right 2WØLX
Upper
Left 2WØ9X
Right 2WØ8X
Face 2WØ1X
Finger
Left 2WØKX
Right 2WØJX
Foot
Left 2WØTX
Right 2WØSX
Genital Tract, Female 2YØ4X5Z
Hand
Left 2WØFX
Right 2WØEX
Head 2WØØX
Inguinal Region
Left 2WØ7X
Right 2WØ6X
Leg
Lower
Left 2WØRX
Right 2WØQX
Upper
Left 2WØPX
Right 2WØNX
Mouth and Pharynx 2YØØX5Z
Nasal 2YØ1X5Z
Neck 2WØ2X
Thumb
Left 2WØHX
Right 2WØGX
Toe
Left 2WØVX
Right 2WØUX
Urethra 2YØ5X5Z
Chemoembolization *see* Introduction of substance in or on
Chemosurgery, Skin 3EØØXTZ
Chemothalamectomy *see* Destruction, Thalamus ØØ59
Chemotherapy, Infusion for cancer *see* Introduction of substance in or on
Chest x-ray *see* Plain Radiography, Chest BWØ3
Chiropractic Manipulation
Abdomen 9WB9X
Cervical 9WB1X
Extremities
Lower 9WB6X
Upper 9WB7X
Head 9WBØX
Lumbar 9WB3X
Pelvis 9WB5X
Rib Cage 9WB8X
Sacrum 9WB4X
Thoracic 9WB2X
Choana *use* Nasopharynx
Cholangiogram
see Fluoroscopy, Hepatobiliary System and Pancreas BF1
see Plain Radiography, Hepatobiliary System and Pancreas BFØ
Cholecystectomy
see Excision, Gallbladder ØFB4
see Resection, Gallbladder ØFT4
Cholecystojejunostomy
see Bypass, Hepatobiliary System and Pancreas ØF1
see Drainage, Hepatobiliary System and Pancreas ØF9
Cholecystopexy
see Repair, Gallbladder ØFQ4
see Reposition, Gallbladder ØFS4

Cholecystoscopy ØFJ44ZZ
Cholecystostomy
see Bypass, Gallbladder ØF14
see Drainage, Gallbladder ØF94
Cholecystotomy *see* Drainage, Gallbladder ØF94
Choledochectomy
see Excision, Hepatobiliary System and Pancreas ØFB
see Resection, Hepatobiliary System and Pancreas ØFT
Choledocholithotomy *see* Extirpation, Duct, Common Bile ØFC9
Choledochoplasty
see Repair, Hepatobiliary System and Pancreas ØFQ
see Replacement, Hepatobiliary System and Pancreas ØFR
see Supplement, Hepatobiliary System and Pancreas ØFU
Choledochoscopy ØFJB8ZZ
Choledochotomy *see* Drainage, Hepatobiliary System and Pancreas ØF9
Cholelithotomy *see* Extirpation, Hepatobiliary System and Pancreas ØFC
Chondrectomy
see Excision, Lower Joints ØSB
see Excision, Upper Joints ØRB
Knee *see* Excision, Lower Joints ØSB
Semilunar cartilage *see* Excision, Lower Joints ØSB
Chondroglossus muscle *use* Muscle, Tongue, Palate, Pharynx
Chorda tympani *use* Nerve, Facial
Chordotomy *see* Division, Central Nervous System ØØ8
Choroid plexus *use* Cerebral Ventricle
Choroidectomy
see Excision, Eye Ø8B
see Resection, Eye Ø8T
Ciliary body
use Eye, Left
use Eye, Right
Ciliary ganglion *use* Nerve, Head and Neck Sympathetic
Circle of Willis *use* Artery, Intracranial
Circumflex iliac artery
use Artery, Femoral, Left
use Artery, Femoral, Right
Clamp and rod internal fixation system (CRIF)
use Internal Fixation Device in Lower Bones
use Internal Fixation Device in Upper Bones
Clamping *see* Occlusion
Claustrum *use* Basal Ganglia
Claviculectomy
see Excision, Upper Bones ØPB
see Resection, Upper Bones ØPT
Claviculotomy
see Division, Upper Bones ØP8
see Drainage, Upper Bones ØP9
Clipping, aneurysm *see* Restriction using Extraluminal Device
Clitorectomy, clitoridectomy
see Excision, Clitoris ØUBJ
see Resection, Clitoris ØUTJ
Clolar *use* Clofarabine
Closure
see Occlusion
see Repair
Clysis *see* Introduction of substance in or on
Coagulation *see* Destruction
CoAxia NeuroFlo catheter *use* Intraluminal Device
Cobalt/chromium head and polyethylene socket *use* Synthetic Substitute, Metal on Polyethylene in ØSR
Cobalt/chromium head and socket *use* Synthetic Substitute, Metal in ØSR
Coccygeal body *use* Coccygeal Glomus
Coccygeus muscle
use Muscle, Trunk, Left
use Muscle, Trunk, Right
Cochlea
use Ear, Inner, Left
use Ear, Inner, Right
Cochlear implant (CI), multiple channel (electrode) *use* Hearing Device, Multiple Channel Cochlear Prosthesis in Ø9H
Cochlear implant (CI), single channel (electrode) *use* Hearing Device, Single Channel Cochlear Prosthesis in Ø9H

- **Cochlear Implant Treatment** FØBZØ
- **Cochlear nerve** *use* Nerve, Acoustic
- **COGNIS® CRT-D** *use* Cardiac Resynchronization Defibrillator Pulse Generator in ØJH
- **Colectomy**
  - *see* Excision, Gastrointestinal System ØDB
  - *see* Resection, Gastrointestinal System ØDT
- **Collapse** *see* Occlusion
- **Collection from**
  - Breast, Breast Milk 8EØHX62
  - Indwelling Device
    - Circulatory System
      - Blood 8CØ2X6K
      - Other Fluid 8CØ2X6L
    - Nervous System
      - Cerebrospinal Fluid 8CØ1X6J
      - Other Fluid 8CØ1X6L
  - Integumentary System, Breast Milk 8EØHX62
  - Reproductive System, Male, Sperm 8EØVX63
- **Colocentesis** *see* Drainage, Gastrointestinal System ØD9
- **Colofixation**
  - *see* Repair, Gastrointestinal System ØDQ
  - *see* Reposition, Gastrointestinal System ØDS
- **Colcolysis** *see* Release, Gastrointestinal System ØDN
- **Colonic Z-Stent®** *use* Intraluminal Device
- **Colonoscopy** ØDJD8ZZ
- **Colopexy**
  - *see* Repair, Gastrointestinal System ØDQ
  - *see* Reposition, Gastrointestinal System ØDS
- **Coloplication** *see* Restriction, Gastrointestinal System ØDV
- **Coloproctectomy**
  - *see* Excision, Gastrointestinal System ØDB
  - *see* Resection, Gastrointestinal System ØDT
- **Coloproctostomy**
  - *see* Bypass, Gastrointestinal System ØD1
  - *see* Drainage, Gastrointestinal System ØD9
- **Colopuncture** *see* Drainage, Gastrointestinal System ØD9
- **Colorrhaphy** *see* Repair, Gastrointestinal System ØDQ
- **Colostomy**
  - *see* Bypass, Gastrointestinal System ØD1
  - *see* Drainage, Gastrointestinal System ØD9
- **Colpectomy**
  - *see* Excision, Vagina ØUBG
  - *see* Resection, Vagina ØUTG
- **Colpocentesis** *see* Drainage, Vagina ØU9G
- **Colpopexy**
  - *see* Repair, Vagina ØUQG
  - *see* Reposition, Vagina ØUSG
- **Colpoplasty**
  - *see* Repair, Vagina ØUQG
  - *see* Supplement, Vagina ØUUG
- **Colporrhaphy** *see* Repair, Vagina ØUQG
- **Colposcopy** ØUJH8ZZ
- **Columella** *use* Nose
- **Common digital vein**
  - *use* Vein, Foot, Left
  - *use* Vein, Foot, Right
- **Common facial vein**
  - *use* Vein, Face, Left
  - *use* Vein, Face, Right
- **Common fibular nerve** *use* Nerve, Peroneal
- **Common hepatic artery** *use* Artery, Hepatic
- **Common iliac (subaortic) lymph node** *use* Lymphatic, Pelvis
- **Common interosseous artery**
  - *use* Artery, Ulnar, Left
  - *use* Artery, Ulnar, Right
- **Common peroneal nerve** *use* Nerve, Peroneal
- **Complete (SE) stent** *use* Intraluminal Device
- **Compression**
  - *see* Restriction
  - Abdominal Wall 2W13X
  - Arm
    - Lower
      - Left 2W1DX
      - Right 2W1CX
    - Upper
      - Left 2W1BX
      - Right 2W1AX
  - Back 2W15X
  - Chest Wall 2W14X
- **Compression** — continued
  - Extremity
    - Lower
      - Left 2W1MX
      - Right 2W1LX
    - Upper
      - Left 2W19X
      - Right 2W18X
  - Face 2W11X
  - Finger
    - Left 2W1KX
    - Right 2W1JX
  - Foot
    - Left 2W1TX
    - Right 2W1SX
  - Hand
    - Left 2W1FX
    - Right 2W1EX
  - Head 2W1ØX
  - Inguinal Region
    - Left 2W17X
    - Right 2W16X
  - Leg
    - Lower
      - Left 2W1RX
      - Right 2W1QX
    - Upper
      - Left 2W1PX
      - Right 2W1NX
  - Neck 2W12X
  - Thumb
    - Left 2W1HX
    - Right 2W1GX
  - Toe
    - Left 2W1VX
    - Right 2W1UX
- **Computer Assisted Procedure**
  - Extremity
    - Lower
      - With Computerized Tomography 8EØYXBG
      - With Fluoroscopy 8EØYXBF
      - With Magnetic Resonance Imaging 8EØYXBH
      - No Qualifier 8EØYXBZ
    - Upper
      - With Computerized Tomography 8EØXXBG
      - With Fluoroscopy 8EØXXBF
      - With Magnetic Resonance Imaging 8EØXXBH
      - No Qualifier 8EØXXBZ
  - Head and Neck Region
    - With Computerized Tomography 8EØ9XBG
    - With Fluoroscopy 8EØ9XBF
    - With Magnetic Resonance Imaging 8EØ9XBH
    - No Qualifier 8EØ9XBZ
  - Trunk Region
    - With Computerized Tomography 8EØWXBG
    - With Fluoroscopy 8EØWXBF
    - With Magnetic Resonance Imaging 8EØWXBH
    - No Qualifier 8EØWXBZ
- **Computerized Tomography (CT Scan)**
  - Abdomen BW2Ø
    - Chest and Pelvis BW25
  - Abdomen and Chest BW24
  - Abdomen and Pelvis BW21
  - Airway, Trachea BB2F
  - Ankle
    - Left BQ2H
    - Right BQ2G
  - Aorta
    - Abdominal B42Ø
      - Intravascular Optical Coherence B42ØZ2Z
    - Thoracic B32Ø
      - Intravascular Optical Coherence B32ØZ2Z
  - Arm
    - Left BP2F
    - Right BP2E
  - Artery
    - Celiac B421
      - Intravascular Optical Coherence B421Z2Z
    - Common Carotid
      - Bilateral B325
      - Intravascular Optical Coherence B325Z2Z
    - Coronary
      - Bypass Graft
        - Intravascular Optical Coherence B223Z2Z
        - Multiple B223
      - Multiple B221
- **Computerized Tomography (CT Scan)** — continued
  - Artery — continued
    - Coronary — continued
      - Multiple — continued
        - Intravascular Optical Coherence B221Z2Z
    - Internal Carotid
      - Bilateral B328
      - Intravascular Optical Coherence B328Z2Z
    - Intracranial B32R
      - Intravascular Optical Coherence B32RZ2Z
    - Lower Extremity
      - Bilateral B42H
        - Intravascular Optical Coherence B42HZ2Z
      - Left B42G
        - Intravascular Optical Coherence B42GZ2Z
      - Right B42F
        - Intravascular Optical Coherence B42FZ2Z
    - Pelvic B42C
      - Intravascular Optical Coherence B42CZ2Z
    - Pulmonary
      - Left B32T
        - Intravascular Optical Coherence B32TZ2Z
      - Right B32S
        - Intravascular Optical Coherence B32SZ2Z
    - Renal
      - Bilateral B428
        - Intravascular Optical Coherence B428Z2Z
      - Transplant B42M
        - Intravascular Optical Coherence B42MZ2Z
    - Superior Mesenteric B424
      - Intravascular Optical Coherence B424Z2Z
    - Vertebral
      - Bilateral B32G
      - Intravascular Optical Coherence B32GZ2Z
  - Bladder BT2Ø
  - Bone
    - Facial BN25
    - Temporal BN2F
  - Brain BØ2Ø
  - Calcaneus
    - Left BQ2K
    - Right BQ2J
  - Cerebral Ventricle BØ28
  - Chest, Abdomen and Pelvis BW25
  - Chest and Abdomen BW24
  - Cisterna BØ27
  - Clavicle
    - Left BP25
    - Right BP24
  - Coccyx BR2F
  - Colon BD24
  - Ear B92Ø
  - Elbow
    - Left BP2H
    - Right BP2G
  - Extremity
    - Lower
      - Left BQ2S
      - Right BQ2R
    - Upper
      - Bilateral BP2V
      - Left BP2U
      - Right BP2T
  - Eye
    - Bilateral B827
    - Left B826
    - Right B825
  - Femur
    - Left BQ24
    - Right BQ23
  - Fibula
    - Left BQ2C
    - Right BQ2B
  - Finger
    - Left BP2S
    - Right BP2R
  - Foot
    - Left BQ2M
    - Right BQ2L
  - Forearm
    - Left BP2K
    - Right BP2J
  - Gland
    - Adrenal, Bilateral BG22
    - Parathyroid BG23

Computerized Tomography (CT Scan) — continued
  Gland — continued
    Parotid, Bilateral B926
    Salivary, Bilateral B92D
    Submandibular, Bilateral B929
    Thyroid BG24
  Hand
    Left BP2P
    Right BP2N
  Hands and Wrists, Bilateral BP2Q
  Head BW28
  Head and Neck BW29
  Heart
    Intravascular Optical Coherence B226Z2Z
    Right and Left B226
  Hepatobiliary System, All BF2C
  Hip
    Left BQ21
    Right BQ2Ø
  Humerus
    Left BP2B
    Right BP2A
  Intracranial Sinus B522
    Intravascular Optical Coherence B522Z2Z
  Joint
    Acromioclavicular, Bilateral BP23
    Finger
      Left BP2DZZZ
      Right BP2CZZZ
    Foot
      Left BQ2Y
      Right BQ2X
    Hand
      Left BP2DZZZ
      Right BP2CZZZ
    Sacroiliac BR2D
    Sternoclavicular
      Bilateral BP22
      Left BP21
      Right BP2Ø
    Temporomandibular, Bilateral BN29
    Toe
      Left BQ2Y
      Right BQ2X
  Kidney
    Bilateral BT23
    Left BT22
    Right BT21
    Transplant BT29
  Knee
    Left BQ28
    Right BQ27
  Larynx B92J
  Leg
    Left BQ2F
    Right BQ2D
  Liver BF25
  Liver and Spleen BF26
  Lung, Bilateral BB24
  Mandible BN26
  Nasopharynx B92F
  Neck BW2F
  Neck and Head BW29
  Orbit, Bilateral BN23
  Oropharynx B92F
  Pancreas BF27
  Patella
    Left BQ2W
    Right BQ2V
  Pelvic Region BW2G
  Pelvis BR2C
    Chest and Abdomen BW25
  Pelvis and Abdomen BW21
  Pituitary Gland BØ29
  Prostate BV23
  Ribs
    Left BP2Y
    Right BP2X
  Sacrum BR2F
  Scapula
    Left BP27
    Right BP26
  Sella Turcica BØ29
  Shoulder
    Left BP29

Computerized Tomography (CT Scan) — continued
  Shoulder — continued
    Right BP28
  Sinus
    Intracranial B522
      Intravascular Optical Coherence B522Z2Z
    Paranasal B922
  Skull BN2Ø
  Spinal Cord BØ2B
  Spine
    Cervical BR2Ø
    Lumbar BR29
    Thoracic BR27
  Spleen and Liver BF26
  Thorax BP2W
  Tibia
    Left BQ2C
    Right BQ2B
  Toe
    Left BQ2Q
    Right BQ2P
  Trachea BB2F
  Tracheobronchial Tree
    Bilateral BB29
    Left BB28
    Right BB27
  Vein
    Pelvic (Iliac)
      Left B52G
        Intravascular Optical Coherence B52GZ2Z
      Right B52F
        Intravascular Optical Coherence B52FZ2Z
    Pelvic (Iliac) Bilateral B52H
      Intravascular Optical Coherence B52HZ2Z
    Portal B52T
      Intravascular Optical Coherence B52TZ2Z
    Pulmonary
      Bilateral B52S
        Intravascular Optical Coherence B52SZ2Z
      Left B52R
        Intravascular Optical Coherence B52RZ2Z
      Right B52Q
        Intravascular Optical Coherence B52QZ2Z
    Renal
      Bilateral B52L
        Intravascular Optical Coherence B52LZ2Z
      Left B52K
        Intravascular Optical Coherence B52KZ2Z
      Right B52J
        Intravascular Optical Coherence B52JZ2Z
    Spanchnic B52T
      Intravascular Optical Coherence B52TZ2Z
  Vena Cava
    Inferior B529
      Intravascular Optical Coherence B529Z2Z
    Superior B528
      Intravascular Optical Coherence B528Z2Z
  Ventricle, Cerebral BØ28
  Wrist
    Left BP2M
    Right BP2L
Concerto II CRT-D *use* Cardiac Resynchronization Defibrillator Pulse Generator in ØJH
Condylectomy
  see Excision, Head and Facial Bones ØNB
  see Excision, Lower Bones ØQB
  see Excision, Upper Bones ØPB
Condyloid process
  use Mandible, Left
  use Mandible, Right
Condylotomy
  see Division, Head and Facial Bones ØN8
  see Division, Lower Bones ØQ8
  see Division, Upper Bones ØP8
  see Drainage, Head and Facial Bones ØN9
  see Drainage, Lower Bones ØQ9
  see Drainage, Upper Bones ØP9
Condylysis
  see Release, Head and Facial Bones ØNN
  see Release, Lower Bones ØQN
  see Release, Upper Bones ØPN
Conization, cervix *see* Excision, Uterus ØUB9
Conjunctivoplasty
  see Repair, Eye Ø8Q
  see Replacement, Eye Ø8R

CONSERVE® PLUS Total Resurfacing Hip System *use* Resurfacing Device in Lower Joints
Construction
  Auricle, ear *see* Replacement, Ear, Nose, Sinus Ø9R
  Ileal conduit *see* Bypass, Urinary System ØT1
Consulta CRT-D *use* Cardiac Resynchronization Defibrillator Pulse Generator in ØJH
Consulta CRT-P *use* Cardiac Resynchronization Pacemaker Pulse Generator in ØJH
Contact Radiation
  Abdomen DWY37ZZ
  Adrenal Gland DGY27ZZ
  Bile Ducts DFY27ZZ
  Bladder DTY27ZZ
  Bone, Other DPYC7ZZ
  Brain DØYØ7ZZ
  Brain Stem DØY17ZZ
  Breast
    Left DMYØ7ZZ
    Right DMY17ZZ
  Bronchus DBY17ZZ
  Cervix DUY17ZZ
  Chest DWY27ZZ
  Chest Wall DBY77ZZ
  Colon DDY57ZZ
  Diaphragm DBY87ZZ
  Duodenum DDY27ZZ
  Ear D9YØ7ZZ
  Esophagus DDYØ7ZZ
  Eye D8YØ7ZZ
  Femur DPY97ZZ
  Fibula DPYB7ZZ
  Gallbladder DFY17ZZ
  Gland
    Adrenal DGY27ZZ
    Parathyroid DGY47ZZ
    Pituitary DGYØ7ZZ
    Thyroid DGY57ZZ
  Glands, Salivary D9Y67ZZ
  Head and Neck DWY17ZZ
  Hemibody DWY47ZZ
  Humerus DPY67ZZ
  Hypopharynx D9Y37ZZ
  Ileum DDY47ZZ
  Jejunum DDY37ZZ
  Kidney DTYØ7ZZ
  Larynx D9YB7ZZ
  Liver DFYØ7ZZ
  Lung DBY27ZZ
  Mandible DPY37ZZ
  Maxilla DPY27ZZ
  Mediastinum DBY67ZZ
  Mouth D9Y47ZZ
  Nasopharynx D9YD7ZZ
  Neck and Head DWY17ZZ
  Nerve, Peripheral DØY77ZZ
  Nose D9Y17ZZ
  Oropharynx D9YF7ZZ
  Ovary DUYØ7ZZ
  Palate
    Hard D9Y87ZZ
    Soft D9Y97ZZ
  Pancreas DFY37ZZ
  Parathyroid Gland DGY47ZZ
  Pelvic Bones DPY87ZZ
  Pelvic Region DWY67ZZ
  Pineal Body DGY17ZZ
  Pituitary Gland DGYØ7ZZ
  Pleura DBY57ZZ
  Prostate DVYØ7ZZ
  Radius DPY77ZZ
  Rectum DDY77ZZ
  Rib DPY57ZZ
  Sinuses D9Y77ZZ
  Skin
    Abdomen DHY87ZZ
    Arm DHY47ZZ
    Back DHY77ZZ
    Buttock DHY97ZZ
    Chest DHY67ZZ
    Face DHY27ZZ
    Leg DHYB7ZZ
    Neck DHY37ZZ
  Skull DPYØ7ZZ
  Spinal Cord DØY67ZZ
  Sternum DPY47ZZ

Contact Radiation — continued
Stomach DDY17ZZ
Testis DVY17ZZ
Thyroid Gland DGY57ZZ
Tibia DPYB7ZZ
Tongue D9Y57ZZ
Trachea DBY07ZZ
Ulna DPY77ZZ
Ureter DTY17ZZ
Urethra DTY37ZZ
Uterus DUY27ZZ
Whole Body DWY57ZZ
CONTAK RENEWAL® 3 RF (HE) CRT-D *use* Cardiac Resynchronization Defibrillator Pulse Generator in 0JH
Continuous Glucose Monitoring (CGM) device *use* Monitoring Device
Continuous Negative Airway Pressure
24-96 Consecutive Hours, Ventilation 5A09459
Greater than 96 Consecutive Hours, Ventilation 5A09559
Less than 24 Consecutive Hours, Ventilation 5A09359
Continuous Positive Airway Pressure
24-96 Consecutive Hours, Ventilation 5A09457
Greater than 96 Consecutive Hours, Ventilation 5A09557
Less than 24 Consecutive Hours, Ventilation 5A09357
Contraceptive Device
Change device in, Uterus and Cervix 0U2DXHZ
Insertion of device in
Cervix 0UHC
Subcutaneous Tissue and Fascia
Abdomen 0JH8
Chest 0JH6
Lower Arm
Left 0JHH
Right 0JHG
Lower Leg
Left 0JHP
Right 0JHN
Upper Arm
Left 0JHF
Right 0JHD
Upper Leg
Left 0JHM
Right 0JHL
Uterus 0UH9
Removal of device from
Subcutaneous Tissue and Fascia
Lower Extremity 0JPW
Trunk 0JPT
Upper Extremity 0JPV
Uterus and Cervix 0UPD
Revision of device in
Subcutaneous Tissue and Fascia
Lower Extremity 0JWW
Trunk 0JWT
Upper Extremity 0JWV
Uterus and Cervix 0UWD
Contractility Modulation Device
Abdomen 0JH8
Chest 0JH6
Control postprocedural bleeding in
Abdominal Wall 0W3F
Ankle Region
Left 0Y3L
Right 0Y3K
Arm
Lower
Left 0X3F
Right 0X3D
Upper
Left 0X39
Right 0X38
Axilla
Left 0X35
Right 0X34
Back
Lower 0W3L
Upper 0W3K
Buttock
Left 0Y31
Right 0Y30
Cavity, Cranial 0W31
Chest Wall 0W38

Control postprocedural bleeding in — continued
Elbow Region
Left 0X3C
Right 0X3B
Extremity
Lower
Left 0Y3B
Right 0Y39
Upper
Left 0X37
Right 0X36
Face 0W32
Femoral Region
Left 0Y38
Right 0Y37
Foot
Left 0Y3N
Right 0Y3M
Gastrointestinal Tract 0W3P
Genitourinary Tract 0W3R
Hand
Left 0X3K
Right 0X3J
Head 0W30
Inguinal Region
Left 0Y36
Right 0Y35
Jaw
Lower 0W35
Upper 0W34
Knee Region
Left 0Y3G
Right 0Y3F
Leg
Lower
Left 0Y3J
Right 0Y3H
Upper
Left 0Y3D
Right 0Y3C
Mediastinum 0W3C
Neck 0W36
Oral Cavity and Throat 0W33
Pelvic Cavity 0W3J
Pericardial Cavity 0W3D
Perineum
Female 0W3N
Male 0W3M
Peritoneal Cavity 0W3G
Pleural Cavity
Left 0W3B
Right 0W39
Respiratory Tract 0W3Q
Retroperitoneum 0W3H
Shoulder Region
Left 0X33
Right 0X32
Wrist Region
Left 0X3H
Right 0X3G
Conus arteriosus *use* Ventricle, Right
Conus medullaris *use* Spinal Cord, Lumbar
Conversion
Cardiac rhythm 5A2204Z
Gastrostomy to jejunostomy feeding device *see* Insertion of device in, Jejunum 0DHA
Coracoacromial ligament
use Bursa and Ligament, Shoulder, Left
use Bursa and Ligament, Shoulder, Right
Coracobrachialis muscle
use Muscle, Upper Arm, Left
use Muscle, Upper Arm, Right
Coracoclavicular ligament
use Bursa and Ligament, Shoulder, Left
use Bursa and Ligament, Shoulder, Right
Coracohumeral ligament
use Bursa and Ligament, Shoulder, Left
use Bursa and Ligament, Shoulder, Right
Coracoid process
use Scapula, Left
use Scapula, Right
Cordotomy *see* Division, Central Nervous System 008
Core needle biopsy *see* Excision with qualifier Diagnostic
Cormet Hip Resurfacing System *use* Resurfacing Device in Lower Joints

Corniculate cartilage *use* Larynx
CoRoent® XL *use* Interbody Fusion Device in Lower Joints
Coronary arteriography
see Fluoroscopy, Heart B21
see Plain Radiography, Heart B20
Corox (OTW) Bipolar Lead
use Cardiac Lead, Defibrillator in 02H
use Cardiac Lead, Pacemaker in 02H
Corpus callosum *use* Brain
Corpus cavernosum *use* Penis
Corpus spongiosum *use* Penis
Corpus striatum *use* Basal Ganglia
Corrugator supercilii muscle *use* Muscle, Facial
Cortical strip neurostimulator lead *use* Neurostimulator Lead in Central Nervous System
Costatectomy
see Excision, Upper Bones 0PB
see Resection, Upper Bones 0PT
Costectomy
see Excision, Upper Bones 0PB
see Resection, Upper Bones 0PT
Costocervical trunk
use Artery, Subclavian, Left
use Artery, Subclavian, Right
Costochondrectomy
see Excision, Upper Bones 0PB
see Resection, Upper Bones 0PT
Costoclavicular ligament
use Bursa and Ligament, Shoulder, Left
use Bursa and Ligament, Shoulder, Right
Costosternoplasty
see Repair, Upper Bones 0PQ
see Replacement, Upper Bones 0PR
see Supplement, Upper Bones 0PU
Costotomy
see Division, Upper Bones 0P8
see Drainage, Upper Bones 0P9
Costotransverse joint *use* Joint, Thoracic Vertebral
Costotransverse ligament
use Bursa and Ligament, Thorax, Left
use Bursa and Ligament, Thorax, Right
Costovertebral joint *use* Joint, Thoracic Vertebral
Costoxiphoid ligament
use Bursa and Ligament, Thorax, Left
use Bursa and Ligament, Thorax, Right
Counseling
Family, for substance abuse, Other Family Counseling HZ63ZZZ
Group
12-Step HZ43ZZZ
Behavioral HZ41ZZZ
Cognitive HZ40ZZZ
Cognitive-Behavioral HZ42ZZZ
Confrontational HZ48ZZZ
Continuing Care HZ49ZZZ
Infectious Disease
Post-Test HZ4CZZZ
Pre-Test HZ4CZZZ
Interpersonal HZ44ZZZ
Motivational Enhancement HZ47ZZZ
Psychoeducation HZ46ZZZ
Spiritual HZ4BZZZ
Vocational HZ45ZZZ
Individual
12-Step HZ33ZZZ
Behavioral HZ31ZZZ
Cognitive HZ30ZZZ
Cognitive-Behavioral HZ32ZZZ
Confrontational HZ38ZZZ
Continuing Care HZ39ZZZ
Infectious Disease
Post-Test HZ3CZZZ
Pre-Test HZ3CZZZ
Interpersonal HZ34ZZZ
Motivational Enhancement HZ37ZZZ
Psychoeducation HZ36ZZZ
Spiritual HZ3BZZZ
Vocational HZ35ZZZ
Mental Health Services
Educational GZ60ZZZ
Other Counseling GZ63ZZZ
Vocational GZ61ZZZ
Countershock, cardiac 5A2204Z
Cowper's (bulbourethral) gland *use* Urethra

CPAP (continuous positive airway pressure) *see* Assistance, Respiratory 5A09
Cranial dura mater *use* Dura Mater
Cranial epidural space *use* Epidural Space
Cranial subarachnoid space *use* Subarachnoid Space
Cranial subdural space *use* Subdural Space
Craniectomy
see Excision, Head and Facial Bones 0NB
see Resection, Head and Facial Bones 0NT
Cranioplasty
see Repair, Head and Facial Bones 0NQ
see Replacement, Head and Facial Bones 0NR
see Supplement, Head and Facial Bones 0NU
Craniotomy
see Division, Head and Facial Bones 0N8
see Drainage, Central Nervous System 009
see Drainage, Head and Facial Bones 0N9
Creation
Female 0W4N0
Male 0W4M0
Cremaster muscle *use* Muscle, Perineum
Cribriform plate
use Bone, Ethmoid, Left
use Bone, Ethmoid, Right
Cricoid cartilage *use* Larynx
Cricoidectomy *see* Excision, Larynx 0CBS
Cricothyroid artery
use Artery, Thyroid, Left
use Artery, Thyroid, Right
Cricothyroid muscle
use Muscle, Neck, Left
use Muscle, Neck, Right
Crisis Intervention GZ2ZZZZ
Crural fascia
use Subcutaneous Tissue and Fascia, Upper Leg, Left
use Subcutaneous Tissue and Fascia, Upper Leg, Right
Crushing, nerve
Cranial *see* Destruction, Central Nervous System 005
Peripheral *see* Destruction, Peripheral Nervous System 015
Cryoablation *see* Destruction
Cryotherapy *see* Destruction
Cryptorchidectomy
see Excision, Male Reproductive System 0VB
see Resection, Male Reproductive System 0VT
Cryptorchiectomy
see Excision, Male Reproductive System 0VB
see Resection, Male Reproductive System 0VT
Cryptotomy
see Division, Gastrointestinal System 0D8
see Drainage, Gastrointestinal System 0D9
CT scan *see* Computerized Tomography (CT Scan)
CT sialogram *see* Computerized Tomography (CT Scan), Ear, Nose, Mouth and Throat B92
Cubital lymph node
use Lymphatic, Upper Extremity, Left
use Lymphatic, Upper Extremity, Right
Cubital nerve *use* Nerve, Ulnar
Cuboid bone
use Tarsal, Left
use Tarsal, Right
Cuboideonavicular joint
use Joint, Tarsal, Left
use Joint, Tarsal, Right
Culdocentesis *see* Drainage, Cul-de-sac 0U9F
Culdoplasty
see Repair, Cul-de-sac 0UQF
see Supplement, Cul-de-sac 0UUF
Culdoscopy 0UJH8ZZ
Culdotomy *see* Drainage, Cul-de-sac 0U9F
Culmen *use* Cerebellum
Cultured epidermal cell autograft *use* Autologous Tissue Substitute
Cuneiform cartilage *use* Larynx
Cuneonavicular joint
use Joint, Tarsal, Left
use Joint, Tarsal, Right
Cuneonavicular ligament
use Bursa and Ligament, Foot, Left
use Bursa and Ligament, Foot, Right
Curettage
see Excision
see Extraction
Cutaneous (transverse) cervical nerve *use* Nerve, Cervical Plexus
CVP (central venous pressure) *see* Measurement, Venous 4A04
Cyclodiathermy *see* Destruction, Eye 085
Cyclophotocoagulation *see* Destruction, Eye 085
CYPHER® Stent *use* Intraluminal Device, Drug-eluting in Heart and Great Vessels
Cystectomy
see Excision, Bladder 0TBB
see Resection, Bladder 0TTB
Cystocele repair *see* Repair, Subcutaneous Tissue and Fascia, Pelvic Region 0JQC
Cystography
see Fluoroscopy, Urinary System BT1
see Plain Radiography, Urinary System BT0
Cystolithotomy *see* Extirpation, Bladder 0TCB
Cystopexy
see Repair, Bladder 0TQB
see Reposition, Bladder 0TSB
Cystoplasty
see Repair, Bladder 0TQB
see Replacement, Bladder 0TRB
see Supplement, Bladder 0TUB
Cystorrhaphy *see* Repair, Bladder 0TQB
Cystoscopy 0TJB8ZZ
Cystostomy *see* Bypass, Bladder 0T1B
Cystostomy tube *use* Drainage Device
Cystotomy *see* Drainage, Bladder 0T9B
Cystourethrography
see Fluoroscopy, Urinary System BT1
see Plain Radiography, Urinary System BT0
Cystourethroplasty
see Repair, Urinary System 0TQ
see Replacement, Urinary System 0TR
see Supplement, Urinary System 0TU

DBS lead *use* Neurostimulator Lead in Central Nervous System
DeBakey Left Ventricular Assist Device *use* Implantable Heart Assist System in Heart and Great Vessels
Debridement
Excisional *see* Excision
Non-excisional *see* Extraction
Decompression, Circulatory 6A15
Decortication, lung *see* Extraction, Respiratory System 0BD
Deep brain neurostimulator lead *use* Neurostimulator Lead in Central Nervous System
Deep cervical fascia *use* Subcutaneous Tissue and Fascia, Neck, Anterior
Deep cervical vein
use Vein, Vertebral, Left
use Vein, Vertebral, Right
Deep circumflex iliac artery
use Artery, External Iliac, Left
use Artery, External Iliac, Right
Deep facial vein
use Vein, Face, Left
use Vein, Face, Right
Deep femoral artery
use Artery, Femoral, Left
use Artery, Femoral, Right
Deep femoral (profunda femoris) vein
use Vein, Femoral, Left
use Vein, Femoral, Right
Deep Inferior Epigastric Artery Perforator Flap
Bilateral 0HRV077
Left 0HRU077
Right 0HRT077
Deep palmar arch
use Artery, Hand, Left
use Artery, Hand, Right
Deep transverse perineal muscle *use* Muscle, Perineum
Deferential artery
use Artery, Internal Iliac, Left
use Artery, Internal Iliac, Right
Defibrillator Generator
Abdomen 0JH8
Chest 0JH6
Delivery
Cesarean *see* Extraction, Products of Conception 10D0
Forceps *see* Extraction, Products of Conception 10D0
Manually assisted 10E0XZZ
Products of Conception 10E0XZZ
Vacuum assisted *see* Extraction, Products of Conception 10D0
Delta frame external fixator
use External Fixation Device, Hybrid in 0PS
use External Fixation Device, Hybrid in 0QH
use External Fixation Device, Hybrid in 0QS
use External Fixation Device, Hybrid in 0PH
Delta III Reverse shoulder prosthesis *use* Synthetic Substitute, Reverse Ball and Socket in 0RR
Deltoid fascia
use Subcutaneous Tissue and Fascia, Upper Arm, Left
use Subcutaneous Tissue and Fascia, Upper Arm, Right
Deltoid ligament
use Bursa and Ligament, Ankle, Left
use Bursa and Ligament, Ankle, Right
Deltoid muscle
use Muscle, Shoulder, Left
use Muscle, Shoulder, Right
Deltopectoral (infraclavicular) lymph node
use Lymphatic, Upper Extremity, Left
use Lymphatic, Upper Extremity, Right
Denervation
Cranial nerve *see* Destruction, Central Nervous System 005
Peripheral nerve *see* Destruction, Peripheral Nervous System 015
Densitometry
Plain Radiography
Femur
Left BQ04ZZ1
Right BQ03ZZ1
Hip
Left BQ01ZZ1
Right BQ00ZZ1
Spine
Cervical BR00ZZ1
Lumbar BR09ZZ1
Thoracic BR07ZZ1
Whole BR0GZZ1
Ultrasonography
Elbow
Left BP4HZZ1
Right BP4GZZ1
Hand
Left BP4PZZ1
Right BP4NZZ1
Shoulder
Left BP49ZZ1
Right BP48ZZ1
Wrist
Left BP4MZZ1
Right BP4LZZ1
Dentate ligament *use* Dura Mater
Denticulate ligament *use* Spinal Meninges
Depressor anguli oris muscle *use* Muscle, Facial
Depressor labii inferioris muscle *use* Muscle, Facial
Depressor septi nasi muscle *use* Muscle, Facial
Depressor supercilii muscle *use* Muscle, Facial
Dermabrasion *see* Extraction, Skin and Breast 0HD
Dermis *use* Skin
Descending genicular artery
use Artery, Femoral, Left
use Artery, Femoral, Right
Destruction
Acetabulum
Left 0Q55
Right 0Q54
Adenoids 0C5Q
Ampulla of Vater 0F5C
Anal Sphincter 0D5R
Anterior Chamber
Left 08533ZZ
Right 08523ZZ
Anus 0D5Q
Aorta
Abdominal 0450
Thoracic 025W
Aortic Body 0G5D
Appendix 0D5J

Destruction — continued
Artery
Anterior Tibial
Left Ø45Q
Right Ø45P
Axillary
Left Ø356
Right Ø355
Brachial
Left Ø358
Right Ø357
Celiac Ø451
Colic
Left Ø457
Middle Ø458
Right Ø456
Common Carotid
Left Ø35J
Right Ø35H
Common Iliac
Left Ø45D
Right Ø45C
External Carotid
Left Ø35N
Right Ø35M
External Iliac
Left Ø45J
Right Ø45H
Face Ø35R
Femoral
Left Ø45L
Right Ø45K
Foot
Left Ø45W
Right Ø45V
Gastric Ø452
Hand
Left Ø35F
Right Ø35D
Hepatic Ø453
Inferior Mesenteric Ø45B
Innominate Ø352
Internal Carotid
Left Ø35L
Right Ø35K
Internal Iliac
Left Ø45F
Right Ø45E
Internal Mammary
Left Ø351
Right Ø35Ø
Intracranial Ø35G
Lower Ø45Y
Peroneal
Left Ø45U
Right Ø45T
Popliteal
Left Ø45N
Right Ø45M
Posterior Tibial
Left Ø45S
Right Ø45R
Pulmonary
Left Ø25R
Right Ø25Q
Pulmonary Trunk Ø25P
Radial
Left Ø35C
Right Ø35B
Renal
Left Ø45A
Right Ø459
Splenic Ø454
Subclavian
Left Ø354
Right Ø353
Superior Mesenteric Ø455
Temporal
Left Ø35T
Right Ø35S
Thyroid
Left Ø35V
Right Ø35U
Ulnar
Left Ø35A
Right Ø359

Destruction — continued
Artery — continued
Upper Ø35Y
Vertebral
Left Ø35Q
Right Ø35P
Atrium
Left Ø257
Right Ø256
Auditory Ossicle
Left Ø95AØZZ
Right Ø959ØZZ
Basal Ganglia ØØ58
Bladder ØT5B
Bladder Neck ØT5C
Bone
Ethmoid
Left ØN5G
Right ØN5F
Frontal
Left ØN52
Right ØN51
Hyoid ØN5X
Lacrimal
Left ØN5J
Right ØN5H
Nasal ØN5B
Occipital
Left ØN58
Right ØN57
Palatine
Left ØN5L
Right ØN5K
Parietal
Left ØN54
Right ØN53
Pelvic
Left ØQ53
Right ØQ52
Sphenoid
Left ØN5D
Right ØN5C
Temporal
Left ØN56
Right ØN55
Zygomatic
Left ØN5N
Right ØN5M
Brain ØØ5Ø
Breast
Bilateral ØH5V
Left ØH5U
Right ØH5T
Bronchus
Lingula ØB59
Lower Lobe
Left ØB5B
Right ØB56
Main
Left ØB57
Right ØB53
Middle Lobe, Right ØB55
Upper Lobe
Left ØB58
Right ØB54
Buccal Mucosa ØC54
Bursa and Ligament
Abdomen
Left ØM5J
Right ØM5H
Ankle
Left ØM5R
Right ØM5Q
Elbow
Left ØM54
Right ØM53
Foot
Left ØM5T
Right ØM5S
Hand
Left ØM58
Right ØM57
Head and Neck ØM5Ø
Hip
Left ØM5M
Right ØM5L

Destruction — continued
Bursa and Ligament — continued
Knee
Left ØM5P
Right ØM5N
Lower Extremity
Left ØM5W
Right ØM5V
Perineum ØM5K
Shoulder
Left ØM52
Right ØM51
Thorax
Left ØM5G
Right ØM5F
Trunk
Left ØM5D
Right ØM5C
Upper Extremity
Left ØM5B
Right ØM59
Wrist
Left ØM56
Right ØM55
Carina ØB52
Carotid Bodies, Bilateral ØG58
Carotid Body
Left ØG56
Right ØG57
Carpal
Left ØP5N
Right ØP5M
Cecum ØD5H
Cerebellum ØØ5C
Cerebral Hemisphere ØØ57
Cerebral Meninges ØØ51
Cerebral Ventricle ØØ56
Cervix ØU5C
Chordae Tendineae Ø259
Choroid
Left Ø85B
Right Ø85A
Cisterna Chyli Ø75L
Clavicle
Left ØP5B
Right ØP59
Clitoris ØU5J
Coccygeal Glomus ØG5B
Coccyx ØQ5S
Colon
Ascending ØD5K
Descending ØD5M
Sigmoid ØD5N
Transverse ØD5L
Conduction Mechanism Ø258
Conjunctiva
Left Ø85TXZZ
Right Ø85SXZZ
Cord
Bilateral ØV5H
Left ØV5G
Right ØV5F
Cornea
Left Ø859XZZ
Right Ø858XZZ
Cul-de-sac ØU5F
Diaphragm
Left ØB5S
Right ØB5R
Disc
Cervical Vertebral ØR53
Cervicothoracic Vertebral ØR55
Lumbar Vertebral ØS52
Lumbosacral ØS54
Thoracic Vertebral ØR59
Thoracolumbar Vertebral ØR5B
Duct
Common Bile ØF59
Cystic ØF58
Hepatic
Left ØF56
Right ØF55
Lacrimal
Left Ø85Y
Right Ø85X
Pancreatic ØF5D

Destruction — continued
Duct — continued
Pancreatic — continued
Accessory ØF5F
Parotid
Left ØC5C
Right ØC5B
Duodenum ØD59
Dura Mater ØØ52
Ear
External
Left Ø951
Right Ø95Ø
External Auditory Canal
Left Ø954
Right Ø953
Inner
Left Ø95EØZZ
Right Ø95DØZZ
Middle
Left Ø956ØZZ
Right Ø955ØZZ
Endometrium ØU5B
Epididymis
Bilateral ØV5L
Left ØV5K
Right ØV5J
Epiglottis ØC5R
Esophagogastric Junction ØD54
Esophagus ØD55
Lower ØD53
Middle ØD52
Upper ØD51
Eustachian Tube
Left Ø95G
Right Ø95F
Eye
Left Ø851XZZ
Right Ø85ØXZZ
Eyelid
Lower
Left Ø85R
Right Ø85Q
Upper
Left Ø85P
Right Ø85N
Fallopian Tube
Left ØU56
Right ØU55
Fallopian Tubes, Bilateral ØU57
Femoral Shaft
Left ØQ59
Right ØQ58
Femur
Lower
Left ØQ5C
Right ØQ5B
Upper
Left ØQ57
Right ØQ56
Fibula
Left ØQ5K
Right ØQ5J
Finger Nail ØH5QXZZ
Gallbladder ØF54
Gingiva
Lower ØC56
Upper ØC55
Gland
Adrenal
Bilateral ØG54
Left ØG52
Right ØG53
Lacrimal
Left Ø85W
Right Ø85V
Minor Salivary ØC5J
Parotid
Left ØC59
Right ØC58
Pituitary ØG5Ø
Sublingual
Left ØC5F
Right ØC5D
Submaxillary
Left ØC5H

Destruction — continued
Gland — continued
Submaxillary — continued
Right ØC5G
Vestibular ØU5L
Glenoid Cavity
Left ØP58
Right ØP57
Glomus Jugulare ØG5C
Humeral Head
Left ØP5D
Right ØP5C
Humeral Shaft
Left ØP5G
Right ØP5F
Hymen ØU5K
Hypothalamus ØØ5A
Ileocecal Valve ØD5C
Ileum ØD5B
Intestine
Large ØD5E
Left ØD5G
Right ØD5F
Small ØD58
Iris
Left Ø85D3ZZ
Right Ø85C3ZZ
Jejunum ØD5A
Joint
Acromioclavicular
Left ØR5H
Right ØR5G
Ankle
Left ØS5G
Right ØS5F
Carpal
Left ØR5R
Right ØR5Q
Cervical Vertebral ØR51
Cervicothoracic Vertebral ØR54
Coccygeal ØS56
Elbow
Left ØR5M
Right ØR5L
Finger Phalangeal
Left ØR5X
Right ØR5W
Hip
Left ØS5B
Right ØS59
Knee
Left ØS5D
Right ØS5C
Lumbar Vertebral ØS5Ø
Lumbosacral ØS53
Metacarpocarpal
Left ØR5T
Right ØR5S
Metacarpophalangeal
Left ØR5V
Right ØR5U
Metatarsal-Phalangeal
Left ØS5N
Right ØS5M
Metatarsal-Tarsal
Left ØS5L
Right ØS5K
Occipital-cervical ØR5Ø
Sacrococcygeal ØS55
Sacroiliac
Left ØS58
Right ØS57
Shoulder
Left ØR5K
Right ØR5J
Sternoclavicular
Left ØR5F
Right ØR5E
Tarsal
Left ØS5J
Right ØS5H
Temporomandibular
Left ØR5D
Right ØR5C
Thoracic Vertebral ØR56
Thoracolumbar Vertebral ØR5A

Destruction — continued
Joint — continued
Toe Phalangeal
Left ØS5Q
Right ØS5P
Wrist
Left ØR5P
Right ØR5N
Kidney
Left ØT51
Right ØT5Ø
Kidney Pelvis
Left ØT54
Right ØT53
Larynx ØC5S
Lens
Left Ø85K3ZZ
Right Ø85J3ZZ
Lip
Lower ØC51
Upper ØC5Ø
Liver ØF5Ø
Left Lobe ØF52
Right Lobe ØF51
Lung
Bilateral ØB5M
Left ØB5L
Lower Lobe
Left ØB5J
Right ØB5F
Middle Lobe, Right ØB5D
Right ØB5K
Upper Lobe
Left ØB5G
Right ØB5C
Lung Lingula ØB5H
Lymphatic
Aortic Ø75D
Axillary
Left Ø756
Right Ø755
Head Ø75Ø
Inguinal
Left Ø75J
Right Ø75H
Internal Mammary
Left Ø759
Right Ø758
Lower Extremity
Left Ø75G
Right Ø75F
Mesenteric Ø75B
Neck
Left Ø752
Right Ø751
Pelvis Ø75C
Thoracic Duct Ø75K
Thorax Ø757
Upper Extremity
Left Ø754
Right Ø753
Mandible
Left ØN5V
Right ØN5T
Maxilla
Left ØN5S
Right ØN5R
Medulla Oblongata ØØ5D
Mesentery ØD5V
Metacarpal
Left ØP5Q
Right ØP5P
Metatarsal
Left ØQ5P
Right ØQ5N
Muscle
Abdomen
Left ØK5L
Right ØK5K
Extraocular
Left Ø85M
Right Ø85L
Facial ØK51
Foot
Left ØK5W
Right ØK5V

Subterms under main terms may continue to next column or page

Destruction — continued
Muscle — continued
Hand
Left ØK5D
Right ØK5C
Head ØK5Ø
Hip
Left ØK5P
Right ØK5N
Lower Arm and Wrist
Left ØK5B
Right ØK59
Lower Leg
Left ØK5T
Right ØK5S
Neck
Left ØK53
Right ØK52
Papillary Ø25D
Perineum ØK5M
Shoulder
Left ØK56
Right ØK55
Thorax
Left ØK5J
Right ØK5H
Tongue, Palate, Pharynx ØK54
Trunk
Left ØK5G
Right ØK5F
Upper Arm
Left ØK58
Right ØK57
Upper Leg
Left ØK5R
Right ØK5Q
Nasopharynx Ø95N
Nerve
Abdominal Sympathetic Ø15M
Abducens ØØ5L
Accessory ØØ5R
Acoustic ØØ5N
Brachial Plexus Ø153
Cervical Ø151
Cervical Plexus Ø15Ø
Facial ØØ5M
Femoral Ø15D
Glossopharyngeal ØØ5P
Head and Neck Sympathetic Ø15K
Hypoglossal ØØ5S
Lumbar Ø15B
Lumbar Plexus Ø159
Lumbar Sympathetic Ø15N
Lumbosacral Plexus Ø15A
Median Ø155
Oculomotor ØØ5H
Olfactory ØØ5F
Optic ØØ5G
Peroneal Ø15H
Phrenic Ø152
Pudendal Ø15C
Radial Ø156
Sacral Ø15R
Sacral Plexus Ø15Q
Sacral Sympathetic Ø15P
Sciatic Ø15F
Thoracic Ø158
Thoracic Sympathetic Ø15L
Tibial Ø15G
Trigeminal ØØ5K
Trochlear ØØ5J
Ulnar Ø154
Vagus ØØ5Q
Nipple
Left ØH5X
Right ØH5W
Nose Ø95K
Omentum
Greater ØD5S
Lesser ØD5T
Orbit
Left ØN5Q
Right ØN5P
Ovary
Bilateral ØU52
Left ØU51

Destruction — continued
Ovary — continued
Right ØU5Ø
Palate
Hard ØC52
Soft ØC53
Pancreas ØF5G
Para-aortic Body ØG59
Paraganglion Extremity ØG5F
Parathyroid Gland ØG5R
Inferior
Left ØG5P
Right ØG5N
Multiple ØG5Q
Superior
Left ØG5M
Right ØG5L
Patella
Left ØQ5F
Right ØQ5D
Penis ØV5S
Pericardium Ø25N
Peritoneum ØD5W
Phalanx
Finger
Left ØP5V
Right ØP5T
Thumb
Left ØP5S
Right ØP5R
Toe
Left ØQ5R
Right ØQ5Q
Pharynx ØC5M
Pineal Body ØG51
Pleura
Left ØB5P
Right ØB5N
Pons ØØ5B
Prepuce ØV5T
Prostate ØV5Ø
Radius
Left ØP5J
Right ØP5H
Rectum ØD5P
Retina
Left Ø85F3ZZ
Right Ø85E3ZZ
Retinal Vessel
Left Ø85H3ZZ
Right Ø85G3ZZ
Rib
Left ØP52
Right ØP51
Sacrum ØQ51
Scapula
Left ØP56
Right ØP55
Sclera
Left Ø857XZZ
Right Ø856XZZ
Scrotum ØV55
Septum
Atrial Ø255
Nasal Ø95M
Ventricular Ø25M
Sinus
Accessory Ø95P
Ethmoid
Left Ø95V
Right Ø95U
Frontal
Left Ø95T
Right Ø95S
Mastoid
Left Ø95C
Right Ø95B
Maxillary
Left Ø95R
Right Ø95Q
Sphenoid
Left Ø95X
Right Ø95W
Skin
Abdomen ØH57XZ
Back ØH56XZ

Destruction — continued
Skin — continued
Buttock ØH58XZ
Chest ØH55XZ
Ear
Left ØH53XZ
Right ØH52XZ
Face ØH51XZ
Foot
Left ØH5NXZ
Right ØH5MXZ
Genitalia ØH5AXZ
Hand
Left ØH5GXZ
Right ØH5FXZ
Lower Arm
Left ØH5EXZ
Right ØH5DXZ
Lower Leg
Left ØH5LXZ
Right ØH5KXZ
Neck ØH54XZ
Perineum ØH59XZ
Scalp ØH5ØXZ
Upper Arm
Left ØH5CXZ
Right ØH5BXZ
Upper Leg
Left ØH5JXZ
Right ØH5HXZ
Skull ØN5Ø
Spinal Cord
Cervical ØØ5W
Lumbar ØØ5Y
Thoracic ØØ5X
Spinal Meninges ØØ5T
Spleen Ø75P
Sternum ØP5Ø
Stomach ØD56
Pylorus ØD57
Subcutaneous Tissue and Fascia
Abdomen ØJ58
Back ØJ57
Buttock ØJ59
Chest ØJ56
Face ØJ51
Foot
Left ØJ5R
Right ØJ5Q
Hand
Left ØJ5K
Right ØJ5J
Lower Arm
Left ØJ5H
Right ØJ5G
Lower Leg
Left ØJ5P
Right ØJ5N
Neck
Anterior ØJ54
Posterior ØJ55
Pelvic Region ØJ5C
Perineum ØJ5B
Scalp ØJ5Ø
Upper Arm
Left ØJ5F
Right ØJ5D
Upper Leg
Left ØJ5M
Right ØJ5L
Tarsal
Left ØQ5M
Right ØQ5L
Tendon
Abdomen
Left ØL5G
Right ØL5F
Ankle
Left ØL5T
Right ØL5S
Foot
Left ØL5W
Right ØL5V
Hand
Left ØL58
Right ØL57

Destruction — continued
Tendon — continued
Head and Neck ØL5Ø
Hip
Left ØL5K
Right ØL5J
Knee
Left ØL5R
Right ØL5Q
Lower Arm and Wrist
Left ØL56
Right ØL55
Lower Leg
Left ØL5P
Right ØL5N
Perineum ØL5H
Shoulder
Left ØL52
Right ØL51
Thorax
Left ØL5D
Right ØL5C
Trunk
Left ØL5B
Right ØL59
Upper Arm
Left ØL54
Right ØL53
Upper Leg
Left ØL5M
Right ØL5L
Testis
Bilateral ØV5C
Left ØV5B
Right ØV59
Thalamus ØØ59
Thymus Ø75M
Thyroid Gland ØG5K
Left Lobe ØG5G
Right Lobe ØG5H
Tibia
Left ØQ5H
Right ØQ5G
Toe Nail ØH5RXZZ
Tongue ØC57
Tonsils ØC5P
Tooth
Lower ØC5X
Upper ØC5W
Trachea ØB51
Tunica Vaginalis
Left ØV57
Right ØV56
Turbinate, Nasal Ø95L
Tympanic Membrane
Left Ø958
Right Ø957
Ulna
Left ØP5L
Right ØP5K
Ureter
Left ØT57
Right ØT56
Urethra ØT5D
Uterine Supporting Structure ØU54
Uterus ØU59
Uvula ØC5N
Vagina ØU5G
Valve
Aortic Ø25F
Mitral Ø25G
Pulmonary Ø25H
Tricuspid Ø25J
Vas Deferens
Bilateral ØV5Q
Left ØV5P
Right ØV5N
Vein
Axillary
Left Ø558
Right Ø557
Azygos Ø55Ø
Basilic
Left Ø55C
Right Ø55B

Destruction — continued
Vein — continued
Brachial
Left Ø55A
Right Ø559
Cephalic
Left Ø55F
Right Ø55D
Colic Ø657
Common Iliac
Left Ø65D
Right Ø65C
Coronary Ø254
Esophageal Ø653
External Iliac
Left Ø65G
Right Ø65F
External Jugular
Left Ø55Q
Right Ø55P
Face
Left Ø55V
Right Ø55T
Femoral
Left Ø65N
Right Ø65M
Foot
Left Ø65V
Right Ø65T
Gastric Ø652
Greater Saphenous
Left Ø65Q
Right Ø65P
Hand
Left Ø55H
Right Ø55G
Hemiazygos Ø551
Hepatic Ø654
Hypogastric
Left Ø65J
Right Ø65H
Inferior Mesenteric Ø656
Innominate
Left Ø554
Right Ø553
Internal Jugular
Left Ø55N
Right Ø55M
Intracranial Ø55L
Lesser Saphenous
Left Ø65S
Right Ø65R
Lower Ø65Y
Portal Ø658
Pulmonary
Left Ø25T
Right Ø25S
Renal
Left Ø65B
Right Ø659
Splenic Ø651
Subclavian
Left Ø556
Right Ø555
Superior Mesenteric Ø655
Upper Ø55Y
Vertebral
Left Ø55S
Right Ø55R
Vena Cava
Inferior Ø65Ø
Superior Ø25V
Ventricle
Left Ø25L
Right Ø25K
Vertebra
Cervical ØP53
Lumbar ØQ5Ø
Thoracic ØP54
Vesicle
Bilateral ØV53
Left ØV52
Right ØV51
Vitreous
Left Ø8553ZZ
Right Ø8543ZZ

Destruction — continued
Vocal Cord
Left ØC5V
Right ØC5T
Vulva ØU5M
Detachment
Arm
Lower
Left ØX6FØZ
Right ØX6DØZ
Upper
Left ØX69ØZ
Right ØX68ØZ
Elbow Region
Left ØX6CØZZ
Right ØX6BØZZ
Femoral Region
Left ØY68ØZZ
Right ØY67ØZZ
Finger
Index
Left ØX6PØZ
Right ØX6NØZ
Little
Left ØX6WØZ
Right ØX6VØZ
Middle
Left ØX6RØZ
Right ØX6QØZ
Ring
Left ØX6TØZ
Right ØX6SØZ
Foot
Left ØY6NØZ
Right ØY6MØZ
Forequarter
Left ØX61ØZZ
Right ØX6ØØZZ
Hand
Left ØX6KØZ
Right ØX6JØZ
Hindquarter
Bilateral ØY64ØZZ
Left ØY63ØZZ
Right ØY62ØZZ
Knee Region
Left ØY6GØZZ
Right ØY6FØZZ
Leg
Lower
Left ØY6JØZ
Right ØY6HØZ
Upper
Left ØY6DØZ
Right ØY6CØZ
Shoulder Region
Left ØX63ØZZ
Right ØX62ØZZ
Thumb
Left ØX6MØZ
Right ØX6LØZ
Toe
1st
Left ØY6QØZ
Right ØY6PØZ
2nd
Left ØY6SØZ
Right ØY6RØZ
3rd
Left ØY6UØZ
Right ØY6TØZ
4th
Left ØY6WØZ
Right ØY6VØZ
5th
Left ØY6YØZ
Right ØY6XØZ
Determination, Mental status GZ14ZZZ
Detorsion
see Release
see Reposition
Detoxification Services, for substance abuse HZ2ZZZZ
Device Fitting FØDZ
Diagnostic Audiology *see* Audiology, Diagnostic
Diagnostic imaging *see* Imaging, Diagnostic

- **Diagnostic radiology** *see* Imaging, Diagnostic
- **Dialysis**
  - Hemodialysis 5A1DØØZ
  - Peritoneal 3E1M39Z
- **Diaphragma sellae** *use* Dura Mater
- **Diaphragmatic pacemaker generator** *use* Stimulator Generator in Subcutaneous Tissue and Fascia
- **Diaphragmatic Pacemaker Lead**
  - Insertion of device in
    - Left ØBHS
    - Right ØBHR
  - Removal of device from, Diaphragm ØBPT
  - Revision of device in, Diaphragm ØBWT
- **Digital radiography, plain** *see* Plain Radiography
- **Dilation**
  - Ampulla of Vater ØF7C
  - Anus ØD7Q
  - Aorta
    - Abdominal Ø47Ø
    - Thoracic Ø27W
  - Artery
    - Anterior Tibial
      - Left Ø47Q
      - Right Ø47P
    - Axillary
      - Left Ø376
      - Right Ø375
    - Brachial
      - Left Ø378
      - Right Ø377
    - Celiac Ø471
    - Colic
      - Left Ø477
      - Middle Ø478
      - Right Ø476
    - Common Carotid
      - Left Ø37J
      - Right Ø37H
    - Common Iliac
      - Left Ø47D
      - Right Ø47C
    - Coronary
      - Four or More Sites Ø273
      - One Site Ø27Ø
      - Three Sites Ø272
      - Two Sites Ø271
    - External Carotid
      - Left Ø37N
      - Right Ø37M
    - External Iliac
      - Left Ø47J
      - Right Ø47H
    - Face Ø37R
    - Femoral
      - Left Ø47L
      - Right Ø47K
    - Foot
      - Left Ø47W
      - Right Ø47V
    - Gastric Ø472
    - Hand
      - Left Ø37F
      - Right Ø37D
    - Hepatic Ø473
    - Inferior Mesenteric Ø47B
    - Innominate Ø372
    - Internal Carotid
      - Left Ø37L
      - Right Ø37K
    - Internal Iliac
      - Left Ø47F
      - Right Ø47E
    - Internal Mammary
      - Left Ø371
      - Right Ø37Ø
    - Intracranial Ø37G
    - Lower Ø47Y
    - Peroneal
      - Left Ø47U
      - Right Ø47T
    - Popliteal
      - Left Ø47N
      - Right Ø47M
    - Posterior Tibial
      - Left Ø47S
      - Right Ø47R

Dilation — continued
  - Artery — continued
    - Pulmonary
      - Left Ø27R
      - Right Ø27Q
    - Pulmonary Trunk Ø27P
    - Radial
      - Left Ø37C
      - Right Ø37B
    - Renal
      - Left Ø47A
      - Right Ø479
    - Splenic Ø474
    - Subclavian
      - Left Ø374
      - Right Ø373
    - Superior Mesenteric Ø475
    - Temporal
      - Left Ø37T
      - Right Ø37S
    - Thyroid
      - Left Ø37V
      - Right Ø37U
    - Ulnar
      - Left Ø37A
      - Right Ø379
    - Upper Ø37Y
    - Vertebral
      - Left Ø37Q
      - Right Ø37P
  - Bladder ØT7B
  - Bladder Neck ØT7C
  - Bronchus
    - Lingula ØB79
    - Lower Lobe
      - Left ØB7B
      - Right ØB76
    - Main
      - Left ØB77
      - Right ØB73
    - Middle Lobe, Right ØB75
    - Upper Lobe
      - Left ØB78
      - Right ØB74
  - Carina ØB72
  - Cecum ØD7H
  - Cervix ØU7C
  - Colon
    - Ascending ØD7K
    - Descending ØD7M
    - Sigmoid ØD7N
    - Transverse ØD7L
  - Duct
    - Common Bile ØF79
    - Cystic ØF78
    - Hepatic
      - Left ØF76
      - Right ØF75
    - Lacrimal
      - Left Ø87Y
      - Right Ø87X
    - Pancreatic ØF7D
      - Accessory ØF7F
    - Parotid
      - Left ØC7C
      - Right ØC7B
  - Duodenum ØD79
  - Esophagogastric Junction ØD74
  - Esophagus ØD75
    - Lower ØD73
    - Middle ØD72
    - Upper ØD71
  - Eustachian Tube
    - Left Ø97G
    - Right Ø97F
  - Fallopian Tube
    - Left ØU76
    - Right ØU75
  - Fallopian Tubes, Bilateral ØU77
  - Hymen ØU7K
  - Ileocecal Valve ØD7C
  - Ileum ØD7B
  - Intestine
    - Large ØD7E
      - Left ØD7G
      - Right ØD7F

Dilation — continued
  - Intestine — continued
    - Small ØD78
  - Jejunum ØD7A
  - Kidney Pelvis
    - Left ØT74
    - Right ØT73
  - Larynx ØC7S
  - Pharynx ØC7M
  - Rectum ØD7P
  - Stomach ØD76
    - Pylorus ØD77
  - Trachea ØB71
  - Ureter
    - Left ØT77
    - Right ØT76
  - Ureters, Bilateral ØT78
  - Urethra ØT7D
  - Uterus ØU79
  - Vagina ØU7G
  - Valve
    - Aortic Ø27F
    - Mitral Ø27G
    - Pulmonary Ø27H
    - Tricuspid Ø27J
  - Vas Deferens
    - Bilateral ØV7Q
    - Left ØV7P
    - Right ØV7N
  - Vein
    - Axillary
      - Left Ø578
      - Right Ø577
    - Azygos Ø57Ø
    - Basilic
      - Left Ø57C
      - Right Ø57B
    - Brachial
      - Left Ø57A
      - Right Ø579
    - Cephalic
      - Left Ø57F
      - Right Ø57D
    - Colic Ø677
    - Common Iliac
      - Left Ø67D
      - Right Ø67C
    - Esophageal Ø673
    - External Iliac
      - Left Ø67G
      - Right Ø67F
    - External Jugular
      - Left Ø57Q
      - Right Ø57P
    - Face
      - Left Ø57V
      - Right Ø57T
    - Femoral
      - Left Ø67N
      - Right Ø67M
    - Foot
      - Left Ø67V
      - Right Ø67T
    - Gastric Ø672
    - Greater Saphenous
      - Left Ø67Q
      - Right Ø67P
    - Hand
      - Left Ø57H
      - Right Ø57G
    - Hemiazygos Ø571
    - Hepatic Ø674
    - Hypogastric
      - Left Ø67J
      - Right Ø67H
    - Inferior Mesenteric Ø676
    - Innominate
      - Left Ø574
      - Right Ø573
    - Internal Jugular
      - Left Ø57N
      - Right Ø57M
    - Intracranial Ø57L
    - Lesser Saphenous
      - Left Ø67S
      - Right Ø67R

Dilation — continued
Vein — continued
Lower Ø67Y
Portal Ø678
Pulmonary
Left Ø27T
Right Ø27S
Renal
Left Ø67B
Right Ø679
Splenic Ø671
Subclavian
Left Ø576
Right Ø575
Superior Mesenteric Ø675
Upper Ø57Y
Vertebral
Left Ø57S
Right Ø57R
Vena Cava
Inferior Ø67Ø
Superior Ø27V
Ventricle, Right Ø27K
Direct Lateral Interbody Fusion (DLIF) device *use* Interbody Fusion Device in Lower Joints
Disarticulation *see* Detachment
Discectomy, diskectomy
see Excision, Lower Joints ØSB
see Excision, Upper Joints ØRB
see Resection, Lower Joints ØST
see Resection, Upper Joints ØRT
Discography
see Fluoroscopy, Axial Skeleton, Except Skull and Facial Bones BR1
see Plain Radiography, Axial Skeleton, Except Skull and Facial Bones BRØ
Distal humerus
use Humeral Shaft, Left
use Humeral Shaft, Right
Distal humerus, involving joint
use Joint, Elbow, Left
use Joint, Elbow, Right
Distal radioulnar joint
use Joint, Wrist, Left
use Joint, Wrist, Right
Diversion *see* Bypass
Diverticulectomy *see* Excision, Gastrointestinal System ØDB
Division
Acetabulum
Left ØQ85
Right ØQ84
Anal Sphincter ØD8R
Basal Ganglia ØØ88
Bladder Neck ØT8C
Bone
Ethmoid
Left ØN8G
Right ØN8F
Frontal
Left ØN82
Right ØN81
Hyoid ØN8X
Lacrimal
Left ØN8J
Right ØN8H
Nasal ØN8B
Occipital
Left ØN88
Right ØN87
Palatine
Left ØN8L
Right ØN8K
Parietal
Left ØN84
Right ØN83
Pelvic
Left ØQ83
Right ØQ82
Sphenoid
Left ØN8D
Right ØN8C
Temporal
Left ØN86
Right ØN85

Division — continued
Bone — continued
Zygomatic
Left ØN8N
Right ØN8M
Brain ØØ8Ø
Bursa and Ligament
Abdomen
Left ØM8J
Right ØM8H
Ankle
Left ØM8R
Right ØM8Q
Elbow
Left ØM84
Right ØM83
Foot
Left ØM8T
Right ØM8S
Hand
Left ØM88
Right ØM87
Head and Neck ØM8Ø
Hip
Left ØM8M
Right ØM8L
Knee
Left ØM8P
Right ØM8N
Lower Extremity
Left ØM8W
Right ØM8V
Perineum ØM8K
Shoulder
Left ØM82
Right ØM81
Thorax
Left ØM8G
Right ØM8F
Trunk
Left ØM8D
Right ØM8C
Upper Extremity
Left ØM8B
Right ØM89
Wrist
Left ØM86
Right ØM85
Carpal
Left ØP8N
Right ØP8M
Cerebral Hemisphere ØØ87
Chordae Tendineae Ø289
Clavicle
Left ØP8B
Right ØP89
Coccyx ØQ8S
Conduction Mechanism Ø288
Esophagogastric Junction ØD84
Femoral Shaft
Left ØQ89
Right ØQ88
Femur
Lower
Left ØQ8C
Right ØQ8B
Upper
Left ØQ87
Right ØQ86
Fibula
Left ØQ8K
Right ØQ8J
Gland, Pituitary ØG8Ø
Glenoid Cavity
Left ØP88
Right ØP87
Humeral Head
Left ØP8D
Right ØP8C
Humeral Shaft
Left ØP8G
Right ØP8F
Hymen ØU8K
Kidneys, Bilateral ØT82
Mandible
Left ØN8V

Division — continued
Mandible — continued
Right ØN8T
Maxilla
Left ØN8S
Right ØN8R
Metacarpal
Left ØP8Q
Right ØP8P
Metatarsal
Left ØQ8P
Right ØQ8N
Muscle
Abdomen
Left ØK8L
Right ØK8K
Facial ØK81
Foot
Left ØK8W
Right ØK8V
Hand
Left ØK8D
Right ØK8C
Head ØK8Ø
Hip
Left ØK8P
Right ØK8N
Lower Arm and Wrist
Left ØK8B
Right ØK89
Lower Leg
Left ØK8T
Right ØK8S
Neck
Left ØK83
Right ØK82
Papillary Ø28D
Perineum ØK8M
Shoulder
Left ØK86
Right ØK85
Thorax
Left ØK8J
Right ØK8H
Tongue, Palate, Pharynx ØK84
Trunk
Left ØK8G
Right ØK8F
Upper Arm
Left ØK88
Right ØK87
Upper Leg
Left ØK8R
Right ØK8Q
Nerve
Abdominal Sympathetic Ø18M
Abducens ØØ8L
Accessory ØØ8R
Acoustic ØØ8N
Brachial Plexus Ø183
Cervical Ø181
Cervical Plexus Ø18Ø
Facial ØØ8M
Femoral Ø18D
Glossopharyngeal ØØ8P
Head and Neck Sympathetic Ø18K
Hypoglossal ØØ8S
Lumbar Ø18B
Lumbar Plexus Ø189
Lumbar Sympathetic Ø18N
Lumbosacral Plexus Ø18A
Median Ø185
Oculomotor ØØ8H
Olfactory ØØ8F
Optic ØØ8G
Peroneal Ø18H
Phrenic Ø182
Pudendal Ø18C
Radial Ø186
Sacral Ø18R
Sacral Plexus Ø18Q
Sacral Sympathetic Ø18P
Sciatic Ø18F
Thoracic Ø188
Thoracic Sympathetic Ø18L
Tibial Ø18G

Division — continued
- Nerve — continued
  - Trigeminal ØØ8K
  - Trochlear ØØ8J
  - Ulnar Ø184
  - Vagus ØØ8Q
- Orbit
  - Left ØN8Q
  - Right ØN8P
- Ovary
  - Bilateral ØU82
  - Left ØU81
  - Right ØU8Ø
- Pancreas ØF8G
- Patella
  - Left ØQ8F
  - Right ØQ8D
- Perineum, Female ØW8NXZZ
- Phalanx
  - Finger
    - Left ØP8V
    - Right ØP8T
  - Thumb
    - Left ØP8S
    - Right ØP8R
  - Toe
    - Left ØQ8R
    - Right ØQ8Q
- Radius
  - Left ØP8J
  - Right ØP8H
- Rib
  - Left ØP82
  - Right ØP81
- Sacrum ØQ81
- Scapula
  - Left ØP86
  - Right ØP85
- Skin
  - Abdomen ØH87XZZ
  - Back ØH86XZZ
  - Buttock ØH88XZZ
  - Chest ØH85XZZ
  - Ear
    - Left ØH83XZZ
    - Right ØH82XZZ
  - Face ØH81XZZ
  - Foot
    - Left ØH8NXZZ
    - Right ØH8MXZZ
  - Genitalia ØH8AXZZ
  - Hand
    - Left ØH8GXZZ
    - Right ØH8FXZZ
  - Lower Arm
    - Left ØH8EXZZ
    - Right ØH8DXZZ
  - Lower Leg
    - Left ØH8LXZZ
    - Right ØH8KXZZ
  - Neck ØH84XZZ
  - Perineum ØH89XZZ
  - Scalp ØH8ØXZZ
  - Upper Arm
    - Left ØH8CXZZ
    - Right ØH8BXZZ
  - Upper Leg
    - Left ØH8JXZZ
    - Right ØH8HXZZ
- Skull ØN8Ø
- Spinal Cord
  - Cervical ØØ8W
  - Lumbar ØØ8Y
  - Thoracic ØØ8X
- Sternum ØP8Ø
- Stomach, Pylorus ØD87
- Subcutaneous Tissue and Fascia
  - Abdomen ØJ88
  - Back ØJ87
  - Buttock ØJ89
  - Chest ØJ86
  - Face ØJ81
  - Foot
    - Left ØJ8R
    - Right ØJ8Q

Division — continued
- Subcutaneous Tissue and Fascia — continued
  - Hand
    - Left ØJ8K
    - Right ØJ8J
  - Head and Neck ØJ8S
  - Lower Arm
    - Left ØJ8H
    - Right ØJ8G
  - Lower Extremity ØJ8W
  - Lower Leg
    - Left ØJ8P
    - Right ØJ8N
  - Neck
    - Anterior ØJ84
    - Posterior ØJ85
  - Pelvic Region ØJ8C
  - Perineum ØJ8B
  - Scalp ØJ8Ø
  - Trunk ØJ8T
  - Upper Arm
    - Left ØJ8F
    - Right ØJ8D
  - Upper Extremity ØJ8V
  - Upper Leg
    - Left ØJ8M
    - Right ØJ8L
- Tarsal
  - Left ØQ8M
  - Right ØQ8L
- Tendon
  - Abdomen
    - Left ØL8G
    - Right ØL8F
  - Ankle
    - Left ØL8T
    - Right ØL8S
  - Foot
    - Left ØL8W
    - Right ØL8V
  - Hand
    - Left ØL88
    - Right ØL87
  - Head and Neck ØL8Ø
  - Hip
    - Left ØL8K
    - Right ØL8J
  - Knee
    - Left ØL8R
    - Right ØL8Q
  - Lower Arm and Wrist
    - Left ØL86
    - Right ØL85
  - Lower Leg
    - Left ØL8P
    - Right ØL8N
  - Perineum ØL8H
  - Shoulder
    - Left ØL82
    - Right ØL81
  - Thorax
    - Left ØL8D
    - Right ØL8C
  - Trunk
    - Left ØL8B
    - Right ØL89
  - Upper Arm
    - Left ØL84
    - Right ØL83
  - Upper Leg
    - Left ØL8M
    - Right ØL8L
- Thyroid Gland Isthmus ØG8J
- Tibia
  - Left ØQ8H
  - Right ØQ8G
- Turbinate, Nasal Ø98L
- Ulna
  - Left ØP8L
  - Right ØP8K
- Uterine Supporting Structure ØU84
- Vertebra
  - Cervical ØP83
  - Lumbar ØQ8Ø
  - Thoracic ØP84

Doppler study *see* Ultrasonography

Dorsal digital nerve *use* Nerve, Radial

Dorsal metacarpal vein
- *use* Vein, Hand, Left
- *use* Vein, Hand, Right

Dorsal metatarsal artery
- *use* Artery, Foot, Left
- *use* Artery, Foot, Right

Dorsal metatarsal vein
- *use* Vein, Foot, Left
- *use* Vein, Foot, Right

Dorsal scapular artery
- *use* Artery, Subclavian, Left
- *use* Artery, Subclavian, Right

Dorsal scapular nerve *use* Nerve, Brachial Plexus

Dorsal venous arch
- *use* Vein, Foot, Left
- *use* Vein, Foot, Right

Dorsalis pedis artery
- *use* Artery, Anterior Tibial, Left
- *use* Artery, Anterior Tibial, Right

Drainage
- Abdominal Wall ØW9F
- Acetabulum
  - Left ØQ95
  - Right ØQ94
- Adenoids ØC9Q
- Ampulla of Vater ØF9C
- Anal Sphincter ØD9R
- Ankle Region
  - Left ØY9L
  - Right ØY9K
- Anterior Chamber
  - Left Ø893
  - Right Ø892
- Anus ØD9Q
- Aorta, Abdominal Ø49Ø
- Aortic Body ØG9D
- Appendix ØD9J
- Arm
  - Lower
    - Left ØX9F
    - Right ØX9D
  - Upper
    - Left ØX99
    - Right ØX98
- Artery
  - Anterior Tibial
    - Left Ø49Q
    - Right Ø49P
  - Axillary
    - Left Ø396
    - Right Ø395
  - Brachial
    - Left Ø398
    - Right Ø397
  - Celiac Ø491
  - Colic
    - Left Ø497
    - Middle Ø498
    - Right Ø496
  - Common Carotid
    - Left Ø39J
    - Right Ø39H
  - Common Iliac
    - Left Ø49D
    - Right Ø49C
  - External Carotid
    - Left Ø39N
    - Right Ø39M
  - External Iliac
    - Left Ø49J
    - Right Ø49H
  - Face Ø39R
  - Femoral
    - Left Ø49L
    - Right Ø49K
  - Foot
    - Left Ø49W
    - Right Ø49V
  - Gastric Ø492
  - Hand
    - Left Ø39F
    - Right Ø39D
  - Hepatic Ø493
  - Inferior Mesenteric Ø49B
  - Innominate Ø392

Subterms under main terms may continue to next column or page

Drainage — continued
Artery — continued
Internal Carotid
Left Ø39L
Right Ø39K
Internal Iliac
Left Ø49F
Right Ø49E
Internal Mammary
Left Ø391
Right Ø39Ø
Intracranial Ø39G
Lower Ø49Y
Peroneal
Left Ø49U
Right Ø49T
Popliteal
Left Ø49N
Right Ø49M
Posterior Tibial
Left Ø49S
Right Ø49R
Radial
Left Ø39C
Right Ø39B
Renal
Left Ø49A
Right Ø499
Splenic Ø494
Subclavian
Left Ø394
Right Ø393
Superior Mesenteric Ø495
Temporal
Left Ø39T
Right Ø39S
Thyroid
Left Ø39V
Right Ø39U
Ulnar
Left Ø39A
Right Ø399
Upper Ø39Y
Vertebral
Left Ø39Q
Right Ø39P
Auditory Ossicle
Left Ø99A
Right Ø999
Axilla
Left ØX95
Right ØX94
Back
Lower ØW9L
Upper ØW9K
Basal Ganglia ØØ98
Bladder ØT9B
Bladder Neck ØT9C
Bone
Ethmoid
Left ØN9G
Right ØN9F
Frontal
Left ØN92
Right ØN91
Hyoid ØN9X
Lacrimal
Left ØN9J
Right ØN9H
Nasal ØN9B
Occipital
Left ØN98
Right ØN97
Palatine
Left ØN9L
Right ØN9K
Parietal
Left ØN94
Right ØN93
Pelvic
Left ØQ93
Right ØQ92
Sphenoid
Left ØN9D
Right ØN9C

Drainage — continued
Bone — continued
Temporal
Left ØN96
Right ØN95
Zygomatic
Left ØN9N
Right ØN9M
Bone Marrow Ø79T
Brain ØØ9Ø
Breast
Bilateral ØH9V
Left ØH9U
Right ØH9T
Bronchus
Lingula ØB99
Lower Lobe
Left ØB9B
Right ØB96
Main
Left ØB97
Right ØB93
Middle Lobe, Right ØB95
Upper Lobe
Left ØB98
Right ØB94
Buccal Mucosa ØC94
Bursa and Ligament
Abdomen
Left ØM9J
Right ØM9H
Ankle
Left ØM9R
Right ØM9Q
Elbow
Left ØM94
Right ØM93
Foot
Left ØM9T
Right ØM9S
Hand
Left ØM98
Right ØM97
Head and Neck ØM9Ø
Hip
Left ØM9M
Right ØM9L
Knee
Left ØM9P
Right ØM9N
Lower Extremity
Left ØM9W
Right ØM9V
Perineum ØM9K
Shoulder
Left ØM92
Right ØM91
Thorax
Left ØM9G
Right ØM9F
Trunk
Left ØM9D
Right ØM9C
Upper Extremity
Left ØM9B
Right ØM99
Wrist
Left ØM96
Right ØM95
Buttock
Left ØY91
Right ØY9Ø
Carina ØB92
Carotid Bodies, Bilateral ØG98
Carotid Body
Left ØG96
Right ØG97
Carpal
Left ØP9N
Right ØP9M
Cavity, Cranial ØW91
Cecum ØD9H
Cerebellum ØØ9C
Cerebral Hemisphere ØØ97
Cerebral Meninges ØØ91
Cerebral Ventricle ØØ96

Drainage — continued
Cervix ØU9C
Chest Wall ØW98
Choroid
Left Ø89B
Right Ø89A
Cisterna Chyli Ø79L
Clavicle
Left ØP9B
Right ØP99
Clitoris ØU9J
Coccygeal Glomus ØG9B
Coccyx ØQ9S
Colon
Ascending ØD9K
Descending ØD9M
Sigmoid ØD9N
Transverse ØD9L
Conjunctiva
Left Ø89T
Right Ø89S
Cord
Bilateral ØV9H
Left ØV9G
Right ØV9F
Cornea
Left Ø899
Right Ø898
Cul-de-sac ØU9F
Diaphragm
Left ØB9S
Right ØB9R
Disc
Cervical Vertebral ØR93
Cervicothoracic Vertebral ØR95
Lumbar Vertebral ØS92
Lumbosacral ØS94
Thoracic Vertebral ØR99
Thoracolumbar Vertebral ØR9B
Duct
Common Bile ØF99
Cystic ØF98
Hepatic
Left ØF96
Right ØF95
Lacrimal
Left Ø89Y
Right Ø89X
Pancreatic ØF9D
Accessory ØF9F
Parotid
Left ØC9C
Right ØC9B
Duodenum ØD99
Dura Mater ØØ92
Ear
External
Left Ø991
Right Ø99Ø
External Auditory Canal
Left Ø994
Right Ø993
Inner
Left Ø99E
Right Ø99D
Middle
Left Ø996
Right Ø995
Elbow Region
Left ØX9C
Right ØX9B
Epididymis
Bilateral ØV9L
Left ØV9K
Right ØV9J
Epidural Space ØØ93
Epiglottis ØC9R
Esophagogastric Junction ØD94
Esophagus ØD95
Lower ØD93
Middle ØD92
Upper ØD91
Eustachian Tube
Left Ø99G
Right Ø99F

Drainage — continued
Extremity
Lower
Left ØY9B
Right ØY99
Upper
Left ØX97
Right ØX96
Eye
Left Ø891
Right Ø89Ø
Eyelid
Lower
Left Ø89R
Right Ø89Q
Upper
Left Ø89P
Right Ø89N
Face ØW92
Fallopian Tube
Left ØU96
Right ØU95
Fallopian Tubes, Bilateral ØU97
Femoral Region
Left ØY98
Right ØY97
Femoral Shaft
Left ØQ99
Right ØQ98
Femur
Lower
Left ØQ9C
Right ØQ9B
Upper
Left ØQ97
Right ØQ96
Fibula
Left ØQ9K
Right ØQ9J
Finger Nail ØH9Q
Foot
Left ØY9N
Right ØY9M
Gallbladder ØF94
Gingiva
Lower ØC96
Upper ØC95
Gland
Adrenal
Bilateral ØG94
Left ØG92
Right ØG93
Lacrimal
Left Ø89W
Right Ø89V
Minor Salivary ØC9J
Parotid
Left ØC99
Right ØC98
Pituitary ØG9Ø
Sublingual
Left ØC9F
Right ØC9D
Submaxillary
Left ØC9H
Right ØC9G
Vestibular ØU9L
Glenoid Cavity
Left ØP98
Right ØP97
Glomus Jugulare ØG9C
Hand
Left ØX9K
Right ØX9J
Head ØW9Ø
Humeral Head
Left ØP9D
Right ØP9C
Humeral Shaft
Left ØP9G
Right ØP9F
Hymen ØU9K
Hypothalamus ØØ9A
Ileocecal Valve ØD9C
Ileum ØD9B

Drainage — continued
Inguinal Region
Left ØY96
Right ØY95
Intestine
Large ØD9E
Left ØD9G
Right ØD9F
Small ØD98
Iris
Left Ø89D
Right Ø89C
Jaw
Lower ØW95
Upper ØW94
Jejunum ØD9A
Joint
Acromioclavicular
Left ØR9H
Right ØR9G
Ankle
Left ØS9G
Right ØS9F
Carpal
Left ØR9R
Right ØR9Q
Cervical Vertebral ØR91
Cervicothoracic Vertebral ØR94
Coccygeal ØS96
Elbow
Left ØR9M
Right ØR9L
Finger Phalangeal
Left ØR9X
Right ØR9W
Hip
Left ØS9B
Right ØS99
Knee
Left ØS9D
Right ØS9C
Lumbar Vertebral ØS9Ø
Lumbosacral ØS93
Metacarpocarpal
Left ØR9T
Right ØR9S
Metacarpophalangeal
Left ØR9V
Right ØR9U
Metatarsal-Phalangeal
Left ØS9N
Right ØS9M
Metatarsal-Tarsal
Left ØS9L
Right ØS9K
Occipital-cervical ØR9Ø
Sacrococcygeal ØS95
Sacroiliac
Left ØS98
Right ØS97
Shoulder
Left ØR9K
Right ØR9J
Sternoclavicular
Left ØR9F
Right ØR9E
Tarsal
Left ØS9J
Right ØS9H
Temporomandibular
Left ØR9D
Right ØR9C
Thoracic Vertebral ØR96
Thoracolumbar Vertebral ØR9A
Toe Phalangeal
Left ØS9Q
Right ØS9P
Wrist
Left ØR9P
Right ØR9N
Kidney
Left ØT91
Right ØT9Ø
Kidney Pelvis
Left ØT94
Right ØT93

Drainage — continued
Knee Region
Left ØY9G
Right ØY9F
Larynx ØC9S
Leg
Lower
Left ØY9J
Right ØY9H
Upper
Left ØY9D
Right ØY9C
Lens
Left Ø89K
Right Ø89J
Lip
Lower ØC91
Upper ØC9Ø
Liver ØF9Ø
Left Lobe ØF92
Right Lobe ØF91
Lung
Bilateral ØB9M
Left ØB9L
Lower Lobe
Left ØB9J
Right ØB9F
Middle Lobe, Right ØB9D
Right ØB9K
Upper Lobe
Left ØB9G
Right ØB9C
Lung Lingula ØB9H
Lymphatic
Aortic Ø79D
Axillary
Left Ø796
Right Ø795
Head Ø79Ø
Inguinal
Left Ø79J
Right Ø79H
Internal Mammary
Left Ø799
Right Ø798
Lower Extremity
Left Ø79G
Right Ø79F
Mesenteric Ø79B
Neck
Left Ø792
Right Ø791
Pelvis Ø79C
Thoracic Duct Ø79K
Thorax Ø797
Upper Extremity
Left Ø794
Right Ø793
Mandible
Left ØN9V
Right ØN9T
Maxilla
Left ØN9S
Right ØN9R
Mediastinum ØW9C
Medulla Oblongata ØØ9D
Mesentery ØD9V
Metacarpal
Left ØP9Q
Right ØP9P
Metatarsal
Left ØQ9P
Right ØQ9N
Muscle
Abdomen
Left ØK9L
Right ØK9K
Extraocular
Left Ø89M
Right Ø89L
Facial ØK91
Foot
Left ØK9W
Right ØK9V
Hand
Left ØK9D

Subterms under main terms may continue to next column or page

Drainage — continued
Muscle — continued
Hand — continued
Right ØK9C
Head ØK9Ø
Hip
Left ØK9P
Right ØK9N
Lower Arm and Wrist
Left ØK9B
Right ØK99
Lower Leg
Left ØK9T
Right ØK9S
Neck
Left ØK93
Right ØK92
Perineum ØK9M
Shoulder
Left ØK96
Right ØK95
Thorax
Left ØK9J
Right ØK9H
Tongue, Palate, Pharynx ØK94
Trunk
Left ØK9G
Right ØK9F
Upper Arm
Left ØK98
Right ØK97
Upper Leg
Left ØK9R
Right ØK9Q
Nasopharynx Ø99N
Neck ØW96
Nerve
Abdominal Sympathetic Ø19M
Abducens ØØ9L
Accessory ØØ9R
Acoustic ØØ9N
Brachial Plexus Ø193
Cervical Ø191
Cervical Plexus Ø19Ø
Facial ØØ9M
Femoral Ø19D
Glossopharyngeal ØØ9P
Head and Neck Sympathetic Ø19K
Hypoglossal ØØ9S
Lumbar Ø19B
Lumbar Plexus Ø199
Lumbar Sympathetic Ø19N
Lumbosacral Plexus Ø19A
Median Ø195
Oculomotor ØØ9H
Olfactory ØØ9F
Optic ØØ9G
Peroneal Ø19H
Phrenic Ø192
Pudendal Ø19C
Radial Ø196
Sacral Ø19R
Sacral Plexus Ø19Q
Sacral Sympathetic Ø19P
Sciatic Ø19F
Thoracic Ø198
Thoracic Sympathetic Ø19L
Tibial Ø19G
Trigeminal ØØ9K
Trochlear ØØ9J
Ulnar Ø194
Vagus ØØ9Q
Nipple
Left ØH9X
Right ØH9W
Nose Ø99K
Omentum
Greater ØD9S
Lesser ØD9T
Oral Cavity and Throat ØW93
Orbit
Left ØN9Q
Right ØN9P
Ovary
Bilateral ØU92
Left ØU91

Drainage — continued
Ovary — continued
Right ØU9Ø
Palate
Hard ØC92
Soft ØC93
Pancreas ØF9G
Para-aortic Body ØG99
Paraganglion Extremity ØG9F
Parathyroid Gland ØG9R
Inferior
Left ØG9P
Right ØG9N
Multiple ØG9Q
Superior
Left ØG9M
Right ØG9L
Patella
Left ØQ9F
Right ØQ9D
Pelvic Cavity ØW9J
Penis ØV9S
Pericardial Cavity ØW9D
Perineum
Female ØW9N
Male ØW9M
Peritoneal Cavity ØW9G
Peritoneum ØD9W
Phalanx
Finger
Left ØP9V
Right ØP9T
Thumb
Left ØP9S
Right ØP9R
Toe
Left ØQ9R
Right ØQ9Q
Pharynx ØC9M
Pineal Body ØG91
Pleura
Left ØB9P
Right ØB9N
Pleural Cavity
Left ØW9B
Right ØW99
Pons ØØ9B
Prepuce ØV9T
Products of Conception
Amniotic Fluid
Diagnostic 1Ø9Ø
Therapeutic 1Ø9Ø
Fetal Blood 1Ø9Ø
Fetal Cerebrospinal Fluid 1Ø9Ø
Fetal Fluid, Other 1Ø9Ø
Fluid, Other 1Ø9Ø
Prostate ØV9Ø
Radius
Left ØP9J
Right ØP9H
Rectum ØD9P
Retina
Left Ø89F
Right Ø89E
Retinal Vessel
Left Ø89H
Right Ø89G
Retroperitoneum ØW9H
Rib
Left ØP92
Right ØP91
Sacrum ØQ91
Scapula
Left ØP96
Right ØP95
Sclera
Left Ø897
Right Ø896
Scrotum ØV95
Septum, Nasal Ø99M
Shoulder Region
Left ØX93
Right ØX92
Sinus
Accessory Ø99P

Drainage — continued
Sinus — continued
Ethmoid
Left Ø99V
Right Ø99U
Frontal
Left Ø99T
Right Ø99S
Mastoid
Left Ø99C
Right Ø99B
Maxillary
Left Ø99R
Right Ø99Q
Sphenoid
Left Ø99X
Right Ø99W
Skin
Abdomen ØH97
Back ØH96
Buttock ØH98
Chest ØH95
Ear
Left ØH93
Right ØH92
Face ØH91
Foot
Left ØH9N
Right ØH9M
Genitalia ØH9A
Hand
Left ØH9G
Right ØH9F
Lower Arm
Left ØH9E
Right ØH9D
Lower Leg
Left ØH9L
Right ØH9K
Neck ØH94
Perineum ØH99
Scalp ØH9Ø
Upper Arm
Left ØH9C
Right ØH9B
Upper Leg
Left ØH9J
Right ØH9H
Skull ØN9Ø
Spinal Canal ØØ9U
Spinal Cord
Cervical ØØ9W
Lumbar ØØ9Y
Thoracic ØØ9X
Spinal Meninges ØØ9T
Spleen Ø79P
Sternum ØP9Ø
Stomach ØD96
Pylorus ØD97
Subarachnoid Space ØØ95
Subcutaneous Tissue and Fascia
Abdomen ØJ98
Back ØJ97
Buttock ØJ99
Chest ØJ96
Face ØJ91
Foot
Left ØJ9R
Right ØJ9Q
Hand
Left ØJ9K
Right ØJ9J
Lower Arm
Left ØJ9H
Right ØJ9G
Lower Leg
Left ØJ9P
Right ØJ9N
Neck
Anterior ØJ94
Posterior ØJ95
Pelvic Region ØJ9C
Perineum ØJ9B
Scalp ØJ9Ø
Upper Arm
Left ØJ9F

Drainage — continued
Subcutaneous Tissue and Fascia — continued
Upper Arm — continued
Right ØJ9D
Upper Leg
Left ØJ9M
Right ØJ9L
Subdural Space ØØ94
Tarsal
Left ØQ9M
Right ØQ9L
Tendon
Abdomen
Left ØL9G
Right ØL9F
Ankle
Left ØL9T
Right ØL9S
Foot
Left ØL9W
Right ØL9V
Hand
Left ØL98
Right ØL97
Head and Neck ØL9Ø
Hip
Left ØL9K
Right ØL9J
Knee
Left ØL9R
Right ØL9Q
Lower Arm and Wrist
Left ØL96
Right ØL95
Lower Leg
Left ØL9P
Right ØL9N
Perineum ØL9H
Shoulder
Left ØL92
Right ØL91
Thorax
Left ØL9D
Right ØL9C
Trunk
Left ØL9B
Right ØL99
Upper Arm
Left ØL94
Right ØL93
Upper Leg
Left ØL9M
Right ØL9L
Testis
Bilateral ØV9C
Left ØV9B
Right ØV99
Thalamus ØØ99
Thymus Ø79M
Thyroid Gland ØG9K
Left Lobe ØG9G
Right Lobe ØG9H
Tibia
Left ØQ9H
Right ØQ9G
Toe Nail ØH9R
Tongue ØC97
Tonsils ØC9P
Tooth
Lower ØC9X
Upper ØC9W
Trachea ØB91
Tunica Vaginalis
Left ØV97
Right ØV96
Turbinate, Nasal Ø99L
Tympanic Membrane
Left Ø998
Right Ø997
Ulna
Left ØP9L
Right ØP9K
Ureter
Left ØT97
Right ØT96
Ureters, Bilateral ØT98

Drainage — continued
Urethra ØT9D
Uterine Supporting Structure ØU94
Uterus ØU99
Uvula ØC9N
Vagina ØU9G
Vas Deferens
Bilateral ØV9Q
Left ØV9P
Right ØV9N
Vein
Axillary
Left Ø598
Right Ø597
Azygos Ø59Ø
Basilic
Left Ø59C
Right Ø59B
Brachial
Left Ø59A
Right Ø599
Cephalic
Left Ø59F
Right Ø59D
Colic Ø697
Common Iliac
Left Ø69D
Right Ø69C
Esophageal Ø693
External Iliac
Left Ø69G
Right Ø69F
External Jugular
Left Ø59Q
Right Ø59P
Face
Left Ø59V
Right Ø59T
Femoral
Left Ø69N
Right Ø69M
Foot
Left Ø69V
Right Ø69T
Gastric Ø692
Greater Saphenous
Left Ø69Q
Right Ø69P
Hand
Left Ø59H
Right Ø59G
Hemiazygos Ø591
Hepatic Ø694
Hypogastric
Left Ø69J
Right Ø69H
Inferior Mesenteric Ø696
Innominate
Left Ø594
Right Ø593
Internal Jugular
Left Ø59N
Right Ø59M
Intracranial Ø59L
Lesser Saphenous
Left Ø69S
Right Ø69R
Lower Ø69Y
Portal Ø698
Renal
Left Ø69B
Right Ø699
Splenic Ø691
Subclavian
Left Ø596
Right Ø595
Superior Mesenteric Ø695
Upper Ø59Y
Vertebral
Left Ø59S
Right Ø59R
Vena Cava, Inferior Ø69Ø
Vertebra
Cervical ØP93
Lumbar ØQ9Ø
Thoracic ØP94

Drainage — continued
Vesicle
Bilateral ØV93
Left ØV92
Right ØV91
Vitreous
Left Ø895
Right Ø894
Vocal Cord
Left ØC9V
Right ØC9T
Vulva ØU9M
Wrist Region
Left ØX9H
Right ØX9G
Dressing
Abdominal Wall 2W23X4Z
Arm
Lower
Left 2W2DX4Z
Right 2W2CX4Z
Upper
Left 2W2BX4Z
Right 2W2AX4Z
Back 2W25X4Z
Chest Wall 2W24X4Z
Extremity
Lower
Left 2W2MX4Z
Right 2W2LX4Z
Upper
Left 2W29X4Z
Right 2W28X4Z
Face 2W21X4Z
Finger
Left 2W2KX4Z
Right 2W2JX4Z
Foot
Left 2W2TX4Z
Right 2W2SX4Z
Hand
Left 2W2FX4Z
Right 2W2EX4Z
Head 2W2ØX4Z
Inguinal Region
Left 2W27X4Z
Right 2W26X4Z
Leg
Lower
Left 2W2RX4Z
Right 2W2QX4Z
Upper
Left 2W2PX4Z
Right 2W2NX4Z
Neck 2W22X4Z
Thumb
Left 2W2HX4Z
Right 2W2GX4Z
Toe
Left 2W2VX4Z
Right 2W2UX4Z
Driver stent (RX) (OTW) *use* Intraluminal Device
Drotrecogin alfa *see* Introduction of Recombinant Human-activated Protein C
Duct of Santorini *use* Duct, Pancreatic, Accessory
Duct of Wirsung *use* Duct, Pancreatic
Ductogram, mammary *see* Plain Radiography, Skin, Subcutaneous Tissue and Breast BHØ
Ductography, mammary *see* Plain Radiography, Skin, Subcutaneous Tissue and Breast BHØ
Ductus deferens
use Vas Deferens
use Vas Deferens, Bilateral
use Vas Deferens, Left
use Vas Deferens, Right
Duodenal ampulla *use* Ampulla of Vater
Duodenectomy
see Excision, Duodenum ØDB9
see Resection, Duodenum ØDT9
Duodenocholedochotomy *see* Drainage, Gallbladder ØF94
Duodenocystostomy
see Bypass, Gallbladder ØF14
see Drainage, Gallbladder ØF94
Duodenoenterostomy
see Bypass, Gastrointestinal System ØD1

Duodenoenterostomy — continued
see Drainage, Gastrointestinal System ØD9
Duodenojejunal flexure *use* Jejunum
Duodenolysis *see* Release, Duodenum ØDN9
Duodenorrhaphy *see* Repair, Duodenum ØDQ9
Duodenostomy
see Bypass, Duodenum ØD19
see Drainage, Duodenum ØD99
Duodenotomy *see* Drainage, Duodenum ØD99
DuraHeart Left Ventricular Assist System *use* Implantable Heart Assist System in Heart and Great Vessels
Dural venous sinus *use* Vein, Intracranial
Durata® Defibrillation Lead *use* Cardiac Lead, Defibrillator in Ø2H
Dynesys® Dynamic Stabilization System
use Spinal Stabilization Device, Pedicle-Based in ØSH
use Spinal Stabilization Device, Pedicle-Based in ØRH

E

Earlobe
use Ear, External, Bilateral
use Ear, External, Left
use Ear, External, Right
Echocardiogram *see* Ultrasonography, Heart B24
Echography *see* Ultrasonography
ECMO *see* Performance, Circulatory 5A15
EEG (electroencephalogram) *see* Measurement, Central Nervous 4AØØ
EGD (esophagogastroduodenscopy) ØDJØ8ZZ
Eighth cranial nerve *use* Nerve, Acoustic
Ejaculatory duct
use Vas Deferens
use Vas Deferens, Bilateral
use Vas Deferens, Left
use Vas Deferens, Right
EKG (electrocardiogram) *see* Measurement, Cardiac 4AØ2
Electrical bone growth stimulator (EBGS)
use Bone Growth Stimulator in Head and Facial Bones
use Bone Growth Stimulator in Lower Bones
use Bone Growth Stimulator in Upper Bones
Electrical muscle stimulation (EMS) lead *use* Stimulator Lead in Muscles
Electrocautery
Destruction *see* Destruction
Repair *see* Repair
Electroconvulsive Therapy
Bilateral-Multiple Seizure GZB3ZZZ
Bilateral-Single Seizure GZB2ZZZ
Electroconvulsive Therapy, Other GZB4ZZZ
Unilateral-Multiple Seizure GZB1ZZZ
Unilateral-Single Seizure GZBØZZZ
Electroencephalogram (EEG) *see* Measurement, Central Nervous 4AØØ
Electromagnetic Therapy
Central Nervous 6A22
Urinary 6A21
Electronic muscle stimulator lead *use* Stimulator Lead in Muscles
Electrophysiologic stimulation (EPS) *see* Measurement, Cardiac 4AØ2
Electroshock therapy *see* Electroconvulsive Therapy
Elevation, bone fragments, skull *see* Reposition, Head and Facial Bones ØNS
Eleventh cranial nerve *use* Nerve, Accessory
E-Luminexx™ (Biliary) (Vascular) Stent *use* Intraluminal Device
Embolectomy *see* Extirpation
Embolization
see Occlusion
see Restriction
Embolization coil(s) *use* Intraluminal Device
EMG (electromyogram) *see* Measurement, Musculoskeletal 4AØF
Encephalon *use* Brain
Endarterectomy
see Extirpation, Lower Arteries Ø4C
see Extirpation, Upper Arteries Ø3C
Endeavor® (III) (IV) (Sprint) Zotarolimus-eluting Coronary Stent System *use* Intraluminal Device, Drug-eluting in Heart and Great Vessels
EndoSure® sensor *use* Monitoring Device, Pressure Sensor in Ø2H
ENDOTAK RELIANCE® (G) Defibrillation Lead *use* Cardiac Lead, Defibrillator in Ø2H
Endotracheal tube (cuffed) (double-lumen) *use* Intraluminal Device, Endotracheal Airway in Respiratory System
Endurant® Endovascular Stent Graft *use* Intraluminal Device
Enlargement
see Dilation
see Repair
EnRhythm *use* Pacemaker, Dual Chamber in ØJH
Enterorrhaphy *see* Repair, Gastrointestinal System ØDQ
Enterra gastric neurostimulator *use* Stimulator Generator, Multiple Array in ØJH
Enucleation
Eyeball *see* Resection, Eye Ø8T
Eyeball with prosthetic implant *see* Replacement, Eye Ø8R
Ependyma *use* Cerebral Ventricle
Epicel® cultured epidermal autograft *use* Autologous Tissue Substitute
Epic™ Stented Tissue Valve (aortic) *use* Zooplastic Tissue in Heart and Great Vessels
Epidermis *use* Skin
Epididymectomy
see Excision, Male Reproductive System ØVB
see Resection, Male Reproductive System ØVT
Epididymoplasty
see Repair, Male Reproductive System ØVQ
see Supplement, Male Reproductive System ØVU
Epididymorrhaphy *see* Repair, Male Reproductive System ØVQ
Epididymotomy *see* Drainage, Male Reproductive System ØV9
Epiphysiodesis
see Fusion, Lower Joints ØSG
see Fusion, Upper Joints ØRG
Epiploic foramen *use* Peritoneum
Epiretinal Visual Prosthesis
use Epiretinal Visual Prosthesis in Eye
Insertion of device in
Left Ø8H1Ø5Z
Right Ø8HØØ5Z
Episiorrhaphy *see* Repair, Perineum, Female ØWQN
Episiotomy *see* Division, Perineum, Female ØW8N
Epithalamus *use* Thalamus
Epitrochlear lymph node
use Lymphatic, Upper Extremity, Left
use Lymphatic, Upper Extremity, Right
EPS (electrophysiologic stimulation) *see* Measurement, Cardiac 4AØ2
Eptifibatide, infusion *see* Introduction of Platelet Inhibitor
ERCP (endoscopic retrograde cholangiopancreatography) *see* Fluoroscopy, Hepatobiliary System and Pancreas BF1
Erector spinae muscle
use Muscle, Trunk, Left
use Muscle, Trunk, Right
Esophageal artery *use* Aorta, Thoracic
Esophageal obturator airway (EOA) *use* Intraluminal Device, Airway in Gastrointestinal System
Esophageal plexus *use* Nerve, Thoracic Sympathetic
Esophagectomy
see Excision, Gastrointestinal System ØDB
see Resection, Gastrointestinal System ØDT
Esophagocoloplasty
see Repair, Gastrointestinal System ØDQ
see Supplement, Gastrointestinal System ØDU
Esophagoenterostomy
see Bypass, Gastrointestinal System ØD1
see Drainage, Gastrointestinal System ØD9
Esophagoesophagostomy
see Bypass, Gastrointestinal System ØD1
see Drainage, Gastrointestinal System ØD9
Esophagogastrectomy
see Excision, Gastrointestinal System ØDB
see Resection, Gastrointestinal System ØDT
Esophagogastroduodenoscopy (EGD) ØDJØ8ZZ
Esophagogastroplasty
see Repair, Gastrointestinal System ØDQ
see Supplement, Gastrointestinal System ØDU
Esophagogastroscopy ØDJ68ZZ
Esophagogastrostomy
see Bypass, Gastrointestinal System ØD1
see Drainage, Gastrointestinal System ØD9
Esophagojejunoplasty *see* Supplement, Gastrointestinal System ØDU
Esophagojejunostomy
see Bypass, Gastrointestinal System ØD1
see Drainage, Gastrointestinal System ØD9
Esophagomyotomy *see* Division, Esophagogastric Junction ØD84
Esophagoplasty
see Repair, Gastrointestinal System ØDQ
see Replacement, Esophagus ØDR5
see Supplement, Gastrointestinal System ØDU
Esophagoplication *see* Restriction, Gastrointestinal System ØDV
Esophagorrhaphy *see* Repair, Gastrointestinal System ØDQ
Esophagoscopy ØDJØ8ZZ
Esophagotomy *see* Drainage, Gastrointestinal System ØD9
Esteem® implantable hearing system *use* Hearing Device in Ear, Nose, Sinus
ESWL (extracorporeal shock wave lithotripsy) *see* Fragmentation
Ethmoidal air cell
use Sinus, Ethmoid, Left
use Sinus, Ethmoid, Right
Ethmoidectomy
see Excision, Ear, Nose, Sinus Ø9B
see Excision, Head and Facial Bones ØNB
see Resection, Ear, Nose, Sinus Ø9T
see Resection, Head and Facial Bones ØNT
Ethmoidotomy *see* Drainage, Ear, Nose, Sinus Ø99
Evacuation
Hematoma *see* Extirpation
Other Fluid *see* Drainage
Evera (XT) (S) (DR/VR) *use* Defibrillator Generator in ØJH
Everolimus-eluting coronary stent *use* Intraluminal Device, Drug-eluting in Heart and Great Vessels
Evisceration
Eyeball *see* Resection, Eye Ø8T
Eyeball with prosthetic implant *see* Replacement, Eye Ø8R
Examination *see* Inspection
Exchange *see* Change device in
Excision
Abdominal Wall ØWBF
Acetabulum
Left ØQB5
Right ØQB4
Adenoids ØCBQ
Ampulla of Vater ØFBC
Anal Sphincter ØDBR
Ankle Region
Left ØYBL
Right ØYBK
Anus ØDBQ
Aorta
Abdominal Ø4BØ
Thoracic Ø2BW
Aortic Body ØGBD
Appendix ØDBJ
Arm
Lower
Left ØXBF
Right ØXBD
Upper
Left ØXB9
Right ØXB8
Artery
Anterior Tibial
Left Ø4BQ
Right Ø4BP
Axillary
Left Ø3B6
Right Ø3B5
Brachial
Left Ø3B8
Right Ø3B7
Celiac Ø4B1
Colic
Left Ø4B7

Excision — continued
Artery — continued
Colic — continued
Middle Ø4B8
Right Ø4B6
Common Carotid
Left Ø3BJ
Right Ø3BH
Common Iliac
Left Ø4BD
Right Ø4BC
External Carotid
Left Ø3BN
Right Ø3BM
External Iliac
Left Ø4BJ
Right Ø4BH
Face Ø3BR
Femoral
Left Ø4BL
Right Ø4BK
Foot
Left Ø4BW
Right Ø4BV
Gastric Ø4B2
Hand
Left Ø3BF
Right Ø3BD
Hepatic Ø4B3
Inferior Mesenteric Ø4BB
Innominate Ø3B2
Internal Carotid
Left Ø3BL
Right Ø3BK
Internal Iliac
Left Ø4BF
Right Ø4BE
Internal Mammary
Left Ø3B1
Right Ø3BØ
Intracranial Ø3BG
Lower Ø4BY
Peroneal
Left Ø4BU
Right Ø4BT
Popliteal
Left Ø4BN
Right Ø4BM
Posterior Tibial
Left Ø4BS
Right Ø4BR
Pulmonary
Left Ø2BR
Right Ø2BQ
Pulmonary Trunk Ø2BP
Radial
Left Ø3BC
Right Ø3BB
Renal
Left Ø4BA
Right Ø4B9
Splenic Ø4B4
Subclavian
Left Ø3B4
Right Ø3B3
Superior Mesenteric Ø4B5
Temporal
Left Ø3BT
Right Ø3BS
Thyroid
Left Ø3BV
Right Ø3BU
Ulnar
Left Ø3BA
Right Ø3B9
Upper Ø3BY
Vertebral
Left Ø3BQ
Right Ø3BP
Atrium
Left Ø2B7
Right Ø2B6
Auditory Ossicle
Left Ø9BAØZ
Right Ø9B9ØZ

Excision — continued
Axilla
Left ØXB5
Right ØXB4
Back
Lower ØWBL
Upper ØWBK
Basal Ganglia ØØB8
Bladder ØTBB
Bladder Neck ØTBC
Bone
Ethmoid
Left ØNBG
Right ØNBF
Frontal
Left ØNB2
Right ØNB1
Hyoid ØNBX
Lacrimal
Left ØNBJ
Right ØNBH
Nasal ØNBB
Occipital
Left ØNB8
Right ØNB7
Palatine
Left ØNBL
Right ØNBK
Parietal
Left ØNB4
Right ØNB3
Pelvic
Left ØQB3
Right ØQB2
Sphenoid
Left ØNBD
Right ØNBC
Temporal
Left ØNB6
Right ØNB5
Zygomatic
Left ØNBN
Right ØNBM
Brain ØØBØ
Breast
Bilateral ØHBV
Left ØHBU
Right ØHBT
Supernumerary ØHBY
Bronchus
Lingula ØBB9
Lower Lobe
Left ØBBB
Right ØBB6
Main
Left ØBB7
Right ØBB3
Middle Lobe, Right ØBB5
Upper Lobe
Left ØBB8
Right ØBB4
Buccal Mucosa ØCB4
Bursa and Ligament
Abdomen
Left ØMBJ
Right ØMBH
Ankle
Left ØMBR
Right ØMBQ
Elbow
Left ØMB4
Right ØMB3
Foot
Left ØMBT
Right ØMBS
Hand
Left ØMB8
Right ØMB7
Head and Neck ØMBØ
Hip
Left ØMBM
Right ØMBL
Knee
Left ØMBP
Right ØMBN

Excision — continued
Bursa and Ligament — continued
Lower Extremity
Left ØMBW
Right ØMBV
Perineum ØMBK
Shoulder
Left ØMB2
Right ØMB1
Thorax
Left ØMBG
Right ØMBF
Trunk
Left ØMBD
Right ØMBC
Upper Extremity
Left ØMBB
Right ØMB9
Wrist
Left ØMB6
Right ØMB5
Buttock
Left ØYB1
Right ØYBØ
Carina ØBB2
Carotid Bodies, Bilateral ØGB8
Carotid Body
Left ØGB6
Right ØGB7
Carpal
Left ØPBN
Right ØPBM
Cecum ØDBH
Cerebellum ØØBC
Cerebral Hemisphere ØØB7
Cerebral Meninges ØØB1
Cerebral Ventricle ØØB6
Cervix ØUBC
Chest Wall ØWB8
Chordae Tendineae Ø2B9
Choroid
Left Ø8BB
Right Ø8BA
Cisterna Chyli Ø7BL
Clavicle
Left ØPBB
Right ØPB9
Clitoris ØUBJ
Coccygeal Glomus ØGBB
Coccyx ØQBS
Colon
Ascending ØDBK
Descending ØDBM
Sigmoid ØDBN
Transverse ØDBL
Conduction Mechanism Ø2B8
Conjunctiva
Left Ø8BTXZ
Right Ø8BSXZ
Cord
Bilateral ØVBH
Left ØVBG
Right ØVBF
Cornea
Left Ø8B9XZ
Right Ø8B8XZ
Cul-de-sac ØUBF
Diaphragm
Left ØBBS
Right ØBBR
Disc
Cervical Vertebral ØRB3
Cervicothoracic Vertebral ØRB5
Lumbar Vertebral ØSB2
Lumbosacral ØSB4
Thoracic Vertebral ØRB9
Thoracolumbar Vertebral ØRBB
Duct
Common Bile ØFB9
Cystic ØFB8
Hepatic
Left ØFB6
Right ØFB5
Lacrimal
Left Ø8BY
Right Ø8BX

Excision — continued
Duct — continued
Pancreatic ØFBD
Accessory ØFBF
Parotid
Left ØCBC
Right ØCBB
Duodenum ØDB9
Dura Mater ØØB2
Ear
External
Left Ø9B1
Right Ø9BØ
External Auditory Canal
Left Ø9B4
Right Ø9B3
Inner
Left Ø9BEØZ
Right Ø9BDØZ
Middle
Left Ø9B6ØZ
Right Ø9B5ØZ
Elbow Region
Left ØXBC
Right ØXBB
Epididymis
Bilateral ØVBL
Left ØVBK
Right ØVBJ
Epiglottis ØCBR
Esophagogastric Junction ØDB4
Esophagus ØDB5
Lower ØDB3
Middle ØDB2
Upper ØDB1
Eustachian Tube
Left Ø9BG
Right Ø9BF
Extremity
Lower
Left ØYBB
Right ØYB9
Upper
Left ØXB7
Right ØXB6
Eye
Left Ø8B1
Right Ø8BØ
Eyelid
Lower
Left Ø8BR
Right Ø8BQ
Upper
Left Ø8BP
Right Ø8BN
Face ØWB2
Fallopian Tube
Left ØUB6
Right ØUB5
Fallopian Tubes, Bilateral ØUB7
Femoral Region
Left ØYB8
Right ØYB7
Femoral Shaft
Left ØQB9
Right ØQB8
Femur
Lower
Left ØQBC
Right ØQBB
Upper
Left ØQB7
Right ØQB6
Fibula
Left ØQBK
Right ØQBJ
Finger Nail ØHBQXZ
Foot
Left ØYBN
Right ØYBM
Gallbladder ØFB4
Gingiva
Lower ØCB6
Upper ØCB5

Excision — continued
Gland
Adrenal
Bilateral ØGB4
Left ØGB2
Right ØGB3
Lacrimal
Left Ø8BW
Right Ø8BV
Minor Salivary ØCBJ
Parotid
Left ØCB9
Right ØCB8
Pituitary ØGBØ
Sublingual
Left ØCBF
Right ØCBD
Submaxillary
Left ØCBH
Right ØCBG
Vestibular ØUBL
Glenoid Cavity
Left ØPB8
Right ØPB7
Glomus Jugulare ØGBC
Hand
Left ØXBK
Right ØXBJ
Head ØWBØ
Humeral Head
Left ØPBD
Right ØPBC
Humeral Shaft
Left ØPBG
Right ØPBF
Hymen ØUBK
Hypothalamus ØØBA
Ileocecal Valve ØDBC
Ileum ØDBB
Inguinal Region
Left ØYB6
Right ØYB5
Intestine
Large ØDBE
Left ØDBG
Right ØDBF
Small ØDB8
Iris
Left Ø8BD3Z
Right Ø8BC3Z
Jaw
Lower ØWB5
Upper ØWB4
Jejunum ØDBA
Joint
Acromioclavicular
Left ØRBH
Right ØRBG
Ankle
Left ØSBG
Right ØSBF
Carpal
Left ØRBR
Right ØRBQ
Cervical Vertebral ØRB1
Cervicothoracic Vertebral ØRB4
Coccygeal ØSB6
Elbow
Left ØRBM
Right ØRBL
Finger Phalangeal
Left ØRBX
Right ØRBW
Hip
Left ØSBB
Right ØSB9
Knee
Left ØSBD
Right ØSBC
Lumbar Vertebral ØSBØ
Lumbosacral ØSB3
Metacarpocarpal
Left ØRBT
Right ØRBS
Metacarpophalangeal
Left ØRBV

Excision — continued
Joint — continued
Metacarpophalangeal — continued
Right ØRBU
Metatarsal-Phalangeal
Left ØSBN
Right ØSBM
Metatarsal-Tarsal
Left ØSBL
Right ØSBK
Occipital-cervical ØRBØ
Sacrococcygeal ØSB5
Sacroiliac
Left ØSB8
Right ØSB7
Shoulder
Left ØRBK
Right ØRBJ
Sternoclavicular
Left ØRBF
Right ØRBE
Tarsal
Left ØSBJ
Right ØSBH
Temporomandibular
Left ØRBD
Right ØRBC
Thoracic Vertebral ØRB6
Thoracolumbar Vertebral ØRBA
Toe Phalangeal
Left ØSBQ
Right ØSBP
Wrist
Left ØRBP
Right ØRBN
Kidney
Left ØTB1
Right ØTBØ
Kidney Pelvis
Left ØTB4
Right ØTB3
Knee Region
Left ØYBG
Right ØYBF
Larynx ØCBS
Leg
Lower
Left ØYBJ
Right ØYBH
Upper
Left ØYBD
Right ØYBC
Lens
Left Ø8BK3Z
Right Ø8BJ3Z
Lip
Lower ØCB1
Upper ØCBØ
Liver ØFBØ
Left Lobe ØFB2
Right Lobe ØFB1
Lung
Bilateral ØBBM
Left ØBBL
Lower Lobe
Left ØBBJ
Right ØBBF
Middle Lobe, Right ØBBD
Right ØBBK
Upper Lobe
Left ØBBG
Right ØBBC
Lung Lingula ØBBH
Lymphatic
Aortic Ø7BD
Axillary
Left Ø7B6
Right Ø7B5
Head Ø7BØ
Inguinal
Left Ø7BJ
Right Ø7BH
Internal Mammary
Left Ø7B9
Right Ø7B8

Excision — continued
Lymphatic — continued
Lower Extremity
Left Ø7BG
Right Ø7BF
Mesenteric Ø7BB
Neck
Left Ø7B2
Right Ø7B1
Pelvis Ø7BC
Thoracic Duct Ø7BK
Thorax Ø7B7
Upper Extremity
Left Ø7B4
Right Ø7B3
Mandible
Left ØNBV
Right ØNBT
Maxilla
Left ØNBS
Right ØNBR
Mediastinum ØWBC
Medulla Oblongata ØØBD
Mesentery ØDBV
Metacarpal
Left ØPBQ
Right ØPBP
Metatarsal
Left ØQBP
Right ØQBN
Muscle
Abdomen
Left ØKBL
Right ØKBK
Extraocular
Left Ø8BM
Right Ø8BL
Facial ØKB1
Foot
Left ØKBW
Right ØKBV
Hand
Left ØKBD
Right ØKBC
Head ØKBØ
Hip
Left ØKBP
Right ØKBN
Lower Arm and Wrist
Left ØKBB
Right ØKB9
Lower Leg
Left ØKBT
Right ØKBS
Neck
Left ØKB3
Right ØKB2
Papillary Ø2BD
Perineum ØKBM
Shoulder
Left ØKB6
Right ØKB5
Thorax
Left ØKBJ
Right ØKBH
Tongue, Palate, Pharynx ØKB4
Trunk
Left ØKBG
Right ØKBF
Upper Arm
Left ØKB8
Right ØKB7
Upper Leg
Left ØKBR
Right ØKBQ
Nasopharynx Ø9BN
Neck ØWB6
Nerve
Abdominal Sympathetic Ø1BM
Abducens ØØBL
Accessory ØØBR
Acoustic ØØBN
Brachial Plexus Ø1B3
Cervical Ø1B1
Cervical Plexus Ø1BØ
Facial ØØBM

Excision — continued
Nerve — continued
Femoral Ø1BD
Glossopharyngeal ØØBP
Head and Neck Sympathetic Ø1BK
Hypoglossal ØØBS
Lumbar Ø1BB
Lumbar Plexus Ø1B9
Lumbar Sympathetic Ø1BN
Lumbosacral Plexus Ø1BA
Median Ø1B5
Oculomotor ØØBH
Olfactory ØØBF
Optic ØØBG
Peroneal Ø1BH
Phrenic Ø1B2
Pudendal Ø1BC
Radial Ø1B6
Sacral Ø1BR
Sacral Plexus Ø1BQ
Sacral Sympathetic Ø1BP
Sciatic Ø1BF
Thoracic Ø1B8
Thoracic Sympathetic Ø1BL
Tibial Ø1BG
Trigeminal ØØBK
Trochlear ØØBJ
Ulnar Ø1B4
Vagus ØØBQ
Nipple
Left ØHBX
Right ØHBW
Nose Ø9BK
Omentum
Greater ØDBS
Lesser ØDBT
Orbit
Left ØNBQ
Right ØNBP
Ovary
Bilateral ØUB2
Left ØUB1
Right ØUBØ
Palate
Hard ØCB2
Soft ØCB3
Pancreas ØFBG
Para-aortic Body ØGB9
Paraganglion Extremity ØGBF
Parathyroid Gland ØGBR
Inferior
Left ØGBP
Right ØGBN
Multiple ØGBQ
Superior
Left ØGBM
Right ØGBL
Patella
Left ØQBF
Right ØQBD
Penis ØVBS
Pericardium Ø2BN
Perineum
Female ØWBN
Male ØWBM
Peritoneum ØDBW
Phalanx
Finger
Left ØPBV
Right ØPBT
Thumb
Left ØPBS
Right ØPBR
Toe
Left ØQBR
Right ØQBQ
Pharynx ØCBM
Pineal Body ØGB1
Pleura
Left ØBBP
Right ØBBN
Pons ØØBB
Prepuce ØVBT
Prostate ØVBØ
Radius
Left ØPBJ

Excision — continued
Radius — continued
Right ØPBH
Rectum ØDBP
Retina
Left Ø8BF3Z
Right Ø8BE3Z
Retroperitoneum ØWBH
Rib
Left ØPB2
Right ØPB1
Sacrum ØQB1
Scapula
Left ØPB6
Right ØPB5
Sclera
Left Ø8B7XZ
Right Ø8B6XZ
Scrotum ØVB5
Septum
Atrial Ø2B5
Nasal Ø9BM
Ventricular Ø2BM
Shoulder Region
Left ØXB3
Right ØXB2
Sinus
Accessory Ø9BP
Ethmoid
Left Ø9BV
Right Ø9BU
Frontal
Left Ø9BT
Right Ø9BS
Mastoid
Left Ø9BC
Right Ø9BB
Maxillary
Left Ø9BR
Right Ø9BQ
Sphenoid
Left Ø9BX
Right Ø9BW
Skin
Abdomen ØHB7XZ
Back ØHB6XZ
Buttock ØHB8XZ
Chest ØHB5XZ
Ear
Left ØHB3XZ
Right ØHB2XZ
Face ØHB1XZ
Foot
Left ØHBNXZ
Right ØHBMXZ
Genitalia ØHBAXZ
Hand
Left ØHBGXZ
Right ØHBFXZ
Lower Arm
Left ØHBEXZ
Right ØHBDXZ
Lower Leg
Left ØHBLXZ
Right ØHBKXZ
Neck ØHB4XZ
Perineum ØHB9XZ
Scalp ØHBØXZ
Upper Arm
Left ØHBCXZ
Right ØHBBXZ
Upper Leg
Left ØHBJXZ
Right ØHBHXZ
Skull ØNBØ
Spinal Cord
Cervical ØØBW
Lumbar ØØBY
Thoracic ØØBX
Spinal Meninges ØØBT
Spleen Ø7BP
Sternum ØPBØ
Stomach ØDB6
Pylorus ØDB7
Subcutaneous Tissue and Fascia
Abdomen ØJB8

Subterms under main terms may continue to next column or page

Excision — continued
Subcutaneous Tissue and Fascia — continued
Back ØJB7
Buttock ØJB9
Chest ØJB6
Face ØJB1
Foot
Left ØJBR
Right ØJBQ
Hand
Left ØJBK
Right ØJBJ
Lower Arm
Left ØJBH
Right ØJBG
Lower Leg
Left ØJBP
Right ØJBN
Neck
Anterior ØJB4
Posterior ØJB5
Pelvic Region ØJBC
Perineum ØJBB
Scalp ØJBØ
Upper Arm
Left ØJBF
Right ØJBD
Upper Leg
Left ØJBM
Right ØJBL
Tarsal
Left ØQBM
Right ØQBL
Tendon
Abdomen
Left ØLBG
Right ØLBF
Ankle
Left ØLBT
Right ØLBS
Foot
Left ØLBW
Right ØLBV
Hand
Left ØLB8
Right ØLB7
Head and Neck ØLBØ
Hip
Left ØLBK
Right ØLBJ
Knee
Left ØLBR
Right ØLBQ
Lower Arm and Wrist
Left ØLB6
Right ØLB5
Lower Leg
Left ØLBP
Right ØLBN
Perineum ØLBH
Shoulder
Left ØLB2
Right ØLB1
Thorax
Left ØLBD
Right ØLBC
Trunk
Left ØLBB
Right ØLB9
Upper Arm
Left ØLB4
Right ØLB3
Upper Leg
Left ØLBM
Right ØLBL
Testis
Bilateral ØVBC
Left ØVBB
Right ØVB9
Thalamus ØØB9
Thymus Ø7BM
Thyroid Gland
Left Lobe ØGBG
Right Lobe ØGBH
Tibia
Left ØQBH

Excision — continued
Tibia — continued
Right ØQBG
Toe Nail ØHBRXZ
Tongue ØCB7
Tonsils ØCBP
Tooth
Lower ØCBX
Upper ØCBW
Trachea ØBB1
Tunica Vaginalis
Left ØVB7
Right ØVB6
Turbinate, Nasal Ø9BL
Tympanic Membrane
Left Ø9B8
Right Ø9B7
Ulna
Left ØPBL
Right ØPBK
Ureter
Left ØTB7
Right ØTB6
Urethra ØTBD
Uterine Supporting Structure ØUB4
Uterus ØUB9
Uvula ØCBN
Vagina ØUBG
Valve
Aortic Ø2BF
Mitral Ø2BG
Pulmonary Ø2BH
Tricuspid Ø2BJ
Vas Deferens
Bilateral ØVBQ
Left ØVBP
Right ØVBN
Vein
Axillary
Left Ø5B8
Right Ø5B7
Azygos Ø5BØ
Basilic
Left Ø5BC
Right Ø5BB
Brachial
Left Ø5BA
Right Ø5B9
Cephalic
Left Ø5BF
Right Ø5BD
Colic Ø6B7
Common Iliac
Left Ø6BD
Right Ø6BC
Coronary Ø2B4
Esophageal Ø6B3
External Iliac
Left Ø6BG
Right Ø6BF
External Jugular
Left Ø5BQ
Right Ø5BP
Face
Left Ø5BV
Right Ø5BT
Femoral
Left Ø6BN
Right Ø6BM
Foot
Left Ø6BV
Right Ø6BT
Gastric Ø6B2
Greater Saphenous
Left Ø6BQ
Right Ø6BP
Hand
Left Ø5BH
Right Ø5BG
Hemiazygos Ø5B1
Hepatic Ø6B4
Hypogastric
Left Ø6BJ
Right Ø6BH
Inferior Mesenteric Ø6B6

Excision — continued
Vein — continued
Innominate
Left Ø5B4
Right Ø5B3
Internal Jugular
Left Ø5BN
Right Ø5BM
Intracranial Ø5BL
Lesser Saphenous
Left Ø6BS
Right Ø6BR
Lower Ø6BY
Portal Ø6B8
Pulmonary
Left Ø2BT
Right Ø2BS
Renal
Left Ø6BB
Right Ø6B9
Splenic Ø6B1
Subclavian
Left Ø5B6
Right Ø5B5
Superior Mesenteric Ø6B5
Upper Ø5BY
Vertebral
Left Ø5BS
Right Ø5BR
Vena Cava
Inferior Ø6BØ
Superior Ø2BV
Ventricle
Left Ø2BL
Right Ø2BK
Vertebra
Cervical ØPB3
Lumbar ØQBØ
Thoracic ØPB4
Vesicle
Bilateral ØVB3
Left ØVB2
Right ØVB1
Vitreous
Left Ø8B53Z
Right Ø8B43Z
Vocal Cord
Left ØCBV
Right ØCBT
Vulva ØUBM
Wrist Region
Left ØXBH
Right ØXBG
Exclusion, Left atrial appendage (LAA) *see* Occlusion, Atrium, Left Ø2L7
Exercise, rehabilitation *see* Motor Treatment, Rehabilitation FØ7
Exploration *see* Inspection
Express® Biliary SD Monorail® Premounted Stent System *use* Intraluminal Device
Express® (LD) Premounted Stent System *use* Intraluminal Device
Express® SD Renal Monorail® Premounted Stent System *use* Intraluminal Device
Ex-PRESS™ mini glaucoma shunt *use* Synthetic Substitute
Extensor carpi radialis muscle
use Muscle, Lower Arm and Wrist, Left
use Muscle, Lower Arm and Wrist, Right
Extensor carpi ulnaris muscle
use Muscle, Lower Arm and Wrist, Left
use Muscle, Lower Arm and Wrist, Right
Extensor digitorum brevis muscle
use Muscle, Foot, Left
use Muscle, Foot, Right
Extensor digitorum longus muscle
use Muscle, Lower Leg, Left
use Muscle, Lower Leg, Right
Extensor hallucis brevis muscle
use Muscle, Foot, Left
use Muscle, Foot, Right
Extensor hallucis longus muscle
use Muscle, Lower Leg, Left
use Muscle, Lower Leg, Right
External anal sphincter *use* Anal Sphincter

External auditory meatus
use Ear, External Auditory Canal, Left
use Ear, External Auditory Canal, Right
External fixator
use External Fixation Device in Head and Facial Bones
use External Fixation Device in Lower Bones
use External Fixation Device in Lower Joints
use External Fixation Device in Upper Bones
use External Fixation Device in Upper Joints
External maxillary artery *use* Artery, Face
External naris *use* Nose
External oblique aponeurosis *use* Subcutaneous Tissue and Fascia, Trunk
External oblique muscle
use Muscle, Abdomen, Left
use Muscle, Abdomen, Right
External popliteal nerve *use* Nerve, Peroneal
External pudendal artery
use Artery, Femoral, Left
use Artery, Femoral, Right
External pudendal vein
use Vein, Greater Saphenous, Left
use Vein, Greater Saphenous, Right
External urethral sphincter *use* Urethra
Extirpation
Acetabulum
Left ØQC5
Right ØQC4
Adenoids ØCCQ
Ampulla of Vater ØFCC
Anal Sphincter ØDCR
Anterior Chamber
Left Ø8C3
Right Ø8C2
Anus ØDCQ
Aorta
Abdominal Ø4CØ
Thoracic Ø2CW
Aortic Body ØGCD
Appendix ØDCJ
Artery
Anterior Tibial
Left Ø4CQ
Right Ø4CP
Axillary
Left Ø3C6
Right Ø3C5
Brachial
Left Ø3C8
Right Ø3C7
Celiac Ø4C1
Colic
Left Ø4C7
Middle Ø4C8
Right Ø4C6
Common Carotid
Left Ø3CJ
Right Ø3CH
Common Iliac
Left Ø4CD
Right Ø4CC
Coronary
Four or More Sites Ø2C3
One Site Ø2CØ
Three Sites Ø2C2
Two Sites Ø2C1
External Carotid
Left Ø3CN
Right Ø3CM
External Iliac
Left Ø4CJ
Right Ø4CH
Face Ø3CR
Femoral
Left Ø4CL
Right Ø4CK
Foot
Left Ø4CW
Right Ø4CV
Gastric Ø4C2
Hand
Left Ø3CF
Right Ø3CD
Hepatic Ø4C3
Inferior Mesenteric Ø4CB
Innominate Ø3C2

Extirpation — continued
Artery — continued
Internal Carotid
Left Ø3CL
Right Ø3CK
Internal Iliac
Left Ø4CF
Right Ø4CE
Internal Mammary
Left Ø3C1
Right Ø3CØ
Intracranial Ø3CG
Lower Ø4CY
Peroneal
Left Ø4CU
Right Ø4CT
Popliteal
Left Ø4CN
Right Ø4CM
Posterior Tibial
Left Ø4CS
Right Ø4CR
Pulmonary
Left Ø2CR
Right Ø2CQ
Pulmonary Trunk Ø2CP
Radial
Left Ø3CC
Right Ø3CB
Renal
Left Ø4CA
Right Ø4C9
Splenic Ø4C4
Subclavian
Left Ø3C4
Right Ø3C3
Superior Mesenteric Ø4C5
Temporal
Left Ø3CT
Right Ø3CS
Thyroid
Left Ø3CV
Right Ø3CU
Ulnar
Left Ø3CA
Right Ø3C9
Upper Ø3CY
Vertebral
Left Ø3CQ
Right Ø3CP
Atrium
Left Ø2C7
Right Ø2C6
Auditory Ossicle
Left Ø9CAØZZ
Right Ø9C9ØZZ
Basal Ganglia ØØC8
Bladder ØTCB
Bladder Neck ØTCC
Bone
Ethmoid
Left ØNCG
Right ØNCF
Frontal
Left ØNC2
Right ØNC1
Hyoid ØNCX
Lacrimal
Left ØNCJ
Right ØNCH
Nasal ØNCB
Occipital
Left ØNC8
Right ØNC7
Palatine
Left ØNCL
Right ØNCK
Parietal
Left ØNC4
Right ØNC3
Pelvic
Left ØQC3
Right ØQC2
Sphenoid
Left ØNCD
Right ØNCC

Extirpation — continued
Bone — continued
Temporal
Left ØNC6
Right ØNC5
Zygomatic
Left ØNCN
Right ØNCM
Brain ØØCØ
Breast
Bilateral ØHCV
Left ØHCU
Right ØHCT
Bronchus
Lingula ØBC9
Lower Lobe
Left ØBCB
Right ØBC6
Main
Left ØBC7
Right ØBC3
Middle Lobe, Right ØBC5
Upper Lobe
Left ØBC8
Right ØBC4
Buccal Mucosa ØCC4
Bursa and Ligament
Abdomen
Left ØMCJ
Right ØMCH
Ankle
Left ØMCR
Right ØMCQ
Elbow
Left ØMC4
Right ØMC3
Foot
Left ØMCT
Right ØMCS
Hand
Left ØMC8
Right ØMC7
Head and Neck ØMCØ
Hip
Left ØMCM
Right ØMCL
Knee
Left ØMCP
Right ØMCN
Lower Extremity
Left ØMCW
Right ØMCV
Perineum ØMCK
Shoulder
Left ØMC2
Right ØMC1
Thorax
Left ØMCG
Right ØMCF
Trunk
Left ØMCD
Right ØMCC
Upper Extremity
Left ØMCB
Right ØMC9
Wrist
Left ØMC6
Right ØMC5
Carina ØBC2
Carotid Bodies, Bilateral ØGC8
Carotid Body
Left ØGC6
Right ØGC7
Carpal
Left ØPCN
Right ØPCM
Cavity, Cranial ØWC1
Cecum ØDCH
Cerebellum ØØCC
Cerebral Hemisphere ØØC7
Cerebral Meninges ØØC1
Cerebral Ventricle ØØC6
Cervix ØUCC
Chordae Tendineae Ø2C9
Choroid
Left Ø8CB

Extirpation — continued
Choroid — continued
Right Ø8CA
Cisterna Chyli Ø7CL
Clavicle
Left ØPCB
Right ØPC9
Clitoris ØUCJ
Coccygeal Glomus ØGCB
Coccyx ØQCS
Colon
Ascending ØDCK
Descending ØDCM
Sigmoid ØDCN
Transverse ØDCL
Conduction Mechanism Ø2C8
Conjunctiva
Left Ø8CTXZZ
Right Ø8CSXZZ
Cord
Bilateral ØVCH
Left ØVCG
Right ØVCF
Cornea
Left Ø8C9XZZ
Right Ø8C8XZZ
Cul-de-sac ØUCF
Diaphragm
Left ØBCS
Right ØBCR
Disc
Cervical Vertebral ØRC3
Cervicothoracic Vertebral ØRC5
Lumbar Vertebral ØSC2
Lumbosacral ØSC4
Thoracic Vertebral ØRC9
Thoracolumbar Vertebral ØRCB
Duct
Common Bile ØFC9
Cystic ØFC8
Hepatic
Left ØFC6
Right ØFC5
Lacrimal
Left Ø8CY
Right Ø8CX
Pancreatic ØFCD
Accessory ØFCF
Parotid
Left ØCCC
Right ØCCB
Duodenum ØDC9
Dura Mater ØØC2
Ear
External
Left Ø9C1
Right Ø9CØ
External Auditory Canal
Left Ø9C4
Right Ø9C3
Inner
Left Ø9CEØZZ
Right Ø9CDØZZ
Middle
Left Ø9C6ØZZ
Right Ø9C5ØZZ
Endometrium ØUCB
Epididymis
Bilateral ØVCL
Left ØVCK
Right ØVCJ
Epidural Space ØØC3
Epiglottis ØCCR
Esophagogastric Junction ØDC4
Esophagus ØDC5
Lower ØDC3
Middle ØDC2
Upper ØDC1
Eustachian Tube
Left Ø9CG
Right Ø9CF
Eye
Left Ø8C1XZZ
Right Ø8CØXZZ

Extirpation — continued
Eyelid
Lower
Left Ø8CR
Right Ø8CQ
Upper
Left Ø8CP
Right Ø8CN
Fallopian Tube
Left ØUC6
Right ØUC5
Fallopian Tubes, Bilateral ØUC7
Femoral Shaft
Left ØQC9
Right ØQC8
Femur
Lower
Left ØQCC
Right ØQCB
Upper
Left ØQC7
Right ØQC6
Fibula
Left ØQCK
Right ØQCJ
Finger Nail ØHCQXZZ
Gallbladder ØFC4
Gastrointestinal Tract ØWCP
Genitourinary Tract ØWCR
Gingiva
Lower ØCC6
Upper ØCC5
Gland
Adrenal
Bilateral ØGC4
Left ØGC2
Right ØGC3
Lacrimal
Left Ø8CW
Right Ø8CV
Minor Salivary ØCCJ
Parotid
Left ØCC9
Right ØCC8
Pituitary ØGCØ
Sublingual
Left ØCCF
Right ØCCD
Submaxillary
Left ØCCH
Right ØCCG
Vestibular ØUCL
Glenoid Cavity
Left ØPC8
Right ØPC7
Glomus Jugulare ØGCC
Humeral Head
Left ØPCD
Right ØPCC
Humeral Shaft
Left ØPCG
Right ØPCF
Hymen ØUCK
Hypothalamus ØØCA
Ileocecal Valve ØDCC
Ileum ØDCB
Intestine
Large ØDCE
Left ØDCG
Right ØDCF
Small ØDC8
Iris
Left Ø8CD
Right Ø8CC
Jejunum ØDCA
Joint
Acromioclavicular
Left ØRCH
Right ØRCG
Ankle
Left ØSCG
Right ØSCF
Carpal
Left ØRCR
Right ØRCQ
Cervical Vertebral ØRC1

Extirpation — continued
Joint — continued
Cervicothoracic Vertebral ØRC4
Coccygeal ØSC6
Elbow
Left ØRCM
Right ØRCL
Finger Phalangeal
Left ØRCX
Right ØRCW
Hip
Left ØSCB
Right ØSC9
Knee
Left ØSCD
Right ØSCC
Lumbar Vertebral ØSCØ
Lumbosacral ØSC3
Metacarpocarpal
Left ØRCT
Right ØRCS
Metacarpophalangeal
Left ØRCV
Right ØRCU
Metatarsal-Phalangeal
Left ØSCN
Right ØSCM
Metatarsal-Tarsal
Left ØSCL
Right ØSCK
Occipital-cervical ØRCØ
Sacrococcygeal ØSC5
Sacroiliac
Left ØSC8
Right ØSC7
Shoulder
Left ØRCK
Right ØRCJ
Sternoclavicular
Left ØRCF
Right ØRCE
Tarsal
Left ØSCJ
Right ØSCH
Temporomandibular
Left ØRCD
Right ØRCC
Thoracic Vertebral ØRC6
Thoracolumbar Vertebral ØRCA
Toe Phalangeal
Left ØSCQ
Right ØSCP
Wrist
Left ØRCP
Right ØRCN
Kidney
Left ØTC1
Right ØTCØ
Kidney Pelvis
Left ØTC4
Right ØTC3
Larynx ØCCS
Lens
Left Ø8CK
Right Ø8CJ
Lip
Lower ØCC1
Upper ØCCØ
Liver ØFCØ
Left Lobe ØFC2
Right Lobe ØFC1
Lung
Bilateral ØBCM
Left ØBCL
Lower Lobe
Left ØBCJ
Right ØBCF
Middle Lobe, Right ØBCD
Right ØBCK
Upper Lobe
Left ØBCG
Right ØBCC
Lung Lingula ØBCH
Lymphatic
Aortic Ø7CD

Extirpation — continued
Lymphatic — continued
Axillary
Left Ø7C6
Right Ø7C5
Head Ø7CØ
Inguinal
Left Ø7CJ
Right Ø7CH
Internal Mammary
Left Ø7C9
Right Ø7C8
Lower Extremity
Left Ø7CG
Right Ø7CF
Mesenteric Ø7CB
Neck
Left Ø7C2
Right Ø7C1
Pelvis Ø7CC
Thoracic Duct Ø7CK
Thorax Ø7C7
Upper Extremity
Left Ø7C4
Right Ø7C3
Mandible
Left ØNCV
Right ØNCT
Maxilla
Left ØNCS
Right ØNCR
Mediastinum ØWCC
Medulla Oblongata ØØCD
Mesentery ØDCV
Metacarpal
Left ØPCQ
Right ØPCP
Metatarsal
Left ØQCP
Right ØQCN
Muscle
Abdomen
Left ØKCL
Right ØKCK
Extraocular
Left Ø8CM
Right Ø8CL
Facial ØKC1
Foot
Left ØKCW
Right ØKCV
Hand
Left ØKCD
Right ØKCC
Head ØKCØ
Hip
Left ØKCP
Right ØKCN
Lower Arm and Wrist
Left ØKCB
Right ØKC9
Lower Leg
Left ØKCT
Right ØKCS
Neck
Left ØKC3
Right ØKC2
Papillary Ø2CD
Perineum ØKCM
Shoulder
Left ØKC6
Right ØKC5
Thorax
Left ØKCJ
Right ØKCH
Tongue, Palate, Pharynx ØKC4
Trunk
Left ØKCG
Right ØKCF
Upper Arm
Left ØKC8
Right ØKC7
Upper Leg
Left ØKCR
Right ØKCQ
Nasopharynx Ø9CN

Extirpation — continued
Nerve
Abdominal Sympathetic Ø1CM
Abducens ØØCL
Accessory ØØCR
Acoustic ØØCN
Brachial Plexus Ø1C3
Cervical Ø1C1
Cervical Plexus Ø1CØ
Facial ØØCM
Femoral Ø1CD
Glossopharyngeal ØØCP
Head and Neck Sympathetic Ø1CK
Hypoglossal ØØCS
Lumbar Ø1CB
Lumbar Plexus Ø1C9
Lumbar Sympathetic Ø1CN
Lumbosacral Plexus Ø1CA
Median Ø1C5
Oculomotor ØØCH
Olfactory ØØCF
Optic ØØCG
Peroneal Ø1CH
Phrenic Ø1C2
Pudendal Ø1CC
Radial Ø1C6
Sacral Ø1CR
Sacral Plexus Ø1CQ
Sacral Sympathetic Ø1CP
Sciatic Ø1CF
Thoracic Ø1C8
Thoracic Sympathetic Ø1CL
Tibial Ø1CG
Trigeminal ØØCK
Trochlear ØØCJ
Ulnar Ø1C4
Vagus ØØCQ
Nipple
Left ØHCX
Right ØHCW
Nose Ø9CK
Omentum
Greater ØDCS
Lesser ØDCT
Oral Cavity and Throat ØWC3
Orbit
Left ØNCQ
Right ØNCP
Ovary
Bilateral ØUC2
Left ØUC1
Right ØUCØ
Palate
Hard ØCC2
Soft ØCC3
Pancreas ØFCG
Para-aortic Body ØGC9
Paraganglion Extremity ØGCF
Parathyroid Gland ØGCR
Inferior
Left ØGCP
Right ØGCN
Multiple ØGCQ
Superior
Left ØGCM
Right ØGCL
Patella
Left ØQCF
Right ØQCD
Pelvic Cavity ØWCJ
Penis ØVCS
Pericardial Cavity ØWCD
Pericardium Ø2CN
Peritoneal Cavity ØWCG
Peritoneum ØDCW
Phalanx
Finger
Left ØPCV
Right ØPCT
Thumb
Left ØPCS
Right ØPCR
Toe
Left ØQCR
Right ØQCQ
Pharynx ØCCM

Extirpation — continued
Pineal Body ØGC1
Pleura
Left ØBCP
Right ØBCN
Pleural Cavity
Left ØWCB
Right ØWC9
Pons ØØCB
Prepuce ØVCT
Prostate ØVCØ
Radius
Left ØPCJ
Right ØPCH
Rectum ØDCP
Respiratory Tract ØWCQ
Retina
Left Ø8CF
Right Ø8CE
Retinal Vessel
Left Ø8CH
Right Ø8CG
Rib
Left ØPC2
Right ØPC1
Sacrum ØQC1
Scapula
Left ØPC6
Right ØPC5
Sclera
Left Ø8C7XZZ
Right Ø8C6XZZ
Scrotum ØVC5
Septum
Atrial Ø2C5
Nasal Ø9CM
Ventricular Ø2CM
Sinus
Accessory Ø9CP
Ethmoid
Left Ø9CV
Right Ø9CU
Frontal
Left Ø9CT
Right Ø9CS
Mastoid
Left Ø9CC
Right Ø9CB
Maxillary
Left Ø9CR
Right Ø9CQ
Sphenoid
Left Ø9CX
Right Ø9CW
Skin
Abdomen ØHC7XZZ
Back ØHC6XZZ
Buttock ØHC8XZZ
Chest ØHC5XZZ
Ear
Left ØHC3XZZ
Right ØHC2XZZ
Face ØHC1XZZ
Foot
Left ØHCNXZZ
Right ØHCMXZZ
Genitalia ØHCAXZZ
Hand
Left ØHCGXZZ
Right ØHCFXZZ
Lower Arm
Left ØHCEXZZ
Right ØHCDXZZ
Lower Leg
Left ØHCLXZZ
Right ØHCKXZZ
Neck ØHC4XZZ
Perineum ØHC9XZZ
Scalp ØHCØXZZ
Upper Arm
Left ØHCCXZZ
Right ØHCBXZZ
Upper Leg
Left ØHCJXZZ
Right ØHCHXZZ

Subterms under main terms may continue to next column or page

Extirpation — continued
Spinal Cord
Cervical ØØCW
Lumbar ØØCY
Thoracic ØØCX
Spinal Meninges ØØCT
Spleen Ø7CP
Sternum ØPCØ
Stomach ØDC6
Pylorus ØDC7
Subarachnoid Space ØØC5
Subcutaneous Tissue and Fascia
Abdomen ØJC8
Back ØJC7
Buttock ØJC9
Chest ØJC6
Face ØJC1
Foot
Left ØJCR
Right ØJCQ
Hand
Left ØJCK
Right ØJCJ
Lower Arm
Left ØJCH
Right ØJCG
Lower Leg
Left ØJCP
Right ØJCN
Neck
Anterior ØJC4
Posterior ØJC5
Pelvic Region ØJCC
Perineum ØJCB
Scalp ØJCØ
Upper Arm
Left ØJCF
Right ØJCD
Upper Leg
Left ØJCM
Right ØJCL
Subdural Space ØØC4
Tarsal
Left ØQCM
Right ØQCL
Tendon
Abdomen
Left ØLCG
Right ØLCF
Ankle
Left ØLCT
Right ØLCS
Foot
Left ØLCW
Right ØLCV
Hand
Left ØLC8
Right ØLC7
Head and Neck ØLCØ
Hip
Left ØLCK
Right ØLCJ
Knee
Left ØLCR
Right ØLCQ
Lower Arm and Wrist
Left ØLC6
Right ØLC5
Lower Leg
Left ØLCP
Right ØLCN
Perineum ØLCH
Shoulder
Left ØLC2
Right ØLC1
Thorax
Left ØLCD
Right ØLCC
Trunk
Left ØLCB
Right ØLC9
Upper Arm
Left ØLC4
Right ØLC3
Upper Leg
Left ØLCM

Extirpation — continued
Tendon — continued
Upper Leg — continued
Right ØLCL
Testis
Bilateral ØVCC
Left ØVCB
Right ØVC9
Thalamus ØØC9
Thymus Ø7CM
Thyroid Gland ØGCK
Left Lobe ØGCG
Right Lobe ØGCH
Tibia
Left ØQCH
Right ØQCG
Toe Nail ØHCRXZZ
Tongue ØCC7
Tonsils ØCCP
Tooth
Lower ØCCX
Upper ØCCW
Trachea ØBC1
Tunica Vaginalis
Left ØVC7
Right ØVC6
Turbinate, Nasal Ø9CL
Tympanic Membrane
Left Ø9C8
Right Ø9C7
Ulna
Left ØPCL
Right ØPCK
Ureter
Left ØTC7
Right ØTC6
Urethra ØTCD
Uterine Supporting Structure ØUC4
Uterus ØUC9
Uvula ØCCN
Vagina ØUCG
Valve
Aortic Ø2CF
Mitral Ø2CG
Pulmonary Ø2CH
Tricuspid Ø2CJ
Vas Deferens
Bilateral ØVCQ
Left ØVCP
Right ØVCN
Vein
Axillary
Left Ø5C8
Right Ø5C7
Azygos Ø5CØ
Basilic
Left Ø5CC
Right Ø5CB
Brachial
Left Ø5CA
Right Ø5C9
Cephalic
Left Ø5CF
Right Ø5CD
Colic Ø6C7
Common Iliac
Left Ø6CD
Right Ø6CC
Coronary Ø2C4
Esophageal Ø6C3
External Iliac
Left Ø6CG
Right Ø6CF
External Jugular
Left Ø5CQ
Right Ø5CP
Face
Left Ø5CV
Right Ø5CT
Femoral
Left Ø6CN
Right Ø6CM
Foot
Left Ø6CV
Right Ø6CT
Gastric Ø6C2

Extirpation — continued
Vein — continued
Greater Saphenous
Left Ø6CQ
Right Ø6CP
Hand
Left Ø5CH
Right Ø5CG
Hemiazygos Ø5C1
Hepatic Ø6C4
Hypogastric
Left Ø6CJ
Right Ø6CH
Inferior Mesenteric Ø6C6
Innominate
Left Ø5C4
Right Ø5C3
Internal Jugular
Left Ø5CN
Right Ø5CM
Intracranial Ø5CL
Lesser Saphenous
Left Ø6CS
Right Ø6CR
Lower Ø6CY
Portal Ø6C8
Pulmonary
Left Ø2CT
Right Ø2CS
Renal
Left Ø6CB
Right Ø6C9
Splenic Ø6C1
Subclavian
Left Ø5C6
Right Ø5C5
Superior Mesenteric Ø6C5
Upper Ø5CY
Vertebral
Left Ø5CS
Right Ø5CR
Vena Cava
Inferior Ø6CØ
Superior Ø2CV
Ventricle
Left Ø2CL
Right Ø2CK
Vertebra
Cervical ØPC3
Lumbar ØQCØ
Thoracic ØPC4
Vesicle
Bilateral ØVC3
Left ØVC2
Right ØVC1
Vitreous
Left Ø8C5
Right Ø8C4
Vocal Cord
Left ØCCV
Right ØCCT
Vulva ØUCM
Extracorporeal shock wave lithotripsy *see* Fragmentation
Extracranial-intracranial bypass (EC-IC) *see* Bypass, Upper Arteries Ø31
Extraction
Auditory Ossicle
Left Ø9DAØZZ
Right Ø9D9ØZZ
Bone Marrow
Iliac Ø7DR
Sternum Ø7DQ
Vertebral Ø7DS
Bursa and Ligament
Abdomen
Left ØMDJ
Right ØMDH
Ankle
Left ØMDR
Right ØMDQ
Elbow
Left ØMD4
Right ØMD3
Foot
Left ØMDT

- **Extraction** — continued
  - Bursa and Ligament — continued
    - Foot — continued
      - Right ØMDS
    - Hand
      - Left ØMD8
      - Right ØMD7
    - Head and Neck ØMDØ
    - Hip
      - Left ØMDM
      - Right ØMDL
    - Knee
      - Left ØMDP
      - Right ØMDN
    - Lower Extremity
      - Left ØMDW
      - Right ØMDV
    - Perineum ØMDK
    - Shoulder
      - Left ØMD2
      - Right ØMD1
    - Thorax
      - Left ØMDG
      - Right ØMDF
    - Trunk
      - Left ØMDD
      - Right ØMDC
    - Upper Extremity
      - Left ØMDB
      - Right ØMD9
    - Wrist
      - Left ØMD6
      - Right ØMD5
  - Cerebral Meninges ØØD1
  - Cornea
    - Left Ø8D9XZ
    - Right Ø8D8XZ
  - Dura Mater ØØD2
  - Endometrium ØUDB
  - Finger Nail ØHDQXZZ
  - Hair ØHDSXZZ
  - Kidney
    - Left ØTD1
    - Right ØTDØ
  - Lens
    - Left Ø8DK3ZZ
    - Right Ø8DJ3ZZ
  - Nerve
    - Abdominal Sympathetic Ø1DM
    - Abducens ØØDL
    - Accessory ØØDR
    - Acoustic ØØDN
    - Brachial Plexus Ø1D3
    - Cervical Ø1D1
    - Cervical Plexus Ø1DØ
    - Facial ØØDM
    - Femoral Ø1DD
    - Glossopharyngeal ØØDP
    - Head and Neck Sympathetic Ø1DK
    - Hypoglossal ØØDS
    - Lumbar Ø1DB
    - Lumbar Plexus Ø1D9
    - Lumbar Sympathetic Ø1DN
    - Lumbosacral Plexus Ø1DA
    - Median Ø1D5
    - Oculomotor ØØDH
    - Olfactory ØØDF
    - Optic ØØDG
    - Peroneal Ø1DH
    - Phrenic Ø1D2
    - Pudendal Ø1DC
    - Radial Ø1D6
    - Sacral Ø1DR
    - Sacral Plexus Ø1DQ
    - Sacral Sympathetic Ø1DP
    - Sciatic Ø1DF
    - Thoracic Ø1D8
    - Thoracic Sympathetic Ø1DL
    - Tibial Ø1DG
    - Trigeminal ØØDK
    - Trochlear ØØDJ
    - Ulnar Ø1D4
    - Vagus ØØDQ
  - Ova ØUDN
  - Pleura
    - Left ØBDP

- **Extraction** — continued
  - Pleura — continued
    - Right ØBDN
  - Products of Conception
    - Classical 1ØDØØZØ
    - Ectopic 1ØD2
    - Extraperitoneal 1ØDØØZ2
    - High Forceps 1ØDØ7Z5
    - Internal Version 1ØDØ7Z7
    - Low Cervical 1ØDØØZ1
    - Low Forceps 1ØDØ7Z3
    - Mid Forceps 1ØDØ7Z4
    - Other 1ØDØ7Z8
    - Retained 1ØD1
    - Vacuum 1ØDØ7Z6
  - Septum, Nasal Ø9DM
  - Sinus
    - Accessory Ø9DP
    - Ethmoid
      - Left Ø9DV
      - Right Ø9DU
    - Frontal
      - Left Ø9DT
      - Right Ø9DS
    - Mastoid
      - Left Ø9DC
      - Right Ø9DB
    - Maxillary
      - Left Ø9DR
      - Right Ø9DQ
    - Sphenoid
      - Left Ø9DX
      - Right Ø9DW
  - Skin
    - Abdomen ØHD7XZZ
    - Back ØHD6XZZ
    - Buttock ØHD8XZZ
    - Chest ØHD5XZZ
    - Ear
      - Left ØHD3XZZ
      - Right ØHD2XZZ
    - Face ØHD1XZZ
    - Foot
      - Left ØHDNXZZ
      - Right ØHDMXZZ
    - Genitalia ØHDAXZZ
    - Hand
      - Left ØHDGXZZ
      - Right ØHDFXZZ
    - Lower Arm
      - Left ØHDEXZZ
      - Right ØHDDXZZ
    - Lower Leg
      - Left ØHDLXZZ
      - Right ØHDKXZZ
    - Neck ØHD4XZZ
    - Perineum ØHD9XZZ
    - Scalp ØHDØXZZ
    - Upper Arm
      - Left ØHDCXZZ
      - Right ØHDBXZZ
    - Upper Leg
      - Left ØHDJXZZ
      - Right ØHDHXZZ
  - Spinal Meninges ØØDT
  - Subcutaneous Tissue and Fascia
    - Abdomen ØJD8
    - Back ØJD7
    - Buttock ØJD9
    - Chest ØJD6
    - Face ØJD1
    - Foot
      - Left ØJDR
      - Right ØJDQ
    - Hand
      - Left ØJDK
      - Right ØJDJ
    - Lower Arm
      - Left ØJDH
      - Right ØJDG
    - Lower Leg
      - Left ØJDP
      - Right ØJDN
    - Neck
      - Anterior ØJD4
      - Posterior ØJD5

- **Extraction** — continued
  - Subcutaneous Tissue and Fascia — continued
    - Pelvic Region ØJDC
    - Perineum ØJDB
    - Scalp ØJDØ
    - Upper Arm
      - Left ØJDF
      - Right ØJDD
    - Upper Leg
      - Left ØJDM
      - Right ØJDL
  - Toe Nail ØHDRXZZ
  - Tooth
    - Lower ØCDXXZ
    - Upper ØCDWXZ
  - Turbinate, Nasal Ø9DL
  - Tympanic Membrane
    - Left Ø9D8
    - Right Ø9D7
  - Vein
    - Basilic
      - Left Ø5DC
      - Right Ø5DB
    - Brachial
      - Left Ø5DA
      - Right Ø5D9
    - Cephalic
      - Left Ø5DF
      - Right Ø5DD
    - Femoral
      - Left Ø6DN
      - Right Ø6DM
    - Foot
      - Left Ø6DV
      - Right Ø6DT
    - Greater Saphenous
      - Left Ø6DQ
      - Right Ø6DP
    - Hand
      - Left Ø5DH
      - Right Ø5DG
    - Lesser Saphenous
      - Left Ø6DS
      - Right Ø6DR
    - Lower Ø6DY
    - Upper Ø5DY
  - Vocal Cord
    - Left ØCDV
    - Right ØCDT
- **Extradural space** *use* Epidural Space
- **EXtreme Lateral Interbody Fusion (XLIF) device** *use* Interbody Fusion Device in Lower Joints

F

- **Face lift** *see* Alteration, Face ØWØ2
- **Facet replacement spinal stabilization device**
  - *use* Spinal Stabilization Device, Facet Replacement in ØRH
  - *use* Spinal Stabilization Device, Facet Replacement in ØSH
- **Facial artery** *use* Artery, Face
- **False vocal cord** *use* Larynx
- **Falx cerebri** *use* Dura Mater
- **Fascia lata**
  - *use* Subcutaneous Tissue and Fascia, Upper Leg, Left
  - *use* Subcutaneous Tissue and Fascia, Upper Leg, Right
- **Fasciaplasty, fascioplasty**
  - *see* Repair, Subcutaneous Tissue and Fascia ØJQ
  - *see* Replacement, Subcutaneous Tissue and Fascia ØJR
- **Fasciectomy** *see* Excision, Subcutaneous Tissue and Fascia ØJB
- **Fasciorrhaphy** *see* Repair, Subcutaneous Tissue and Fascia ØJQ
- **Fasciotomy**
  - *see* Division, Subcutaneous Tissue and Fascia ØJ8
  - *see* Drainage, Subcutaneous Tissue and Fascia ØJ9
- **Feeding Device**
  - Change device in
    - Lower ØD2DXUZ
    - Upper ØD2ØXUZ
  - Insertion of device in
    - Duodenum ØDH9
    - Esophagus ØDH5

Feeding Device — continued
Insertion of device in — continued
Ileum ØDHB
Intestine, Small ØDH8
Jejunum ØDHA
Stomach ØDH6
Removal of device from
Esophagus ØDP5
Intestinal Tract
Lower ØDPD
Upper ØDPØ
Stomach ØDP6
Revision of device in
Intestinal Tract
Lower ØDWD
Upper ØDWØ
Stomach ØDW6
Femoral head
use Femur, Upper, Left
use Femur, Upper, Right
Femoral lymph node
use Lymphatic, Lower Extremity, Left
use Lymphatic, Lower Extremity, Right
Femoropatellar joint
use Joint, Knee, Left
use Joint, Knee, Left, Tibial Surface
use Joint, Knee, Right
use Joint, Knee, Right, Femoral Surface
Femorotibial joint
use Joint, Knee, Left
use Joint, Knee, Left, Tibial Surface
use Joint, Knee, Right
use Joint, Knee, Right, Tibial Surface
Fibular artery
use Artery, Peroneal, Left
use Artery, Peroneal, Right
Fibularis brevis muscle
use Muscle, Lower Leg, Left
use Muscle, Lower Leg, Right
Fibularis longus muscle
use Muscle, Lower Leg, Left
use Muscle, Lower Leg, Right
Fifth cranial nerve *use* Nerve, Trigeminal
Fimbriectomy
see Excision, Female Reproductive System ØUB
see Resection, Female Reproductive System ØUT
First cranial nerve *use* Nerve, Olfactory
First intercostal nerve *use* Nerve, Brachial Plexus
Fistulization
see Bypass
see Drainage
see Repair
Fitting
Arch bars, for fracture reduction *see* Reposition, Mouth and Throat ØCS
Arch bars, for immobilization *see* Immobilization, Face 2W31
Artificial limb *see* Device Fitting, Rehabilitation FØD
Hearing aid *see* Device Fitting, Rehabilitation FØD
Ocular prosthesis FØDZ8UZ
Prosthesis, limb *see* Device Fitting, Rehabilitation FØD
Prosthesis, ocular FØDZ8UZ
Fixation, bone
External, with fracture reduction *see* Reposition
External, without fracture reduction *see* Insertion
Internal, with fracture reduction *see* Reposition
Internal, without fracture reduction *see* Insertion
FLAIR® Endovascular Stent Graft *use* Intraluminal Device
Flexible Composite Mesh *use* Synthetic Substitute
Flexor carpi radialis muscle
use Muscle, Lower Arm and Wrist, Left
use Muscle, Lower Arm and Wrist, Right
Flexor carpi ulnaris muscle
use Muscle, Lower Arm and Wrist, Left
use Muscle, Lower Arm and Wrist, Right
Flexor digitorum brevis muscle
use Muscle, Foot, Left
use Muscle, Foot, Right
Flexor digitorum longus muscle
use Muscle, Lower Leg, Left
use Muscle, Lower Leg, Right
Flexor hallucis brevis muscle
use Muscle, Foot, Left
Flexor hallucis brevis muscle — continued
use Muscle, Foot, Right
Flexor hallucis longus muscle
use Muscle, Lower Leg, Left
use Muscle, Lower Leg, Right
Flexor pollicis longus muscle
use Muscle, Lower Arm and Wrist, Left
use Muscle, Lower Arm and Wrist, Right
Fluoroscopy
Abdomen and Pelvis BW11
Airway, Upper BB1DZZZ
Ankle
Left BQ1H
Right BQ1G
Aorta
Abdominal B41Ø
Laser, Intraoperative B41Ø
Thoracic B31Ø
Laser, Intraoperative B31Ø
Thoraco-Abdominal B31P
Laser, Intraoperative B31P
Aorta and Bilateral Lower Extremity Arteries B41D
Laser, Intraoperative B41D
Arm
Left BP1FZZZ
Right BP1EZZZ
Artery
Brachiocephalic-Subclavian
Laser, Intraoperative B311
Right B311
Bronchial B31L
Laser, Intraoperative B31L
Bypass Graft, Other B21F
Cervico-Cerebral Arch B31Q
Laser, Intraoperative B31Q
Common Carotid
Bilateral B315
Laser, Intraoperative B315
Left B314
Laser, Intraoperative B314
Right B313
Laser, Intraoperative B313
Coronary
Bypass Graft
Multiple B213
Laser, Intraoperative B213
Single B212
Laser, Intraoperative B212
Multiple B211
Laser, Intraoperative B211
Single B21Ø
Laser, Intraoperative B21Ø
External Carotid
Bilateral B31C
Laser, Intraoperative B31C
Left B31B
Laser, Intraoperative B31B
Right B319
Laser, Intraoperative B319
Hepatic B412
Laser, Intraoperative B412
Inferior Mesenteric B415
Laser, Intraoperative B415
Intercostal B31L
Laser, Intraoperative B31L
Internal Carotid
Bilateral B318
Laser, Intraoperative B318
Left B317
Laser, Intraoperative B317
Right B316
Laser, Intraoperative B316
Internal Mammary Bypass Graft
Left B218
Right B217
Intra-Abdominal
Laser, Intraoperative B41B
Other B41B
Intracranial B31R
Laser, Intraoperative B31R
Lower
Laser, Intraoperative B41J
Other B41J
Lower Extremity
Bilateral and Aorta B41D
Laser, Intraoperative B41D
Fluoroscopy — continued
Artery — continued
Lower Extremity — continued
Left B41G
Laser, Intraoperative B41G
Right B41F
Laser, Intraoperative B41F
Lumbar B419
Laser, Intraoperative B419
Pelvic B41C
Laser, Intraoperative B41C
Pulmonary
Left B31T
Laser, Intraoperative B31T
Right B31S
Laser, Intraoperative B31S
Renal
Bilateral B418
Laser, Intraoperative B418
Left B417
Laser, Intraoperative B417
Right B416
Laser, Intraoperative B416
Spinal B31M
Laser, Intraoperative B31M
Splenic B413
Laser, Intraoperative B413
Subclavian
Laser, Intraoperative B312
Left B312
Superior Mesenteric B414
Laser, Intraoperative B414
Upper
Laser, Intraoperative B31N
Other B31N
Upper Extremity
Bilateral B31K
Laser, Intraoperative B31K
Left B31J
Laser, Intraoperative B31J
Right B31H
Laser, Intraoperative B31H
Vertebral
Bilateral B31G
Laser, Intraoperative B31G
Left B31F
Laser, Intraoperative B31F
Right B31D
Laser, Intraoperative B31D
Bile Duct BF1Ø
Pancreatic Duct and Gallbladder BF14
Bile Duct and Gallbladder BF13
Biliary Duct BF11
Bladder BT1Ø
Kidney and Ureter BT14
Left BT1F
Right BT1D
Bladder and Urethra BT1B
Bowel, Small BD1
Calcaneus
Left BQ1KZZZ
Right BQ1JZZZ
Clavicle
Left BP15ZZZ
Right BP14ZZZ
Coccyx BR1F
Colon BD14
Corpora Cavernosa BV1Ø
Dialysis Fistula B51W
Dialysis Shunt B51W
Diaphragm BB16ZZZ
Disc
Cervical BR11
Lumbar BR13
Thoracic BR12
Duodenum BD19
Elbow
Left BP1H
Right BP1G
Epiglottis B91G
Esophagus BD11
Extremity
Lower BW1C
Upper BW1J
Facet Joint
Cervical BR14

- **Fluoroscopy** — continued
  - Facet Joint — continued
    - Lumbar BR16
    - Thoracic BR15
  - Fallopian Tube
    - Bilateral BU12
    - Left BU11
    - Right BU1Ø
  - Fallopian Tube and Uterus BU18
  - Femur
    - Left BQ14ZZZ
    - Right BQ13ZZZ
  - Finger
    - Left BP1SZZZ
    - Right BP1RZZZ
  - Foot
    - Left BQ1MZZZ
    - Right BQ1LZZZ
  - Forearm
    - Left BP1KZZZ
    - Right BP1JZZZ
  - Gallbladder BF12
    - Bile Duct and Pancreatic Duct BF14
  - Gallbladder and Bile Duct BF13
  - Gastrointestinal, Upper BD1
  - Hand
    - Left BP1PZZZ
    - Right BP1NZZZ
  - Head and Neck BW19
  - Heart
    - Left B215
    - Right B214
    - Right and Left B216
  - Hip
    - Left BQ11
    - Right BQ1Ø
  - Humerus
    - Left BP1BZZZ
    - Right BP1AZZZ
  - Ileal Diversion Loop BT1C
  - Ileal Loop, Ureters and Kidney BT1G
  - Intracranial Sinus B512
  - Joint
    - Acromioclavicular, Bilateral BP13ZZZ
    - Finger
      - Left BP1D
      - Right BP1C
    - Foot
      - Left BQ1Y
      - Right BQ1X
    - Hand
      - Left BP1D
      - Right BP1C
    - Lumbosacral BR1B
    - Sacroiliac BR1D
    - Sternoclavicular
      - Bilateral BP12ZZZ
      - Left BP11ZZZ
      - Right BP1ØZZZ
    - Temporomandibular
      - Bilateral BN19
      - Left BN18
      - Right BN17
    - Thoracolumbar BR18
    - Toe
      - Left BQ1Y
      - Right BQ1X
  - Kidney
    - Bilateral BT13
    - Ileal Loop and Ureter BT1G
    - Left BT12
    - Right BT11
    - Ureter and Bladder BT14
      - Left BT1F
      - Right BT1D
  - Knee
    - Left BQ18
    - Right BQ17
  - Larynx B91J
  - Leg
    - Left BQ1FZZZ
    - Right BQ1DZZZ
  - Lung
    - Bilateral BB14ZZZ
    - Left BB13ZZZ
    - Right BB12ZZZ

- **Fluoroscopy** — continued
  - Mediastinum BB1CZZZ
  - Mouth BD1B
  - Neck and Head BW19
  - Oropharynx BD1B
  - Pancreatic Duct BF1
    - Gallbladder and Bile Buct BF14
  - Patella
    - Left BQ1WZZZ
    - Right BQ1VZZZ
  - Pelvis BR1C
  - Pelvis and Abdomen BW11
  - Pharynix B91G
  - Ribs
    - Left BP1YZZZ
    - Right BP1XZZZ
  - Sacrum BR1F
  - Scapula
    - Left BP17ZZZ
    - Right BP16ZZZ
  - Shoulder
    - Left BP19
    - Right BP18
  - Sinus, Intracranial B512
  - Spinal Cord BØ1B
  - Spine
    - Cervical BR1Ø
    - Lumbar BR19
    - Thoracic BR17
    - Whole BR1G
  - Sternum BR1H
  - Stomach BD12
  - Toe
    - Left BQ1QZZZ
    - Right BQ1PZZZ
  - Tracheobronchial Tree
    - Bilateral BB19YZZ
    - Left BB18YZZ
    - Right BB17YZZ
  - Ureter
    - Ileal Loop and Kidney BT1G
    - Kidney and Bladder BT14
      - Left BT1F
      - Right BT1D
    - Left BT17
    - Right BT16
  - Urethra BT15
  - Urethra and Bladder BT1B
  - Uterus BU16
  - Uterus and Fallopian Tube BU18
  - Vagina BU19
  - Vasa Vasorum BV18
  - Vein
    - Cerebellar B511
    - Cerebral B511
    - Epidural B51Ø
    - Jugular
      - Bilateral B515
      - Left B514
      - Right B513
    - Lower Extremity
      - Bilateral B51D
      - Left B51C
      - Right B51B
    - Other B51V
    - Pelvic (Iliac)
      - Left B51G
      - Right B51F
    - Pelvic (Iliac) Bilateral B51H
    - Portal B51T
    - Pulmonary
      - Bilateral B51S
      - Left B51R
      - Right B51Q
    - Renal
      - Bilateral B51L
      - Left B51K
      - Right B51J
    - Spanchnic B51T
    - Subclavian
      - Left B517
      - Right B516
    - Upper Extremity
      - Bilateral B51P
      - Left B51N
      - Right B51M

- **Fluoroscopy** — continued
  - Vena Cava
    - Inferior B519
    - Superior B518
  - Wrist
    - Left BP1M
    - Right BP1L
- **Flushing** *see* Irrigation
- **Foley catheter** *use* Drainage Device
- **Foramen magnum**
  - *use* Bone, Occipital, Left
  - *use* Bone, Occipital, Right
- **Foramen of Monro (intraventricular)** *use* Cerebral Ventricle
- **Foreskin** *use* Prepuce
- **Formula™ Balloon-Expandable Renal Stent System** *use* Intraluminal Device
- **Fossa of Rosenmuller** *use* Nasopharynx
- **Fourth cranial nerve** *use* Nerve, Trochlear
- **Fourth ventricle** *use* Cerebral Ventricle
- **Fovea**
  - *use* Retina, Left
  - *use* Retina, Right
- **Fragmentation**
  - Ampulla of Vater ØFFC
  - Anus ØDFQ
  - Appendix ØDFJ
  - Bladder ØTFB
  - Bladder Neck ØTFC
  - Bronchus
    - Lingula ØBF9
    - Lower Lobe
      - Left ØBFB
      - Right ØBF6
    - Main
      - Left ØBF7
      - Right ØBF3
    - Middle Lobe, Right ØBF5
    - Upper Lobe
      - Left ØBF8
      - Right ØBF4
  - Carina ØBF2
  - Cavity, Cranial ØWF1
  - Cecum ØDFH
  - Cerebral Ventricle ØØF6
  - Colon
    - Ascending ØDFK
    - Descending ØDFM
    - Sigmoid ØDFN
    - Transverse ØDFL
  - Duct
    - Common Bile ØFF9
    - Cystic ØFF8
    - Hepatic
      - Left ØFF6
      - Right ØFF5
    - Pancreatic ØFFD
      - Accessory ØFFF
    - Parotid
      - Left ØCFC
      - Right ØCFB
  - Duodenum ØDF9
  - Epidural Space ØØF3
  - Esophagus ØDF5
  - Fallopian Tube
    - Left ØUF6
    - Right ØUF5
  - Fallopian Tubes, Bilateral ØUF7
  - Gallbladder ØFF4
  - Gastrointestinal Tract ØWFP
  - Genitourinary Tract ØWFR
  - Ileum ØDFB
  - Intestine
    - Large ØDFE
      - Left ØDFG
      - Right ØDFF
    - Small ØDF8
  - Jejunum ØDFA
  - Kidney Pelvis
    - Left ØTF4
    - Right ØTF3
  - Mediastinum ØWFC
  - Oral Cavity and Throat ØWF3
  - Pelvic Cavity ØWFJ
  - Pericardial Cavity ØWFD
  - Pericardium Ø2FN

Fragmentation — continued
Peritoneal Cavity ØWFG
Pleural Cavity
Left ØWFB
Right ØWF9
Rectum ØDFP
Respiratory Tract ØWFQ
Spinal Canal ØØFU
Stomach ØDF6
Subarachnoid Space ØØF5
Subdural Space ØØF4
Trachea ØBF1
Ureter
Left ØTF7
Right ØTF6
Urethra ØTFD
Uterus ØUF9
Vitreous
Left Ø8F5
Right Ø8F4
Freestyle (Stentless) Aortic Root Bioprosthesis *use* Zooplastic Tissue in Heart and Great Vessels
Frenectomy
see Excision, Mouth and Throat ØCB
see Resection, Mouth and Throat ØCT
Frenoplasty, frenuloplasty
see Repair, Mouth and Throat ØCQ
see Replacement, Mouth and Throat ØCR
see Supplement, Mouth and Throat ØCU
Frenotomy
see Drainage, Mouth and Throat ØC9
see Release, Mouth and Throat ØCN
Frenulotomy
see Drainage, Mouth and Throat ØC9
see Release, Mouth and Throat ØCN
Frenulum labii inferioris *use* Lip, Lower
Frenulum labii superioris *use* Lip, Upper
Frenulum linguae *use* Tongue
Frenulumectomy
see Excision, Mouth and Throat ØCB
see Resection, Mouth and Throat ØCT
Frontal lobe *use* Cerebral Hemisphere
Frontal vein
use Vein, Face, Left
use Vein, Face, Right
Fulguration *see* Destruction
Fundoplication, gastroesophageal *see* Restriction, Esophagogastric Junction ØDV4
Fundus uteri *use* Uterus
Fusion
Acromioclavicular
Left ØRGH
Right ØRGG
Ankle
Left ØSGG
Right ØSGF
Carpal
Left ØRGR
Right ØRGQ
Cervical Vertebral ØRG1
2 or more ØRG2
Cervicothoracic Vertebral ØRG4
Coccygeal ØSG6
Elbow
Left ØRGM
Right ØRGL
Finger Phalangeal
Left ØRGX
Right ØRGW
Hip
Left ØSGB
Right ØSG9
Knee
Left ØSGD
Right ØSGC
Lumbar Vertebral ØSGØ
2 or more ØSG1
Lumbosacral ØSG3
Metacarpocarpal
Left ØRGT
Right ØRGS
Metacarpophalangeal
Left ØRGV
Right ØRGU
Metatarsal-Phalangeal
Left ØSGN

Fusion — continued
Metatarsal-Phalangeal — continued
Right ØSGM
Metatarsal-Tarsal
Left ØSGL
Right ØSGK
Occipital-cervical ØRGØ
Sacrococcygeal ØSG5
Sacroiliac
Left ØSG8
Right ØSG7
Shoulder
Left ØRGK
Right ØRGJ
Sternoclavicular
Left ØRGF
Right ØRGE
Tarsal
Left ØSGJ
Right ØSGH
Temporomandibular
Left ØRGD
Right ØRGC
Thoracic Vertebral ØRG6
2 to 7 ØRG7
8 or more ØRG8
Thoracolumbar Vertebral ØRGA
Toe Phalangeal
Left ØSGQ
Right ØSGP
Wrist
Left ØRGP
Right ØRGN
Fusion screw (compression) (lag) (locking)
use Internal Fixation Device in Lower Joints
use Internal Fixation Device in Upper Joints

G

Gait training *see* Motor Treatment, Rehabilitation FØ7
Galea aponeurotica *use* Subcutaneous Tissue and Fascia, Scalp
Ganglion impar (ganglion of Walther) *use* Nerve, Sacral Sympathetic
Ganglionectomy
Destruction of lesion *see* Destruction
Excision of lesion *see* Excision
Gasserian ganglion *use* Nerve, Trigeminal
Gastrectomy
Partial *see* Excision, Stomach ØDB6
Total *see* Resection, Stomach ØDT6
Vertical (sleeve) *see* Excision, Stomach ØDB6
Gastric electrical stimulation (GES) lead *use* Stimulator Lead in Gastrointestinal System
Gastric lymph node *use* Lymphatic, Aortic
Gastric pacemaker lead *use* Stimulator Lead in Gastrointestinal System
Gastric plexus *use* Nerve, Abdominal Sympathetic
Gastrocnemius muscle
use Muscle, Lower Leg, Left
use Muscle, Lower Leg, Right
Gastrocolic ligament *use* Omentum, Greater
Gastrocolic omentum *use* Omentum, Greater
Gastrocolostomy
see Bypass, Gastrointestinal System ØD1
see Drainage, Gastrointestinal System ØD9
Gastroduodenal artery *use* Artery, Hepatic
Gastroduodenectomy
see Excision, Gastrointestinal System ØDB
see Resection, Gastrointestinal System ØDT
Gastroduodenoscopy ØDJØ8ZZ
Gastroenteroplasty
see Repair, Gastrointestinal System ØDQ
see Supplement, Gastrointestinal System ØDU
Gastroenterostomy
see Bypass, Gastrointestinal System ØD1
see Drainage, Gastrointestinal System ØD9
Gastroesophageal (GE) junction *use* Esophagogastric Junction
Gastrogastrostomy
see Bypass, Stomach ØD16
see Drainage, Stomach ØD96
Gastrohepatic omentum *use* Omentum, Lesser
Gastrojejunostomy
see Bypass, Stomach ØD16
see Drainage, Stomach ØD96
Gastrolysis *see* Release, Stomach ØDN6
Gastropexy
see Repair, Stomach ØDQ6
see Reposition, Stomach ØDS6
Gastrophrenic ligament *use* Omentum, Greater
Gastroplasty
see Repair, Stomach ØDQ6
see Supplement, Stomach ØDU6
Gastroplication *see* Restriction, Stomach ØDV6
Gastropylorectomy *see* Excision, Gastrointestinal System ØDB
Gastrorrhaphy *see* Repair, Stomach ØDQ6
Gastroscopy ØDJ68ZZ
Gastrosplenic ligament *use* Omentum, Greater
Gastrostomy
see Bypass, Stomach ØD16
see Drainage, Stomach ØD96
Gastrotomy *see* Drainage, Stomach ØD96
Gemellus muscle
use Muscle, Hip, Left
use Muscle, Hip, Right
Geniculate ganglion *use* Nerve, Facial
Geniculate nucleus *use* Thalamus
Genioglossus muscle *use* Muscle, Tongue, Palate, Pharynx
Genioplasty *see* Alteration, Jaw, Lower ØWØ5
Genitofemoral nerve *use* Nerve, Lumbar Plexus
Gingivectomy *see* Excision, Mouth and Throat ØCB
Gingivoplasty
see Repair, Mouth and Throat ØCQ
see Replacement, Mouth and Throat ØCR
see Supplement, Mouth and Throat ØCU
Glans penis *use* Prepuce
Glenohumeral joint
use Joint, Shoulder, Left
use Joint, Shoulder, Right
Glenohumeral ligament
use Bursa and Ligament, Shoulder, Left
use Bursa and Ligament, Shoulder, Right
Glenoid fossa (of scapula)
use Glenoid Cavity, Left
use Glenoid Cavity, Right
Glenoid ligament (labrum)
use Bursa and Ligament, Shoulder, Left
use Bursa and Ligament, Shoulder, Right
Globus pallidus *use* Basal Ganglia
Glomectomy
see Excision, Endocrine System ØGB
see Resection, Endocrine System ØGT
Glossectomy
see Excision, Tongue ØCB7
see Resection, Tongue ØCT7
Glossoepiglottic fold *use* Epiglottis
Glossopexy
see Repair, Tongue ØCQ7
see Reposition, Tongue ØCS7
Glossoplasty
see Repair, Tongue ØCQ7
see Replacement, Tongue ØCR7
see Supplement, Tongue ØCU7
Glossorrhaphy *see* Repair, Tongue ØCQ7
Glossotomy *see* Drainage, Tongue ØC97
Glottis *use* Larynx
Gluteal Artery Perforator Flap
Bilateral ØHRVØ79
Left ØHRUØ79
Right ØHRTØ79
Gluteal lymph node *use* Lymphatic, Pelvis
Gluteal vein
use Vein, Hypogastric, Left
use Vein, Hypogastric, Right
Gluteus maximus muscle
use Muscle, Hip, Left
use Muscle, Hip, Right
Gluteus medius muscle
use Muscle, Hip, Left
use Muscle, Hip, Right
Gluteus minimus muscle
use Muscle, Hip, Left
use Muscle, Hip, Right
GORE® DUALMESH® *use* Synthetic Substitute

Gracilis muscle
use Muscle, Upper Leg, Left
use Muscle, Upper Leg, Right
Graft
see Replacement
see Supplement
Great auricular nerve *use* Nerve, Cervical Plexus
Great cerebral vein *use* Vein, Intracranial
Great saphenous vein
use Vein, Greater Saphenous, Left
use Vein, Greater Saphenous, Right
Greater alar cartilage *use* Nose
Greater occipital nerve *use* Nerve, Cervical
Greater splanchnic nerve *use* Nerve, Thoracic Sympathetic
Greater superficial petrosal nerve *use* Nerve, Facial
Greater trochanter
use Femur, Upper, Left
use Femur, Upper, Right
Greater tuberosity
use Humeral Head, Left
use Humeral Head, Right
Greater vestibular (Bartholin's) gland *use* Gland, Vestibular
Greater wing
use Bone, Sphenoid, Left
use Bone, Sphenoid, Right
Guedel airway *use* Intraluminal Device, Airway in Mouth and Throat
Guidance, catheter placement
EKG *see* Measurement, Physiological Systems 4AØ
Fluoroscopy *see* Fluoroscopy, Veins B51
Ultrasound *see* Ultrasonography, Veins B54

Hallux
use Toe, 1st, Left
use Toe, 1st, Right
Hamate bone
use Carpal, Left
use Carpal, Right
Hancock Bioprosthesis (aortic) (mitral) valve *use* Zooplastic Tissue in Heart and Great Vessels
Hancock Bioprosthetic Valved Conduit *use* Zooplastic Tissue in Heart and Great Vessels
Harvesting, stem cells *see* Pheresis, Circulatory 6A55
Head of fibula
use Fibula, Left
use Fibula, Right
Hearing Aid Assessment F14Z
Hearing Assessment F13Z
Hearing Device
Bone Conduction
Left Ø9HE
Right Ø9HD
Insertion of device in
Left ØNH6
Right ØNH5
Multiple Channel Cochlear Prosthesis
Left Ø9HE
Right Ø9HD
Removal of device from, Skull ØNPØ
Revision of device in, Skull ØNWØ
Single Channel Cochlear Prosthesis
Left Ø9HE
Right Ø9HD
Hearing Treatment FØ9Z
Heart Assist System
External
Insertion of device in, Heart Ø2HA
Removal of device from, Heart Ø2PA
Revision of device in, Heart Ø2WA
Implantable
Insertion of device in, Heart Ø2HA
Removal of device from, Heart Ø2PA
Revision of device in, Heart Ø2WA
HeartMate II® Left Ventricular Assist Device (LVAD) *use* Implantable Heart Assist System in Heart and Great Vessels
HeartMate XVE® Left Ventricular Assist Device (LVAD) *use* Implantable Heart Assist System in Heart and Great Vessels
HeartMate® implantable heart assist system *see* Insertion of device in, Heart Ø2HA
Helix
use Ear, External, Bilateral
use Ear, External, Left
use Ear, External, Right
Hemicolectomy *see* Resection, Gastrointestinal System ØDT
Hemicystectomy *see* Excision, Urinary System ØTB
Hemigastrectomy *see* Excision, Gastrointestinal System ØDB
Hemiglossectomy *see* Excision, Mouth and Throat ØCB
Hemilaminectomy
see Excision, Lower Bones ØQB
see Excision, Upper Bones ØPB
Hemilaminotomy
see Drainage, Lower Bones ØQ9
see Drainage, Upper Bones ØP9
see Excision, Lower Bones ØQB
see Excision, Upper Bones ØPB
see Release, Central Nervous System ØØN
see Release, Lower Bones ØQN
see Release, Peripheral Nervous System Ø1N
see Release, Upper Bones ØPN
Hemilaryngectomy *see* Excision, Larynx ØCBS
Hemimandibulectomy *see* Excision, Head and Facial Bones ØNB
Hemimaxillectomy *see* Excision, Head and Facial Bones ØNB
Hemipylorectomy *see* Excision, Gastrointestinal System ØDB
Hemispherectomy
see Excision, Central Nervous System ØØB
see Resection, Central Nervous System ØØT
Hemithyroidectomy
see Excision, Endocrine System ØGB
see Resection, Endocrine System ØGT
Hemodialysis 5A1DØØZ
Hepatectomy
see Excision, Hepatobiliary System and Pancreas ØFB
see Resection, Hepatobiliary System and Pancreas ØFT
Hepatic artery proper *use* Artery, Hepatic
Hepatic flexure *use* Colon, Ascending
Hepatic lymph node *use* Lymphatic, Aortic
Hepatic plexus *use* Nerve, Abdominal Sympathetic
Hepatic portal vein *use* Vein, Portal
Hepaticoduodenostomy
see Bypass, Hepatobiliary System and Pancreas ØF1
see Drainage, Hepatobiliary System and Pancreas ØF9
Hepaticotomy *see* Drainage, Hepatobiliary System and Pancreas ØF9
Hepatocholedochostomy *see* Drainage, Duct, Common Bile ØF99
Hepatogastric ligament *use* Omentum, Lesser
Hepatopancreatic ampulla *use* Ampulla of Vater
Hepatopexy
see Repair, Hepatobiliary System and Pancreas ØFQ
see Reposition, Hepatobiliary System and Pancreas ØFS
Hepatorrhaphy *see* Repair, Hepatobiliary System and Pancreas ØFQ
Hepatotomy *see* Drainage, Hepatobiliary System and Pancreas ØF9
Herculink (RX) Elite Renal Stent System *use* Intraluminal Device
Herniorrhaphy
with synthetic substitute
see Supplement, Anatomical Regions, General ØWU
see Supplement, Anatomical Regions, Lower Extremities ØYU
see Repair, Anatomical Regions, General ØWQ
see Repair, Anatomical Regions, Lower Extremities ØYQ
Hip (joint) liner *use* Liner in Lower Joints
Holter monitoring 4A12X45
Holter valve ventricular shunt *use* Synthetic Substitute
Humeroradial joint
use Joint, Elbow, Left
use Joint, Elbow, Right
Humeroulnar joint
use Joint, Elbow, Left
Humeroulnar joint — continued
use Joint, Elbow, Right
Humerus, distal
use Humeral Shaft, Left
use Humeral Shaft, Right
Hydrocelectomy *see* Excision, Male Reproductive System ØVB
Hydrotherapy
Assisted exercise in pool *see* Motor Treatment, Rehabilitation FØ7
Whirlpool *see* Activities of Daily Living Treatment, Rehabilitation FØ8
Hymenectomy
see Excision, Hymen ØUBK
see Resection, Hymen ØUTK
Hymenoplasty
see Repair, Hymen ØUQK
see Supplement, Hymen ØUUK
Hymenorrhaphy *see* Repair, Hymen ØUQK
Hymenotomy
see Division, Hymen ØU8K
see Drainage, Hymen ØU9K
Hyoglossus muscle *use* Muscle, Tongue, Palate, Pharynx
Hyoid artery
use Artery, Thyroid, Left
use Artery, Thyroid, Right
Hyperalimentation *see* Introduction of substance in or on
Hyperbaric oxygenation
Decompression sickness treatment *see* Decompression, Circulatory 6A15
Wound treatment *see* Assistance, Circulatory 5AØ5
Hyperthermia
Radiation Therapy
Abdomen DWY38ZZ
Adrenal Gland DGY28ZZ
Bile Ducts DFY28ZZ
Bladder DTY28ZZ
Bone Marrow D7YØ8ZZ
Bone, Other DPYC8ZZ
Brain DØYØ8ZZ
Brain Stem DØY18ZZ
Breast
Left DMYØ8ZZ
Right DMY18ZZ
Bronchus DBY18ZZ
Cervix DUY18ZZ
Chest DWY28ZZ
Chest Wall DBY78ZZ
Colon DDY58ZZ
Diaphragm DBY88ZZ
Duodenum DDY28ZZ
Ear D9YØ8ZZ
Esophagus DDYØ8ZZ
Eye D8YØ8ZZ
Femur DPY98ZZ
Fibula DPYB8ZZ
Gallbladder DFY18ZZ
Gland
Adrenal DGY28ZZ
Parathyroid DGY48ZZ
Pituitary DGYØ8ZZ
Thyroid DGY58ZZ
Glands, Salivary D9Y68ZZ
Head and Neck DWY18ZZ
Hemibody DWY48ZZ
Humerus DPY68ZZ
Hypopharynx D9Y38ZZ
Ileum DDY48ZZ
Jejunum DDY38ZZ
Kidney DTYØ8ZZ
Larynx D9YB8ZZ
Liver DFYØ8ZZ
Lung DBY28ZZ
Lymphatics
Abdomen D7Y68ZZ
Axillary D7Y48ZZ
Inguinal D7Y88ZZ
Neck D7Y38ZZ
Pelvis D7Y78ZZ
Thorax D7Y58ZZ
Mandible DPY38ZZ
Maxilla DPY28ZZ
Mediastinum DBY68ZZ
Mouth D9Y48ZZ
Nasopharynx D9YD8ZZ

Hyperthermia — continued
Radiation Therapy — continued
Neck and Head DWY18ZZ
Nerve, Peripheral DØY78ZZ
Nose D9Y18ZZ
Oropharynx D9YF8ZZ
Ovary DUYØ8ZZ
Palate
Hard D9Y88ZZ
Soft D9Y98ZZ
Pancreas DFY38ZZ
Parathyroid Gland DGY48ZZ
Pelvic Bones DPY88ZZ
Pelvic Region DWY68ZZ
Pineal Body DGY18ZZ
Pituitary Gland DGYØ8ZZ
Pleura DBY58ZZ
Prostate DVYØ8ZZ
Radius DPY78ZZ
Rectum DDY78ZZ
Rib DPY58ZZ
Sinuses D9Y78ZZ
Skin
Abdomen DHY88ZZ
Arm DHY48ZZ
Back DHY78ZZ
Buttock DHY98ZZ
Chest DHY68ZZ
Face DHY28ZZ
Leg DHYB8ZZ
Neck DHY38ZZ
Skull DPYØ8ZZ
Spinal Cord DØY68ZZ
Spleen D7Y28ZZ
Sternum DPY48ZZ
Stomach DDY18ZZ
Testis DVY18ZZ
Thymus D7Y18ZZ
Thyroid Gland DGY58ZZ
Tibia DPYB8ZZ
Tongue D9Y58ZZ
Trachea DBYØ8ZZ
Ulna DPY78ZZ
Ureter DTY18ZZ
Urethra DTY38ZZ
Uterus DUY28ZZ
Whole Body DWY58ZZ
Whole Body 6A3Z
Hypnosis GZFZZZZ
Hypogastric artery
use Artery, Internal Iliac, Left
use Artery, Internal Iliac, Right
Hypopharynx *use* Pharynx
Hypophysectomy
see Excision, Gland, Pituitary ØGBØ
see Resection, Gland, Pituitary ØGTØ
Hypophysis *use* Gland, Pituitary
Hypothalamotomy *see* Destruction, Thalamus ØØ59
Hypothenar muscle
use Muscle, Hand, Left
use Muscle, Hand, Right
Hypothermia, Whole Body 6A4Z
Hysterectomy
see Excision, Uterus ØUB9
see Resection, Uterus ØUT9
Hysterolysis *see* Release, Uterus ØUN9
Hysteropexy
see Repair, Uterus ØUQ9
see Reposition, Uterus ØUS9
Hysteroplasty *see* Repair, Uterus ØUQ9
Hysterorrhaphy *see* Repair, Uterus ØUQ9
Hysteroscopy ØUJD8ZZ
Hysterotomy *see* Drainage, Uterus ØU99
Hysterotrachelectomy *see* Resection, Uterus ØUT9
Hysterotracheloplasty *see* Repair, Uterus ØUQ9
Hysterotrachelorrhaphy *see* Repair, Uterus ØUQ9

I

IABP (Intra-aortic balloon pump) *see* Assistance, Cardiac 5AØ2
IAEMT (Intraoperative anesthetic effect monitoring and titration) *see* Monitoring, Central Nervous 4A1Ø
Ileal artery *use* Artery, Superior Mesenteric
Ileectomy
see Excision, Ileum ØDBB
see Resection, Ileum ØDTB
Ileocolic artery *use* Artery, Superior Mesenteric
Ileocolic vein *use* Vein, Colic
Ileopexy
see Repair, Ileum ØDQB
see Reposition, Ileum ØDSB
Ileorrhaphy *see* Repair, Ileum ØDQB
Ileoscopy ØDJD8ZZ
Ileostomy
see Bypass, Ileum ØD1B
see Drainage, Ileum ØD9B
Ileotomy *see* Drainage, Ileum ØD9B
Ileoureterostomy *see* Bypass, Urinary System ØT1
Iliac crest
use Bone, Pelvic, Left
use Bone, Pelvic, Right
Iliac fascia
use Subcutaneous Tissue and Fascia, Upper Leg, Left
use Subcutaneous Tissue and Fascia, Upper Leg, Right
Iliac lymph node *use* Lymphatic, Pelvis
Iliacus muscle
use Muscle, Hip, Left
use Muscle, Hip, Right
Iliofemoral ligament
use Bursa and Ligament, Hip, Left
use Bursa and Ligament, Hip, Right
Iliohypogastric nerve *use* Nerve, Lumbar Plexus
Ilioinguinal nerve *use* Nerve, Lumbar Plexus
Iliolumbar artery
use Artery, Internal Iliac, Left
use Artery, Internal Iliac, Right
Iliolumbar ligament
use Bursa and Ligament, Trunk, Left
use Bursa and Ligament, Trunk, Right
Iliotibial tract (band)
use Subcutaneous Tissue and Fascia, Upper Leg, Left
use Subcutaneous Tissue and Fascia, Upper Leg, Right
Ilium
use Bone, Pelvic, Left
use Bone, Pelvic, Right
Ilizarov external fixator
use External Fixation Device, Ring in ØPH
use External Fixation Device, Ring in ØQS
use External Fixation Device, Ring in ØQH
use External Fixation Device, Ring in ØPS
Ilizarov-Vecklich device
use External Fixation Device, Limb Lengthening in ØPH
use External Fixation Device, Limb Lengthening in ØQH
Imaging, diagnostic
see Computerized Tomography (CT Scan)
see Fluoroscopy
see Magnetic Resonance Imaging (MRI)
see Plain Radiography
see Ultrasonography
Immobilization
Abdominal Wall 2W33X
Arm
Lower
Left 2W3DX
Right 2W3CX
Upper
Left 2W3BX
Right 2W3AX
Back 2W35X
Chest Wall 2W34X
Extremity
Lower
Left 2W3MX
Right 2W3LX
Upper
Left 2W39X
Right 2W38X
Face 2W31X
Finger
Left 2W3KX
Right 2W3JX
Foot
Left 2W3TX
Right 2W3SX
Hand
Left 2W3FX
Immobilization — continued
Hand — continued
Right 2W3EX
Head 2W3ØX
Inguinal Region
Left 2W37X
Right 2W36X
Leg
Lower
Left 2W3RX
Right 2W3QX
Upper
Left 2W3PX
Right 2W3NX
Neck 2W32X
Thumb
Left 2W3HX
Right 2W3GX
Toe
Left 2W3VX
Right 2W3UX
Immunization *see* Introduction of Serum, Toxoid, and Vaccine
Immunotherapy *see* Introduction of Immunotherapeutic Substance
Immunotherapy, antineoplastic
Interferon *see* Introduction of Low-dose Interleukin-2
Interleukin-2, high-dose *see* Introduction of High-dose Interleukin-2
Interleukin-2, low-dose *see* Introduction of Low-dose Interleukin-2
Monoclonal antibody *see* Introduction of Monoclonal Antibody
Proleukin, high-dose *see* Introduction of High-dose Interleukin-2
Proleukin, low-dose *see* Introduction of Low-dose Interleukin-2
Impeller Pump
Continuous, Output 5AØ221D
Intermittent, Output 5AØ211D
Implantable cardioverter-defibrillator (ICD) *use* Defibrillator Generator in ØJH
Implantable drug infusion pump (anti-spasmodic) (chemotherapy) (pain) *use* Infusion Device, Pump in Subcutaneous Tissue and Fascia
Implantable glucose monitoring device *use* Monitoring Device
Implantable hemodynamic monitor (IHM) *use* Monitoring Device, Hemodynamic in ØJH
Implantable hemodynamic monitoring system (IHMS) *use* Monitoring Device, Hemodynamic in ØJH
Implantable Miniature Telescope™ (IMT) *use* Synthetic Substitute, Intraocular Telescope in Ø8R
Implantation
see Insertion
see Replacement
Implanted (venous)(access) port *use* Vascular Access Device, Reservoir in Subcutaneous Tissue and Fascia
IMV (intermittent mandatory ventilation) *see* Assistance, Respiratory 5AØ9
In Vitro Fertilization 8EØZXY1
Incision, abscess *see* Drainage
Incudectomy
see Excision, Ear, Nose, Sinus Ø9B
see Resection, Ear, Nose, Sinus Ø9T
Incudopexy
see Repair, Ear, Nose, Sinus Ø9Q
see Reposition, Ear, Nose, Sinus Ø9S
Incus
use Auditory Ossicle, Left
use Auditory Ossicle, Right
Induction of labor
Artificial rupture of membranes *see* Drainage, Pregnancy 1Ø9
Oxytocin *see* Introduction of Hormone
InDura, intrathecal catheter (1P) (spinal) *use* Infusion Device
Inferior cardiac nerve *use* Nerve, Thoracic Sympathetic
Inferior cerebellar vein *use* Vein, Intracranial
Inferior cerebral vein *use* Vein, Intracranial
Inferior epigastric artery
use Artery, External Iliac, Left

Inferior epigastric artery — continued
use Artery, External Iliac, Right
Inferior epigastric lymph node *use* Lymphatic, Pelvis
Inferior genicular artery
use Artery, Popliteal, Left
use Artery, Popliteal, Right
Inferior gluteal artery
use Artery, Internal Iliac, Left
use Artery, Internal Iliac, Right
Inferior gluteal nerve *use* Nerve, Sacral Plexus
Inferior hypogastric plexus *use* Nerve, Abdominal Sympathetic
Inferior labial artery *use* Artery, Face
Inferior longitudinal muscle *use* Muscle, Tongue, Palate, Pharynx
Inferior mesenteric ganglion *use* Nerve, Abdominal Sympathetic
Inferior mesenteric lymph node *use* Lymphatic, Mesenteric
Inferior mesenteric plexus *use* Nerve, Abdominal Sympathetic
Inferior oblique muscle
use Muscle, Extraocular, Left
use Muscle, Extraocular, Right
Inferior pancreaticoduodenal artery *use* Artery, Superior Mesenteric
Inferior phrenic artery *use* Aorta, Abdominal
Inferior rectus muscle
use Muscle, Extraocular, Left
use Muscle, Extraocular, Right
Inferior suprarenal artery
use Artery, Renal, Left
use Artery, Renal, Right
Inferior tarsal plate
use Eyelid, Lower, Left
use Eyelid, Lower, Right
Inferior thyroid vein
use Vein, Innominate, Left
use Vein, Innominate, Right
Inferior tibiofibular joint
use Joint, Ankle, Left
use Joint, Ankle, Right
Inferior turbinate *use* Turbinate, Nasal
Inferior ulnar collateral artery
use Artery, Brachial, Left
use Artery, Brachial, Right
Inferior vesical artery
use Artery, Internal Iliac, Left
use Artery, Internal Iliac, Right
Infraauricular lymph node *use* Lymphatic, Head
Infraclavicular (deltopectoral) lymph node
use Lymphatic, Upper Extremity, Left
use Lymphatic, Upper Extremity, Right
Infrahyoid muscle
use Muscle, Neck, Left
use Muscle, Neck, Right
Infraparotid lymph node *use* Lymphatic, Head
Infraspinatus fascia
use Subcutaneous Tissue and Fascia, Upper Arm, Left
use Subcutaneous Tissue and Fascia, Upper Arm, Right
Infraspinatus muscle
use Muscle, Shoulder, Left
use Muscle, Shoulder, Right
Infundibulopelvic ligament *use* Uterine Supporting Structure
Infusion *see* Introduction of substance in or on
Infusion Device, Pump
Insertion of device in
Abdomen ØJH8
Back ØJH7
Chest ØJH6
Lower Arm
Left ØJHH
Right ØJHG
Lower Leg
Left ØJHP
Right ØJHN
Trunk ØJHT
Upper Arm
Left ØJHF
Right ØJHD
Upper Leg
Left ØJHM
Right ØJHL

Infusion Device, Pump — continued
Removal of device from
Lower Extremity ØJPW
Trunk ØJPT
Upper Extremity ØJPV
Revision of device in
Lower Extremity ØJWW
Trunk ØJWT
Upper Extremity ØJWV
Infusion, glucarpidase
Central Vein 3EØ43GQ
Peripheral Vein 3EØ33GQ
Inguinal canal
use Inguinal Region, Bilateral
use Inguinal Region, Left
use Inguinal Region, Right
Inguinal triangle
use Inguinal Region, Bilateral
use Inguinal Region, Left
use Inguinal Region, Right
Injection *see* Introduction of substance in or on
Injection reservoir *use* Vascular Access Device, Reservoir in Subcutaneous Tissue and Fascia
Insemination, artificial 3EØP7LZ
Insertion
Antimicrobial envelope *see* Introduction of Anti-infective
Aqueous drainage shunt
see Bypass, Eye Ø81
see Drainage, Eye Ø89
Products of Conception 1ØHØ
Spinal Stabilization Device
see Insertion of device in, Lower Joints ØSH
see Insertion of device in, Upper Joints ØRH
Insertion of device in
Abdominal Wall ØWHF
Acetabulum
Left ØQH5
Right ØQH4
Anal Sphincter ØDHR
Ankle Region
Left ØYHL
Right ØYHK
Anus ØDHQ
Aorta
Abdominal Ø4HØ
Thoracic Ø2HW
Arm
Lower
Left ØXHF
Right ØXHD
Upper
Left ØXH9
Right ØXH8
Artery
Anterior Tibial
Left Ø4HQ
Right Ø4HP
Axillary
Left Ø3H6
Right Ø3H5
Brachial
Left Ø3H8
Right Ø3H7
Celiac Ø4H1
Colic
Left Ø4H7
Middle Ø4H8
Right Ø4H6
Common Carotid
Left Ø3HJ
Right Ø3HH
Common Iliac
Left Ø4HD
Right Ø4HC
External Carotid
Left Ø3HN
Right Ø3HM
External Iliac
Left Ø4HJ
Right Ø4HH
Face Ø3HR
Femoral
Left Ø4HL
Right Ø4HK

Insertion of device in — continued
Artery — continued
Foot
Left Ø4HW
Right Ø4HV
Gastric Ø4H2
Hand
Left Ø3HF
Right Ø3HD
Hepatic Ø4H3
Inferior Mesenteric Ø4HB
Innominate Ø3H2
Internal Carotid
Left Ø3HL
Right Ø3HK
Internal Iliac
Left Ø4HF
Right Ø4HE
Internal Mammary
Left Ø3H1
Right Ø3HØ
Intracranial Ø3HG
Lower Ø4HY
Peroneal
Left Ø4HU
Right Ø4HT
Popliteal
Left Ø4HN
Right Ø4HM
Posterior Tibial
Left Ø4HS
Right Ø4HR
Pulmonary
Left Ø2HR
Right Ø2HQ
Pulmonary Trunk Ø2HP
Radial
Left Ø3HC
Right Ø3HB
Renal
Left Ø4HA
Right Ø4H9
Splenic Ø4H4
Subclavian
Left Ø3H4
Right Ø3H3
Superior Mesenteric Ø4H5
Temporal
Left Ø3HT
Right Ø3HS
Thyroid
Left Ø3HV
Right Ø3HU
Ulnar
Left Ø3HA
Right Ø3H9
Upper Ø3HY
Vertebral
Left Ø3HQ
Right Ø3HP
Atrium
Left Ø2H7
Right Ø2H6
Axilla
Left ØXH5
Right ØXH4
Back
Lower ØWHL
Upper ØWHK
Bladder ØTHB
Bladder Neck ØTHC
Bone
Ethmoid
Left ØNHG
Right ØNHF
Facial ØNHW
Frontal
Left ØNH2
Right ØNH1
Hyoid ØNHX
Lacrimal
Left ØNHJ
Right ØNHH
Lower ØQHY
Nasal ØNHB

Insertion of device in — continued
Bone — continued
Occipital
Left ØNH8
Right ØNH7
Palatine
Left ØNHL
Right ØNHK
Parietal
Left ØNH4
Right ØNH3
Pelvic
Left ØQH3
Right ØQH2
Sphenoid
Left ØNHD
Right ØNHC
Temporal
Left ØNH6
Right ØNH5
Upper ØPHY
Zygomatic
Left ØNHN
Right ØNHM
Brain ØØHØ
Breast
Bilateral ØHHV
Left ØHHU
Right ØHHT
Bronchus
Lingula ØBH9
Lower Lobe
Left ØBHB
Right ØBH6
Main
Left ØBH7
Right ØBH3
Middle Lobe, Right ØBH5
Upper Lobe
Left ØBH8
Right ØBH4
Buttock
Left ØYH1
Right ØYHØ
Carpal
Left ØPHN
Right ØPHM
Cavity, Cranial ØWH1
Cerebral Ventricle ØØH6
Cervix ØUHC
Chest Wall ØWH8
Cisterna Chyli Ø7HL
Clavicle
Left ØPHB
Right ØPH9
Coccyx ØQHS
Cul-de-sac ØUHF
Diaphragm
Left ØBHS
Right ØBHR
Disc
Cervical Vertebral ØRH3
Cervicothoracic Vertebral ØRH5
Lumbar Vertebral ØSH2
Lumbosacral ØSH4
Thoracic Vertebral ØRH9
Thoracolumbar Vertebral ØRHB
Duct
Hepatobiliary ØFHB
Pancreatic ØFHD
Duodenum ØDH9
Ear
Left Ø9HE
Right Ø9HD
Elbow Region
Left ØXHC
Right ØXHB
Epididymis and Spermatic Cord ØVHM
Esophagus ØDH5
Extremity
Lower
Left ØYHB
Right ØYH9
Upper
Left ØXH7
Right ØXH6

Insertion of device in — continued
Eye
Left Ø8H1
Right Ø8HØ
Face ØWH2
Fallopian Tube ØUH8
Femoral Region
Left ØYH8
Right ØYH7
Femoral Shaft
Left ØQH9
Right ØQH8
Femur
Lower
Left ØQHC
Right ØQHB
Upper
Left ØQH7
Right ØQH6
Fibula
Left ØQHK
Right ØQHJ
Foot
Left ØYHN
Right ØYHM
Gallbladder ØFH4
Gastrointestinal Tract ØWHP
Genitourinary Tract ØWHR
Gland, Endocrine ØGHS
Glenoid Cavity
Left ØPH8
Right ØPH7
Hand
Left ØXHK
Right ØXHJ
Head ØWHØ
Heart Ø2HA
Humeral Head
Left ØPHD
Right ØPHC
Humeral Shaft
Left ØPHG
Right ØPHF
Ileum ØDHB
Inguinal Region
Left ØYH6
Right ØYH5
Intestine
Large ØDHE
Small ØDH8
Jaw
Lower ØWH5
Upper ØWH4
Jejunum ØDHA
Joint
Acromioclavicular
Left ØRHH
Right ØRHG
Ankle
Left ØSHG
Right ØSHF
Carpal
Left ØRHR
Right ØRHQ
Cervical Vertebral ØRH1
Cervicothoracic Vertebral ØRH4
Coccygeal ØSH6
Elbow
Left ØRHM
Right ØRHL
Finger Phalangeal
Left ØRHX
Right ØRHW
Hip
Left ØSHB
Right ØSH9
Knee
Left ØSHD
Right ØSHC
Lumbar Vertebral ØSHØ
Lumbosacral ØSH3
Metacarpocarpal
Left ØRHT
Right ØRHS
Metacarpophalangeal
Left ØRHV

Insertion of device in — continued
Joint — continued
Metacarpophalangeal — continued
Right ØRHU
Metatarsal-Phalangeal
Left ØSHN
Right ØSHM
Metatarsal-Tarsal
Left ØSHL
Right ØSHK
Occipital-cervical ØRHØ
Sacrococcygeal ØSH5
Sacroiliac
Left ØSH8
Right ØSH7
Shoulder
Left ØRHK
Right ØRHJ
Sternoclavicular
Left ØRHF
Right ØRHE
Tarsal
Left ØSHJ
Right ØSHH
Temporomandibular
Left ØRHD
Right ØRHC
Thoracic Vertebral ØRH6
Thoracolumbar Vertebral ØRHA
Toe Phalangeal
Left ØSHQ
Right ØSHP
Wrist
Left ØRHP
Right ØRHN
Kidney ØTH5
Knee Region
Left ØYHG
Right ØYHF
Leg
Lower
Left ØYHJ
Right ØYHH
Upper
Left ØYHD
Right ØYHC
Liver ØFHØ
Left Lobe ØFH2
Right Lobe ØFH1
Lung
Left ØBHL
Right ØBHK
Lymphatic Ø7HN
Thoracic Duct Ø7HK
Mandible
Left ØNHV
Right ØNHT
Maxilla
Left ØNHS
Right ØNHR
Mediastinum ØWHC
Metacarpal
Left ØPHQ
Right ØPHP
Metatarsal
Left ØQHP
Right ØQHN
Mouth and Throat ØCHY
Muscle
Lower ØKHY
Upper ØKHX
Nasopharynx Ø9HN
Neck ØWH6
Nerve
Cranial ØØHE
Peripheral Ø1HY
Nipple
Left ØHHX
Right ØHHW
Oral Cavity and Throat ØWH3
Orbit
Left ØNHQ
Right ØNHP
Ovary ØUH3
Pancreas ØFHG

Insertion of device in — continued
- Patella
  - Left ØQHF
  - Right ØQHD
- Pelvic Cavity ØWHJ
- Penis ØVHS
- Pericardial Cavity ØWHD
- Pericardium Ø2HN
- Perineum
  - Female ØWHN
  - Male ØWHM
- Peritoneal Cavity ØWHG
- Phalanx
  - Finger
    - Left ØPHV
    - Right ØPHT
  - Thumb
    - Left ØPHS
    - Right ØPHR
  - Toe
    - Left ØQHR
    - Right ØQHQ
- Pleural Cavity
  - Left ØWHB
  - Right ØWH9
- Prostate ØVHØ
- Prostate and Seminal Vesicles ØVH4
- Radius
  - Left ØPHJ
  - Right ØPHH
- Rectum ØDHP
- Respiratory Tract ØWHQ
- Retroperitoneum ØWHH
- Rib
  - Left ØPH2
  - Right ØPH1
- Sacrum ØQH1
- Scapula
  - Left ØPH6
  - Right ØPH5
- Scrotum and Tunica Vaginalis ØVH8
- Shoulder Region
  - Left ØXH3
  - Right ØXH2
- Skull ØNHØ
- Spinal Canal ØØHU
- Spinal Cord ØØHV
- Spleen Ø7HP
- Sternum ØPHØ
- Stomach ØDH6
- Subcutaneous Tissue and Fascia
  - Abdomen ØJH8
  - Back ØJH7
  - Buttock ØJH9
  - Chest ØJH6
  - Face ØJH1
  - Foot
    - Left ØJHR
    - Right ØJHQ
  - Hand
    - Left ØJHK
    - Right ØJHJ
  - Head and Neck ØJHS
  - Lower Arm
    - Left ØJHH
    - Right ØJHG
  - Lower Extremity ØJHW
  - Lower Leg
    - Left ØJHP
    - Right ØJHN
  - Neck
    - Anterior ØJH4
    - Posterior ØJH5
  - Pelvic Region ØJHC
  - Perineum ØJHB
  - Scalp ØJHØ
  - Trunk ØJHT
  - Upper Arm
    - Left ØJHF
    - Right ØJHD
  - Upper Extremity ØJHV
  - Upper Leg
    - Left ØJHM
    - Right ØJHL
- Tarsal
  - Left ØQHM

Insertion of device in — continued
- Tarsal — continued
  - Right ØQHL
- Testis ØVHD
- Thymus Ø7HM
- Tibia
  - Left ØQHH
  - Right ØQHG
- Tongue ØCH7
- Trachea ØBH1
- Tracheobronchial Tree ØBHØ
- Ulna
  - Left ØPHL
  - Right ØPHK
- Ureter ØTH9
- Urethra ØTHD
- Uterus ØUH9
- Uterus and Cervix ØUHD
- Vagina ØUHG
- Vagina and Cul-de-sac ØUHH
- Vas Deferens ØVHR
- Vein
  - Axillary
    - Left Ø5H8
    - Right Ø5H7
  - Azygos Ø5HØ
  - Basilic
    - Left Ø5HC
    - Right Ø5HB
  - Brachial
    - Left Ø5HA
    - Right Ø5H9
  - Cephalic
    - Left Ø5HF
    - Right Ø5HD
  - Colic Ø6H7
  - Common Iliac
    - Left Ø6HD
    - Right Ø6HC
  - Coronary Ø2H4
  - Esophageal Ø6H3
  - External Iliac
    - Left Ø6HG
    - Right Ø6HF
  - External Jugular
    - Left Ø5HQ
    - Right Ø5HP
  - Face
    - Left Ø5HV
    - Right Ø5HT
  - Femoral
    - Left Ø6HN
    - Right Ø6HM
  - Foot
    - Left Ø6HV
    - Right Ø6HT
  - Gastric Ø6H2
  - Greater Saphenous
    - Left Ø6HQ
    - Right Ø6HP
  - Hand
    - Left Ø5HH
    - Right Ø5HG
  - Hemiazygos Ø5H1
  - Hepatic Ø6H4
  - Hypogastric
    - Left Ø6HJ
    - Right Ø6HH
  - Inferior Mesenteric Ø6H6
  - Innominate
    - Left Ø5H4
    - Right Ø5H3
  - Internal Jugular
    - Left Ø5HN
    - Right Ø5HM
  - Intracranial Ø5HL
  - Lesser Saphenous
    - Left Ø6HS
    - Right Ø6HR
  - Lower Ø6HY
  - Portal Ø6H8
  - Pulmonary
    - Left Ø2HT
    - Right Ø2HS
  - Renal
    - Left Ø6HB

Insertion of device in — continued
- Vein — continued
  - Renal — continued
    - Right Ø6H9
  - Splenic Ø6H1
  - Subclavian
    - Left Ø5H6
    - Right Ø5H5
  - Superior Mesenteric Ø6H5
  - Upper Ø5HY
  - Vertebral
    - Left Ø5HS
    - Right Ø5HR
- Vena Cava
  - Inferior Ø6HØ
  - Superior Ø2HV
- Ventricle
  - Left Ø2HL
  - Right Ø2HK
- Vertebra
  - Cervical ØPH3
  - Lumbar ØQHØ
  - Thoracic ØPH4
- Wrist Region
  - Left ØXHH
  - Right ØXHG

Inspection
- Abdominal Wall ØWJF
- Ankle Region
  - Left ØYJL
  - Right ØYJK
- Arm
  - Lower
    - Left ØXJF
    - Right ØXJD
  - Upper
    - Left ØXJ9
    - Right ØXJ8
- Artery
  - Lower Ø4JY
  - Upper Ø3JY
- Axilla
  - Left ØXJ5
  - Right ØXJ4
- Back
  - Lower ØWJL
  - Upper ØWJK
- Bladder ØTJB
- Bone
  - Facial ØNJW
  - Lower ØQJY
  - Nasal ØNJB
  - Upper ØPJY
- Bone Marrow Ø7JT
- Brain ØØJØ
- Breast
  - Left ØHJU
  - Right ØHJT
- Bursa and Ligament
  - Lower ØMJY
  - Upper ØMJX
- Buttock
  - Left ØYJ1
  - Right ØYJØ
- Cavity, Cranial ØWJ1
- Chest Wall ØWJ8
- Cisterna Chyli Ø7JL
- Diaphragm ØBJT
- Disc
  - Cervical Vertebral ØRJ3
  - Cervicothoracic Vertebral ØRJ5
  - Lumbar Vertebral ØSJ2
  - Lumbosacral ØSJ4
  - Thoracic Vertebral ØRJ9
  - Thoracolumbar Vertebral ØRJB
- Duct
  - Hepatobiliary ØFJB
  - Pancreatic ØFJD
- Ear
  - Inner
    - Left Ø9JE
    - Right Ø9JD
  - Left Ø9JJ
  - Right Ø9JH
- Elbow Region
  - Left ØXJC

Subterms under main terms may continue to next column or page

Inspection — continued
Elbow Region — continued
Right ØXJB
Epididymis and Spermatic Cord ØVJM
Extremity
Lower
Left ØYJB
Right ØYJ9
Upper
Left ØXJ7
Right ØXJ6
Eye
Left Ø8J1XZZ
Right Ø8JØXZZ
Face ØWJ2
Fallopian Tube ØUJ8
Femoral Region
Bilateral ØYJE
Left ØYJ8
Right ØYJ7
Finger Nail ØHJQXZZ
Foot
Left ØYJN
Right ØYJM
Gallbladder ØFJ4
Gastrointestinal Tract ØWJP
Genitourinary Tract ØWJR
Gland
Adrenal ØGJ5
Endocrine ØGJS
Pituitary ØGJØ
Salivary ØCJA
Great Vessel Ø2JY
Hand
Left ØXJK
Right ØXJJ
Head ØWJØ
Heart Ø2JA
Inguinal Region
Bilateral ØYJA
Left ØYJ6
Right ØYJ5
Intestinal Tract
Lower ØDJD
Upper ØDJØ
Jaw
Lower ØWJ5
Upper ØWJ4
Joint
Acromioclavicular
Left ØRJH
Right ØRJG
Ankle
Left ØSJG
Right ØSJF
Carpal
Left ØRJR
Right ØRJQ
Cervical Vertebral ØRJ1
Cervicothoracic Vertebral ØRJ4
Coccygeal ØSJ6
Elbow
Left ØRJM
Right ØRJL
Finger Phalangeal
Left ØRJX
Right ØRJW
Hip
Left ØSJB
Right ØSJ9
Knee
Left ØSJD
Right ØSJC
Lumbar Vertebral ØSJØ
Lumbosacral ØSJ3
Metacarpocarpal
Left ØRJT
Right ØRJS
Metacarpophalangeal
Left ØRJV
Right ØRJU
Metatarsal-Phalangeal
Left ØSJN
Right ØSJM
Metatarsal-Tarsal
Left ØSJL

Inspection — continued
Joint — continued
Metatarsal-Tarsal — continued
Right ØSJK
Occipital-cervical ØRJØ
Sacrococcygeal ØSJ5
Sacroiliac
Left ØSJ8
Right ØSJ7
Shoulder
Left ØRJK
Right ØRJJ
Sternoclavicular
Left ØRJF
Right ØRJE
Tarsal
Left ØSJJ
Right ØSJH
Temporomandibular
Left ØRJD
Right ØRJC
Thoracic Vertebral ØRJ6
Thoracolumbar Vertebral ØRJA
Toe Phalangeal
Left ØSJQ
Right ØSJP
Wrist
Left ØRJP
Right ØRJN
Kidney ØTJ5
Knee Region
Left ØYJG
Right ØYJF
Larynx ØCJS
Leg
Lower
Left ØYJJ
Right ØYJH
Upper
Left ØYJD
Right ØYJC
Lens
Left Ø8JKXZZ
Right Ø8JJXZZ
Liver ØFJØ
Lung
Left ØBJL
Right ØBJK
Lymphatic Ø7JN
Thoracic Duct Ø7JK
Mediastinum ØWJC
Mesentery ØDJV
Mouth and Throat ØCJY
Muscle
Extraocular
Left Ø8JM
Right Ø8JL
Lower ØKJY
Upper ØKJX
Neck ØWJ6
Nerve
Cranial ØØJE
Peripheral Ø1JY
Nose Ø9JK
Omentum ØDJU
Oral Cavity and Throat ØWJ3
Ovary ØUJ3
Pancreas ØFJG
Parathyroid Gland ØGJR
Pelvic Cavity ØWJJ
Penis ØVJS
Pericardial Cavity ØWJD
Perineum
Female ØWJN
Male ØWJM
Peritoneal Cavity ØWJG
Peritoneum ØDJW
Pineal Body ØGJ1
Pleura ØBJQ
Pleural Cavity
Left ØWJB
Right ØWJ9
Products of Conception 1ØJØ
Ectopic 1ØJ2
Retained 1ØJ1
Prostate and Seminal Vesicles ØVJ4

Inspection — continued
Respiratory Tract ØWJQ
Retroperitoneum ØWJH
Scrotum and Tunica Vaginalis ØVJ8
Shoulder Region
Left ØXJ3
Right ØXJ2
Sinus Ø9JY
Skin ØHJPXZZ
Skull ØNJØ
Spinal Canal ØØJU
Spinal Cord ØØJV
Spleen Ø7JP
Stomach ØDJ6
Subcutaneous Tissue and Fascia
Head and Neck ØJJS
Lower Extremity ØJJW
Trunk ØJJT
Upper Extremity ØJJV
Tendon
Lower ØLJY
Upper ØLJX
Testis ØVJD
Thymus Ø7JM
Thyroid Gland ØGJK
Toe Nail ØHJRXZZ
Trachea ØBJ1
Tracheobronchial Tree ØBJØ
Tympanic Membrane
Left Ø9J8
Right Ø9J7
Ureter ØTJ9
Urethra ØTJD
Uterus and Cervix ØUJD
Vagina and Cul-de-sac ØUJH
Vas Deferens ØVJR
Vein
Lower Ø6JY
Upper Ø5JY
Vulva ØUJM
Wrist Region
Left ØXJH
Right ØXJG
Instillation *see* Introduction of substance in or on
Insufflation *see* Introduction of substance in or on
Interatrial septum *use* Septum, Atrial
Interbody fusion (spine) cage
use Interbody Fusion Device in Lower Joints
use Interbody Fusion Device in Upper Joints
Intercarpal joint
use Joint, Carpal, Left
use Joint, Carpal, Right
Intercarpal ligament
use Bursa and Ligament, Hand, Left
use Bursa and Ligament, Hand, Right
Interclavicular ligament
use Bursa and Ligament, Shoulder, Left
use Bursa and Ligament, Shoulder, Right
Intercostal lymph node *use* Lymphatic, Thorax
Intercostal muscle
use Muscle, Thorax, Left
use Muscle, Thorax, Right
Intercostal nerve *use* Nerve, Thoracic
Intercostobrachial nerve *use* Nerve, Thoracic
Intercuneiform joint
use Joint, Tarsal, Left
use Joint, Tarsal, Right
Intercuneiform ligament
use Bursa and Ligament, Foot, Left
use Bursa and Ligament, Foot, Right
Intermediate cuneiform bone
use Tarsal, Left
use Tarsal, Right
Intermittent mandatory ventilation *see* Assistance, Respiratory 5AØ9
Intermittent Negative Airway Pressure
24-96 Consecutive Hours, Ventilation 5AØ945B
Greater than 96 Consecutive Hours, Ventilation 5AØ955B
Less than 24 Consecutive Hours, Ventilation 5AØ935B
Intermittent Positive Airway Pressure
24-96 Consecutive Hours, Ventilation 5AØ9458
Greater than 96 Consecutive Hours, Ventilation 5AØ9558
Less than 24 Consecutive Hours, Ventilation 5AØ9358

Intermittent positive pressure breathing *see* Assistance, Respiratory 5AØ9
Internal anal sphincter *use* Anal Sphincter
Internal carotid plexus *use* Nerve, Head and Neck Sympathetic
Internal (basal) cerebral vein *use* Vein, Intracranial
Internal iliac vein
use Vein, Hypogastric, Left
use Vein, Hypogastric, Right
Internal maxillary artery
use Artery, External Carotid, Left
use Artery, External Carotid, Right
Internal naris *use* Nose
Internal oblique muscle
use Muscle, Abdomen, Left
use Muscle, Abdomen, Right
Internal pudendal artery
use Artery, Internal Iliac, Left
use Artery, Internal Iliac, Right
Internal pudendal vein
use Vein, Hypogastric, Left
use Vein, Hypogastric, Right
Internal thoracic artery
use Artery, Internal Mammary, Left
use Artery, Internal Mammary, Right
use Artery, Subclavian, Left
use Artery, Subclavian, Right
Internal urethral sphincter *use* Urethra
Interphalangeal (IP) joint
use Joint, Finger Phalangeal, Left
use Joint, Finger Phalangeal, Right
use Joint, Toe Phalangeal, Left
use Joint, Toe Phalangeal, Right
Interphalangeal ligament
use Bursa and Ligament, Foot, Left
use Bursa and Ligament, Foot, Right
use Bursa and Ligament, Hand, Left
use Bursa and Ligament, Hand, Right
Interrogation, cardiac rhythm related device
With cardiac function testing *see* Measurement, Cardiac 4AØ2
Interrogation only *see* Measurement, Cardiac 4BØ2
Interruption *see* Occlusion
Interspinalis muscle
use Muscle, Trunk, Left
use Muscle, Trunk, Right
Interspinous ligament
use Bursa and Ligament, Trunk, Left
use Bursa and Ligament, Trunk, Right
Interspinous process spinal stabilization device
use Spinal Stabilization Device, Interspinous Process in ØRH
use Spinal Stabilization Device, Interspinous Process in ØSH
InterStim® Therapy lead *use* Neurostimulator Lead in Peripheral Nervous System
InterStim® Therapy neurostimulator *use* Stimulator Generator, Single Array in ØJH
Intertransversarius muscle
use Muscle, Trunk, Left
use Muscle, Trunk, Right
Intertransverse ligament
use Bursa and Ligament, Trunk, Left
use Bursa and Ligament, Trunk, Right
Interventricular foramen (Monro) *use* Cerebral Ventricle
Interventricular septum *use* Septum, Ventricular
Intestinal lymphatic trunk *use* Cisterna Chyli
Intraluminal Device
Airway
Esophagus ØDH5
Mouth and Throat ØCHY
Nasopharynx Ø9HN
Bioactive
Occlusion
Common Carotid
Left Ø3LJ
Right Ø3LH
External Carotid
Left Ø3LN
Right Ø3LM
Internal Carotid
Left Ø3LL
Right Ø3LK
Intracranial Ø3LG
Intraluminal Device — continued
Bioactive — continued
Occlusion — continued
Vertebral
Left Ø3LQ
Right Ø3LP
Restriction
Common Carotid
Left Ø3VJ
Right Ø3VH
External Carotid
Left Ø3VN
Right Ø3VM
Internal Carotid
Left Ø3VL
Right Ø3VK
Intracranial Ø3VG
Vertebral
Left Ø3VQ
Right Ø3VP
Endobronchial Valve
Lingula ØBH9
Lower Lobe
Left ØBHB
Right ØBH6
Main
Left ØBH7
Right ØBH3
Middle Lobe, Right ØBH5
Upper Lobe
Left ØBH8
Right ØBH4
Endotracheal Airway
Change device in, Trachea ØB21XEZ
Insertion of device in, Trachea ØBH1
Pessary
Change device in, Vagina and Cul-de-sac ØU2HXGZ
Insertion of device in
Cul-de-sac ØUHF
Vagina ØUHG
Intramedullary (IM) rod (nail)
use Internal Fixation Device, Intramedullary in Lower Bones
use Internal Fixation Device, Intramedullary in Upper Bones
Intramedullary skeletal kinetic distractor (ISKD)
use Internal Fixation Device, Intramedullary in Lower Bones
use Internal Fixation Device, Intramedullary in Upper Bones
Intraocular Telescope
Left Ø8RK3ØZ
Right Ø8RJ3ØZ
Intraoperative Radiation Therapy (IORT)
Anus DDY8CZZ
Bile Ducts DFY2CZZ
Bladder DTY2CZZ
Cervix DUY1CZZ
Colon DDY5CZZ
Duodenum DDY2CZZ
Gallbladder DFY1CZZ
Ileum DDY4CZZ
Jejunum DDY3CZZ
Kidney DTYØCZZ
Larynx D9YBCZZ
Liver DFYØCZZ
Mouth D9Y4CZZ
Nasopharynx D9YDCZZ
Ovary DUYØCZZ
Pancreas DFY3CZZ
Pharynx D9YCCZZ
Prostate DVYØCZZ
Rectum DDY7CZZ
Stomach DDY1CZZ
Ureter DTY1CZZ
Urethra DTY3CZZ
Uterus DUY2CZZ
Intrauterine Device (IUD) *use* Contraceptive Device in Female Reproductive System
Introduction of substance in or on
Artery
Central 3EØ6
Analgesics 3EØ6
Anesthetic, Intracirculatory 3EØ6
Antiarrhythmic 3EØ6
Introduction of substance in or on — continued
Artery — continued
Central — continued
Anti-infective 3EØ6
Anti-inflammatory 3EØ6
Antineoplastic 3EØ6
Destructive Agent 3EØ6
Diagnostic Substance, Other 3EØ6
Electrolytic Substance 3EØ6
Hormone 3EØ6
Hypnotics 3EØ6
Immunotherapeutic 3EØ6
Nutritional Substance 3EØ6
Platelet Inhibitor 3EØ6
Radioactive Substance 3EØ6
Sedatives 3EØ6
Serum 3EØ6
Thrombolytic 3EØ6
Toxoid 3EØ6
Vaccine 3EØ6
Vasopressor 3EØ6
Water Balance Substance 3EØ6
Coronary 3EØ7
Diagnostic Substance, Other 3EØ7
Platelet Inhibitor 3EØ7
Thrombolytic 3EØ7
Peripheral 3EØ5
Analgesics 3EØ5
Anesthetic, Intracirculatory 3EØ5
Antiarrhythmic 3EØ5
Anti-infective 3EØ5
Anti-inflammatory 3EØ5
Antineoplastic 3EØ5
Destructive Agent 3EØ5
Diagnostic Substance, Other 3EØ5
Electrolytic Substance 3EØ5
Hormone 3EØ5
Hypnotics 3EØ5
Immunotherapeutic 3EØ5
Nutritional Substance 3EØ5
Platelet Inhibitor 3EØ5
Radioactive Substance 3EØ5
Sedatives 3EØ5
Serum 3EØ5
Thrombolytic 3EØ5
Toxoid 3EØ5
Vaccine 3EØ5
Vasopressor 3EØ5
Water Balance Substance 3EØ5
Biliary Tract 3EØJ
Analgesics 3EØJ
Anesthetic, Local 3EØJ
Anti-infective 3EØJ
Anti-inflammatory 3EØJ
Antineoplastic 3EØJ
Destructive Agent 3EØJ
Diagnostic Substance, Other 3EØJ
Electrolytic Substance 3EØJ
Gas 3EØJ
Hypnotics 3EØJ
Islet Cells, Pancreatic 3EØJ
Nutritional Substance 3EØJ
Radioactive Substance 3EØJ
Sedatives 3EØJ
Water Balance Substance 3EØJ
Bone 3EØV
Analgesics 3EØV3NZ
Anesthetic, Local 3EØV3BZ
Anti-infective 3EØV32
Anti-inflammatory 3EØV33Z
Antineoplastic 3EØV3Ø
Destructive Agent 3EØV3TZ
Diagnostic Substance, Other 3EØV3KZ
Electrolytic Substance 3EØV37Z
Hypnotics 3EØV3NZ
Nutritional Substance 3EØV36Z
Radioactive Substance 3EØV3HZ
Sedatives 3EØV3NZ
Water Balance Substance 3EØV37Z
Bone Marrow 3EØA3GC
Antineoplastic 3EØA3Ø
Brain 3EØQ3GC
Analgesics 3EØQ3NZ
Anesthetic, Local 3EØQ3BZ
Anti-infective 3EØQ32
Anti-inflammatory 3EØQ33Z

Introduction of substance in or on — continued
  Brain — continued
    Antineoplastic 3EØQ
    Destructive Agent 3EØQ3TZ
    Diagnostic Substance, Other 3EØQ3KZ
    Electrolytic Substance 3EØQ37Z
    Gas 3EØQ
    Hypnotics 3EØQ3NZ
    Nutritional Substance 3EØQ36Z
    Radioactive Substance 3EØQ3HZ
    Sedatives 3EØQ3NZ
    Stem Cells
      Embryonic 3EØQ
      Somatic 3EØQ
    Water Balance Substance 3EØQ37Z
  Cranial Cavity 3EØQ3GC
    Analgesics 3EØQ3NZ
    Anesthetic, Local 3EØQ3BZ
    Anti-infective 3EØQ32
    Anti-inflammatory 3EØQ33Z
    Antineoplastic 3EØQ
    Destructive Agent 3EØQ3TZ
    Diagnostic Substance, Other 3EØQ3KZ
    Electrolytic Substance 3EØQ37Z
    Gas 3EØQ
    Hypnotics 3EØQ3NZ
    Nutritional Substance 3EØQ36Z
    Radioactive Substance 3EØQ3HZ
    Sedatives 3EØQ3NZ
    Stem Cells
      Embryonic 3EØQ
      Somatic 3EØQ
    Water Balance Substance 3EØQ37Z
  Ear 3EØB
    Analgesics 3EØB
    Anesthetic, Local 3EØB
    Anti-infective 3EØB
    Anti-inflammatory 3EØB
    Antineoplastic 3EØB
    Destructive Agent 3EØB
    Diagnostic Substance, Other 3EØB
    Hypnotics 3EØB
    Radioactive Substance 3EØB
    Sedatives 3EØB
  Epidural Space 3EØS3GC
    Analgesics 3EØS3NZ
    Anesthetic
      Local 3EØS3BZ
      Regional 3EØS3CZ
    Anti-infective 3EØS32
    Anti-inflammatory 3EØS33Z
    Antineoplastic 3EØS3Ø
    Destructive Agent 3EØS3TZ
    Diagnostic Substance, Other 3EØS3KZ
    Electrolytic Substance 3EØS37Z
    Gas 3EØS
    Hypnotics 3EØS3NZ
    Nutritional Substance 3EØS36Z
    Radioactive Substance 3EØS3HZ
    Sedatives 3EØS3NZ
    Water Balance Substance 3EØS37Z
  Eye 3EØC
    Analgesics 3EØC
    Anesthetic, Local 3EØC
    Anti-infective 3EØC
    Anti-inflammatory 3EØC
    Antineoplastic 3EØC
    Destructive Agent 3EØC
    Diagnostic Substance, Other 3EØC
    Gas 3EØC
    Hypnotics 3EØC
    Pigment 3EØC
    Radioactive Substance 3EØC
    Sedatives 3EØC
  Gastrointestinal Tract
    Lower 3EØH
      Analgesics 3EØH
      Anesthetic, Local 3EØH
      Anti-infective 3EØH
      Anti-inflammatory 3EØH
      Antineoplastic 3EØH
      Destructive Agent 3EØH
      Diagnostic Substance, Other 3EØH
      Electrolytic Substance 3EØH
      Gas 3EØH
      Hypnotics 3EØH

Introduction of substance in or on — continued
  Gastrointestinal Tract — continued
    Lower — continued
      Nutritional Substance 3EØH
      Radioactive Substance 3EØH
      Sedatives 3EØH
      Water Balance Substance 3EØH
    Upper 3EØG
      Analgesics 3EØG
      Anesthetic, Local 3EØG
      Anti-infective 3EØG
      Anti-inflammatory 3EØG
      Antineoplastic 3EØG
      Destructive Agent 3EØG
      Diagnostic Substance, Other 3EØG
      Electrolytic Substance 3EØG
      Gas 3EØG
      Hypnotics 3EØG
      Nutritional Substance 3EØG
      Radioactive Substance 3EØG
      Sedatives 3EØG
      Water Balance Substance 3EØG
  Genitourinary Tract 3EØK
    Analgesics 3EØK
    Anesthetic, Local 3EØK
    Anti-infective 3EØK
    Anti-inflammatory 3EØK
    Antineoplastic 3EØK
    Destructive Agent 3EØK
    Diagnostic Substance, Other 3EØK
    Electrolytic Substance 3EØK
    Gas 3EØK
    Hypnotics 3EØK
    Nutritional Substance 3EØK
    Radioactive Substance 3EØK
    Sedatives 3EØK
    Water Balance Substance 3EØK
  Heart 3EØ8
    Diagnostic Substance, Other 3EØ8
    Platelet Inhibitor 3EØ8
    Thrombolytic 3EØ8
  Joint 3EØU
    Analgesics 3EØU3NZ
    Anesthetic, Local 3EØU3BZ
    Anti-infective 3EØU
    Anti-inflammatory 3EØU33Z
    Antineoplastic 3EØU3Ø
    Destructive Agent 3EØU3TZ
    Diagnostic Substance, Other 3EØU3KZ
    Electrolytic Substance 3EØU37Z
    Gas 3EØU3SF
    Hypnotics 3EØU3NZ
    Nutritional Substance 3EØU36Z
    Radioactive Substance 3EØU3HZ
    Sedatives 3EØU3NZ
    Water Balance Substance 3EØU37Z
  Lymphatic 3EØW3GC
    Analgesics 3EØW3NZ
    Anesthetic, Local 3EØW3BZ
    Anti-infective 3EØW32
    Anti-inflammatory 3EØW33Z
    Antineoplastic 3EØW3Ø
    Destructive Agent 3EØW3TZ
    Diagnostic Substance, Other 3EØW3KZ
    Electrolytic Substance 3EØW37Z
    Hypnotics 3EØW3NZ
    Nutritional Substance 3EØW36Z
    Radioactive Substance 3EØW3HZ
    Sedatives 3EØW3NZ
    Water Balance Substance 3EØW37Z
  Mouth 3EØD
    Analgesics 3EØD
    Anesthetic, Local 3EØD
    Antiarrhythmic 3EØD
    Anti-infective 3EØD
    Anti-inflammatory 3EØD
    Antineoplastic 3EØD
    Destructive Agent 3EØD
    Diagnostic Substance, Other 3EØD
    Electrolytic Substance 3EØD
    Hypnotics 3EØD
    Nutritional Substance 3EØD
    Radioactive Substance 3EØD
    Sedatives 3EØD
    Serum 3EØD
    Toxoid 3EØD

Introduction of substance in or on — continued
  Mouth — continued
    Vaccine 3EØD
    Water Balance Substance 3EØD
  Mucous Membrane 3EØØXGC
    Analgesics 3EØØXNZ
    Anesthetic, Local 3EØØXBZ
    Anti-infective 3EØØX2
    Anti-inflammatory 3EØØX3Z
    Antineoplastic 3EØØXØ
    Destructive Agent 3EØØXTZ
    Diagnostic Substance, Other 3EØØXKZ
    Hypnotics 3EØØXNZ
    Pigment 3EØØXMZ
    Sedatives 3EØØXNZ
    Serum 3EØØX4Z
    Toxoid 3EØØX4Z
    Vaccine 3EØØX4Z
  Muscle 3EØ23GC
    Analgesics 3EØ23NZ
    Anesthetic, Local 3EØ23BZ
    Anti-infective 3EØ232
    Anti-inflammatory 3EØ233Z
    Antineoplastic 3EØ23Ø
    Destructive Agent 3EØ23TZ
    Diagnostic Substance, Other 3EØ23KZ
    Electrolytic Substance 3EØ237Z
    Hypnotics 3EØ23NZ
    Nutritional Substance 3EØ236Z
    Radioactive Substance 3EØ23HZ
    Sedatives 3EØ23NZ
    Serum 3EØ234Z
    Toxoid 3EØ234Z
    Vaccine 3EØ234Z
    Water Balance Substance 3EØ237Z
  Nerve
    Cranial 3EØX3GC
      Anesthetic
        Local 3EØX3BZ
        Regional 3EØX3CZ
      Anti-inflammatory 3EØX33Z
      Destructive Agent 3EØX3TZ
    Peripheral 3EØT3GC
      Anesthetic
        Local 3EØT3BZ
        Regional 3EØT3CZ
      Anti-inflammatory 3EØT33Z
      Destructive Agent 3EØT3TZ
    Plexus 3EØT3GC
      Anesthetic
        Local 3EØT3BZ
        Regional 3EØT3CZ
      Anti-inflammatory 3EØT33Z
      Destructive Agent 3EØT3TZ
  Nose 3EØ9
    Analgesics 3EØ9
    Anesthetic, Local 3EØ9
    Anti-infective 3EØ9
    Anti-inflammatory 3EØ9
    Antineoplastic 3EØ9
    Destructive Agent 3EØ9
    Diagnostic Substance, Other 3EØ9
    Hypnotics 3EØ9
    Radioactive Substance 3EØ9
    Sedatives 3EØ9
    Serum 3EØ9
    Toxoid 3EØ9
    Vaccine 3EØ9
  Pancreatic Tract 3EØJ
    Analgesics 3EØJ
    Anesthetic, Local 3EØJ
    Anti-infective 3EØJ
    Anti-inflammatory 3EØJ
    Antineoplastic 3EØJ
    Destructive Agent 3EØJ
    Diagnostic Substance, Other 3EØJ
    Electrolytic Substance 3EØJ
    Gas 3EØJ
    Hypnotics 3EØJ
    Islet Cells, Pancreatic 3EØJ
    Nutritional Substance 3EØJ
    Radioactive Substance 3EØJ
    Sedatives 3EØJ
    Water Balance Substance 3EØJ
  Pericardial Cavity 3EØY3GC
    Analgesics 3EØY3NZ

Introduction of substance in or on — continued
Pericardial Cavity — continued
Anesthetic, Local 3EØY3BZ
Anti-infective 3EØY32
Anti-inflammatory 3EØY33Z
Antineoplastic 3EØY
Destructive Agent 3EØY3TZ
Diagnostic Substance, Other 3EØY3KZ
Electrolytic Substance 3EØY37Z
Gas 3EØY
Hypnotics 3EØY3NZ
Nutritional Substance 3EØY36Z
Radioactive Substance 3EØY3HZ
Sedatives 3EØY3NZ
Water Balance Substance 3EØY37Z
Peritoneal Cavity 3EØM3GC
Adhesion Barrier 3EØMØ5Z
Analgesics 3EØM3NZ
Anesthetic, Local 3EØM3BZ
Anti-infective 3EØM32
Anti-inflammatory 3EØM33Z
Antineoplastic 3EØM
Destructive Agent 3EØM3TZ
Diagnostic Substance, Other 3EØM3KZ
Electrolytic Substance 3EØM37Z
Gas 3EØM
Hypnotics 3EØM3NZ
Nutritional Substance 3EØM36Z
Radioactive Substance 3EØM3HZ
Sedatives 3EØM3NZ
Water Balance Substance 3EØM37Z
Pharynx 3EØD
Analgesics 3EØD
Anesthetic, Local 3EØD
Antiarrhythmic 3EØD
Anti-infective 3EØD
Anti-inflammatory 3EØD
Antineoplastic 3EØD
Destructive Agent 3EØD
Diagnostic Substance, Other 3EØD
Electrolytic Substance 3EØD
Hypnotics 3EØD
Nutritional Substance 3EØD
Radioactive Substance 3EØD
Sedatives 3EØD
Serum 3EØD
Toxoid 3EØD
Vaccine 3EØD
Water Balance Substance 3EØD
Pleural Cavity 3EØL3GC
Adhesion Barrier 3EØLØ5Z
Analgesics 3EØL3NZ
Anesthetic, Local 3EØL3BZ
Anti-infective 3EØL32
Anti-inflammatory 3EØL33Z
Antineoplastic 3EØL
Destructive Agent 3EØL3TZ
Diagnostic Substance, Other 3EØL3KZ
Electrolytic Substance 3EØL37Z
Gas 3EØL
Hypnotics 3EØL3NZ
Nutritional Substance 3EØL36Z
Radioactive Substance 3EØL3HZ
Sedatives 3EØL3NZ
Water Balance Substance 3EØL37Z
Products of Conception 3EØE
Analgesics 3EØE
Anesthetic, Local 3EØE
Anti-infective 3EØE
Anti-inflammatory 3EØE
Antineoplastic 3EØE
Destructive Agent 3EØE
Diagnostic Substance, Other 3EØE
Electrolytic Substance 3EØE
Gas 3EØE
Hypnotics 3EØE
Nutritional Substance 3EØE
Radioactive Substance 3EØE
Sedatives 3EØE
Water Balance Substance 3EØE
Reproductive
Female 3EØP
Adhesion Barrier 3EØPØ5Z
Analgesics 3EØP
Anesthetic, Local 3EØP
Anti-infective 3EØP

Introduction of substance in or on — continued
Reproductive — continued
Female — continued
Anti-inflammatory 3EØP
Antineoplastic 3EØP
Destructive Agent 3EØP
Diagnostic Substance, Other 3EØP
Electrolytic Substance 3EØP
Gas 3EØP
Hypnotics 3EØP
Nutritional Substance 3EØP
Ovum, Fertilized 3EØP
Radioactive Substance 3EØP
Sedatives 3EØP
Sperm 3EØP
Water Balance Substance 3EØP
Male 3EØN
Analgesics 3EØN
Anesthetic, Local 3EØN
Anti-infective 3EØN
Anti-inflammatory 3EØN
Antineoplastic 3EØN
Destructive Agent 3EØN
Diagnostic Substance, Other 3EØN
Electrolytic Substance 3EØN
Gas 3EØN
Hypnotics 3EØN
Nutritional Substance 3EØN
Radioactive Substance 3EØN
Sedatives 3EØN
Water Balance Substance 3EØN
Respiratory Tract 3EØF
Analgesics 3EØF
Anesthetic
Inhalation 3EØF
Local 3EØF
Anti-infective 3EØF
Anti-inflammatory 3EØF
Antineoplastic 3EØF
Destructive Agent 3EØF
Diagnostic Substance, Other 3EØF
Electrolytic Substance 3EØF
Gas 3EØF
Hypnotics 3EØF
Nutritional Substance 3EØF
Radioactive Substance 3EØF
Sedatives 3EØF
Water Balance Substance 3EØF
Skin 3EØØXGC
Analgesics 3EØØXNZ
Anesthetic, Local 3EØØXBZ
Anti-infective 3EØØX2
Anti-inflammatory 3EØØX3Z
Antineoplastic 3EØØXØ
Destructive Agent 3EØØXTZ
Diagnostic Substance, Other 3EØØXKZ
Hypnotics 3EØØXNZ
Pigment 3EØØXMZ
Sedatives 3EØØXNZ
Serum 3EØØX4Z
Toxoid 3EØØX4Z
Vaccine 3EØØX4Z
Spinal Canal 3EØR3GC
Analgesics 3EØR3NZ
Anesthetic
Local 3EØR3BZ
Regional 3EØR3CZ
Anti-infective 3EØR32
Anti-inflammatory 3EØR33Z
Antineoplastic 3EØR3Ø
Destructive Agent 3EØR3TZ
Diagnostic Substance, Other 3EØR3KZ
Electrolytic Substance 3EØR37Z
Gas 3EØR
Hypnotics 3EØR3NZ
Nutritional Substance 3EØR36Z
Radioactive Substance 3EØR3HZ
Sedatives 3EØR3NZ
Stem Cells
Embryonic 3EØR
Somatic 3EØR
Water Balance Substance 3EØR37Z
Subcutaneous Tissue 3EØ13GC
Analgesics 3EØ13NZ
Anesthetic, Local 3EØ13BZ
Anti-infective 3EØ1

Introduction of substance in or on — continued
Subcutaneous Tissue — continued
Anti-inflammatory 3EØ133Z
Antineoplastic 3EØ13Ø
Destructive Agent 3EØ13TZ
Diagnostic Substance, Other 3EØ13KZ
Electrolytic Substance 3EØ137Z
Hormone 3EØ13V
Hypnotics 3EØ13NZ
Nutritional Substance 3EØ136Z
Radioactive Substance 3EØ13HZ
Sedatives 3EØ13NZ
Serum 3EØ134Z
Toxoid 3EØ134Z
Vaccine 3EØ134Z
Water Balance Substance 3EØ137Z
Vein
Central 3EØ4
Analgesics 3EØ4
Anesthetic, Intracirculatory 3EØ4
Antiarrhythmic 3EØ4
Anti-infective 3EØ4
Anti-inflammatory 3EØ4
Antineoplastic 3EØ4
Destructive Agent 3EØ4
Diagnostic Substance, Other 3EØ4
Electrolytic Substance 3EØ4
Hormone 3EØ4
Hypnotics 3EØ4
Immunotherapeutic 3EØ4
Nutritional Substance 3EØ4
Platelet Inhibitor 3EØ4
Radioactive Substance 3EØ4
Sedatives 3EØ4
Serum 3EØ4
Thrombolytic 3EØ4
Toxoid 3EØ4
Vaccine 3EØ4
Vasopressor 3EØ4
Water Balance Substance 3EØ4
Peripheral 3EØ3
Analgesics 3EØ3
Anesthetic, Intracirculatory 3EØ3
Antiarrhythmic 3EØ3
Anti-infective 3EØ3
Anti-inflammatory 3EØ3
Antineoplastic 3EØ3
Destructive Agent 3EØ3
Diagnostic Substance, Other 3EØ3
Electrolytic Substance 3EØ3
Hormone 3EØ3
Hypnotics 3EØ3
Immunotherapeutic 3EØ3
Islet Cells, Pancreatic 3EØ3
Nutritional Substance 3EØ3
Platelet Inhibitor 3EØ3
Radioactive Substance 3EØ3
Sedatives 3EØ3
Serum 3EØ3
Thrombolytic 3EØ3
Toxoid 3EØ3
Vaccine 3EØ3
Vasopressor 3EØ3
Water Balance Substance 3EØ3
Intubation
Airway
see Insertion of device in, Esophagus ØDH5
see Insertion of device in, Mouth and Throat ØCHY
see Insertion of device in, Trachea ØBH1
Drainage device *see* Drainage
Feeding Device *see* Insertion of device in, Gastrointestinal System ØDH
IPPB (intermittent positive pressure breathing) *see* Assistance, Respiratory 5AØ9
Iridectomy
see Excision, Eye Ø8B
see Resection, Eye Ø8T
Iridoplasty
see Repair, Eye Ø8Q
see Replacement, Eye Ø8R
see Supplement, Eye Ø8U
Iridotomy *see* Drainage, Eye Ø89
Irrigation
Biliary Tract, Irrigating Substance 3E1J
Brain, Irrigating Substance 3E1Q38Z
Cranial Cavity, Irrigating Substance 3E1Q38Z

Irrigation — continued
Ear, Irrigating Substance 3E1B
Epidural Space, Irrigating Substance 3E1S38Z
Eye, Irrigating Substance 3E1C
Gastrointestinal Tract
Lower, Irrigating Substance 3E1H
Upper, Irrigating Substance 3E1G
Genitourinary Tract, Irrigating Substance 3E1K
Irrigating Substance 3C1ZX8Z
Joint, Irrigating Substance 3E1U38Z
Mucous Membrane, Irrigating Substance 3E1Ø
Nose, Irrigating Substance 3E19
Pancreatic Tract, Irrigating Substance 3E1J
Pericardial Cavity, Irrigating Substance 3E1Y38Z
Peritoneal Cavity
Dialysate 3E1M39Z
Irrigating Substance 3E1M38Z
Pleural Cavity, Irrigating Substance 3E1L38Z
Reproductive
Female, Irrigating Substance 3E1P
Male, Irrigating Substance 3E1N
Respiratory Tract, Irrigating Substance 3E1F
Skin, Irrigating Substance 3E1Ø
Spinal Canal, Irrigating Substance 3E1R38Z
Ischiatic nerve *use* Nerve, Sciatic
Ischiocavernosus muscle *use* Muscle, Perineum
Ischiofemoral ligament
use Bursa and Ligament, Hip, Left
use Bursa and Ligament, Hip, Right
Ischium
use Bone, Pelvic, Left
use Bone, Pelvic, Right
Isolation 8EØZXY6
Isotope Administration, Whole Body DWY5G
Itrel (3) (4) neurostimulator *use* Stimulator Generator, Single Array ØJH

J

Jejunal artery *use* Artery, Superior Mesenteric
Jejunectomy
see Excision, Jejunum ØDBA
see Resection, Jejunum ØDTA
Jejunocolostomy
see Bypass, Gastrointestinal System ØD1
see Drainage, Gastrointestinal System ØD9
Jejunopexy
see Repair, Jejunum ØDQA
see Reposition, Jejunum ØDSA
Jejunostomy
see Bypass, Jejunum ØD1A
see Drainage, Jejunum ØD9A
Jejunotomy *see* Drainage, Jejunum ØD9A
Joint fixation plate
use Internal Fixation Device in Lower Joints
use Internal Fixation Device in Upper Joints
Joint liner (insert) *use* Liner in Lower Joints
Joint spacer (antibiotic)
use Spacer in Lower Joints
use Spacer in Upper Joints
Jugular body *use* Glomus Jugulare
Jugular lymph node
use Lymphatic, Neck, Left
use Lymphatic, Neck, Right

K

Kappa *use* Pacemaker, Dual Chamber in ØJH
Kcentra *use* 4-Factor Prothrombin Complex Concentrate
Keratectomy, kerectomy
see Excision, Eye Ø8B
see Resection, Eye Ø8T
Keratocentesis *see* Drainage, Eye Ø89
Keratoplasty
see Repair, Eye Ø8Q
see Replacement, Eye Ø8R
see Supplement, Eye Ø8U
Keratotomy
see Drainage, Eye Ø89
see Repair, Eye Ø8Q
Kirschner wire (K-wire)
use Internal Fixation Device in Head and Facial Bones
use Internal Fixation Device in Lower Bones
Kirschner wire (K-wire) — continued
use Internal Fixation Device in Lower Joints
use Internal Fixation Device in Upper Bones
use Internal Fixation Device in Upper Joints
Knee (implant) insert *use* Liner in Lower Joints
KUB x-ray *see* Plain Radiography, Kidney, Ureter and Bladder BTØ4
Kuntscher nail
use Internal Fixation Device, Intramedullary in Lower Bones
use Internal Fixation Device, Intramedullary in Upper Bones

L

Labia majora *use* Vulva
Labia minora *use* Vulva
Labial gland
use Lip, Lower
use Lip, Upper
Labiectomy
see Excision, Female Reproductive System ØUB
see Resection, Female Reproductive System ØUT
Lacrimal canaliculus
use Duct, Lacrimal, Left
use Duct, Lacrimal, Right
Lacrimal punctum
use Duct, Lacrimal, Left
use Duct, Lacrimal, Right
Lacrimal sac
use Duct, Lacrimal, Left
use Duct, Lacrimal, Right
Laminectomy
see Excision, Lower Bones ØQB
see Excision, Upper Bones ØPB
Laminotomy
see Drainage, Lower Bones ØQ9
see Drainage, Upper Bones ØP9
see Excision, Lower Bones ØQB
see Excision, Upper Bones ØPB
see Release, Central Nervous System ØØN
see Release, Lower Bones ØQN
see Release, Peripheral Nervous System Ø1N
see Release, Upper Bones ØPN
Laparoscopy *see* Inspection
Laparotomy
Drainage *see* Drainage, Peritoneal Cavity ØW9G
Exploratory *see* Inspection, Peritoneal Cavity ØWJG
LAP-BAND® Adjustable Gastric Banding System *use* Extraluminal Device
Laryngectomy
see Excision, Larynx ØCBS
see Resection, Larynx ØCTS
Laryngocentesis *see* Drainage, Larynx ØC9S
Laryngogram *see* Fluoroscopy, Larynx B91J
Laryngopexy *see* Repair, Larynx ØCQS
Laryngopharynx *use* Pharynx
Laryngoplasty
see Repair, Larynx ØCQS
see Replacement, Larynx ØCRS
see Supplement, Larynx ØCUS
Laryngorrhaphy *see* Repair, Larynx ØCQS
Laryngoscopy ØCJS8ZZ
Laryngotomy *see* Drainage, Larynx ØC9S
Laser Interstitial Thermal Therapy
Adrenal Gland DGY2KZZ
Anus DDY8KZZ
Bile Ducts DFY2KZZ
Brain DØYØKZZ
Brain Stem DØY1KZZ
Breast
Left DMYØKZZ
Right DMY1KZZ
Bronchus DBY1KZZ
Chest Wall DBY7KZZ
Colon DDY5KZZ
Diaphragm DBY8KZZ
Duodenum DDY2KZZ
Esophagus DDYØKZZ
Gallbladder DFY1KZZ
Gland
Adrenal DGY2KZZ
Parathyroid DGY4KZZ
Pituitary DGYØKZZ
Laser Interstitial Thermal Therapy — continued
Gland — continued
Thyroid DGY5KZZ
Ileum DDY4KZZ
Jejunum DDY3KZZ
Liver DFYØKZZ
Lung DBY2KZZ
Mediastinum DBY6KZZ
Nerve, Peripheral DØY7KZZ
Pancreas DFY3KZZ
Parathyroid Gland DGY4KZZ
Pineal Body DGY1KZZ
Pituitary Gland DGYØKZZ
Pleura DBY5KZZ
Prostate DVYØKZZ
Rectum DDY7KZZ
Spinal Cord DØY6KZZ
Stomach DDY1KZZ
Thyroid Gland DGY5KZZ
Trachea DBYØKZZ
Lateral canthus
use Eyelid, Upper, Left
use Eyelid, Upper, Right
Lateral collateral ligament (LCL)
use Bursa and Ligament, Knee, Left
use Bursa and Ligament, Knee, Right
Lateral condyle of femur
use Femur, Lower, Left
use Femur, Lower, Right
Lateral condyle of tibia
use Tibia, Left
use Tibia, Right
Lateral cuneiform bone
use Tarsal, Left
use Tarsal, Right
Lateral epicondyle of femur
use Femur, Lower, Left
use Femur, Lower, Right
Lateral epicondyle of humerus
use Humeral Shaft, Left
use Humeral Shaft, Right
Lateral femoral cutaneous nerve *use* Nerve, Lumbar Plexus
Lateral (brachial) lymph node
use Lymphatic, Axillary, Left
use Lymphatic, Axillary, Right
Lateral malleolus
use Fibula, Left
use Fibula, Right
Lateral meniscus
use Joint, Knee, Left
use Joint, Knee, Right
Lateral nasal cartilage *use* Nose
Lateral plantar artery
use Artery, Foot, Left
use Artery, Foot, Right
Lateral plantar nerve *use* Nerve, Tibial
Lateral rectus muscle
use Muscle, Extraocular, Left
use Muscle, Extraocular, Right
Lateral sacral artery
use Artery, Internal Iliac, Left
use Artery, Internal Iliac, Right
Lateral sacral vein
use Vein, Hypogastric, Left
use Vein, Hypogastric, Right
Lateral sural cutaneous nerve *use* Nerve, Peroneal
Lateral tarsal artery
use Artery, Foot, Left
use Artery, Foot, Right
Lateral temporomandibular ligament *use* Bursa and Ligament, Head and Neck
Lateral thoracic artery
use Artery, Axillary, Left
use Artery, Axillary, Right
Latissimus dorsi muscle
use Muscle, Trunk, Left
use Muscle, Trunk, Right
Latissimus Dorsi Myocutaneous Flap
Bilateral ØHRVØ75
Left ØHRUØ75
Right ØHRTØ75
Lavage
see Irrigation

Lavage — continued
Bronchial alveolar, diagnostic *see* Drainage, Respiratory System ØB9
Least splanchnic nerve *use* Nerve, Thoracic Sympathetic
Left ascending lumbar vein *use* Vein, Hemiazygos
Left atrioventricular valve *use* Valve, Mitral
Left auricular appendix *use* Atrium, Left
Left colic vein *use* Vein, Colic
Left coronary sulcus *use* Heart, Left
Left gastric artery *use* Artery, Gastric
Left gastroepiploic artery *use* Artery, Splenic
Left gastroepiploic vein *use* Vein, Splenic
Left inferior phrenic vein *use* Vein, Renal, Left
Left inferior pulmonary vein *use* Vein, Pulmonary, Left
Left jugular trunk *use* Lymphatic, Thoracic Duct
Left lateral ventricle *use* Cerebral Ventricle
Left ovarian vein *use* Vein, Renal, Left
Left second lumbar vein *use* Vein, Renal, Left
Left subclavian trunk *use* Lymphatic, Thoracic Duct
Left subcostal vein *use* Vein, Hemiazygos
Left superior pulmonary vein *use* Vein, Pulmonary, Left
Left suprarenal vein *use* Vein, Renal, Left
Left testicular vein *use* Vein, Renal, Left
Lengthening
Bone, with device *see* Insertion of Limb Lengthening Device
Muscle, by incision *see* Division, Muscles ØK8
Tendon, by incision *see* Division, Tendons ØL8
Leptomeninges
use Cerebral Meninges
use Spinal Meninges
Lesser alar cartilage *use* Nose
Lesser occipital nerve *use* Nerve, Cervical Plexus
Lesser splanchnic nerve *use* Nerve, Thoracic Sympathetic
Lesser trochanter
use Femur, Upper, Left
use Femur, Upper, Right
Lesser tuberosity
use Humeral Head, Left
use Humeral Head, Right
Lesser wing
use Bone, Sphenoid, Left
use Bone, Sphenoid, Right
Leukopheresis, therapeutic *see* Pheresis, Circulatory 6A55
Levator anguli oris muscle *use* Muscle, Facial
Levator ani muscle
use Muscle, Trunk, Left
use Muscle, Trunk, Right
Levator labii superioris alaeque nasi muscle *use* Muscle, Facial
Levator labii superioris muscle *use* Muscle, Facial
Levator palpebrae superioris muscle
use Eyelid, Upper, Left
use Eyelid, Upper, Right
Levator scapulae muscle
use Muscle, Neck, Left
use Muscle, Neck, Right
Levator veli palatini muscle *use* Muscle, Tongue, Palate, Pharynx
Levatores costarum muscle
use Muscle, Thorax, Left
use Muscle, Thorax, Right
LifeStent® (Flexstar) (XL) Vascular Stent System *use* Intraluminal Device
Ligament of head of fibula
use Bursa and Ligament, Knee, Left
use Bursa and Ligament, Knee, Right
Ligament of the lateral malleolus
use Bursa and Ligament, Ankle, Left
use Bursa and Ligament, Ankle, Right
Ligamentum flavum
use Bursa and Ligament, Trunk, Left
use Bursa and Ligament, Trunk, Right
Ligation *see* Occlusion
Ligation, hemorrhoid *see* Occlusion, Lower Veins, Hemorrhoidal Plexus
Light Therapy GZJZZZZ
Liner
Removal of device from
Hip
Left ØSPBØ9Z
Right ØSP9Ø9Z
Knee
Left ØSPDØ9Z
Right ØSPCØ9Z
Revision of device in
Hip
Left ØSWBØ9Z
Right ØSW9Ø9Z
Knee
Left ØSWDØ9Z
Right ØSWCØ9Z
Supplement
Hip
Left ØSUBØ9Z
Acetabular Surface ØSUEØ9Z
Femoral Surface ØSUSØ9Z
Right ØSU9Ø9Z
Acetabular Surface ØSUAØ9Z
Femoral Surface ØSURØ9Z
Knee
Left ØSUDØ9
Femoral Surface ØSUUØ9Z
Tibial Surface ØSUWØ9Z
Right ØSUCØ9
Femoral Surface ØSUTØ9Z
Tibial Surface ØSUVØ9Z
Lingual artery
use Artery, External Carotid, Left
use Artery, External Carotid, Right
Lingual tonsil *use* Tongue
Lingulectomy, lung
see Excision, Lung Lingula ØBBH
see Resection, Lung Lingula ØBTH
Lithotripsy
With removal of fragments *see* Extirpation
see Fragmentation
LIVIAN™ CRT-D *use* Cardiac Resynchronization Defibrillator Pulse Generator in ØJH
Lobectomy
see Excision, Central Nervous System ØØB
see Excision, Endocrine System ØGB
see Excision, Hepatobiliary System and Pancreas ØFB
see Excision, Respiratory System ØBB
see Resection, Endocrine System ØGT
see Resection, Hepatobiliary System and Pancreas ØFT
see Resection, Respiratory System ØBT
Lobotomy *see* Division, Brain ØØ8Ø
Localization
see Imaging
see Map
Locus ceruleus *use* Pons
Long thoracic nerve *use* Nerve, Brachial Plexus
Loop ileostomy *see* Bypass, Ileum ØD1B
Loop recorder, implantable *use* Monitoring Device
Lower GI series *see* Fluoroscopy, Colon BD14
Lumbar artery *use* Aorta, Abdominal
Lumbar facet joint *use* Joint, Lumbar Vertebral
Lumbar ganglion *use* Nerve, Lumbar Sympathetic
Lumbar lymph node *use* Lymphatic, Aortic
Lumbar lymphatic trunk *use* Cisterna Chyli
Lumbar splanchnic nerve *use* Nerve, Lumbar Sympathetic
Lumbosacral facet joint *use* Joint, Lumbosacral
Lumbosacral trunk *use* Nerve, Lumbar
Lumpectomy *see* Excision
Lunate bone
use Carpal, Left
use Carpal, Right
Lunotriquetral ligament
use Bursa and Ligament, Hand, Left
use Bursa and Ligament, Hand, Right
Lymphadenectomy
see Excision, Lymphatic and Hemic Systems Ø7B
see Resection, Lymphatic and Hemic Systems Ø7T
Lymphadenotomy *see* Drainage, Lymphatic and Hemic Systems Ø79
Lymphangiectomy
see Excision, Lymphatic and Hemic Systems Ø7B
see Resection, Lymphatic and Hemic Systems Ø7T
Lymphangiogram *see* Plain Radiography, Lymphatic System B7Ø
Lymphangioplasty
see Repair, Lymphatic and Hemic Systems Ø7Q
see Supplement, Lymphatic and Hemic Systems Ø7U
Lymphangiorrhaphy *see* Repair, Lymphatic and Hemic Systems Ø7Q
Lymphangiotomy *see* Drainage, Lymphatic and Hemic Systems Ø79
Lysis *see* Release

M

Macula
use Retina, Left
use Retina, Right
Magnet extraction, ocular foreign body *see* Extirpation, Eye Ø8C
Magnetic Resonance Imaging (MRI)
Abdomen BW3Ø
Ankle
Left BQ3H
Right BQ3G
Aorta
Abdominal B43Ø
Thoracic B33Ø
Arm
Left BP3F
Right BP3E
Artery
Celiac B431
Cervico-Cerebral Arch B33Q
Common Carotid, Bilateral B335
Coronary
Bypass Graft, Multiple B233
Multiple B231
Internal Carotid, Bilateral B338
Intracranial B33R
Lower Extremity
Bilateral B43H
Left B43G
Right B43F
Pelvic B43C
Renal, Bilateral B438
Spinal B33M
Superior Mesenteric B434
Upper Extremity
Bilateral B33K
Left B33J
Right B33H
Vertebral, Bilateral B33G
Bladder BT3Ø
Brachial Plexus BW3P
Brain BØ3Ø
Breast
Bilateral BH32
Left BH31
Right BH3Ø
Calcaneus
Left BQ3K
Right BQ3J
Chest BW33Y
Coccyx BR3F
Connective Tissue
Lower Extremity BL31
Upper Extremity BL3Ø
Corpora Cavernosa BV3Ø
Disc
Cervical BR31
Lumbar BR33
Thoracic BR32
Ear B93Ø
Elbow
Left BP3H
Right BP3G
Eye
Bilateral B837
Left B836
Right B835
Femur
Left BQ34
Right BQ33
Fetal Abdomen BY33
Fetal Extremity BY35
Fetal Head BY3Ø

Magnetic Resonance Imaging (MRI) — continued
Fetal Heart BY31
Fetal Spine BY34
Fetal Thorax BY32
Fetus, Whole BY36
Foot
Left BQ3M
Right BQ3L
Forearm
Left BP3K
Right BP3J
Gland
Adrenal, Bilateral BG32
Parathyroid BG33
Parotid, Bilateral B936
Salivary, Bilateral B93D
Submandibular, Bilateral B939
Thyroid BG34
Head BW38
Heart, Right and Left B236
Hip
Left BQ31
Right BQ3Ø
Intracranial Sinus B532
Joint
Finger
Left BP3D
Right BP3C
Hand
Left BP3D
Right BP3C
Temporomandibular, Bilateral BN39
Kidney
Bilateral BT33
Left BT32
Right BT31
Transplant BT39
Knee
Left BQ38
Right BQ37
Larynx B93J
Leg
Left BQ3F
Right BQ3D
Liver BF35
Liver and Spleen BF36
Lung Apices BB3G
Nasopharynx B93F
Neck BW3F
Nerve
Acoustic BØ3C
Brachial Plexus BW3P
Oropharynx B93F
Ovary
Bilateral BU35
Left BU34
Right BU33
Ovary and Uterus BU3C
Pancreas BF37
Patella
Left BQ3W
Right BQ3V
Pelvic Region BW3G
Pelvis BR3C
Pituitary Gland BØ39
Plexus, Brachial BW3P
Prostate BV33
Retroperitoneum BW3H
Sacrum BR3F
Scrotum BV34
Sella Turcica BØ39
Shoulder
Left BP39
Right BP38
Sinus
Intracranial B532
Paranasal B932
Spinal Cord BØ3B
Spine
Cervical BR3Ø
Lumbar BR39
Thoracic BR37
Spleen and Liver BF36
Subcutaneous Tissue
Abdomen BH3H

Magnetic Resonance Imaging (MRI) — continued
Subcutaneous Tissue — continued
Extremity
Lower BH3J
Upper BH3F
Head BH3D
Neck BH3D
Pelvis BH3H
Thorax BH3G
Tendon
Lower Extremity BL33
Upper Extremity BL32
Testicle
Bilateral BV37
Left BV36
Right BV35
Toe
Left BQ3Q
Right BQ3P
Uterus BU36
Pregnant BU3B
Uterus and Ovary BU3C
Vagina BU39
Vein
Cerebellar B531
Cerebral B531
Jugular, Bilateral B535
Lower Extremity
Bilateral B53D
Left B53C
Right B53B
Other B53V
Pelvic (Iliac) Bilateral B53H
Portal B53T
Pulmonary, Bilateral B53S
Renal, Bilateral B53L
Spanchnic B53T
Upper Extremity
Bilateral B53P
Left B53N
Right B53M
Vena Cava
Inferior B539
Superior B538
Wrist
Left BP3M
Right BP3L
Malleotomy *see* Drainage, Ear, Nose, Sinus Ø99
Malleus
use Auditory Ossicle, Left
use Auditory Ossicle, Right
Mammaplasty, mammoplasty
see Alteration, Skin and Breast ØHØ
see Repair, Skin and Breast ØHQ
see Replacement, Skin and Breast ØHR
see Supplement, Skin and Breast ØHU
Mammary duct
use Breast, Bilateral
use Breast, Left
use Breast, Right
Mammary gland
use Breast, Bilateral
use Breast, Left
use Breast, Right
Mammectomy
see Excision, Skin and Breast ØHB
see Resection, Skin and Breast ØHT
Mammillary body *use* Hypothalamus
Mammography *see* Plain Radiography, Skin, Subcutaneous Tissue and Breast BHØ
Mammotomy *see* Drainage, Skin and Breast ØH9
Mandibular nerve *use* Nerve, Trigeminal
Mandibular notch
use Mandible, Left
use Mandible, Right
Mandibulectomy
see Excision, Head and Facial Bones ØNB
see Resection, Head and Facial Bones ØNT
Manipulation
Adhesions *see* Release
Chiropractic *see* Chiropractic Manipulation
Manubrium *use* Sternum
Map
Basal Ganglia ØØK8
Brain ØØKØ

Map — continued
Cerebellum ØØKC
Cerebral Hemisphere ØØK7
Conduction Mechanism Ø2K8
Hypothalamus ØØKA
Medulla Oblongata ØØKD
Pons ØØKB
Thalamus ØØK9
Mapping
Doppler ultrasound *see* Ultrasonography
Electrocardiogram only *see* Measurement, Cardiac 4AØ2
Mark IV Breathing Pacemaker System *use* Stimulator Generator in Subcutaneous Tissue and Fascia
Marsupialization
see Drainage
see Excision
Massage, cardiac
External 5A12Ø12
Open Ø2QAØZZ
Masseter muscle *use* Muscle, Head
Masseteric fascia *use* Subcutaneous Tissue and Fascia, Face
Mastectomy
see Excision, Skin and Breast ØHB
see Resection, Skin and Breast ØHT
Mastoid air cells
use Sinus, Mastoid, Left
use Sinus, Mastoid, Right
Mastoid (postauricular) lymph node
use Lymphatic, Neck, Left
use Lymphatic, Neck, Right
Mastoid process
use Bone, Temporal, Left
use Bone, Temporal, Right
Mastoidectomy
see Excision, Ear, Nose, Sinus Ø9B
see Resection, Ear, Nose, Sinus Ø9T
Mastoidotomy *see* Drainage, Ear, Nose, Sinus Ø99
Mastopexy
see Repair, Skin and Breast ØHQ
see Reposition, Skin and Breast ØHS
Mastorrhaphy *see* Repair, Skin and Breast ØHQ
Mastotomy *see* Drainage, Skin and Breast ØH9
Maxillary artery
use Artery, External Carotid, Left
use Artery, External Carotid, Right
Maxillary nerve *use* Nerve, Trigeminal
Maximo II DR (VR) *use* Defibrillator Generator in ØJH
Maximo II DR CRT-D *use* Cardiac Resynchronization Defibrillator Pulse Generator in ØJH
Measurement
Arterial
Flow
Coronary 4AØ3
Peripheral 4AØ3
Pulmonary 4AØ3
Pressure
Coronary 4AØ3
Peripheral 4AØ3
Pulmonary 4AØ3
Thoracic, Other 4AØ3
Pulse
Coronary 4AØ3
Peripheral 4AØ3
Pulmonary 4AØ3
Saturation, Peripheral 4AØ3
Sound, Peripheral 4AØ3
Biliary
Flow 4AØC
Pressure 4AØC
Cardiac
Action Currents 4AØ2
Defibrillator 4BØ2XTZ
Electrical Activity 4AØ2
Guidance 4AØ2X4A
No Qualifier 4AØ2X4Z
Output 4AØ2
Pacemaker 4BØ2XSZ
Rate 4AØ2
Rhythm 4AØ2
Sampling and Pressure
Bilateral 4AØ2
Left Heart 4AØ2
Right Heart 4AØ2

Measurement — continued
Cardiac — continued
Sound 4AØ2
Total Activity, Stress 4AØ2XM4
Central Nervous
Conductivity 4AØØ
Electrical Activity 4AØØ
Pressure 4AØØØBZ
Intracranial 4AØØ
Saturation, Intracranial 4AØØ
Stimulator 4BØØXVZ
Temperature, Intracranial 4AØØ
Circulatory, Volume 4AØ5XLZ
Gastrointestinal
Motility 4AØB
Pressure 4AØB
Secretion 4AØB
Lymphatic
Flow 4AØ6
Pressure 4AØ6
Metabolism 4AØZ
Musculoskeletal
Contractility 4AØF
Stimulator 4BØFXVZ
Olfactory, Acuity 4AØ8XØZ
Peripheral Nervous
Conductivity
Motor 4AØ1
Sensory 4AØ1
Electrical Activity 4AØ1
Stimulator 4BØ1XVZ
Products of Conception
Cardiac
Electrical Activity 4AØH
Rate 4AØH
Rhythm 4AØH
Sound 4AØH
Nervous
Conductivity 4AØJ
Electrical Activity 4AØJ
Pressure 4AØJ
Respiratory
Capacity 4AØ9
Flow 4AØ9
Pacemaker 4BØ9XSZ
Rate 4AØ9
Resistance 4AØ9
Total Activity 4AØ9
Volume 4AØ9
Sleep 4AØZXQZ
Temperature 4AØZ
Urinary
Contractility 4AØD73Z
Flow 4AØD75Z
Pressure 4AØD7BZ
Resistance 4AØD7DZ
Volume 4AØD7LZ
Venous
Flow
Central 4AØ4
Peripheral 4AØ4
Portal 4AØ4
Pulmonary 4AØ4
Pressure
Central 4AØ4
Peripheral 4AØ4
Portal 4AØ4
Pulmonary 4AØ4
Pulse
Central 4AØ4
Peripheral 4AØ4
Portal 4AØ4
Pulmonary 4AØ4
Saturation, Peripheral 4AØ4
Visual
Acuity 4AØ7XØZ
Mobility 4AØ7X7Z
Pressure 4AØ7XBZ
Meatoplasty, urethra *see* Repair, Urethra ØTQD
Meatotomy *see* Drainage, Urinary System ØT9
Mechanical ventilation *see* Performance, Respiratory 5A19
Medial canthus
use Eyelid, Lower, Left
use Eyelid, Lower, Right
Medial collateral ligament (MCL)
use Bursa and Ligament, Knee, Left
use Bursa and Ligament, Knee, Right
Medial condyle of femur
use Femur, Lower, Left
use Femur, Lower, Right
Medial condyle of tibia
use Tibia, Left
use Tibia, Right
Medial cuneiform bone
use Tarsal, Left
use Tarsal, Right
Medial epicondyle of femur
use Femur, Lower, Left
use Femur, Lower, Right
Medial epicondyle of humerus
use Humeral Shaft, Left
use Humeral Shaft, Right
Medial malleolus
use Tibia, Left
use Tibia, Right
Medial meniscus
use Joint, Knee, Left
use Joint, Knee, Right
Medial plantar artery
use Artery, Foot, Left
use Artery, Foot, Right
Medial plantar nerve *use* Nerve, Tibial
Medial popliteal nerve *use* Nerve, Tibial
Medial rectus muscle
use Muscle, Extraocular, Left
use Muscle, Extraocular, Right
Medial sural cutaneous nerve *use* Nerve, Tibial
Median antebrachial vein
use Vein, Basilic, Left
use Vein, Basilic, Right
Median cubital vein
use Vein, Basilic, Left
use Vein, Basilic, Right
Median sacral artery *use* Aorta, Abdominal
Mediastinal lymph node *use* Lymphatic, Thorax
Mediastinoscopy ØWJC4ZZ
Medication Management GZ3ZZZZ
for substance abuse
Antabuse HZ83ZZZ
Bupropion HZ87ZZZ
Clonidine HZ86ZZZ
Levo-alpha-acetyl-methadol (LAAM) HZ82ZZZ
Methadone Maintenance HZ81ZZZ
Naloxone HZ85ZZZ
Naltrexone HZ84ZZZ
Nicotine Replacement HZ8ØZZZ
Other Replacement Medication HZ89ZZZ
Psychiatric Medication HZ88ZZZ
Meditation 8EØZXY5
Meissner's (submucous) plexus *use* Nerve, Abdominal Sympathetic
Melody® transcatheter pulmonary valve *use* Zooplastic Tissue in Heart and Great Vessels
Membranous urethra *use* Urethra
Meningeorrhaphy
see Repair, Cerebral Meninges ØØQ1
see Repair, Spinal Meninges ØØQT
Meniscectomy
see Excision, Lower Joints ØSB
see Resection, Lower Joints ØST
Mental foramen
use Mandible, Left
use Mandible, Right
Mentalis muscle *use* Muscle, Facial
Mentoplasty *see* Alteration, Jaw, Lower ØWØ5
Mesenterectomy *see* Excision, Mesentery ØDBV
Mesenteriorrhaphy, mesenterorrhaphy *see* Repair, Mesentery ØDQV
Mesenteriplication *see* Repair, Mesentery ØDQV
Mesoappendix *use* Mesentery
Mesocolon *use* Mesentery
Metacarpal ligament
use Bursa and Ligament, Hand, Left
use Bursa and Ligament, Hand, Right
Metacarpophalangeal ligament
use Bursa and Ligament, Hand, Left
use Bursa and Ligament, Hand, Right
Metatarsal ligament
use Bursa and Ligament, Foot, Left
use Bursa and Ligament, Foot, Right
Metatarsectomy
see Excision, Lower Bones ØQB
see Resection, Lower Bones ØQT
Metatarsophalangeal (MTP) joint
use Joint, Metatarsal-Phalangeal, Left
use Joint, Metatarsal-Phalangeal, Right
Metatarsophalangeal ligament
use Bursa and Ligament, Foot, Left
use Bursa and Ligament, Foot, Right
Metathalamus *use* Thalamus
Micro-Driver stent (RX) (OTW) *use* Intraluminal Device
MicroMed HeartAssist *use* Implantable Heart Assist System in Heart and Great Vessels
Micrus CERECYTE Microcoil *use* Intraluminal Device, Bioactive in Upper Arteries
Midcarpal joint
use Joint, Carpal, Left
use Joint, Carpal, Right
Middle cardiac nerve *use* Nerve, Thoracic Sympathetic
Middle cerebral artery *use* Artery, Intracranial
Middle cerebral vein *use* Vein, Intracranial
Middle colic vein *use* Vein, Colic
Middle genicular artery
use Artery, Popliteal, Left
use Artery, Popliteal, Right
Middle hemorrhoidal vein
use Vein, Hypogastric, Left
use Vein, Hypogastric, Right
Middle rectal artery
use Artery, Internal Iliac, Left
use Artery, Internal Iliac, Right
Middle suprarenal artery *use* Aorta, Abdominal
Middle temporal artery
use Artery, Temporal, Left
use Artery, Temporal, Right
Middle turbinate *use* Turbinate, Nasal
MitraClip valve repair system *use* Synthetic Substitute
Mitral annulus *use* Valve, Mitral
Mitroflow® Aortic Pericardial Heart Valve *use* Zooplastic Tissue in Heart and Great Vessels
Mobilization, adhesions *see* Release
Molar gland *use* Buccal Mucosa
Monitoring
Arterial
Flow
Coronary 4A13
Peripheral 4A13
Pulmonary 4A13
Pressure
Coronary 4A13
Peripheral 4A13
Pulmonary 4A13
Pulse
Coronary 4A13
Peripheral 4A13
Pulmonary 4A13
Saturation, Peripheral 4A13
Sound, Peripheral 4A13
Cardiac
Electrical Activity 4A12
Ambulatory 4A12X45
No Qualifier 4A12X4Z
Output 4A12
Rate 4A12
Rhythm 4A12
Sound 4A12
Total Activity, Stress 4A12XM4
Central Nervous
Conductivity 4A1Ø
Electrical Activity
Intraoperative 4A1Ø
No Qualifier 4A1Ø
Pressure 4A1ØØBZ
Intracranial 4A1Ø
Saturation, Intracranial 4A1Ø
Temperature, Intracranial 4A1Ø
Gastrointestinal
Motility 4A1B
Pressure 4A1B
Secretion 4A1B
Lymphatic
Flow 4A16

Subterms under main terms may continue to next column or page

Monitoring — continued
Lymphatic — continued
Pressure 4A16
Peripheral Nervous
Conductivity
Motor 4A11
Sensory 4A11
Electrical Activity
Intraoperative 4A11
No Qualifier 4A11
Products of Conception
Cardiac
Electrical Activity 4A1H
Rate 4A1H
Rhythm 4A1H
Sound 4A1H
Nervous
Conductivity 4A1J
Electrical Activity 4A1J
Pressure 4A1J
Respiratory
Capacity 4A19
Flow 4A19
Rate 4A19
Resistance 4A19
Volume 4A19
Sleep 4A1ZXQZ
Temperature 4A1Z
Urinary
Contractility 4A1D73Z
Flow 4A1D75Z
Pressure 4A1D7BZ
Resistance 4A1D7DZ
Volume 4A1D7LZ
Venous
Flow
Central 4A14
Peripheral 4A14
Portal 4A14
Pulmonary 4A14
Pressure
Central 4A14
Peripheral 4A14
Portal 4A14
Pulmonary 4A14
Pulse
Central 4A14
Peripheral 4A14
Portal 4A14
Pulmonary 4A14
Saturation
Central 4A14
Portal 4A14
Pulmonary 4A14
Monitoring Device, Hemodynamic
Abdomen ØJH8
Chest ØJH6
Mosaic Bioprosthesis (aortic) (mitral) valve *use* Zooplastic Tissue in Heart and Great Vessels
Motor Function Assessment FØ1
Motor Treatment FØ7
MR Angiography
see Magnetic Resonance Imaging (MRI), Heart B23
see Magnetic Resonance Imaging (MRI), Lower Arteries B43
see Magnetic Resonance Imaging (MRI), Upper Arteries B33
MULTI-LINK (VISION) (MINI-VISION) (ULTRA) Coronary Stent System *use* Intraluminal Device
Multiple sleep latency test 4AØZXQZ
Musculocutaneous nerve *use* Nerve, Brachial Plexus
Musculopexy
see Repair, Muscles ØKQ
see Reposition, Muscles ØKS
Musculophrenic artery
use Artery, Internal Mammary, Left
use Artery, Internal Mammary, Right
Musculoplasty
see Repair, Muscles ØKQ
see Supplement, Muscles ØKU
Musculorrhaphy *see* Repair, Muscles ØKQ
Musculospiral nerve *use* Nerve, Radial
Myectomy
see Excision, Muscles ØKB
see Resection, Muscles ØKT
Myelencephalon *use* Medulla Oblongata
Myelogram
CT *see* Computerized Tomography (CT Scan), Central Nervous System BØ2
MRI *see* Magnetic Resonance Imaging (MRI), Central Nervous System BØ3
Myenteric (Auerbach's) plexus *use* Nerve, Abdominal Sympathetic
Myomectomy *see* Excision, Female Reproductive System ØUB
Myometrium *use* Uterus
Myopexy
see Repair, Muscles ØKQ
see Reposition, Muscles ØKS
Myoplasty
see Repair, Muscles ØKQ
see Supplement, Muscles ØKU
Myorrhaphy *see* Repair, Muscles ØKQ
Myoscopy *see* Inspection, Muscles ØKJ
Myotomy
see Division, Muscles ØK8
see Drainage, Muscles ØK9
Myringectomy
see Excision, Ear, Nose, Sinus Ø9B
see Resection, Ear, Nose, Sinus Ø9T
Myringoplasty
see Repair, Ear, Nose, Sinus Ø9Q
see Replacement, Ear, Nose, Sinus Ø9R
see Supplement, Ear, Nose, Sinus Ø9U
Myringostomy *see* Drainage, Ear, Nose, Sinus Ø99
Myringotomy *see* Drainage, Ear, Nose, Sinus Ø99

N

Nail bed
use Finger Nail
use Toe Nail
Nail plate
use Finger Nail
use Toe Nail
Narcosynthesis GZGZZZZ
Nasal cavity *use* Nose
Nasal concha *use* Turbinate, Nasal
Nasalis muscle *use* Muscle, Facial
Nasolacrimal duct
use Duct, Lacrimal, Left
use Duct, Lacrimal, Right
Nasopharyngeal airway (NPA) *use* Intraluminal Device, Airway in Ear, Nose, Sinus
Navicular bone
use Tarsal, Left
use Tarsal, Right
Near Infrared Spectroscopy, Circulatory System 8EØ23DZ
Neck of femur
use Femur, Upper, Left
use Femur, Upper, Right
Neck of humerus (anatomical) (surgical)
use Humeral Head, Left
use Humeral Head, Right
Nephrectomy
see Excision, Urinary System ØTB
see Resection, Urinary System ØTT
Nephrolithotomy *see* Extirpation, Urinary System ØTC
Nephrolysis *see* Release, Urinary System ØTN
Nephropexy
see Repair, Urinary System ØTQ
see Reposition, Urinary System ØTS
Nephroplasty
see Repair, Urinary System ØTQ
see Supplement, Urinary System ØTU
Nephropyeloureterostomy
see Bypass, Urinary System ØT1
see Drainage, Urinary System ØT9
Nephrorrhaphy *see* Repair, Urinary System ØTQ
Nephroscopy, transurethral ØTJ58ZZ
Nephrostomy
see Bypass, Urinary System ØT1
see Drainage, Urinary System ØT9
Nephrotomography
see Fluoroscopy, Urinary System BT1
see Plain Radiography, Urinary System BTØ
Nephrotomy
see Division, Urinary System ØT8
Nephrotomy — continued
see Drainage, Urinary System ØT9
Nerve conduction study
see Measurement, Central Nervous 4AØØ
see Measurement, Peripheral Nervous 4AØ1
Nerve Function Assessment FØ1
Nerve to the stapedius *use* Nerve, Facial
Nesiritide *use* Human B-type Natriuretic Peptide
Neurectomy
see Excision, Central Nervous System ØØB
see Excision, Peripheral Nervous System Ø1B
Neurexeresis
see Extraction, Central Nervous System ØØD
see Extraction, Peripheral Nervous System Ø1D
Neurohypophysis *use* Gland, Pituitary
Neurolysis
see Release, Central Nervous System ØØN
see Release, Peripheral Nervous System Ø1N
Neuromuscular electrical stimulation (NEMS) lead *use* Stimulator Lead in Muscles
Neurophysiologic monitoring *see* Monitoring, Central Nervous 4A1Ø
Neuroplasty
see Repair, Central Nervous System ØØQ
see Repair, Peripheral Nervous System Ø1Q
see Supplement, Central Nervous System ØØU
see Supplement, Peripheral Nervous System Ø1U
Neurorrhaphy
see Repair, Central Nervous System ØØQ
see Repair, Peripheral Nervous System Ø1Q
Neurostimulator Generator
Insertion of device in, Skull ØNHØØNZ
Removal of device from, Skull ØNPØØNZ
Revision of device in, Skull ØNWØØNZ
Neurostimulator generator, multiple channel *use* Stimulator Generator, Multiple Array in ØJH
Neurostimulator generator, multiple channel rechargeable *use* Stimulator Generator, Multiple Array Rechargeable in ØJH
Neurostimulator generator, single channel *use* Stimulator Generator, Single Array in ØJH
Neurostimulator generator, single channel rechargeable *use* Stimulator Generator, Single Array Rechargeable in ØJH
Neurostimulator Lead
Insertion of device in
Brain ØØHØ
Cerebral Ventricle ØØH6
Nerve
Cranial ØØHE
Peripheral Ø1HY
Spinal Canal ØØHU
Spinal Cord ØØHV
Removal of device from
Brain ØØPØ
Cerebral Ventricle ØØP6
Nerve
Cranial ØØPE
Peripheral Ø1PY
Spinal Canal ØØPU
Spinal Cord ØØPV
Revision of device in
Brain ØØWØ
Cerebral Ventricle ØØW6
Nerve
Cranial ØØWE
Peripheral Ø1WY
Spinal Canal ØØWU
Spinal Cord ØØWV
Neurotomy
see Division, Central Nervous System ØØ8
see Division, Peripheral Nervous System Ø18
Neurotripsy
see Destruction, Central Nervous System ØØ5
see Destruction, Peripheral Nervous System Ø15
Neutralization plate
use Internal Fixation Device in Head and Facial Bones
use Internal Fixation Device in Lower Bones
use Internal Fixation Device in Upper Bones
Ninth cranial nerve *use* Nerve, Glossopharyngeal
Nitinol framed polymer mesh *use* Synthetic Substitute
Nonimaging Nuclear Medicine Assay
Bladder, Kidneys and Ureters CT63
Blood C763
Kidneys, Ureters and Bladder CT63

Nonimaging Nuclear Medicine Assay — continued
Lymphatics and Hematologic System C76YYZZ
Ureters, Kidneys and Bladder CT63
Urinary System CT6YYZZ
Nonimaging Nuclear Medicine Probe CP5YYZZ
Abdomen CW5Ø
Abdomen and Chest CW54
Abdomen and Pelvis CW51
Brain CØ5Ø
Central Nervous System CØ5YYZZ
Chest CW53
Chest and Abdomen CW54
Chest and Neck CW56
Extremity
Lower CP5
Upper CP5
Head and Neck CW5B
Heart C25YYZZ
Right and Left C256
Lymphatics
Head C75J
Head and Neck C755
Lower Extremity C75P
Neck C75K
Pelvic C75D
Trunk C75M
Upper Chest C75L
Upper Extremity C75N
Lymphatics and Hematologic System C75YYZZ
Neck and Chest CW56
Neck and Head CW5B
Pelvic Region CW5J
Pelvis and Abdomen CW51
Spine CP55ZZZ
Nonimaging Nuclear Medicine Uptake
Endocrine System CG4YYZZ
Gland, Thyroid CG42
Non-tunneled central venous catheter *use* Infusion Device
Nostril *use* Nose
Novacor Left Ventricular Assist Device *use* Implantable Heart Assist System in Heart and Great Vessels
Novation® Ceramic AHS® (Articulation Hip System) *use* Synthetic Substitute, Ceramic in ØSR
Nuclear medicine
see Nonimaging Nuclear Medicine Assay
see Nonimaging Nuclear Medicine Probe
see Nonimaging Nuclear Medicine Uptake
see Planar Nuclear Medicine Imaging
see Positron Emission Tomographic (PET) Imaging
see Systemic Nuclear Medicine Therapy
see Tomographic (Tomo) Nuclear Medicine Imaging
Nuclear scintigraphy *see* Nuclear Medicine
Nutrition, concentrated substances
Enteral infusion 3EØG36Z
Parenteral (peripheral) infusion *see* Introduction of Nutritional Substance

O

Obliteration *see* Destruction
Obturator artery
use Artery, Internal Iliac, Left
use Artery, Internal Iliac, Right
Obturator lymph node *use* Lymphatic, Pelvis
Obturator muscle
use Muscle, Hip, Left
use Muscle, Hip, Right
Obturator nerve *use* Nerve, Lumbar Plexus
Obturator vein
use Vein, Hypogastric, Left
use Vein, Hypogastric, Right
Obtuse margin *use* Heart, Left
Occipital artery
use Artery, External Carotid, Left
use Artery, External Carotid, Right
Occipital lobe *use* Cerebral Hemisphere
Occipital lymph node
use Lymphatic, Neck, Left
use Lymphatic, Neck, Right
Occipitofrontalis muscle *use* Muscle, Facial
Occlusion
Ampulla of Vater ØFLC
Anus ØDLQ
Aorta, Abdominal Ø4LØ
Artery
Anterior Tibial
Left Ø4LQ
Right Ø4LP
Axillary
Left Ø3L6
Right Ø3L5
Brachial
Left Ø3L8
Right Ø3L7
Celiac Ø4L1
Colic
Left Ø4L7
Middle Ø4L8
Right Ø4L6
Common Carotid
Left Ø3LJ
Right Ø3LH
Common Iliac
Left Ø4LD
Right Ø4LC
External Carotid
Left Ø3LN
Right Ø3LM
External Iliac
Left Ø4LJ
Right Ø4LH
Face Ø3LR
Femoral
Left Ø4LL
Right Ø4LK
Foot
Left Ø4LW
Right Ø4LV
Gastric Ø4L2
Hand
Left Ø3LF
Right Ø3LD
Hepatic Ø4L3
Inferior Mesenteric Ø4LB
Innominate Ø3L2
Internal Carotid
Left Ø3LL
Right Ø3LK
Internal Iliac
Left, Uterine Artery, Left Ø4LF
Right, Uterine Artery, Right Ø4LE
Internal Mammary
Left Ø3L1
Right Ø3LØ
Intracranial Ø3LG
Lower Ø4LY
Peroneal
Left Ø4LU
Right Ø4LT
Popliteal
Left Ø4LN
Right Ø4LM
Posterior Tibial
Left Ø4LS
Right Ø4LR
Pulmonary, Left Ø2LR
Radial
Left Ø3LC
Right Ø3LB
Renal
Left Ø4LA
Right Ø4L9
Splenic Ø4L4
Subclavian
Left Ø3L4
Right Ø3L3
Superior Mesenteric Ø4L5
Temporal
Left Ø3LT
Right Ø3LS
Thyroid
Left Ø3LV
Right Ø3LU
Ulnar
Left Ø3LA
Right Ø3L9
Occlusion — continued
Artery — continued
Upper Ø3LY
Vertebral
Left Ø3LQ
Right Ø3LP
Atrium, Left Ø2L7
Bladder ØTLB
Bladder Neck ØTLC
Bronchus
Lingula ØBL9
Lower Lobe
Left ØBLB
Right ØBL6
Main
Left ØBL7
Right ØBL3
Middle Lobe, Right ØBL5
Upper Lobe
Left ØBL8
Right ØBL4
Carina ØBL2
Cecum ØDLH
Cisterna Chyli Ø7LL
Colon
Ascending ØDLK
Descending ØDLM
Sigmoid ØDLN
Transverse ØDLL
Cord
Bilateral ØVLH
Left ØVLG
Right ØVLF
Cul-de-sac ØULF
Duct
Common Bile ØFL9
Cystic ØFL8
Hepatic
Left ØFL6
Right ØFL5
Lacrimal
Left Ø8LY
Right Ø8LX
Pancreatic ØFLD
Accessory ØFLF
Parotid
Left ØCLC
Right ØCLB
Duodenum ØDL9
Esophagogastric Junction ØDL4
Esophagus ØDL5
Lower ØDL3
Middle ØDL2
Upper ØDL1
Fallopian Tube
Left ØUL6
Right ØUL5
Fallopian Tubes, Bilateral ØUL7
Ileocecal Valve ØDLC
Ileum ØDLB
Intestine
Large ØDLE
Left ØDLG
Right ØDLF
Small ØDL8
Jejunum ØDLA
Kidney Pelvis
Left ØTL4
Right ØTL3
Left atrial appendage (LAA) *see* Occlusion, Atrium, Left Ø2L7
Lymphatic
Aortic Ø7LD
Axillary
Left Ø7L6
Right Ø7L5
Head Ø7LØ
Inguinal
Left Ø7LJ
Right Ø7LH
Internal Mammary
Left Ø7L9
Right Ø7L8
Lower Extremity
Left Ø7LG
Right Ø7LF

Occlusion — continued
Lymphatic — continued
Mesenteric Ø7LB
Neck
Left Ø7L2
Right Ø7L1
Pelvis Ø7LC
Thoracic Duct Ø7LK
Thorax Ø7L7
Upper Extremity
Left Ø7L4
Right Ø7L3
Rectum ØDLP
Stomach ØDL6
Pylorus ØDL7
Trachea ØBL1
Ureter
Left ØTL7
Right ØTL6
Urethra ØTLD
Vagina ØULG
Vas Deferens
Bilateral ØVLQ
Left ØVLP
Right ØVLN
Vein
Axillary
Left Ø5L8
Right Ø5L7
Azygos Ø5LØ
Basilic
Left Ø5LC
Right Ø5LB
Brachial
Left Ø5LA
Right Ø5L9
Cephalic
Left Ø5LF
Right Ø5LD
Colic Ø6L7
Common Iliac
Left Ø6LD
Right Ø6LC
Esophageal Ø6L3
External Iliac
Left Ø6LG
Right Ø6LF
External Jugular
Left Ø5LQ
Right Ø5LP
Face
Left Ø5LV
Right Ø5LT
Femoral
Left Ø6LN
Right Ø6LM
Foot
Left Ø6LV
Right Ø6LT
Gastric Ø6L2
Greater Saphenous
Left Ø6LQ
Right Ø6LP
Hand
Left Ø5LH
Right Ø5LG
Hemiazygos Ø5L1
Hepatic Ø6L4
Hypogastric
Left Ø6LJ
Right Ø6LH
Inferior Mesenteric Ø6L6
Innominate
Left Ø5L4
Right Ø5L3
Internal Jugular
Left Ø5LN
Right Ø5LM
Intracranial Ø5LL
Lesser Saphenous
Left Ø6LS
Right Ø6LR
Lower Ø6LY
Portal Ø6L8
Pulmonary
Left Ø2LT

Occlusion — continued
Vein — continued
Pulmonary — continued
Right Ø2LS
Renal
Left Ø6LB
Right Ø6L9
Splenic Ø6L1
Subclavian
Left Ø5L6
Right Ø5L5
Superior Mesenteric Ø6L5
Upper Ø5LY
Vertebral
Left Ø5LS
Right Ø5LR
Vena Cava
Inferior Ø6LØ
Superior Ø2LV
Occupational therapy *see* Activities of Daily Living Treatment, Rehabilitation FØ8
Odentectomy
see Excision, Mouth and Throat ØCB
see Resection, Mouth and Throat ØCT
Olecranon bursa
use Bursa and Ligament, Elbow, Left
use Bursa and Ligament, Elbow, Right
Olecranon process
use Ulna, Left
use Ulna, Right
Olfactory bulb *use* Nerve, Olfactory
Omentectomy, omentumectomy
see Excision, Gastrointestinal System ØDB
see Resection, Gastrointestinal System ØDT
Omentofixation *see* Repair, Gastrointestinal System ØDQ
Omentoplasty
see Repair, Gastrointestinal System ØDQ
see Replacement, Gastrointestinal System ØDR
see Supplement, Gastrointestinal System ØDU
Omentorrhaphy *see* Repair, Gastrointestinal System ØDQ
Omentotomy *see* Drainage, Gastrointestinal System ØD9
Omnilink Elite Vascular Balloon Expandable Stent System *use* Intraluminal Device
Onychectomy
see Excision, Skin and Breast ØHB
see Resection, Skin and Breast ØHT
Onychoplasty
see Repair, Skin and Breast ØHQ
see Replacement, Skin and Breast ØHR
Onychotomy *see* Drainage, Skin and Breast ØH9
Oophorectomy
see Excision, Female Reproductive System ØUB
see Resection, Female Reproductive System ØUT
Oophoropexy
see Repair, Female Reproductive System ØUQ
see Reposition, Female Reproductive System ØUS
Oophoroplasty
see Repair, Female Reproductive System ØUQ
see Supplement, Female Reproductive System ØUU
Oophororrhaphy *see* Repair, Female Reproductive System ØUQ
Oophorostomy *see* Drainage, Female Reproductive System ØU9
Oophorotomy
see Division, Female Reproductive System ØU8
see Drainage, Female Reproductive System ØU9
Oophorrhaphy *see* Repair, Female Reproductive System ØUQ
Open Pivot Aortic Valve Graft (AVG) *use* Synthetic Substitute
Open Pivot (mechanical) Valve *use* Synthetic Substitute
Ophthalmic artery
use Artery, Internal Carotid, Left
use Artery, Internal Carotid, Right
Ophthalmic nerve *use* Nerve, Trigeminal
Ophthalmic vein *use* Vein, Intracranial
Opponensplasty
Tendon replacement *see* Replacement, Tendons ØLR
Tendon transfer *see* Transfer, Tendons ØLX
Optic chiasma *use* Nerve, Optic

Optic disc
use Retina, Left
use Retina, Right
Optic foramen
use Bone, Sphenoid, Left
use Bone, Sphenoid, Right
Optical coherence tomography, intravascular *see* Computerized Tomography (CT Scan)
Optimizer™ III implantable pulse generator *use* Contractility Modulation Device in ØJH
Orbicularis oculi muscle
use Eyelid, Upper, Left
use Eyelid, Upper, Right
Orbicularis oris muscle *use* Muscle, Facial
Orbital fascia *use* Subcutaneous Tissue and Fascia, Face
Orbital portion of ethmoid bone
use Orbit, Left
use Orbit, Right
Orbital portion of frontal bone
use Orbit, Left
use Orbit, Right
Orbital portion of lacrimal bone
use Orbit, Left
use Orbit, Right
Orbital portion of maxilla
use Orbit, Left
use Orbit, Right
Orbital portion of palatine bone
use Orbit, Left
use Orbit, Right
Orbital portion of sphenoid bone
use Orbit, Left
use Orbit, Right
Orbital portion of zygomatic bone
use Orbit, Left
use Orbit, Right
Orchectomy, orchidectomy, orchiectomy
see Excision, Male Reproductive System ØVB
see Resection, Male Reproductive System ØVT
Orchidoplasty, orchioplasty
see Repair, Male Reproductive System ØVQ
see Replacement, Male Reproductive System ØVR
see Supplement, Male Reproductive System ØVU
Orchidorrhaphy, orchiorrhaphy *see* Repair, Male Reproductive System ØVQ
Orchidotomy, orchiotomy, orchotomy *see* Drainage, Male Reproductive System ØV9
Orchiopexy
see Repair, Male Reproductive System ØVQ
see Reposition, Male Reproductive System ØVS
Oropharyngeal airway (OPA) *use* Intraluminal Device, Airway in Mouth and Throat
Oropharynx *use* Pharynx
Ossicular chain
use Auditory Ossicle, Left
use Auditory Ossicle, Right
Ossiculectomy
see Excision, Ear, Nose, Sinus Ø9B
see Resection, Ear, Nose, Sinus Ø9T
Ossiculotomy *see* Drainage, Ear, Nose, Sinus Ø99
Ostectomy
see Excision, Head and Facial Bones ØNB
see Excision, Lower Bones ØQB
see Excision, Upper Bones ØPB
see Resection, Head and Facial Bones ØNT
see Resection, Lower Bones ØQT
see Resection, Upper Bones ØPT
Osteoclasis
see Division, Head and Facial Bones ØN8
see Division, Lower Bones ØQ8
see Division, Upper Bones ØP8
Osteolysis
see Release, Head and Facial Bones ØNN
see Release, Lower Bones ØQN
see Release, Upper Bones ØPN
Osteopathic Treatment
Abdomen 7WØ9X
Cervical 7WØ1X
Extremity
Lower 7WØ6X
Upper 7WØ7X
Head 7WØØX
Lumbar 7WØ3X
Pelvis 7WØ5X

Osteopathic Treatment — continued
Rib Cage 7W08X
Sacrum 7W04X
Thoracic 7W02X
Osteopexy
see Repair, Head and Facial Bones 0NQ
see Repair, Lower Bones 0QQ
see Repair, Upper Bones 0PQ
see Reposition, Head and Facial Bones 0NS
see Reposition, Lower Bones 0QS
see Reposition, Upper Bones 0PS
Osteoplasty
see Repair, Head and Facial Bones 0NQ
see Repair, Lower Bones 0QQ
see Repair, Upper Bones 0PQ
see Replacement, Head and Facial Bones 0NR
see Replacement, Lower Bones 0QR
see Replacement, Upper Bones 0PR
see Supplement, Head and Facial Bones 0NU
see Supplement, Lower Bones 0QU
see Supplement, Upper Bones 0PU
Osteorrhaphy
see Repair, Head and Facial Bones 0NQ
see Repair, Lower Bones 0QQ
see Repair, Upper Bones 0PQ
Osteotomy, ostotomy
see Division, Head and Facial Bones 0N8
see Division, Lower Bones 0Q8
see Division, Upper Bones 0P8
see Drainage, Head and Facial Bones 0N9
see Drainage, Lower Bones 0Q9
see Drainage, Upper Bones 0P9
Otic ganglion *use* Nerve, Head and Neck Sympathetic
Otoplasty
see Repair, Ear, Nose, Sinus 09Q
see Replacement, Ear, Nose, Sinus 09R
see Supplement, Ear, Nose, Sinus 09U
Otoscopy *see* Inspection, Ear, Nose, Sinus 09J
Oval window
use Ear, Middle, Left
use Ear, Middle, Right
Ovarian artery *use* Aorta, Abdominal
Ovarian ligament *use* Uterine Supporting Structure
Ovariectomy
see Excision, Female Reproductive System 0UB
see Resection, Female Reproductive System 0UT
Ovariocentesis *see* Drainage, Female Reproductive System 0U9
Ovariopexy
see Repair, Female Reproductive System 0UQ
see Reposition, Female Reproductive System 0US
Ovariotomy
see Division, Female Reproductive System 0U8
see Drainage, Female Reproductive System 0U9
Ovatio™ CRT-D *use* Cardiac Resynchronization Defibrillator Pulse Generator in 0JH
Oversewing
Gastrointestinal ulcer *see* Repair, Gastrointestinal System 0DQ
Pleural bleb *see* Repair, Respiratory System 0BQ
Oviduct
use Fallopian Tube, Left
use Fallopian Tube, Right
Oxidized zirconium ceramic hip bearing surface *use* Synthetic Substitute, Ceramic on Polyethylene in 0SR
Oximetry, Fetal pulse 10H073Z
Oxygenation
Extracorporeal membrane (ECMO) *see* Performance, Circulatory 5A15
Hyperbaric *see* Assistance, Circulatory 5A05
Supersaturated *see* Assistance, Circulatory 5A05

P

Pacemaker
Dual Chamber
Abdomen 0JH8
Chest 0JH6
Single Chamber
Abdomen 0JH8
Chest 0JH6
Single Chamber Rate Responsive
Abdomen 0JH8
Pacemaker — continued
Single Chamber Rate Responsive — continued
Chest 0JH6
Packing
Abdominal Wall 2W43X5Z
Anorectal 2Y43X5Z
Arm
Lower
Left 2W4DX5Z
Right 2W4CX5Z
Upper
Left 2W4BX5Z
Right 2W4AX5Z
Back 2W45X5Z
Chest Wall 2W44X5Z
Ear 2Y42X5Z
Extremity
Lower
Left 2W4MX5Z
Right 2W4LX5Z
Upper
Left 2W49X5Z
Right 2W48X5Z
Face 2W41X5Z
Finger
Left 2W4KX5Z
Right 2W4JX5Z
Foot
Left 2W4TX5Z
Right 2W4SX5Z
Genital Tract, Female 2Y44X5Z
Hand
Left 2W4FX5Z
Right 2W4EX5Z
Head 2W40X5Z
Inguinal Region
Left 2W47X5Z
Right 2W46X5Z
Leg
Lower
Left 2W4RX5Z
Right 2W4QX5Z
Upper
Left 2W4PX5Z
Right 2W4NX5Z
Mouth and Pharynx 2Y40X5Z
Nasal 2Y41X5Z
Neck 2W42X5Z
Thumb
Left 2W4HX5Z
Right 2W4GX5Z
Toe
Left 2W4VX5Z
Right 2W4UX5Z
Urethra 2Y45X5Z
Paclitaxel-eluting coronary stent *use* Intraluminal Device, Drug-eluting in Heart and Great Vessels
Paclitaxel-eluting peripheral stent
use Intraluminal Device, Drug-eluting in Lower Arteries
use Intraluminal Device, Drug-eluting in Upper Arteries
Palatine gland *use* Buccal Mucosa
Palatine tonsil *use* Tonsils
Palatine uvula *use* Uvula
Palatoglossal muscle *use* Muscle, Tongue, Palate, Pharynx
Palatopharyngeal muscle *use* Muscle, Tongue, Palate, Pharynx
Palatoplasty
see Repair, Mouth and Throat 0CQ
see Replacement, Mouth and Throat 0CR
see Supplement, Mouth and Throat 0CU
Palatorrhaphy *see* Repair, Mouth and Throat 0CQ
Palmar cutaneous nerve
use Nerve, Median
use Nerve, Radial
Palmar (volar) digital vein
use Vein, Hand, Left
use Vein, Hand, Right
Palmar fascia (aponeurosis)
use Subcutaneous Tissue and Fascia, Hand, Left
use Subcutaneous Tissue and Fascia, Hand, Right
Palmar interosseous muscle
use Muscle, Hand, Left
use Muscle, Hand, Right
Palmar (volar) metacarpal vein
use Vein, Hand, Left
use Vein, Hand, Right
Palmar ulnocarpal ligament
use Bursa and Ligament, Wrist, Left
use Bursa and Ligament, Wrist, Right
Palmaris longus muscle
use Muscle, Lower Arm and Wrist, Left
use Muscle, Lower Arm and Wrist, Right
Pancreatectomy
see Excision, Pancreas 0FBG
see Resection, Pancreas 0FTG
Pancreatic artery *use* Artery, Splenic
Pancreatic plexus *use* Nerve, Abdominal Sympathetic
Pancreatic vein *use* Vein, Splenic
Pancreaticoduodenostomy *see* Bypass, Hepatobiliary System and Pancreas 0F1
Pancreaticosplenic lymph node *use* Lymphatic, Aortic
Pancreatogram, endoscopic retrograde *see* Fluoroscopy, Pancreatic Duct BF18
Pancreatolithotomy *see* Extirpation, Pancreas 0FCG
Pancreatotomy
see Division, Pancreas 0F8G
see Drainage, Pancreas 0F9G
Panniculectomy
see Excision, Abdominal Wall 0WBF
see Excision, Skin, Abdomen 0HB7
Paraaortic lymph node *use* Lymphatic, Aortic
Paracentesis
Eye *see* Drainage, Eye 089
Peritoneal Cavity *see* Drainage, Peritoneal Cavity 0W9G
Tympanum *see* Drainage, Ear, Nose, Sinus 099
Pararectal lymph node *use* Lymphatic, Mesenteric
Parasternal lymph node *use* Lymphatic, Thorax
Parathyroidectomy
see Excision, Endocrine System 0GB
see Resection, Endocrine System 0GT
Paratracheal lymph node *use* Lymphatic, Thorax
Paraurethral (Skene's) gland *use* Gland, Vestibular
Parenteral nutrition, total *see* Introduction of Nutritional Substance
Parietal lobe *use* Cerebral Hemisphere
Parotid lymph node *use* Lymphatic, Head
Parotid plexus *use* Nerve, Facial
Parotidectomy
see Excision, Mouth and Throat 0CB
see Resection, Mouth and Throat 0CT
Pars flaccida
use Tympanic Membrane, Left
use Tympanic Membrane, Right
Partial joint replacement
Hip *see* Replacement, Lower Joints 0SR
Knee *see* Replacement, Lower Joints 0SR
Shoulder *see* Replacement, Upper Joints 0RR
Partially absorbable mesh *use* Synthetic Substitute
Patch, blood, spinal 3E0S3GC
Patellapexy
see Repair, Lower Bones 0QQ
see Reposition, Lower Bones 0QS
Patellaplasty
see Repair, Lower Bones 0QQ
see Replacement, Lower Bones 0QR
see Supplement, Lower Bones 0QU
Patellar ligament
use Bursa and Ligament, Knee, Left
use Bursa and Ligament, Knee, Right
Patellar tendon
use Tendon, Knee, Left
use Tendon, Knee, Right
Patellectomy
see Excision, Lower Bones 0QB
see Resection, Lower Bones 0QT
Patellofemoral joint
use Joint, Knee, Left
use Joint, Knee, Left, Femoral Surface
use Joint, Knee, Right
use Joint, Knee, Right, Femoral Surface
Pectineus muscle
use Muscle, Upper Leg, Left
use Muscle, Upper Leg, Right
Pectoral fascia *use* Subcutaneous Tissue and Fascia, Chest

Subterms under main terms may continue to next column or page

Pectoral (anterior) lymph node
use Lymphatic, Axillary, Left
use Lymphatic, Axillary, Right
Pectoralis major muscle
use Muscle, Thorax, Left
use Muscle, Thorax, Right
Pectoralis minor muscle
use Muscle, Thorax, Left
use Muscle, Thorax, Right
Pedicle-based dynamic stabilization device
use Spinal Stabilization Device, Pedicle-Based in ØRH
use Spinal Stabilization Device, Pedicle-Based in ØSH
PEEP (positive end expiratory pressure) *see* Assistance, Respiratory 5AØ9
PEG (percutaneous endoscopic gastrostomy) ØDH64UZ
PEJ (percutaneous endoscopic jejunostomy) ØDHA4UZ
Pelvic splanchnic nerve
use Nerve, Abdominal Sympathetic
use Nerve, Sacral Sympathetic
Penectomy
see Excision, Male Reproductive System ØVB
see Resection, Male Reproductive System ØVT
Penile urethra *use* Urethra
Percutaneous endoscopic gastrojejunostomy (PEG/J) tube *use* Feeding Device in Gastrointestinal System
Percutaneous endoscopic gastrostomy (PEG) tube *use* Feeding Device in Gastrointestinal System
Percutaneous nephrostomy catheter *use* Drainage Device
Percutaneous transluminal coronary angioplasty (PTCA) *see* Dilation, Heart and Great Vessels Ø27
Performance
Biliary
Multiple, Filtration 5A1C6ØZ
Single, Filtration 5A1CØØZ
Cardiac
Continuous
Output 5A1221Z
Pacing 5A1223Z
Intermittent, Pacing 5A1213Z
Single, Output, Manual 5A12Ø12
Circulatory, Continuous, Oxygenation, Membrane 5A15223
Respiratory
24-96 Consecutive Hours, Ventilation 5A1945Z
Greater than 96 Consecutive Hours, Ventilation 5A1955Z
Less than 24 Consecutive Hours, Ventilation 5A1935Z
Single, Ventilation, Nonmechanical 5A19Ø54
Urinary
Multiple, Filtration 5A1D6ØZ
Single, Filtration 5A1DØØZ
Perfusion *see* Introduction of substance in or on
Pericardiectomy
see Excision, Pericardium Ø2BN
see Resection, Pericardium Ø2TN
Pericardiocentesis *see* Drainage, Pericardial Cavity ØW9D
Pericardiolysis *see* Release, Pericardium Ø2NN
Pericardiophrenic artery
use Artery, Internal Mammary, Left
use Artery, Internal Mammary, Right
Pericardioplasty
see Repair, Pericardium Ø2QN
see Replacement, Pericardium Ø2RN
see Supplement, Pericardium Ø2UN
Pericardiorrhaphy *see* Repair, Pericardium Ø2QN
Pericardiostomy *see* Drainage, Pericardial Cavity ØW9D
Pericardiotomy *see* Drainage, Pericardial Cavity ØW9D
Perimetrium *use* Uterus
Peripheral parenteral nutrition *see* Introduction of Nutritional Substance
Peripherally inserted central catheter (PICC) *use* Infusion Device
Peritoneal dialysis 3E1M39Z
Peritoneocentesis
see Drainage, Peritoneal Cavity ØW9G
see Drainage, Peritoneum ØD9W
Peritoneoplasty
see Repair, Peritoneum ØDQW
see Replacement, Peritoneum ØDRW
Peritoneoplasty — continued
see Supplement, Peritoneum ØDUW
Peritoneoscopy ØDJW4ZZ
Peritoneotomy *see* Drainage, Peritoneum ØD9W
Peritoneumectomy *see* Excision, Peritoneum ØDBW
Peroneus brevis muscle
use Muscle, Lower Leg, Left
use Muscle, Lower Leg, Right
Peroneus longus muscle
use Muscle, Lower Leg, Left
use Muscle, Lower Leg, Right
Pessary ring *use* Intraluminal Device, Pessary in Female Reproductive System
PET scan *see* Positron Emission Tomographic (PET) Imaging
Petrous part of temoporal bone
use Bone, Temporal, Left
use Bone, Temporal, Right
Phacoemulsification, lens
With IOL implant *see* Replacement, Eye Ø8R
Without IOL implant *see* Extraction, Eye Ø8D
Phalangectomy
see Excision, Lower Bones ØQB
see Excision, Upper Bones ØPB
see Resection, Lower Bones ØQT
see Resection, Upper Bones ØPT
Phallectomy
see Excision, Penis ØVBS
see Resection, Penis ØVTS
Phalloplasty
see Repair, Penis ØVQS
see Supplement, Penis ØVUS
Phallotomy *see* Drainage, Penis ØV9S
Pharmacotherapy, for substance abuse
Antabuse HZ93ZZZ
Bupropion HZ97ZZZ
Clonidine HZ96ZZZ
Levo-alpha-acetyl-methadol (LAAM) HZ92ZZZ
Methadone Maintenance HZ91ZZZ
Naloxone HZ95ZZZ
Naltrexone HZ94ZZZ
Nicotine Replacement HZ9ØZZZ
Psychiatric Medication HZ98ZZZ
Replacement Medication, Other HZ99ZZZ
Pharyngeal constrictor muscle *use* Muscle, Tongue, Palate, Pharynx
Pharyngeal plexus *use* Nerve, Vagus
Pharyngeal recess *use* Nasopharynx
Pharyngeal tonsil *use* Adenoids
Pharyngogram *see* Fluoroscopy, Pharynix B91G
Pharyngoplasty
see Repair, Mouth and Throat ØCQ
see Replacement, Mouth and Throat ØCR
see Supplement, Mouth and Throat ØCU
Pharyngorrhaphy *see* Repair, Mouth and Throat ØCQ
Pharyngotomy *see* Drainage, Mouth and Throat ØC9
Pharyngotympanic tube
use Eustachian Tube, Left
use Eustachian Tube, Right
Pheresis
Erythrocytes 6A55
Leukocytes 6A55
Plasma 6A55
Platelets 6A55
Stem Cells
Cord Blood 6A55
Hematopoietic 6A55
Phlebectomy
see Excision, Lower Veins Ø6B
see Excision, Upper Veins Ø5B
see Extraction, Lower Veins Ø6D
see Extraction, Upper Veins Ø5D
Phlebography
see Plain Radiography, Veins B5Ø
Impedance 4AØ4X51
Phleborrhaphy
see Repair, Lower Veins Ø6Q
see Repair, Upper Veins Ø5Q
Phlebotomy
see Drainage, Lower Veins Ø69
see Drainage, Upper Veins Ø59
Photocoagulation
for Destruction *see* Destruction
for Repair *see* Repair
Photopheresis, therapeutic *see* Phototherapy, Circulatory 6A65
Phototherapy
Circulatory 6A65
Skin 6A6Ø
Phrenectomy, phrenoneurectomy *see* Excision, Nerve, Phrenic Ø1B2
Phrenemphraxis *see* Destruction, Nerve, Phrenic Ø152
Phrenic nerve stimulator generator *use* Stimulator Generator in Subcutaneous Tissue and Fascia
Phrenic nerve stimulator lead *use* Diaphragmatic Pacemaker Lead in Respiratory System
Phreniclasis *see* Destruction, Nerve, Phrenic Ø152
Phrenicoexeresis *see* Extraction, Nerve, Phrenic Ø1D2
Phrenicotomy *see* Division, Nerve, Phrenic Ø182
Phrenicotripsy *see* Destruction, Nerve, Phrenic Ø152
Phrenoplasty
see Repair, Respiratory System ØBQ
see Supplement, Respiratory System ØBU
Phrenotomy *see* Drainage, Respiratory System ØB9
Physiatry *see* Motor Treatment, Rehabilitation FØ7
Physical medicine *see* Motor Treatment, Rehabilitation FØ7
Physical therapy *see* Motor Treatment, Rehabilitation FØ7
PHYSIOMESH™ Flexible Composite Mesh *use* Synthetic Substitute
Pia mater
use Cerebral Meninges
use Spinal Meninges
Pinealectomy
see Excision, Pineal Body ØGB1
see Resection, Pineal Body ØGT1
Pinealoscopy ØGJ14ZZ
Pinealotomy *see* Drainage, Pineal Body ØG91
Pinna
use Ear, External, Bilateral
use Ear, External, Left
use Ear, External, Right
Pipeline™ Embolization device (PED) *use* Intraluminal Device
Piriform recess (sinus) *use* Pharynx
Piriformis muscle
use Muscle, Hip, Left
use Muscle, Hip, Right
Pisiform bone
use Carpal, Left
use Carpal, Right
Pisohamate ligament
use Bursa and Ligament, Hand, Left
use Bursa and Ligament, Hand, Right
Pisometacarpal ligament
use Bursa and Ligament, Hand, Left
use Bursa and Ligament, Hand, Right
Pituitectomy
see Excision, Gland, Pituitary ØGBØ
see Resection, Gland, Pituitary ØGTØ
Plain film radiology *see* Plain Radiography
Plain Radiography
Abdomen BWØØZZZ
Abdomen and Pelvis BWØ1ZZZ
Abdominal Lymphatic
Bilateral B7Ø1
Unilateral B7ØØ
Airway, Upper BBØDZZZ
Ankle
Left BQØH
Right BQØG
Aorta
Abdominal B4ØØ
Thoracic B3ØØ
Thoraco-Abdominal B3ØP
Aorta and Bilateral Lower Extremity Arteries B4ØD
Arch
Bilateral BNØDZZZ
Left BNØCZZZ
Right BNØBZZZ
Arm
Left BPØFZZZ
Right BPØEZZZ
Artery
Brachiocephalic-Subclavian, Right B3Ø1
Bronchial B3ØL
Bypass Graft, Other B2ØF
Cervico-Cerebral Arch B3ØQ

Subterms under main terms may continue to next column or page

- Plain Radiography — continued
  - Artery — continued
    - Common Carotid
      - Bilateral B3Ø5
      - Left B3Ø4
      - Right B3Ø3
    - Coronary
      - Bypass Graft
        - Multiple B2Ø3
        - Single B2Ø2
      - Multiple B2Ø1
      - Single B2ØØ
    - External Carotid
      - Bilateral B3ØC
      - Left B3ØB
      - Right B3Ø9
    - Hepatic B4Ø2
    - Inferior Mesenteric B4Ø5
    - Intercostal B3ØL
    - Internal Carotid
      - Bilateral B3Ø8
      - Left B3Ø7
      - Right B3Ø6
    - Internal Mammary Bypass Graft
      - Left B2Ø8
      - Right B2Ø7
    - Intra-Abdominal, Other B4ØB
    - Intracranial B3ØR
    - Lower Extremity
      - Bilateral and Aorta B4ØD
      - Left B4ØG
      - Right B4ØF
    - Lower, Other B4ØJ
    - Lumbar B4Ø9
    - Pelvic B4ØC
    - Pulmonary
      - Left B3ØT
      - Right B3ØS
    - Renal
      - Bilateral B4Ø8
      - Left B4Ø7
      - Right B4Ø6
      - Transplant B4ØM
    - Spinal B3ØM
    - Splenic B4Ø3
    - Subclavian, Left B3Ø2
    - Superior Mesenteric B4Ø4
    - Upper Extremity
      - Bilateral B3ØK
      - Left B3ØJ
      - Right B3ØH
    - Upper, Other B3ØN
    - Vertebral
      - Bilateral B3ØG
      - Left B3ØF
      - Right B3ØD
  - Bile Duct BFØØ
  - Bile Duct and Gallbladder BFØ3
  - Bladder BTØØ
    - Kidney and Ureter BTØ4
  - Bladder and Urethra BTØB
  - Bone
    - Facial BNØ5ZZZ
    - Nasal BNØ4ZZZ
  - Bones, Long, All BWØBZZZ
  - Breast
    - Bilateral BHØ2ZZZ
    - Left BHØ1ZZZ
    - Right BHØØZZZ
  - Calcaneus
    - Left BQØKZZZ
    - Right BQØJZZZ
  - Chest BWØ3ZZZ
  - Clavicle
    - Left BPØ5ZZZ
    - Right BPØ4ZZZ
  - Coccyx BRØFZZZ
  - Corpora Cavernosa BVØØ
  - Dialysis Fistula B5ØW
  - Dialysis Shunt B5ØW
  - Disc
    - Cervical BRØ1
    - Lumbar BRØ3
    - Thoracic BRØ2

- Plain Radiography — continued
  - Duct
    - Lacrimal
      - Bilateral B8Ø2
      - Left B8Ø1
      - Right B8ØØ
    - Mammary
      - Multiple
        - Left BHØ6
        - Right BHØ5
      - Single
        - Left BHØ4
        - Right BHØ3
  - Elbow
    - Left BPØH
    - Right BPØG
  - Epididymis
    - Left BVØ2
    - Right BVØ1
  - Extremity
    - Lower BWØCZZZ
    - Upper BWØJZZZ
  - Eye
    - Bilateral B8Ø7ZZZ
    - Left B8Ø6ZZZ
    - Right B8Ø5ZZZ
  - Facet Joint
    - Cervical BRØ4
    - Lumbar BRØ6
    - Thoracic BRØ5
  - Fallopian Tube
    - Bilateral BUØ2
    - Left BUØ1
    - Right BUØØ
  - Fallopian Tube and Uterus BUØ8
  - Femur
    - Left, Densitometry BQØ4ZZ1
    - Right, Densitometry BQØ3ZZ1
  - Finger
    - Left BPØSZZZ
    - Right BPØRZZZ
  - Foot
    - Left BQØMZZZ
    - Right BQØLZZZ
  - Forearm
    - Left BPØKZZZ
    - Right BPØJZZZ
  - Gallbladder and Bile Duct BFØ3
  - Gland
    - Parotid
      - Bilateral B9Ø6
      - Left B9Ø5
      - Right B9Ø4
    - Salivary
      - Bilateral B9ØD
      - Left B9ØC
      - Right B9ØB
    - Submandibular
      - Bilateral B9Ø9
      - Left B9Ø8
      - Right B9Ø7
  - Hand
    - Left BPØPZZZ
    - Right BPØNZZZ
  - Heart
    - Left B2Ø5
    - Right B2Ø4
    - Right and Left B2Ø6
  - Hepatobiliary System, All BFØC
  - Hip
    - Left BQØ1
      - Densitometry BQØ1ZZ1
    - Right BQØØ
      - Densitometry BQØØZZ1
  - Humerus
    - Left BPØBZZZ
    - Right BPØAZZZ
  - Ileal Diversion Loop BTØC
  - Intracranial Sinus B5Ø2
  - Joint
    - Acromioclavicular, Bilateral BPØ3ZZZ
    - Finger
      - Left BPØD
      - Right BPØC
    - Foot
      - Left BQØY

- Plain Radiography — continued
  - Joint — continued
    - Foot — continued
      - Right BQØX
    - Hand
      - Left BPØD
      - Right BPØC
    - Lumbosacral BRØBZZZ
    - Sacroiliac BRØD
    - Sternoclavicular
      - Bilateral BPØ2ZZZ
      - Left BPØ1ZZZ
      - Right BPØØZZZ
    - Temporomandibular
      - Bilateral BNØ9
      - Left BNØ8
      - Right BNØ7
    - Thoracolumbar BRØ8ZZZ
    - Toe
      - Left BQØY
      - Right BQØX
  - Kidney
    - Bilateral BTØ3
    - Left BTØ2
    - Right BTØ1
    - Ureter and Bladder BTØ4
  - Knee
    - Left BQØ8
    - Right BQØ7
  - Leg
    - Left BQØFZZZ
    - Right BQØDZZZ
  - Lymphatic
    - Head B7Ø4
    - Lower Extremity
      - Bilateral B7ØB
      - Left B7Ø9
      - Right B7Ø8
    - Neck B7Ø4
    - Pelvic B7ØC
    - Upper Extremity
      - Bilateral B7Ø7
      - Left B7Ø6
      - Right B7Ø5
  - Mandible BNØ6ZZZ
  - Mastoid B9ØHZZZ
  - Nasopharynx B9ØFZZZ
  - Optic Foramina
    - Left B8Ø4ZZZ
    - Right B8Ø3ZZZ
  - Orbit
    - Bilateral BNØ3ZZZ
    - Left BNØ2ZZZ
    - Right BNØ1ZZZ
  - Oropharynx B9ØFZZZ
  - Patella
    - Left BQØWZZZ
    - Right BQØVZZZ
  - Pelvis BRØCZZZ
  - Pelvis and Abdomen BWØ1ZZZ
  - Prostate BVØ3
  - Retroperitoneal Lymphatic
    - Bilateral B7Ø1
    - Unilateral B7ØØ
  - Ribs
    - Left BPØYZZZ
    - Right BPØXZZZ
  - Sacrum BRØFZZZ
  - Scapula
    - Left BPØ7ZZZ
    - Right BPØ6ZZZ
  - Shoulder
    - Left BPØ9
    - Right BPØ8
  - Sinus
    - Intracranial B5Ø2
    - Paranasal B9Ø2ZZZ
  - Skull BNØØZZZ
  - Spinal Cord BØØB
  - Spine
    - Cervical, Densitometry BRØØZZ1
    - Lumbar, Densitometry BRØ9ZZ1
    - Thoracic, Densitometry BRØ7ZZ1
    - Whole, Densitometry BRØGZZ1
  - Sternum BRØHZZZ

Plain Radiography — continued
Teeth
All BNØJZZZ
Multiple BNØHZZZ
Testicle
Left BVØ6
Right BVØ5
Toe
Left BQØQZZZ
Right BQØPZZZ
Tooth, Single BNØGZZZ
Tracheobronchial Tree
Bilateral BBØ9YZZ
Left BBØ8YZZ
Right BBØ7YZZ
Ureter
Bilateral BTØ8
Kidney and Bladder BTØ4
Left BTØ7
Right BTØ6
Urethra BTØ5
Urethra and Bladder BTØB
Uterus BUØ6
Uterus and Fallopian Tube BUØ8
Vagina BUØ9
Vasa Vasorum BVØ8
Vein
Cerebellar B5Ø1
Cerebral B5Ø1
Epidural B5ØØ
Jugular
Bilateral B5Ø5
Left B5Ø4
Right B5Ø3
Lower Extremity
Bilateral B5ØD
Left B5ØC
Right B5ØB
Other B5ØV
Pelvic (Iliac)
Left B5ØG
Right B5ØF
Pelvic (Iliac) Bilateral B5ØH
Portal B5ØT
Pulmonary
Bilateral B5ØS
Left B5ØR
Right B5ØQ
Renal
Bilateral B5ØL
Left B5ØK
Right B5ØJ
Spanchnic B5ØT
Subclavian
Left B5Ø7
Right B5Ø6
Upper Extremity
Bilateral B5ØP
Left B5ØN
Right B5ØM
Vena Cava
Inferior B5Ø9
Superior B5Ø8
Whole Body BWØKZZZ
Infant BWØMZZZ
Whole Skeleton BWØLZZZ
Wrist
Left BPØM
Right BPØL
Planar Nuclear Medicine Imaging CP1
Abdomen CW1Ø
Abdomen and Chest CW14
Abdomen and Pelvis CW11
Anatomical Regions, Multiple CW1YYZZ
Bladder and Ureters CT1H
Bladder, Kidneys and Ureters CT13
Blood C713
Bone Marrow C71Ø
Brain CØ1Ø
Breast CH1YYZZ
Bilateral CH12
Left CH11
Right CH1Ø
Bronchi and Lungs CB12
Central Nervous System CØ1YYZZ
Cerebrospinal Fluid CØ15
Planar Nuclear Medicine Imaging — continued
Chest CW13
Chest and Abdomen CW14
Chest and Neck CW16
Digestive System CD1YYZZ
Ducts, Lacrimal, Bilateral C819
Ear, Nose, Mouth and Throat C91YYZZ
Endocrine System CG1YYZZ
Extremity
Lower CW1D
Bilateral CP1F
Left CP1D
Right CP1C
Upper CW1M
Bilateral CP1B
Left CP19
Right CP18
Eye C81YYZZ
Gallbladder CF14
Gastrointestinal Tract CD17
Upper CD15
Gland
Adrenal, Bilateral CG14
Parathyroid CG11
Thyroid CG12
Glands, Salivary, Bilateral C91B
Head and Neck CW1B
Heart C21YYZZ
Right and Left C216
Hepatobiliary System, All CF1C
Hepatobiliary System and Pancreas CF1YYZZ
Kidneys, Ureters and Bladder CT13
Liver CF15
Liver and Spleen CF16
Lungs and Bronchi CB12
Lymphatics
Head C71J
Head and Neck C715
Lower Extremity C71P
Neck C71K
Pelvic C71D
Trunk C71M
Upper Chest C71L
Upper Extremity C71N
Lymphatics and Hematologic System C71YYZZ
Musculoskeletal System, All CP1Z
Myocardium C21G
Neck and Chest CW16
Neck and Head CW1B
Pancreas and Hepatobiliary System CF1YYZZ
Pelvic Region CW1J
Pelvis CP16
Pelvis and Abdomen CW11
Pelvis and Spine CP17
Reproductive System, Male CV1YYZZ
Respiratory System CB1YYZZ
Skin CH1YYZZ
Skull CP11
Spine CP15
Spine and Pelvis CP17
Spleen C712
Spleen and Liver CF16
Subcutaneous Tissue CH1YYZZ
Testicles, Bilateral CV19
Thorax CP14
Ureters and Bladder CT1H
Ureters, Kidneys and Bladder CT13
Urinary System CT1YYZZ
Veins C51YYZZ
Central C51R
Lower Extremity
Bilateral C51D
Left C51C
Right C51B
Upper Extremity
Bilateral C51Q
Left C51P
Right C51N
Whole Body CW1N
Plantar digital vein
use Vein, Foot, Left
use Vein, Foot, Right
Plantar fascia (aponeurosis)
use Subcutaneous Tissue and Fascia, Foot, Left
use Subcutaneous Tissue and Fascia, Foot, Right
Plantar metatarsal vein
use Vein, Foot, Left
use Vein, Foot, Right
Plantar venous arch
use Vein, Foot, Left
use Vein, Foot, Right
Plaque Radiation
Abdomen DWY3FZZ
Adrenal Gland DGY2FZZ
Anus DDY8FZZ
Bile Ducts DFY2FZZ
Bladder DTY2FZZ
Bone Marrow D7YØFZZ
Bone, Other DPYCFZZ
Brain DØYØFZZ
Brain Stem DØY1FZZ
Breast
Left DMYØFZZ
Right DMY1FZZ
Bronchus DBY1FZZ
Cervix DUY1FZZ
Chest DWY2FZZ
Chest Wall DBY7FZZ
Colon DDY5FZZ
Diaphragm DBY8FZZ
Duodenum DDY2FZZ
Ear D9YØFZZ
Esophagus DDYØFZZ
Eye D8YØFZZ
Femur DPY9FZZ
Fibula DPYBFZZ
Gallbladder DFY1FZZ
Gland
Adrenal DGY2FZZ
Parathyroid DGY4FZZ
Pituitary DGYØFZZ
Thyroid DGY5FZZ
Glands, Salivary D9Y6FZZ
Head and Neck DWY1FZZ
Hemibody DWY4FZZ
Humerus DPY6FZZ
Ileum DDY4FZZ
Jejunum DDY3FZZ
Kidney DTYØFZZ
Larynx D9YBFZZ
Liver DFYØFZZ
Lung DBY2FZZ
Lymphatics
Abdomen D7Y6FZZ
Axillary D7Y4FZZ
Inguinal D7Y8FZZ
Neck D7Y3FZZ
Pelvis D7Y7FZZ
Thorax D7Y5FZZ
Mandible DPY3FZZ
Maxilla DPY2FZZ
Mediastinum DBY6FZZ
Mouth D9Y4FZZ
Nasopharynx D9YDFZZ
Neck and Head DWY1FZZ
Nerve, Peripheral DØY7FZZ
Nose D9Y1FZZ
Ovary DUYØFZZ
Palate
Hard D9Y8FZZ
Soft D9Y9FZZ
Pancreas DFY3FZZ
Parathyroid Gland DGY4FZZ
Pelvic Bones DPY8FZZ
Pelvic Region DWY6FZZ
Pharynx D9YCFZZ
Pineal Body DGY1FZZ
Pituitary Gland DGYØFZZ
Pleura DBY5FZZ
Prostate DVYØFZZ
Radius DPY7FZZ
Rectum DDY7FZZ
Rib DPY5FZZ
Sinuses D9Y7FZZ
Skin
Abdomen DHY8FZZ
Arm DHY4FZZ
Back DHY7FZZ
Buttock DHY9FZZ
Chest DHY6FZZ
Face DHY2FZZ

Plaque Radiation — continued
  Skin — continued
    Foot DHYCFZZ
    Hand DHY5FZZ
    Leg DHYBFZZ
    Neck DHY3FZZ
  Skull DPYØFZZ
  Spinal Cord DØY6FZZ
  Spleen D7Y2FZZ
  Sternum DPY4FZZ
  Stomach DDY1FZZ
  Testis DVY1FZZ
  Thymus D7Y1FZZ
  Thyroid Gland DGY5FZZ
  Tibia DPYBFZZ
  Tongue D9Y5FZZ
  Trachea DBYØFZZ
  Ulna DPY7FZZ
  Ureter DTY1FZZ
  Urethra DTY3FZZ
  Uterus DUY2FZZ
  Whole Body DWY5FZZ
Plasmapheresis, therapeutic 6A55ØZ3
Plateletpheresis, therapeutic 6A55ØZ2
Platysma muscle
  use Muscle, Neck, Left
  use Muscle, Neck, Right
Pleurectomy
  see Excision, Respiratory System ØBB
  see Resection, Respiratory System ØBT
Pleurocentesis *see* Drainage, Anatomical Regions, General ØW9
Pleurodesis, pleurosclerosis
  Chemical injection *see* Introduction of Substance in or on, Pleural Cavity 3EØL
  Surgical *see* Destruction, Respiratory System ØB5
Pleurolysis *see* Release, Respiratory System ØBN
Pleuroscopy ØBJQ4ZZ
Pleurotomy *see* Drainage, Respiratory System ØB9
Plica semilunaris
  use Conjunctiva, Left
  use Conjunctiva, Right
Plication *see* Restriction
Pneumectomy
  see Excision, Respiratory System ØBB
  see Resection, Respiratory System ØBT
Pneumocentesis *see* Drainage, Respiratory System ØB9
Pneumogastric nerve *use* Nerve, Vagus
Pneumolysis *see* Release, Respiratory System ØBN
Pneumonectomy *see* Resection, Respiratory System ØBT
Pneumonolysis *see* Release, Respiratory System ØBN
Pneumonopexy
  see Repair, Respiratory System ØBQ
  see Reposition, Respiratory System ØBS
Pneumonorrhaphy *see* Repair, Respiratory System ØBQ
Pneumonotomy *see* Drainage, Respiratory System ØB9
Pneumotaxic center *use* Pons
Pneumotomy *see* Drainage, Respiratory System ØB9
Pollicization *see* Transfer, Anatomical Regions, Upper Extremities ØXX
Polyethylene socket *use* Synthetic Substitute, Polyethylene in ØSR
Polymethylmethacrylate (PMMA) *use* Synthetic Substitute
Polypectomy, gastrointestinal *see* Excision, Gastrointestinal System ØDB
Polypropylene mesh *use* Synthetic Substitute
Polysomnogram 4A1ZXQZ
Pontine tegmentum *use* Pons
Popliteal ligament
  use Bursa and Ligament, Knee, Left
  use Bursa and Ligament, Knee, Right
Popliteal lymph node
  use Lymphatic, Lower Extremity, Left
  use Lymphatic, Lower Extremity, Right
Popliteal vein
  use Vein, Femoral, Left
  use Vein, Femoral, Right
Popliteus muscle
  use Muscle, Lower Leg, Left
  use Muscle, Lower Leg, Right
Porcine (bioprosthetic) valve *use* Zooplastic Tissue in Heart and Great Vessels
Positive end expiratory pressure *see* Performance, Respiratory 5A19
Positron Emission Tomographic (PET) Imaging
  Brain CØ3Ø
  Bronchi and Lungs CB32
  Central Nervous System CØ3YYZZ
  Heart C23YYZZ
  Lungs and Bronchi CB32
  Myocardium C23G
  Respiratory System CB3YYZZ
  Whole Body CW3NYZZ
Positron emission tomography *see* Positron Emission Tomographic (PET) Imaging
Postauricular (mastoid) lymph node
  use Lymphatic, Neck, Left
  use Lymphatic, Neck, Right
Postcava *use* Vena Cava, Inferior
Posterior auricular artery
  use Artery, External Carotid, Left
  use Artery, External Carotid, Right
Posterior auricular nerve *use* Nerve, Facial
Posterior auricular vein
  use Vein, External Jugular, Left
  use Vein, External Jugular, Right
Posterior cerebral artery *use* Artery, Intracranial
Posterior chamber
  use Eye, Left
  use Eye, Right
Posterior circumflex humeral artery
  use Artery, Axillary, Left
  use Artery, Axillary, Right
Posterior communicating artery *use* Artery, Intracranial
Posterior cruciate ligament (PCL)
  use Bursa and Ligament, Knee, Left
  use Bursa and Ligament, Knee, Right
Posterior facial (retromandibular) vein
  use Vein, Face, Left
  use Vein, Face, Right
Posterior femoral cutaneous nerve *use* Nerve, Sacral Plexus
Posterior inferior cerebellar artery (PICA) *use* Artery, Intracranial
Posterior interosseous nerve *use* Nerve, Radial
Posterior labial nerve *use* Nerve, Pudendal
Posterior (subscapular) lymph node
  use Lymphatic, Axillary, Left
  use Lymphatic, Axillary, Right
Posterior scrotal nerve *use* Nerve, Pudendal
Posterior spinal artery
  use Artery, Vertebral, Left
  use Artery, Vertebral, Right
Posterior tibial recurrent artery
  use Artery, Anterior Tibial, Left
  use Artery, Anterior Tibial, Right
Posterior ulnar recurrent artery
  use Artery, Ulnar, Left
  use Artery, Ulnar, Right
Posterior vagal trunk *use* Nerve, Vagus
PPN (peripheral parenteral nutrition) *see* Introduction of Nutritional Substance
Preauricular lymph node *use* Lymphatic, Head
Precava *use* Vena Cava, Superior
Prepatellar bursa
  use Bursa and Ligament, Knee, Left
  use Bursa and Ligament, Knee, Right
Preputiotomy *see* Drainage, Male Reproductive System ØV9
Pressure support ventilation *see* Performance, Respiratory 5A19
PRESTIGE® Cervical Disc *use* Synthetic Substitute
Pretracheal fascia *use* Subcutaneous Tissue and Fascia, Neck, Anterior
Prevertebral fascia *use* Subcutaneous Tissue and Fascia, Neck, Posterior
PrimeAdvanced neurostimulator (SureScan) (MRI Safe) *use* Stimulator Generator, Multiple Array in ØJH
Princeps pollicis artery
  use Artery, Hand, Left
  use Artery, Hand, Right
Probing, duct
  Diagnostic *see* Inspection
  Dilation *see* Dilation
PROCEED™ Ventral Patch *use* Synthetic Substitute
Procerus muscle *use* Muscle, Facial
Proctectomy
  see Excision, Rectum ØDBP
  see Resection, Rectum ØDTP
Proctoclysis *see* Introduction of substance in or on, Gastrointestinal Tract, Lower 3EØH
Proctocolectomy
  see Excision, Gastrointestinal System ØDB
  see Resection, Gastrointestinal System ØDT
Proctocolpoplasty
  see Repair, Gastrointestinal System ØDQ
  see Supplement, Gastrointestinal System ØDU
Proctoperineoplasty
  see Repair, Gastrointestinal System ØDQ
  see Supplement, Gastrointestinal System ØDU
Proctoperineorrhaphy *see* Repair, Gastrointestinal System ØDQ
Proctopexy
  see Repair, Rectum ØDQP
  see Reposition, Rectum ØDSP
Proctoplasty
  see Repair, Rectum ØDQP
  see Supplement, Rectum ØDUP
Proctorrhaphy *see* Repair, Rectum ØDQP
Proctoscopy ØDJD8ZZ
Proctosigmoidectomy
  see Excision, Gastrointestinal System ØDB
  see Resection, Gastrointestinal System ØDT
Proctosigmoidoscopy ØDJD8ZZ
Proctostomy *see* Drainage, Rectum ØD9P
Proctotomy *see* Drainage, Rectum ØD9P
Prodisc-C *use* Synthetic Substitute
Prodisc-L *use* Synthetic Substitute
Production, atrial septal defect *see* Excision, Septum, Atrial Ø2B5
Profunda brachii
  use Artery, Brachial, Left
  use Artery, Brachial, Right
Profunda femoris (deep femoral) vein
  use Vein, Femoral, Left
  use Vein, Femoral, Right
PROLENE Polypropylene Hernia System (PHS) *use* Synthetic Substitute
Pronator quadratus muscle
  use Muscle, Lower Arm and Wrist, Left
  use Muscle, Lower Arm and Wrist, Right
Pronator teres muscle
  use Muscle, Lower Arm and Wrist, Left
  use Muscle, Lower Arm and Wrist, Right
Prostatectomy
  see Excision, Prostate ØVBØ
  see Resection, Prostate ØVTØ
Prostatic urethra *use* Urethra
Prostatomy, prostatotomy *see* Drainage, Prostate ØV9Ø
Protecta XT CRT-D *use* Cardiac Resynchronization Defibrillator Pulse Generator in ØJH
Protecta XT DR (XT VR) *use* Defibrillator Generator in ØJH
Protégé® RX Carotid Stent System *use* Intraluminal Device
Proximal radioulnar joint
  use Joint, Elbow, Left
  use Joint, Elbow, Right
Psoas muscle
  use Muscle, Hip, Left
  use Muscle, Hip, Right
PSV (pressure support ventilation) *see* Performance, Respiratory 5A19
Psychoanalysis GZ54ZZZ
Psychological Tests
  Cognitive Status GZ14ZZZ
  Developmental GZ1ØZZZ
  Intellectual and Psychoeducational GZ12ZZZ
  Neurobehavioral Status GZ14ZZZ
  Neuropsychological GZ13ZZZ
  Personality and Behavioral GZ11ZZZ
Psychotherapy
  Family, Mental Health Services GZ72ZZZ
  Group GZHZZZZ
    Mental Health Services GZHZZZZ

Subterms under main terms may continue to next column or page

Psychotherapy — continued
  Individual
    see Psychotherapy, Individual, Mental Health Services
    for substance abuse
      12-Step HZ53ZZZ
      Behavioral HZ51ZZZ
      Cognitive HZ50ZZZ
      Cognitive-Behavioral HZ52ZZZ
      Confrontational HZ58ZZZ
      Interactive HZ55ZZZ
      Interpersonal HZ54ZZZ
      Motivational Enhancement HZ57ZZZ
      Psychoanalysis HZ5BZZZ
      Psychodynamic HZ5CZZZ
      Psychoeducation HZ56ZZZ
      Psychophysiological HZ5DZZZ
      Supportive HZ59ZZZ
    Mental Health Services
      Behavioral GZ51ZZZ
      Cognitive GZ52ZZZ
      Cognitive-Behavioral GZ58ZZZ
      Interactive GZ50ZZZ
      Interpersonal GZ53ZZZ
      Psychoanalysis GZ54ZZZ
      Psychodynamic GZ55ZZZ
      Psychophysiological GZ59ZZZ
      Supportive GZ56ZZZ
PTCA (percutaneous transluminal coronary angioplasty) *see* Dilation, Heart and Great Vessels 027
Pterygoid muscle *use* Muscle, Head
Pterygoid process
  use Bone, Sphenoid, Left
  use Bone, Sphenoid, Right
Pterygopalatine (sphenopalatine) ganglion *use* Nerve, Head and Neck Sympathetic
Pubic ligament
  use Bursa and Ligament, Trunk, Left
  use Bursa and Ligament, Trunk, Right
Pubis
  use Bone, Pelvic, Left
  use Bone, Pelvic, Right
Pubofemoral ligament
  use Bursa and Ligament, Hip, Left
  use Bursa and Ligament, Hip, Right
Pudendal nerve *use* Nerve, Sacral Plexus
Pull-through, rectal *see* Resection, Rectum 0DTP
Pulmoaortic canal *use* Artery, Pulmonary, Left
Pulmonary annulus *use* Valve, Pulmonary
Pulmonary artery wedge monitoring *see* Monitoring, Arterial 4A13
Pulmonary plexus
  use Nerve, Thoracic Sympathetic
  use Nerve, Vagus
Pulmonic valve *use* Valve, Pulmonary
Pulpectomy *see* Excision, Mouth and Throat 0CB
Pulverization *see* Fragmentation
Pulvinar *use* Thalamus
Pump reservoir *use* Infusion Device, Pump in Subcutaneous Tissue and Fascia
Punch biopsy *see* Excision with qualifier Diagnostic
Puncture *see* Drainage
Puncture, lumbar *see* Drainage, Spinal Canal 009U
Pyelography
  see Fluoroscopy, Urinary System BT1
  see Plain Radiography, Urinary System BT0
Pyeloileostomy, urinary diversion *see* Bypass, Urinary System 0T1
Pyeloplasty
  see Repair, Urinary System 0TQ
  see Replacement, Urinary System 0TR
  see Supplement, Urinary System 0TU
Pyelorrhaphy *see* Repair, Urinary System 0TQ
Pyeloscopy 0TJ58ZZ
Pyelostomy
  see Bypass, Urinary System 0T1
  see Drainage, Urinary System 0T9
Pyelotomy *see* Drainage, Urinary System 0T9
Pylorectomy
  see Excision, Stomach, Pylorus 0DB7
  see Resection, Stomach, Pylorus 0DT7
Pyloric antrum *use* Stomach, Pylorus
Pyloric canal *use* Stomach, Pylorus
Pyloric sphincter *use* Stomach, Pylorus
Pylorodiosis *see* Dilation, Stomach, Pylorus 0D77
Pylorogastrectomy
  see Excision, Gastrointestinal System 0DB
  see Resection, Gastrointestinal System 0DT
Pyloroplasty
  see Repair, Stomach, Pylorus 0DQ7
  see Supplement, Stomach, Pylorus 0DU7
Pyloroscopy 0DJ68ZZ
Pylorotomy *see* Drainage, Stomach, Pylorus 0D97
Pyramidalis muscle
  use Muscle, Abdomen, Left
  use Muscle, Abdomen, Right

Q

Quadrangular cartilage *use* Septum, Nasal
Quadrant resection of breast *see* Excision, Skin and Breast 0HB
Quadrate lobe *use* Liver
Quadratus femoris muscle
  use Muscle, Hip, Left
  use Muscle, Hip, Right
Quadratus lumborum muscle
  use Muscle, Trunk, Left
  use Muscle, Trunk, Right
Quadratus plantae muscle
  use Muscle, Foot, Left
  use Muscle, Foot, Right
Quadriceps (femoris)
  use Muscle, Upper Leg, Left
  use Muscle, Upper Leg, Right
Quarantine 8E0ZXY6

R

Radial collateral carpal ligament
  use Bursa and Ligament, Wrist, Left
  use Bursa and Ligament, Wrist, Right
Radial collateral ligament
  use Bursa and Ligament, Elbow, Left
  use Bursa and Ligament, Elbow, Right
Radial notch
  use Ulna, Left
  use Ulna, Right
Radial recurrent artery
  use Artery, Radial, Left
  use Artery, Radial, Right
Radial vein
  use Vein, Brachial, Left
  use Vein, Brachial, Right
Radialis indicis
  use Artery, Hand, Left
  use Artery, Hand, Right
Radiation Therapy
  see Beam Radiation
  see Brachytherapy
Radiation treatment *see* Radiation Oncology
Radiocarpal joint
  use Joint, Wrist, Left
  use Joint, Wrist, Right
Radiocarpal ligament
  use Bursa and Ligament, Wrist, Left
  use Bursa and Ligament, Wrist, Right
Radiography *see* Plain Radiography
Radiology, analog *see* Plain Radiography
Radiology, diagnostic *see* Imaging, Diagnostic
Radioulnar ligament
  use Bursa and Ligament, Wrist, Left
  use Bursa and Ligament, Wrist, Right
Range of motion testing *see* Motor Function Assessment, Rehabilitation F01
REALIZE® Adjustable Gastric Band *use* Extraluminal Device
Reattachment
  Abdominal Wall 0WMF0ZZ
  Ampulla of Vater 0FMC
  Ankle Region
    Left 0YML0ZZ
    Right 0YMK0ZZ
  Arm
    Lower
      Left 0XMF0ZZ
      Right 0XMD0ZZ
Reattachment — continued
  Arm — continued
    Upper
      Left 0XM90ZZ
      Right 0XM80ZZ
  Axilla
    Left 0XM50ZZ
    Right 0XM40ZZ
  Back
    Lower 0WML0ZZ
    Upper 0WMK0ZZ
  Bladder 0TMB
  Bladder Neck 0TMC
  Breast
    Bilateral 0HMVXZZ
    Left 0HMUXZZ
    Right 0HMTXZZ
  Bronchus
    Lingula 0BM90ZZ
    Lower Lobe
      Left 0BMB0ZZ
      Right 0BM60ZZ
    Main
      Left 0BM70ZZ
      Right 0BM30ZZ
    Middle Lobe, Right 0BM50ZZ
    Upper Lobe
      Left 0BM80ZZ
      Right 0BM40ZZ
  Bursa and Ligament
    Abdomen
      Left 0MMJ
      Right 0MMH
    Ankle
      Left 0MMR
      Right 0MMQ
    Elbow
      Left 0MM4
      Right 0MM3
    Foot
      Left 0MMT
      Right 0MMS
    Hand
      Left 0MM8
      Right 0MM7
    Head and Neck 0MM0
    Hip
      Left 0MMM
      Right 0MML
    Knee
      Left 0MMP
      Right 0MMN
    Lower Extremity
      Left 0MMW
      Right 0MMV
    Perineum 0MMK
    Shoulder
      Left 0MM2
      Right 0MM1
    Thorax
      Left 0MMG
      Right 0MMF
    Trunk
      Left 0MMD
      Right 0MMC
    Upper Extremity
      Left 0MMB
      Right 0MM9
    Wrist
      Left 0MM6
      Right 0MM5
  Buttock
    Left 0YM10ZZ
    Right 0YM00ZZ
  Carina 0BM20ZZ
  Cecum 0DMH
  Cervix 0UMC
  Chest Wall 0WM80ZZ
  Clitoris 0UMJXZZ
  Colon
    Ascending 0DMK
    Descending 0DMM
    Sigmoid 0DMN
    Transverse 0DML
  Cord
    Bilateral 0VMH

Reattachment — continued
Cord — continued
Left ØVMG
Right ØVMF
Cul-de-sac ØUMF
Diaphragm
Left ØBMSØZZ
Right ØBMRØZZ
Duct
Common Bile ØFM9
Cystic ØFM8
Hepatic
Left ØFM6
Right ØFM5
Pancreatic ØFMD
Accessory ØFMF
Duodenum ØDM9
Ear
Left Ø9M1XZZ
Right Ø9MØXZZ
Elbow Region
Left ØXMCØZZ
Right ØXMBØZZ
Esophagus ØDM5
Extremity
Lower
Left ØYMBØZZ
Right ØYM9ØZZ
Upper
Left ØXM7ØZZ
Right ØXM6ØZZ
Eyelid
Lower
Left Ø8MRXZZ
Right Ø8MQXZZ
Upper
Left Ø8MPXZZ
Right Ø8MNXZZ
Face ØWM2ØZZ
Fallopian Tube
Left ØUM6
Right ØUM5
Fallopian Tubes, Bilateral ØUM7
Femoral Region
Left ØYM8ØZZ
Right ØYM7ØZZ
Finger
Index
Left ØXMPØZZ
Right ØXMNØZZ
Little
Left ØXMWØZZ
Right ØXMVØZZ
Middle
Left ØXMRØZZ
Right ØXMQØZZ
Ring
Left ØXMTØZZ
Right ØXMSØZZ
Foot
Left ØYMNØZZ
Right ØYMMØZZ
Forequarter
Left ØXM1ØZZ
Right ØXMØØZZ
Gallbladder ØFM4
Gland
Left ØGM2
Right ØGM3
Hand
Left ØXMKØZZ
Right ØXMJØZZ
Hindquarter
Bilateral ØYM4ØZZ
Left ØYM3ØZZ
Right ØYM2ØZZ
Hymen ØUMK
Ileum ØDMB
Inguinal Region
Left ØYM6ØZZ
Right ØYM5ØZZ
Intestine
Large ØDME
Left ØDMG
Right ØDMF
Small ØDM8

Reattachment — continued
Jaw
Lower ØWM5ØZZ
Upper ØWM4ØZZ
Jejunum ØDMA
Kidney
Left ØTM1
Right ØTMØ
Kidney Pelvis
Left ØTM4
Right ØTM3
Kidneys, Bilateral ØTM2
Knee Region
Left ØYMGØZZ
Right ØYMFØZZ
Leg
Lower
Left ØYMJØZZ
Right ØYMHØZZ
Upper
Left ØYMDØZZ
Right ØYMCØZZ
Lip
Lower ØCM1ØZZ
Upper ØCMØØZZ
Liver ØFMØ
Left Lobe ØFM2
Right Lobe ØFM1
Lung
Left ØBMLØZZ
Lower Lobe
Left ØBMJØZZ
Right ØBMFØZZ
Middle Lobe, Right ØBMDØZZ
Right ØBMKØZZ
Upper Lobe
Left ØBMGØZZ
Right ØBMCØZZ
Lung Lingula ØBMHØZZ
Muscle
Abdomen
Left ØKML
Right ØKMK
Facial ØKM1
Foot
Left ØKMW
Right ØKMV
Hand
Left ØKMD
Right ØKMC
Head ØKMØ
Hip
Left ØKMP
Right ØKMN
Lower Arm and Wrist
Left ØKMB
Right ØKM9
Lower Leg
Left ØKMT
Right ØKMS
Neck
Left ØKM3
Right ØKM2
Perineum ØKMM
Shoulder
Left ØKM6
Right ØKM5
Thorax
Left ØKMJ
Right ØKMH
Tongue, Palate, Pharynx ØKM4
Trunk
Left ØKMG
Right ØKMF
Upper Arm
Left ØKM8
Right ØKM7
Upper Leg
Left ØKMR
Right ØKMQ
Neck ØWM6ØZZ
Nipple
Left ØHMXXZZ
Right ØHMWXZZ
Nose Ø9MKXZZ

Reattachment — continued
Ovary
Bilateral ØUM2
Left ØUM1
Right ØUMØ
Palate, Soft ØCM3ØZZ
Pancreas ØFMG
Parathyroid Gland ØGMR
Inferior
Left ØGMP
Right ØGMN
Multiple ØGMQ
Superior
Left ØGMM
Right ØGML
Penis ØVMSXZZ
Perineum
Female ØWMNØZZ
Male ØWMMØZZ
Rectum ØDMP
Scrotum ØVM5XZZ
Shoulder Region
Left ØXM3ØZZ
Right ØXM2ØZZ
Skin
Abdomen ØHM7XZZ
Back ØHM6XZZ
Buttock ØHM8XZZ
Chest ØHM5XZZ
Ear
Left ØHM3XZZ
Right ØHM2XZZ
Face ØHM1XZZ
Foot
Left ØHMNXZZ
Right ØHMMXZZ
Genitalia ØHMAXZZ
Hand
Left ØHMGXZZ
Right ØHMFXZZ
Lower Arm
Left ØHMEXZZ
Right ØHMDXZZ
Lower Leg
Left ØHMLXZZ
Right ØHMKXZZ
Neck ØHM4XZZ
Perineum ØHM9XZZ
Scalp ØHMØXZZ
Upper Arm
Left ØHMCXZZ
Right ØHMBXZZ
Upper Leg
Left ØHMJXZZ
Right ØHMHXZZ
Stomach ØDM6
Tendon
Abdomen
Left ØLMG
Right ØLMF
Ankle
Left ØLMT
Right ØLMS
Foot
Left ØLMW
Right ØLMV
Hand
Left ØLM8
Right ØLM7
Head and Neck ØLMØ
Hip
Left ØLMK
Right ØLMJ
Knee
Left ØLMR
Right ØLMQ
Lower Arm and Wrist
Left ØLM6
Right ØLM5
Lower Leg
Left ØLMP
Right ØLMN
Perineum ØLMH
Shoulder
Left ØLM2
Right ØLM1

Subterms under main terms may continue to next column or page

Reattachment — continued
Tendon — continued
Thorax
Left ØLMD
Right ØLMC
Trunk
Left ØLMB
Right ØLM9
Upper Arm
Left ØLM4
Right ØLM3
Upper Leg
Left ØLMM
Right ØLML
Testis
Bilateral ØVMC
Left ØVMB
Right ØVM9
Thumb
Left ØXMMØZZ
Right ØXMLØZZ
Thyroid Gland
Left Lobe ØGMG
Right Lobe ØGMH
Toe
1st
Left ØYMQØZZ
Right ØYMPØZZ
2nd
Left ØYMSØZZ
Right ØYMRØZZ
3rd
Left ØYMUØZZ
Right ØYMTØZZ
4th
Left ØYMWØZZ
Right ØYMVØZZ
5th
Left ØYMYØZZ
Right ØYMXØZZ
Tongue ØCM7ØZZ
Tooth
Lower ØCMX
Upper ØCMW
Trachea ØBM1ØZZ
Tunica Vaginalis
Left ØVM7
Right ØVM6
Ureter
Left ØTM7
Right ØTM6
Ureters, Bilateral ØTM8
Urethra ØTMD
Uterine Supporting Structure ØUM4
Uterus ØUM9
Uvula ØCMNØZZ
Vagina ØUMG
Vulva ØUMMXZZ
Wrist Region
Left ØXMHØZZ
Right ØXMGØZZ
Rebound HRD® (Hernia Repair Device) *use* Synthetic Substitute
Recession
see Repair
see Reposition
Reclosure, disrupted abdominal wall ØWQFXZZ
Reconstruction
see Repair
see Replacement
see Supplement
Rectectomy
see Excision, Rectum ØDBP
see Resection, Rectum ØDTP
Rectocele repair *see* Repair, Subcutaneous Tissue and Fascia, Pelvic Region ØJQC
Rectopexy
see Repair, Gastrointestinal System ØDQ
see Reposition, Gastrointestinal System ØDS
Rectoplasty
see Repair, Gastrointestinal System ØDQ
see Supplement, Gastrointestinal System ØDU
Rectorrhaphy *see* Repair, Gastrointestinal System ØDQ
Rectoscopy ØDJD8ZZ
Rectosigmoid junction *use* Colon, Sigmoid
Rectosigmoidectomy
see Excision, Gastrointestinal System ØDB
see Resection, Gastrointestinal System ØDT
Rectostomy *see* Drainage, Rectum ØD9P
Rectotomy *see* Drainage, Rectum ØD9P
Rectus abdominis muscle
use Muscle, Abdomen, Left
use Muscle, Abdomen, Right
Rectus femoris muscle
use Muscle, Upper Leg, Left
use Muscle, Upper Leg, Right
Recurrent laryngeal nerve *use* Nerve, Vagus
Reduction
Dislocation *see* Reposition
Fracture *see* Reposition
Intussusception, intestinal *see* Reposition, Gastrointestinal System ØDS
Mammoplasty *see* Excision, Skin and Breast ØHB
Prolapse *see* Reposition
Torsion *see* Reposition
Volvulus, gastrointestinal *see* Reposition, Gastrointestinal System ØDS
Refusion *see* Fusion
Reimplantation
see Reattachment
see Reposition
see Transfer
Reinforcement
see Repair
see Supplement
Relaxation, scar tissue *see* Release
Release
Acetabulum
Left ØQN5
Right ØQN4
Adenoids ØCNQ
Ampulla of Vater ØFNC
Anal Sphincter ØDNR
Anterior Chamber
Left Ø8N33ZZ
Right Ø8N23ZZ
Anus ØDNQ
Aorta
Abdominal Ø4NØ
Thoracic Ø2NW
Aortic Body ØGND
Appendix ØDNJ
Artery
Anterior Tibial
Left Ø4NQ
Right Ø4NP
Axillary
Left Ø3N6
Right Ø3N5
Brachial
Left Ø3N8
Right Ø3N7
Celiac Ø4N1
Colic
Left Ø4N7
Middle Ø4N8
Right Ø4N6
Common Carotid
Left Ø3NJ
Right Ø3NH
Common Iliac
Left Ø4ND
Right Ø4NC
External Carotid
Left Ø3NN
Right Ø3NM
External Iliac
Left Ø4NJ
Right Ø4NH
Face Ø3NR
Femoral
Left Ø4NL
Right Ø4NK
Foot
Left Ø4NW
Right Ø4NV
Gastric Ø4N2
Hand
Left Ø3NF
Right Ø3ND
Hepatic Ø4N3
Release — continued
Artery — continued
Inferior Mesenteric Ø4NB
Innominate Ø3N2
Internal Carotid
Left Ø3NL
Right Ø3NK
Internal Iliac
Left Ø4NF
Right Ø4NE
Internal Mammary
Left Ø3N1
Right Ø3NØ
Intracranial Ø3NG
Lower Ø4NY
Peroneal
Left Ø4NU
Right Ø4NT
Popliteal
Left Ø4NN
Right Ø4NM
Posterior Tibial
Left Ø4NS
Right Ø4NR
Pulmonary
Left Ø2NR
Right Ø2NQ
Pulmonary Trunk Ø2NP
Radial
Left Ø3NC
Right Ø3NB
Renal
Left Ø4NA
Right Ø4N9
Splenic Ø4N4
Subclavian
Left Ø3N4
Right Ø3N3
Superior Mesenteric Ø4N5
Temporal
Left Ø3NT
Right Ø3NS
Thyroid
Left Ø3NV
Right Ø3NU
Ulnar
Left Ø3NA
Right Ø3N9
Upper Ø3NY
Vertebral
Left Ø3NQ
Right Ø3NP
Atrium
Left Ø2N7
Right Ø2N6
Auditory Ossicle
Left Ø9NAØZZ
Right Ø9N9ØZZ
Basal Ganglia ØØN8
Bladder ØTNB
Bladder Neck ØTNC
Bone
Ethmoid
Left ØNNG
Right ØNNF
Frontal
Left ØNN2
Right ØNN1
Hyoid ØNNX
Lacrimal
Left ØNNJ
Right ØNNH
Nasal ØNNB
Occipital
Left ØNN8
Right ØNN7
Palatine
Left ØNNL
Right ØNNK
Parietal
Left ØNN4
Right ØNN3
Pelvic
Left ØQN3
Right ØQN2

- **Release** — continued
  - Bone — continued
    - Sphenoid
      - Left ØNND
      - Right ØNNC
    - Temporal
      - Left ØNN6
      - Right ØNN5
    - Zygomatic
      - Left ØNNN
      - Right ØNNM
  - Brain ØØNØ
  - Breast
    - Bilateral ØHNV
    - Left ØHNU
    - Right ØHNT
  - Bronchus
    - Lingula ØBN9
    - Lower Lobe
      - Left ØBNB
      - Right ØBN6
    - Main
      - Left ØBN7
      - Right ØBN3
    - Middle Lobe, Right ØBN5
    - Upper Lobe
      - Left ØBN8
      - Right ØBN4
  - Buccal Mucosa ØCN4
  - Bursa and Ligament
    - Abdomen
      - Left ØMNJ
      - Right ØMNH
    - Ankle
      - Left ØMNR
      - Right ØMNQ
    - Elbow
      - Left ØMN4
      - Right ØMN3
    - Foot
      - Left ØMNT
      - Right ØMNS
    - Hand
      - Left ØMN8
      - Right ØMN7
    - Head and Neck ØMNØ
    - Hip
      - Left ØMNM
      - Right ØMNL
    - Knee
      - Left ØMNP
      - Right ØMNN
    - Lower Extremity
      - Left ØMNW
      - Right ØMNV
    - Perineum ØMNK
    - Shoulder
      - Left ØMN2
      - Right ØMN1
    - Thorax
      - Left ØMNG
      - Right ØMNF
    - Trunk
      - Left ØMND
      - Right ØMNC
    - Upper Extremity
      - Left ØMNB
      - Right ØMN9
    - Wrist
      - Left ØMN6
      - Right ØMN5
  - Carina ØBN2
  - Carotid Bodies, Bilateral ØGN8
  - Carotid Body
    - Left ØGN6
    - Right ØGN7
  - Carpal
    - Left ØPNN
    - Right ØPNM
  - Cecum ØDNH
  - Cerebellum ØØNC
  - Cerebral Hemisphere ØØN7
  - Cerebral Meninges ØØN1
  - Cerebral Ventricle ØØN6
  - Cervix ØUNC
  - Chordae Tendineae Ø2N9

- **Release** — continued
  - Choroid
    - Left Ø8NB
    - Right Ø8NA
  - Cisterna Chyli Ø7NL
  - Clavicle
    - Left ØPNB
    - Right ØPN9
  - Clitoris ØUNJ
  - Coccygeal Glomus ØGNB
  - Coccyx ØQNS
  - Colon
    - Ascending ØDNK
    - Descending ØDNM
    - Sigmoid ØDNN
    - Transverse ØDNL
  - Conduction Mechanism Ø2N8
  - Conjunctiva
    - Left Ø8NTXZZ
    - Right Ø8NSXZZ
  - Cord
    - Bilateral ØVNH
    - Left ØVNG
    - Right ØVNF
  - Cornea
    - Left Ø8N9XZZ
    - Right Ø8N8XZZ
  - Cul-de-sac ØUNF
  - Diaphragm
    - Left ØBNS
    - Right ØBNR
  - Disc
    - Cervical Vertebral ØRN3
    - Cervicothoracic Vertebral ØRN5
    - Lumbar Vertebral ØSN2
    - Lumbosacral ØSN4
    - Thoracic Vertebral ØRN9
    - Thoracolumbar Vertebral ØRNB
  - Duct
    - Common Bile ØFN9
    - Cystic ØFN8
    - Hepatic
      - Left ØFN6
      - Right ØFN5
    - Lacrimal
      - Left Ø8NY
      - Right Ø8NX
    - Pancreatic ØFND
      - Accessory ØFNF
    - Parotid
      - Left ØCNC
      - Right ØCNB
  - Duodenum ØDN9
  - Dura Mater ØØN2
  - Ear
    - External
      - Left Ø9N1
      - Right Ø9NØ
    - External Auditory Canal
      - Left Ø9N4
      - Right Ø9N3
    - Inner
      - Left Ø9NEØZZ
      - Right Ø9NDØZZ
    - Middle
      - Left Ø9N6ØZZ
      - Right Ø9N5ØZZ
  - Epididymis
    - Bilateral ØVNL
    - Left ØVNK
    - Right ØVNJ
  - Epiglottis ØCNR
  - Esophagogastric Junction ØDN4
  - Esophagus ØDN5
    - Lower ØDN3
    - Middle ØDN2
    - Upper ØDN1
  - Eustachian Tube
    - Left Ø9NG
    - Right Ø9NF
  - Eye
    - Left Ø8N1XZZ
    - Right Ø8NØXZZ
  - Eyelid
    - Lower
      - Left Ø8NR

- **Release** — continued
  - Eyelid — continued
    - Lower — continued
      - Right Ø8NQ
    - Upper
      - Left Ø8NP
      - Right Ø8NN
  - Fallopian Tube
    - Left ØUN6
    - Right ØUN5
  - Fallopian Tubes, Bilateral ØUN7
  - Femoral Shaft
    - Left ØQN9
    - Right ØQN8
  - Femur
    - Lower
      - Left ØQNC
      - Right ØQNB
    - Upper
      - Left ØQN7
      - Right ØQN6
  - Fibula
    - Left ØQNK
    - Right ØQNJ
  - Finger Nail ØHNQXZZ
  - Gallbladder ØFN4
  - Gingiva
    - Lower ØCN6
    - Upper ØCN5
  - Gland
    - Adrenal
      - Bilateral ØGN4
      - Left ØGN2
      - Right ØGN3
    - Lacrimal
      - Left Ø8NW
      - Right Ø8NV
    - Minor Salivary ØCNJ
    - Parotid
      - Left ØCN9
      - Right ØCN8
    - Pituitary ØGNØ
    - Sublingual
      - Left ØCNF
      - Right ØCND
    - Submaxillary
      - Left ØCNH
      - Right ØCNG
    - Vestibular ØUNL
  - Glenoid Cavity
    - Left ØPN8
    - Right ØPN7
  - Glomus Jugulare ØGNC
  - Humeral Head
    - Left ØPND
    - Right ØPNC
  - Humeral Shaft
    - Left ØPNG
    - Right ØPNF
  - Hymen ØUNK
  - Hypothalamus ØØNA
  - Ileocecal Valve ØDNC
  - Ileum ØDNB
  - Intestine
    - Large ØDNE
      - Left ØDNG
      - Right ØDNF
    - Small ØDN8
  - Iris
    - Left Ø8ND3ZZ
    - Right Ø8NC3ZZ
  - Jejunum ØDNA
  - Joint
    - Acromioclavicular
      - Left ØRNH
      - Right ØRNG
    - Ankle
      - Left ØSNG
      - Right ØSNF
    - Carpal
      - Left ØRNR
      - Right ØRNQ
    - Cervical Vertebral ØRN1
    - Cervicothoracic Vertebral ØRN4
    - Coccygeal ØSN6

Release — continued
Joint — continued
Elbow
Left ØRNM
Right ØRNL
Finger Phalangeal
Left ØRNX
Right ØRNW
Hip
Left ØSNB
Right ØSN9
Knee
Left ØSND
Right ØSNC
Lumbar Vertebral ØSNØ
Lumbosacral ØSN3
Metacarpocarpal
Left ØRNT
Right ØRNS
Metacarpophalangeal
Left ØRNV
Right ØRNU
Metatarsal-Phalangeal
Left ØSNN
Right ØSNM
Metatarsal-Tarsal
Left ØSNL
Right ØSNK
Occipital-cervical ØRNØ
Sacrococcygeal ØSN5
Sacroiliac
Left ØSN8
Right ØSN7
Shoulder
Left ØRNK
Right ØRNJ
Sternoclavicular
Left ØRNF
Right ØRNE
Tarsal
Left ØSNJ
Right ØSNH
Temporomandibular
Left ØRND
Right ØRNC
Thoracic Vertebral ØRN6
Thoracolumbar Vertebral ØRNA
Toe Phalangeal
Left ØSNQ
Right ØSNP
Wrist
Left ØRNP
Right ØRNN
Kidney
Left ØTN1
Right ØTNØ
Kidney Pelvis
Left ØTN4
Right ØTN3
Larynx ØCNS
Lens
Left Ø8NK3ZZ
Right Ø8NJ3ZZ
Lip
Lower ØCN1
Upper ØCNØ
Liver ØFNØ
Left Lobe ØFN2
Right Lobe ØFN1
Lung
Bilateral ØBNM
Left ØBNL
Lower Lobe
Left ØBNJ
Right ØBNF
Middle Lobe, Right ØBND
Right ØBNK
Upper Lobe
Left ØBNG
Right ØBNC
Lung Lingula ØBNH
Lymphatic
Aortic Ø7ND
Axillary
Left Ø7N6
Right Ø7N5

Release — continued
Lymphatic — continued
Head Ø7NØ
Inguinal
Left Ø7NJ
Right Ø7NH
Internal Mammary
Left Ø7N9
Right Ø7N8
Lower Extremity
Left Ø7NG
Right Ø7NF
Mesenteric Ø7NB
Neck
Left Ø7N2
Right Ø7N1
Pelvis Ø7NC
Thoracic Duct Ø7NK
Thorax Ø7N7
Upper Extremity
Left Ø7N4
Right Ø7N3
Mandible
Left ØNNV
Right ØNNT
Maxilla
Left ØNNS
Right ØNNR
Medulla Oblongata ØØND
Mesentery ØDNV
Metacarpal
Left ØPNQ
Right ØPNP
Metatarsal
Left ØQNP
Right ØQNN
Muscle
Abdomen
Left ØKNL
Right ØKNK
Extraocular
Left Ø8NM
Right Ø8NL
Facial ØKN1
Foot
Left ØKNW
Right ØKNV
Hand
Left ØKND
Right ØKNC
Head ØKNØ
Hip
Left ØKNP
Right ØKNN
Lower Arm and Wrist
Left ØKNB
Right ØKN9
Lower Leg
Left ØKNT
Right ØKNS
Neck
Left ØKN3
Right ØKN2
Papillary Ø2ND
Perineum ØKNM
Shoulder
Left ØKN6
Right ØKN5
Thorax
Left ØKNJ
Right ØKNH
Tongue, Palate, Pharynx ØKN4
Trunk
Left ØKNG
Right ØKNF
Upper Arm
Left ØKN8
Right ØKN7
Upper Leg
Left ØKNR
Right ØKNQ
Nasopharynx Ø9NN
Nerve
Abdominal Sympathetic Ø1NM
Abducens ØØNL
Accessory ØØNR

Release — continued
Nerve — continued
Acoustic ØØNN
Brachial Plexus Ø1N3
Cervical Ø1N1
Cervical Plexus Ø1NØ
Facial ØØNM
Femoral Ø1ND
Glossopharyngeal ØØNP
Head and Neck Sympathetic Ø1NK
Hypoglossal ØØNS
Lumbar Ø1NB
Lumbar Plexus Ø1N9
Lumbar Sympathetic Ø1NN
Lumbosacral Plexus Ø1NA
Median Ø1N5
Oculomotor ØØNH
Olfactory ØØNF
Optic ØØNG
Peroneal Ø1NH
Phrenic Ø1N2
Pudendal Ø1NC
Radial Ø1N6
Sacral Ø1NR
Sacral Plexus Ø1NQ
Sacral Sympathetic Ø1NP
Sciatic Ø1NF
Thoracic Ø1N8
Thoracic Sympathetic Ø1NL
Tibial Ø1NG
Trigeminal ØØNK
Trochlear ØØNJ
Ulnar Ø1N4
Vagus ØØNQ
Nipple
Left ØHNX
Right ØHNW
Nose Ø9NK
Omentum
Greater ØDNS
Lesser ØDNT
Orbit
Left ØNNQ
Right ØNNP
Ovary
Bilateral ØUN2
Left ØUN1
Right ØUNØ
Palate
Hard ØCN2
Soft ØCN3
Pancreas ØFNG
Para-aortic Body ØGN9
Paraganglion Extremity ØGNF
Parathyroid Gland ØGNR
Inferior
Left ØGNP
Right ØGNN
Multiple ØGNQ
Superior
Left ØGNM
Right ØGNL
Patella
Left ØQNF
Right ØQND
Penis ØVNS
Pericardium Ø2NN
Peritoneum ØDNW
Phalanx
Finger
Left ØPNV
Right ØPNT
Thumb
Left ØPNS
Right ØPNR
Toe
Left ØQNR
Right ØQNQ
Pharynx ØCNM
Pineal Body ØGN1
Pleura
Left ØBNP
Right ØBNN
Pons ØØNB
Prepuce ØVNT
Prostate ØVNØ

Release — continued
Radius
Left ØPNJ
Right ØPNH
Rectum ØDNP
Retina
Left Ø8NF3ZZ
Right Ø8NE3ZZ
Retinal Vessel
Left Ø8NH3ZZ
Right Ø8NG3ZZ
Rib
Left ØPN2
Right ØPN1
Sacrum ØQN1
Scapula
Left ØPN6
Right ØPN5
Sclera
Left Ø8N7XZZ
Right Ø8N6XZZ
Scrotum ØVN5
Septum
Atrial Ø2N5
Nasal Ø9NM
Ventricular Ø2NM
Sinus
Accessory Ø9NP
Ethmoid
Left Ø9NV
Right Ø9NU
Frontal
Left Ø9NT
Right Ø9NS
Mastoid
Left Ø9NC
Right Ø9NB
Maxillary
Left Ø9NR
Right Ø9NQ
Sphenoid
Left Ø9NX
Right Ø9NW
Skin
Abdomen ØHN7XZZ
Back ØHN6XZZ
Buttock ØHN8XZZ
Chest ØHN5XZZ
Ear
Left ØHN3XZZ
Right ØHN2XZZ
Face ØHN1XZZ
Foot
Left ØHNNXZZ
Right ØHNMXZZ
Genitalia ØHNAXZZ
Hand
Left ØHNGXZZ
Right ØHNFXZZ
Lower Arm
Left ØHNEXZZ
Right ØHNDXZZ
Lower Leg
Left ØHNLXZZ
Right ØHNKXZZ
Neck ØHN4XZZ
Perineum ØHN9XZZ
Scalp ØHNØXZZ
Upper Arm
Left ØHNCXZZ
Right ØHNBXZZ
Upper Leg
Left ØHNJXZZ
Right ØHNHXZZ
Spinal Cord
Cervical ØØNW
Lumbar ØØNY
Thoracic ØØNX
Spinal Meninges ØØNT
Spleen Ø7NP
Sternum ØPNØ
Stomach ØDN6
Pylorus ØDN7
Subcutaneous Tissue and Fascia
Abdomen ØJN8
Back ØJN7

Release — continued
Subcutaneous Tissue and Fascia — continued
Buttock ØJN9
Chest ØJN6
Face ØJN1
Foot
Left ØJNR
Right ØJNQ
Hand
Left ØJNK
Right ØJNJ
Lower Arm
Left ØJNH
Right ØJNG
Lower Leg
Left ØJNP
Right ØJNN
Neck
Anterior ØJN4
Posterior ØJN5
Pelvic Region ØJNC
Perineum ØJNB
Scalp ØJNØ
Upper Arm
Left ØJNF
Right ØJND
Upper Leg
Left ØJNM
Right ØJNL
Tarsal
Left ØQNM
Right ØQNL
Tendon
Abdomen
Left ØLNG
Right ØLNF
Ankle
Left ØLNT
Right ØLNS
Foot
Left ØLNW
Right ØLNV
Hand
Left ØLN8
Right ØLN7
Head and Neck ØLNØ
Hip
Left ØLNK
Right ØLNJ
Knee
Left ØLNR
Right ØLNQ
Lower Arm and Wrist
Left ØLN6
Right ØLN5
Lower Leg
Left ØLNP
Right ØLNN
Perineum ØLNH
Shoulder
Left ØLN2
Right ØLN1
Thorax
Left ØLND
Right ØLNC
Trunk
Left ØLNB
Right ØLN9
Upper Arm
Left ØLN4
Right ØLN3
Upper Leg
Left ØLNM
Right ØLNL
Testis
Bilateral ØVNC
Left ØVNB
Right ØVN9
Thalamus ØØN9
Thymus Ø7NM
Thyroid Gland ØGNK
Left Lobe ØGNG
Right Lobe ØGNH
Tibia
Left ØQNH
Right ØQNG

Release — continued
Toe Nail ØHNRXZZ
Tongue ØCN7
Tonsils ØCNP
Tooth
Lower ØCNX
Upper ØCNW
Trachea ØBN1
Tunica Vaginalis
Left ØVN7
Right ØVN6
Turbinate, Nasal Ø9NL
Tympanic Membrane
Left Ø9N8
Right Ø9N7
Ulna
Left ØPNL
Right ØPNK
Ureter
Left ØTN7
Right ØTN6
Urethra ØTND
Uterine Supporting Structure ØUN4
Uterus ØUN9
Uvula ØCNN
Vagina ØUNG
Valve
Aortic Ø2NF
Mitral Ø2NG
Pulmonary Ø2NH
Tricuspid Ø2NJ
Vas Deferens
Bilateral ØVNQ
Left ØVNP
Right ØVNN
Vein
Axillary
Left Ø5N8
Right Ø5N7
Azygos Ø5NØ
Basilic
Left Ø5NC
Right Ø5NB
Brachial
Left Ø5NA
Right Ø5N9
Cephalic
Left Ø5NF
Right Ø5ND
Colic Ø6N7
Common Iliac
Left Ø6ND
Right Ø6NC
Coronary Ø2N4
Esophageal Ø6N3
External Iliac
Left Ø6NG
Right Ø6NF
External Jugular
Left Ø5NQ
Right Ø5NP
Face
Left Ø5NV
Right Ø5NT
Femoral
Left Ø6NN
Right Ø6NM
Foot
Left Ø6NV
Right Ø6NT
Gastric Ø6N2
Greater Saphenous
Left Ø6NQ
Right Ø6NP
Hand
Left Ø5NH
Right Ø5NG
Hemiazygos Ø5N1
Hepatic Ø6N4
Hypogastric
Left Ø6NJ
Right Ø6NH
Inferior Mesenteric Ø6N6
Innominate
Left Ø5N4
Right Ø5N3

Subterms under main terms may continue to next column or page

Release — continued
Vein — continued
Internal Jugular
Left Ø5NN
Right Ø5NM
Intracranial Ø5NL
Lesser Saphenous
Left Ø6NS
Right Ø6NR
Lower Ø6NY
Portal Ø6N8
Pulmonary
Left Ø2NT
Right Ø2NS
Renal
Left Ø6NB
Right Ø6N9
Splenic Ø6N1
Subclavian
Left Ø5N6
Right Ø5N5
Superior Mesenteric Ø6N5
Upper Ø5NY
Vertebral
Left Ø5NS
Right Ø5NR
Vena Cava
Inferior Ø6NØ
Superior Ø2NV
Ventricle
Left Ø2NL
Right Ø2NK
Vertebra
Cervical ØPN3
Lumbar ØQNØ
Thoracic ØPN4
Vesicle
Bilateral ØVN3
Left ØVN2
Right ØVN1
Vitreous
Left Ø8N53ZZ
Right Ø8N43ZZ
Vocal Cord
Left ØCNV
Right ØCNT
Vulva ØUNM
Relocation *see* Reposition
Removal
Abdominal Wall 2W53X
Anorectal 2Y53X5Z
Arm
Lower
Left 2W5DX
Right 2W5CX
Upper
Left 2W5BX
Right 2W5AX
Back 2W55X
Chest Wall 2W54X
Ear 2Y52X5Z
Extremity
Lower
Left 2W5MX
Right 2W5LX
Upper
Left 2W59X
Right 2W58X
Face 2W51X
Finger
Left 2W5KX
Right 2W5JX
Foot
Left 2W5TX
Right 2W5SX
Genital Tract, Female 2Y54X5Z
Hand
Left 2W5FX
Right 2W5EX
Head 2W5ØX
Inguinal Region
Left 2W57X
Right 2W56X
Leg
Lower
Left 2W5RX
Removal — continued
Leg — continued
Lower — continued
Right 2W5QX
Upper
Left 2W5PX
Right 2W5NX
Mouth and Pharynx 2Y5ØX5Z
Nasal 2Y51X5Z
Neck 2W52X
Thumb
Left 2W5HX
Right 2W5GX
Toe
Left 2W5VX
Right 2W5UX
Urethra 2Y55X5Z
Removal of device from
Abdominal Wall ØWPF
Acetabulum
Left ØQP5
Right ØQP4
Anal Sphincter ØDPR
Anus ØDPQ
Artery
Lower Ø4PY
Upper Ø3PY
Back
Lower ØWPL
Upper ØWPK
Bladder ØTPB
Bone
Facial ØNPW
Lower ØQPY
Nasal ØNPB
Pelvic
Left ØQP3
Right ØQP2
Upper ØPPY
Bone Marrow Ø7PT
Brain ØØPØ
Breast
Left ØHPU
Right ØHPT
Bursa and Ligament
Lower ØMPY
Upper ØMPX
Carpal
Left ØPPN
Right ØPPM
Cavity, Cranial ØWP1
Cerebral Ventricle ØØP6
Chest Wall ØWP8
Cisterna Chyli Ø7PL
Clavicle
Left ØPPB
Right ØPP9
Coccyx ØQPS
Diaphragm ØBPT
Disc
Cervical Vertebral ØRP3
Cervicothoracic Vertebral ØRP5
Lumbar Vertebral ØSP2
Lumbosacral ØSP4
Thoracic Vertebral ØRP9
Thoracolumbar Vertebral ØRPB
Duct
Hepatobiliary ØFPB
Pancreatic ØFPD
Ear
Inner
Left Ø9PE
Right Ø9PD
Left Ø9PJ
Right Ø9PH
Epididymis and Spermatic Cord ØVPM
Esophagus ØDP5
Extremity
Lower
Left ØYPB
Right ØYP9
Upper
Left ØXP7
Right ØXP6
Eye
Left Ø8P1
Removal of device from — continued
Eye — continued
Right Ø8PØ
Face ØWP2
Fallopian Tube ØUP8
Femoral Shaft
Left ØQP9
Right ØQP8
Femur
Lower
Left ØQPC
Right ØQPB
Upper
Left ØQP7
Right ØQP6
Fibula
Left ØQPK
Right ØQPJ
Finger Nail ØHPQX
Gallbladder ØFP4
Gastrointestinal Tract ØWPP
Genitourinary Tract ØWPR
Gland
Adrenal ØGP5
Endocrine ØGPS
Pituitary ØGPØ
Salivary ØCPA
Glenoid Cavity
Left ØPP8
Right ØPP7
Great Vessel Ø2PY
Hair ØHPSX
Head ØWPØ
Heart Ø2PA
Humeral Head
Left ØPPD
Right ØPPC
Humeral Shaft
Left ØPPG
Right ØPPF
Intestinal Tract
Lower ØDPD
Upper ØDPØ
Jaw
Lower ØWP5
Upper ØWP4
Joint
Acromioclavicular
Left ØRPH
Right ØRPG
Ankle
Left ØSPG
Right ØSPF
Carpal
Left ØRPR
Right ØRPQ
Cervical Vertebral ØRP1
Cervicothoracic Vertebral ØRP4
Coccygeal ØSP6
Elbow
Left ØRPM
Right ØRPL
Finger Phalangeal
Left ØRPX
Right ØRPW
Hip
Left ØSPB
Right ØSP9
Knee
Left ØSPD
Right ØSPC
Lumbar Vertebral ØSPØ
Lumbosacral ØSP3
Metacarpocarpal
Left ØRPT
Right ØRPS
Metacarpophalangeal
Left ØRPV
Right ØRPU
Metatarsal-Phalangeal
Left ØSPN
Right ØSPM
Metatarsal-Tarsal
Left ØSPL
Right ØSPK
Occipital-cervical ØRPØ

Removal of device from — continued
Joint — continued
Sacrococcygeal ØSP5
Sacroiliac
Left ØSP8
Right ØSP7
Shoulder
Left ØRPK
Right ØRPJ
Sternoclavicular
Left ØRPF
Right ØRPE
Tarsal
Left ØSPJ
Right ØSPH
Temporomandibular
Left ØRPD
Right ØRPC
Thoracic Vertebral ØRP6
Thoracolumbar Vertebral ØRPA
Toe Phalangeal
Left ØSPQ
Right ØSPP
Wrist
Left ØRPP
Right ØRPN
Kidney ØTP5
Larynx ØCPS
Lens
Left Ø8PK3JZ
Right Ø8PJ3JZ
Liver ØFPØ
Lung
Left ØBPL
Right ØBPK
Lymphatic Ø7PN
Thoracic Duct Ø7PK
Mediastinum ØWPC
Mesentery ØDPV
Metacarpal
Left ØPPQ
Right ØPPP
Metatarsal
Left ØQPP
Right ØQPN
Mouth and Throat ØCPY
Muscle
Extraocular
Left Ø8PM
Right Ø8PL
Lower ØKPY
Upper ØKPX
Neck ØWP6
Nerve
Cranial ØØPE
Peripheral Ø1PY
Nose Ø9PK
Omentum ØDPU
Ovary ØUP3
Pancreas ØFPG
Parathyroid Gland ØGPR
Patella
Left ØQPF
Right ØQPD
Pelvic Cavity ØWPJ
Penis ØVPS
Pericardial Cavity ØWPD
Perineum
Female ØWPN
Male ØWPM
Peritoneal Cavity ØWPG
Peritoneum ØDPW
Phalanx
Finger
Left ØPPV
Right ØPPT
Thumb
Left ØPPS
Right ØPPR
Toe
Left ØQPR
Right ØQPQ
Pineal Body ØGP1
Pleura ØBPQ
Pleural Cavity
Left ØWPB

Removal of device from — continued
Pleural Cavity — continued
Right ØWP9
Products of Conception 1ØPØ
Prostate and Seminal Vesicles ØVP4
Radius
Left ØPPJ
Right ØPPH
Rectum ØDPP
Respiratory Tract ØWPQ
Retroperitoneum ØWPH
Rib
Left ØPP2
Right ØPP1
Sacrum ØQP1
Scapula
Left ØPP6
Right ØPP5
Scrotum and Tunica Vaginalis ØVP8
Sinus Ø9PY
Skin ØHPPX
Skull ØNPØ
Spinal Canal ØØPU
Spinal Cord ØØPV
Spleen Ø7PP
Sternum ØPPØ
Stomach ØDP6
Subcutaneous Tissue and Fascia
Head and Neck ØJPS
Lower Extremity ØJPW
Trunk ØJPT
Upper Extremity ØJPV
Tarsal
Left ØQPM
Right ØQPL
Tendon
Lower ØLPY
Upper ØLPX
Testis ØVPD
Thymus Ø7PM
Thyroid Gland ØGPK
Tibia
Left ØQPH
Right ØQPG
Toe Nail ØHPRX
Trachea ØBP1
Tracheobronchial Tree ØBPØ
Tympanic Membrane
Left Ø9P8
Right Ø9P7
Ulna
Left ØPPL
Right ØPPK
Ureter ØTP9
Urethra ØTPD
Uterus and Cervix ØUPD
Vagina and Cul-de-sac ØUPH
Vas Deferens ØVPR
Vein
Lower Ø6PY
Upper Ø5PY
Vertebra
Cervical ØPP3
Lumbar ØQPØ
Thoracic ØPP4
Vulva ØUPM
Renal calyx
use Kidney
use Kidney, Left
use Kidney, Right
use Kidneys, Bilateral
Renal capsule
use Kidney
use Kidney, Left
use Kidney, Right
use Kidneys, Bilateral
Renal cortex
use Kidney
use Kidney, Left
use Kidney, Right
use Kidneys, Bilateral
Renal dialysis *see* Performance, Urinary 5A1D
Renal plexus *use* Nerve, Abdominal Sympathetic
Renal segment
use Kidney
use Kidney, Left

Renal segment — continued
use Kidney, Right
use Kidneys, Bilateral
Renal segmental artery
use Artery, Renal, Left
use Artery, Renal, Right
Reopening, operative site
Control of bleeding *see* Control postprocedural bleeding in
Inspection only *see* Inspection
Repair
Abdominal Wall ØWQF
Acetabulum
Left ØQQ5
Right ØQQ4
Adenoids ØCQQ
Ampulla of Vater ØFQC
Anal Sphincter ØDQR
Ankle Region
Left ØYQL
Right ØYQK
Anterior Chamber
Left Ø8Q33ZZ
Right Ø8Q23ZZ
Anus ØDQQ
Aorta
Abdominal Ø4QØ
Thoracic Ø2QW
Aortic Body ØGQD
Appendix ØDQJ
Arm
Lower
Left ØXQF
Right ØXQD
Upper
Left ØXQ9
Right ØXQ8
Artery
Anterior Tibial
Left Ø4QQ
Right Ø4QP
Axillary
Left Ø3Q6
Right Ø3Q5
Brachial
Left Ø3Q8
Right Ø3Q7
Celiac Ø4Q1
Colic
Left Ø4Q7
Middle Ø4Q8
Right Ø4Q6
Common Carotid
Left Ø3QJ
Right Ø3QH
Common Iliac
Left Ø4QD
Right Ø4QC
Coronary
Four or More Sites Ø2Q3
One Site Ø2QØ
Three Sites Ø2Q2
Two Sites Ø2Q1
External Carotid
Left Ø3QN
Right Ø3QM
External Iliac
Left Ø4QJ
Right Ø4QH
Face Ø3QR
Femoral
Left Ø4QL
Right Ø4QK
Foot
Left Ø4QW
Right Ø4QV
Gastric Ø4Q2
Hand
Left Ø3QF
Right Ø3QD
Hepatic Ø4Q3
Inferior Mesenteric Ø4QB
Innominate Ø3Q2
Internal Carotid
Left Ø3QL
Right Ø3QK

Repair — continued
- Artery — continued
  - Internal Iliac
    - Left Ø4QF
    - Right Ø4QE
  - Internal Mammary
    - Left Ø3Q1
    - Right Ø3QØ
  - Intracranial Ø3QG
  - Lower Ø4QY
  - Peroneal
    - Left Ø4QU
    - Right Ø4QT
  - Popliteal
    - Left Ø4QN
    - Right Ø4QM
  - Posterior Tibial
    - Left Ø4QS
    - Right Ø4QR
  - Pulmonary
    - Left Ø2QR
    - Right Ø2QQ
  - Pulmonary Trunk Ø2QP
  - Radial
    - Left Ø3QC
    - Right Ø3QB
  - Renal
    - Left Ø4QA
    - Right Ø4Q9
  - Splenic Ø4Q4
  - Subclavian
    - Left Ø3Q4
    - Right Ø3Q3
  - Superior Mesenteric Ø4Q5
  - Temporal
    - Left Ø3QT
    - Right Ø3QS
  - Thyroid
    - Left Ø3QV
    - Right Ø3QU
  - Ulnar
    - Left Ø3QA
    - Right Ø3Q9
  - Upper Ø3QY
  - Vertebral
    - Left Ø3QQ
    - Right Ø3QP
- Atrium
  - Left Ø2Q7
  - Right Ø2Q6
- Auditory Ossicle
  - Left Ø9QAØZZ
  - Right Ø9Q9ØZZ
- Axilla
  - Left ØXQ5
  - Right ØXQ4
- Back
  - Lower ØWQL
  - Upper ØWQK
- Basal Ganglia ØØQ8
- Bladder ØTQB
- Bladder Neck ØTQC
- Bone
  - Ethmoid
    - Left ØNQG
    - Right ØNQF
  - Frontal
    - Left ØNQ2
    - Right ØNQ1
  - Hyoid ØNQX
  - Lacrimal
    - Left ØNQJ
    - Right ØNQH
  - Nasal ØNQB
  - Occipital
    - Left ØNQ8
    - Right ØNQ7
  - Palatine
    - Left ØNQL
    - Right ØNQK
  - Parietal
    - Left ØNQ4
    - Right ØNQ3
  - Pelvic
    - Left ØQQ3
    - Right ØQQ2

Repair — continued
- Bone — continued
  - Sphenoid
    - Left ØNQD
    - Right ØNQC
  - Temporal
    - Left ØNQ6
    - Right ØNQ5
  - Zygomatic
    - Left ØNQN
    - Right ØNQM
- Brain ØØQØ
- Breast
  - Bilateral ØHQV
  - Left ØHQU
  - Right ØHQT
  - Supernumerary ØHQY
- Bronchus
  - Lingula ØBQ9
  - Lower Lobe
    - Left ØBQB
    - Right ØBQ6
  - Main
    - Left ØBQ7
    - Right ØBQ3
  - Middle Lobe, Right ØBQ5
  - Upper Lobe
    - Left ØBQ8
    - Right ØBQ4
- Buccal Mucosa ØCQ4
- Bursa and Ligament
  - Abdomen
    - Left ØMQJ
    - Right ØMQH
  - Ankle
    - Left ØMQR
    - Right ØMQQ
  - Elbow
    - Left ØMQ4
    - Right ØMQ3
  - Foot
    - Left ØMQT
    - Right ØMQS
  - Hand
    - Left ØMQ8
    - Right ØMQ7
  - Head and Neck ØMQØ
  - Hip
    - Left ØMQM
    - Right ØMQL
  - Knee
    - Left ØMQP
    - Right ØMQN
  - Lower Extremity
    - Left ØMQW
    - Right ØMQV
  - Perineum ØMQK
  - Shoulder
    - Left ØMQ2
    - Right ØMQ1
  - Thorax
    - Left ØMQG
    - Right ØMQF
  - Trunk
    - Left ØMQD
    - Right ØMQC
  - Upper Extremity
    - Left ØMQB
    - Right ØMQ9
  - Wrist
    - Left ØMQ6
    - Right ØMQ5
- Buttock
  - Left ØYQ1
  - Right ØYQØ
- Carina ØBQ2
- Carotid Bodies, Bilateral ØGQ8
- Carotid Body
  - Left ØGQ6
  - Right ØGQ7
- Carpal
  - Left ØPQN
  - Right ØPQM
- Cecum ØDQH
- Cerebellum ØØQC
- Cerebral Hemisphere ØØQ7

Repair — continued
- Cerebral Meninges ØØQ1
- Cerebral Ventricle ØØQ6
- Cervix ØUQC
- Chest Wall ØWQ8
- Chordae Tendineae Ø2Q9
- Choroid
  - Left Ø8QB
  - Right Ø8QA
- Cisterna Chyli Ø7QL
- Clavicle
  - Left ØPQB
  - Right ØPQ9
- Clitoris ØUQJ
- Coccygeal Glomus ØGQB
- Coccyx ØQQS
- Colon
  - Ascending ØDQK
  - Descending ØDQM
  - Sigmoid ØDQN
  - Transverse ØDQL
- Conduction Mechanism Ø2Q8
- Conjunctiva
  - Left Ø8QTXZZ
  - Right Ø8QSXZZ
- Cord
  - Bilateral ØVQH
  - Left ØVQG
  - Right ØVQF
- Cornea
  - Left Ø8Q9XZZ
  - Right Ø8Q8XZZ
- Cul-de-sac ØUQF
- Diaphragm
  - Left ØBQS
  - Right ØBQR
- Disc
  - Cervical Vertebral ØRQ3
  - Cervicothoracic Vertebral ØRQ5
  - Lumbar Vertebral ØSQ2
  - Lumbosacral ØSQ4
  - Thoracic Vertebral ØRQ9
  - Thoracolumbar Vertebral ØRQB
- Duct
  - Common Bile ØFQ9
  - Cystic ØFQ8
  - Hepatic
    - Left ØFQ6
    - Right ØFQ5
  - Lacrimal
    - Left Ø8QY
    - Right Ø8QX
  - Pancreatic ØFQD
    - Accessory ØFQF
  - Parotid
    - Left ØCQC
    - Right ØCQB
- Duodenum ØDQ9
- Dura Mater ØØQ2
- Ear
  - External
    - Bilateral Ø9Q2
    - Left Ø9Q1
    - Right Ø9QØ
  - External Auditory Canal
    - Left Ø9Q4
    - Right Ø9Q3
  - Inner
    - Left Ø9QEØZZ
    - Right Ø9QDØZZ
  - Middle
    - Left Ø9Q6ØZZ
    - Right Ø9Q5ØZZ
- Elbow Region
  - Left ØXQC
  - Right ØXQB
- Epididymis
  - Bilateral ØVQL
  - Left ØVQK
  - Right ØVQJ
- Epiglottis ØCQR
- Esophagogastric Junction ØDQ4
- Esophagus ØDQ5
  - Lower ØDQ3
  - Middle ØDQ2
  - Upper ØDQ1

Repair — continued
Eustachian Tube
Left Ø9QG
Right Ø9QF
Extremity
Lower
Left ØYQB
Right ØYQ9
Upper
Left ØXQ7
Right ØXQ6
Eye
Left Ø8Q1XZZ
Right Ø8QØXZZ
Eyelid
Lower
Left Ø8QR
Right Ø8QQ
Upper
Left Ø8QP
Right Ø8QN
Face ØWQ2
Fallopian Tube
Left ØUQ6
Right ØUQ5
Fallopian Tubes, Bilateral ØUQ7
Femoral Region
Bilateral ØYQE
Left ØYQ8
Right ØYQ7
Femoral Shaft
Left ØQQ9
Right ØQQ8
Femur
Lower
Left ØQQC
Right ØQQB
Upper
Left ØQQ7
Right ØQQ6
Fibula
Left ØQQK
Right ØQQJ
Finger
Index
Left ØXQP
Right ØXQN
Little
Left ØXQW
Right ØXQV
Middle
Left ØXQR
Right ØXQQ
Ring
Left ØXQT
Right ØXQS
Finger Nail ØHQQXZZ
Foot
Left ØYQN
Right ØYQM
Gallbladder ØFQ4
Gingiva
Lower ØCQ6
Upper ØCQ5
Gland
Adrenal
Bilateral ØGQ4
Left ØGQ2
Right ØGQ3
Lacrimal
Left Ø8QW
Right Ø8QV
Minor Salivary ØCQJ
Parotid
Left ØCQ9
Right ØCQ8
Pituitary ØGQØ
Sublingual
Left ØCQF
Right ØCQD
Submaxillary
Left ØCQH
Right ØCQG
Vestibular ØUQL
Glenoid Cavity
Left ØPQ8

Repair — continued
Glenoid Cavity — continued
Right ØPQ7
Glomus Jugulare ØGQC
Hand
Left ØXQK
Right ØXQJ
Head ØWQØ
Heart Ø2QA
Left Ø2QC
Right Ø2QB
Humeral Head
Left ØPQD
Right ØPQC
Humeral Shaft
Left ØPQG
Right ØPQF
Hymen ØUQK
Hypothalamus ØØQA
Ileocecal Valve ØDQC
Ileum ØDQB
Inguinal Region
Bilateral ØYQA
Left ØYQ6
Right ØYQ5
Intestine
Large ØDQE
Left ØDQG
Right ØDQF
Small ØDQ8
Iris
Left Ø8QD3ZZ
Right Ø8QC3ZZ
Jaw
Lower ØWQ5
Upper ØWQ4
Jejunum ØDQA
Joint
Acromioclavicular
Left ØRQH
Right ØRQG
Ankle
Left ØSQG
Right ØSQF
Carpal
Left ØRQR
Right ØRQQ
Cervical Vertebral ØRQ1
Cervicothoracic Vertebral ØRQ4
Coccygeal ØSQ6
Elbow
Left ØRQM
Right ØRQL
Finger Phalangeal
Left ØRQX
Right ØRQW
Hip
Left ØSQB
Right ØSQ9
Knee
Left ØSQD
Right ØSQC
Lumbar Vertebral ØSQØ
Lumbosacral ØSQ3
Metacarpocarpal
Left ØRQT
Right ØRQS
Metacarpophalangeal
Left ØRQV
Right ØRQU
Metatarsal-Phalangeal
Left ØSQN
Right ØSQM
Metatarsal-Tarsal
Left ØSQL
Right ØSQK
Occipital-cervical ØRQØ
Sacrococcygeal ØSQ5
Sacroiliac
Left ØSQ8
Right ØSQ7
Shoulder
Left ØRQK
Right ØRQJ
Sternoclavicular
Left ØRQF

Repair — continued
Joint — continued
Sternoclavicular — continued
Right ØRQE
Tarsal
Left ØSQJ
Right ØSQH
Temporomandibular
Left ØRQD
Right ØRQC
Thoracic Vertebral ØRQ6
Thoracolumbar Vertebral ØRQA
Toe Phalangeal
Left ØSQQ
Right ØSQP
Wrist
Left ØRQP
Right ØRQN
Kidney
Left ØTQ1
Right ØTQØ
Kidney Pelvis
Left ØTQ4
Right ØTQ3
Knee Region
Left ØYQG
Right ØYQF
Larynx ØCQS
Leg
Lower
Left ØYQJ
Right ØYQH
Upper
Left ØYQD
Right ØYQC
Lens
Left Ø8QK3ZZ
Right Ø8QJ3ZZ
Lip
Lower ØCQ1
Upper ØCQØ
Liver ØFQØ
Left Lobe ØFQ2
Right Lobe ØFQ1
Lung
Bilateral ØBQM
Left ØBQL
Lower Lobe
Left ØBQJ
Right ØBQF
Middle Lobe, Right ØBQD
Right ØBQK
Upper Lobe
Left ØBQG
Right ØBQC
Lung Lingula ØBQH
Lymphatic
Aortic Ø7QD
Axillary
Left Ø7Q6
Right Ø7Q5
Head Ø7QØ
Inguinal
Left Ø7QJ
Right Ø7QH
Internal Mammary
Left Ø7Q9
Right Ø7Q8
Lower Extremity
Left Ø7QG
Right Ø7QF
Mesenteric Ø7QB
Neck
Left Ø7Q2
Right Ø7Q1
Pelvis Ø7QC
Thoracic Duct Ø7QK
Thorax Ø7Q7
Upper Extremity
Left Ø7Q4
Right Ø7Q3
Mandible
Left ØNQV
Right ØNQT
Maxilla
Left ØNQS

Repair — continued
Maxilla — continued
Right ØNQR
Mediastinum ØWQC
Medulla Oblongata ØØQD
Mesentery ØDQV
Metacarpal
Left ØPQQ
Right ØPQP
Metatarsal
Left ØQQP
Right ØQQN
Muscle
Abdomen
Left ØKQL
Right ØKQK
Extraocular
Left Ø8QM
Right Ø8QL
Facial ØKQ1
Foot
Left ØKQW
Right ØKQV
Hand
Left ØKQD
Right ØKQC
Head ØKQØ
Hip
Left ØKQP
Right ØKQN
Lower Arm and Wrist
Left ØKQB
Right ØKQ9
Lower Leg
Left ØKQT
Right ØKQS
Neck
Left ØKQ3
Right ØKQ2
Papillary Ø2QD
Perineum ØKQM
Shoulder
Left ØKQ6
Right ØKQ5
Thorax
Left ØKQJ
Right ØKQH
Tongue, Palate, Pharynx ØKQ4
Trunk
Left ØKQG
Right ØKQF
Upper Arm
Left ØKQ8
Right ØKQ7
Upper Leg
Left ØKQR
Right ØKQQ
Nasopharynx Ø9QN
Neck ØWQ6
Nerve
Abdominal Sympathetic Ø1QM
Abducens ØØQL
Accessory ØØQR
Acoustic ØØQN
Brachial Plexus Ø1Q3
Cervical Ø1Q1
Cervical Plexus Ø1QØ
Facial ØØQM
Femoral Ø1QD
Glossopharyngeal ØØQP
Head and Neck Sympathetic Ø1QK
Hypoglossal ØØQS
Lumbar Ø1QB
Lumbar Plexus Ø1Q9
Lumbar Sympathetic Ø1QN
Lumbosacral Plexus Ø1QA
Median Ø1Q5
Oculomotor ØØQH
Olfactory ØØQF
Optic ØØQG
Peroneal Ø1QH
Phrenic Ø1Q2
Pudendal Ø1QC
Radial Ø1Q6
Sacral Ø1QR
Sacral Plexus Ø1QQ

Repair — continued
Nerve — continued
Sacral Sympathetic Ø1QP
Sciatic Ø1QF
Thoracic Ø1Q8
Thoracic Sympathetic Ø1QL
Tibial Ø1QG
Trigeminal ØØQK
Trochlear ØØQJ
Ulnar Ø1Q4
Vagus ØØQQ
Nipple
Left ØHQX
Right ØHQW
Nose Ø9QK
Omentum
Greater ØDQS
Lesser ØDQT
Orbit
Left ØNQQ
Right ØNQP
Ovary
Bilateral ØUQ2
Left ØUQ1
Right ØUQØ
Palate
Hard ØCQ2
Soft ØCQ3
Pancreas ØFQG
Para-aortic Body ØGQ9
Paraganglion Extremity ØGQF
Parathyroid Gland ØGQR
Inferior
Left ØGQP
Right ØGQN
Multiple ØGQQ
Superior
Left ØGQM
Right ØGQL
Patella
Left ØQQF
Right ØQQD
Penis ØVQS
Pericardium Ø2QN
Perineum
Female ØWQN
Male ØWQM
Peritoneum ØDQW
Phalanx
Finger
Left ØPQV
Right ØPQT
Thumb
Left ØPQS
Right ØPQR
Toe
Left ØQQR
Right ØQQQ
Pharynx ØCQM
Pineal Body ØGQ1
Pleura
Left ØBQP
Right ØBQN
Pons ØØQB
Prepuce ØVQT
Products of Conception 1ØQØ
Prostate ØVQØ
Radius
Left ØPQJ
Right ØPQH
Rectum ØDQP
Retina
Left Ø8QF3ZZ
Right Ø8QE3ZZ
Retinal Vessel
Left Ø8QH3ZZ
Right Ø8QG3ZZ
Rib
Left ØPQ2
Right ØPQ1
Sacrum ØQQ1
Scapula
Left ØPQ6
Right ØPQ5
Sclera
Left Ø8Q7XZZ

Repair — continued
Sclera — continued
Right Ø8Q6XZZ
Scrotum ØVQ5
Septum
Atrial Ø2Q5
Nasal Ø9QM
Ventricular Ø2QM
Shoulder Region
Left ØXQ3
Right ØXQ2
Sinus
Accessory Ø9QP
Ethmoid
Left Ø9QV
Right Ø9QU
Frontal
Left Ø9QT
Right Ø9QS
Mastoid
Left Ø9QC
Right Ø9QB
Maxillary
Left Ø9QR
Right Ø9QQ
Sphenoid
Left Ø9QX
Right Ø9QW
Skin
Abdomen ØHQ7XZZ
Back ØHQ6XZZ
Buttock ØHQ8XZZ
Chest ØHQ5XZZ
Ear
Left ØHQ3XZZ
Right ØHQ2XZZ
Face ØHQ1XZZ
Foot
Left ØHQNXZZ
Right ØHQMXZZ
Genitalia ØHQAXZZ
Hand
Left ØHQGXZZ
Right ØHQFXZZ
Lower Arm
Left ØHQEXZZ
Right ØHQDXZZ
Lower Leg
Left ØHQLXZZ
Right ØHQKXZZ
Neck ØHQ4XZZ
Perineum ØHQ9XZZ
Scalp ØHQØXZZ
Upper Arm
Left ØHQCXZZ
Right ØHQBXZZ
Upper Leg
Left ØHQJXZZ
Right ØHQHXZZ
Skull ØNQØ
Spinal Cord
Cervical ØØQW
Lumbar ØØQY
Thoracic ØØQX
Spinal Meninges ØØQT
Spleen Ø7QP
Sternum ØPQØ
Stomach ØDQ6
Pylorus ØDQ7
Subcutaneous Tissue and Fascia
Abdomen ØJQ8
Back ØJQ7
Buttock ØJQ9
Chest ØJQ6
Face ØJQ1
Foot
Left ØJQR
Right ØJQQ
Hand
Left ØJQK
Right ØJQJ
Lower Arm
Left ØJQH
Right ØJQG
Lower Leg
Left ØJQP

Repair — continued
  Subcutaneous Tissue and Fascia — continued
    Lower Leg — continued
      Right ØJQN
    Neck
      Anterior ØJQ4
      Posterior ØJQ5
    Pelvic Region ØJQC
    Perineum ØJQB
    Scalp ØJQØ
    Upper Arm
      Left ØJQF
      Right ØJQD
    Upper Leg
      Left ØJQM
      Right ØJQL
  Tarsal
    Left ØQQM
    Right ØQQL
  Tendon
    Abdomen
      Left ØLQG
      Right ØLQF
    Ankle
      Left ØLQT
      Right ØLQS
    Foot
      Left ØLQW
      Right ØLQV
    Hand
      Left ØLQ8
      Right ØLQ7
    Head and Neck ØLQØ
    Hip
      Left ØLQK
      Right ØLQJ
    Knee
      Left ØLQR
      Right ØLQQ
    Lower Arm and Wrist
      Left ØLQ6
      Right ØLQ5
    Lower Leg
      Left ØLQP
      Right ØLQN
    Perineum ØLQH
    Shoulder
      Left ØLQ2
      Right ØLQ1
    Thorax
      Left ØLQD
      Right ØLQC
    Trunk
      Left ØLQB
      Right ØLQ9
    Upper Arm
      Left ØLQ4
      Right ØLQ3
    Upper Leg
      Left ØLQM
      Right ØLQL
  Testis
    Bilateral ØVQC
    Left ØVQB
    Right ØVQ9
  Thalamus ØØQ9
  Thumb
    Left ØXQM
    Right ØXQL
  Thymus Ø7QM
  Thyroid Gland ØGQK
    Left Lobe ØGQG
    Right Lobe ØGQH
  Thyroid Gland Isthmus ØGQJ
  Tibia
    Left ØQQH
    Right ØQQG
  Toe
    1st
      Left ØYQQ
      Right ØYQP
    2nd
      Left ØYQS
      Right ØYQR
    3rd
      Left ØYQU

Repair — continued
  Toe — continued
    3rd — continued
      Right ØYQT
    4th
      Left ØYQW
      Right ØYQV
    5th
      Left ØYQY
      Right ØYQX
  Toe Nail ØHQRXZZ
  Tongue ØCQ7
  Tonsils ØCQP
  Tooth
    Lower ØCQX
    Upper ØCQW
  Trachea ØBQ1
  Tunica Vaginalis
    Left ØVQ7
    Right ØVQ6
  Turbinate, Nasal Ø9QL
  Tympanic Membrane
    Left Ø9Q8
    Right Ø9Q7
  Ulna
    Left ØPQL
    Right ØPQK
  Ureter
    Left ØTQ7
    Right ØTQ6
  Urethra ØTQD
  Uterine Supporting Structure ØUQ4
  Uterus ØUQ9
  Uvula ØCQN
  Vagina ØUQG
  Valve
    Aortic Ø2QF
    Mitral Ø2QG
    Pulmonary Ø2QH
    Tricuspid Ø2QJ
  Vas Deferens
    Bilateral ØVQQ
    Left ØVQP
    Right ØVQN
  Vein
    Axillary
      Left Ø5Q8
      Right Ø5Q7
    Azygos Ø5QØ
    Basilic
      Left Ø5QC
      Right Ø5QB
    Brachial
      Left Ø5QA
      Right Ø5Q9
    Cephalic
      Left Ø5QF
      Right Ø5QD
    Colic Ø6Q7
    Common Iliac
      Left Ø6QD
      Right Ø6QC
    Coronary Ø2Q4
    Esophageal Ø6Q3
    External Iliac
      Left Ø6QG
      Right Ø6QF
    External Jugular
      Left Ø5QQ
      Right Ø5QP
    Face
      Left Ø5QV
      Right Ø5QT
    Femoral
      Left Ø6QN
      Right Ø6QM
    Foot
      Left Ø6QV
      Right Ø6QT
    Gastric Ø6Q2
    Greater Saphenous
      Left Ø6QQ
      Right Ø6QP
    Hand
      Left Ø5QH
      Right Ø5QG

Repair — continued
  Vein — continued
    Hemiazygos Ø5Q1
    Hepatic Ø6Q4
    Hypogastric
      Left Ø6QJ
      Right Ø6QH
    Inferior Mesenteric Ø6Q6
    Innominate
      Left Ø5Q4
      Right Ø5Q3
    Internal Jugular
      Left Ø5QN
      Right Ø5QM
    Intracranial Ø5QL
    Lesser Saphenous
      Left Ø6QS
      Right Ø6QR
    Lower Ø6QY
    Portal Ø6Q8
    Pulmonary
      Left Ø2QT
      Right Ø2QS
    Renal
      Left Ø6QB
      Right Ø6Q9
    Splenic Ø6Q1
    Subclavian
      Left Ø5Q6
      Right Ø5Q5
    Superior Mesenteric Ø6Q5
    Upper Ø5QY
    Vertebral
      Left Ø5QS
      Right Ø5QR
  Vena Cava
    Inferior Ø6QØ
    Superior Ø2QV
  Ventricle
    Left Ø2QL
    Right Ø2QK
  Vertebra
    Cervical ØPQ3
    Lumbar ØQQØ
    Thoracic ØPQ4
  Vesicle
    Bilateral ØVQ3
    Left ØVQ2
    Right ØVQ1
  Vitreous
    Left Ø8Q53ZZ
    Right Ø8Q43ZZ
  Vocal Cord
    Left ØCQV
    Right ØCQT
  Vulva ØUQM
  Wrist Region
    Left ØXQH
    Right ØXQG
Replacement
  Acetabulum
    Left ØQR5
    Right ØQR4
  Ampulla of Vater ØFRC
  Anal Sphincter ØDRR
  Aorta
    Abdominal Ø4RØ
    Thoracic Ø2RW
  Artery
    Anterior Tibial
      Left Ø4RQ
      Right Ø4RP
    Axillary
      Left Ø3R6
      Right Ø3R5
    Brachial
      Left Ø3R8
      Right Ø3R7
    Celiac Ø4R1
    Colic
      Left Ø4R7
      Middle Ø4R8
      Right Ø4R6
    Common Carotid
      Left Ø3RJ
      Right Ø3RH

Subterms under main terms may continue to next column or page

Replacement — continued
Artery — continued
Common Iliac
Left Ø4RD
Right Ø4RC
External Carotid
Left Ø3RN
Right Ø3RM
External Iliac
Left Ø4RJ
Right Ø4RH
Face Ø3RR
Femoral
Left Ø4RL
Right Ø4RK
Foot
Left Ø4RW
Right Ø4RV
Gastric Ø4R2
Hand
Left Ø3RF
Right Ø3RD
Hepatic Ø4R3
Inferior Mesenteric Ø4RB
Innominate Ø3R2
Internal Carotid
Left Ø3RL
Right Ø3RK
Internal Iliac
Left Ø4RF
Right Ø4RE
Internal Mammary
Left Ø3R1
Right Ø3RØ
Intracranial Ø3RG
Lower Ø4RY
Peroneal
Left Ø4RU
Right Ø4RT
Popliteal
Left Ø4RN
Right Ø4RM
Posterior Tibial
Left Ø4RS
Right Ø4RR
Pulmonary
Left Ø2RR
Right Ø2RQ
Pulmonary Trunk Ø2RP
Radial
Left Ø3RC
Right Ø3RB
Renal
Left Ø4RA
Right Ø4R9
Splenic Ø4R4
Subclavian
Left Ø3R4
Right Ø3R3
Superior Mesenteric Ø4R5
Temporal
Left Ø3RT
Right Ø3RS
Thyroid
Left Ø3RV
Right Ø3RU
Ulnar
Left Ø3RA
Right Ø3R9
Upper Ø3RY
Vertebral
Left Ø3RQ
Right Ø3RP
Atrium
Left Ø2R7
Right Ø2R6
Auditory Ossicle
Left Ø9RAØ
Right Ø9R9Ø
Bladder ØTRB
Bladder Neck ØTRC
Bone
Ethmoid
Left ØNRG
Right ØNRF

Replacement — continued
Bone — continued
Frontal
Left ØNR2
Right ØNR1
Hyoid ØNRX
Lacrimal
Left ØNRJ
Right ØNRH
Nasal ØNRB
Occipital
Left ØNR8
Right ØNR7
Palatine
Left ØNRL
Right ØNRK
Parietal
Left ØNR4
Right ØNR3
Pelvic
Left ØQR3
Right ØQR2
Sphenoid
Left ØNRD
Right ØNRC
Temporal
Left ØNR6
Right ØNR5
Zygomatic
Left ØNRN
Right ØNRM
Breast
Bilateral ØHRV
Left ØHRU
Right ØHRT
Buccal Mucosa ØCR4
Carpal
Left ØPRN
Right ØPRM
Chordae Tendineae Ø2R9
Choroid
Left Ø8RB
Right Ø8RA
Clavicle
Left ØPRB
Right ØPR9
Coccyx ØQRS
Conjunctiva
Left Ø8RTX
Right Ø8RSX
Cornea
Left Ø8R9
Right Ø8R8
Disc
Cervical Vertebral ØRR3Ø
Cervicothoracic Vertebral ØRR5Ø
Lumbar Vertebral ØSR2Ø
Lumbosacral ØSR4Ø
Thoracic Vertebral ØRR9Ø
Thoracolumbar Vertebral ØRRBØ
Duct
Common Bile ØFR9
Cystic ØFR8
Hepatic
Left ØFR6
Right ØFR5
Lacrimal
Left Ø8RY
Right Ø8RX
Pancreatic ØFRD
Accessory ØFRF
Parotid
Left ØCRC
Right ØCRB
Ear
External
Bilateral Ø9R2
Left Ø9R1
Right Ø9RØ
Inner
Left Ø9REØ
Right Ø9RDØ
Middle
Left Ø9R6Ø
Right Ø9R5Ø
Epiglottis ØCRR

Replacement — continued
Esophagus ØDR5
Eye
Left Ø8R1
Right Ø8RØ
Eyelid
Lower
Left Ø8RR
Right Ø8RQ
Upper
Left Ø8RP
Right Ø8RN
Femoral Shaft
Left ØQR9
Right ØQR8
Femur
Lower
Left ØQRC
Right ØQRB
Upper
Left ØQR7
Right ØQR6
Fibula
Left ØQRK
Right ØQRJ
Finger Nail ØHRQX
Gingiva
Lower ØCR6
Upper ØCR5
Glenoid Cavity
Left ØPR8
Right ØPR7
Hair ØHRSX
Humeral Head
Left ØPRD
Right ØPRC
Humeral Shaft
Left ØPRG
Right ØPRF
Iris
Left Ø8RD3
Right Ø8RC3
Joint
Acromioclavicular
Left ØRRHØ
Right ØRRGØ
Ankle
Left ØSRG
Right ØSRF
Carpal
Left ØRRRØ
Right ØRRQØ
Cervical Vertebral ØRR1Ø
Cervicothoracic Vertebral ØRR4Ø
Coccygeal ØSR6Ø
Elbow
Left ØRRMØ
Right ØRRLØ
Finger Phalangeal
Left ØRRXØ
Right ØRRWØ
Hip
Left ØSRB
Acetabular Surface ØSRE
Femoral Surface ØSRS
Right ØSR9
Acetabular Surface ØSRA
Femoral Surface ØSRR
Knee
Left ØSRD
Femoral Surface ØSRU
Tibial Surface ØSRW
Right ØSRC
Femoral Surface ØSRT
Tibial Surface ØSRV
Lumbar Vertebral ØSRØØ
Lumbosacral ØSR3Ø
Metacarpocarpal
Left ØRRTØ
Right ØRRSØ
Metacarpophalangeal
Left ØRRVØ
Right ØRRUØ
Metatarsal-Phalangeal
Left ØSRNØ
Right ØSRMØ

Replacement — continued
Joint — continued
Metatarsal-Tarsal
Left ØSRLØ
Right ØSRKØ
Occipital-cervical ØRRØØ
Sacrococcygeal ØSR5Ø
Sacroiliac
Left ØSR8Ø
Right ØSR7Ø
Shoulder
Left ØRRK
Right ØRRJ
Sternoclavicular
Left ØRRFØ
Right ØRREØ
Tarsal
Left ØSRJØ
Right ØSRHØ
Temporomandibular
Left ØRRDØ
Right ØRRCØ
Thoracic Vertebral ØRR6Ø
Thoracolumbar Vertebral ØRRAØ
Toe Phalangeal
Left ØSRQØ
Right ØSRPØ
Wrist
Left ØRRPØ
Right ØRRNØ
Kidney Pelvis
Left ØTR4
Right ØTR3
Larynx ØCRS
Lens
Left Ø8RK3ØZ
Right Ø8RJ3ØZ
Lip
Lower ØCR1
Upper ØCRØ
Mandible
Left ØNRV
Right ØNRT
Maxilla
Left ØNRS
Right ØNRR
Mesentery ØDRV
Metacarpal
Left ØPRQ
Right ØPRP
Metatarsal
Left ØQRP
Right ØQRN
Muscle, Papillary Ø2RD
Nasopharynx Ø9RN
Nipple
Left ØHRX
Right ØHRW
Nose Ø9RK
Omentum
Greater ØDRS
Lesser ØDRT
Orbit
Left ØNRQ
Right ØNRP
Palate
Hard ØCR2
Soft ØCR3
Patella
Left ØQRF
Right ØQRD
Pericardium Ø2RN
Peritoneum ØDRW
Phalanx
Finger
Left ØPRV
Right ØPRT
Thumb
Left ØPRS
Right ØPRR
Toe
Left ØQRR
Right ØQRQ
Pharynx ØCRM
Radius
Left ØPRJ

Replacement — continued
Radius — continued
Right ØPRH
Retinal Vessel
Left Ø8RH3
Right Ø8RG3
Rib
Left ØPR2
Right ØPR1
Sacrum ØQR1
Scapula
Left ØPR6
Right ØPR5
Sclera
Left Ø8R7X
Right Ø8R6X
Septum
Atrial Ø2R5
Nasal Ø9RM
Ventricular Ø2RM
Skin
Abdomen ØHR7
Back ØHR6
Buttock ØHR8
Chest ØHR5
Ear
Left ØHR3
Right ØHR2
Face ØHR1
Foot
Left ØHRN
Right ØHRM
Genitalia ØHRA
Hand
Left ØHRG
Right ØHRF
Lower Arm
Left ØHRE
Right ØHRD
Lower Leg
Left ØHRL
Right ØHRK
Neck ØHR4
Perineum ØHR9
Scalp ØHRØ
Upper Arm
Left ØHRC
Right ØHRB
Upper Leg
Left ØHRJ
Right ØHRH
Skull ØNRØ
Sternum ØPRØ
Subcutaneous Tissue and Fascia
Abdomen ØJR8
Back ØJR7
Buttock ØJR9
Chest ØJR6
Face ØJR1
Foot
Left ØJRR
Right ØJRQ
Hand
Left ØJRK
Right ØJRJ
Lower Arm
Left ØJRH
Right ØJRG
Lower Leg
Left ØJRP
Right ØJRN
Neck
Anterior ØJR4
Posterior ØJR5
Pelvic Region ØJRC
Perineum ØJRB
Scalp ØJRØ
Upper Arm
Left ØJRF
Right ØJRD
Upper Leg
Left ØJRM
Right ØJRL
Tarsal
Left ØQRM
Right ØQRL

Replacement — continued
Tendon
Abdomen
Left ØLRG
Right ØLRF
Ankle
Left ØLRT
Right ØLRS
Foot
Left ØLRW
Right ØLRV
Hand
Left ØLR8
Right ØLR7
Head and Neck ØLRØ
Hip
Left ØLRK
Right ØLRJ
Knee
Left ØLRR
Right ØLRQ
Lower Arm and Wrist
Left ØLR6
Right ØLR5
Lower Leg
Left ØLRP
Right ØLRN
Perineum ØLRH
Shoulder
Left ØLR2
Right ØLR1
Thorax
Left ØLRD
Right ØLRC
Trunk
Left ØLRB
Right ØLR9
Upper Arm
Left ØLR4
Right ØLR3
Upper Leg
Left ØLRM
Right ØLRL
Testis
Bilateral ØVRCØJZ
Left ØVRBØJZ
Right ØVR9ØJZ
Thumb
Left ØXRM
Right ØXRL
Tibia
Left ØQRH
Right ØQRG
Toe Nail ØHRRX
Tongue ØCR7
Tooth
Lower ØCRX
Upper ØCRW
Turbinate, Nasal Ø9RL
Tympanic Membrane
Left Ø9R8
Right Ø9R7
Ulna
Left ØPRL
Right ØPRK
Ureter
Left ØTR7
Right ØTR6
Urethra ØTRD
Uvula ØCRN
Valve
Aortic Ø2RF
Mitral Ø2RG
Pulmonary Ø2RH
Tricuspid Ø2RJ
Vein
Axillary
Left Ø5R8
Right Ø5R7
Azygos Ø5RØ
Basilic
Left Ø5RC
Right Ø5RB
Brachial
Left Ø5RA
Right Ø5R9

Replacement — continued
Vein — continued
Cephalic
Left Ø5RF
Right Ø5RD
Colic Ø6R7
Common Iliac
Left Ø6RD
Right Ø6RC
Esophageal Ø6R3
External Iliac
Left Ø6RG
Right Ø6RF
External Jugular
Left Ø5RQ
Right Ø5RP
Face
Left Ø5RV
Right Ø5RT
Femoral
Left Ø6RN
Right Ø6RM
Foot
Left Ø6RV
Right Ø6RT
Gastric Ø6R2
Greater Saphenous
Left Ø6RQ
Right Ø6RP
Hand
Left Ø5RH
Right Ø5RG
Hemiazygos Ø5R1
Hepatic Ø6R4
Hypogastric
Left Ø6RJ
Right Ø6RH
Inferior Mesenteric Ø6R6
Innominate
Left Ø5R4
Right Ø5R3
Internal Jugular
Left Ø5RN
Right Ø5RM
Intracranial Ø5RL
Lesser Saphenous
Left Ø6RS
Right Ø6RR
Lower Ø6RY
Portal Ø6R8
Pulmonary
Left Ø2RT
Right Ø2RS
Renal
Left Ø6RB
Right Ø6R9
Splenic Ø6R1
Subclavian
Left Ø5R6
Right Ø5R5
Superior Mesenteric Ø6R5
Upper Ø5RY
Vertebral
Left Ø5RS
Right Ø5RR
Vena Cava
Inferior Ø6RØ
Superior Ø2RV
Ventricle
Left Ø2RL
Right Ø2RK
Vertebra
Cervical ØPR3
Lumbar ØQRØ
Thoracic ØPR4
Vitreous
Left Ø8R53
Right Ø8R43
Vocal Cord
Left ØCRV
Right ØCRT
Replantation *see* Reposition
Replantation, scalp *see* Reattachment, Skin, Scalp ØHMØ
Reposition
Acetabulum
Left ØQS5
Right ØQS4
Ampulla of Vater ØFSC
Anus ØDSQ
Aorta
Abdominal Ø4SØ
Thoracic Ø2SWØZZ
Artery
Anterior Tibial
Left Ø4SQ
Right Ø4SP
Axillary
Left Ø3S6
Right Ø3S5
Brachial
Left Ø3S8
Right Ø3S7
Celiac Ø4S1
Colic
Left Ø4S7
Middle Ø4S8
Right Ø4S6
Common Carotid
Left Ø3SJ
Right Ø3SH
Common Iliac
Left Ø4SD
Right Ø4SC
External Carotid
Left Ø3SN
Right Ø3SM
External Iliac
Left Ø4SJ
Right Ø4SH
Face Ø3SR
Femoral
Left Ø4SL
Right Ø4SK
Foot
Left Ø4SW
Right Ø4SV
Gastric Ø4S2
Hand
Left Ø3SF
Right Ø3SD
Hepatic Ø4S3
Inferior Mesenteric Ø4SB
Innominate Ø3S2
Internal Carotid
Left Ø3SL
Right Ø3SK
Internal Iliac
Left Ø4SF
Right Ø4SE
Internal Mammary
Left Ø3S1
Right Ø3SØ
Intracranial Ø3SG
Lower Ø4SY
Peroneal
Left Ø4SU
Right Ø4ST
Popliteal
Left Ø4SN
Right Ø4SM
Posterior Tibial
Left Ø4SS
Right Ø4SR
Pulmonary
Left Ø2SRØZZ
Right Ø2SQØZZ
Pulmonary Trunk Ø2SPØZZ
Radial
Left Ø3SC
Right Ø3SB
Renal
Left Ø4SA
Right Ø4S9
Splenic Ø4S4
Subclavian
Left Ø3S4
Right Ø3S3
Superior Mesenteric Ø4S5
Reposition — continued
Artery — continued
Temporal
Left Ø3ST
Right Ø3SS
Thyroid
Left Ø3SV
Right Ø3SU
Ulnar
Left Ø3SA
Right Ø3S9
Upper Ø3SY
Vertebral
Left Ø3SQ
Right Ø3SP
Auditory Ossicle
Left Ø9SA
Right Ø9S9
Bladder ØTSB
Bladder Neck ØTSC
Bone
Ethmoid
Left ØNSG
Right ØNSF
Frontal
Left ØNS2
Right ØNS1
Hyoid ØNSX
Lacrimal
Left ØNSJ
Right ØNSH
Nasal ØNSB
Occipital
Left ØNS8
Right ØNS7
Palatine
Left ØNSL
Right ØNSK
Parietal
Left ØNS4
Right ØNS3
Pelvic
Left ØQS3
Right ØQS2
Sphenoid
Left ØNSD
Right ØNSC
Temporal
Left ØNS6
Right ØNS5
Zygomatic
Left ØNSN
Right ØNSM
Breast
Bilateral ØHSVØZZ
Left ØHSUØZZ
Right ØHSTØZZ
Bronchus
Lingula ØBS9ØZZ
Lower Lobe
Left ØBSBØZZ
Right ØBS6ØZZ
Main
Left ØBS7ØZZ
Right ØBS3ØZZ
Middle Lobe, Right ØBS5ØZZ
Upper Lobe
Left ØBS8ØZZ
Right ØBS4ØZZ
Bursa and Ligament
Abdomen
Left ØMSJ
Right ØMSH
Ankle
Left ØMSR
Right ØMSQ
Elbow
Left ØMS4
Right ØMS3
Foot
Left ØMST
Right ØMSS
Hand
Left ØMS8
Right ØMS7
Head and Neck ØMSØ

- **Reposition** — continued
  - Bursa and Ligament — continued
    - Hip
      - Left ØMSM
      - Right ØMSL
    - Knee
      - Left ØMSP
      - Right ØMSN
    - Lower Extremity
      - Left ØMSW
      - Right ØMSV
    - Perineum ØMSK
    - Shoulder
      - Left ØMS2
      - Right ØMS1
    - Thorax
      - Left ØMSG
      - Right ØMSF
    - Trunk
      - Left ØMSD
      - Right ØMSC
    - Upper Extremity
      - Left ØMSB
      - Right ØMS9
    - Wrist
      - Left ØMS6
      - Right ØMS5
  - Carina ØBS2ØZZ
  - Carpal
    - Left ØPSN
    - Right ØPSM
  - Cecum ØDSH
  - Cervix ØUSC
  - Clavicle
    - Left ØPSB
    - Right ØPS9
  - Coccyx ØQSS
  - Colon
    - Ascending ØDSK
    - Descending ØDSM
    - Sigmoid ØDSN
    - Transverse ØDSL
  - Cord
    - Bilateral ØVSH
    - Left ØVSG
    - Right ØVSF
  - Cul-de-sac ØUSF
  - Diaphragm
    - Left ØBSSØZZ
    - Right ØBSRØZZ
  - Duct
    - Common Bile ØFS9
    - Cystic ØFS8
    - Hepatic
      - Left ØFS6
      - Right ØFS5
    - Lacrimal
      - Left Ø8SY
      - Right Ø8SX
    - Pancreatic ØFSD
      - Accessory ØFSF
    - Parotid
      - Left ØCSC
      - Right ØCSB
  - Duodenum ØDS9
  - Ear
    - Bilateral Ø9S2
    - Left Ø9S1
    - Right Ø9SØ
  - Epiglottis ØCSR
  - Esophagus ØDS5
  - Eustachian Tube
    - Left Ø9SG
    - Right Ø9SF
  - Eyelid
    - Lower
      - Left Ø8SR
      - Right Ø8SQ
    - Upper
      - Left Ø8SP
      - Right Ø8SN
  - Fallopian Tube
    - Left ØUS6
    - Right ØUS5
  - Fallopian Tubes, Bilateral ØUS7
- **Reposition** — continued
  - Femoral Shaft
    - Left ØQS9
    - Right ØQS8
  - Femur
    - Lower
      - Left ØQSC
      - Right ØQSB
    - Upper
      - Left ØQS7
      - Right ØQS6
  - Fibula
    - Left ØQSK
    - Right ØQSJ
  - Gallbladder ØFS4
  - Gland
    - Adrenal
      - Left ØGS2
      - Right ØGS3
    - Lacrimal
      - Left Ø8SW
      - Right Ø8SV
  - Glenoid Cavity
    - Left ØPS8
    - Right ØPS7
  - Hair ØHSSXZZ
  - Humeral Head
    - Left ØPSD
    - Right ØPSC
  - Humeral Shaft
    - Left ØPSG
    - Right ØPSF
  - Ileum ØDSB
  - Iris
    - Left Ø8SD3ZZ
    - Right Ø8SC3ZZ
  - Jejunum ØDSA
  - Joint
    - Acromioclavicular
      - Left ØRSH
      - Right ØRSG
    - Ankle
      - Left ØSSG
      - Right ØSSF
    - Carpal
      - Left ØRSR
      - Right ØRSQ
    - Cervical Vertebral ØRS1
    - Cervicothoracic Vertebral ØRS4
    - Coccygeal ØSS6
    - Elbow
      - Left ØRSM
      - Right ØRSL
    - Finger Phalangeal
      - Left ØRSX
      - Right ØRSW
    - Hip
      - Left ØSSB
      - Right ØSS9
    - Knee
      - Left ØSSD
      - Right ØSSC
    - Lumbar Vertebral ØSSØ
    - Lumbosacral ØSS3
    - Metacarpocarpal
      - Left ØRST
      - Right ØRSS
    - Metacarpophalangeal
      - Left ØRSV
      - Right ØRSU
    - Metatarsal-Phalangeal
      - Left ØSSN
      - Right ØSSM
    - Metatarsal-Tarsal
      - Left ØSSL
      - Right ØSSK
    - Occipital-cervical ØRSØ
    - Sacrococcygeal ØSS5
    - Sacroiliac
      - Left ØSS8
      - Right ØSS7
    - Shoulder
      - Left ØRSK
      - Right ØRSJ
    - Sternoclavicular
      - Left ØRSF
- **Reposition** — continued
  - Joint — continued
    - Sternoclavicular — continued
      - Right ØRSE
    - Tarsal
      - Left ØSSJ
      - Right ØSSH
    - Temporomandibular
      - Left ØRSD
      - Right ØRSC
    - Thoracic Vertebral ØRS6
    - Thoracolumbar Vertebral ØRSA
    - Toe Phalangeal
      - Left ØSSQ
      - Right ØSSP
    - Wrist
      - Left ØRSP
      - Right ØRSN
  - Kidney
    - Left ØTS1
    - Right ØTSØ
  - Kidney Pelvis
    - Left ØTS4
    - Right ØTS3
  - Kidneys, Bilateral ØTS2
  - Lens
    - Left Ø8SK3ZZ
    - Right Ø8SJ3ZZ
  - Lip
    - Lower ØCS1
    - Upper ØCSØ
  - Liver ØFSØ
  - Lung
    - Left ØBSLØZZ
    - Lower Lobe
      - Left ØBSJØZZ
      - Right ØBSFØZZ
    - Middle Lobe, Right ØBSDØZZ
    - Right ØBSKØZZ
    - Upper Lobe
      - Left ØBSGØZZ
      - Right ØBSCØZZ
  - Lung Lingula ØBSHØZZ
  - Mandible
    - Left ØNSV
    - Right ØNST
  - Maxilla
    - Left ØNSS
    - Right ØNSR
  - Metacarpal
    - Left ØPSQ
    - Right ØPSP
  - Metatarsal
    - Left ØQSP
    - Right ØQSN
  - Muscle
    - Abdomen
      - Left ØKSL
      - Right ØKSK
    - Extraocular
      - Left Ø8SM
      - Right Ø8SL
    - Facial ØKS1
    - Foot
      - Left ØKSW
      - Right ØKSV
    - Hand
      - Left ØKSD
      - Right ØKSC
    - Head ØKSØ
    - Hip
      - Left ØKSP
      - Right ØKSN
    - Lower Arm and Wrist
      - Left ØKSB
      - Right ØKS9
    - Lower Leg
      - Left ØKST
      - Right ØKSS
    - Neck
      - Left ØKS3
      - Right ØKS2
    - Perineum ØKSM
    - Shoulder
      - Left ØKS6
      - Right ØKS5

Reposition — continued
- Muscle — continued
  - Thorax
    - Left ØKSJ
    - Right ØKSH
  - Tongue, Palate, Pharynx ØKS4
  - Trunk
    - Left ØKSG
    - Right ØKSF
  - Upper Arm
    - Left ØKS8
    - Right ØKS7
  - Upper Leg
    - Left ØKSR
    - Right ØKSQ
- Nerve
  - Abducens ØØSL
  - Accessory ØØSR
  - Acoustic ØØSN
  - Brachial Plexus Ø1S3
  - Cervical Ø1S1
  - Cervical Plexus Ø1SØ
  - Facial ØØSM
  - Femoral Ø1SD
  - Glossopharyngeal ØØSP
  - Hypoglossal ØØSS
  - Lumbar Ø1SB
  - Lumbar Plexus Ø1S9
  - Lumbosacral Plexus Ø1SA
  - Median Ø1S5
  - Oculomotor ØØSH
  - Olfactory ØØSF
  - Optic ØØSG
  - Peroneal Ø1SH
  - Phrenic Ø1S2
  - Pudendal Ø1SC
  - Radial Ø1S6
  - Sacral Ø1SR
  - Sacral Plexus Ø1SQ
  - Sciatic Ø1SF
  - Thoracic Ø1S8
  - Tibial Ø1SG
  - Trigeminal ØØSK
  - Trochlear ØØSJ
  - Ulnar Ø1S4
  - Vagus ØØSQ
- Nipple
  - Left ØHSXXZZ
  - Right ØHSWXZZ
- Nose Ø9SK
- Orbit
  - Left ØNSQ
  - Right ØNSP
- Ovary
  - Bilateral ØUS2
  - Left ØUS1
  - Right ØUSØ
- Palate
  - Hard ØCS2
  - Soft ØCS3
- Pancreas ØFSG
- Parathyroid Gland ØGSR
  - Inferior
    - Left ØGSP
    - Right ØGSN
  - Multiple ØGSQ
  - Superior
    - Left ØGSM
    - Right ØGSL
- Patella
  - Left ØQSF
  - Right ØQSD
- Phalanx
  - Finger
    - Left ØPSV
    - Right ØPST
  - Thumb
    - Left ØPSS
    - Right ØPSR
  - Toe
    - Left ØQSR
    - Right ØQSQ
- Products of Conception 1ØSØ
  - Ectopic 1ØS2
- Radius
  - Left ØPSJ

Reposition — continued
- Radius — continued
  - Right ØPSH
- Rectum ØDSP
- Retinal Vessel
  - Left Ø8SH3ZZ
  - Right Ø8SG3ZZ
- Rib
  - Left ØPS2
  - Right ØPS1
- Sacrum ØQS1
- Scapula
  - Left ØPS6
  - Right ØPS5
- Septum, Nasal Ø9SM
- Skull ØNSØ
- Spinal Cord
  - Cervical ØØSW
  - Lumbar ØØSY
  - Thoracic ØØSX
- Spleen Ø7SPØZZ
- Sternum ØPSØ
- Stomach ØDS6
- Tarsal
  - Left ØQSM
  - Right ØQSL
- Tendon
  - Abdomen
    - Left ØLSG
    - Right ØLSF
  - Ankle
    - Left ØLST
    - Right ØLSS
  - Foot
    - Left ØLSW
    - Right ØLSV
  - Hand
    - Left ØLS8
    - Right ØLS7
  - Head and Neck ØLSØ
  - Hip
    - Left ØLSK
    - Right ØLSJ
  - Knee
    - Left ØLSR
    - Right ØLSQ
  - Lower Arm and Wrist
    - Left ØLS6
    - Right ØLS5
  - Lower Leg
    - Left ØLSP
    - Right ØLSN
  - Perineum ØLSH
  - Shoulder
    - Left ØLS2
    - Right ØLS1
  - Thorax
    - Left ØLSD
    - Right ØLSC
  - Trunk
    - Left ØLSB
    - Right ØLS9
  - Upper Arm
    - Left ØLS4
    - Right ØLS3
  - Upper Leg
    - Left ØLSM
    - Right ØLSL
- Testis
  - Bilateral ØVSC
  - Left ØVSB
  - Right ØVS9
- Thymus Ø7SMØZZ
- Thyroid Gland
  - Left Lobe ØGSG
  - Right Lobe ØGSH
- Tibia
  - Left ØQSH
  - Right ØQSG
- Tongue ØCS7
- Tooth
  - Lower ØCSX
  - Upper ØCSW
- Trachea ØBS1ØZZ
- Turbinate, Nasal Ø9SL

Reposition — continued
- Tympanic Membrane
  - Left Ø9S8
  - Right Ø9S7
- Ulna
  - Left ØPSL
  - Right ØPSK
- Ureter
  - Left ØTS7
  - Right ØTS6
- Ureters, Bilateral ØTS8
- Urethra ØTSD
- Uterine Supporting Structure ØUS4
- Uterus ØUS9
- Uvula ØCSN
- Vagina ØUSG
- Vein
  - Axillary
    - Left Ø5S8
    - Right Ø5S7
  - Azygos Ø5SØ
  - Basilic
    - Left Ø5SC
    - Right Ø5SB
  - Brachial
    - Left Ø5SA
    - Right Ø5S9
  - Cephalic
    - Left Ø5SF
    - Right Ø5SD
  - Colic Ø6S7
  - Common Iliac
    - Left Ø6SD
    - Right Ø6SC
  - Esophageal Ø6S3
  - External Iliac
    - Left Ø6SG
    - Right Ø6SF
  - External Jugular
    - Left Ø5SQ
    - Right Ø5SP
  - Face
    - Left Ø5SV
    - Right Ø5ST
  - Femoral
    - Left Ø6SN
    - Right Ø6SM
  - Foot
    - Left Ø6SV
    - Right Ø6ST
  - Gastric Ø6S2
  - Greater Saphenous
    - Left Ø6SQ
    - Right Ø6SP
  - Hand
    - Left Ø5SH
    - Right Ø5SG
  - Hemiazygos Ø5S1
  - Hepatic Ø6S4
  - Hypogastric
    - Left Ø6SJ
    - Right Ø6SH
  - Inferior Mesenteric Ø6S6
  - Innominate
    - Left Ø5S4
    - Right Ø5S3
  - Internal Jugular
    - Left Ø5SN
    - Right Ø5SM
  - Intracranial Ø5SL
  - Lesser Saphenous
    - Left Ø6SS
    - Right Ø6SR
  - Lower Ø6SY
  - Portal Ø6S8
  - Pulmonary
    - Left Ø2STØZZ
    - Right Ø2SSØZZ
  - Renal
    - Left Ø6SB
    - Right Ø6S9
  - Splenic Ø6S1
  - Subclavian
    - Left Ø5S6
    - Right Ø5S5
  - Superior Mesenteric Ø6S5

Reposition — continued
Vein — continued
Upper Ø5SY
Vertebral
Left Ø5SS
Right Ø5SR
Vena Cava
Inferior Ø6SØ
Superior Ø2SVØZZ
Vertebra
Cervical ØPS3
Lumbar ØQSØ
Thoracic ØPS4
Vocal Cord
Left ØCSV
Right ØCST
Resection
Acetabulum
Left ØQT5ØZZ
Right ØQT4ØZZ
Adenoids ØCTQ
Ampulla of Vater ØFTC
Anal Sphincter ØDTR
Anus ØDTQ
Aortic Body ØGTD
Appendix ØDTJ
Auditory Ossicle
Left Ø9TAØZZ
Right Ø9T9ØZZ
Bladder ØTTB
Bladder Neck ØTTC
Bone
Ethmoid
Left ØNTGØZZ
Right ØNTFØZZ
Frontal
Left ØNT2ØZZ
Right ØNT1ØZZ
Hyoid ØNTXØZZ
Lacrimal
Left ØNTJØZZ
Right ØNTHØZZ
Nasal ØNTBØZZ
Occipital
Left ØNT8ØZZ
Right ØNT7ØZZ
Palatine
Left ØNTLØZZ
Right ØNTKØZZ
Parietal
Left ØNT4ØZZ
Right ØNT3ØZZ
Pelvic
Left ØQT3ØZZ
Right ØQT2ØZZ
Sphenoid
Left ØNTDØZZ
Right ØNTCØZZ
Temporal
Left ØNT6ØZZ
Right ØNT5ØZZ
Zygomatic
Left ØNTNØZZ
Right ØNTMØZZ
Breast
Bilateral ØHTVØZZ
Left ØHTUØZZ
Right ØHTTØZZ
Supernumerary ØHTYØZZ
Bronchus
Lingula ØBT9
Lower Lobe
Left ØBTB
Right ØBT6
Main
Left ØBT7
Right ØBT3
Middle Lobe, Right ØBT5
Upper Lobe
Left ØBT8
Right ØBT4
Bursa and Ligament
Abdomen
Left ØMTJ
Right ØMTH

Resection — continued
Bursa and Ligament — continued
Ankle
Left ØMTR
Right ØMTQ
Elbow
Left ØMT4
Right ØMT3
Foot
Left ØMTT
Right ØMTS
Hand
Left ØMT8
Right ØMT7
Head and Neck ØMTØ
Hip
Left ØMTM
Right ØMTL
Knee
Left ØMTP
Right ØMTN
Lower Extremity
Left ØMTW
Right ØMTV
Perineum ØMTK
Shoulder
Left ØMT2
Right ØMT1
Thorax
Left ØMTG
Right ØMTF
Trunk
Left ØMTD
Right ØMTC
Upper Extremity
Left ØMTB
Right ØMT9
Wrist
Left ØMT6
Right ØMT5
Carina ØBT2
Carotid Bodies, Bilateral ØGT8
Carotid Body
Left ØGT6
Right ØGT7
Carpal
Left ØPTNØZZ
Right ØPTMØZZ
Cecum ØDTH
Cerebral Hemisphere ØØT7
Cervix ØUTC
Chordae Tendineae Ø2T9
Cisterna Chyli Ø7TL
Clavicle
Left ØPTBØZZ
Right ØPT9ØZZ
Clitoris ØUTJ
Coccygeal Glomus ØGTB
Coccyx ØQTSØZZ
Colon
Ascending ØDTK
Descending ØDTM
Sigmoid ØDTN
Transverse ØDTL
Conduction Mechanism Ø2T8
Cord
Bilateral ØVTH
Left ØVTG
Right ØVTF
Cornea
Left Ø8T9XZZ
Right Ø8T8XZZ
Cul-de-sac ØUTF
Diaphragm
Left ØBTS
Right ØBTR
Disc
Cervical Vertebral ØRT3ØZZ
Cervicothoracic Vertebral ØRT5ØZZ
Lumbar Vertebral ØST2ØZZ
Lumbosacral ØST4ØZZ
Thoracic Vertebral ØRT9ØZZ
Thoracolumbar Vertebral ØRTBØZZ
Duct
Common Bile ØFT9
Cystic ØFT8

Resection — continued
Duct — continued
Hepatic
Left ØFT6
Right ØFT5
Lacrimal
Left Ø8TY
Right Ø8TX
Pancreatic ØFTD
Accessory ØFTF
Parotid
Left ØCTCØZZ
Right ØCTBØZZ
Duodenum ØDT9
Ear
External
Left Ø9T1
Right Ø9TØ
Inner
Left Ø9TEØZZ
Right Ø9TDØZZ
Middle
Left Ø9T6ØZZ
Right Ø9T5ØZZ
Epididymis
Bilateral ØVTL
Left ØVTK
Right ØVTJ
Epiglottis ØCTR
Esophagogastric Junction ØDT4
Esophagus ØDT5
Lower ØDT3
Middle ØDT2
Upper ØDT1
Eustachian Tube
Left Ø9TG
Right Ø9TF
Eye
Left Ø8T1XZZ
Right Ø8TØXZZ
Eyelid
Lower
Left Ø8TR
Right Ø8TQ
Upper
Left Ø8TP
Right Ø8TN
Fallopian Tube
Left ØUT6
Right ØUT5
Fallopian Tubes, Bilateral ØUT7
Femoral Shaft
Left ØQT9ØZZ
Right ØQT8ØZZ
Femur
Lower
Left ØQTCØZZ
Right ØQTBØZZ
Upper
Left ØQT7ØZZ
Right ØQT6ØZZ
Fibula
Left ØQTKØZZ
Right ØQTJØZZ
Finger Nail ØHTQXZZ
Gallbladder ØFT4
Gland
Adrenal
Bilateral ØGT4
Left ØGT2
Right ØGT3
Lacrimal
Left Ø8TW
Right Ø8TV
Minor Salivary ØCTJØZZ
Parotid
Left ØCT9ØZZ
Right ØCT8ØZZ
Pituitary ØGTØ
Sublingual
Left ØCTFØZZ
Right ØCTDØZZ
Submaxillary
Left ØCTHØZZ
Right ØCTGØZZ
Vestibular ØUTL

Resection — continued
- Glenoid Cavity
  - Left ØPT8ØZZ
  - Right ØPT7ØZZ
- Glomus Jugulare ØGTC
- Humeral Head
  - Left ØPTDØZZ
  - Right ØPTCØZZ
- Humeral Shaft
  - Left ØPTGØZZ
  - Right ØPTFØZZ
- Hymen ØUTK
- Ileocecal Valve ØDTC
- Ileum ØDTB
- Intestine
  - Large ØDTE
    - Left ØDTG
    - Right ØDTF
  - Small ØDT8
- Iris
  - Left Ø8TD3ZZ
  - Right Ø8TC3ZZ
- Jejunum ØDTA
- Joint
  - Acromioclavicular
    - Left ØRTHØZZ
    - Right ØRTGØZZ
  - Ankle
    - Left ØSTGØZZ
    - Right ØSTFØZZ
  - Carpal
    - Left ØRTRØZZ
    - Right ØRTQØZZ
  - Cervicothoracic Vertebral ØRT4ØZZ
  - Coccygeal ØST6ØZZ
  - Elbow
    - Left ØRTMØZZ
    - Right ØRTLØZZ
  - Finger Phalangeal
    - Left ØRTXØZZ
    - Right ØRTWØZZ
  - Hip
    - Left ØSTBØZZ
    - Right ØST9ØZZ
  - Knee
    - Left ØSTDØZZ
    - Right ØSTCØZZ
  - Metacarpocarpal
    - Left ØRTTØZZ
    - Right ØRTSØZZ
  - Metacarpophalangeal
    - Left ØRTVØZZ
    - Right ØRTUØZZ
  - Metatarsal-Phalangeal
    - Left ØSTNØZZ
    - Right ØSTMØZZ
  - Metatarsal-Tarsal
    - Left ØSTLØZZ
    - Right ØSTKØZZ
  - Sacrococcygeal ØST5ØZZ
  - Sacroiliac
    - Left ØST8ØZZ
    - Right ØST7ØZZ
  - Shoulder
    - Left ØRTKØZZ
    - Right ØRTJØZZ
  - Sternoclavicular
    - Left ØRTFØZZ
    - Right ØRTEØZZ
  - Tarsal
    - Left ØSTJØZZ
    - Right ØSTHØZZ
  - Temporomandibular
    - Left ØRTDØZZ
    - Right ØRTCØZZ
  - Toe Phalangeal
    - Left ØSTQØZZ
    - Right ØSTPØZZ
  - Wrist
    - Left ØRTPØZZ
    - Right ØRTNØZZ
- Kidney
  - Left ØTT1
  - Right ØTTØ
- Kidney Pelvis
  - Left ØTT4

Resection — continued
- Kidney Pelvis — continued
  - Right ØTT3
- Kidneys, Bilateral ØTT2
- Larynx ØCTS
- Lens
  - Left Ø8TK3ZZ
  - Right Ø8TJ3ZZ
- Lip
  - Lower ØCT1
  - Upper ØCTØ
- Liver ØFTØ
  - Left Lobe ØFT2
  - Right Lobe ØFT1
- Lung
  - Bilateral ØBTM
  - Left ØBTL
  - Lower Lobe
    - Left ØBTJ
    - Right ØBTF
  - Middle Lobe, Right ØBTD
  - Right ØBTK
  - Upper Lobe
    - Left ØBTG
    - Right ØBTC
- Lung Lingula ØBTH
- Lymphatic
  - Aortic Ø7TD
  - Axillary
    - Left Ø7T6
    - Right Ø7T5
  - Head Ø7TØ
  - Inguinal
    - Left Ø7TJ
    - Right Ø7TH
  - Internal Mammary
    - Left Ø7T9
    - Right Ø7T8
  - Lower Extremity
    - Left Ø7TG
    - Right Ø7TF
  - Mesenteric Ø7TB
  - Neck
    - Left Ø7T2
    - Right Ø7T1
  - Pelvis Ø7TC
  - Thoracic Duct Ø7TK
  - Thorax Ø7T7
  - Upper Extremity
    - Left Ø7T4
    - Right Ø7T3
- Mandible
  - Left ØNTVØZZ
  - Right ØNTTØZZ
- Maxilla
  - Left ØNTSØZZ
  - Right ØNTRØZZ
- Metacarpal
  - Left ØPTQØZZ
  - Right ØPTPØZZ
- Metatarsal
  - Left ØQTPØZZ
  - Right ØQTNØZZ
- Muscle
  - Abdomen
    - Left ØKTL
    - Right ØKTK
  - Extraocular
    - Left Ø8TM
    - Right Ø8TL
  - Facial ØKT1
  - Foot
    - Left ØKTW
    - Right ØKTV
  - Hand
    - Left ØKTD
    - Right ØKTC
  - Head ØKTØ
  - Hip
    - Left ØKTP
    - Right ØKTN
  - Lower Arm and Wrist
    - Left ØKTB
    - Right ØKT9
  - Lower Leg
    - Left ØKTT

Resection — continued
- Muscle — continued
  - Lower Leg — continued
    - Right ØKTS
  - Neck
    - Left ØKT3
    - Right ØKT2
  - Papillary Ø2TD
  - Perineum ØKTM
  - Shoulder
    - Left ØKT6
    - Right ØKT5
  - Thorax
    - Left ØKTJ
    - Right ØKTH
  - Tongue, Palate, Pharynx ØKT4
  - Trunk
    - Left ØKTG
    - Right ØKTF
  - Upper Arm
    - Left ØKT8
    - Right ØKT7
  - Upper Leg
    - Left ØKTR
    - Right ØKTQ
- Nasopharynx Ø9TN
- Nipple
  - Left ØHTXXZZ
  - Right ØHTWXZZ
- Nose Ø9TK
- Omentum
  - Greater ØDTS
  - Lesser ØDTT
- Orbit
  - Left ØNTQØZZ
  - Right ØNTPØZZ
- Ovary
  - Bilateral ØUT2
  - Left ØUT1
  - Right ØUTØ
- Palate
  - Hard ØCT2
  - Soft ØCT3
- Pancreas ØFTG
- Para-aortic Body ØGT9
- Paraganglion Extremity ØGTF
- Parathyroid Gland ØGTR
  - Inferior
    - Left ØGTP
    - Right ØGTN
  - Multiple ØGTQ
  - Superior
    - Left ØGTM
    - Right ØGTL
- Patella
  - Left ØQTFØZZ
  - Right ØQTDØZZ
- Penis ØVTS
- Pericardium Ø2TN
- Phalanx
  - Finger
    - Left ØPTVØZZ
    - Right ØPTTØZZ
  - Thumb
    - Left ØPTSØZZ
    - Right ØPTRØZZ
  - Toe
    - Left ØQTRØZZ
    - Right ØQTQØZZ
- Pharynx ØCTM
- Pineal Body ØGT1
- Prepuce ØVTT
- Products of Conception, Ectopic 1ØT2
- Prostate ØVTØ
- Radius
  - Left ØPTJØZZ
  - Right ØPTHØZZ
- Rectum ØDTP
- Rib
  - Left ØPT2ØZZ
  - Right ØPT1ØZZ
- Scapula
  - Left ØPT6ØZZ
  - Right ØPT5ØZZ
- Scrotum ØVT5

Resection — continued
Septum
Atrial Ø2T5
Nasal Ø9TM
Ventricular Ø2TM
Sinus
Accessory Ø9TP
Ethmoid
Left Ø9TV
Right Ø9TU
Frontal
Left Ø9TT
Right Ø9TS
Mastoid
Left Ø9TC
Right Ø9TB
Maxillary
Left Ø9TR
Right Ø9TQ
Sphenoid
Left Ø9TX
Right Ø9TW
Spleen Ø7TP
Sternum ØPTØØZZ
Stomach ØDT6
Pylorus ØDT7
Tarsal
Left ØQTMØZZ
Right ØQTLØZZ
Tendon
Abdomen
Left ØLTG
Right ØLTF
Ankle
Left ØLTT
Right ØLTS
Foot
Left ØLTW
Right ØLTV
Hand
Left ØLT8
Right ØLT7
Head and Neck ØLTØ
Hip
Left ØLTK
Right ØLTJ
Knee
Left ØLTR
Right ØLTQ
Lower Arm and Wrist
Left ØLT6
Right ØLT5
Lower Leg
Left ØLTP
Right ØLTN
Perineum ØLTH
Shoulder
Left ØLT2
Right ØLT1
Thorax
Left ØLTD
Right ØLTC
Trunk
Left ØLTB
Right ØLT9
Upper Arm
Left ØLT4
Right ØLT3
Upper Leg
Left ØLTM
Right ØLTL
Testis
Bilateral ØVTC
Left ØVTB
Right ØVT9
Thymus Ø7TM
Thyroid Gland ØGTK
Left Lobe ØGTG
Right Lobe ØGTH
Tibia
Left ØQTHØZZ
Right ØQTGØZZ
Toe Nail ØHTRXZZ
Tongue ØCT7
Tonsils ØCTP

Resection — continued
Tooth
Lower ØCTXØZ
Upper ØCTWØZ
Trachea ØBT1
Tunica Vaginalis
Left ØVT7
Right ØVT6
Turbinate, Nasal Ø9TL
Tympanic Membrane
Left Ø9T8
Right Ø9T7
Ulna
Left ØPTLØZZ
Right ØPTKØZZ
Ureter
Left ØTT7
Right ØTT6
Urethra ØTTD
Uterine Supporting Structure ØUT4
Uterus ØUT9
Uvula ØCTN
Vagina ØUTG
Valve, Pulmonary Ø2TH
Vas Deferens
Bilateral ØVTQ
Left ØVTP
Right ØVTN
Vesicle
Bilateral ØVT3
Left ØVT2
Right ØVT1
Vitreous
Left Ø8T53ZZ
Right Ø8T43ZZ
Vocal Cord
Left ØCTV
Right ØCTT
Vulva ØUTM
Restoration, Cardiac, Single, Rhythm 5A22Ø4Z
RestoreAdvanced neurostimulator (SureScan) (MRI Safe) *use* Stimulator Generator, Multiple Array Rechargeable in ØJH
RestoreSensor neurostimulator (SureScan) (MRI Safe) *use* Stimulator Generator, Multiple Array Rechargeable in ØJH
RestoreUltra neurostimulator (SureScan) (MRI Safe) *use* Simulator Generator, Multiple Array Rechargeable in ØJH
Restriction
Ampulla of Vater ØFVC
Anus ØDVQ
Aorta
Abdominal Ø4VØ
Thoracic Ø2VW
Artery
Anterior Tibial
Left Ø4VQ
Right Ø4VP
Axillary
Left Ø3V6
Right Ø3V5
Brachial
Left Ø3V8
Right Ø3V7
Celiac Ø4V1
Colic
Left Ø4V7
Middle Ø4V8
Right Ø4V6
Common Carotid
Left Ø3VJ
Right Ø3VH
Common Iliac
Left Ø4VD
Right Ø4VC
External Carotid
Left Ø3VN
Right Ø3VM
External Iliac
Left Ø4VJ
Right Ø4VH
Face Ø3VR
Femoral
Left Ø4VL
Right Ø4VK

Restriction — continued
Artery — continued
Foot
Left Ø4VW
Right Ø4VV
Gastric Ø4V2
Hand
Left Ø3VF
Right Ø3VD
Hepatic Ø4V3
Inferior Mesenteric Ø4VB
Innominate Ø3V2
Internal Carotid
Left Ø3VL
Right Ø3VK
Internal Iliac
Left Ø4VF
Right Ø4VE
Internal Mammary
Left Ø3V1
Right Ø3VØ
Intracranial Ø3VG
Lower Ø4VY
Peroneal
Left Ø4VU
Right Ø4VT
Popliteal
Left Ø4VN
Right Ø4VM
Posterior Tibial
Left Ø4VS
Right Ø4VR
Pulmonary
Left Ø2VR
Right Ø2VQ
Pulmonary Trunk Ø2VP
Radial
Left Ø3VC
Right Ø3VB
Renal
Left Ø4VA
Right Ø4V9
Splenic Ø4V4
Subclavian
Left Ø3V4
Right Ø3V3
Superior Mesenteric Ø4V5
Temporal
Left Ø3VT
Right Ø3VS
Thyroid
Left Ø3VV
Right Ø3VU
Ulnar
Left Ø3VA
Right Ø3V9
Upper Ø3VY
Vertebral
Left Ø3VQ
Right Ø3VP
Bladder ØTVB
Bladder Neck ØTVC
Bronchus
Lingula ØBV9
Lower Lobe
Left ØBVB
Right ØBV6
Main
Left ØBV7
Right ØBV3
Middle Lobe, Right ØBV5
Upper Lobe
Left ØBV8
Right ØBV4
Carina ØBV2
Cecum ØDVH
Cervix ØUVC
Cisterna Chyli Ø7VL
Colon
Ascending ØDVK
Descending ØDVM
Sigmoid ØDVN
Transverse ØDVL
Duct
Common Bile ØFV9
Cystic ØFV8

Restriction — continued
Duct — continued
Hepatic
Left ØFV6
Right ØFV5
Lacrimal
Left Ø8VY
Right Ø8VX
Pancreatic ØFVD
Accessory ØFVF
Parotid
Left ØCVC
Right ØCVB
Duodenum ØDV9
Esophagogastric Junction ØDV4
Esophagus ØDV5
Lower ØDV3
Middle ØDV2
Upper ØDV1
Heart Ø2VA
Ileocecal Valve ØDVC
Ileum ØDVB
Intestine
Large ØDVE
Left ØDVG
Right ØDVF
Small ØDV8
Jejunum ØDVA
Kidney Pelvis
Left ØTV4
Right ØTV3
Lymphatic
Aortic Ø7VD
Axillary
Left Ø7V6
Right Ø7V5
Head Ø7VØ
Inguinal
Left Ø7VJ
Right Ø7VH
Internal Mammary
Left Ø7V9
Right Ø7V8
Lower Extremity
Left Ø7VG
Right Ø7VF
Mesenteric Ø7VB
Neck
Left Ø7V2
Right Ø7V1
Pelvis Ø7VC
Thoracic Duct Ø7VK
Thorax Ø7V7
Upper Extremity
Left Ø7V4
Right Ø7V3
Rectum ØDVP
Stomach ØDV6
Pylorus ØDV7
Trachea ØBV1
Ureter
Left ØTV7
Right ØTV6
Urethra ØTVD
Vein
Axillary
Left Ø5V8
Right Ø5V7
Azygos Ø5VØ
Basilic
Left Ø5VC
Right Ø5VB
Brachial
Left Ø5VA
Right Ø5V9
Cephalic
Left Ø5VF
Right Ø5VD
Colic Ø6V7
Common Iliac
Left Ø6VD
Right Ø6VC
Esophageal Ø6V3
External Iliac
Left Ø6VG
Right Ø6VF

Restriction — continued
Vein — continued
External Jugular
Left Ø5VQ
Right Ø5VP
Face
Left Ø5VV
Right Ø5VT
Femoral
Left Ø6VN
Right Ø6VM
Foot
Left Ø6VV
Right Ø6VT
Gastric Ø6V2
Greater Saphenous
Left Ø6VQ
Right Ø6VP
Hand
Left Ø5VH
Right Ø5VG
Hemiazygos Ø5V1
Hepatic Ø6V4
Hypogastric
Left Ø6VJ
Right Ø6VH
Inferior Mesenteric Ø6V6
Innominate
Left Ø5V4
Right Ø5V3
Internal Jugular
Left Ø5VN
Right Ø5VM
Intracranial Ø5VL
Lesser Saphenous
Left Ø6VS
Right Ø6VR
Lower Ø6VY
Portal Ø6V8
Pulmonary
Left Ø2VT
Right Ø2VS
Renal
Left Ø6VB
Right Ø6V9
Splenic Ø6V1
Subclavian
Left Ø5V6
Right Ø5V5
Superior Mesenteric Ø6V5
Upper Ø5VY
Vertebral
Left Ø5VS
Right Ø5VR
Vena Cava
Inferior Ø6VØ
Superior Ø2VV
Resurfacing Device
Removal of device from
Left ØSPBØBZ
Right ØSP9ØBZ
Revision of device in
Left ØSWBØBZ
Right ØSW9ØBZ
Supplement
Left ØSUBØBZ
Acetabular Surface ØSUEØBZ
Femoral Surface ØSUSØBZ
Right ØSU9ØBZ
Acetabular Surface ØSUAØBZ
Femoral Surface ØSURØBZ
Resuscitation
Cardiopulmonary *see* Assistance, Cardiac 5AØ2
Cardioversion 5A22Ø4Z
Defibrillation 5A22Ø4Z
Endotracheal intubation *see* Insertion of device in, Trachea ØBH1
External chest compression 5A12Ø12
Pulmonary 5A19Ø54
Resuture, Heart valve prosthesis *see* Revision of device in, Heart and Great Vessels Ø2W
Retraining
Cardiac *see* Motor Treatment, Rehabilitation FØ7
Vocational *see* Activities of Daily Living Treatment, Rehabilitation FØ8

Retrogasserian rhizotomy *see* Division, Nerve, Trigeminal ØØ8K
Retroperitoneal lymph node *use* Lymphatic, Aortic
Retroperitoneal space *use* Retroperitoneum
Retropharyngeal lymph node
use Lymphatic, Neck, Left
use Lymphatic, Neck, Right
Retropubic space *use* Pelvic Cavity
Reveal (DX) (XT) *use* Monitoring Device
Reverse total shoulder replacement *see* Replacement, Upper Joints ØRR
Reverse® Shoulder Prosthesis *use* Synthetic Substitute, Reverse Ball and Socket in ØRR
Revision of device in
Abdominal Wall ØWWF
Acetabulum
Left ØQW5
Right ØQW4
Anal Sphincter ØDWR
Anus ØDWQ
Artery
Lower Ø4WY
Upper Ø3WY
Auditory Ossicle
Left Ø9WA
Right Ø9W9
Back
Lower ØWWL
Upper ØWWK
Bladder ØTWB
Bone
Facial ØNWW
Lower ØQWY
Nasal ØNWB
Pelvic
Left ØQW3
Right ØQW2
Upper ØPWY
Bone Marrow Ø7WT
Brain ØØWØ
Breast
Left ØHWU
Right ØHWT
Bursa and Ligament
Lower ØMWY
Upper ØMWX
Carpal
Left ØPWN
Right ØPWM
Cavity, Cranial ØWW1
Cerebral Ventricle ØØW6
Chest Wall ØWW8
Cisterna Chyli Ø7WL
Clavicle
Left ØPWB
Right ØPW9
Coccyx ØQWS
Diaphragm ØBWT
Disc
Cervical Vertebral ØRW3
Cervicothoracic Vertebral ØRW5
Lumbar Vertebral ØSW2
Lumbosacral ØSW4
Thoracic Vertebral ØRW9
Thoracolumbar Vertebral ØRWB
Duct
Hepatobiliary ØFWB
Pancreatic ØFWD
Ear
Inner
Left Ø9WE
Right Ø9WD
Left Ø9WJ
Right Ø9WH
Epididymis and Spermatic Cord ØVWM
Esophagus ØDW5
Extremity
Lower
Left ØYWB
Right ØYW9
Upper
Left ØXW7
Right ØXW6
Eye
Left Ø8W1
Right Ø8WØ

Revision of device in — continued
- Face ØWW2
- Fallopian Tube ØUW8
- Femoral Shaft
  - Left ØQW9
  - Right ØQW8
- Femur
  - Lower
    - Left ØQWC
    - Right ØQWB
  - Upper
    - Left ØQW7
    - Right ØQW6
- Fibula
  - Left ØQWK
  - Right ØQWJ
- Finger Nail ØHWQX
- Gallbladder ØFW4
- Gastrointestinal Tract ØWWP
- Genitourinary Tract ØWWR
- Gland
  - Adrenal ØGW5
  - Endocrine ØGWS
  - Pituitary ØGWØ
  - Salivary ØCWA
- Glenoid Cavity
  - Left ØPW8
  - Right ØPW7
- Great Vessel Ø2WY
- Hair ØHWSX
- Head ØWWØ
- Heart Ø2WA
- Humeral Head
  - Left ØPWD
  - Right ØPWC
- Humeral Shaft
  - Left ØPWG
  - Right ØPWF
- Intestinal Tract
  - Lower ØDWD
  - Upper ØDWØ
- Intestine
  - Large ØDWE
  - Small ØDW8
- Jaw
  - Lower ØWW5
  - Upper ØWW4
- Joint
  - Acromioclavicular
    - Left ØRWH
    - Right ØRWG
  - Ankle
    - Left ØSWG
    - Right ØSWF
  - Carpal
    - Left ØRWR
    - Right ØRWQ
  - Cervical Vertebral ØRW1
  - Cervicothoracic Vertebral ØRW4
  - Coccygeal ØSW6
  - Elbow
    - Left ØRWM
    - Right ØRWL
  - Finger Phalangeal
    - Left ØRWX
    - Right ØRWW
  - Hip
    - Left ØSWB
    - Right ØSW9
  - Knee
    - Left ØSWD
    - Right ØSWC
  - Lumbar Vertebral ØSWØ
  - Lumbosacral ØSW3
  - Metacarpocarpal
    - Left ØRWT
    - Right ØRWS
  - Metacarpophalangeal
    - Left ØRWV
    - Right ØRWU
  - Metatarsal-Phalangeal
    - Left ØSWN
    - Right ØSWM
  - Metatarsal-Tarsal
    - Left ØSWL
    - Right ØSWK

Revision of device in — continued
- Joint — continued
  - Occipital-cervical ØRWØ
  - Sacrococcygeal ØSW5
  - Sacroiliac
    - Left ØSW8
    - Right ØSW7
  - Shoulder
    - Left ØRWK
    - Right ØRWJ
  - Sternoclavicular
    - Left ØRWF
    - Right ØRWE
  - Tarsal
    - Left ØSWJ
    - Right ØSWH
  - Temporomandibular
    - Left ØRWD
    - Right ØRWC
  - Thoracic Vertebral ØRW6
  - Thoracolumbar Vertebral ØRWA
  - Toe Phalangeal
    - Left ØSWQ
    - Right ØSWP
  - Wrist
    - Left ØRWP
    - Right ØRWN
- Kidney ØTW5
- Larynx ØCWS
- Lens
  - Left Ø8WK
  - Right Ø8WJ
- Liver ØFWØ
- Lung
  - Left ØBWL
  - Right ØBWK
- Lymphatic Ø7WN
  - Thoracic Duct Ø7WK
- Mediastinum ØWWC
- Mesentery ØDWV
- Metacarpal
  - Left ØPWQ
  - Right ØPWP
- Metatarsal
  - Left ØQWP
  - Right ØQWN
- Mouth and Throat ØCWY
- Muscle
  - Extraocular
    - Left Ø8WM
    - Right Ø8WL
  - Lower ØKWY
  - Upper ØKWX
- Neck ØWW6
- Nerve
  - Cranial ØØWE
  - Peripheral Ø1WY
- Nose Ø9WK
- Omentum ØDWU
- Ovary ØUW3
- Pancreas ØFWG
- Parathyroid Gland ØGWR
- Patella
  - Left ØQWF
  - Right ØQWD
- Pelvic Cavity ØWWJ
- Penis ØVWS
- Pericardial Cavity ØWWD
- Perineum
  - Female ØWWN
  - Male ØWWM
- Peritoneal Cavity ØWWG
- Peritoneum ØDWW
- Phalanx
  - Finger
    - Left ØPWV
    - Right ØPWT
  - Thumb
    - Left ØPWS
    - Right ØPWR
  - Toe
    - Left ØQWR
    - Right ØQWQ
- Pineal Body ØGW1
- Pleura ØBWQ

Revision of device in — continued
- Pleural Cavity
  - Left ØWWB
  - Right ØWW9
- Prostate and Seminal Vesicles ØVW4
- Radius
  - Left ØPWJ
  - Right ØPWH
- Respiratory Tract ØWWQ
- Retroperitoneum ØWWH
- Rib
  - Left ØPW2
  - Right ØPW1
- Sacrum ØQW1
- Scapula
  - Left ØPW6
  - Right ØPW5
- Scrotum and Tunica Vaginalis ØVW8
- Septum
  - Atrial Ø2W5
  - Ventricular Ø2WM
- Sinus Ø9WY
- Skin ØHWPX
- Skull ØNWØ
- Spinal Canal ØØWU
- Spinal Cord ØØWV
- Spleen Ø7WP
- Sternum ØPWØ
- Stomach ØDW6
- Subcutaneous Tissue and Fascia
  - Head and Neck ØJWS
  - Lower Extremity ØJWW
  - Trunk ØJWT
  - Upper Extremity ØJWV
- Tarsal
  - Left ØQWM
  - Right ØQWL
- Tendon
  - Lower ØLWY
  - Upper ØLWX
- Testis ØVWD
- Thymus Ø7WM
- Thyroid Gland ØGWK
- Tibia
  - Left ØQWH
  - Right ØQWG
- Toe Nail ØHWRX
- Trachea ØBW1
- Tracheobronchial Tree ØBWØ
- Tympanic Membrane
  - Left Ø9W8
  - Right Ø9W7
- Ulna
  - Left ØPWL
  - Right ØPWK
- Ureter ØTW9
- Urethra ØTWD
- Uterus and Cervix ØUWD
- Vagina and Cul-de-sac ØUWH
- Valve
  - Aortic Ø2WF
  - Mitral Ø2WG
  - Pulmonary Ø2WH
  - Tricuspid Ø2WJ
- Vas Deferens ØVWR
- Vein
  - Lower Ø6WY
  - Upper Ø5WY
- Vertebra
  - Cervical ØPW3
  - Lumbar ØQWØ
  - Thoracic ØPW4
- Vulva ØUWM

Revo MRI™ SureScan® pacemaker *use* Pacemaker, Dual Chamber in ØJH

rhBMP-2 *use* Recombinant Bone Morphogenetic Protein

Rheos® System device *use* Stimulator Generator in Subcutaneous Tissue and Fascia

Rheos® System lead *use* Stimulator Lead in Upper Arteries

Rhinopharynx *use* Nasopharynx

Rhinoplasty
- *see* Alteration, Nose Ø9ØK
- *see* Repair, Nose Ø9QK
- *see* Replacement, Nose Ø9RK
- *see* Supplement, Nose Ø9UK

Rhinorrhaphy *see* Repair, Nose Ø9QK
Rhinoscopy Ø9JKXZZ
Rhizotomy
see Division, Central Nervous System ØØ8
see Division, Peripheral Nervous System Ø18
Rhomboid major muscle
use Muscle, Trunk, Left
use Muscle, Trunk, Right
Rhomboid minor muscle
use Muscle, Trunk, Left
use Muscle, Trunk, Right
Rhythm electrocardiogram *see* Measurement, Cardiac 4AØ2
Rhytidectomy *see* Face lift
Right ascending lumbar vein *use* Vein, Azygos
Right atrioventricular valve *use* Valve, Tricuspid
Right auricular appendix *use* Atrium, Right
Right colic vein *use* Vein, Colic
Right coronary sulcus *use* Heart, Right
Right gastric artery *use* Artery, Gastric
Right gastroepiploic vein *use* Vein, Superior Mesenteric
Right inferior phrenic vein *use* Vena Cava, Inferior
Right inferior pulmonary vein *use* Vein, Pulmonary, Right
Right jugular trunk *use* Lymphatic, Neck, Right
Right lateral ventricle *use* Cerebral Ventricle
Right lymphatic duct *use* Lymphatic, Neck, Right
Right ovarian vein *use* Vena Cava, Inferior
Right second lumbar vein *use* Vena Cava, Inferior
Right subclavian trunk *use* Lymphatic, Neck, Right
Right subcostal vein *use* Vein, Azygos
Right superior pulmonary vein *use* Vein, Pulmonary, Right
Right suprarenal vein *use* Vena Cava, Inferior
Right testicular vein *use* Vena Cava, Inferior
Rima glottidis *use* Larynx
Risorius muscle *use* Muscle, Facial
RNS System lead *use* Neurostimulator Lead in Central Nervous System
RNS system neurostimulator generator *use* Neurostimulator Generator in Head and Facial Bones
Robotic Assisted Procedure
Extremity
Lower 8EØY
Upper 8EØX
Head and Neck Region 8EØ9
Trunk Region 8EØW
Rotation of fetal head
Forceps 1ØSØ7ZZ
Manual 1ØSØXZZ
Round ligament of uterus *use* Uterine Supporting Structure
Round window
use Ear, Inner, Left
use Ear, Inner, Right
Roux-en-Y operation
see Bypass, Gastrointestinal System ØD1
see Bypass, Hepatobiliary System and Pancreas ØF1
Rupture
Adhesions *see* Release
Fluid collection *see* Drainage

S

Sacral ganglion *use* Nerve, Sacral Sympathetic
Sacral lymph node *use* Lymphatic, Pelvis
Sacral nerve modulation (SNM) lead *use* Stimulator Lead in Urinary System
Sacral neuromodulation lead *use* Stimulator Lead in Urinary System
Sacral splanchnic nerve *use* Nerve, Sacral Sympathetic
Sacrectomy *see* Excision, Lower Bones ØQB
Sacrococcygeal ligament
use Bursa and Ligament, Trunk, Left
use Bursa and Ligament, Trunk, Right
Sacrococcygeal symphysis *use* Joint, Sacrococcygeal
Sacroiliac ligament
use Bursa and Ligament, Trunk, Left
use Bursa and Ligament, Trunk, Right
Sacrospinous ligament
use Bursa and Ligament, Trunk, Left
use Bursa and Ligament, Trunk, Right
Sacrotuberous ligament
use Bursa and Ligament, Trunk, Left
use Bursa and Ligament, Trunk, Right
Salpingectomy
see Excision, Female Reproductive System ØUB
see Resection, Female Reproductive System ØUT
Salpingolysis *see* Release, Female Reproductive System ØUN
Salpingopexy
see Repair, Female Reproductive System ØUQ
see Reposition, Female Reproductive System ØUS
Salpingopharyngeus muscle *use* Muscle, Tongue, Palate, Pharynx
Salpingoplasty
see Repair, Female Reproductive System ØUQ
see Supplement, Female Reproductive System ØUU
Salpingorrhaphy *see* Repair, Female Reproductive System ØUQ
Salpingoscopy ØUJ88ZZ
Salpingostomy *see* Drainage, Female Reproductive System ØU9
Salpingotomy *see* Drainage, Female Reproductive System ØU9
Salpinx
use Fallopian Tube, Left
use Fallopian Tube, Right
Saphenous nerve *use* Nerve, Femoral
SAPIEN transcatheter aortic valve *use* Zooplastic Tissue in Heart and Great Vessels
Sartorius muscle
use Muscle, Upper Leg, Left
use Muscle, Upper Leg, Right
Scalene muscle
use Muscle, Neck, Left
use Muscle, Neck, Right
Scan
Computerized Tomography (CT) *see* Computerized Tomography (CT Scan)
Radioisotope *see* Planar Nuclear Medicine Imaging
Scaphoid bone
use Carpal, Left
use Carpal, Right
Scapholunate ligament
use Bursa and Ligament, Hand, Left
use Bursa and Ligament, Hand, Right
Scaphotrapezium ligament
use Bursa and Ligament, Hand, Left
use Bursa and Ligament, Hand, Right
Scapulectomy
see Excision, Upper Bones ØPB
see Resection, Upper Bones ØPT
Scapulopexy
see Repair, Upper Bones ØPQ
see Reposition, Upper Bones ØPS
Scarpa's (vestibular) ganglion *use* Nerve, Acoustic
Sclerectomy *see* Excision, Eye Ø8B
Sclerotherapy, mechanical *see* Destruction
Sclerotomy *see* Drainage, Eye Ø89
Scrotectomy
see Excision, Male Reproductive System ØVB
see Resection, Male Reproductive System ØVT
Scrotoplasty
see Repair, Male Reproductive System ØVQ
see Supplement, Male Reproductive System ØVU
Scrotorrhaphy *see* Repair, Male Reproductive System ØVQ
Scrototomy *see* Drainage, Male Reproductive System ØV9
Sebaceous gland *use* Skin
Second cranial nerve *use* Nerve, Optic
Section, cesarean *see* Extraction, Pregnancy 1ØD
Secura (DR) (VR) *use* Defibrillator Generator in ØJH
Sella Turcica
use Bone, Sphenoid, Left
use Bone, Sphenoid, Right
Semicircular canal
use Ear, Inner, Left
use Ear, Inner, Right
Semimembranosus muscle
use Muscle, Upper Leg, Left
use Muscle, Upper Leg, Right
Semitendinosus muscle
use Muscle, Upper Leg, Left
use Muscle, Upper Leg, Right
Seprafilm *use* Adhesion Barrier
Septal cartilage *use* Septum, Nasal
Septectomy
see Excision, Ear, Nose, Sinus Ø9B
see Excision, Heart and Great Vessels Ø2B
see Resection, Ear, Nose, Sinus Ø9T
see Resection, Heart and Great Vessels Ø2T
Septoplasty
see Repair, Ear, Nose, Sinus Ø9Q
see Repair, Heart and Great Vessels Ø2Q
see Replacement, Ear, Nose, Sinus Ø9R
see Replacement, Heart and Great Vessels Ø2R
see Reposition, Ear, Nose, Sinus Ø9S
see Supplement, Ear, Nose, Sinus Ø9U
see Supplement, Heart and Great Vessels Ø2U
Septotomy *see* Drainage, Ear, Nose, Sinus Ø99
Sequestrectomy, bone *see* Extirpation
Serratus anterior muscle
use Muscle, Thorax, Left
use Muscle, Thorax, Right
Serratus posterior muscle
use Muscle, Trunk, Left
use Muscle, Trunk, Right
Seventh cranial nerve *use* Nerve, Facial
Sheffield hybrid external fixator
use External Fixation Device, Hybrid in ØQH
use External Fixation Device, Hybrid in ØQS
use External Fixation Device, Hybrid in ØPS
use External Fixation Device, Hybrid in ØPH
Sheffield ring external fixator
use External Fixation Device, Ring in ØPS
use External Fixation Device, Ring in ØQS
use External Fixation Device, Ring in ØQH
use External Fixation Device, Ring in ØPH
Shirodkar cervical cerclage ØUVC7ZZ
Shock Wave Therapy, Musculoskeletal 6A93
Short gastric artery *use* Artery, Splenic
Shortening
see Excision
see Repair
see Reposition
Shunt creation *see* Bypass
Sialoadenectomy
Complete *see* Resection, Mouth and Throat ØCT
Partial *see* Excision, Mouth and Throat ØCB
Sialodochoplasty
see Repair, Mouth and Throat ØCQ
see Replacement, Mouth and Throat ØCR
see Supplement, Mouth and Throat ØCU
Sialoectomy
see Excision, Mouth and Throat ØCB
see Resection, Mouth and Throat ØCT
Sialography *see* Plain Radiography, Ear, Nose, Mouth and Throat B9Ø
Sialolithotomy *see* Extirpation, Mouth and Throat ØCC
Sigmoid artery *use* Artery, Inferior Mesenteric
Sigmoid flexure *use* Colon, Sigmoid
Sigmoid vein *use* Vein, Inferior Mesenteric
Sigmoidectomy
see Excision, Gastrointestinal System ØDB
see Resection, Gastrointestinal System ØDT
Sigmoidorrhaphy *see* Repair, Gastrointestinal System ØDQ
Sigmoidoscopy ØDJD8ZZ
Sigmoidotomy *see* Drainage, Gastrointestinal System ØD9
Single lead pacemaker (atrium) (ventricle) *use* Pacemaker, Single Chamber in ØJH
Single lead rate responsive pacemaker (atrium) (ventricle) *use* Pacemaker, Single Chamber Rate Responsive in ØJH
Sinoatrial node *use* Conduction Mechanism
Sinogram
Abdominal Wall *see* Fluoroscopy, Abdomen and Pelvis BW11
Chest Wall *see* Plain Radiography, Chest BWØ3
Retroperitoneum *see* Fluoroscopy, Abdomen and Pelvis BW11
Sinus venosus *use* Atrium, Right
Sinusectomy
see Excision, Ear, Nose, Sinus Ø9B
see Resection, Ear, Nose, Sinus Ø9T
Sinusoscopy Ø9JY4ZZ
Sinusotomy *see* Drainage, Ear, Nose, Sinus Ø99

Sirolimus-eluting coronary stent *use* Intraluminal Device, Drug-eluting in Heart and Great Vessels
Sixth cranial nerve *use* Nerve, Abducens
Size reduction, breast *see* Excision, Skin and Breast ØHB
SJM Biocor® Stented Valve System *use* Zooplastic Tissue in Heart and Great Vessels
Skene's (paraurethral) gland *use* Gland, Vestibular
Sling
  Fascial, orbicularis muscle (mouth) *see* Supplement, Muscle, Facial ØKU1
  Levator muscle, for urethral suspension *see* Reposition, Bladder Neck ØTSC
  Pubococcygeal, for urethral suspension *see* Reposition, Bladder Neck ØTSC
  Rectum *see* Reposition, Rectum ØDSP
Small bowel series *see* Fluoroscopy, Bowel, Small BD13
Small saphenous vein
  use Vein, Lesser Saphenous, Left
  use Vein, Lesser Saphenous, Right
Snaring, polyp, colon *see* Excision, Gastrointestinal System ØDB
Solar (celiac) plexus *use* Nerve, Abdominal Sympathetic
Soletra® single-channel neurostimulator *use* Stimulator Generator, Single Array in ØJH
Soleus muscle
  use Muscle, Lower Leg, Left
  use Muscle, Lower Leg, Right
Spacer
  Insertion of device in
    Disc
      Lumbar Vertebral ØSH2
      Lumbosacral ØSH4
    Joint
      Acromioclavicular
        Left ØRHH
        Right ØRHG
      Ankle
        Left ØSHG
        Right ØSHF
      Carpal
        Left ØRHR
        Right ØRHQ
      Cervical Vertebral ØRH1
      Cervicothoracic Vertebral ØRH4
      Coccygeal ØSH6
      Elbow
        Left ØRHM
        Right ØRHL
      Finger Phalangeal
        Left ØRHX
        Right ØRHW
      Hip
        Left ØSHB
        Right ØSH9
      Knee
        Left ØSHD
        Right ØSHC
      Lumbar Vertebral ØSHØ
      Lumbosacral ØSH3
      Metacarpocarpal
        Left ØRHT
        Right ØRHS
      Metacarpophalangeal
        Left ØRHV
        Right ØRHU
      Metatarsal-Phalangeal
        Left ØSHN
        Right ØSHM
      Metatarsal-Tarsal
        Left ØSHL
        Right ØSHK
      Occipital-cervical ØRHØ
      Sacrococcygeal ØSH5
      Sacroiliac
        Left ØSH8
        Right ØSH7
      Shoulder
        Left ØRHK
        Right ØRHJ
      Sternoclavicular
        Left ØRHF
        Right ØRHE
      Tarsal
        Left ØSHJ
        Right ØSHH

Spacer — continued
  Insertion of device in — continued
    Joint — continued
      Temporomandibular
        Left ØRHD
        Right ØRHC
      Thoracic Vertebral ØRH6
      Thoracolumbar Vertebral ØRHA
      Toe Phalangeal
        Left ØSHQ
        Right ØSHP
      Wrist
        Left ØRHP
        Right ØRHN
  Removal of device from
    Acromioclavicular
      Left ØRPH
      Right ØRPG
    Ankle
      Left ØSPG
      Right ØSPF
    Carpal
      Left ØRPR
      Right ØRPQ
    Cervical Vertebral ØRP1
    Cervicothoracic Vertebral ØRP4
    Coccygeal ØSP6
    Elbow
      Left ØRPM
      Right ØRPL
    Finger Phalangeal
      Left ØRPX
      Right ØRPW
    Hip
      Left ØSPB
      Right ØSP9
    Knee
      Left ØSPD
      Right ØSPC
    Lumbar Vertebral ØSPØ
    Lumbosacral ØSP3
    Metacarpocarpal
      Left ØRPT
      Right ØRPS
    Metacarpophalangeal
      Left ØRPV
      Right ØRPU
    Metatarsal-Phalangeal
      Left ØSPN
      Right ØSPM
    Metatarsal-Tarsal
      Left ØSPL
      Right ØSPK
    Occipital-cervical ØRPØ
    Sacrococcygeal ØSP5
    Sacroiliac
      Left ØSP8
      Right ØSP7
    Shoulder
      Left ØRPK
      Right ØRPJ
    Sternoclavicular
      Left ØRPF
      Right ØRPE
    Tarsal
      Left ØSPJ
      Right ØSPH
    Temporomandibular
      Left ØRPD
      Right ØRPC
    Thoracic Vertebral ØRP6
    Thoracolumbar Vertebral ØRPA
    Toe Phalangeal
      Left ØSPQ
      Right ØSPP
    Wrist
      Left ØRPP
      Right ØRPN
  Revision of device in
    Acromioclavicular
      Left ØRWH
      Right ØRWG
    Ankle
      Left ØSWG
      Right ØSWF

Spacer — continued
  Revision of device in — continued
    Carpal
      Left ØRWR
      Right ØRWQ
    Cervical Vertebral ØRW1
    Cervicothoracic Vertebral ØRW4
    Coccygeal ØSW6
    Elbow
      Left ØRWM
      Right ØRWL
    Finger Phalangeal
      Left ØRWX
      Right ØRWW
    Hip
      Left ØSWB
      Right ØSW9
    Knee
      Left ØSWD
      Right ØSWC
    Lumbar Vertebral ØSWØ
    Lumbosacral ØSW3
    Metacarpocarpal
      Left ØRWT
      Right ØRWS
    Metacarpophalangeal
      Left ØRWV
      Right ØRWU
    Metatarsal-Phalangeal
      Left ØSWN
      Right ØSWM
    Metatarsal-Tarsal
      Left ØSWL
      Right ØSWK
    Occipital-cervical ØRWØ
    Sacrococcygeal ØSW5
    Sacroiliac
      Left ØSW8
      Right ØSW7
    Shoulder
      Left ØRWK
      Right ØRWJ
    Sternoclavicular
      Left ØRWF
      Right ØRWE
    Tarsal
      Left ØSWJ
      Right ØSWH
    Temporomandibular
      Left ØRWD
      Right ØRWC
    Thoracic Vertebral ØRW6
    Thoracolumbar Vertebral ØRWA
    Toe Phalangeal
      Left ØSWQ
      Right ØSWP
    Wrist
      Left ØRWP
      Right ØRWN
Spectroscopy
  Intravascular 8EØ23DZ
  Near infrared 8EØ23DZ
Speech Assessment FØØ
Speech therapy *see* Speech Treatment, Rehabilitation FØ6
Speech Treatment FØ6
Sphenoidectomy
  see Excision, Ear, Nose, Sinus Ø9B
  see Excision, Head and Facial Bones ØNB
  see Resection, Ear, Nose, Sinus Ø9T
  see Resection, Head and Facial Bones ØNT
Sphenoidotomy *see* Drainage, Ear, Nose, Sinus Ø99
Sphenomandibular ligament *use* Bursa and Ligament, Head and Neck
Sphenopalatine (pterygopalatine) ganglion *use* Nerve, Head and Neck Sympathetic
Sphincterorrhaphy, anal *see* Repair, Anal Sphincter ØDQR
Sphincterotomy, anal
  see Division, Anal Sphincter ØD8R
  see Drainage, Anal Sphincter ØD9R
Spinal cord neurostimulator lead *use* Neurostimulator Lead in Central Nervous System
Spinal dura mater *use* Dura Mater
Spinal epidural space *use* Epidural Space
Spinal nerve, cervical *use* Nerve, Cervical

Spinal nerve, lumbar *use* Nerve, Lumbar
Spinal nerve, sacral *use* Nerve, Sacral
Spinal nerve, thoracic *use* Nerve, Thoracic
Spinal Stabilization Device
  Facet Replacement
    Cervical Vertebral ØRH1
    Cervicothoracic Vertebral ØRH4
    Lumbar Vertebral ØSHØ
    Lumbosacral ØSH3
    Occipital-cervical ØRHØ
    Thoracic Vertebral ØRH6
    Thoracolumbar Vertebral ØRHA
  Interspinous Process
    Cervical Vertebral ØRH1
    Cervicothoracic Vertebral ØRH4
    Lumbar Vertebral ØSHØ
    Lumbosacral ØSH3
    Occipital-cervical ØRHØ
    Thoracic Vertebral ØRH6
    Thoracolumbar Vertebral ØRHA
  Pedicle-Based
    Cervical Vertebral ØRH1
    Cervicothoracic Vertebral ØRH4
    Lumbar Vertebral ØSHØ
    Lumbosacral ØSH3
    Occipital-cervical ØRHØ
    Thoracic Vertebral ØRH6
    Thoracolumbar Vertebral ØRHA
Spinal subarachnoid space *use* Subarachnoid Space
Spinal subdural space *use* Subdural Space
Spinous process
  use Vertebra, Cervical
  use Vertebra, Lumbar
  use Vertebra, Thoracic
Spiral ganglion *use* Nerve, Acoustic
Spiration IBV™ Valve System *use* Intraluminal Device, Endobronchial Valve in Respiratory System
Splenectomy
  see Excision, Lymphatic and Hemic Systems Ø7B
  see Resection, Lymphatic and Hemic Systems Ø7T
Splenic flexure *use* Colon, Transverse
Splenic plexus *use* Nerve, Abdominal Sympathetic
Splenius capitis muscle *use* Muscle, Head
Splenius cervicis muscle
  use Muscle, Neck, Left
  use Muscle, Neck, Right
Splenolysis *see* Release, Lymphatic and Hemic Systems Ø7N
Splenopexy
  see Repair, Lymphatic and Hemic Systems Ø7Q
  see Reposition, Lymphatic and Hemic Systems Ø7S
Splenoplasty *see* Repair, Lymphatic and Hemic Systems Ø7Q
Splenorrhaphy *see* Repair, Lymphatic and Hemic Systems Ø7Q
Splenotomy *see* Drainage, Lymphatic and Hemic Systems Ø79
Splinting, musculoskeletal *see* Immobilization, Anatomical Regions 2W3
Stapedectomy
  see Excision, Ear, Nose, Sinus Ø9B
  see Resection, Ear, Nose, Sinus Ø9T
Stapediolysis *see* Release, Ear, Nose, Sinus Ø9N
Stapedioplasty
  see Repair, Ear, Nose, Sinus Ø9Q
  see Replacement, Ear, Nose, Sinus Ø9R
  see Supplement, Ear, Nose, Sinus Ø9U
Stapedotomy *see* Drainage, Ear, Nose, Sinus Ø99
Stapes
  use Auditory Ossicle, Left
  use Auditory Ossicle, Right
Stellate ganglion *use* Nerve, Head and Neck Sympathetic
Stensen's duct
  use Duct, Parotid, Left
  use Duct, Parotid, Right
Stent, intraluminal (cardiovascular) (gastrointestinal) (hepatobiliary) (urinary) *use* Intraluminal Device
Stented tissue valve *use* Zooplastic Tissue in Heart and Great Vessels
Stereotactic Radiosurgery
  Gamma Beam
    Abdomen DW23JZZ
    Adrenal Gland DG22JZZ

Stereotactic Radiosurgery — continued
  Gamma Beam — continued
    Bile Ducts DF22JZZ
    Bladder DT22JZZ
    Bone Marrow D72ØJZZ
    Brain DØ2ØJZZ
    Brain Stem DØ21JZZ
    Breast
      Left DM2ØJZZ
      Right DM21JZZ
    Bronchus DB21JZZ
    Cervix DU21JZZ
    Chest DW22JZZ
    Chest Wall DB27JZZ
    Colon DD25JZZ
    Diaphragm DB28JZZ
    Duodenum DD22JZZ
    Ear D92ØJZZ
    Esophagus DD2ØJZZ
    Eye D82ØJZZ
    Gallbladder DF21JZZ
    Gland
      Adrenal DG22JZZ
      Parathyroid DG24JZZ
      Pituitary DG2ØJZZ
      Thyroid DG25JZZ
    Glands, Salivary D926JZZ
    Head and Neck DW21JZZ
    Ileum DD24JZZ
    Jejunum DD23JZZ
    Kidney DT2ØJZZ
    Larynx D92BJZZ
    Liver DF2ØJZZ
    Lung DB22JZZ
    Lymphatics
      Abdomen D726JZZ
      Axillary D724JZZ
      Inguinal D728JZZ
      Neck D723JZZ
      Pelvis D727JZZ
      Thorax D725JZZ
    Mediastinum DB26JZZ
    Mouth D924JZZ
    Nasopharynx D92DJZZ
    Neck and Head DW21JZZ
    Nerve, Peripheral DØ27JZZ
    Nose D921JZZ
    Ovary DU2ØJZZ
    Palate
      Hard D928JZZ
      Soft D929JZZ
    Pancreas DF23JZZ
    Parathyroid Gland DG24JZZ
    Pelvic Region DW26JZZ
    Pharynx D92CJZZ
    Pineal Body DG21JZZ
    Pituitary Gland DG2ØJZZ
    Pleura DB25JZZ
    Prostate DV2ØJZZ
    Rectum DD27JZZ
    Sinuses D927JZZ
    Spinal Cord DØ26JZZ
    Spleen D722JZZ
    Stomach DD21JZZ
    Testis DV21JZZ
    Thymus D721JZZ
    Thyroid Gland DG25JZZ
    Tongue D925JZZ
    Trachea DB2ØJZZ
    Ureter DT21JZZ
    Urethra DT23JZZ
    Uterus DU22JZZ
  Other Photon
    Abdomen DW23DZZ
    Adrenal Gland DG22DZZ
    Bile Ducts DF22DZZ
    Bladder DT22DZZ
    Bone Marrow D72ØDZZ
    Brain DØ2ØDZZ
    Brain Stem DØ21DZZ
    Breast
      Left DM2ØDZZ
      Right DM21DZZ
    Bronchus DB21DZZ
    Cervix DU21DZZ
    Chest DW22DZZ

Stereotactic Radiosurgery — continued
  Other Photon — continued
    Chest Wall DB27DZZ
    Colon DD25DZZ
    Diaphragm DB28DZZ
    Duodenum DD22DZZ
    Ear D92ØDZZ
    Esophagus DD2ØDZZ
    Eye D82ØDZZ
    Gallbladder DF21DZZ
    Gland
      Adrenal DG22DZZ
      Parathyroid DG24DZZ
      Pituitary DG2ØDZZ
      Thyroid DG25DZZ
    Glands, Salivary D926DZZ
    Head and Neck DW21DZZ
    Ileum DD24DZZ
    Jejunum DD23DZZ
    Kidney DT2ØDZZ
    Larynx D92BDZZ
    Liver DF2ØDZZ
    Lung DB22DZZ
    Lymphatics
      Abdomen D726DZZ
      Axillary D724DZZ
      Inguinal D728DZZ
      Neck D723DZZ
      Pelvis D727DZZ
      Thorax D725DZZ
    Mediastinum DB26DZZ
    Mouth D924DZZ
    Nasopharynx D92DDZZ
    Neck and Head DW21DZZ
    Nerve, Peripheral DØ27DZZ
    Nose D921DZZ
    Ovary DU2ØDZZ
    Palate
      Hard D928DZZ
      Soft D929DZZ
    Pancreas DF23DZZ
    Parathyroid Gland DG24DZZ
    Pelvic Region DW26DZZ
    Pharynx D92CDZZ
    Pineal Body DG21DZZ
    Pituitary Gland DG2ØDZZ
    Pleura DB25DZZ
    Prostate DV2ØDZZ
    Rectum DD27DZZ
    Sinuses D927DZZ
    Spinal Cord DØ26DZZ
    Spleen D722DZZ
    Stomach DD21DZZ
    Testis DV21DZZ
    Thymus D721DZZ
    Thyroid Gland DG25DZZ
    Tongue D925DZZ
    Trachea DB2ØDZZ
    Ureter DT21DZZ
    Urethra DT23DZZ
    Uterus DU22DZZ
  Particulate
    Abdomen DW23HZZ
    Adrenal Gland DG22HZZ
    Bile Ducts DF22HZZ
    Bladder DT22HZZ
    Bone Marrow D72ØHZZ
    Brain DØ2ØHZZ
    Brain Stem DØ21HZZ
    Breast
      Left DM2ØHZZ
      Right DM21HZZ
    Bronchus DB21HZZ
    Cervix DU21HZZ
    Chest DW22HZZ
    Chest Wall DB27HZZ
    Colon DD25HZZ
    Diaphragm DB28HZZ
    Duodenum DD22HZZ
    Ear D92ØHZZ
    Esophagus DD2ØHZZ
    Eye D82ØHZZ
    Gallbladder DF21HZZ
    Gland
      Adrenal DG22HZZ
      Parathyroid DG24HZZ

Stereotactic Radiosurgery — continued
Particulate — continued
Gland — continued
Pituitary DG2ØHZZ
Thyroid DG25HZZ
Glands, Salivary D926HZZ
Head and Neck DW21HZZ
Ileum DD24HZZ
Jejunum DD23HZZ
Kidney DT2ØHZZ
Larynx D92BHZZ
Liver DF2ØHZZ
Lung DB22HZZ
Lymphatics
Abdomen D726HZZ
Axillary D724HZZ
Inguinal D728HZZ
Neck D723HZZ
Pelvis D727HZZ
Thorax D725HZZ
Mediastinum DB26HZZ
Mouth D924HZZ
Nasopharynx D92DHZZ
Neck and Head DW21HZZ
Nerve, Peripheral DØ27HZZ
Nose D921HZZ
Ovary DU2ØHZZ
Palate
Hard D928HZZ
Soft D929HZZ
Pancreas DF23HZZ
Parathyroid Gland DG24HZZ
Pelvic Region DW26HZZ
Pharynx D92CHZZ
Pineal Body DG21HZZ
Pituitary Gland DG2ØHZZ
Pleura DB25HZZ
Prostate DV2ØHZZ
Rectum DD27HZZ
Sinuses D927HZZ
Spinal Cord DØ26HZZ
Spleen D722HZZ
Stomach DD21HZZ
Testis DV21HZZ
Thymus D721HZZ
Thyroid Gland DG25HZZ
Tongue D925HZZ
Trachea DB2ØHZZ
Ureter DT21HZZ
Urethra DT23HZZ
Uterus DU22HZZ
Sternoclavicular ligament
use Bursa and Ligament, Shoulder, Left
use Bursa and Ligament, Shoulder, Right
Sternocleidomastoid artery
use Artery, Thyroid, Left
use Artery, Thyroid, Right
Sternocleidomastoid muscle
use Muscle, Neck, Left
use Muscle, Neck, Right
Sternocostal ligament
use Bursa and Ligament, Thorax, Left
use Bursa and Ligament, Thorax, Right
Sternotomy
see Division, Sternum ØP8Ø
see Drainage, Sternum ØP9Ø
Stimulation, cardiac
Cardioversion 5A22Ø4Z
Electrophysiologic testing *see* Measurement, Cardiac 4AØ2
Stimulator Generator
Insertion of device in
Abdomen ØJH8
Back ØJH7
Chest ØJH6
Multiple Array
Abdomen ØJH8
Back ØJH7
Chest ØJH6
Multiple Array Rechargeable
Abdomen ØJH8
Back ØJH7
Chest ØJH6
Removal of device from, Subcutaneous Tissue and Fascia, Trunk ØJPT
Stimulator Generator — continued
Revision of device in, Subcutaneous Tissue and Fascia, Trunk ØJWT
Single Array
Abdomen ØJH8
Back ØJH7
Chest ØJH6
Single Array Rechargeable
Abdomen ØJH8
Back ØJH7
Chest ØJH6
Stimulator Lead
Insertion of device in
Anal Sphincter ØDHR
Artery
Left Ø3HL
Right Ø3HK
Bladder ØTHB
Muscle
Lower ØKHY
Upper ØKHX
Stomach ØDH6
Ureter ØTH9
Removal of device from
Anal Sphincter ØDPR
Artery, Upper Ø3PY
Bladder ØTPB
Muscle
Lower ØKPY
Upper ØKPX
Stomach ØDP6
Ureter ØTP9
Revision of device in
Anal Sphincter ØDWR
Artery, Upper Ø3WY
Bladder ØTWB
Muscle
Lower ØKWY
Upper ØKWX
Stomach ØDW6
Ureter ØTW9
Stoma
Excision
Abdominal Wall ØWBFXZ2
Neck ØWB6XZ2
Repair
Abdominal Wall ØWQFXZ2
Neck ØWQ6XZ2
Stomatoplasty
see Repair, Mouth and Throat ØCQ
see Replacement, Mouth and Throat ØCR
see Supplement, Mouth and Throat ØCU
Stomatorrhaphy *see* Repair, Mouth and Throat ØCQ
Stratos LV *use* Cardiac Resynchronization Pacemaker Pulse Generator in ØJH
Stress test 4A12XM4
Stripping *see* Extraction
Study
Electrophysiologic stimulation, cardiac *see* Measurement, Cardiac 4AØ2
Ocular motility 4AØ7X7Z
Pulmonary airway flow measurement *see* Measurement, Respiratory 4AØ9
Visual acuity 4AØ7XØZ
Styloglossus muscle *use* Muscle, Tongue, Palate, Pharynx
Stylomandibular ligament *use* Bursa and Ligament, Head and Neck
Stylopharyngeus muscle *use* Muscle, Tongue, Palate, Pharynx
Subacromial bursa
use Bursa and Ligament, Shoulder, Left
use Bursa and Ligament, Shoulder, Right
Subaortic (common iliac) lymph node *use* Lymphatic, Pelvis
Subclavicular (apical) lymph node
use Lymphatic, Axillary, Left
use Lymphatic, Axillary, Right
Subclavius muscle
use Muscle, Thorax, Left
use Muscle, Thorax, Right
Subclavius nerve *use* Nerve, Brachial Plexus
Subcostal artery *use* Aorta, Thoracic
Subcostal muscle
use Muscle, Thorax, Left
Subcostal muscle — continued
use Muscle, Thorax, Right
Subcostal nerve *use* Nerve, Thoracic
Subcutaneous injection reservoir, port *use* Vascular Access Device, Reservoir in Subcutaneous Tissue and Fascia
Subcutaneous injection reservoir, pump *use* Infusion Device, Pump in Subcutaneous Tissue and Fascia
Subdermal progesterone implant *use* Contraceptive Device in Subcutaneous Tissue and Fascia
Submandibular ganglion
use Nerve, Facial
use Nerve, Head and Neck Sympathetic
Submandibular gland
use Gland, Submaxillary, Left
use Gland, Submaxillary, Right
Submandibular lymph node *use* Lymphatic, Head
Submaxillary ganglion *use* Nerve, Head and Neck Sympathetic
Submaxillary lymph node *use* Lymphatic, Head
Submental artery *use* Artery, Face
Submental lymph node *use* Lymphatic, Head
Submucous (Meissner's) plexus *use* Nerve, Abdominal Sympathetic
Suboccipital nerve *use* Nerve, Cervical
Suboccipital venous plexus
use Vein, Vertebral, Left
use Vein, Vertebral, Right
Subparotid lymph node *use* Lymphatic, Head
Subscapular aponeurosis
use Subcutaneous Tissue and Fascia, Upper Arm, Left
use Subcutaneous Tissue and Fascia, Upper Arm, Right
Subscapular artery
use Artery, Axillary, Left
use Artery, Axillary, Right
Subscapular (posterior) lymph node
use Lymphatic, Axillary, Left
use Lymphatic, Axillary, Right
Subscapularis muscle
use Muscle, Shoulder, Left
use Muscle, Shoulder, Right
Substance Abuse Treatment
Counseling
Family, for substance abuse, Other Family Counseling HZ63ZZZ
Group
12-Step HZ43ZZZ
Behavioral HZ41ZZZ
Cognitive HZ4ØZZZ
Cognitive-Behavioral HZ42ZZZ
Confrontational HZ48ZZZ
Continuing Care HZ49ZZZ
Infectious Disease
Post-Test HZ4CZZZ
Pre-Test HZ4CZZZ
Interpersonal HZ44ZZZ
Motivational Enhancement HZ47ZZZ
Psychoeducation HZ46ZZZ
Spiritual HZ4BZZZ
Vocational HZ45ZZZ
Individual
12-Step HZ33ZZZ
Behavioral HZ31ZZZ
Cognitive HZ3ØZZZ
Cognitive-Behavioral HZ32ZZZ
Confrontational HZ38ZZZ
Continuing Care HZ39ZZZ
Infectious Disease
Post-Test HZ3CZZZ
Pre-Test HZ3CZZZ
Interpersonal HZ34ZZZ
Motivational Enhancement HZ37ZZZ
Psychoeducation HZ36ZZZ
Spiritual HZ3BZZZ
Vocational HZ35ZZZ
Detoxification Services, for substance abuse HZ2ZZZZ
Medication Management
Antabuse HZ83ZZZ
Bupropion HZ87ZZZ
Clonidine HZ86ZZZ
Levo-alpha-acetyl-methadol (LAAM) HZ82ZZZ
Methadone Maintenance HZ81ZZZ
Naloxone HZ85ZZZ
Naltrexone HZ84ZZZ

Substance Abuse Treatment — continued
Medication Management — continued
Nicotine Replacement HZ80ZZZ
Other Replacement Medication HZ89ZZZ
Psychiatric Medication HZ88ZZZ
Pharmacotherapy
Antabuse HZ93ZZZ
Bupropion HZ97ZZZ
Clonidine HZ96ZZZ
Levo-alpha-acetyl-methadol (LAAM) HZ92ZZZ
Methadone Maintenance HZ91ZZZ
Naloxone HZ95ZZZ
Naltrexone HZ94ZZZ
Nicotine Replacement HZ90ZZZ
Psychiatric Medication HZ98ZZZ
Replacement Medication, Other HZ99ZZZ
Psychotherapy
12-Step HZ53ZZZ
Behavioral HZ51ZZZ
Cognitive HZ50ZZZ
Cognitive-Behavioral HZ52ZZZ
Confrontational HZ58ZZZ
Interactive HZ55ZZZ
Interpersonal HZ54ZZZ
Motivational Enhancement HZ57ZZZ
Psychoanalysis HZ5BZZZ
Psychodynamic HZ5CZZZ
Psychoeducation HZ56ZZZ
Psychophysiological HZ5DZZZ
Supportive HZ59ZZZ
Substantia nigra *use* Basal Ganglia
Subtalar (talocalcaneal) joint
use Joint, Tarsal, Left
use Joint, Tarsal, Right
Subtalar ligament
use Bursa and Ligament, Foot, Left
use Bursa and Ligament, Foot, Right
Subthalamic nucleus *use* Basal Ganglia
Suction *see* Drainage
Suction curettage (D&C), nonobstetric *see* Extraction, Endometrium 0UDB
Suction curettage, obstetric post-delivery *see* Extraction, Products of Conception, Retained 10D1
Superficial circumflex iliac vein
use Vein, Greater Saphenous, Left
use Vein, Greater Saphenous, Right
Superficial epigastric artery
use Artery, Femoral, Left
use Artery, Femoral, Right
Superficial epigastric vein
use Vein, Greater Saphenous, Left
use Vein, Greater Saphenous, Right
Superficial Inferior Epigastric Artery Flap
Bilateral 0HRV078
Left 0HRU078
Right 0HRT078
Superficial palmar arch
use Artery, Hand, Left
use Artery, Hand, Right
Superficial palmar venous arch
use Vein, Hand, Left
use Vein, Hand, Right
Superficial temporal artery
use Artery, Temporal, Left
use Artery, Temporal, Right
Superficial transverse perineal muscle *use* Muscle, Perineum
Superior cardiac nerve *use* Nerve, Thoracic Sympathetic
Superior cerebellar vein *use* Vein, Intracranial
Superior cerebral vein *use* Vein, Intracranial
Superior clunic (cluneal) nerve *use* Nerve, Lumbar
Superior epigastric artery
use Artery, Internal Mammary, Left
use Artery, Internal Mammary, Right
Superior genicular artery
use Artery, Popliteal, Left
use Artery, Popliteal, Right
Superior gluteal artery
use Artery, Internal Iliac, Left
use Artery, Internal Iliac, Right
Superior gluteal nerve *use* Nerve, Lumbar Plexus
Superior hypogastric plexus *use* Nerve, Abdominal Sympathetic
Superior labial artery *use* Artery, Face
Superior laryngeal artery
use Artery, Thyroid, Left
use Artery, Thyroid, Right
Superior laryngeal nerve *use* Nerve, Vagus
Superior longitudinal muscle *use* Muscle, Tongue, Palate, Pharynx
Superior mesenteric ganglion *use* Nerve, Abdominal Sympathetic
Superior mesenteric lymph node *use* Lymphatic, Mesenteric
Superior mesenteric plexus *use* Nerve, Abdominal Sympathetic
Superior oblique muscle
use Muscle, Extraocular, Left
use Muscle, Extraocular, Right
Superior olivary nucleus *use* Pons
Superior rectal artery *use* Artery, Inferior Mesenteric
Superior rectal vein *use* Vein, Inferior Mesenteric
Superior rectus muscle
use Muscle, Extraocular, Left
use Muscle, Extraocular, Right
Superior tarsal plate
use Eyelid, Upper, Left
use Eyelid, Upper, Right
Superior thoracic artery
use Artery, Axillary, Left
use Artery, Axillary, Right
Superior thyroid artery
use Artery, External Carotid, Left
use Artery, External Carotid, Right
use Artery, Thyroid, Left
use Artery, Thyroid, Right
Superior turbinate *use* Turbinate, Nasal
Superior ulnar collateral artery
use Artery, Brachial, Left
use Artery, Brachial, Right
Supplement
Abdominal Wall 0WUF
Acetabulum
Left 0QU5
Right 0QU4
Ampulla of Vater 0FUC
Anal Sphincter 0DUR
Ankle Region
Left 0YUL
Right 0YUK
Anus 0DUQ
Aorta
Abdominal 04U0
Thoracic 02UW
Arm
Lower
Left 0XUF
Right 0XUD
Upper
Left 0XU9
Right 0XU8
Artery
Anterior Tibial
Left 04UQ
Right 04UP
Axillary
Left 03U6
Right 03U5
Brachial
Left 03U8
Right 03U7
Celiac 04U1
Colic
Left 04U7
Middle 04U8
Right 04U6
Common Carotid
Left 03UJ
Right 03UH
Common Iliac
Left 04UD
Right 04UC
External Carotid
Left 03UN
Right 03UM
External Iliac
Left 04UJ
Right 04UH
Face 03UR
Supplement — continued
Artery — continued
Femoral
Left 04UL
Right 04UK
Foot
Left 04UW
Right 04UV
Gastric 04U2
Hand
Left 03UF
Right 03UD
Hepatic 04U3
Inferior Mesenteric 04UB
Innominate 03U2
Internal Carotid
Left 03UL
Right 03UK
Internal Iliac
Left 04UF
Right 04UE
Internal Mammary
Left 03U1
Right 03U0
Intracranial 03UG
Lower 04UY
Peroneal
Left 04UU
Right 04UT
Popliteal
Left 04UN
Right 04UM
Posterior Tibial
Left 04US
Right 04UR
Pulmonary
Left 02UR
Right 02UQ
Pulmonary Trunk 02UP
Radial
Left 03UC
Right 03UB
Renal
Left 04UA
Right 04U9
Splenic 04U4
Subclavian
Left 03U4
Right 03U3
Superior Mesenteric 04U5
Temporal
Left 03UT
Right 03US
Thyroid
Left 03UV
Right 03UU
Ulnar
Left 03UA
Right 03U9
Upper 03UY
Vertebral
Left 03UQ
Right 03UP
Atrium
Left 02U7
Right 02U6
Auditory Ossicle
Left 09UA0
Right 09U90
Axilla
Left 0XU5
Right 0XU4
Back
Lower 0WUL
Upper 0WUK
Bladder 0TUB
Bladder Neck 0TUC
Bone
Ethmoid
Left 0NUG
Right 0NUF
Frontal
Left 0NU2
Right 0NU1
Hyoid 0NUX

Supplement — continued
Bone — continued
Lacrimal
Left ØNUJ
Right ØNUH
Nasal ØNUB
Occipital
Left ØNU8
Right ØNU7
Palatine
Left ØNUL
Right ØNUK
Parietal
Left ØNU4
Right ØNU3
Pelvic
Left ØQU3
Right ØQU2
Sphenoid
Left ØNUD
Right ØNUC
Temporal
Left ØNU6
Right ØNU5
Zygomatic
Left ØNUN
Right ØNUM
Breast
Bilateral ØHUV
Left ØHUU
Right ØHUT
Bronchus
Lingula ØBU9
Lower Lobe
Left ØBUB
Right ØBU6
Main
Left ØBU7
Right ØBU3
Middle Lobe, Right ØBU5
Upper Lobe
Left ØBU8
Right ØBU4
Buccal Mucosa ØCU4
Bursa and Ligament
Abdomen
Left ØMUJ
Right ØMUH
Ankle
Left ØMUR
Right ØMUQ
Elbow
Left ØMU4
Right ØMU3
Foot
Left ØMUT
Right ØMUS
Hand
Left ØMU8
Right ØMU7
Head and Neck ØMUØ
Hip
Left ØMUM
Right ØMUL
Knee
Left ØMUP
Right ØMUN
Lower Extremity
Left ØMUW
Right ØMUV
Perineum ØMUK
Shoulder
Left ØMU2
Right ØMU1
Thorax
Left ØMUG
Right ØMUF
Trunk
Left ØMUD
Right ØMUC
Upper Extremity
Left ØMUB
Right ØMU9
Wrist
Left ØMU6
Right ØMU5

Supplement — continued
Buttock
Left ØYU1
Right ØYUØ
Carina ØBU2
Carpal
Left ØPUN
Right ØPUM
Cecum ØDUH
Cerebral Meninges ØØU1
Chest Wall ØWU8
Chordae Tendineae Ø2U9
Cisterna Chyli Ø7UL
Clavicle
Left ØPUB
Right ØPU9
Clitoris ØUUJ
Coccyx ØQUS
Colon
Ascending ØDUK
Descending ØDUM
Sigmoid ØDUN
Transverse ØDUL
Cord
Bilateral ØVUH
Left ØVUG
Right ØVUF
Cornea
Left Ø8U9
Right Ø8U8
Cul-de-sac ØUUF
Diaphragm
Left ØBUS
Right ØBUR
Disc
Cervical Vertebral ØRU3
Cervicothoracic Vertebral ØRU5
Lumbar Vertebral ØSU2
Lumbosacral ØSU4
Thoracic Vertebral ØRU9
Thoracolumbar Vertebral ØRUB
Duct
Common Bile ØFU9
Cystic ØFU8
Hepatic
Left ØFU6
Right ØFU5
Lacrimal
Left Ø8UY
Right Ø8UX
Pancreatic ØFUD
Accessory ØFUF
Duodenum ØDU9
Dura Mater ØØU2
Ear
External
Bilateral Ø9U2
Left Ø9U1
Right Ø9UØ
Inner
Left Ø9UEØ
Right Ø9UDØ
Middle
Left Ø9U6Ø
Right Ø9U5Ø
Elbow Region
Left ØXUC
Right ØXUB
Epididymis
Bilateral ØVUL
Left ØVUK
Right ØVUJ
Epiglottis ØCUR
Esophagogastric Junction ØDU4
Esophagus ØDU5
Lower ØDU3
Middle ØDU2
Upper ØDU1
Extremity
Lower
Left ØYUB
Right ØYU9
Upper
Left ØXU7
Right ØXU6

Supplement — continued
Eye
Left Ø8U1
Right Ø8UØ
Eyelid
Lower
Left Ø8UR
Right Ø8UQ
Upper
Left Ø8UP
Right Ø8UN
Face ØWU2
Fallopian Tube
Left ØUU6
Right ØUU5
Fallopian Tubes, Bilateral ØUU7
Femoral Region
Bilateral ØYUE
Left ØYU8
Right ØYU7
Femoral Shaft
Left ØQU9
Right ØQU8
Femur
Lower
Left ØQUC
Right ØQUB
Upper
Left ØQU7
Right ØQU6
Fibula
Left ØQUK
Right ØQUJ
Finger
Index
Left ØXUP
Right ØXUN
Little
Left ØXUW
Right ØXUV
Middle
Left ØXUR
Right ØXUQ
Ring
Left ØXUT
Right ØXUS
Foot
Left ØYUN
Right ØYUM
Gingiva
Lower ØCU6
Upper ØCU5
Glenoid Cavity
Left ØPU8
Right ØPU7
Hand
Left ØXUK
Right ØXUJ
Head ØWUØ
Heart Ø2UA
Humeral Head
Left ØPUD
Right ØPUC
Humeral Shaft
Left ØPUG
Right ØPUF
Hymen ØUUK
Ileocecal Valve ØDUC
Ileum ØDUB
Inguinal Region
Bilateral ØYUA
Left ØYU6
Right ØYU5
Intestine
Large ØDUE
Left ØDUG
Right ØDUF
Small ØDU8
Iris
Left Ø8UD
Right Ø8UC
Jaw
Lower ØWU5
Upper ØWU4
Jejunum ØDUA

Supplement — continued
Joint
Acromioclavicular
Left ØRUH
Right ØRUG
Ankle
Left ØSUG
Right ØSUF
Carpal
Left ØRUR
Right ØRUQ
Cervical Vertebral ØRU1
Cervicothoracic Vertebral ØRU4
Coccygeal ØSU6
Elbow
Left ØRUM
Right ØRUL
Finger Phalangeal
Left ØRUX
Right ØRUW
Hip
Left ØSUB
Acetabular Surface ØSUE
Femoral Surface ØSUS
Right ØSU9
Acetabular Surface ØSUA
Femoral Surface ØSUR
Knee
Left ØSUD
Femoral Surface ØSUUØ9Z
Tibial Surface ØSUWØ9Z
Right ØSUC
Femoral Surface ØSUTØ9Z
Tibial Surface ØSUVØ9Z
Lumbar Vertebral ØSUØ
Lumbosacral ØSU3
Metacarpocarpal
Left ØRUT
Right ØRUS
Metacarpophalangeal
Left ØRUV
Right ØRUU
Metatarsal-Phalangeal
Left ØSUN
Right ØSUM
Metatarsal-Tarsal
Left ØSUL
Right ØSUK
Occipital-cervical ØRUØ
Sacrococcygeal ØSU5
Sacroiliac
Left ØSU8
Right ØSU7
Shoulder
Left ØRUK
Right ØRUJ
Sternoclavicular
Left ØRUF
Right ØRUE
Tarsal
Left ØSUJ
Right ØSUH
Temporomandibular
Left ØRUD
Right ØRUC
Thoracic Vertebral ØRU6
Thoracolumbar Vertebral ØRUA
Toe Phalangeal
Left ØSUQ
Right ØSUP
Wrist
Left ØRUP
Right ØRUN
Kidney Pelvis
Left ØTU4
Right ØTU3
Knee Region
Left ØYUG
Right ØYUF
Larynx ØCUS
Leg
Lower
Left ØYUJ
Right ØYUH
Upper
Left ØYUD

Supplement — continued
Leg — continued
Upper — continued
Right ØYUC
Lip
Lower ØCU1
Upper ØCUØ
Lymphatic
Aortic Ø7UD
Axillary
Left Ø7U6
Right Ø7U5
Head Ø7UØ
Inguinal
Left Ø7UJ
Right Ø7UH
Internal Mammary
Left Ø7U9
Right Ø7U8
Lower Extremity
Left Ø7UG
Right Ø7UF
Mesenteric Ø7UB
Neck
Left Ø7U2
Right Ø7U1
Pelvis Ø7UC
Thoracic Duct Ø7UK
Thorax Ø7U7
Upper Extremity
Left Ø7U4
Right Ø7U3
Mandible
Left ØNUV
Right ØNUT
Maxilla
Left ØNUS
Right ØNUR
Mediastinum ØWUC
Mesentery ØDUV
Metacarpal
Left ØPUQ
Right ØPUP
Metatarsal
Left ØQUP
Right ØQUN
Muscle
Abdomen
Left ØKUL
Right ØKUK
Extraocular
Left Ø8UM
Right Ø8UL
Facial ØKU1
Foot
Left ØKUW
Right ØKUV
Hand
Left ØKUD
Right ØKUC
Head ØKUØ
Hip
Left ØKUP
Right ØKUN
Lower Arm and Wrist
Left ØKUB
Right ØKU9
Lower Leg
Left ØKUT
Right ØKUS
Neck
Left ØKU3
Right ØKU2
Papillary Ø2UD
Perineum ØKUM
Shoulder
Left ØKU6
Right ØKU5
Thorax
Left ØKUJ
Right ØKUH
Tongue, Palate, Pharynx ØKU4
Trunk
Left ØKUG
Right ØKUF

Supplement — continued
Muscle — continued
Upper Arm
Left ØKU8
Right ØKU7
Upper Leg
Left ØKUR
Right ØKUQ
Nasopharynx Ø9UN
Neck ØWU6
Nerve
Abducens ØØUL
Accessory ØØUR
Acoustic ØØUN
Cervical Ø1U1
Facial ØØUM
Femoral Ø1UD
Glossopharyngeal ØØUP
Hypoglossal ØØUS
Lumbar Ø1UB
Median Ø1U5
Oculomotor ØØUH
Olfactory ØØUF
Optic ØØUG
Peroneal Ø1UH
Phrenic Ø1U2
Pudendal Ø1UC
Radial Ø1U6
Sacral Ø1UR
Sciatic Ø1UF
Thoracic Ø1U8
Tibial Ø1UG
Trigeminal ØØUK
Trochlear ØØUJ
Ulnar Ø1U4
Vagus ØØUQ
Nipple
Left ØHUX
Right ØHUW
Nose Ø9UK
Omentum
Greater ØDUS
Lesser ØDUT
Orbit
Left ØNUQ
Right ØNUP
Palate
Hard ØCU2
Soft ØCU3
Patella
Left ØQUF
Right ØQUD
Penis ØVUS
Pericardium Ø2UN
Perineum
Female ØWUN
Male ØWUM
Peritoneum ØDUW
Phalanx
Finger
Left ØPUV
Right ØPUT
Thumb
Left ØPUS
Right ØPUR
Toe
Left ØQUR
Right ØQUQ
Pharynx ØCUM
Prepuce ØVUT
Radius
Left ØPUJ
Right ØPUH
Rectum ØDUP
Retina
Left Ø8UF
Right Ø8UE
Retinal Vessel
Left Ø8UH
Right Ø8UG
Rib
Left ØPU2
Right ØPU1
Sacrum ØQU1
Scapula
Left ØPU6

Supplement — continued
Scapula — continued
Right ØPU5
Scrotum ØVU5
Septum
Atrial Ø2U5
Nasal Ø9UM
Ventricular Ø2UM
Shoulder Region
Left ØXU3
Right ØXU2
Skull ØNUØ
Spinal Meninges ØØUT
Sternum ØPUØ
Stomach ØDU6
Pylorus ØDU7
Subcutaneous Tissue and Fascia
Abdomen ØJU8
Back ØJU7
Buttock ØJU9
Chest ØJU6
Face ØJU1
Foot
Left ØJUR
Right ØJUQ
Hand
Left ØJUK
Right ØJUJ
Lower Arm
Left ØJUH
Right ØJUG
Lower Leg
Left ØJUP
Right ØJUN
Neck
Anterior ØJU4
Posterior ØJU5
Pelvic Region ØJUC
Perineum ØJUB
Scalp ØJUØ
Upper Arm
Left ØJUF
Right ØJUD
Upper Leg
Left ØJUM
Right ØJUL
Tarsal
Left ØQUM
Right ØQUL
Tendon
Abdomen
Left ØLUG
Right ØLUF
Ankle
Left ØLUT
Right ØLUS
Foot
Left ØLUW
Right ØLUV
Hand
Left ØLU8
Right ØLU7
Head and Neck ØLUØ
Hip
Left ØLUK
Right ØLUJ
Knee
Left ØLUR
Right ØLUQ
Lower Arm and Wrist
Left ØLU6
Right ØLU5
Lower Leg
Left ØLUP
Right ØLUN
Perineum ØLUH
Shoulder
Left ØLU2
Right ØLU1
Thorax
Left ØLUD
Right ØLUC
Trunk
Left ØLUB
Right ØLU9

Supplement — continued
Tendon — continued
Upper Arm
Left ØLU4
Right ØLU3
Upper Leg
Left ØLUM
Right ØLUL
Testis
Bilateral ØVUCØ
Left ØVUBØ
Right ØVU9Ø
Thumb
Left ØXUM
Right ØXUL
Tibia
Left ØQUH
Right ØQUG
Toe
1st
Left ØYUQ
Right ØYUP
2nd
Left ØYUS
Right ØYUR
3rd
Left ØYUU
Right ØYUT
4th
Left ØYUW
Right ØYUV
5th
Left ØYUY
Right ØYUX
Tongue ØCU7
Trachea ØBU1
Tunica Vaginalis
Left ØVU7
Right ØVU6
Turbinate, Nasal Ø9UL
Tympanic Membrane
Left Ø9U8
Right Ø9U7
Ulna
Left ØPUL
Right ØPUK
Ureter
Left ØTU7
Right ØTU6
Urethra ØTUD
Uterine Supporting Structure ØUU4
Uvula ØCUN
Vagina ØUUG
Valve
Aortic Ø2UF
Mitral Ø2UG
Pulmonary Ø2UH
Tricuspid Ø2UJ
Vas Deferens
Bilateral ØVUQ
Left ØVUP
Right ØVUN
Vein
Axillary
Left Ø5U8
Right Ø5U7
Azygos Ø5UØ
Basilic
Left Ø5UC
Right Ø5UB
Brachial
Left Ø5UA
Right Ø5U9
Cephalic
Left Ø5UF
Right Ø5UD
Colic Ø6U7
Common Iliac
Left Ø6UD
Right Ø6UC
Esophageal Ø6U3
External Iliac
Left Ø6UG
Right Ø6UF
External Jugular
Left Ø5UQ

Supplement — continued
Vein — continued
External Jugular — continued
Right Ø5UP
Face
Left Ø5UV
Right Ø5UT
Femoral
Left Ø6UN
Right Ø6UM
Foot
Left Ø6UV
Right Ø6UT
Gastric Ø6U2
Greater Saphenous
Left Ø6UQ
Right Ø6UP
Hand
Left Ø5UH
Right Ø5UG
Hemiazygos Ø5U1
Hepatic Ø6U4
Hypogastric
Left Ø6UJ
Right Ø6UH
Inferior Mesenteric Ø6U6
Innominate
Left Ø5U4
Right Ø5U3
Internal Jugular
Left Ø5UN
Right Ø5UM
Intracranial Ø5UL
Lesser Saphenous
Left Ø6US
Right Ø6UR
Lower Ø6UY
Portal Ø6U8
Pulmonary
Left Ø2UT
Right Ø2US
Renal
Left Ø6UB
Right Ø6U9
Splenic Ø6U1
Subclavian
Left Ø5U6
Right Ø5U5
Superior Mesenteric Ø6U5
Upper Ø5UY
Vertebral
Left Ø5US
Right Ø5UR
Vena Cava
Inferior Ø6UØ
Superior Ø2UV
Ventricle
Left Ø2UL
Right Ø2UK
Vertebra
Cervical ØPU3
Lumbar ØQUØ
Thoracic ØPU4
Vesicle
Bilateral ØVU3
Left ØVU2
Right ØVU1
Vocal Cord
Left ØCUV
Right ØCUT
Vulva ØUUM
Wrist Region
Left ØXUH
Right ØXUG
Supraclavicular (Virchow's) lymph node
use Lymphatic, Neck, Left
use Lymphatic, Neck, Right
Supraclavicular nerve *use* Nerve, Cervical Plexus
Suprahyoid lymph node *use* Lymphatic, Head
Suprahyoid muscle
use Muscle, Neck, Left
use Muscle, Neck, Right
Suprainguinal lymph node *use* Lymphatic, Pelvis
Supraorbital vein
use Vein, Face, Left
use Vein, Face, Right

Suprarenal gland
use Gland, Adrenal
use Gland, Adrenal, Bilateral
use Gland, Adrenal, Left
use Gland, Adrenal, Right
Suprarenal plexus *use* Nerve, Abdominal Sympathetic
Suprascapular nerve *use* Nerve, Brachial Plexus
Supraspinatus fascia
use Subcutaneous Tissue and Fascia, Upper Arm, Left
use Subcutaneous Tissue and Fascia, Upper Arm, Right
Supraspinatus muscle
use Muscle, Shoulder, Left
use Muscle, Shoulder, Right
Supraspinous ligament
use Bursa and Ligament, Trunk, Left
use Bursa and Ligament, Trunk, Right
Suprasternal notch *use* Sternum
Supratrochlear lymph node
use Lymphatic, Upper Extremity, Left
use Lymphatic, Upper Extremity, Right
Sural artery
use Artery, Popliteal, Left
use Artery, Popliteal, Right
Suspension
Bladder Neck *see* Reposition, Bladder Neck ØTSC
Kidney *see* Reposition, Urinary System ØTS
Urethra *see* Reposition, Urinary System ØTS
Urethrovesical *see* Reposition, Bladder Neck ØTSC
Uterus *see* Reposition, Uterus ØUS9
Vagina *see* Reposition, Vagina ØUSG
Suture
Laceration repair *see* Repair
Ligation *see* Occlusion
Suture Removal
Extremity
Lower 8EØYXY8
Upper 8EØXXY8
Head and Neck Region 8EØ9XY8
Trunk Region 8EØWXY8
Sweat gland *use* Skin
Sympathectomy *see* Excision, Peripheral Nervous System Ø1B
SynCardia Total Artificial Heart *use* Synthetic Substitute
Synchra CRT-P *use* Cardiac Resynchronization Pacemaker Pulse Generator in ØJH
SynchroMed pump *use* Infusion Device, Pump in Subcutaneous Tissue and Fascia
Synechiotomy, iris *see* Release, Eye Ø8N
Synovectomy
Lower joint *see* Excision, Lower Joints ØSB
Upper joint *see* Excision, Upper Joints ØRB
Systemic Nuclear Medicine Therapy
Abdomen CW7Ø
Anatomical Regions, Multiple CW7YYZZ
Chest CW73
Thyroid CW7G
Whole Body CW7N

T

Takedown
Arteriovenous shunt *see* Removal of device from, Upper Arteries Ø3P
Arteriovenous shunt, with creation of new shunt *see* Bypass, Upper Arteries Ø31
Stoma *see* Repair
Talent® Converter *use* Intraluminal Device
Talent® Occluder *use* Intraluminal Device
Talent® Stent Graft (abdominal) (thoracic) *use* Intraluminal Device
Talocalcaneal (subtalar) joint
use Joint, Tarsal, Left
use Joint, Tarsal, Right
Talocalcaneal ligament
use Bursa and Ligament, Foot, Left
use Bursa and Ligament, Foot, Right
Talocalcaneonavicular joint
use Joint, Tarsal, Left
use Joint, Tarsal, Right
Talocalcaneonavicular ligament
use Bursa and Ligament, Foot, Left
use Bursa and Ligament, Foot, Right
Talocrural joint
use Joint, Ankle, Left
use Joint, Ankle, Right
Talofibular ligament
use Bursa and Ligament, Ankle, Left
use Bursa and Ligament, Ankle, Right
Talus bone
use Tarsal, Left
use Tarsal, Right
TandemHeart® System *use* External Heart Assist System in Heart and Great Vessels
Tarsectomy
see Excision, Lower Bones ØQB
see Resection, Lower Bones ØQT
Tarsometatarsal joint
use Joint, Metatarsal-Tarsal, Left
use Joint, Metatarsal-Tarsal, Right
Tarsometatarsal ligament
use Bursa and Ligament, Foot, Left
use Bursa and Ligament, Foot, Right
Tarsorrhaphy *see* Repair, Eye Ø8Q
Tattooing
Cornea 3EØCXMZ
Skin *see* Introduction of substance in or on, Skin 3EØØ
TAXUS® Liberté® Paclitaxel-eluting Coronary Stent System *use* Intraluminal Device, Drug-eluting in Heart and Great Vessels
TBNA (transbronchial needle aspiration) *see* Drainage, Respiratory System ØB9
Telemetry 4A12X4Z
Ambulatory 4A12X45
Temperature gradient study 4AØZXKZ
Temporal lobe *use* Cerebral Hemisphere
Temporalis muscle *use* Muscle, Head
Temporoparietalis muscle *use* Muscle, Head
Tendolysis *see* Release, Tendons ØLN
Tendonectomy
see Excision, Tendons ØLB
see Resection, Tendons ØLT
Tendonoplasty, tenoplasty
see Repair, Tendons ØLQ
see Replacement, Tendons ØLR
see Supplement, Tendons ØLU
Tendorrhaphy *see* Repair, Tendons ØLQ
Tendototomy
see Division, Tendons ØL8
see Drainage, Tendons ØL9
Tenectomy, tenonectomy
see Excision, Tendons ØLB
see Resection, Tendons ØLT
Tenolysis *see* Release, Tendons ØLN
Tenontorrhaphy *see* Repair, Tendons ØLQ
Tenontotomy
see Division, Tendons ØL8
see Drainage, Tendons ØL9
Tenorrhaphy *see* Repair, Tendons ØLQ
Tenosynovectomy
see Excision, Tendons ØLB
see Resection, Tendons ØLT
Tenotomy
see Division, Tendons ØL8
see Drainage, Tendons ØL9
Tensor fasciae latae muscle
use Muscle, Hip, Left
use Muscle, Hip, Right
Tensor veli palatini muscle *use* Muscle, Tongue, Palate, Pharynx
Tenth cranial nerve *use* Nerve, Vagus
Tentorium cerebelli *use* Dura Mater
Teres major muscle
use Muscle, Shoulder, Left
use Muscle, Shoulder, Right
Teres minor muscle
use Muscle, Shoulder, Left
use Muscle, Shoulder, Right
Termination of pregnancy
Aspiration curettage 1ØAØ7ZZ
Dilation and curettage 1ØAØ7ZZ
Hysterotomy 1ØAØØZZ
Intra-amniotic injection 1ØAØ3ZZ
Laminaria 1ØAØ7ZW
Vacuum 1ØAØ7Z6
Testectomy
see Excision, Male Reproductive System ØVB
Testectomy — continued
see Resection, Male Reproductive System ØVT
Testicular artery *use* Aorta, Abdominal
Testing
Glaucoma 4AØ7XBZ
Hearing *see* Hearing Assessment, Diagnostic Audiology F13
Mental health *see* Psychological Tests
Muscle function, electromyography (EMG) *see* Measurement, Musculoskeletal 4AØF
Muscle function, manual *see* Motor Function Assessment, Rehabilitation FØ1
Neurophysiologic monitoring, intra-operative *see* Monitoring, Physiological Systems 4A1
Range of motion *see* Motor Function Assessment, Rehabilitation FØ1
Vestibular function *see* Vestibular Assessment, Diagnostic Audiology F15
Thalamectomy *see* Excision, Thalamus ØØB9
Thalamotomy *see* Drainage, Thalamus ØØ99
Thenar muscle
use Muscle, Hand, Left
use Muscle, Hand, Right
Therapeutic Massage
Musculoskeletal System 8EØKX1Z
Reproductive System
Prostate 8EØVX1C
Rectum 8EØVX1D
Therapeutic occlusion coil(s) *use* Intraluminal Device
Thermography 4AØZXKZ
Thermotherapy, prostate *see* Destruction, Prostate ØV5Ø
Third cranial nerve *use* Nerve, Oculomotor
Third occipital nerve *use* Nerve, Cervical
Third ventricle *use* Cerebral Ventricle
Thoracectomy *see* Excision, Anatomical Regions, General ØWB
Thoracentesis *see* Drainage, Anatomical Regions, General ØW9
Thoracic aortic plexus *use* Nerve, Thoracic Sympathetic
Thoracic esophagus *use* Esophagus, Middle
Thoracic facet joint *use* Joint, Thoracic Vertebral
Thoracic ganglion *use* Nerve, Thoracic Sympathetic
Thoracoacromial artery
use Artery, Axillary, Left
use Artery, Axillary, Right
Thoracocentesis *see* Drainage, Anatomical Regions, General ØW9
Thoracolumbar facet joint *use* Joint, Thoracolumbar Vertebral
Thoracoplasty
see Repair, Anatomical Regions, General ØWQ
see Supplement, Anatomical Regions, General ØWU
Thoracostomy, for lung collapse *see* Drainage, Respiratory System ØB9
Thoracostomy tube *use* Drainage Device
Thoracotomy *see* Drainage, Anatomical Regions, General ØW9
Thoratec IVAD (Implantable Ventricular Assist Device) *use* Implantable Heart Assist System in Heart and Great Vessels
Thoratec Paracorporeal Ventricular Assist Device
use External Heart Assist System in Heart and Great Vessels
Thrombectomy *see* Extirpation
Thymectomy
see Excision, Lymphatic and Hemic Systems Ø7B
see Resection, Lymphatic and Hemic Systems Ø7T
Thymopexy
see Repair, Lymphatic and Hemic Systems Ø7Q
see Reposition, Lymphatic and Hemic Systems Ø7S
Thymus gland *use* Thymus
Thyroarytenoid muscle
use Muscle, Neck, Left
use Muscle, Neck, Right
Thyrocervical trunk
use Artery, Thyroid, Left
use Artery, Thyroid, Right
Thyroid cartilage *use* Larynx
Thyroidectomy
see Excision, Endocrine System ØGB
see Resection, Endocrine System ØGT
Thyroidorrhaphy *see* Repair, Endocrine System ØGQ
Thyroidoscopy ØGJK4ZZ

Thyroidotomy *see* Drainage, Endocrine System ØG9
Tibialis anterior muscle
use Muscle, Lower Leg, Left
use Muscle, Lower Leg, Right
Tibialis posterior muscle
use Muscle, Lower Leg, Left
use Muscle, Lower Leg, Right
Tibiofemoral joint
use Joint, Knee, Left
use Joint, Knee, Left, Tibial Surface
use Joint, Knee, Right
use Joint, Knee, Right, Tibial Surface
TigerPaw® system for closure of left atrial appendage *use* Extraluminal Device
Tissue bank graft *use* Nonautologous Tissue Substitute
Tissue Expander
Insertion of device in
Breast
Bilateral ØHHV
Left ØHHU
Right ØHHT
Nipple
Left ØHHX
Right ØHHW
Subcutaneous Tissue and Fascia
Abdomen ØJH8
Back ØJH7
Buttock ØJH9
Chest ØJH6
Face ØJH1
Foot
Left ØJHR
Right ØJHQ
Hand
Left ØJHK
Right ØJHJ
Lower Arm
Left ØJHH
Right ØJHG
Lower Leg
Left ØJHP
Right ØJHN
Neck
Anterior ØJH4
Posterior ØJH5
Pelvic Region ØJHC
Perineum ØJHB
Scalp ØJHØ
Upper Arm
Left ØJHF
Right ØJHD
Upper Leg
Left ØJHM
Right ØJHL
Removal of device from
Breast
Left ØHPU
Right ØHPT
Subcutaneous Tissue and Fascia
Head and Neck ØJPS
Lower Extremity ØJPW
Trunk ØJPT
Upper Extremity ØJPV
Revision of device in
Breast
Left ØHWU
Right ØHWT
Subcutaneous Tissue and Fascia
Head and Neck ØJWS
Lower Extremity ØJWW
Trunk ØJWT
Upper Extremity ØJWV
Tissue expander (inflatable) (injectable)
use Tissue Expander in Skin and Breast
use Tissue Expander in Subcutaneous Tissue and Fascia
Tissue Plasminogen Activator (tPA) (r-tPA) *use* Thrombolytic, Other
Titanium Sternal Fixation System (TSFS)
use Internal Fixation Device, Rigid Plate in ØPH
use Internal Fixation Device, Rigid Plate in ØPS
Tomographic (Tomo) Nuclear Medicine Imaging CP2YYZZ
Abdomen CW2Ø
Abdomen and Chest CW24
Abdomen and Pelvis CW21
Tomographic (Tomo) Nuclear Medicine Imaging — continued
Anatomical Regions, Multiple CW2YYZZ
Bladder, Kidneys and Ureters CT23
Brain CØ2Ø
Breast CH2YYZZ
Bilateral CH22
Left CH21
Right CH2Ø
Bronchi and Lungs CB22
Central Nervous System CØ2YYZZ
Cerebrospinal Fluid CØ25
Chest CW23
Chest and Abdomen CW24
Chest and Neck CW26
Digestive System CD2YYZZ
Endocrine System CG2YYZZ
Extremity
Lower CW2D
Bilateral CP2F
Left CP2D
Right CP2C
Upper CW2M
Bilateral CP2B
Left CP29
Right CP28
Gallbladder CF24
Gastrointestinal Tract CD27
Gland, Parathyroid CG21
Head and Neck CW2B
Heart C22YYZZ
Right and Left C226
Hepatobiliary System and Pancreas CF2YYZZ
Kidneys, Ureters and Bladder CT23
Liver CF25
Liver and Spleen CF26
Lungs and Bronchi CB22
Lymphatics and Hematologic System C72YYZZ
Myocardium C22G
Neck and Chest CW26
Neck and Head CW2B
Pancreas and Hepatobiliary System CF2YYZZ
Pelvic Region CW2J
Pelvis CP26
Pelvis and Abdomen CW21
Pelvis and Spine CP27
Respiratory System CB2YYZZ
Skin CH2YYZZ
Skull CP21
Skull and Cervical Spine CP23
Spine
Cervical CP22
Cervical and Skull CP23
Lumbar CP2H
Thoracic CP2G
Thoracolumbar CP2J
Spine and Pelvis CP27
Spleen C722
Spleen and Liver CF26
Subcutaneous Tissue CH2YYZZ
Thorax CP24
Ureters, Kidneys and Bladder CT23
Urinary System CT2YYZZ
Tomography, computerized *see* Computerized Tomography (CT Scan)
Tonometry 4AØ7XBZ
Tonsillectomy
see Excision, Mouth and Throat ØCB
see Resection, Mouth and Throat ØCT
Tonsillotomy *see* Drainage, Mouth and Throat ØC9
Total artificial (replacement) heart *use* Synthetic Substitute
Total parenteral nutrition (TPN) *see* Introduction of Nutritional Substance
Trachectomy
see Excision, Trachea ØBB1
see Resection, Trachea ØBT1
Trachelectomy
see Excision, Cervix ØUBC
see Resection, Cervix ØUTC
Trachelopexy
see Repair, Cervix ØUQC
see Reposition, Cervix ØUSC
Tracheloplasty *see* Repair, Cervix ØUQC
Trachelorrhaphy *see* Repair, Cervix ØUQC
Trachelotomy *see* Drainage, Cervix ØU9C
Tracheobronchial lymph node *use* Lymphatic, Thorax
Tracheoesophageal fistulization ØB11ØD6
Tracheolysis *see* Release, Respiratory System ØBN
Tracheoplasty
see Repair, Respiratory System ØBQ
see Supplement, Respiratory System ØBU
Tracheorrhaphy *see* Repair, Respiratory System ØBQ
Tracheoscopy ØBJ18ZZ
Tracheostomy *see* Bypass, Respiratory System ØB1
Tracheostomy Device
Bypass, Trachea ØB11
Change device in, Trachea ØB21XFZ
Removal of device from, Trachea ØBP1
Revision of device in, Trachea ØBW1
Tracheostomy tube *use* Tracheostomy Device in Respiratory System
Tracheotomy *see* Drainage, Respiratory System ØB9
Traction
Abdominal Wall 2W63X
Arm
Lower
Left 2W6DX
Right 2W6CX
Upper
Left 2W6BX
Right 2W6AX
Back 2W65X
Chest Wall 2W64X
Extremity
Lower
Left 2W6MX
Right 2W6LX
Upper
Left 2W69X
Right 2W68X
Face 2W61X
Finger
Left 2W6KX
Right 2W6JX
Foot
Left 2W6TX
Right 2W6SX
Hand
Left 2W6FX
Right 2W6EX
Head 2W6ØX
Inguinal Region
Left 2W67X
Right 2W66X
Leg
Lower
Left 2W6RX
Right 2W6QX
Upper
Left 2W6PX
Right 2W6NX
Neck 2W62X
Thumb
Left 2W6HX
Right 2W6GX
Toe
Left 2W6VX
Right 2W6UX
Tractotomy *see* Division, Central Nervous System ØØ8
Tragus
use Ear, External, Bilateral
use Ear, External, Left
use Ear, External, Right
Training, caregiver *see* Caregiver Training
TRAM (transverse rectus abdominis myocutaneous) flap reconstruction
Free *see* Replacement, Skin and Breast ØHR
Pedicled *see* Transfer, Muscles ØKX
Transection *see* Division
Transfer
Buccal Mucosa ØCX4
Bursa and Ligament
Abdomen
Left ØMXJ
Right ØMXH
Ankle
Left ØMXR
Right ØMXQ
Elbow
Left ØMX4
Right ØMX3

Subterms under main terms may continue to next column or page

Transfer — continued
Bursa and Ligament — continued
Foot
Left ØMXT
Right ØMXS
Hand
Left ØMX8
Right ØMX7
Head and Neck ØMXØ
Hip
Left ØMXM
Right ØMXL
Knee
Left ØMXP
Right ØMXN
Lower Extremity
Left ØMXW
Right ØMXV
Perineum ØMXK
Shoulder
Left ØMX2
Right ØMX1
Thorax
Left ØMXG
Right ØMXF
Trunk
Left ØMXD
Right ØMXC
Upper Extremity
Left ØMXB
Right ØMX9
Wrist
Left ØMX6
Right ØMX5
Finger
Left ØXXPØZM
Right ØXXNØZL
Gingiva
Lower ØCX6
Upper ØCX5
Intestine
Large ØDXE
Small ØDX8
Lip
Lower ØCX1
Upper ØCXØ
Muscle
Abdomen
Left ØKXL
Right ØKXK
Extraocular
Left Ø8XM
Right Ø8XL
Facial ØKX1
Foot
Left ØKXW
Right ØKXV
Hand
Left ØKXD
Right ØKXC
Head ØKXØ
Hip
Left ØKXP
Right ØKXN
Lower Arm and Wrist
Left ØKXB
Right ØKX9
Lower Leg
Left ØKXT
Right ØKXS
Neck
Left ØKX3
Right ØKX2
Perineum ØKXM
Shoulder
Left ØKX6
Right ØKX5
Thorax
Left ØKXJ
Right ØKXH
Tongue, Palate, Pharynx ØKX4
Trunk
Left ØKXG
Right ØKXF
Upper Arm
Left ØKX8

Transfer — continued
Muscle — continued
Upper Arm — continued
Right ØKX7
Upper Leg
Left ØKXR
Right ØKXQ
Nerve
Abducens ØØXL
Accessory ØØXR
Acoustic ØØXN
Cervical Ø1X1
Facial ØØXM
Femoral Ø1XD
Glossopharyngeal ØØXP
Hypoglossal ØØXS
Lumbar Ø1XB
Median Ø1X5
Oculomotor ØØXH
Olfactory ØØXF
Optic ØØXG
Peroneal Ø1XH
Phrenic Ø1X2
Pudendal Ø1XC
Radial Ø1X6
Sciatic Ø1XF
Thoracic Ø1X8
Tibial Ø1XG
Trigeminal ØØXK
Trochlear ØØXJ
Ulnar Ø1X4
Vagus ØØXQ
Palate, Soft ØCX3
Skin
Abdomen ØHX7XZZ
Back ØHX6XZZ
Buttock ØHX8XZZ
Chest ØHX5XZZ
Ear
Left ØHX3XZZ
Right ØHX2XZZ
Face ØHX1XZZ
Foot
Left ØHXNXZZ
Right ØHXMXZZ
Genitalia ØHXAXZZ
Hand
Left ØHXGXZZ
Right ØHXFXZZ
Lower Arm
Left ØHXEXZZ
Right ØHXDXZZ
Lower Leg
Left ØHXLXZZ
Right ØHXKXZZ
Neck ØHX4XZZ
Perineum ØHX9XZZ
Scalp ØHXØXZZ
Upper Arm
Left ØHXCXZZ
Right ØHXBXZZ
Upper Leg
Left ØHXJXZZ
Right ØHXHXZZ
Stomach ØDX6
Subcutaneous Tissue and Fascia
Abdomen ØJX8
Back ØJX7
Buttock ØJX9
Chest ØJX6
Face ØJX1
Foot
Left ØJXR
Right ØJXQ
Hand
Left ØJXK
Right ØJXJ
Lower Arm
Left ØJXH
Right ØJXG
Lower Leg
Left ØJXP
Right ØJXN
Neck
Anterior ØJX4
Posterior ØJX5

Transfer — continued
Subcutaneous Tissue and Fascia — continued
Pelvic Region ØJXC
Perineum ØJXB
Scalp ØJXØ
Upper Arm
Left ØJXF
Right ØJXD
Upper Leg
Left ØJXM
Right ØJXL
Tendon
Abdomen
Left ØLXG
Right ØLXF
Ankle
Left ØLXT
Right ØLXS
Foot
Left ØLXW
Right ØLXV
Hand
Left ØLX8
Right ØLX7
Head and Neck ØLXØ
Hip
Left ØLXK
Right ØLXJ
Knee
Left ØLXR
Right ØLXQ
Lower Arm and Wrist
Left ØLX6
Right ØLX5
Lower Leg
Left ØLXP
Right ØLXN
Perineum ØLXH
Shoulder
Left ØLX2
Right ØLX1
Thorax
Left ØLXD
Right ØLXC
Trunk
Left ØLXB
Right ØLX9
Upper Arm
Left ØLX4
Right ØLX3
Upper Leg
Left ØLXM
Right ØLXL
Tongue ØCX7
Transfusion
Artery
Central
Antihemophilic Factors 3Ø26
Blood
Platelets 3Ø26
Red Cells 3Ø26
Frozen 3Ø26
White Cells 3Ø26
Whole 3Ø26
Bone Marrow 3Ø26
Factor IX 3Ø26
Fibrinogen 3Ø26
Globulin 3Ø26
Plasma
Fresh 3Ø26
Frozen 3Ø26
Plasma Cryoprecipitate 3Ø26
Serum Albumin 3Ø26
Stem Cells
Cord Blood 3Ø26
Hematopoietic 3Ø26
Peripheral
Antihemophilic Factors 3Ø25
Blood
Platelets 3Ø25
Red Cells 3Ø25
Frozen 3Ø25
White Cells 3Ø25
Whole 3Ø25
Bone Marrow 3Ø25
Factor IX 3Ø25

Transfusion — continued
- Artery — continued
  - Peripheral — continued
    - Fibrinogen 3Ø25
    - Globulin 3Ø25
    - Plasma
      - Fresh 3Ø25
      - Frozen 3Ø25
    - Plasma Cryoprecipitate 3Ø25
    - Serum Albumin 3Ø25
    - Stem Cells
      - Cord Blood 3Ø25
      - Hematopoietic 3Ø25
- Products of Conception
  - Antihemophilic Factors 3Ø27
  - Blood
    - Platelets 3Ø27
    - Red Cells 3Ø27
      - Frozen 3Ø27
    - White Cells 3Ø27
    - Whole 3Ø27
  - Factor IX 3Ø27
  - Fibrinogen 3Ø27
  - Globulin 3Ø27
  - Plasma
    - Fresh 3Ø27
    - Frozen 3Ø27
  - Plasma Cryoprecipitate 3Ø27
  - Serum Albumin 3Ø27
- Vein
  - 4-Factor Prothrombin Complex Concentrate 3Ø28ØB1
  - Central
    - Antihemophilic Factors 3Ø24
    - Blood
      - Platelets 3Ø24
      - Red Cells 3Ø24
        - Frozen 3Ø24
      - White Cells 3Ø24
      - Whole 3Ø24
    - Bone Marrow 3Ø24
    - Factor IX 3Ø24
    - Fibrinogen 3Ø24
    - Globulin 3Ø24
    - Plasma
      - Fresh 3Ø24
      - Frozen 3Ø24
    - Plasma Cryoprecipitate 3Ø24
    - Serum Albumin 3Ø24
    - Stem Cells
      - Cord Blood 3Ø24
      - Embryonic 3Ø24
      - Hematopoietic 3Ø24
  - Peripheral
    - Antihemophilic Factors 3Ø23
    - Blood
      - Platelets 3Ø23
      - Red Cells 3Ø23
        - Frozen 3Ø23
      - White Cells 3Ø23
      - Whole 3Ø23
    - Bone Marrow 3Ø23
    - Factor IX 3Ø23
    - Fibrinogen 3Ø23
    - Globulin 3Ø23
    - Plasma
      - Fresh 3Ø23
      - Frozen 3Ø23
    - Plasma Cryoprecipitate 3Ø23
    - Serum Albumin 3Ø23
    - Stem Cells
      - Cord Blood 3Ø23
      - Embryonic 3Ø23
      - Hematopoietic 3Ø23

Transplantation
- Esophagus ØDY5ØZ
- Heart Ø2YAØZ
- Intestine
  - Large ØDYEØZ
  - Small ØDY8ØZ
- Kidney
  - Left ØTY1ØZ
  - Right ØTYØØZ
- Liver ØFYØØZ
- Lung
  - Bilateral ØBYMØZ

Transplantation — continued
- Lung — continued
  - Left ØBYLØZ
  - Lower Lobe
    - Left ØBYJØZ
    - Right ØBYFØZ
  - Middle Lobe, Right ØBYDØZ
  - Right ØBYKØZ
  - Upper Lobe
    - Left ØBYGØZ
    - Right ØBYCØZ
- Lung Lingula ØBYHØZ
- Ovary
  - Left ØUY1ØZ
  - Right ØUYØØZ
- Pancreas ØFYGØZ
- Products of Conception 1ØYØ
- Spleen Ø7YPØZ
- Stomach ØDY6ØZ
- Thymus Ø7YMØZ

Transposition
- *see* Reposition
- *see* Transfer

Transversalis fascia *use* Subcutaneous Tissue and Fascia, Trunk

Transverse acetabular ligament
- *use* Bursa and Ligament, Hip, Left
- *use* Bursa and Ligament, Hip, Right

Transverse (cutaneous) cervical nerve *use* Nerve, Cervical Plexus

Transverse facial artery
- *use* Artery, Temporal, Left
- *use* Artery, Temporal, Right

Transverse humeral ligament
- *use* Bursa and Ligament, Shoulder, Left
- *use* Bursa and Ligament, Shoulder, Right

Transverse ligament of atlas *use* Bursa and Ligament, Head and Neck

Transverse Rectus Abdominis Myocutaneous Flap
- Replacement
  - Bilateral ØHRVØ76
  - Left ØHRUØ76
  - Right ØHRTØ76
- Transfer
  - Left ØKXL
  - Right ØKXK

Transverse scapular ligament
- *use* Bursa and Ligament, Shoulder, Left
- *use* Bursa and Ligament, Shoulder, Right

Transverse thoracis muscle
- *use* Muscle, Thorax, Left
- *use* Muscle, Thorax, Right

Transversospinalis muscle
- *use* Muscle, Trunk, Left
- *use* Muscle, Trunk, Right

Transversus abdominis muscle
- *use* Muscle, Abdomen, Left
- *use* Muscle, Abdomen, Right

Trapezium bone
- *use* Carpal, Left
- *use* Carpal, Right

Trapezius muscle
- *use* Muscle, Trunk, Left
- *use* Muscle, Trunk, Right

Trapezoid bone
- *use* Carpal, Left
- *use* Carpal, Right

Triceps brachii muscle
- *use* Muscle, Upper Arm, Left
- *use* Muscle, Upper Arm, Right

Tricuspid annulus *use* Valve, Tricuspid

Trifacial nerve *use* Nerve, Trigeminal

Trifecta™ Valve (aortic) *use* Zooplastic Tissue in Heart and Great Vessels

Trigone of bladder *use* Bladder

Trimming, excisional *see* Excision

Triquetral bone
- *use* Carpal, Left
- *use* Carpal, Right

Trochanteric bursa
- *use* Bursa and Ligament, Hip, Left
- *use* Bursa and Ligament, Hip, Right

TUMT (transurethral microwave thermotherapy of prostate) ØV5Ø7ZZ

TUNA (transurethral needle ablation of prostate) ØV5Ø7ZZ

Tunneled central venous catheter *use* Vascular Access Device in Subcutaneous Tissue and Fascia

Tunneled spinal (intrathecal) catheter *use* Infusion Device

Turbinectomy
- *see* Excision, Ear, Nose, Sinus Ø9B
- *see* Resection, Ear, Nose, Sinus Ø9T

Turbinoplasty
- *see* Repair, Ear, Nose, Sinus Ø9Q
- *see* Replacement, Ear, Nose, Sinus Ø9R
- *see* Supplement, Ear, Nose, Sinus Ø9U

Turbinotomy
- *see* Division, Ear, Nose, Sinus Ø98
- *see* Drainage, Ear, Nose, Sinus Ø99

TURP (transurethral resection of prostate)
- *see* Excision, Prostate ØVBØ
- *see* Resection, Prostate ØVTØ

Twelfth cranial nerve *use* Nerve, Hypoglossal

Two lead pacemaker *use* Pacemaker, Dual Chamber in ØJH

Tympanic cavity
- *use* Ear, Middle, Left
- *use* Ear, Middle, Right

Tympanic nerve *use* Nerve, Glossopharyngeal

Tympanic part of temoporal bone
- *use* Bone, Temporal, Left
- *use* Bone, Temporal, Right

Tympanogram *see* Hearing Assessment, Diagnostic Audiology F13

Tympanoplasty
- *see* Repair, Ear, Nose, Sinus Ø9Q
- *see* Replacement, Ear, Nose, Sinus Ø9R
- *see* Supplement, Ear, Nose, Sinus Ø9U

Tympanosympathectomy *see* Excision, Nerve, Head and Neck Sympathetic Ø1BK

Tympanotomy *see* Drainage, Ear, Nose, Sinus Ø99

U

Ulnar collateral carpal ligament
- *use* Bursa and Ligament, Wrist, Left
- *use* Bursa and Ligament, Wrist, Right

Ulnar collateral ligament
- *use* Bursa and Ligament, Elbow, Left
- *use* Bursa and Ligament, Elbow, Right

Ulnar notch
- *use* Radius, Left
- *use* Radius, Right

Ulnar vein
- *use* Vein, Brachial, Left
- *use* Vein, Brachial, Right

Ultrafiltration
- Hemodialysis *see* Performance, Urinary 5A1D
- Therapeutic plasmapheresis *see* Pheresis, Circulatory 6A55

Ultraflex™ Precision Colonic Stent System *use* Intraluminal Device

ULTRAPRO Hernia System (UHS) *use* Synthetic Substitute

ULTRAPRO Partially Absorbable Lightweight Mesh *use* Synthetic Substitute

ULTRAPRO Plug *use* Synthetic Substitute

Ultrasonic osteogenic stimulator
- *use* Bone Growth Stimulator in Head and Facial Bones
- *use* Bone Growth Stimulator in Lower Bones
- *use* Bone Growth Stimulator in Upper Bones

Ultrasonography
- Abdomen BW4ØZZZ
- Abdomen and Pelvis BW41ZZZ
- Abdominal Wall BH49ZZZ
- Aorta
  - Abdominal, Intravascular B44ØZZ3
  - Thoracic, Intravascular B34ØZZ3
- Appendix BD48ZZZ
- Artery
  - Brachiocephalic-Subclavian, Right, Intravascular B341ZZ3
  - Celiac and Mesenteric, Intravascular B44KZZ3
  - Common Carotid
    - Bilateral, Intravascular B345ZZ3
    - Left, Intravascular B344ZZ3
    - Right, Intravascular B343ZZ3

- **Ultrasonography** — continued
  - Artery — continued
    - Coronary
      - Multiple B241YZZ
        - Intravascular B241ZZ3
        - Transesophageal B241ZZ4
      - Single B240YZZ
        - Intravascular B240ZZ3
        - Transesophageal B240ZZ4
    - Femoral, Intravascular B44LZZ3
    - Inferior Mesenteric, Intravascular B445ZZ3
    - Internal Carotid
      - Bilateral, Intravascular B348ZZ3
      - Left, Intravascular B347ZZ3
      - Right, Intravascular B346ZZ3
    - Intra-Abdominal, Other, Intravascular B44BZZ3
    - Intracranial, Intravascular B34RZZ3
    - Lower Extremity
      - Bilateral, Intravascular B44HZZ3
      - Left, Intravascular B44GZZ3
      - Right, Intravascular B44FZZ3
    - Mesenteric and Celiac, Intravascular B44KZZ3
    - Ophthalmic, Intravascular B34VZZ3
    - Penile, Intravascular B44NZZ3
    - Pulmonary
      - Left, Intravascular B34TZZ3
      - Right, Intravascular B34SZZ3
    - Renal
      - Bilateral, Intravascular B448ZZ3
      - Left, Intravascular B447ZZ3
      - Right, Intravascular B446ZZ3
    - Subclavian, Left, Intravascular B342ZZ3
    - Superior Mesenteric, Intravascular B444ZZ3
    - Upper Extremity
      - Bilateral, Intravascular B34KZZ3
      - Left, Intravascular B34JZZ3
      - Right, Intravascular B34HZZ3
  - Bile Duct BF40ZZZ
  - Bile Duct and Gallbladder BF43ZZZ
  - Bladder BT40ZZZ
    - and Kidney BT4JZZZ
  - Brain B040ZZZ
  - Breast
    - Bilateral BH42ZZZ
    - Left BH41ZZZ
    - Right BH40ZZZ
  - Chest Wall BH4BZZZ
  - Coccyx BR4FZZZ
  - Connective Tissue
    - Lower Extremity BL41ZZZ
    - Upper Extremity BL40ZZZ
  - Duodenum BD49ZZZ
  - Elbow
    - Left, Densitometry BP4HZZ1
    - Right, Densitometry BP4GZZ1
  - Esophagus BD41ZZZ
  - Extremity
    - Lower BH48ZZZ
    - Upper BH47ZZZ
  - Eye
    - Bilateral B847ZZZ
    - Left B846ZZZ
    - Right B845ZZZ
  - Fallopian Tube
    - Bilateral BU42
    - Left BU41
    - Right BU40
  - Fetal Umbilical Cord BY47ZZZ
  - Fetus
    - First Trimester, Multiple Gestation BY4BZZZ
    - Second Trimester, Multiple Gestation BY4DZZZ
    - Single
      - First Trimester BY49ZZZ
      - Second Trimester BY4CZZZ
      - Third Trimester BY4FZZZ
    - Third Trimester, Multiple Gestation BY4GZZZ
  - Gallbladder BF42ZZZ
  - Gallbladder and Bile Duct BF43ZZZ
  - Gastrointestinal Tract BD47ZZZ
  - Gland
    - Adrenal
      - Bilateral BG42ZZZ
      - Left BG41ZZZ
      - Right BG40ZZZ
    - Parathyroid BG43ZZZ
    - Thyroid BG44ZZZ
- **Ultrasonography** — continued
  - Hand
    - Left, Densitometry BP4PZZ1
    - Right, Densitometry BP4NZZ1
  - Head and Neck BH4CZZZ
  - Heart
    - Left B245YZZ
      - Intravascular B245ZZ3
      - Transesophageal B245ZZ4
    - Pediatric B24DYZZ
      - Intravascular B24DZZ3
      - Transesophageal B24DZZ4
    - Right B244YZZ
      - Intravascular B244ZZ3
      - Transesophageal B244ZZ4
    - Right and Left B246YZZ
      - Intravascular B246ZZ3
      - Transesophageal B246ZZ4
  - Heart with Aorta B24BYZZ
    - Intravascular B24BZZ3
    - Transesophageal B24BZZ4
  - Hepatobiliary System, All BF4CZZZ
  - Hip
    - Bilateral BQ42ZZZ
    - Left BQ41ZZZ
    - Right BQ40ZZZ
  - Kidney
    - and Bladder BT4JZZZ
    - Bilateral BT43ZZZ
    - Left BT42ZZZ
    - Right BT41ZZZ
    - Transplant BT49ZZZ
  - Knee
    - Bilateral BQ49ZZZ
    - Left BQ48ZZZ
    - Right BQ47ZZZ
  - Liver BF45ZZZ
  - Liver and Spleen BF46ZZZ
  - Mediastinum BB4CZZZ
  - Neck BW4FZZZ
  - Ovary
    - Bilateral BU45
    - Left BU44
    - Right BU43
  - Ovary and Uterus BU4C
  - Pancreas BF47ZZZ
  - Pelvic Region BW4GZZZ
  - Pelvis and Abdomen BW41ZZZ
  - Penis BV4BZZZ
  - Pericardium B24CYZZ
    - Intravascular B24CZZ3
    - Transesophageal B24CZZ4
  - Placenta BY48ZZZ
  - Pleura BB4BZZZ
  - Prostate and Seminal Vesicle BV49ZZZ
  - Rectum BD4CZZZ
  - Sacrum BR4FZZZ
  - Scrotum BV44ZZZ
  - Seminal Vesicle and Prostate BV49ZZZ
  - Shoulder
    - Left, Densitometry BP49ZZ1
    - Right, Densitometry BP48ZZ1
  - Spinal Cord B04BZZZ
  - Spine
    - Cervical BR40ZZZ
    - Lumbar BR49ZZZ
    - Thoracic BR47ZZZ
  - Spleen and Liver BF46ZZZ
  - Stomach BD42ZZZ
  - Tendon
    - Lower Extremity BL43ZZZ
    - Upper Extremity BL42ZZZ
  - Ureter
    - Bilateral BT48ZZZ
    - Left BT47ZZZ
    - Right BT46ZZZ
  - Urethra BT45ZZZ
  - Uterus BU46
  - Uterus and Ovary BU4C
  - Vein
    - Jugular
      - Left, Intravascular B544ZZ3
      - Right, Intravascular B543ZZ3
    - Lower Extremity
      - Bilateral, Intravascular B54DZZ3
      - Left, Intravascular B54CZZ3
- **Ultrasonography** — continued
  - Vein — continued
    - Lower Extremity — continued
      - Right, Intravascular B54BZZ3
    - Portal, Intravascular B54TZZ3
    - Renal
      - Bilateral, Intravascular B54LZZ3
      - Left, Intravascular B54KZZ3
      - Right, Intravascular B54JZZ3
    - Spanchnic, Intravascular B54TZZ3
    - Subclavian
      - Left, Intravascular B547ZZ3
      - Right, Intravascular B546ZZ3
    - Upper Extremity
      - Bilateral, Intravascular B54PZZ3
      - Left, Intravascular B54NZZ3
      - Right, Intravascular B54MZZ3
  - Vena Cava
    - Inferior, Intravascular B549ZZ3
    - Superior, Intravascular B548ZZ3
  - Wrist
    - Left, Densitometry BP4MZZ1
    - Right, Densitometry BP4LZZ1
- **Ultrasound bone healing system**
  - *use* Bone Growth Stimulator in Head and Facial Bones
  - *use* Bone Growth Stimulator in Lower Bones
  - *use* Bone Growth Stimulator in Upper Bones
- **Ultrasound Therapy**
  - Heart 6A75
  - No Qualifier 6A75
  - Vessels
    - Head and Neck 6A75
    - Other 6A75
    - Peripheral 6A75
- **Ultraviolet Light Therapy, Skin** 6A80
- **Umbilical artery**
  - *use* Artery, Internal Iliac, Left
  - *use* Artery, Internal Iliac, Right
- **Uniplanar external fixator**
  - *use* External Fixation Device, Monoplanar in 0QS
  - *use* External Fixation Device, Monoplanar in 0QH
  - *use* External Fixation Device, Monoplanar in 0PH
  - *use* External Fixation Device, Monoplanar in 0PS
- **Upper GI series** *see* Fluoroscopy, Gastrointestinal, Upper BD15
- **Ureteral orifice**
  - *use* Ureter
  - *use* Ureter, Left
  - *use* Ureter, Right
  - *use* Ureters, Bilateral
- **Ureterectomy**
  - *see* Excision, Urinary System 0TB
  - *see* Resection, Urinary System 0TT
- **Ureterocolostomy** *see* Bypass, Urinary System 0T1
- **Ureterocystostomy** *see* Bypass, Urinary System 0T1
- **Ureteroenterostomy** *see* Bypass, Urinary System 0T1
- **Ureteroileostomy** *see* Bypass, Urinary System 0T1
- **Ureterolithotomy** *see* Extirpation, Urinary System 0TC
- **Ureterolysis** *see* Release, Urinary System 0TN
- **Ureteroneocystostomy**
  - *see* Bypass, Urinary System 0T1
  - *see* Reposition, Urinary System 0TS
- **Ureteropelvic junction (UPJ)**
  - *use* Kidney Pelvis, Left
  - *use* Kidney Pelvis, Right
- **Ureteropexy**
  - *see* Repair, Urinary System 0TQ
  - *see* Reposition, Urinary System 0TS
- **Ureteroplasty**
  - *see* Repair, Urinary System 0TQ
  - *see* Replacement, Urinary System 0TR
  - *see* Supplement, Urinary System 0TU
- **Ureteroplication** *see* Restriction, Urinary System 0TV
- **Ureteropyelography** *see* Fluoroscopy, Urinary System BT1
- **Ureterorrhaphy** *see* Repair, Urinary System 0TQ
- **Ureteroscopy** 0TJ98ZZ
- **Ureterostomy**
  - *see* Bypass, Urinary System 0T1
  - *see* Drainage, Urinary System 0T9
- **Ureterotomy** *see* Drainage, Urinary System 0T9
- **Ureteroureterostomy** *see* Bypass, Urinary System 0T1
- **Ureterovesical orifice**
  - *use* Ureter
  - *use* Ureter, Left

Ureterovesical orifice — continued
use Ureter, Right
use Ureters, Bilateral
Urethral catheterization, indwelling ØT9B7ØZ
Urethrectomy
see Excision, Urethra ØTBD
see Resection, Urethra ØTTD
Urethrolithotomy *see* Extirpation, Urethra ØTCD
Urethrolysis *see* Release, Urethra ØTND
Urethropexy
see Repair, Urethra ØTQD
see Reposition, Urethra ØTSD
Urethroplasty
see Repair, Urethra ØTQD
see Replacement, Urethra ØTRD
see Supplement, Urethra ØTUD
Urethrorrhaphy *see* Repair, Urethra ØTQD
Urethroscopy ØTJD8ZZ
Urethrotomy *see* Drainage, Urethra ØT9D
Urinary incontinence stimulator lead *use* Stimulator Lead in Urinary System
Urography *see* Fluoroscopy, Urinary System BT1
Uterine Artery
use Artery, Internal Iliac, Left
use Artery, Internal Iliac, Right
Left, Occlusion, Artery, Internal Iliac, Left Ø4LF
Right, Occlusion, Artery, Internal Iliac, Right Ø4LE
Uterine artery embolization (UAE) *see* Occlusion, Lower Arteries Ø4L
Uterine cornu *use* Uterus
Uterine tube
use Fallopian Tube, Left
use Fallopian Tube, Right
Uterine vein
use Vein, Hypogastric, Left
use Vein, Hypogastric, Right
Uvulectomy
see Excision, Uvula ØCBN
see Resection, Uvula ØCTN
Uvulorrhaphy *see* Repair, Uvula ØCQN
Uvulotomy *see* Drainage, Uvula ØC9N

V

Vaccination *see* Introduction of Serum, Toxoid, and Vaccine
Vacuum extraction, obstetric 1ØDØ7Z6
Vaginal artery
use Artery, Internal Iliac, Left
use Artery, Internal Iliac, Right
Vaginal pessary *use* Intraluminal Device, Pessary in Female Reproductive System
Vaginal vein
use Vein, Hypogastric, Left
use Vein, Hypogastric, Right
Vaginectomy
see Excision, Vagina ØUBG
see Resection, Vagina ØUTG
Vaginofixation
see Repair, Vagina ØUQG
see Reposition, Vagina ØUSG
Vaginoplasty
see Repair, Vagina ØUQG
see Supplement, Vagina ØUUG
Vaginorrhaphy *see* Repair, Vagina ØUQG
Vaginoscopy ØUJH8ZZ
Vaginotomy *see* Drainage, Female Reproductive System ØU9
Vagotomy *see* Division, Nerve, Vagus ØØ8Q
Valiant Thoracic Stent Graft *use* Synthetic Substitute
Valvotomy, valvulotomy
see Division, Heart and Great Vessels Ø28
see Release, Heart and Great Vessels Ø2N
Valvuloplasty
see Repair, Heart and Great Vessels Ø2Q
see Replacement, Heart and Great Vessels Ø2R
see Supplement, Heart and Great Vessels Ø2U
Vascular Access Device
Insertion of device in
Abdomen ØJH8
Chest ØJH6
Lower Arm
Left ØJHH
Right ØJHG
Vascular Access Device — continued
Insertion of device in — continued
Lower Leg
Left ØJHP
Right ØJHN
Upper Arm
Left ØJHF
Right ØJHD
Upper Leg
Left ØJHM
Right ØJHL
Removal of device from
Lower Extremity ØJPW
Trunk ØJPT
Upper Extremity ØJPV
Reservoir
Insertion of device in
Abdomen ØJH8
Chest ØJH6
Lower Arm
Left ØJHH
Right ØJHG
Lower Leg
Left ØJHP
Right ØJHN
Upper Arm
Left ØJHF
Right ØJHD
Upper Leg
Left ØJHM
Right ØJHL
Removal of device from
Lower Extremity ØJPW
Trunk ØJPT
Upper Extremity ØJPV
Revision of device in
Lower Extremity ØJWW
Trunk ØJWT
Upper Extremity ØJWV
Revision of device in
Lower Extremity ØJWW
Trunk ØJWT
Upper Extremity ØJWV
Vasectomy *see* Excision, Male Reproductive System ØVB
Vasography
see Fluoroscopy, Male Reproductive System BV1
see Plain Radiography, Male Reproductive System BVØ
Vasoligation *see* Occlusion, Male Reproductive System ØVL
Vasorrhaphy *see* Repair, Male Reproductive System ØVQ
Vasostomy *see* Bypass, Male Reproductive System ØV1
Vasotomy
With ligation *see* Occlusion, Male Reproductive System ØVL
Drainage *see* Drainage, Male Reproductive System ØV9
Vasovasostomy *see* Repair, Male Reproductive System ØVQ
Vastus intermedius muscle
use Muscle, Upper Leg, Left
use Muscle, Upper Leg, Right
Vastus lateralis muscle
use Muscle, Upper Leg, Left
use Muscle, Upper Leg, Right
Vastus medialis muscle
use Muscle, Upper Leg, Left
use Muscle, Upper Leg, Right
VCG (vectorcardiogram) *see* Measurement, Cardiac 4AØ2
Vectra® Vascular Access Graft *use* Vascular Access Device in Subcutaneous Tissue and Fascia
Venectomy
see Excision, Lower Veins Ø6B
see Excision, Upper Veins Ø5B
Venography
see Fluoroscopy, Veins B51
see Plain Radiography, Veins B5Ø
Venorrhaphy
see Repair, Lower Veins Ø6Q
see Repair, Upper Veins Ø5Q
Venotripsy
see Occlusion, Lower Veins Ø6L
see Occlusion, Upper Veins Ø5L
Ventricular fold *use* Larynx
Ventriculoatriostomy *see* Bypass, Central Nervous System ØØ1
Ventriculocisternostomy *see* Bypass, Central Nervous System ØØ1
Ventriculogram, cardiac
Combined left and right heart *see* Fluoroscopy, Heart, Right and Left B216
Left ventricle *see* Fluoroscopy, Heart, Left B215
Right ventricle *see* Fluoroscopy, Heart, Right B214
Ventriculopuncture, through previously implanted catheter 8CØ1X6J
Ventriculoscopy ØØJØ4ZZ
Ventriculostomy
External drainage *see* Drainage, Cerebral Ventricle ØØ96
Internal shunt *see* Bypass, Cerebral Ventricle ØØ16
Ventriculovenostomy *see* Bypass, Cerebral Ventricle ØØ16
Ventrio™ Hernia Patch *use* Synthetic Substitute
VEP (visual evoked potential) 4AØ7XØZ
Vermiform appendix *use* Appendix
Vermilion border
use Lip, Lower
use Lip, Upper
Versa *use* Pacemaker, Dual Chamber in ØJH
Version, obstetric
External 1ØSØXZZ
Internal 1ØSØ7ZZ
Vertebral arch
use Vertebra, Cervical
use Vertebra, Lumbar
use Vertebra, Thoracic
Vertebral canal *use* Spinal Canal
Vertebral foramen
use Vertebra, Cervical
use Vertebra, Lumbar
use Vertebra, Thoracic
Vertebral lamina
use Vertebra, Cervical
use Vertebra, Lumbar
use Vertebra, Thoracic
Vertebral pedicle
use Vertebra, Cervical
use Vertebra, Lumbar
use Vertebra, Thoracic
Vesical vein
use Vein, Hypogastric, Left
use Vein, Hypogastric, Right
Vesicotomy *see* Drainage, Urinary System ØT9
Vesiculectomy
see Excision, Male Reproductive System ØVB
see Resection, Male Reproductive System ØVT
Vesiculogram, seminal *see* Plain Radiography, Male Reproductive System BVØ
Vesiculotomy *see* Drainage, Male Reproductive System ØV9
Vestibular Assessment F15Z
Vestibular (Scarpa's) ganglion *use* Nerve, Acoustic
Vestibular nerve *use* Nerve, Acoustic
Vestibular Treatment FØC
Vestibulocochlear nerve *use* Nerve, Acoustic
Virchow's (supraclavicular) lymph node
use Lymphatic, Neck, Left
use Lymphatic, Neck, Right
Virtuoso (II) (DR) (VR) *use* Defibrillator Generator in ØJH
Vitrectomy
see Excision, Eye Ø8B
see Resection, Eye Ø8T
Vitreous body
use Vitreous, Left
use Vitreous, Right
Viva (XT) (S) *use* Cardiac Resynchronization Defibrillator Pulse Generator in ØJH
Vocal fold
use Vocal Cord, Left
use Vocal Cord, Right
Vocational
Assessment *see* Activities of Daily Living Assessment, Rehabilitation FØ2
Retraining *see* Activities of Daily Living Treatment, Rehabilitation FØ8
Volar (palmar) digital vein
use Vein, Hand, Left

Subterms under main terms may continue to next column or page

Volar (palmar) digital vein — continued
  use Vein, Hand, Right
Volar (palmar) metacarpal vein
  use Vein, Hand, Left
  use Vein, Hand, Right
Vomer bone *use* Septum, Nasal
Vomer of nasal septum *use* Bone, Nasal
Voraxaze *use* Glucarpidase
Vulvectomy
  see Excision, Female Reproductive System ØUB
  see Resection, Female Reproductive System ØUT

W

WALLSTENT® Endoprosthesis *use* Intraluminal Device
Washing *see* Irrigation
Wedge resection, pulmonary *see* Excision, Respiratory System ØBB
Window *see* Drainage
Wiring, dental 2W31X9Z

Xact Carotid Stent System *use* Intraluminal Device
Xenograft *use* Zooplastic Tissue in Heart and Great Vessels
XIENCE Everolimus Eluting Coronary Stent System
  use Intraluminal Device, Drug-eluting in Heart and Great Vessels
Xiphoid process *use* Sternum
XLIF® System *use* Interbody Fusion Device in Lower Joints
X-ray *see* Plain Radiography
X-STOP® Spacer
  use Spinal Stabilization Device, Interspinous Process in ØRH
  use Spinal Stabilization Device, Interspinous Process in ØSH

Yoga Therapy 8EØZXY4

Z

Zenith Flex® AAA Endovascular Graft *use* Intraluminal Device
Zenith TX2® TAA Endovascular Graft *use* Intraluminal Device
Zenith® Renu™ AAA Ancillary Graft *use* Intraluminal Device
Zilver® PTX® (paclitaxel) Drug-Eluting Peripheral Stent
  use Intraluminal Device, Drug-eluting in Lower Arteries
  use Intraluminal Device, Drug-eluting in Upper Arteries
Zimmer® NexGen® LPS Mobile Bearing Knee *use* Synthetic Substitute
Zimmer® NexGen® LPS-Flex Mobile Knee *use* Synthetic Substitute
Zonule of Zinn
  use Lens, Left
  use Lens, Right
Zotarolimus-eluting coronary stent *use* Intraluminal Device, Drug-eluting in Heart and Great Vessels
Z-plasty, skin for scar contracture *see* Release, Skin and Breast ØHN
Zygomatic process of frontal bone
  use Bone, Frontal, Left
  use Bone, Frontal, Right
Zygomatic process of temporal bone
  use Bone, Temporal, Left
  use Bone, Temporal, Right
Zygomaticus muscle *use* Muscle, Facial
Zyvox *use* Oxazolidinones

ICD-10-PCS Tables

Central Nervous System 001–00X

0 Medical and Surgical
0 Central Nervous System
1 Bypass Altering the route of passage of the contents of a tubular body part

Body Part Character 4	Approach Character 5	Device Character 6	Qualifier Character 7
6 Cerebral Ventricle	0 Open 3 Percutaneous	7 Autologous Tissue Substitute J Synthetic Substitute K Nonautologous Tissue Substitute	0 Nasopharynx 1 Mastoid Sinus 2 Atrium 3 Blood Vessel 4 Pleural Cavity 5 Intestine 6 Peritoneal Cavity 7 Urinary Tract 8 Bone Marrow B Cerebral Cisterns
U Spinal Canal	0 Open 3 Percutaneous	7 Autologous Tissue Substitute J Synthetic Substitute K Nonautologous Tissue Substitute	4 Pleural Cavity 6 Peritoneal Cavity 7 Urinary Tract 9 Fallopian Tube

AHA: 2013, 2Q, 36

0 Medical and Surgical
0 Central Nervous System
2 Change Taking out or off a device from a body part and putting back an identical or similar device in or on the same body part without cutting or puncturing the skin or a mucous membrane

Body Part Character 4	Approach Character 5	Device Character 6	Qualifier Character 7
0 Brain E Cranial Nerve U Spinal Canal	X External	0 Drainage Device Y Other Device	Z No Qualifier

Non-OR For all body part, approach, device, and qualifier values

0 Medical and Surgical
0 Central Nervous System
5 Destruction Physical eradication of all or a portion of a body part by the direct use of energy, force, or a destructive agent

Body Part Character 4	Approach Character 5	Device Character 6	Qualifier Character 7
0 Brain 1 Cerebral Meninges 2 Dura Mater 6 Cerebral Ventricle 7 Cerebral Hemisphere 8 Basal Ganglia 9 Thalamus A Hypothalamus B Pons C Cerebellum D Medulla Oblongata F Olfactory Nerve G Optic Nerve H Oculomotor Nerve J Trochlear Nerve K Trigeminal Nerve L Abducens Nerve M Facial Nerve N Acoustic Nerve P Glossopharyngeal Nerve Q Vagus Nerve R Accessory Nerve S Hypoglossal Nerve T Spinal Meninges W Cervical Spinal Cord X Thoracic Spinal Cord Y Lumbar Spinal Cord	0 Open 3 Percutaneous 4 Percutaneous Endoscopic	Z No Device	Z No Qualifier

Non-OR 005[F,G,H,J,K,L,M,N,P,Q,R,S][0,3,4]ZZ

Ø Medical and Surgical
Ø Central Nervous System
8 Division Cutting into a body part without draining fluids and/or gases from the body part in order to separate or transect a body part

Body Part Character 4	Approach Character 5	Device Character 6	Qualifier Character 7
Ø Brain **7** Cerebral Hemisphere **8** Basal Ganglia **F** Olfactory Nerve **G** Optic Nerve **H** Oculomotor Nerve **J** Trochlear Nerve **K** Trigeminal Nerve **L** Abducens Nerve **M** Facial Nerve **N** Acoustic Nerve **P** Glossopharyngeal Nerve **Q** Vagus Nerve **R** Accessory Nerve **S** Hypoglossal Nerve **W** Cervical Spinal Cord **X** Thoracic Spinal Cord **Y** Lumbar Spinal Cord	**Ø** Open **3** Percutaneous **4** Percutaneous Endoscopic	**Z** No Device	**Z** No Qualifier

Ø Medical and Surgical
Ø Central Nervous System
9 Drainage Taking or letting out fluids and/or gases from a body part

Body Part Character 4	Approach Character 5	Device Character 6	Qualifier Character 7
Ø Brain **1** Cerebral Meninges **2** Dura Mater **3** Epidural Space **4** Subdural Space **5** Subarachnoid Space **6** Cerebral Ventricle **7** Cerebral Hemisphere **8** Basal Ganglia **9** Thalamus **A** Hypothalamus **B** Pons **C** Cerebellum **D** Medulla Oblongata **F** Olfactory Nerve **G** Optic Nerve **H** Oculomotor Nerve **J** Trochlear Nerve **K** Trigeminal Nerve **L** Abducens Nerve **M** Facial Nerve **N** Acoustic Nerve **P** Glossopharyngeal Nerve **Q** Vagus Nerve **R** Accessory Nerve **S** Hypoglossal Nerve **T** Spinal Meninges **U** Spinal Canal **W** Cervical Spinal Cord **X** Thoracic Spinal Cord **Y** Lumbar Spinal Cord	**Ø** Open **3** Percutaneous **4** Percutaneous Endoscopic	**Ø** Drainage Device	**Z** No Qualifier

ØØ9 Continued on next page

Non-OR ØØ9[1,2,4,5,U][3,4]ØZ
AHA: 2Ø14, 1Q, 8

009 Continued

0 Medical and Surgical
0 Central Nervous System
9 Drainage Taking or letting out fluids and/or gases from a body part

Body Part Character 4	Approach Character 5	Device Character 6	Qualifier Character 7
0 Brain **1** Cerebral Meninges **2** Dura Mater **3** Epidural Space **4** Subdural Space **5** Subarachnoid Space **6** Cerebral Ventricle **7** Cerebral Hemisphere **8** Basal Ganglia **9** Thalamus **A** Hypothalamus **B** Pons **C** Cerebellum **D** Medulla Oblongata **F** Olfactory Nerve **G** Optic Nerve **H** Oculomotor Nerve **J** Trochlear Nerve **K** Trigeminal Nerve **L** Abducens Nerve **M** Facial Nerve **N** Acoustic Nerve **P** Glossopharyngeal Nerve **Q** Vagus Nerve **R** Accessory Nerve **S** Hypoglossal Nerve **T** Spinal Meninges **U** Spinal Canal **W** Cervical Spinal Cord **X** Thoracic Spinal Cord **Y** Lumbar Spinal Cord	**0** Open **3** Percutaneous **4** Percutaneous Endoscopic	**Z** No Device	**X** Diagnostic **Z** No Qualifier

Non-OR 009[0,1,2,3,4,5,6,7,8,9,A,B,C,D,F,G,H,J,K,L,M,N,P,Q,R,S,U][3,4]ZX
Non-OR 009[1,2,4,5,6,U][3,4]ZZ
AHA: 2014, 1Q, 8

0 Medical and Surgical
0 Central Nervous System
B Excision Cutting out or off, without replacement, a portion of a body part

Body Part Character 4	Approach Character 5	Device Character 6	Qualifier Character 7
0 Brain **1** Cerebral Meninges **2** Dura Mater **6** Cerebral Ventricle **7** Cerebral Hemisphere **8** Basal Ganglia **9** Thalamus **A** Hypothalamus **B** Pons **C** Cerebellum **D** Medulla Oblongata **F** Olfactory Nerve **G** Optic Nerve **H** Oculomotor Nerve **J** Trochlear Nerve **K** Trigeminal Nerve **L** Abducens Nerve **M** Facial Nerve **N** Acoustic Nerve **P** Glossopharyngeal Nerve **Q** Vagus Nerve **R** Accessory Nerve **S** Hypoglossal Nerve **T** Spinal Meninges **W** Cervical Spinal Cord **X** Thoracic Spinal Cord **Y** Lumbar Spinal Cord	**0** Open **3** Percutaneous **4** Percutaneous Endoscopic	**Z** No Device	**X** Diagnostic **Z** No Qualifier

Non-OR 00B[0,1,2,6,7,8,9,A,B,C,D,F,G,H,J,K,L,M,N,P,Q,R,S][3,4]ZX

Ø Medical and Surgical
Ø Central Nervous System
C Extirpation Taking or cutting out solid matter from a body part

Body Part Character 4	Approach Character 5	Device Character 6	Qualifier Character 7
Ø Brain 1 Cerebral Meninges 2 Dura Mater 3 Epidural Space 4 Subdural Space 5 Subarachnoid Space 6 Cerebral Ventricle 7 Cerebral Hemisphere 8 Basal Ganglia 9 Thalamus A Hypothalamus B Pons C Cerebellum D Medulla Oblongata F Olfactory Nerve G Optic Nerve H Oculomotor Nerve J Trochlear Nerve K Trigeminal Nerve L Abducens Nerve M Facial Nerve N Acoustic Nerve P Glossopharyngeal Nerve Q Vagus Nerve R Accessory Nerve S Hypoglossal Nerve T Spinal Meninges W Cervical Spinal Cord X Thoracic Spinal Cord Y Lumbar Spinal Cord	Ø Open 3 Percutaneous 4 Percutaneous Endoscopic	Z No Device	Z No Qualifier

Ø Medical and Surgical
Ø Central Nervous System
D Extraction Pulling or stripping out or off all or a portion of a body part by the use of force

Body Part Character 4	Approach Character 5	Device Character 6	Qualifier Character 7
1 Cerebral Meninges 2 Dura Mater F Olfactory Nerve G Optic Nerve H Oculomotor Nerve J Trochlear Nerve K Trigeminal Nerve L Abducens Nerve M Facial Nerve N Acoustic Nerve P Glossopharyngeal Nerve Q Vagus Nerve R Accessory Nerve S Hypoglossal Nerve T Spinal Meninges	Ø Open 3 Percutaneous 4 Percutaneous Endoscopic	Z No Device	Z No Qualifier

Ø Medical and Surgical
Ø Central Nervous System
F Fragmentation Breaking solid matter in a body part into pieces

Body Part Character 4	Approach Character 5	Device Character 6	Qualifier Character 7
3 Epidural Space NC 4 Subdural Space NC 5 Subarachnoid Space NC 6 Cerebral Ventricle NC U Spinal Canal	Ø Open 3 Percutaneous 4 Percutaneous Endoscopic X External	Z No Device	Z No Qualifier

Non-OR ØØF[3,4,5,6]XZZ
NC ØØF[3,4,5,6]XZZ

0 Medical and Surgical
0 Central Nervous System
H Insertion Putting in a nonbiological appliance that monitors, assists, performs, or prevents a physiological function but does not physically take the place of a body part

Body Part Character 4	Approach Character 5	Device Character 6	Qualifier Character 7
0 Brain ⊞ 6 Cerebral Ventricle ⊞ E Cranial Nerve ⊞ U Spinal Canal ⊞ V Spinal Cord ⊞	0 Open 3 Percutaneous 4 Percutaneous Endoscopic	2 Monitoring Device 3 Infusion Device M Neurostimulator Lead	Z No Qualifier

Non-OR 00H[U,V][0,3,4]3Z

See Appendix I for Procedure Combinations
⊞ 00H[0,6,E,U,V][0,3,4]MZ

0 Medical and Surgical
0 Central Nervous System
J Inspection Visually and/or manually exploring a body part

Body Part Character 4	Approach Character 5	Device Character 6	Qualifier Character 7
0 Brain E Cranial Nerve U Spinal Canal V Spinal Cord	0 Open 3 Percutaneous 4 Percutaneous Endoscopic	Z No Device	Z No Qualifier

0 Medical and Surgical
0 Central Nervous System
K Map Locating the route of passage of electrical impulses and/or locating functional areas in a body part

Body Part Character 4	Approach Character 5	Device Character 6	Qualifier Character 7
0 Brain 7 Cerebral Hemisphere 8 Basal Ganglia 9 Thalamus A Hypothalamus B Pons C Cerebellum D Medulla Oblongata	0 Open 3 Percutaneous 4 Percutaneous Endoscopic	Z No Device	Z No Qualifier

0 Medical and Surgical
0 Central Nervous System
N Release Freeing a body part from an abnormal physical constraint

Body Part Character 4	Approach Character 5	Device Character 6	Qualifier Character 7
0 Brain 1 Cerebral Meninges 2 Dura Mater 6 Cerebral Ventricle 7 Cerebral Hemisphere 8 Basal Ganglia 9 Thalamus A Hypothalamus B Pons C Cerebellum D Medulla Oblongata F Olfactory Nerve G Optic Nerve H Oculomotor Nerve J Trochlear Nerve K Trigeminal Nerve L Abducens Nerve M Facial Nerve N Acoustic Nerve P Glossopharyngeal Nerve Q Vagus Nerve R Accessory Nerve S Hypoglossal Nerve T Spinal Meninges W Cervical Spinal Cord X Thoracic Spinal Cord Y Lumbar Spinal Cord	0 Open 3 Percutaneous 4 Percutaneous Endoscopic	Z No Device	Z No Qualifier

Ø Medical and Surgical
Ø Central Nervous System
P Removal Taking out or off a device from a body part

Body Part Character 4	Approach Character 5	Device Character 6	Qualifier Character 7
Ø Brain 6 Cerebral Ventricle E Cranial Nerve U Spinal Canal V Spinal Cord	X External	Ø Drainage Device 2 Monitoring Device 3 Infusion Device M Neurostimulator Lead	Z No Qualifier
Ø Brain V Spinal Cord	Ø Open 3 Percutaneous 4 Percutaneous Endoscopic	Ø Drainage Device 2 Monitoring Device 3 Infusion Device 7 Autologous Tissue Substitute J Synthetic Substitute K Nonautologous Tissue Substitute M Neurostimulator Lead	Z No Qualifier
6 Cerebral Ventricle U Spinal Canal	Ø Open 3 Percutaneous 4 Percutaneous Endoscopic	Ø Drainage Device 2 Monitoring Device 3 Infusion Device J Synthetic Substitute M Neurostimulator Lead	Z No Qualifier
E Cranial Nerve	Ø Open 3 Percutaneous 4 Percutaneous Endoscopic	Ø Drainage Device 2 Monitoring Device 3 Infusion Device 7 Autologous Tissue Substitute M Neurostimulator Lead	Z No Qualifier

Non-OR ØØP[Ø,U,V]X[Ø,2,3,M]Z
Non-OR ØØP6X[Ø,3]Z
Non-OR ØØPEX[Ø,2,3]Z

Ø Medical and Surgical
Ø Central Nervous System
Q Repair Restoring, to the extent possible, a body part to its normal anatomic structure and function

Body Part Character 4	Approach Character 5	Device Character 6	Qualifier Character 7
Ø Brain 1 Cerebral Meninges 2 Dura Mater 6 Cerebral Ventricle 7 Cerebral Hemisphere 8 Basal Ganglia 9 Thalamus A Hypothalamus B Pons C Cerebellum D Medulla Oblongata F Olfactory Nerve G Optic Nerve H Oculomotor Nerve J Trochlear Nerve K Trigeminal Nerve L Abducens Nerve M Facial Nerve N Acoustic Nerve P Glossopharyngeal Nerve Q Vagus Nerve R Accessory Nerve S Hypoglossal Nerve T Spinal Meninges W Cervical Spinal Cord X Thoracic Spinal Cord Y Lumbar Spinal Cord	Ø Open 3 Percutaneous 4 Percutaneous Endoscopic	Z No Device	Z No Qualifier

AHA: 2Ø13, 3Q, 25

0 Medical and Surgical
0 Central Nervous System
S Reposition Moving to its normal location or other suitable location all or a portion of a body part

Body Part Character 4	Approach Character 5	Device Character 6	Qualifier Character 7
F Olfactory Nerve G Optic Nerve H Oculomotor Nerve J Trochlear Nerve K Trigeminal Nerve L Abducens Nerve M Facial Nerve N Acoustic Nerve P Glossopharyngeal Nerve Q Vagus Nerve R Accessory Nerve S Hypoglossal Nerve W Cervical Spinal Cord X Thoracic Spinal Cord Y Lumbar Spinal Cord	0 Open 3 Percutaneous 4 Percutaneous Endoscopic	Z No Device	Z No Qualifier

0 Medical and Surgical
0 Central Nervous System
T Resection Cutting out or off, without replacement, all of a body part

Body Part Character 4	Approach Character 5	Device Character 6	Qualifier Character 7
7 Cerebral Hemisphere	0 Open 3 Percutaneous 4 Percutaneous Endoscopic	Z No Device	Z No Qualifier

0 Medical and Surgical
0 Central Nervous System
U Supplement Putting in or on biological or synthetic material that physically reinforces and/or augments the function of a portion of a body part

Body Part Character 4	Approach Character 5	Device Character 6	Qualifier Character 7
1 Cerebral Meninges 2 Dura Mater T Spinal Meninges	0 Open 3 Percutaneous 4 Percutaneous Endoscopic	7 Autologous Tissue Substitute J Synthetic Substitute K Nonautologous Tissue Substitute	Z No Qualifier
F Olfactory Nerve G Optic Nerve H Oculomotor Nerve J Trochlear Nerve K Trigeminal Nerve L Abducens Nerve M Facial Nerve N Acoustic Nerve P Glossopharyngeal Nerve Q Vagus Nerve R Accessory Nerve S Hypoglossal Nerve	0 Open 3 Percutaneous 4 Percutaneous Endoscopic	7 Autologous Tissue Substitute	Z No Qualifier

Ø Medical and Surgical
Ø Central Nervous System
W Revision Correcting, to the extent possible, a portion of a malfunctioning device or the position of a displaced device

Body Part Character 4	Approach Character 5	Device Character 6	Qualifier Character 7
Ø Brain **V** Spinal Cord	**Ø** Open **3** Percutaneous **4** Percutaneous Endoscopic **X** External	**Ø** Drainage Device **2** Monitoring Device **3** Infusion Device **7** Autologous Tissue Substitute **J** Synthetic Substitute **K** Nonautologous Tissue Substitute **M** Neurostimulator Lead	**Z** No Qualifier
6 Cerebral Ventricle **U** Spinal Canal	**Ø** Open **3** Percutaneous **4** Percutaneous Endoscopic **X** External	**Ø** Drainage Device **2** Monitoring Device **3** Infusion Device **J** Synthetic Substitute **M** Neurostimulator Lead	**Z** No Qualifier
E Cranial Nerve	**Ø** Open **3** Percutaneous **4** Percutaneous Endoscopic **X** External	**Ø** Drainage Device **2** Monitoring Device **3** Infusion Device **7** Autologous Tissue Substitute **M** Neurostimulator Lead	**Z** No Qualifier

Non-OR ØØWEX[Ø,2,3,7,M]Z
Non-OR ØØW[6,U]X[Ø,2,3,J,M]Z
Non-OR ØØW[Ø,V]X[Ø,2,3,7,J,K,M]Z

Ø Medical and Surgical
Ø Central Nervous System
X Transfer Moving, without taking out, all or a portion of a body part to another location to take over the function of all or a portion of a body part

Body Part Character 4	Approach Character 5	Device Character 6	Qualifier Character 7
F Olfactory Nerve **G** Optic Nerve **H** Oculomotor Nerve **J** Trochlear Nerve **K** Trigeminal Nerve **L** Abducens Nerve **M** Facial Nerve **N** Acoustic Nerve **P** Glossopharyngeal Nerve **Q** Vagus Nerve **R** Accessory Nerve **S** Hypoglossal Nerve	**Ø** Open **4** Percutaneous Endoscopic	**Z** No Device	**F** Olfactory Nerve **G** Optic Nerve **H** Oculomotor Nerve **J** Trochlear Nerve **K** Trigeminal Nerve **L** Abducens Nerve **M** Facial Nerve **N** Acoustic Nerve **P** Glossopharyngeal Nerve **Q** Vagus Nerve **R** Accessory Nerve **S** Hypoglossal Nerve

Peripheral Nervous System 012–01X

0 Medical and Surgical
1 Peripheral Nervous System
2 Change Taking out or off a device from a body part and putting back an identical or similar device in or on the same body part without cutting or puncturing the skin or a mucous membrane

Body Part Character 4	Approach Character 5	Device Character 6	Qualifier Character 7
Y Peripheral Nerve	X External	0 Drainage Device Y Other Device	Z No Qualifier

Non-OR For all body part, approach, device, and qualifier values

0 Medical and Surgical
1 Peripheral Nervous System
5 Destruction Physical eradication of all or a portion of a body part by the direct use of energy, force, or a destructive agent

Body Part Character 4	Approach Character 5	Device Character 6	Qualifier Character 7
0 Cervical Plexus 1 Cervical Nerve 2 Phrenic Nerve 3 Brachial Plexus 4 Ulnar Nerve 5 Median Nerve 6 Radial Nerve 8 Thoracic Nerve 9 Lumbar Plexus A Lumbosacral Plexus B Lumbar Nerve C Pudendal Nerve D Femoral Nerve F Sciatic Nerve G Tibial Nerve H Peroneal Nerve K Head and Neck Sympathetic Nerve L Thoracic Sympathetic Nerve M Abdominal Sympathetic Nerve N Lumbar Sympathetic Nerve P Sacral Sympathetic Nerve Q Sacral Plexus R Sacral Nerve	0 Open 3 Percutaneous 4 Percutaneous Endoscopic	Z No Device	Z No Qualifier

Non-OR 015[0,2,3,4,5,6,9,A,C,D,F,G,H,Q][0,3,4]ZZ
Non-OR 015[1,8,B,R]3ZZ

0 Medical and Surgical
1 Peripheral Nervous System
8 Division Cutting into a body part without draining fluids and/or gases from the body part in order to separate or transect a body part

Body Part Character 4	Approach Character 5	Device Character 6	Qualifier Character 7
0 Cervical Plexus 1 Cervical Nerve 2 Phrenic Nerve 3 Brachial Plexus 4 Ulnar Nerve 5 Median Nerve 6 Radial Nerve 8 Thoracic Nerve 9 Lumbar Plexus A Lumbosacral Plexus B Lumbar Nerve C Pudendal Nerve D Femoral Nerve F Sciatic Nerve G Tibial Nerve H Peroneal Nerve K Head and Neck Sympathetic Nerve L Thoracic Sympathetic Nerve M Abdominal Sympathetic Nerve N Lumbar Sympathetic Nerve P Sacral Sympathetic Nerve Q Sacral Plexus R Sacral Nerve	0 Open 3 Percutaneous 4 Percutaneous Endoscopic	Z No Device	Z No Qualifier

Ø Medical and Surgical
1 Peripheral Nervous System
9 Drainage Taking or letting out fluids and/or gases from a body part

Body Part Character 4	Approach Character 5	Device Character 6	Qualifier Character 7
Ø Cervical Plexus 1 Cervical Nerve 2 Phrenic Nerve 3 Brachial Plexus 4 Ulnar Nerve 5 Median Nerve 6 Radial Nerve 8 Thoracic Nerve 9 Lumbar Plexus A Lumbosacral Plexus B Lumbar Nerve C Pudendal Nerve D Femoral Nerve F Sciatic Nerve G Tibial Nerve H Peroneal Nerve K Head and Neck Sympathetic Nerve L Thoracic Sympathetic Nerve M Abdominal Sympathetic Nerve N Lumbar Sympathetic Nerve P Sacral Sympathetic Nerve Q Sacral Plexus R Sacral Nerve	Ø Open 3 Percutaneous 4 Percutaneous Endoscopic	Ø Drainage Device	Z No Qualifier
Ø Cervical Plexus 1 Cervical Nerve 2 Phrenic Nerve 3 Brachial Plexus 4 Ulnar Nerve 5 Median Nerve 6 Radial Nerve 8 Thoracic Nerve 9 Lumbar Plexus A Lumbosacral Plexus B Lumbar Nerve C Pudendal Nerve D Femoral Nerve F Sciatic Nerve G Tibial Nerve H Peroneal Nerve K Head and Neck Sympathetic Nerve L Thoracic Sympathetic Nerve M Abdominal Sympathetic Nerve N Lumbar Sympathetic Nerve P Sacral Sympathetic Nerve Q Sacral Plexus R Sacral Nerve	Ø Open 3 Percutaneous 4 Percutaneous Endoscopic	Z No Device	X Diagnostic Z No Qualifier

Non-OR Ø19[Ø,1,2,3,4,5,6,8,9,A,B,C,D,F,G,H,Q,R][3,4]ZX

Ø Medical and Surgical
1 Peripheral Nervous System
B Excision Cutting out or off, without replacement, a portion of a body part

Body Part Character 4	Approach Character 5	Device Character 6	Qualifier Character 7
Ø Cervical Plexus 1 Cervical Nerve 2 Phrenic Nerve 3 Brachial Plexus ⊞ 4 Ulnar Nerve 5 Median Nerve 6 Radial Nerve 8 Thoracic Nerve 9 Lumbar Plexus A Lumbosacral Plexus B Lumbar Nerve C Pudendal Nerve D Femoral Nerve F Sciatic Nerve G Tibial Nerve H Peroneal Nerve K Head and Neck Sympathetic Nerve L Thoracic Sympathetic Nerve ⊞ M Abdominal Sympathetic Nerve N Lumbar Sympathetic Nerve P Sacral Sympathetic Nerve Q Sacral Plexus R Sacral Nerve	Ø Open 3 Percutaneous 4 Percutaneous Endoscopic	Z No Device	X Diagnostic Z No Qualifier

Non-OR Ø1B[Ø,1,2,3,4,5,6,8,9,A,B,C,D,F,G,H,Q,R][3,4]ZX

No Procedure Combinations Specified
⊞ Ø1B[3,L]ØZZ

Ø Medical and Surgical
1 Peripheral Nervous System
C Extirpation Taking or cutting out solid matter from a body part

Body Part Character 4	Approach Character 5	Device Character 6	Qualifier Character 7
Ø Cervical Plexus 1 Cervical Nerve 2 Phrenic Nerve 3 Brachial Plexus 4 Ulnar Nerve 5 Median Nerve 6 Radial Nerve 8 Thoracic Nerve 9 Lumbar Plexus A Lumbosacral Plexus B Lumbar Nerve C Pudendal Nerve D Femoral Nerve F Sciatic Nerve G Tibial Nerve H Peroneal Nerve K Head and Neck Sympathetic Nerve L Thoracic Sympathetic Nerve M Abdominal Sympathetic Nerve N Lumbar Sympathetic Nerve P Sacral Sympathetic Nerve Q Sacral Plexus R Sacral Nerve	Ø Open 3 Percutaneous 4 Percutaneous Endoscopic	Z No Device	Z No Qualifier

Ø Medical and Surgical
1 Peripheral Nervous System
D Extraction Pulling or stripping out or off all or a portion of a body part by the use of force

Body Part Character 4	Approach Character 5	Device Character 6	Qualifier Character 7
Ø Cervical Plexus **1** Cervical Nerve **2** Phrenic Nerve **3** Brachial Plexus **4** Ulnar Nerve **5** Median Nerve **6** Radial Nerve **8** Thoracic Nerve **9** Lumbar Plexus **A** Lumbosacral Plexus **B** Lumbar Nerve **C** Pudendal Nerve **D** Femoral Nerve **F** Sciatic Nerve **G** Tibial Nerve **H** Peroneal Nerve **K** Head and Neck Sympathetic Nerve **L** Thoracic Sympathetic Nerve **M** Abdominal Sympathetic Nerve **N** Lumbar Sympathetic Nerve **P** Sacral Sympathetic Nerve **Q** Sacral Plexus **R** Sacral Nerve	**Ø** Open **3** Percutaneous **4** Percutaneous Endoscopic	**Z** No Device	**Z** No Qualifier

Ø Medical and Surgical
1 Peripheral Nervous System
H Insertion Putting in a nonbiological appliance that monitors, assists, performs, or prevents a physiological function but does not physically take the place of a body part

Body Part Character 4	Approach Character 5	Device Character 6	Qualifier Character 7
Y Peripheral Nerve ⊞	**Ø** Open **3** Percutaneous **4** Percutaneous Endoscopic	**2** Monitoring Device **M** Neurostimulator Lead	**Z** No Qualifier

See Appendix I for Procedure Combinations
⊞ Ø1HY[Ø,3,4]MZ

Ø Medical and Surgical
1 Peripheral Nervous System
J Inspection Visually and/or manually exploring a body part

Body Part Character 4	Approach Character 5	Device Character 6	Qualifier Character 7
Y Peripheral Nerve	**Ø** Open **3** Percutaneous **4** Percutaneous Endoscopic	**Z** No Device	**Z** No Qualifier

0 Medical and Surgical
1 Peripheral Nervous System
N Release Freeing a body part from an abnormal physical constraint

Body Part Character 4	Approach Character 5	Device Character 6	Qualifier Character 7
0 Cervical Plexus 1 Cervical Nerve 2 Phrenic Nerve 3 Brachial Plexus 4 Ulnar Nerve 5 Median Nerve 6 Radial Nerve 8 Thoracic Nerve 9 Lumbar Plexus A Lumbosacral Plexus B Lumbar Nerve C Pudendal Nerve D Femoral Nerve F Sciatic Nerve G Tibial Nerve H Peroneal Nerve K Head and Neck Sympathetic Nerve L Thoracic Sympathetic Nerve M Abdominal Sympathetic Nerve N Lumbar Sympathetic Nerve P Sacral Sympathetic Nerve Q Sacral Plexus R Sacral Nerve	0 Open 3 Percutaneous 4 Percutaneous Endoscopic	Z No Device	Z No Qualifier

0 Medical and Surgical
1 Peripheral Nervous System
P Removal Taking out or off a device from a body part

Body Part Character 4	Approach Character 5	Device Character 6	Qualifier Character 7
Y Peripheral Nerve	0 Open 3 Percutaneous 4 Percutaneous Endoscopic	0 Drainage Device 2 Monitoring Device 7 Autologous Tissue Substitute M Neurostimulator Lead	Z No Qualifier
Y Peripheral Nerve	X External	0 Drainage Device 2 Monitoring Device M Neurostimulator Lead	Z No Qualifier

Non-OR 01PYX[0,2]Z

0 Medical and Surgical
1 Peripheral Nervous System
Q Repair Restoring, to the extent possible, a body part to its normal anatomic structure and function

Body Part Character 4	Approach Character 5	Device Character 6	Qualifier Character 7
0 Cervical Plexus 1 Cervical Nerve 2 Phrenic Nerve 3 Brachial Plexus 4 Ulnar Nerve 5 Median Nerve 6 Radial Nerve 8 Thoracic Nerve 9 Lumbar Plexus A Lumbosacral Plexus B Lumbar Nerve C Pudendal Nerve D Femoral Nerve F Sciatic Nerve G Tibial Nerve H Peroneal Nerve K Head and Neck Sympathetic Nerve L Thoracic Sympathetic Nerve M Abdominal Sympathetic Nerve N Lumbar Sympathetic Nerve P Sacral Sympathetic Nerve Q Sacral Plexus R Sacral Nerve	0 Open 3 Percutaneous 4 Percutaneous Endoscopic	Z No Device	Z No Qualifier

Ø Medical and Surgical
1 Peripheral Nervous System
S Reposition Moving to its normal location or other suitable location all or a portion of a body part

Body Part Character 4	Approach Character 5	Device Character 6	Qualifier Character 7
Ø Cervical Plexus 1 Cervical Nerve 2 Phrenic Nerve 3 Brachial Plexus 4 Ulnar Nerve 5 Median Nerve 6 Radial Nerve 8 Thoracic Nerve 9 Lumbar Plexus A Lumbosacral Plexus B Lumbar Nerve C Pudendal Nerve D Femoral Nerve F Sciatic Nerve G Tibial Nerve H Peroneal Nerve Q Sacral Plexus R Sacral Nerve	Ø Open 3 Percutaneous 4 Percutaneous Endoscopic	Z No Device	Z No Qualifier

Ø Medical and Surgical
1 Peripheral Nervous System
U Supplement Putting in or on biological or synthetic material that physically reinforces and/or augments the function of a portion of a body part

Body Part Character 4	Approach Character 5	Device Character 6	Qualifier Character 7
1 Cervical Nerve 2 Phrenic Nerve 4 Ulnar Nerve 5 Median Nerve 6 Radial Nerve 8 Thoracic Nerve B Lumbar Nerve C Pudendal Nerve D Femoral Nerve F Sciatic Nerve G Tibial Nerve H Peroneal Nerve R Sacral Nerve	Ø Open 3 Percutaneous 4 Percutaneous Endoscopic	7 Autologous Tissue Substitute	Z No Qualifier

Ø Medical and Surgical
1 Peripheral Nervous System
W Revision Correcting, to the extent possible, a portion of a malfunctioning device or the position of a displaced device

Body Part Character 4	Approach Character 5	Device Character 6	Qualifier Character 7
Y Peripheral Nerve	Ø Open 3 Percutaneous 4 Percutaneous Endoscopic X External	Ø Drainage Device 2 Monitoring Device 7 Autologous Tissue Substitute M Neurostimulator Lead	Z No Qualifier

Non-OR Ø1WYX[Ø,2,7,M]Z

Ø Medical and Surgical
1 Peripheral Nervous System
X Transfer Moving, without taking out, all or a portion of a body part to another location to take over the function of all or a portion of a body part

Body Part Character 4	Approach Character 5	Device Character 6	Qualifier Character 7
1 Cervical Nerve 2 Phrenic Nerve	Ø Open 4 Percutaneous Endoscopic	Z No Device	1 Cervical Nerve 2 Phrenic Nerve
4 Ulnar Nerve 5 Median Nerve 6 Radial Nerve	Ø Open 4 Percutaneous Endoscopic	Z No Device	4 Ulnar Nerve 5 Median Nerve 6 Radial Nerve
8 Thoracic Nerve	Ø Open 4 Percutaneous Endoscopic	Z No Device	8 Thoracic Nerve
B Lumbar Nerve C Pudendal Nerve	Ø Open 4 Percutaneous Endoscopic	Z No Device	B Lumbar Nerve C Perineal Nerve
D Femoral Nerve F Sciatic Nerve G Tibial Nerve H Peroneal Nerve	Ø Open 4 Percutaneous Endoscopic	Z No Device	D Femoral Nerve F Sciatic Nerve G Tibial Nerve H Peroneal Nerve

Heart and Great Vessels 021–02Y

0 Medical and Surgical
2 Heart and Great Vessels
1 Bypass Altering the route of passage of the contents of a tubular body part

Body Part Character 4	Approach Character 5	Device Character 6	Qualifier Character 7
0 Coronary Artery, One Site 1 Coronary Artery, Two Sites 2 Coronary Artery, Three Sites 3 Coronary Artery, Four or More Sites	0 Open 4 Percutaneous Endoscopic	9 Autologous Venous Tissue A Autologous Arterial Tissue J Synthetic Substitute K Nonautologous Tissue Substitute	3 Coronary Artery 8 Internal Mammary, Right 9 Internal Mammary, Left C Thoracic Artery F Abdominal Artery W Aorta
0 Coronary Artery, One Site 1 Coronary Artery, Two Sites 2 Coronary Artery, Three Sites 3 Coronary Artery, Four or More Sites	0 Open 4 Percutaneous Endoscopic	Z No Device	3 Coronary Artery 8 Internal Mammary, Right 9 Internal Mammary, Left C Thoracic Artery F Abdominal Artery
0 Coronary Artery, One Site 1 Coronary Artery, Two Sites 2 Coronary Artery, Three Sites 3 Coronary Artery, Four or More Sites	3 Percutaneous 4 Percutaneous Endoscopic	4 Drug-eluting Intraluminal Device D Intraluminal Device	4 Coronary Vein
6 Atrium, Right	0 Open 4 Percutaneous Endoscopic	Z No Device	7 Atrium, Left P Pulmonary Trunk Q Pulmonary Artery, Right R Pulmonary Artery, Left
6 Atrium, Right K Ventricle, Right L Ventricle, Left	0 Open 4 Percutaneous Endoscopic	9 Autologous Venous Tissue A Autologous Arterial Tissue J Synthetic Substitute K Nonautologous Tissue Substitute	P Pulmonary Trunk Q Pulmonary Artery, Right R Pulmonary Artery, Left
7 Atrium, Left ⊞ V Superior Vena Cava	0 Open 4 Percutaneous Endoscopic	9 Autologous Venous Tissue A Autologous Arterial Tissue J Synthetic Substitute K Nonautologous Tissue Substitute Z No Device	P Pulmonary Trunk Q Pulmonary Artery, Right R Pulmonary Artery, Left
K Ventricle, Right L Ventricle, Left	0 Open 4 Percutaneous Endoscopic	Z No Device	5 Coronary Circulation 8 Internal Mammary, Right 9 Internal Mammary, Left C Thoracic Artery F Abdominal Artery P Pulmonary Trunk Q Pulmonary Artery, Right R Pulmonary Artery, Left W Aorta
W Thoracic Aorta	0 Open 4 Percutaneous Endoscopic	9 Autologous Venous Tissue A Autologous Arterial Tissue J Synthetic Substitute K Nonautologous Tissue Substitute Z No Device	B Subclavian D Carotid P Pulmonary Trunk Q Pulmonary Artery, Right R Pulmonary Artery, Left

Non-OR 021[0,1,2,3][3,4][4,D]4
HAC 021[0,1,2,3][0,4][9,A,J,K][3,8,9,C,F,W] when reported with SDx J98.5
HAC 021[0,1,2,3][0,4]Z[3,8,9,C,F] when reported with SDx J98.5
AHA: 2014, 1Q, 10; 2013, 2Q, 37

No Procedure Combinations Specified
⊞ 02170Z[P,Q,R]

Ø Medical and Surgical
2 Heart and Great Vessels
5 Destruction Physical eradication of all or a portion of a body part by the direct use of energy, force, or a destructive agent

Body Part Character 4	Approach Character 5	Device Character 6	Qualifier Character 7
4 Coronary Vein **5** Atrial Septum **6** Atrium, Right **8** Conduction Mechanism **9** Chordae Tendineae **D** Papillary Muscle **F** Aortic Valve **G** Mitral Valve **H** Pulmonary Valve **J** Tricuspid Valve **K** Ventricle, Right **L** Ventricle, Left **M** Ventricular Septum **N** Pericardium **P** Pulmonary Trunk **Q** Pulmonary Artery, Right **R** Pulmonary Artery, Left **S** Pulmonary Vein, Right **T** Pulmonary Vein, Left **V** Superior Vena Cava **W** Thoracic Aorta	**Ø** Open **3** Percutaneous **4** Percutaneous Endoscopic	**Z** No Device	**Z** No Qualifier
7 Atrium, Left	**Ø** Open **3** Percutaneous **4** Percutaneous Endoscopic	**Z** No Device	**K** Left Atrial Appendage **Z** No Qualifier

DRG Non-OR Ø257[Ø,3,4]ZK
AHA: 2Ø13, 2Q, 38

Ø Medical and Surgical
2 Heart and Great Vessels
7 Dilation Expanding an orifice or the lumen of a tubular body part

Body Part Character 4	Approach Character 5	Device Character 6	Qualifier Character 7
Ø Coronary Artery, One Site **1** Coronary Artery, Two Sites **2** Coronary Artery, Three Sites **3** Coronary Artery, Four or More Sites	**Ø** Open **3** Percutaneous **4** Percutaneous Endoscopic	**4** Intraluminal Device, Drug-eluting **D** Intraluminal Device **T** Radioactive Intraluminal Device **Z** No Device	**6** Bifurcation **Z** No Qualifier
F Aortic Valve **G** Mitral Valve **H** Pulmonary Valve **J** Tricuspid Valve **K** Ventricle, Right **P** Pulmonary Trunk **Q** Pulmonary Artery, Right **S** Pulmonary Vein, Right **T** Pulmonary Vein, Left **V** Superior Vena Cava **W** Thoracic Aorta	**Ø** Open **3** Percutaneous **4** Percutaneous Endoscopic	**4** Intraluminal Device, Drug-eluting **D** Intraluminal Device **Z** No Device	**Z** No Qualifier
R Pulmonary Artery, Left	**Ø** Open **3** Percutaneous **4** Percutaneous Endoscopic	**4** Intraluminal Device, Drug-eluting **D** Intraluminal Device **Z** No Device	**T** Ductus Arteriosus **Z** No Qualifier

AHA: 2Ø14, 2Q, 4

Ø Medical and Surgical
2 Heart and Great Vessels
8 Division Cutting into a body part without draining fluids and/or gases from the body part in order to separate or transect a body part

Body Part Character 4	Approach Character 5	Device Character 6	Qualifier Character 7
8 Conduction Mechanism **9** Chordae Tendineae **D** Papillary Muscle	**Ø** Open **3** Percutaneous **4** Percutaneous Endoscopic	**Z** No Device	**Z** No Qualifier

0 Medical and Surgical
2 Heart and Great Vessels
B Excision Cutting out or off, without replacement, a portion of a body part

Body Part Character 4	Approach Character 5	Device Character 6	Qualifier Character 7
4 Coronary Vein 5 Atrial Septum 6 Atrium, Right 7 Atrium, Left 8 Conduction Mechanism 9 Chordae Tendineae D Papillary Muscle F Aortic Valve G Mitral Valve H Pulmonary Valve J Tricuspid Valve K Ventricle, Right ⊞ NC L Ventricle, Left NC M Ventricular Septum N Pericardium P Pulmonary Trunk Q Pulmonary Artery, Right R Pulmonary Artery, Left S Pulmonary Vein, Right T Pulmonary Vein, Left V Superior Vena Cava W Thoracic Aorta	0 Open 3 Percutaneous 4 Percutaneous Endoscopic	Z No Device	X Diagnostic Z No Qualifier
7 Atrium, Left	0 Open 3 Percutaneous 4 Percutaneous Endoscopic	Z No Device	K Left Atrial Appendage

DRG Non-OR 02B7[0,3,4]ZK
Non-OR 02B[4,5,6,7,8,9,D,F,G,H,J,K,L,M][0,3,4]ZX
NC 02BK[0,3,4]ZZ
NC 02BL[0,3,4]ZZ

No Procedure Combinations Specified
⊞ 02BK0ZZ

0 Medical and Surgical
2 Heart and Great Vessels
C Extirpation Taking or cutting out solid matter from a body part

Body Part Character 4	Approach Character 5	Device Character 6	Qualifier Character 7
0 Coronary Artery, One Site 1 Coronary Artery, Two Sites 2 Coronary Artery, Three Sites 3 Coronary Artery, Four or More Sites 4 Coronary Vein 5 Atrial Septum 6 Atrium, Right 7 Atrium, Left 8 Conduction Mechanism 9 Chordae Tendineae D Papillary Muscle F Aortic Valve G Mitral Valve H Pulmonary Valve J Tricuspid Valve K Ventricle, Right L Ventricle, Left M Ventricular Septum N Pericardium P Pulmonary Trunk Q Pulmonary Artery, Right R Pulmonary Artery, Left S Pulmonary Vein, Right T Pulmonary Vein, Left V Superior Vena Cava W Thoracic Aorta	0 Open 3 Percutaneous 4 Percutaneous Endoscopic	Z No Device	Z No Qualifier

Ø Medical and Surgical
2 Heart and Great Vessels
F Fragmentation Breaking solid matter in a body part into pieces

Body Part Character 4	Approach Character 5	Device Character 6	Qualifier Character 7
N Pericardium NC	Ø Open 3 Percutaneous 4 Percutaneous Endoscopic X External	Z No Device	Z No Qualifier

Non-OR Ø2FNXZZ
NC Ø2FNXZZ

Ø Medical and Surgical
2 Heart and Great Vessels
H Insertion Putting in a nonbiological appliance that monitors, assists, performs, or prevents a physiological function but does not physically take the place of a body part

Body Part Character 4	Approach Character 5	Device Character 6	Qualifier Character 7
4 Coronary Vein ⊞ 6 Atrium, Right ⊞ 7 Atrium, Left ⊞ K Ventricle, Right ⊞ L Ventricle, Left ⊞	Ø Open 3 Percutaneous 4 Percutaneous Endoscopic	Ø Monitoring Device, Pressure Sensor 2 Monitoring Device 3 Infusion Device D Intraluminal Device J Cardiac Lead, Pacemaker K Cardiac Lead, Defibrillator M Cardiac Lead	Z No Qualifier
A Heart LC	Ø Open 3 Percutaneous 4 Percutaneous Endoscopic	Q Implantable Heart Assist System	Z No Qualifier
A Heart ⊞	Ø Open 3 Percutaneous 4 Percutaneous Endoscopic	R External Heart Assist System	S Biventricular Z No Qualifier
N Pericardium ⊞	Ø Open 3 Percutaneous 4 Percutaneous Endoscopic	Ø Monitoring Device, Pressure Sensor 2 Monitoring Device J Cardiac Lead, Pacemaker K Cardiac Lead, Defibrillator M Cardiac Lead	Z No Qualifier
P Pulmonary Trunk Q Pulmonary Artery, Right R Pulmonary Artery, Left S Pulmonary Vein, Right T Pulmonary Vein, Left V Superior Vena Cava W Thoracic Aorta	Ø Open 3 Percutaneous 4 Percutaneous Endoscopic	Ø Monitoring Device, Pressure Sensor 2 Monitoring Device 3 Infusion Device D Intraluminal Device	Z No Qualifier

DRG Non-OR Ø2H[4,6,7][Ø,4][J,M]Z
DRG Non-OR Ø2H[6,7]3J
DRG Non-OR Ø2H[K,L][Ø,3,4][J,M]Z
Non-OR Ø2H[6,K]33Z
Non-OR Ø2H[P,Q,R][Ø,3,4][Ø,2,3]Z
Non-OR Ø2H[S,T,V][Ø,3,4]3Z
Non-OR Ø2HW[Ø,3,4][Ø,3]Z
HAC Ø2H43[J,K,M]Z when reported with SDx K68.11 or T81.4XXA or T82.6XXA or T82.7XXA
HAC Ø2H[6,7]3[J,M]Z when reported with SDx K68.11 or T81.4XXA or T82.6XXA or T82.7XXA
HAC Ø2H[K,L]3JZ when reported with SDx K68.11 or T81.4XXA or T82.6XXA or T82.7XXA
HAC Ø2HN[Ø,3,4][J,M]Z when reported with SDx K68.11 or T81.4XXA or T82.6XXA or T82.7XXA
LC Ø2HA[Ø,3,4]QZ
AHA: 2Ø13, 3Q, 18

See Appendix I for Procedure Combinations
Combo-only Ø2H[4,6,7,K,L][Ø,4][J,M]Z
Combo-only Ø2H[K,L]3MZ
⊞ Ø2H[4,6,7,K,L]3[J,M]Z
⊞ Ø2H[4,6,7,L][Ø,3,4]KZ
⊞ Ø2HK[Ø,3,4][Ø,2,K]Z
⊞ Ø2HA[Ø,4]R[S,Z]
⊞ Ø2HA3RS
⊞ Ø2HN[Ø,3,4][J,K,M]Z

Ø Medical and Surgical
2 Heart and Great Vessels
J Inspection Visually and/or manually exploring a body part

Body Part Character 4	Approach Character 5	Device Character 6	Qualifier Character 7
A Heart Y Great Vessel	Ø Open 3 Percutaneous 4 Percutaneous Endoscopic	Z No Device	Z No Qualifier

Non-OR Ø2J[A,Y]3ZZ

0 Medical and Surgical
2 Heart and Great Vessels
K Map Locating the route of passage of electrical impulses and/or locating functional areas in a body part

Body Part Character 4	Approach Character 5	Device Character 6	Qualifier Character 7
8 Conduction Mechanism	0 Open 3 Percutaneous 4 Percutaneous Endoscopic	Z No Device	Z No Qualifier

DRG Non-OR 02K8[0,3,4]ZZ

0 Medical and Surgical
2 Heart and Great Vessels
L Occlusion Completely closing an orifice or the lumen of a tubular body part

Body Part Character 4	Approach Character 5	Device Character 6	Qualifier Character 7
7 Atrium, Left	0 Open 3 Percutaneous 4 Percutaneous Endoscopic	C Extraluminal Device D Intraluminal Device Z No Device	K Left Atrial Appendage
R Pulmonary Artery, Left ⊞	0 Open 3 Percutaneous 4 Percutaneous Endoscopic	C Extraluminal Device D Intraluminal Device Z No Device	T Ductus Arteriosus
S Pulmonary Vein, Right ⊞ T Pulmonary Vein, Left ⊞ V Superior Vena Cava	0 Open 3 Percutaneous 4 Percutaneous Endoscopic	C Extraluminal Device D Intraluminal Device Z No Device	Z No Qualifier

DRG Non-OR 02L7[0,3,4][C,D,Z]K

No Procedure Combinations Specified
⊞ 02LR0ZT
⊞ 02L[S,T]0ZZ

0 Medical and Surgical
2 Heart and Great Vessels
N Release Freeing a body part from an abnormal physical constraint

Body Part Character 4	Approach Character 5	Device Character 6	Qualifier Character 7
4 Coronary Vein 5 Atrial Septum 6 Atrium, Right 7 Atrium, Left 8 Conduction Mechanism 9 Chordae Tendineae D Papillary Muscle F Aortic Valve G Mitral Valve H Pulmonary Valve ⊞ J Tricuspid Valve K Ventricle, Right L Ventricle, Left M Ventricular Septum N Pericardium P Pulmonary Trunk Q Pulmonary Artery, Right R Pulmonary Artery, Left S Pulmonary Vein, Right T Pulmonary Vein, Left V Superior Vena Cava W Thoracic Aorta	0 Open 3 Percutaneous 4 Percutaneous Endoscopic	Z No Device	Z No Qualifier

No Procedure Combinations Specified
⊞ 02NH0ZZ

Ø Medical and Surgical
2 Heart and Great Vessels
P Removal Taking out or off a device from a body part

Body Part Character 4	Approach Character 5	Device Character 6	Qualifier Character 7
A Heart ⊞	Ø Open 3 Percutaneous 4 Percutaneous Endoscopic	2 Monitoring Device 3 Infusion Device 7 Autologous Tissue Substitute 8 Zooplastic Tissue C Extraluminal Device D Intraluminal Device J Synthetic Substitute K Nonautologous Tissue Substitute M Cardiac Lead Q Implantable Heart Assist System R External Heart Assist System	Z No Qualifier
A Heart ⊞	X External	2 Monitoring Device 3 Infusion Device D Intraluminal Device M Cardiac Lead	Z No Qualifier
Y Great Vessel	Ø Open 3 Percutaneous 4 Percutaneous Endoscopic	2 Monitoring Device 3 Infusion Device 7 Autologous Tissue Substitute 8 Zooplastic Tissue C Extraluminal Device D Intraluminal Device J Synthetic Substitute K Nonautologous Tissue Substitute	Z No Qualifier
Y Great Vessel	X External	2 Monitoring Device 3 Infusion Device D Intraluminal Device	Z No Qualifier

Non-OR Ø2PAX[2,3,D]Z
Non-OR Ø2PYX[2,3,D]Z
HAC Ø2PA[Ø,3,4,X]MZ when reported with SDx K68.11 or T81.4XXA or T82.6XXA or T82.7XXA

See Appendix I for Procedure Combinations
⊞ Ø2PA[Ø,3,4][M,R]Z
⊞ Ø2PAXMZ

Ø Medical and Surgical
2 Heart and Great Vessels
Q Repair Restoring, to the extent possible, a body part to its normal anatomic structure and function

Body Part Character 4	Approach Character 5	Device Character 6	Qualifier Character 7
Ø Coronary Artery, One Site 1 Coronary Artery, Two Sites 2 Coronary Artery, Three Sites 3 Coronary Artery, Four or More Sites 4 Coronary Vein 5 Atrial Septum 6 Atrium, Right 7 Atrium, Left 8 Conduction Mechanism 9 Chordae Tendineae A Heart B Heart, Right C Heart, Left D Papillary Muscle F Aortic Valve G Mitral Valve H Pulmonary Valve J Tricuspid Valve K Ventricle, Right L Ventricle, Left M Ventricular Septum N Pericardium P Pulmonary Trunk Q Pulmonary Artery, Right R Pulmonary Artery, Left S Pulmonary Vein, Right T Pulmonary Vein, Left V Superior Vena Cava W Thoracic Aorta	Ø Open 3 Percutaneous 4 Percutaneous Endoscopic	Z No Device	Z No Qualifier

0 Medical and Surgical
2 Heart and Great Vessels
R Replacement Putting in or on biological or synthetic material that physically takes the place and/or function of all or a portion of a body part

Body Part Character 4	Approach Character 5	Device Character 6	Qualifier Character 7
5 Atrial Septum 6 Atrium, Right 7 Atrium, Left 9 Chordae Tendineae D Papillary Muscle J Tricuspid Valve K Ventricle, Right LC NC L Ventricle, Left LC NC M Ventricular Septum ⊞ N Pericardium P Pulmonary Trunk ⊞ Q Pulmonary Artery, Right ⊞ R Pulmonary Artery, Left ⊞ S Pulmonary Vein, Right T Pulmonary Vein, Left V Superior Vena Cava W Thoracic Aorta	0 Open 4 Percutaneous Endoscopic	7 Autologous Tissue Substitute 8 Zooplastic Tissue J Synthetic Substitute K Nonautologous Tissue Substitute	Z No Qualifier
F Aortic Valve G Mitral Valve H Pulmonary Valve	0 Open 4 Percutaneous Endoscopic	7 Autologous Tissue Substitute 8 Zooplastic Tissue J Synthetic Substitute K Nonautologous Tissue Substitute	Z No Qualifier
F Aortic Valve G Mitral Valve H Pulmonary Valve	3 Percutaneous	7 Autologous Tissue Substitute 8 Zooplastic Tissue J Synthetic Substitute K Nonautologous Tissue Substitute	H Transapical Z No Qualifier

LC 02RK0JZ with 02RL0JZ when reported with diagnosis code Z00.6
NC 02RK0JZ except when reported with 02RL0JZ and diagnosis code Z00.6
AHA: 2014, 1Q, 10; 2013, 3Q, 26

No Procedure Combinations Specified
⊞ 02R[M,P]0JZ
⊞ 02R[Q,R]0[7,J]Z

0 Medical and Surgical
2 Heart and Great Vessels
S Reposition Moving to its normal location or other suitable location all or a portion of a body part

Body Part Character 4	Approach Character 5	Device Character 6	Qualifier Character 7
P Pulmonary Trunk ⊞ Q Pulmonary Artery, Right R Pulmonary Artery, Left S Pulmonary Vein, Right T Pulmonary Vein, Left V Superior Vena Cava W Thoracic Aorta ⊞	0 Open	Z No Device	Z No Qualifier

No Procedure Combinations Specified
⊞ 02S[P,W]0ZZ

0 Medical and Surgical
2 Heart and Great Vessels
T Resection Cutting out or off, without replacement, all of a body part

Body Part Character 4	Approach Character 5	Device Character 6	Qualifier Character 7
5 Atrial Septum 8 Conduction Mechanism 9 Chordae Tendineae D Papillary Muscle H Pulmonary Valve M Ventricular Septum N Pericardium	0 Open 3 Percutaneous 4 Percutaneous Endoscopic	Z No Device	Z No Qualifier

Ø Medical and Surgical
2 Heart and Great Vessels
U Supplement Putting in or on biological or synthetic material that physically reinforces and/or augments the function of a portion of a body part

Body Part Character 4	Approach Character 5	Device Character 6	Qualifier Character 7
5 Atrial Septum **6** Atrium, Right **7** Atrium, Left ⊞ **9** Chordae Tendineae **A** Heart **D** Papillary Muscle **F** Aortic Valve **G** Mitral Valve **H** Pulmonary Valve **J** Tricuspid Valve **K** Ventricle, Right **L** Ventricle, Left **M** Ventricular Septum **N** Pericardium **P** Pulmonary Trunk **Q** Pulmonary Artery, Right **R** Pulmonary Artery, Left **S** Pulmonary Vein, Right **T** Pulmonary Vein, Left **V** Superior Vena Cava **W** Thoracic Aorta	**Ø** Open **3** Percutaneous **4** Percutaneous Endoscopic	**7** Autologous Tissue Substitute **8** Zooplastic Tissue **J** Synthetic Substitute **K** Nonautologous Tissue Substitute	**Z** No Qualifier

DRG Non-OR Ø2U7[3,4]JZ

No Procedure Combinations Specified
⊞ Ø2U7ØJZ

Ø Medical and Surgical
2 Heart and Great Vessels
V Restriction Partially closing an orifice or the lumen of a tubular body part

Body Part Character 4	Approach Character 5	Device Character 6	Qualifier Character 7
A Heart	**Ø** Open **3** Percutaneous **4** Percutaneous Endoscopic	**C** Extraluminal Device **Z** No Device	**Z** No Qualifier
P Pulmonary Trunk **Q** Pulmonary Artery, Right **S** Pulmonary Vein, Right **T** Pulmonary Vein, Left **V** Superior Vena Cava **W** Thoracic Aorta	**Ø** Open **3** Percutaneous **4** Percutaneous Endoscopic	**C** Extraluminal Device **D** Intraluminal Device **Z** No Device	**Z** No Qualifier
R Pulmonary Artery, Left ⊞	**Ø** Open **3** Percutaneous **4** Percutaneous Endoscopic	**C** Extraluminal Device **D** Intraluminal Device **Z** No Device	**T** Ductus Arteriosus **Z** No Qualifier

No Procedure Combinations Specified
⊞ Ø2VRØZT

0 Medical and Surgical
2 Heart and Great Vessels
W Revision Correcting, to the extent possible, a portion of a malfunctioning device or the position of a displaced device

Body Part Character 4	Approach Character 5	Device Character 6	Qualifier Character 7
5 Atrial Septum **M** Ventricular Septum	**0** Open **4** Percutaneous Endoscopic	**J** Synthetic Substitute	**Z** No Qualifier
A Heart ⊞ NC	**0** Open **3** Percutaneous **4** Percutaneous Endoscopic **X** External	**2** Monitoring Device **3** Infusion Device **7** Autologous Tissue Substitute **8** Zooplastic Tissue **C** Extraluminal Device **D** Intraluminal Device **J** Synthetic Substitute **K** Nonautologous Tissue Substitute **M** Cardiac Lead **Q** Implantable Heart Assist System **R** External Heart Assist System	**Z** No Qualifier
F Aortic Valve **G** Mitral Valve **H** Pulmonary Valve **J** Tricuspid Valve	**0** Open **4** Percutaneous Endoscopic	**7** Autologous Tissue Substitute **8** Zooplastic Tissue **J** Synthetic Substitute **K** Nonautologous Tissue Substitute	**Z** No Qualifier
Y Great Vessel	**0** Open **3** Percutaneous **4** Percutaneous Endoscopic **X** External	**2** Monitoring Device **3** Infusion Device **7** Autologous Tissue Substitute **8** Zooplastic Tissue **C** Extraluminal Device **D** Intraluminal Device **J** Synthetic Substitute **K** Nonautologous Tissue Substitute	**Z** No Qualifier

Non-OR 02WAX[2,3,7,8,C,D,J,K,M,Q,R]Z
Non-OR 02WYX[2,3,7,8,C,D,J,K]Z
HAC 02WA[0,3,4]MZ when reported with SDx K68.11 or T81.4XXA or T82.6XXA or T82.7XXA
NC 02WA0[J,Q]Z
NC 02WA[3,4]QZ

See Appendix I for Procedure Combinations
⊞ 02WA[0,3,4][Q,R]Z

0 Medical and Surgical
2 Heart and Great Vessels
Y Transplantation Putting in or on all or a portion of a living body part taken from another individual or animal to physically take the place and/or function of all or a portion of a similar body part

Body Part Character 4	Approach Character 5	Device Character 6	Qualifier Character 7
A Heart LC	**0** Open	**Z** No Device	**0** Allogeneic **1** Syngeneic **2** Zooplastic

LC 02YA0Z[0,1,2]
AHA: 2013, 3Q, 18

Upper Arteries Ø31–Ø3W

Ø Medical and Surgical
3 Upper Arteries
1 Bypass Altering the route of passage of the contents of a tubular body part

Body Part Character 4	Approach Character 5	Device Character 6	Qualifier Character 7
2 Innominate Artery 5 Axillary Artery, Right 6 Axillary Artery, Left	Ø Open	9 Autologous Venous Tissue A Autologous Arterial Tissue J Synthetic Substitute K Nonautologous Tissue Substitute Z No Device	Ø Upper Arm Artery, Right 1 Upper Arm Artery, Left 2 Upper Arm Artery, Bilateral 3 Lower Arm Artery, Right 4 Lower Arm Artery, Left 5 Lower Arm Artery, Bilateral 6 Upper Leg Artery, Right 7 Upper Leg Artery, Left 8 Upper Leg Artery, Bilateral 9 Lower Leg Artery, Right B Lower Leg Artery, Left C Lower Leg Artery, Bilateral D Upper Arm Vein F Lower Arm Vein J Extracranial Artery, Right K Extracranial Artery, Left
3 Subclavian Artery, Right 4 Subclavian Artery, Left	Ø Open	9 Autologous Venous Tissue A Autologous Arterial Tissue J Synthetic Substitute K Nonautologous Tissue Substitute Z No Device	Ø Upper Arm Artery, Right 1 Upper Arm Artery, Left 2 Upper Arm Artery, Bilateral 3 Lower Arm Artery, Right 4 Lower Arm Artery, Left 5 Lower Arm Artery, Bilateral 6 Upper Leg Artery, Right 7 Upper Leg Artery, Left 8 Upper Leg Artery, Bilateral 9 Lower Leg Artery, Right B Lower Leg Artery, Left C Lower Leg Artery, Bilateral D Upper Arm Vein F Lower Arm Vein J Extracranial Artery, Right K Extracranial Artery, Left M Pulmonary Artery, Right N Pulmonary Artery, Left
7 Brachial Artery, Right	Ø Open	9 Autologous Venous Tissue A Autologous Arterial Tissue J Synthetic Substitute K Nonautologous Tissue Substitute Z No Device	Ø Upper Arm Artery, Right 3 Lower Arm Artery, Right D Upper Arm Vein F Lower Arm Vein
8 Brachial Artery, Left	Ø Open	9 Autologous Venous Tissue A Autologous Arterial Tissue J Synthetic Substitute K Nonautologous Tissue Substitute Z No Device	1 Upper Arm Artery, Left 4 Lower Arm Artery, Left D Upper Arm Vein F Lower Arm Vein
9 Ulnar Artery, Right B Radial Artery, Right ⊞	Ø Open	9 Autologous Venous Tissue A Autologous Arterial Tissue J Synthetic Substitute K Nonautologous Tissue Substitute Z No Device	3 Lower Arm Artery, Right F Lower Arm Vein
A Ulnar Artery, Left C Radial Artery, Left ⊞	Ø Open	9 Autologous Venous Tissue A Autologous Arterial Tissue J Synthetic Substitute K Nonautologous Tissue Substitute Z No Device	4 Lower Arm Artery, Left F Lower Arm Vein
G Intracranial Artery S Temporal Artery, Right NC T Temporal Artery, Left NC	Ø Open	9 Autologous Venous Tissue A Autologous Arterial Tissue J Synthetic Substitute K Nonautologous Tissue Substitute Z No Device	G Intracranial Artery

Ø31 Continued on next page

NC Ø31SØ[9,A,J,K,Z]G
NC Ø31TØ[9,A,J,K,Z]G
AHA: 2Ø13, 4Q, 125; 2Ø13, 1Q, 27

No Procedure Combinations Specified
⊞ Ø31[B,C]ØJF

031 Continued

0 Medical and Surgical
3 Upper Arteries
1 Bypass Altering the route of passage of the contents of a tubular body part

Body Part Character 4	Approach Character 5	Device Character 6	Qualifier Character 7
H Common Carotid Artery, Right NC	0 Open	9 Autologous Venous Tissue A Autologous Arterial Tissue J Synthetic Substitute K Nonautologous Tissue Substitute Z No Device	G Intracranial Artery J Extracranial Artery, Right
J Common Carotid Artery, Left NC	0 Open	9 Autologous Venous Tissue A Autologous Arterial Tissue J Synthetic Substitute K Nonautologous Tissue Substitute Z No Device	G Intracranial Artery K Extracranial Artery, Left
K Internal Carotid Artery, Right M External Carotid Artery, Right	0 Open	9 Autologous Venous Tissue A Autologous Arterial Tissue J Synthetic Substitute K Nonautologous Tissue Substitute Z No Device	J Extracranial Artery, Right
L Internal Carotid Artery, Left N External Carotid Artery, Left	0 Open	9 Autologous Venous Tissue A Autologous Arterial Tissue J Synthetic Substitute K Nonautologous Tissue Substitute Z No Device	K Extracranial Artery, Left

NC 031H0[9,A,J,K,Z]G
NC 031J0[9,A,J,K,Z]G

0 Medical and Surgical
3 Upper Arteries
5 Destruction Physical eradication of all or a portion of a body part by the direct use of energy, force, or a destructive agent

Body Part Character 4	Approach Character 5	Device Character 6	Qualifier Character 7
0 Internal Mammary Artery, Right 1 Internal Mammary Artery, Left 2 Innominate Artery 3 Subclavian Artery, Right 4 Subclavian Artery, Left 5 Axillary Artery, Right 6 Axillary Artery, Left 7 Brachial Artery, Right 8 Brachial Artery, Left 9 Ulnar Artery, Right A Ulnar Artery, Left B Radial Artery, Right C Radial Artery, Left D Hand Artery, Right F Hand Artery, Left G Intracranial Artery H Common Carotid Artery, Right J Common Carotid Artery, Left K Internal Carotid Artery, Right L Internal Carotid Artery, Left M External Carotid Artery, Right N External Carotid Artery, Left P Vertebral Artery, Right Q Vertebral Artery, Left R Face Artery S Temporal Artery, Right T Temporal Artery, Left U Thyroid Artery, Right V Thyroid Artery, Left Y Upper Artery	0 Open 3 Percutaneous 4 Percutaneous Endoscopic	Z No Device	Z No Qualifier

Ø Medical and Surgical
3 Upper Arteries
7 Dilation Expanding an orifice or the lumen of a tubular body part

Body Part Character 4	Approach Character 5	Device Character 6	Qualifier Character 7
Ø Internal Mammary Artery, Right **1** Internal Mammary Artery, Left **2** Innominate Artery **3** Subclavian Artery, Right **4** Subclavian Artery, Left **5** Axillary Artery, Right **6** Axillary Artery, Left **7** Brachial Artery, Right **8** Brachial Artery, Left **9** Ulnar Artery, Right **A** Ulnar Artery, Left **B** Radial Artery, Right **C** Radial Artery, Left **D** Hand Artery, Right **F** Hand Artery, Left **G** Intracranial Artery NC **H** Common Carotid Artery, Right **J** Common Carotid Artery, Left **K** Internal Carotid Artery, Right **L** Internal Carotid Artery, Left **M** External Carotid Artery, Right **N** External Carotid Artery, Left **P** Vertebral Artery, Right **Q** Vertebral Artery, Left **R** Face Artery **S** Temporal Artery, Right **T** Temporal Artery, Left **U** Thyroid Artery, Right **V** Thyroid Artery, Left **Y** Upper Artery	**Ø** Open **3** Percutaneous **4** Percutaneous Endoscopic	**4** Drug-eluting Intraluminal Device **D** Intraluminal Device **Z** No Device	**Z** No Qualifier

NC Ø37G[3,4]ZZ Noncovered without stent placement

0 Medical and Surgical
3 Upper Arteries
9 Drainage Taking or letting out fluids and/or gases from a body part

Body Part Character 4	Approach Character 5	Device Character 6	Qualifier Character 7
0 Internal Mammary Artery, Right 1 Internal Mammary Artery, Left 2 Innominate Artery 3 Subclavian Artery, Right 4 Subclavian Artery, Left 5 Axillary Artery, Right 6 Axillary Artery, Left 7 Brachial Artery, Right 8 Brachial Artery, Left 9 Ulnar Artery, Right A Ulnar Artery, Left B Radial Artery, Right C Radial Artery, Left D Hand Artery, Right F Hand Artery, Left G Intracranial Artery H Common Carotid Artery, Right J Common Carotid Artery, Left K Internal Carotid Artery, Right L Internal Carotid Artery, Left M External Carotid Artery, Right N External Carotid Artery, Left P Vertebral Artery, Right Q Vertebral Artery, Left R Face Artery S Temporal Artery, Right T Temporal Artery, Left U Thyroid Artery, Right V Thyroid Artery, Left Y Upper Artery	0 Open 3 Percutaneous 4 Percutaneous Endoscopic	0 Drainage Device	Z No Qualifier
0 Internal Mammary Artery, Right 1 Internal Mammary Artery, Left 2 Innominate Artery 3 Subclavian Artery, Right 4 Subclavian Artery, Left 5 Axillary Artery, Right 6 Axillary Artery, Left 7 Brachial Artery, Right 8 Brachial Artery, Left 9 Ulnar Artery, Right A Ulnar Artery, Left B Radial Artery, Right C Radial Artery, Left D Hand Artery, Right F Hand Artery, Left G Intracranial Artery H Common Carotid Artery, Right J Common Carotid Artery, Left K Internal Carotid Artery, Right L Internal Carotid Artery, Left M External Carotid Artery, Right N External Carotid Artery, Left P Vertebral Artery, Right Q Vertebral Artery, Left R Face Artery S Temporal Artery, Right T Temporal Artery, Left U Thyroid Artery, Right V Thyroid Artery, Left Y Upper Artery	0 Open 3 Percutaneous 4 Percutaneous Endoscopic	Z No Device	X Diagnostic Z No Qualifier

Non-OR 039[0,1,2,3,4,5,6,7,8,9,A,B,C,D,F,G,H,J,K,L,M,N,P,Q,R,S,T,U,V,Y][0,3,4]0Z
Non-OR 039[0,1,2,3,4,5,6,7,8,9,A,B,C,D,F,G,H,J,K,L,M,N,P,Q,R,S,T,U,V,Y][0,3,4]ZZ

Ø Medical and Surgical
3 Upper Arteries
B Excision Cutting out or off, without replacement, a portion of a body part

Body Part Character 4	Approach Character 5	Device Character 6	Qualifier Character 7
Ø Internal Mammary Artery, Right **1** Internal Mammary Artery, Left **2** Innominate Artery **3** Subclavian Artery, Right **4** Subclavian Artery, Left **5** Axillary Artery, Right **6** Axillary Artery, Left **7** Brachial Artery, Right **8** Brachial Artery, Left **9** Ulnar Artery, Right **A** Ulnar Artery, Left **B** Radial Artery, Right **C** Radial Artery, Left **D** Hand Artery, Right **F** Hand Artery, Left **G** Intracranial Artery **H** Common Carotid Artery, Right **J** Common Carotid Artery, Left **K** Internal Carotid Artery, Right **L** Internal Carotid Artery, Left **M** External Carotid Artery, Right **N** External Carotid Artery, Left **P** Vertebral Artery, Right **Q** Vertebral Artery, Left **R** Face Artery **S** Temporal Artery, Right **T** Temporal Artery, Left **U** Thyroid Artery, Right **V** Thyroid Artery, Left **Y** Upper Artery	**Ø** Open **3** Percutaneous **4** Percutaneous Endoscopic	**Z** No Device	**X** Diagnostic **Z** No Qualifier

Ø Medical and Surgical
3 Upper Arteries
C Extirpation Taking or cutting out solid matter from a body part

Body Part Character 4	Approach Character 5	Device Character 6	Qualifier Character 7
Ø Internal Mammary Artery, Right **1** Internal Mammary Artery, Left **2** Innominate Artery **3** Subclavian Artery, Right **4** Subclavian Artery, Left **5** Axillary Artery, Right **6** Axillary Artery, Left **7** Brachial Artery, Right **8** Brachial Artery, Left **9** Ulnar Artery, Right **A** Ulnar Artery, Left **B** Radial Artery, Right **C** Radial Artery, Left **D** Hand Artery, Right **F** Hand Artery, Left **G** Intracranial Artery NC **H** Common Carotid Artery, Right **J** Common Carotid Artery, Left **K** Internal Carotid Artery, Right **L** Internal Carotid Artery, Left **M** External Carotid Artery, Right **N** External Carotid Artery, Left **P** Vertebral Artery, Right **Q** Vertebral Artery, Left **R** Face Artery **S** Temporal Artery, Right **T** Temporal Artery, Left **U** Thyroid Artery, Right **V** Thyroid Artery, Left **Y** Upper Artery	**Ø** Open **3** Percutaneous **4** Percutaneous Endoscopic	**Z** No Device	**Z** No Qualifier

NC Ø3CG[3,4]ZZ

Ø Medical and Surgical
3 Upper Arteries
H Insertion Putting in a nonbiological appliance that monitors, assists, performs, or prevents a physiological function but does not physically take the place of a body part

Body Part Character 4	Approach Character 5	Device Character 6	Qualifier Character 7
Ø Internal Mammary Artery, Right **1** Internal Mammary Artery, Left **2** Innominate Artery **3** Subclavian Artery, Right **4** Subclavian Artery, Left **5** Axillary Artery, Right **6** Axillary Artery, Left **7** Brachial Artery, Right **8** Brachial Artery, Left **9** Ulnar Artery, Right **A** Ulnar Artery, Left **B** Radial Artery, Right **C** Radial Artery, Left **D** Hand Artery, Right **F** Hand Artery, Left **G** Intracranial Artery **H** Common Carotid Artery, Right **J** Common Carotid Artery, Left **M** External Carotid Artery, Right **N** External Carotid Artery, Left **P** Vertebral Artery, Right **Q** Vertebral Artery, Left **R** Face Artery **S** Temporal Artery, Right **T** Temporal Artery, Left **U** Thyroid Artery, Right **V** Thyroid Artery, Left	**Ø** Open **3** Percutaneous **4** Percutaneous Endoscopic	**3** Infusion Device **D** Intraluminal Device	**Z** No Qualifier
K Internal Carotid Artery, Right ⊞ **L** Internal Carotid Artery, Left ⊞	**Ø** Open **3** Percutaneous **4** Percutaneous Endoscope	**3** Infusion Device **D** Intraluminal Device **M** Stimulator Lead	**Z** No Qualifier
Y Upper Artery	**Ø** Open **3** Percutaneous **4** Percutaneous Endoscopic	**2** Monitoring Device **3** Infusion Device **D** Intraluminal Device	**Z** No Qualifier

Non-OR Ø3H[Ø,1,2,3,4,5,6,7,8,9,A,B,C,D,F,G,H,J,M,N,P,Q,R,S,T,U,V][Ø,3,4]3Z
Non-OR Ø3H[K,L][Ø,3,4]3Z
Non-OR Ø3HY[Ø,3,4]3Z

No Procedure Combinations Specified
⊞ Ø3H[K,L][Ø,3,4]MZ

Ø Medical and Surgical
3 Upper Arteries
J Inspection Visually and/or manually exploring a body part

Body Part Character 4	Approach Character 5	Device Character 6	Qualifier Character 7
Y Upper Artery	**Ø** Open **3** Percutaneous **4** Percutaneous Endoscopic **X** External	**Z** No Device	**Z** No Qualifier

Non-OR Ø3JY[4,X]ZZ

Ø Medical and Surgical
3 Upper Arteries
L Occlusion Completely closing an orifice or the lumen of a tubular body part

Body Part Character 4	Approach Character 5	Device Character 6	Qualifier Character 7
Ø Internal Mammary Artery, Right **1** Internal Mammary Artery, Left **2** Innominate Artery **3** Subclavian Artery, Right **4** Subclavian Artery, Left **5** Axillary Artery, Right **6** Axillary Artery, Left **7** Brachial Artery, Right **8** Brachial Artery, Left **9** Ulnar Artery, Right **A** Ulnar Artery, Left **B** Radial Artery, Right **C** Radial Artery, Left **D** Hand Artery, Right **F** Hand Artery, Left **R** Face Artery **S** Temporal Artery, Right **T** Temporal Artery, Left **U** Thyroid Artery, Right **V** Thyroid Artery, Left **Y** Upper Artery	**Ø** Open **3** Percutaneous **4** Percutaneous Endoscopic	**C** Extraluminal Device **D** Intraluminal Device **Z** No Device	**Z** No Qualifier
G Intracranial Artery **H** Common Carotid Artery, Right **J** Common Carotid Artery, Left **K** Internal Carotid Artery, Right **L** Internal Carotid Artery, Left **M** External Carotid Artery, Right **N** External Carotid Artery, Left **P** Vertebral Artery, Right **Q** Vertebral Artery, Left	**Ø** Open **3** Percutaneous **4** Percutaneous Endoscopic	**B** Bioactive Intraluminal Device **C** Extraluminal Device **D** Intraluminal Device **Z** No Device	**Z** No Qualifier

Ø Medical and Surgical
3 Upper Arteries
N Release Freeing a body part from an abnormal physical constraint

Body Part Character 4	Approach Character 5	Device Character 6	Qualifier Character 7
Ø Internal Mammary Artery, Right **1** Internal Mammary Artery, Left **2** Innominate Artery **3** Subclavian Artery, Right **4** Subclavian Artery, Left **5** Axillary Artery, Right **6** Axillary Artery, Left **7** Brachial Artery, Right **8** Brachial Artery, Left **9** Ulnar Artery, Right **A** Ulnar Artery, Left **B** Radial Artery, Right **C** Radial Artery, Left **D** Hand Artery, Right **F** Hand Artery, Left **G** Intracranial Artery **H** Common Carotid Artery, Right **J** Common Carotid Artery, Left **K** Internal Carotid Artery, Right **L** Internal Carotid Artery, Left **M** External Carotid Artery, Right **N** External Carotid Artery, Left **P** Vertebral Artery, Right **Q** Vertebral Artery, Left **R** Face Artery **S** Temporal Artery, Right **T** Temporal Artery, Left **U** Thyroid Artery, Right **V** Thyroid Artery, Left **Y** Upper Artery	**Ø** Open **3** Percutaneous **4** Percutaneous Endoscopic	**Z** No Device	**Z** No Qualifier

0 Medical and Surgical
3 Upper Arteries
P Removal Taking out or off a device from a body part

Body Part Character 4	Approach Character 5	Device Character 6	Qualifier Character 7
Y Upper Artery ⊞	0 Open 3 Percutaneous 4 Percutaneous Endoscopic	0 Drainage Device 2 Monitoring Device 3 Infusion Device 7 Autologous Tissue Substitute C Extraluminal Device D Intraluminal Device J Synthetic Substitute K Nonautologous Tissue Substitute M Stimulator Lead	Z No Qualifier
Y Upper Artery	X External	0 Drainage Device 2 Monitoring Device 3 Infusion Device D Intraluminal Device M Stimulator Lead	Z No Qualifier

Non-OR 03PYX[0,2,3,D,M]Z

No Procedure Combinations Specified
⊞ 03PY[0,3,4][J,M]Z

0 Medical and Surgical
3 Upper Arteries
Q Repair Restoring, to the extent possible, a body part to its normal anatomic structure and function

Body Part Character 4	Approach Character 5	Device Character 6	Qualifier Character 7
0 Internal Mammary Artery, Right 1 Internal Mammary Artery, Left 2 Innominate Artery 3 Subclavian Artery, Right 4 Subclavian Artery, Left 5 Axillary Artery, Right 6 Axillary Artery, Left 7 Brachial Artery, Right 8 Brachial Artery, Left 9 Ulnar Artery, Right A Ulnar Artery, Left B Radial Artery, Right C Radial Artery, Left D Hand Artery, Right F Hand Artery, Left G Intracranial Artery H Common Carotid Artery, Right J Common Carotid Artery, Left K Internal Carotid Artery, Right L Internal Carotid Artery, Left M External Carotid Artery, Right N External Carotid Artery, Left P Vertebral Artery, Right Q Vertebral Artery, Left R Face Artery S Temporal Artery, Right T Temporal Artery, Left U Thyroid Artery, Right V Thyroid Artery, Left Y Upper Artery	0 Open 3 Percutaneous 4 Percutaneous Endoscopic	Z No Device	Z No Qualifier

Ø Medical and Surgical
3 Upper Arteries
R Replacement Putting in or on biological or synthetic material that physically takes the place and/or function of all or a portion of a body part

Body Part Character 4	Approach Character 5	Device Character 6	Qualifier Character 7
Ø Internal Mammary Artery, Right **1** Internal Mammary Artery, Left **2** Innominate Artery **3** Subclavian Artery, Right **4** Subclavian Artery, Left **5** Axillary Artery, Right **6** Axillary Artery, Left **7** Brachial Artery, Right **8** Brachial Artery, Left **9** Ulnar Artery, Right **A** Ulnar Artery, Left **B** Radial Artery, Right **C** Radial Artery, Left **D** Hand Artery, Right **F** Hand Artery, Left **G** Intracranial Artery **H** Common Carotid Artery, Right **J** Common Carotid Artery, Left **K** Internal Carotid Artery, Right **L** Internal Carotid Artery, Left **M** External Carotid Artery, Right **N** External Carotid Artery, Left **P** Vertebral Artery, Right **Q** Vertebral Artery, Left **R** Face Artery **S** Temporal Artery, Right **T** Temporal Artery, Left **U** Thyroid Artery, Right **V** Thyroid Artery, Left **Y** Upper Artery	**Ø** Open **4** Percutaneous Endoscopic	**7** Autologous Tissue Substitute **J** Synthetic Substitute **K** Nonautologous Tissue Substitute	**Z** No Qualifier

Ø Medical and Surgical
3 Upper Arteries
S Reposition Moving to its normal location or other suitable location all or a portion of a body part

Body Part Character 4	Approach Character 5	Device Character 6	Qualifier Character 7
Ø Internal Mammary Artery, Right **1** Internal Mammary Artery, Left **2** Innominate Artery **3** Subclavian Artery, Right **4** Subclavian Artery, Left **5** Axillary Artery, Right **6** Axillary Artery, Left **7** Brachial Artery, Right **8** Brachial Artery, Left **9** Ulnar Artery, Right **A** Ulnar Artery, Left **B** Radial Artery, Right **C** Radial Artery, Left **D** Hand Artery, Right **F** Hand Artery, Left **G** Intracranial Artery **H** Common Carotid Artery, Right **J** Common Carotid Artery, Left **K** Internal Carotid Artery, Right **L** Internal Carotid Artery, Left **M** External Carotid Artery, Right **N** External Carotid Artery, Left **P** Vertebral Artery, Right **Q** Vertebral Artery, Left **R** Face Artery **S** Temporal Artery, Right **T** Temporal Artery, Left **U** Thyroid Artery, Right **V** Thyroid Artery, Left **Y** Upper Artery	**Ø** Open **3** Percutaneous **4** Percutaneous Endoscopic	**Z** No Device	**Z** No Qualifier

0 Medical and Surgical
3 Upper Arteries
U Supplement Putting in or on biological or synthetic material that physically reinforces and/or augments the function of a portion of a body part

Body Part Character 4	Approach Character 5	Device Character 6	Qualifier Character 7
0 Internal Mammary Artery, Right **1** Internal Mammary Artery, Left **2** Innominate Artery **3** Subclavian Artery, Right **4** Subclavian Artery, Left **5** Axillary Artery, Right **6** Axillary Artery, Left **7** Brachial Artery, Right **8** Brachial Artery, Left **9** Ulnar Artery, Right **A** Ulnar Artery, Left **B** Radial Artery, Right **C** Radial Artery, Left **D** Hand Artery, Right **F** Hand Artery, Left **G** Intracranial Artery **H** Common Carotid Artery, Right **J** Common Carotid Artery, Left **K** Internal Carotid Artery, Right **L** Internal Carotid Artery, Left **M** External Carotid Artery, Right **N** External Carotid Artery, Left **P** Vertebral Artery, Right **Q** Vertebral Artery, Left **R** Face Artery **S** Temporal Artery, Right **T** Temporal Artery, Left **U** Thyroid Artery, Right **V** Thyroid Artery, Left **Y** Upper Artery	**0** Open **3** Percutaneous **4** Percutaneous Endoscopic	**7** Autologous Tissue Substitute **J** Synthetic Substitute **K** Nonautologous Tissue Substitute	**Z** No Qualifier

0 Medical and Surgical
3 Upper Arteries
V Restriction Partially closing an orifice or the lumen of a tubular body part

Body Part Character 4	Approach Character 5	Device Character 6	Qualifier Character 7
0 Internal Mammary Artery, Right **1** Internal Mammary Artery, Left **2** Innominate Artery **3** Subclavian Artery, Right **4** Subclavian Artery, Left **5** Axillary Artery, Right **6** Axillary Artery, Left **7** Brachial Artery, Right **8** Brachial Artery, Left **9** Ulnar Artery, Right **A** Ulnar Artery, Left **B** Radial Artery, Right **C** Radial Artery, Left **D** Hand Artery, Right **F** Hand Artery, Left **R** Face Artery **S** Temporal Artery, Right **T** Temporal Artery, Left **U** Thyroid Artery, Right **V** Thyroid Artery, Left **Y** Upper Artery	**0** Open **3** Percutaneous **4** Percutaneous Endoscopic	**C** Extraluminal Device **D** Intraluminal Device **Z** No Device	**Z** No Qualifier
G Intracranial Artery **H** Common Carotid Artery, Right **J** Common Carotid Artery, Left **K** Internal Carotid Artery, Right **L** Internal Carotid Artery, Left **M** External Carotid Artery, Right **N** External Carotid Artery, Left **P** Vertebral Artery, Right **Q** Vertebral Artery, Left	**0** Open **3** Percutaneous **4** Percutaneous Endoscopic	**B** Bioactive Intraluminal Device **C** Extraluminal Device **D** Intraluminal Device **Z** No Device	**Z** No Qualifier

Ø Medical and Surgical
3 Upper Arteries
W Revision Correcting, to the extent possible, a portion of a malfunctioning device or the position of a displaced device

Body Part Character 4	Approach Character 5	Device Character 6	Qualifier Character 7
Y Upper Artery	**Ø** Open **3** Percutaneous **4** Percutaneous Endoscopic **X** External	**Ø** Drainage Device **2** Monitoring Device **3** Infusion Device **7** Autologous Tissue Substitute **C** Extraluminal Device **D** Intraluminal Device **J** Synthetic Substitute **K** Nonautologous Tissue Substitute **M** Stimulator Lead	**Z** No Qualifier

Non-OR Ø3WYX[Ø,2,3,7,C,D,J,K,M]Z

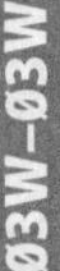

Lower Arteries Ø41–Ø4W

Ø Medical and Surgical
4 Lower Arteries
1 Bypass Altering the route of passage of the contents of a tubular body part

Body Part Character 4	Approach Character 5	Device Character 6	Qualifier Character 7
Ø Abdominal Aorta **C** Common Iliac Artery, Right **D** Common Iliac Artery, Left	**Ø** Open **4** Percutaneous Endoscopic	**9** Autologous Venous Tissue **A** Autologous Arterial Tissue **J** Synthetic Substitute **K** Nonautologous Tissue Substitute **Z** No Device	**Ø** Abdominal Aorta **1** Celiac Artery **2** Mesenteric Artery **3** Renal Artery, Right **4** Renal Artery, Left **5** Renal Artery, Bilateral **6** Common Iliac Artery, Right **7** Common Iliac Artery, Left **8** Common Iliac Arteries, Bilateral **9** Internal Iliac Artery, Right **B** Internal Iliac Artery, Left **C** Internal Iliac Arteries, Bilateral **D** External Iliac Artery, Right **F** External Iliac Artery, Left **G** External Iliac Arteries, Bilateral **H** Femoral Artery, Right **J** Femoral Artery, Left **K** Femoral Arteries, Bilateral **Q** Lower Extremity Artery **R** Lower Artery
4 Splenic Artery	**Ø** Open **4** Percutaneous Endoscopic	**9** Autologous Venous Tissue **A** Autologous Arterial Tissue **J** Synthetic Substitute **K** Nonautologous Tissue Substitute **Z** No Device	**3** Renal Artery, Right **4** Renal Artery, Left **5** Renal Artery, Bilateral
E Internal Iliac Artery, Right **F** Internal Iliac Artery, Left **H** External Iliac Artery, Right **J** External Iliac Artery, Left	**Ø** Open **4** Percutaneous Endoscopic	**9** Autologous Venous Tissue **A** Autologous Arterial Tissue **J** Synthetic Substitute **K** Nonautologous Tissue Substitute **Z** No Device	**9** Internal Iliac Artery, Right **B** Internal Iliac Artery, Left **C** Internal Iliac Arteries, Bilateral **D** External Iliac Artery, Right **F** External Iliac Artery, Left **G** External Iliac Arteries, Bilateral **H** Femoral Artery, Right **J** Femoral Artery, Left **K** Femoral Arteries, Bilateral **P** Foot Artery **Q** Lower Extremity Artery
K Femoral Artery, Right **L** Femoral Artery, Left	**Ø** Open **4** Percutaneous Endoscopic	**9** Autologous Venous Tissue **A** Autologous Arterial Tissue **J** Synthetic Substitute **K** Nonautologous Tissue Substitute **Z** No Device	**H** Femoral Artery, Right **J** Femoral Artery, Left **K** Femoral Arteries, Bilateral **L** Popliteal Artery **M** Peroneal Artery **N** Posterior Tibial Artery **P** Foot Artery **Q** Lower Extremity Artery **S** Lower Extremity Vein
M Popliteal Artery, Right **N** Popliteal Artery, Left	**Ø** Open **4** Percutaneous Endoscopic	**9** Autologous Venous Tissue **A** Autologous Arterial Tissue **J** Synthetic Substitute **K** Nonautologous Tissue Substitute **Z** No Device	**L** Popliteal Artery **M** Peroneal Artery **P** Foot Artery **Q** Lower Extremity Artery **S** Lower Extremity Vein

Ø Medical and Surgical
4 Lower Arteries
5 Destruction Physical eradication of all or a portion of a body part by the direct use of energy, force, or a destructive agent

Body Part Character 4	Approach Character 5	Device Character 6	Qualifier Character 7
Ø Abdominal Aorta	**Ø** Open	**Z** No Device	**Z** No Qualifier
1 Celiac Artery	**3** Percutaneous		
2 Gastric Artery	**4** Percutaneous Endoscopic		
3 Hepatic Artery			
4 Splenic Artery			
5 Superior Mesenteric Artery			
6 Colic Artery, Right			
7 Colic Artery, Left			
8 Colic Artery, Middle			
9 Renal Artery, Right			
A Renal Artery, Left			
B Inferior Mesenteric Artery			
C Common Iliac Artery, Right			
D Common Iliac Artery, Left			
E Internal Iliac Artery, Right			
F Internal Iliac Artery, Left			
H External Iliac Artery, Right			
J External Iliac Artery, Left			
K Femoral Artery, Right			
L Femoral Artery, Left			
M Popliteal Artery, Right			
N Popliteal Artery, Left			
P Anterior Tibial Artery, Right			
Q Anterior Tibial Artery, Left			
R Posterior Tibial Artery, Right			
S Posterior Tibial Artery, Left			
T Peroneal Artery, Right			
U Peroneal Artery, Left			
V Foot Artery, Right			
W Foot Artery, Left			
Y Lower Artery			

Ø Medical and Surgical
4 Lower Arteries
7 Dilation Expanding an orifice or the lumen of a tubular body part

Body Part Character 4	Approach Character 5	Device Character 6	Qualifier Character 7
Ø Abdominal Aorta	**Ø** Open	**4** Drug-eluting Intraluminal Device	**Z** No Qualifier
1 Celiac Artery	**3** Percutaneous	**D** Intraluminal Device	
2 Gastric Artery	**4** Percutaneous Endoscopic	**Z** No Device	
3 Hepatic Artery			
4 Splenic Artery			
5 Superior Mesenteric Artery			
6 Colic Artery, Right			
7 Colic Artery, Left			
8 Colic Artery, Middle			
9 Renal Artery, Right			
A Renal Artery, Left			
B Inferior Mesenteric Artery			
C Common Iliac Artery, Right			
D Common Iliac Artery, Left			
E Internal Iliac Artery, Right			
F Internal Iliac Artery, Left			
H External Iliac Artery, Right			
J External Iliac Artery, Left			
K Femoral Artery, Right			
L Femoral Artery, Left			
M Popliteal Artery, Right			
N Popliteal Artery, Left			
P Anterior Tibial Artery, Right			
Q Anterior Tibial Artery, Left			
R Posterior Tibial Artery, Right			
S Posterior Tibial Artery, Left			
T Peroneal Artery, Right			
U Peroneal Artery, Left			
V Foot Artery, Right			
W Foot Artery, Left			
Y Lower Artery			

Ø Medical and Surgical
4 Lower Arteries
9 Drainage Taking or letting out fluids and/or gases from a body part

Body Part Character 4	Approach Character 5	Device Character 6	Qualifier Character 7
Ø Abdominal Aorta 1 Celiac Artery 2 Gastric Artery 3 Hepatic Artery 4 Splenic Artery 5 Superior Mesenteric Artery 6 Colic Artery, Right 7 Colic Artery, Left 8 Colic Artery, Middle 9 Renal Artery, Right A Renal Artery, Left B Inferior Mesenteric Artery C Common Iliac Artery, Right D Common Iliac Artery, Left E Internal Iliac Artery, Right F Internal Iliac Artery, Left H External Iliac Artery, Right J External Iliac Artery, Left K Femoral Artery, Right L Femoral Artery, Left M Popliteal Artery, Right N Popliteal Artery, Left P Anterior Tibial Artery, Right Q Anterior Tibial Artery, Left R Posterior Tibial Artery, Right S Posterior Tibial Artery, Left T Peroneal Artery, Right U Peroneal Artery, Left V Foot Artery, Right W Foot Artery, Left Y Lower Artery	Ø Open 3 Percutaneous 4 Percutaneous Endoscopic	Ø Drainage Device	Z No Qualifier
Ø Abdominal Aorta 1 Celiac Artery 2 Gastric Artery 3 Hepatic Artery 4 Splenic Artery 5 Superior Mesenteric Artery 6 Colic Artery, Right 7 Colic Artery, Left 8 Colic Artery, Middle 9 Renal Artery, Right A Renal Artery, Left B Inferior Mesenteric Artery C Common Iliac Artery, Right D Common Iliac Artery, Left E Internal Iliac Artery, Right F Internal Iliac Artery, Left H External Iliac Artery, Right J External Iliac Artery, Left K Femoral Artery, Right L Femoral Artery, Left M Popliteal Artery, Right N Popliteal Artery, Left P Anterior Tibial Artery, Right Q Anterior Tibial Artery, Left R Posterior Tibial Artery, Right S Posterior Tibial Artery, Left T Peroneal Artery, Right U Peroneal Artery, Left V Foot Artery, Right W Foot Artery, Left Y Lower Artery	Ø Open 3 Percutaneous 4 Percutaneous Endoscopic	Z No Device	X Diagnostic Z No Qualifier

Non-OR Ø49[Ø,1,2,3,4,5,6,7,8,9,A,B,C,D,E,F,H,J,K,L,M,N,P,Q,R,S,T,U,V,W,Y][Ø,3,4]ØZ
Non-OR Ø49[Ø,1,2,3,4,5,6,7,8,9,A,B,C,D,E,F,H,J,K,L,M,N,P,Q,R,S,T,U,V,W,Y][Ø,3,4]ZZ

Ø Medical and Surgical
4 Lower Arteries
B Excision Cutting out or off, without replacement, a portion of a body part

Body Part Character 4	Approach Character 5	Device Character 6	Qualifier Character 7
Ø Abdominal Aorta **1** Celiac Artery **2** Gastric Artery **3** Hepatic Artery **4** Splenic Artery **5** Superior Mesenteric Artery **6** Colic Artery, Right **7** Colic Artery, Left **8** Colic Artery, Middle **9** Renal Artery, Right **A** Renal Artery, Left **B** Inferior Mesenteric Artery **C** Common Iliac Artery, Right **D** Common Iliac Artery, Left **E** Internal Iliac Artery, Right **F** Internal Iliac Artery, Left **H** External Iliac Artery, Right **J** External Iliac Artery, Left **K** Femoral Artery, Right **L** Femoral Artery, Left **M** Popliteal Artery, Right **N** Popliteal Artery, Left **P** Anterior Tibial Artery, Right **Q** Anterior Tibial Artery, Left **R** Posterior Tibial Artery, Right **S** Posterior Tibial Artery, Left **T** Peroneal Artery, Right **U** Peroneal Artery, Left **V** Foot Artery, Right **W** Foot Artery, Left **Y** Lower Artery	**Ø** Open **3** Percutaneous **4** Percutaneous Endoscopic	**Z** No Device	**X** Diagnostic **Z** No Qualifier

Ø Medical and Surgical
4 Lower Arteries
C Extirpation Taking or cutting out solid matter from a body part

Body Part Character 4	Approach Character 5	Device Character 6	Qualifier Character 7
Ø Abdominal Aorta **1** Celiac Artery **2** Gastric Artery **3** Hepatic Artery **4** Splenic Artery **5** Superior Mesenteric Artery **6** Colic Artery, Right **7** Colic Artery, Left **8** Colic Artery, Middle **9** Renal Artery, Right **A** Renal Artery, Left **B** Inferior Mesenteric Artery **C** Common Iliac Artery, Right **D** Common Iliac Artery, Left **E** Internal Iliac Artery, Right **F** Internal Iliac Artery, Left **H** External Iliac Artery, Right **J** External Iliac Artery, Left **K** Femoral Artery, Right **L** Femoral Artery, Left **M** Popliteal Artery, Right **N** Popliteal Artery, Left **P** Anterior Tibial Artery, Right **Q** Anterior Tibial Artery, Left **R** Posterior Tibial Artery, Right **S** Posterior Tibial Artery, Left **T** Peroneal Artery, Right **U** Peroneal Artery, Left **V** Foot Artery, Right **W** Foot Artery, Left **Y** Lower Artery	**Ø** Open **3** Percutaneous **4** Percutaneous Endoscopic	**Z** No Device	**Z** No Qualifier

0 Medical and Surgical
4 Lower Arteries
H Insertion Putting in a nonbiological appliance that monitors, assists, performs, or prevents a physiological function but does not physically take the place of a body part

Body Part Character 4	Approach Character 5	Device Character 6	Qualifier Character 7
0 Abdominal Aorta Y Lower Artery	0 Open 3 Percutaneous 4 Percutaneous Endoscopic	2 Monitoring Device 3 Infusion Device D Intraluminal Device	Z No Qualifier
1 Celiac Artery 2 Gastric Artery 3 Hepatic Artery 4 Splenic Artery 5 Superior Mesenteric Artery 6 Colic Artery, Right 7 Colic Artery, Left 8 Colic Artery, Middle 9 Renal Artery, Right A Renal Artery, Left B Inferior Mesenteric Artery C Common Iliac Artery, Right D Common Iliac Artery, Left E Internal Iliac Artery, Right F Internal Iliac Artery, Left H External Iliac Artery, Right J External Iliac Artery, Left K Femoral Artery, Right L Femoral Artery, Left M Popliteal Artery, Right N Popliteal Artery, Left P Anterior Tibial Artery, Right Q Anterior Tibial Artery, Left R Posterior Tibial Artery, Right S Posterior Tibial Artery, Left T Peroneal Artery, Right U Peroneal Artery, Left V Foot Artery, Right W Foot Artery, Left	0 Open 3 Percutaneous 4 Percutaneous Endoscopic	3 Infusion Device D Intraluminal Device	Z No Qualifier

Non-OR 04H0[0,3,4][2,3]Z
Non-OR 04HY[0,3,4]3Z
Non-OR 04H[1,2,3,4,5,6,7,8,9,A,B,C,D,E,F,H,J,K,L,M,N,P,Q,R,S,T,U,V,W][0,3,4]3Z

0 Medical and Surgical
4 Lower Arteries
J Inspection Visually and/or manually exploring a body part

Body Part Character 4	Approach Character 5	Device Character 6	Qualifier Character 7
Y Lower Artery	0 Open 3 Percutaneous 4 Percutaneous Endoscopic X External	Z No Device	Z No Qualifier

Non-OR 04JY[4,X]ZZ

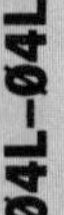

Ø Medical and Surgical
4 Lower Arteries
L Occlusion Completely closing an orifice or the lumen of a tubular body part

Body Part Character 4	Approach Character 5	Device Character 6	Qualifier Character 7
Ø Abdominal Aorta **1** Celiac Artery **2** Gastric Artery **3** Hepatic Artery **4** Splenic Artery **5** Superior Mesenteric Artery **6** Colic Artery, Right **7** Colic Artery, Left **8** Colic Artery, Middle **9** Renal Artery, Right **A** Renal Artery, Left **B** Inferior Mesenteric Artery **C** Common Iliac Artery, Right **D** Common Iliac Artery, Left **H** External Iliac Artery, Right **J** External Iliac Artery, Left **K** Femoral Artery, Right **L** Femoral Artery, Left **M** Popliteal Artery, Right **N** Popliteal Artery, Left **P** Anterior Tibial Artery, Right **Q** Anterior Tibial Artery, Left **R** Posterior Tibial Artery, Right **S** Posterior Tibial Artery, Left **T** Peroneal Artery, Right **U** Peroneal Artery, Left **V** Foot Artery, Right **W** Foot Artery, Left **Y** Lower Artery	**Ø** Open **3** Percutaneous **4** Percutaneous Endoscopic	**C** Extraluminal Device **D** Intraluminal Device **Z** No Device	**Z** No Qualifier
E Internal Iliac Artery, Right	**Ø** Open **3** Percutaneous **4** Percutaneous Endoscopic	**C** Extraluminal Device **D** Intraluminal Device **Z** No Device	**T** Uterine Artery, Right ♀ **Z** No Qualifier
F Internal Iliac Artery, Left	**Ø** Open **3** Percutaneous **4** Percutaneous Endoscopic	**C** Extraluminal Device **D** Intraluminal Device **Z** No Device	**U** Uterine Artery, Left ♀ **Z** No Qualifier

Non-OR Ø4L23DZ
AHA: 2Ø14, 1Q, 24

0 Medical and Surgical
4 Lower Arteries
N Release Freeing a body part from an abnormal physical constraint

Body Part Character 4	Approach Character 5	Device Character 6	Qualifier Character 7
0 Abdominal Aorta 1 Celiac Artery 2 Gastric Artery 3 Hepatic Artery 4 Splenic Artery 5 Superior Mesenteric Artery 6 Colic Artery, Right 7 Colic Artery, Left 8 Colic Artery, Middle 9 Renal Artery, Right A Renal Artery, Left B Inferior Mesenteric Artery C Common Iliac Artery, Right D Common Iliac Artery, Left E Internal Iliac Artery, Right F Internal Iliac Artery, Left H External Iliac Artery, Right J External Iliac Artery, Left K Femoral Artery, Right L Femoral Artery, Left M Popliteal Artery, Right N Popliteal Artery, Left P Anterior Tibial Artery, Right Q Anterior Tibial Artery, Left R Posterior Tibial Artery, Right S Posterior Tibial Artery, Left T Peroneal Artery, Right U Peroneal Artery, Left V Foot Artery, Right W Foot Artery, Left Y Lower Artery	0 Open 3 Percutaneous 4 Percutaneous Endoscopic	Z No Device	Z No Qualifier

0 Medical and Surgical
4 Lower Arteries
P Removal Taking out or off a device from a body part

Body Part Character 4	Approach Character 5	Device Character 6	Qualifier Character 7
Y Lower Artery	0 Open 3 Percutaneous 4 Percutaneous Endoscopic	0 Drainage Device 2 Monitoring Device 3 Infusion Device 7 Autologous Tissue Substitute C Extraluminal Device D Intraluminal Device J Synthetic Substitute K Nonautologous Tissue Substitute	Z No Qualifier
Y Lower Artery	X External	0 Drainage Device 1 Radioactive Element 2 Monitoring Device 3 Infusion Device D Intraluminal Device	Z No Qualifier

Non-OR 04PYX[0,1,2,3,D]Z

Ø Medical and Surgical
4 Lower Arteries
Q Repair Restoring, to the extent possible, a body part to its normal anatomic structure and function

Body Part Character 4	Approach Character 5	Device Character 6	Qualifier Character 7
Ø Abdominal Aorta **1** Celiac Artery **2** Gastric Artery **3** Hepatic Artery **4** Splenic Artery **5** Superior Mesenteric Artery **6** Colic Artery, Right **7** Colic Artery, Left **8** Colic Artery, Middle **9** Renal Artery, Right **A** Renal Artery, Left **B** Inferior Mesenteric Artery **C** Common Iliac Artery, Right **D** Common Iliac Artery, Left **E** Internal Iliac Artery, Right **F** Internal Iliac Artery, Left **H** External Iliac Artery, Right **J** External Iliac Artery, Left **K** Femoral Artery, Right **L** Femoral Artery, Left **M** Popliteal Artery, Right **N** Popliteal Artery, Left **P** Anterior Tibial Artery, Right **Q** Anterior Tibial Artery, Left **R** Posterior Tibial Artery, Right **S** Posterior Tibial Artery, Left **T** Peroneal Artery, Right **U** Peroneal Artery, Left **V** Foot Artery, Right **W** Foot Artery, Left **Y** Lower Artery	**Ø** Open **3** Percutaneous **4** Percutaneous Endoscopic	**Z** No Device	**Z** No Qualifier

AHA: 2Ø14, 1Q, 21

Ø Medical and Surgical
4 Lower Arteries
R Replacement Putting in or on biological or synthetic material that physically takes the place and/or function of all or a portion of a body part

Body Part Character 4	Approach Character 5	Device Character 6	Qualifier Character 7
Ø Abdominal Aorta **1** Celiac Artery **2** Gastric Artery **3** Hepatic Artery **4** Splenic Artery **5** Superior Mesenteric Artery **6** Colic Artery, Right **7** Colic Artery, Left **8** Colic Artery, Middle **9** Renal Artery, Right **A** Renal Artery, Left **B** Inferior Mesenteric Artery **C** Common Iliac Artery, Right **D** Common Iliac Artery, Left **E** Internal Iliac Artery, Right **F** Internal Iliac Artery, Left **H** External Iliac Artery, Right **J** External Iliac Artery, Left **K** Femoral Artery, Right **L** Femoral Artery, Left **M** Popliteal Artery, Right **N** Popliteal Artery, Left **P** Anterior Tibial Artery, Right **Q** Anterior Tibial Artery, Left **R** Posterior Tibial Artery, Right **S** Posterior Tibial Artery, Left **T** Peroneal Artery, Right **U** Peroneal Artery, Left **V** Foot Artery, Right **W** Foot Artery, Left **Y** Lower Artery	**Ø** Open **4** Percutaneous Endoscopic	**7** Autologous Tissue Substitute **J** Synthetic Substitute **K** Nonautologous Tissue Substitute	**Z** No Qualifier

0 Medical and Surgical
4 Lower Arteries
S Reposition Moving to its normal location or other suitable location all or a portion of a body part

Body Part Character 4	Approach Character 5	Device Character 6	Qualifier Character 7
0 Abdominal Aorta 1 Celiac Artery 2 Gastric Artery 3 Hepatic Artery 4 Splenic Artery 5 Superior Mesenteric Artery 6 Colic Artery, Right 7 Colic Artery, Left 8 Colic Artery, Middle 9 Renal Artery, Right A Renal Artery, Left B Inferior Mesenteric Artery C Common Iliac Artery, Right D Common Iliac Artery, Left E Internal Iliac Artery, Right F Internal Iliac Artery, Left H External Iliac Artery, Right J External Iliac Artery, Left K Femoral Artery, Right L Femoral Artery, Left M Popliteal Artery, Right N Popliteal Artery, Left P Anterior Tibial Artery, Right Q Anterior Tibial Artery, Left R Posterior Tibial Artery, Right S Posterior Tibial Artery, Left T Peroneal Artery, Right U Peroneal Artery, Left V Foot Artery, Right W Foot Artery, Left Y Lower Artery	0 Open 3 Percutaneous 4 Percutaneous Endoscopic	Z No Device	Z No Qualifier

0 Medical and Surgical
4 Lower Arteries
U Supplement Putting in or on biological or synthetic material that physically reinforces and/or augments the function of a portion of a body part

Body Part Character 4	Approach Character 5	Device Character 6	Qualifier Character 7
0 Abdominal Aorta 1 Celiac Artery 2 Gastric Artery 3 Hepatic Artery 4 Splenic Artery 5 Superior Mesenteric Artery 6 Colic Artery, Right 7 Colic Artery, Left 8 Colic Artery, Middle 9 Renal Artery, Right A Renal Artery, Left B Inferior Mesenteric Artery C Common Iliac Artery, Right D Common Iliac Artery, Left E Internal Iliac Artery, Right F Internal Iliac Artery, Left H External Iliac Artery, Right J External Iliac Artery, Left K Femoral Artery, Right L Femoral Artery, Left M Popliteal Artery, Right N Popliteal Artery, Left P Anterior Tibial Artery, Right Q Anterior Tibial Artery, Left R Posterior Tibial Artery, Right S Posterior Tibial Artery, Left T Peroneal Artery, Right U Peroneal Artery, Left V Foot Artery, Right W Foot Artery, Left Y Lower Artery	0 Open 3 Percutaneous 4 Percutaneous Endoscopic	7 Autologous Tissue Substitute J Synthetic Substitute K Nonautologous Tissue Substitute	Z No Qualifier

AHA: 2014, 1Q, 22

Ø Medical and Surgical
4 Lower Arteries
V Restriction Partially closing an orifice or the lumen of a tubular body part

Body Part Character 4	Approach Character 5	Device Character 6	Qualifier Character 7
Ø Abdominal Aorta	**Ø** Open **3** Percutaneous **4** Percutaneous Endoscopic	**C** Extraluminal Device **Z** No Device	**Z** No Qualifier
Ø Abdominal Aorta	**Ø** Open **3** Percutaneous **4** Percutaneous Endoscopic	**D** Intraluminal Device	**J** Temporary **Z** No Qualifier
1 Celiac Artery **2** Gastric Artery **3** Hepatic Artery **4** Splenic Artery **5** Superior Mesenteric Artery **6** Colic Artery, Right **7** Colic Artery, Left **8** Colic Artery, Middle **9** Renal Artery, Right **A** Renal Artery, Left **B** Inferior Mesenteric Artery **C** Common Iliac Artery, Right **D** Common Iliac Artery, Left **E** Internal Iliac Artery, Right **F** Internal Iliac Artery, Left **H** External Iliac Artery, Right **J** External Iliac Artery, Left **K** Femoral Artery, Right **L** Femoral Artery, Left **M** Popliteal Artery, Right **N** Popliteal Artery, Left **P** Anterior Tibial Artery, Right **Q** Anterior Tibial Artery, Left **R** Posterior Tibial Artery, Right **S** Posterior Tibial Artery, Left **T** Peroneal Artery, Right **U** Peroneal Artery, Left **V** Foot Artery, Right **W** Foot Artery, Left **Y** Lower Artery	**Ø** Open **3** Percutaneous **4** Percutaneous Endoscopic	**C** Extraluminal Device **D** Intraluminal Device **Z** No Device	**Z** No Qualifier

AHA: 2Ø14, 1Q, 9

Ø Medical and Surgical
4 Lower Arteries
W Revision Correcting, to the extent possible, a portion of a malfunctioning device or the position of a displaced device

Body Part Character 4	Approach Character 5	Device Character 6	Qualifier Character 7
Y Lower Artery	**Ø** Open **3** Percutaneous **4** Percutaneous Endoscopic **X** External	**Ø** Drainage Device **2** Monitoring Device **3** Infusion Device **7** Autologous Tissue Substitute **C** Extraluminal Device **D** Intraluminal Device **J** Synthetic Substitute **K** Nonautologous Tissue Substitute	**Z** No Qualifier

Non-OR Ø4WYX[Ø,2,3,7,C,D,J,K]Z
AHA: 2Ø14, 1Q, 9, 22

Upper Veins 051–05W

0 Medical and Surgical
5 Upper Veins
1 Bypass Altering the route of passage of the contents of a tubular body part

Body Part Character 4	Approach Character 5	Device Character 6	Qualifier Character 7
0 Azygos Vein 1 Hemiazygos Vein 3 Innominate Vein, Right 4 Innominate Vein, Left 5 Subclavian Vein, Right 6 Subclavian Vein, Left 7 Axillary Vein, Right 8 Axillary Vein, Left 9 Brachial Vein, Right A Brachial Vein, Left B Basilic Vein, Right C Basilic Vein, Left D Cephalic Vein, Right F Cephalic Vein, Left G Hand Vein, Right H Hand Vein, Left L Intracranial Vein M Internal Jugular Vein, Right N Internal Jugular Vein, Left P External Jugular Vein, Right Q External Jugular Vein, Left R Vertebral Vein, Right S Vertebral Vein, Left T Face Vein, Right V Face Vein, Left	0 Open 4 Percutaneous Endoscopic	7 Autologous Tissue Substitute 9 Autologous Venous Tissue A Autologous Arterial Tissue J Synthetic Substitute K Nonautologous Tissue Substitute Z No Device	Y Upper Vein

0 Medical and Surgical
5 Upper Veins
5 Destruction Physical eradication of all or a portion of a body part by the direct use of energy, force, or a destructive agent

Body Part Character 4	Approach Character 5	Device Character 6	Qualifier Character 7
0 Azygos Vein 1 Hemiazygos Vein 3 Innominate Vein, Right 4 Innominate Vein, Left 5 Subclavian Vein, Right 6 Subclavian Vein, Left 7 Axillary Vein, Right 8 Axillary Vein, Left 9 Brachial Vein, Right A Brachial Vein, Left B Basilic Vein, Right C Basilic Vein, Left D Cephalic Vein, Right F Cephalic Vein, Left G Hand Vein, Right H Hand Vein, Left L Intracranial Vein M Internal Jugular Vein, Right N Internal Jugular Vein, Left P External Jugular Vein, Right Q External Jugular Vein, Left R Vertebral Vein, Right S Vertebral Vein, Left T Face Vein, Right V Face Vein, Left Y Upper Vein	0 Open 3 Percutaneous 4 Percutaneous Endoscopic	Z No Device	Z No Qualifier

Ø Medical and Surgical
5 Upper Veins
7 Dilation Expanding an orifice or the lumen of a tubular body part

Body Part Character 4	Approach Character 5	Device Character 6	Qualifier Character 7
Ø Azygos Vein **1** Hemiazygos Vein **3** Innominate Vein, Right **4** Innominate Vein, Left **5** Subclavian Vein, Right **6** Subclavian Vein, Left **7** Axillary Vein, Right **8** Axillary Vein, Left **9** Brachial Vein, Right **A** Brachial Vein, Left **B** Basilic Vein, Right **C** Basilic Vein, Left **D** Cephalic Vein, Right **F** Cephalic Vein, Left **G** Hand Vein, Right **H** Hand Vein, Left **L** Intracranial Vein NC **M** Internal Jugular Vein, Right **N** Internal Jugular Vein, Left **P** External Jugular Vein, Right **Q** External Jugular Vein, Left **R** Vertebral Vein, Right **S** Vertebral Vein, Left **T** Face Vein, Right **V** Face Vein, Left **Y** Upper Vein	**Ø** Open **3** Percutaneous **4** Percutaneous Endoscopic	**D** Intraluminal Device **Z** No Device	**Z** No Qualifier

NC Ø57L[3,4]ZZ

0 Medical and Surgical
5 Upper Veins
9 Drainage Taking or letting out fluids and/or gases from a body part

Body Part Character 4	Approach Character 5	Device Character 6	Qualifier Character 7
0 Azygos Vein 1 Hemiazygos Vein 3 Innominate Vein, Right 4 Innominate Vein, Left 5 Subclavian Vein, Right 6 Subclavian Vein, Left 7 Axillary Vein, Right 8 Axillary Vein, Left 9 Brachial Vein, Right A Brachial Vein, Left B Basilic Vein, Right C Basilic Vein, Left D Cephalic Vein, Right F Cephalic Vein, Left G Hand Vein, Right H Hand Vein, Left L Intracranial Vein M Internal Jugular Vein, Right N Internal Jugular Vein, Left P External Jugular Vein, Right Q External Jugular Vein, Left R Vertebral Vein, Right S Vertebral Vein, Left T Face Vein, Right V Face Vein, Left Y Upper Vein	0 Open 3 Percutaneous 4 Percutaneous Endoscopic	0 Drainage Device	Z No Qualifier
0 Azygos Vein 1 Hemiazygos Vein 3 Innominate Vein, Right 4 Innominate Vein, Left 5 Subclavian Vein, Right 6 Subclavian Vein, Left 7 Axillary Vein, Right 8 Axillary Vein, Left 9 Brachial Vein, Right A Brachial Vein, Left B Basilic Vein, Right C Basilic Vein, Left D Cephalic Vein, Right F Cephalic Vein, Left G Hand Vein, Right H Hand Vein, Left L Intracranial Vein M Internal Jugular Vein, Right N Internal Jugular Vein, Left P External Jugular Vein, Right Q External Jugular Vein, Left R Vertebral Vein, Right S Vertebral Vein, Left T Face Vein, Right V Face Vein, Left Y Upper Vein	0 Open 3 Percutaneous 4 Percutaneous Endoscopic	Z No Device	X Diagnostic Z No Qualifier

Non-OR 059[0,1,3,4,5,6,7,8,9,A,B,C,D,F,G,H,L,M,N,P,Q,R,S,T,V,Y][0,3,4]0Z
Non-OR 059[0,1,3,4,5,6,7,8,9,A,B,C,D,F,G,H,L,M,N,P,Q,R,S,T,V,Y][0,3,4]ZZ

Ø Medical and Surgical
5 Upper Veins
B Excision Cutting out or off, without replacement, a portion of a body part

Body Part Character 4	Approach Character 5	Device Character 6	Qualifier Character 7
Ø Azygos Vein 1 Hemiazygos Vein 3 Innominate Vein, Right 4 Innominate Vein, Left 5 Subclavian Vein, Right 6 Subclavian Vein, Left 7 Axillary Vein, Right 8 Axillary Vein, Left 9 Brachial Vein, Right A Brachial Vein, Left B Basilic Vein, Right C Basilic Vein, Left D Cephalic Vein, Right F Cephalic Vein, Left G Hand Vein, Right H Hand Vein, Left L Intracranial Vein M Internal Jugular Vein, Right N Internal Jugular Vein, Left P External Jugular Vein, Right Q External Jugular Vein, Left R Vertebral Vein, Right S Vertebral Vein, Left T Face Vein, Right V Face Vein, Left Y Upper Vein	Ø Open 3 Percutaneous 4 Percutaneous Endoscopic	Z No Device	X Diagnostic Z No Qualifier

Ø Medical and Surgical
5 Upper Veins
C Extirpation Taking or cutting out solid matter from a body part

Body Part Character 4	Approach Character 5	Device Character 6	Qualifier Character 7
Ø Azygos Vein 1 Hemiazygos Vein 3 Innominate Vein, Right 4 Innominate Vein, Left 5 Subclavian Vein, Right 6 Subclavian Vein, Left 7 Axillary Vein, Right 8 Axillary Vein, Left 9 Brachial Vein, Right A Brachial Vein, Left B Basilic Vein, Right C Basilic Vein, Left D Cephalic Vein, Right F Cephalic Vein, Left G Hand Vein, Right H Hand Vein, Left L Intracranial Vein NC M Internal Jugular Vein, Right N Internal Jugular Vein, Left P External Jugular Vein, Right Q External Jugular Vein, Left R Vertebral Vein, Right S Vertebral Vein, Left T Face Vein, Right V Face Vein, Left Y Upper Vein	Ø Open 3 Percutaneous 4 Percutaneous Endoscopic	Z No Device	Z No Qualifier

NC Ø5CL[3,4]ZZ

Ø Medical and Surgical
5 Upper Veins
D Extraction Pulling or stripping out or off all or a portion of a body part by the use of force

Body Part Character 4	Approach Character 5	Device Character 6	Qualifier Character 7
9 Brachial Vein, Right **A** Brachial Vein, Left **B** Basilic Vein, Right **C** Basilic Vein, Left **D** Cephalic Vein, Right **F** Cephalic Vein, Left **G** Hand Vein, Right **H** Hand Vein, Left **Y** Upper Vein	**Ø** Open **3** Percutaneous	**Z** No Device	**Z** No Qualifier

Ø Medical and Surgical
5 Upper Veins
H Insertion Putting in a nonbiological appliance that monitors, assists, performs, or prevents a physiological function but does not physically take the place of a body part

Body Part Character 4	Approach Character 5	Device Character 6	Qualifier Character 7
Ø Azygos Vein **1** Hemiazygos Vein **3** Innominate Vein, Right **4** Innominate Vein, Left **5** Subclavian Vein, Right **6** Subclavian Vein, Left **7** Axillary Vein, Right **8** Axillary Vein, Left **9** Brachial Vein, Right **A** Brachial Vein, Left **B** Basilic Vein, Right **C** Basilic Vein, Left **D** Cephalic Vein, Right **F** Cephalic Vein, Left **G** Hand Vein, Right **H** Hand Vein, Left **L** Intracranial Vein **M** Internal Jugular Vein, Right **N** Internal Jugular Vein, Left **P** External Jugular Vein, Right **Q** External Jugular Vein, Left **R** Vertebral Vein, Right **S** Vertebral Vein, Left **T** Face Vein, Right **V** Face Vein, Left	**Ø** Open **3** Percutaneous **4** Percutaneous Endoscopic	**3** Infusion Device **D** Intraluminal Device	**Z** No Qualifier
Y Upper Vein	**Ø** Open **3** Percutaneous **4** Percutaneous Endoscopic	**2** Monitoring Device **3** Infusion Device **D** Intraluminal Device	**Z** No Qualifier

DRG Non-OR Ø5H[5,6,M,N,P,Q]33Z
Non-OR Ø5H[Ø,1,3,4,7,8,9,A,B,C,D,F,G,H,L,R,S,T,V][Ø,3,4]3Z
Non-OR Ø5H[5,6,M,N,P,Q][Ø,4]3Z
Non-OR Ø5HY[Ø,3,4]3Z
HAC Ø5H[M,N,P,Q]33Z when reported with SDx J95.811

No Procedure Combinations Specified
Combo-only Ø5H[5,6,M,N,P,Q]33Z

Ø Medical and Surgical
5 Upper Veins
J Inspection Visually and/or manually exploring a body part

Body Part Character 4	Approach Character 5	Device Character 6	Qualifier Character 7
Y Upper Vein	**Ø** Open **3** Percutaneous **4** Percutaneous Endoscopic **X** External	**Z** No Device	**Z** No Qualifier

Non-OR Ø5JYXZZ

Ø Medical and Surgical
5 Upper Veins
L Occlusion Completely closing an orifice or the lumen of a tubular body part

Body Part Character 4	Approach Character 5	Device Character 6	Qualifier Character 7
Ø Azygos Vein **1** Hemiazygos Vein **3** Innominate Vein, Right **4** Innominate Vein, Left **5** Subclavian Vein, Right **6** Subclavian Vein, Left **7** Axillary Vein, Right **8** Axillary Vein, Left **9** Brachial Vein, Right **A** Brachial Vein, Left **B** Basilic Vein, Right **C** Basilic Vein, Left **D** Cephalic Vein, Right **F** Cephalic Vein, Left **G** Hand Vein, Right **H** Hand Vein, Left **L** Intracranial Vein **M** Internal Jugular Vein, Right **N** Internal Jugular Vein, Left **P** External Jugular Vein, Right **Q** External Jugular Vein, Left **R** Vertebral Vein, Right **S** Vertebral Vein, Left **T** Face Vein, Right **V** Face Vein, Left **Y** Upper Vein	**Ø** Open **3** Percutaneous **4** Percutaneous Endoscopic	**C** Extraluminal Device **D** Intraluminal Device **Z** No Device	**Z** No Qualifier

Ø Medical and Surgical
5 Upper Veins
N Release Freeing a body part from an abnormal physical constraint

Body Part Character 4	Approach Character 5	Device Character 6	Qualifier Character 7
Ø Azygos Vein **1** Hemiazygos Vein **3** Innominate Vein, Right **4** Innominate Vein, Left **5** Subclavian Vein, Right **6** Subclavian Vein, Left **7** Axillary Vein, Right **8** Axillary Vein, Left **9** Brachial Vein, Right **A** Brachial Vein, Left **B** Basilic Vein, Right **C** Basilic Vein, Left **D** Cephalic Vein, Right **F** Cephalic Vein, Left **G** Hand Vein, Right **H** Hand Vein, Left **L** Intracranial Vein **M** Internal Jugular Vein, Right **N** Internal Jugular Vein, Left **P** External Jugular Vein, Right **Q** External Jugular Vein, Left **R** Vertebral Vein, Right **S** Vertebral Vein, Left **T** Face Vein, Right **V** Face Vein, Left **Y** Upper Vein	**Ø** Open **3** Percutaneous **4** Percutaneous Endoscopic	**Z** No Device	**Z** No Qualifier

0 Medical and Surgical
5 Upper Veins
P Removal Taking out or off a device from a body part

Body Part Character 4	Approach Character 5	Device Character 6	Qualifier Character 7
Y Upper Vein	0 Open 3 Percutaneous 4 Percutaneous Endoscopic	0 Drainage Device 2 Monitoring Device 3 Infusion Device 7 Autologous Tissue Substitute C Extraluminal Device D Intraluminal Device J Synthetic Substitute K Nonautologous Tissue Substitute	Z No Qualifier
Y Upper Vein	X External	0 Drainage Device 2 Monitoring Device 3 Infusion Device D Intraluminal Device	Z No Qualifier

Non-OR 05PYX[0,2,3,D]Z

0 Medical and Surgical
5 Upper Veins
Q Repair Restoring, to the extent possible, a body part to its normal anatomic structure and function

Body Part Character 4	Approach Character 5	Device Character 6	Qualifier Character 7
0 Azygos Vein 1 Hemiazygos Vein 3 Innominate Vein, Right 4 Innominate Vein, Left 5 Subclavian Vein, Right 6 Subclavian Vein, Left 7 Axillary Vein, Right 8 Axillary Vein, Left 9 Brachial Vein, Right A Brachial Vein, Left B Basilic Vein, Right C Basilic Vein, Left D Cephalic Vein, Right F Cephalic Vein, Left G Hand Vein, Right H Hand Vein, Left L Intracranial Vein M Internal Jugular Vein, Right N Internal Jugular Vein, Left P External Jugular Vein, Right Q External Jugular Vein, Left R Vertebral Vein, Right S Vertebral Vein, Left T Face Vein, Right V Face Vein, Left Y Upper Vein	0 Open 3 Percutaneous 4 Percutaneous Endoscopic	Z No Device	Z No Qualifier

Ø Medical and Surgical
5 Upper Veins
R Replacement Putting in or on biological or synthetic material that physically takes the place and/or function of all or a portion of a body part

Body Part Character 4	Approach Character 5	Device Character 6	Qualifier Character 7
Ø Azygos Vein 1 Hemiazygos Vein 3 Innominate Vein, Right 4 Innominate Vein, Left 5 Subclavian Vein, Right 6 Subclavian Vein, Left 7 Axillary Vein, Right 8 Axillary Vein, Left 9 Brachial Vein, Right A Brachial Vein, Left B Basilic Vein, Right C Basilic Vein, Left D Cephalic Vein, Right F Cephalic Vein, Left G Hand Vein, Right H Hand Vein, Left L Intracranial Vein M Internal Jugular Vein, Right N Internal Jugular Vein, Left P External Jugular Vein, Right Q External Jugular Vein, Left R Vertebral Vein, Right S Vertebral Vein, Left T Face Vein, Right V Face Vein, Left Y Upper Vein	Ø Open 4 Percutaneous Endoscopic	7 Autologous Tissue Substitute J Synthetic Substitute K Nonautologous Tissue Substitute	Z No Qualifier

Ø Medical and Surgical
5 Upper Veins
S Reposition Moving to its normal location or other suitable location all or a portion of a body part

Body Part Character 4	Approach Character 5	Device Character 6	Qualifier Character 7
Ø Azygos Vein 1 Hemiazygos Vein 3 Innominate Vein, Right 4 Innominate Vein, Left 5 Subclavian Vein, Right 6 Subclavian Vein, Left 7 Axillary Vein, Right 8 Axillary Vein, Left 9 Brachial Vein, Right A Brachial Vein, Left B Basilic Vein, Right C Basilic Vein, Left D Cephalic Vein, Right F Cephalic Vein, Left G Hand Vein, Right H Hand Vein, Left L Intracranial Vein M Internal Jugular Vein, Right N Internal Jugular Vein, Left P External Jugular Vein, Right Q External Jugular Vein, Left R Vertebral Vein, Right S Vertebral Vein, Left T Face Vein, Right V Face Vein, Left Y Upper Vein	Ø Open 3 Percutaneous 4 Percutaneous Endoscopic	Z No Device	Z No Qualifier

AHA: 2Ø13, 4Q, 125

0 Medical and Surgical
5 Upper Veins
U Supplement Putting in or on biological or synthetic material that physically reinforces and/or augments the function of a portion of a body part

Body Part Character 4	Approach Character 5	Device Character 6	Qualifier Character 7
0 Azygos Vein 1 Hemiazygos Vein 3 Innominate Vein, Right 4 Innominate Vein, Left 5 Subclavian Vein, Right 6 Subclavian Vein, Left 7 Axillary Vein, Right 8 Axillary Vein, Left 9 Brachial Vein, Right A Brachial Vein, Left B Basilic Vein, Right C Basilic Vein, Left D Cephalic Vein, Right F Cephalic Vein, Left G Hand Vein, Right H Hand Vein, Left L Intracranial Vein M Internal Jugular Vein, Right N Internal Jugular Vein, Left P External Jugular Vein, Right Q External Jugular Vein, Left R Vertebral Vein, Right S Vertebral Vein, Left T Face Vein, Right V Face Vein, Left Y Upper Vein	0 Open 3 Percutaneous 4 Percutaneous Endoscopic	7 Autologous Tissue Substitute J Synthetic Substitute K Nonautologous Tissue Substitute	Z No Qualifier

0 Medical and Surgical
5 Upper Veins
V Restriction Partially closing an orifice or the lumen of a tubular body part

Body Part Character 4	Approach Character 5	Device Character 6	Qualifier Character 7
0 Azygos Vein 1 Hemiazygos Vein 3 Innominate Vein, Right 4 Innominate Vein, Left 5 Subclavian Vein, Right 6 Subclavian Vein, Left 7 Axillary Vein, Right 8 Axillary Vein, Left 9 Brachial Vein, Right A Brachial Vein, Left B Basilic Vein, Right C Basilic Vein, Left D Cephalic Vein, Right F Cephalic Vein, Left G Hand Vein, Right H Hand Vein, Left L Intracranial Vein M Internal Jugular Vein, Right N Internal Jugular Vein, Left P External Jugular Vein, Right Q External Jugular Vein, Left R Vertebral Vein, Right S Vertebral Vein, Left T Face Vein, Right V Face Vein, Left Y Upper Vein	0 Open 3 Percutaneous 4 Percutaneous Endoscopic	C Extraluminal Device D Intraluminal Device Z No Device	Z No Qualifier

Ø Medical and Surgical
5 Upper Veins
W Revision Correcting, to the extent possible, a portion of a malfunctioning device or the position of a displaced device

Body Part Character 4	Approach Character 5	Device Character 6	Qualifier Character 7
Y Upper Vein	**Ø** Open **3** Percutaneous **4** Percutaneous Endoscopic **X** External	**Ø** Drainage Device **2** Monitoring Device **3** Infusion Device **7** Autologous Tissue Substitute **C** Extraluminal Device **D** Intraluminal Device **J** Synthetic Substitute **K** Nonautologous Tissue Substitute	**Z** No Qualifier

Non-OR Ø5WYX[Ø,2,3,7,C,D,J,K]Z

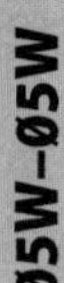

Lower Veins 061–06W

0 Medical and Surgical
6 Lower Veins
1 Bypass Altering the route of passage of the contents of a tubular body part

Body Part Character 4	Approach Character 5	Device Character 6	Qualifier Character 7
0 Inferior Vena Cava	**0** Open **4** Percutaneous Endoscopic	**7** Autologous Tissue Substitute **9** Autologous Venous Tissue **A** Autologous Arterial Tissue **J** Synthetic Substitute **K** Nonautologous Tissue Substitute **Z** No Device	**5** Superior Mesenteric Vein **6** Inferior Mesenteric Vein **Y** Lower Vein
1 Splenic Vein **8** Portal Vein	**0** Open **4** Percutaneous Endoscopic	**7** Autologous Tissue Substitute **9** Autologous Venous Tissue **A** Autologous Arterial Tissue **J** Synthetic Substitute **K** Nonautologous Tissue Substitute **Z** No Device	**9** Renal Vein, Right **B** Renal Vein, Left **Y** Lower Vein
2 Gastric Vein **3** Esophageal Vein **4** Hepatic Vein **5** Superior Mesenteric Vein **6** Inferior Mesenteric Vein **7** Colic Vein **9** Renal Vein, Right **B** Renal Vein, Left **C** Common Iliac Vein, Right **D** Common Iliac Vein, Left **F** External Iliac Vein, Right **G** External Iliac Vein, Left **H** Hypogastric Vein, Right **J** Hypogastric Vein, Left **M** Femoral Vein, Right **N** Femoral Vein, Left **P** Greater Saphenous Vein, Right **Q** Greater Saphenous Vein, Left **R** Lesser Saphenous Vein, Right **S** Lesser Saphenous Vein, Left **T** Foot Vein, Right **V** Foot Vein, Left	**0** Open **4** Percutaneous Endoscopic	**7** Autologous Tissue Substitute **9** Autologous Venous Tissue **A** Autologous Arterial Tissue **J** Synthetic Substitute **K** Nonautologous Tissue Substitute **Z** No Device	**Y** Lower Vein
8 Portal Vein	**3** Percutaneous **4** Percutaneous Endoscopic	**D** Intraluminal Device	**Y** Lower Vein

Ø Medical and Surgical
6 Lower Veins
5 Destruction Physical eradication of all or a portion of a body part by the direct use of energy, force, or a destructive agent

Body Part Character 4	Approach Character 5	Device Character 6	Qualifier Character 7
Ø Inferior Vena Cava 1 Splenic Vein 2 Gastric Vein 3 Esophageal Vein 4 Hepatic Vein 5 Superior Mesenteric Vein 6 Inferior Mesenteric Vein 7 Colic Vein 8 Portal Vein 9 Renal Vein, Right B Renal Vein, Left C Common Iliac Vein, Right D Common Iliac Vein, Left F External Iliac Vein, Right G External Iliac Vein, Left H Hypogastric Vein, Right J Hypogastric Vein, Left M Femoral Vein, Right N Femoral Vein, Left P Greater Saphenous Vein, Right Q Greater Saphenous Vein, Left R Lesser Saphenous Vein, Right S Lesser Saphenous Vein, Left T Foot Vein, Right V Foot Vein, Left	Ø Open 3 Percutaneous 4 Percutaneous Endoscopic	Z No Device	Z No Qualifier
Y Lower Vein	Ø Open 3 Percutaneous 4 Percutaneous Endoscopic	Z No Device	C Hemorrhoidal Plexus Z No Qualifier

Ø Medical and Surgical
6 Lower Veins
7 Dilation Expanding an orifice or the lumen of a tubular body part

Body Part Character 4	Approach Character 5	Device Character 6	Qualifier Character 7
Ø Inferior Vena Cava 1 Splenic Vein 2 Gastric Vein 3 Esophageal Vein 4 Hepatic Vein 5 Superior Mesenteric Vein 6 Inferior Mesenteric Vein 7 Colic Vein 8 Portal Vein 9 Renal Vein, Right B Renal Vein, Left C Common Iliac Vein, Right D Common Iliac Vein, Left F External Iliac Vein, Right G External Iliac Vein, Left H Hypogastric Vein, Right J Hypogastric Vein, Left M Femoral Vein, Right N Femoral Vein, Left P Greater Saphenous Vein, Right Q Greater Saphenous Vein, Left R Lesser Saphenous Vein, Right S Lesser Saphenous Vein, Left T Foot Vein, Right V Foot Vein, Left Y Lower Vein	Ø Open 3 Percutaneous 4 Percutaneous Endoscopic	D Intraluminal Device Z No Device	Z No Qualifier

0 Medical and Surgical
6 Lower Veins
9 Drainage Taking or letting out fluids and/or gases from a body part

Body Part Character 4	Approach Character 5	Device Character 6	Qualifier Character 7
0 Inferior Vena Cava 1 Splenic Vein 2 Gastric Vein 3 Esophageal Vein 4 Hepatic Vein 5 Superior Mesenteric Vein 6 Inferior Mesenteric Vein 7 Colic Vein 8 Portal Vein 9 Renal Vein, Right B Renal Vein, Left C Common Iliac Vein, Right D Common Iliac Vein, Left F External Iliac Vein, Right G External Iliac Vein, Left H Hypogastric Vein, Right J Hypogastric Vein, Left M Femoral Vein, Right N Femoral Vein, Left P Greater Saphenous Vein, Right Q Greater Saphenous Vein, Left R Lesser Saphenous Vein, Right S Lesser Saphenous Vein, Left T Foot Vein, Right V Foot Vein, Left Y Lower Vein	0 Open 3 Percutaneous 4 Percutaneous Endoscopic	0 Drainage Device	Z No Qualifier
0 Inferior Vena Cava 1 Splenic Vein 2 Gastric Vein 3 Esophageal Vein 4 Hepatic Vein 5 Superior Mesenteric Vein 6 Inferior Mesenteric Vein 7 Colic Vein 8 Portal Vein 9 Renal Vein, Right B Renal Vein, Left C Common Iliac Vein, Right D Common Iliac Vein, Left F External Iliac Vein, Right G External Iliac Vein, Left H Hypogastric Vein, Right J Hypogastric Vein, Left M Femoral Vein, Right N Femoral Vein, Left P Greater Saphenous Vein, Right Q Greater Saphenous Vein, Left R Lesser Saphenous Vein, Right S Lesser Saphenous Vein, Left T Foot Vein, Right V Foot Vein, Left Y Lower Vein	0 Open 3 Percutaneous 4 Percutaneous Endoscopic	Z No Device	X Diagnostic Z No Qualifier

Non-OR 069[0,1,2,4,5,6,7,8,9,B,C,D,F,G,H,J,M,N,P,Q,R,S,T,V,Y][0,3,4]0Z
Non-OR 069[0,1,2,4,5,6,7,8,9,B,C,D,F,G,H,J,M,N,P,Q,R,S,T,V,Y][0,3,4]ZZ

Ø Medical and Surgical
6 Lower Veins
B Excision Cutting out or off, without replacement, a portion of a body part

Body Part Character 4	Approach Character 5	Device Character 6	Qualifier Character 7
Ø Inferior Vena Cava 1 Splenic Vein 2 Gastric Vein 3 Esophageal Vein 4 Hepatic Vein 5 Superior Mesenteric Vein 6 Inferior Mesenteric Vein 7 Colic Vein 8 Portal Vein 9 Renal Vein, Right B Renal Vein, Left C Common Iliac Vein, Right D Common Iliac Vein, Left F External Iliac Vein, Right G External Iliac Vein, Left H Hypogastric Vein, Right J Hypogastric Vein, Left M Femoral Vein, Right N Femoral Vein, Left P Greater Saphenous Vein, Right Q Greater Saphenous Vein, Left R Lesser Saphenous Vein, Right S Lesser Saphenous Vein, Left T Foot Vein, Right V Foot Vein, Left	Ø Open 3 Percutaneous 4 Percutaneous Endoscopic	Z No Device	X Diagnostic Z No Qualifier
Y Lower Vein	Ø Open 3 Percutaneous 4 Percutaneous Endoscopic	Z No Device	C Hemorrhoidal Plexus X Diagnostic Z No Qualifier

AHA: 2Ø14, 1Q, 1Ø

Ø Medical and Surgical
6 Lower Veins
C Extirpation Taking or cutting out solid matter from a body part

Body Part Character 4	Approach Character 5	Device Character 6	Qualifier Character 7
Ø Inferior Vena Cava 1 Splenic Vein 2 Gastric Vein 3 Esophageal Vein 4 Hepatic Vein 5 Superior Mesenteric Vein 6 Inferior Mesenteric Vein 7 Colic Vein 8 Portal Vein 9 Renal Vein, Right B Renal Vein, Left C Common Iliac Vein, Right D Common Iliac Vein, Left F External Iliac Vein, Right G External Iliac Vein, Left H Hypogastric Vein, Right J Hypogastric Vein, Left M Femoral Vein, Right N Femoral Vein, Left P Greater Saphenous Vein, Right Q Greater Saphenous Vein, Left R Lesser Saphenous Vein, Right S Lesser Saphenous Vein, Left T Foot Vein, Right V Foot Vein, Left Y Lower Vein	Ø Open 3 Percutaneous 4 Percutaneous Endoscopic	Z No Device	Z No Qualifier

Ø Medical and Surgical
6 Lower Veins
D Extraction Pulling or stripping out or off all or a portion of a body part by the use of force

Body Part Character 4	Approach Character 5	Device Character 6	Qualifier Character 7
M Femoral Vein, Right N Femoral Vein, Left P Greater Saphenous Vein, Right Q Greater Saphenous Vein, Left R Lesser Saphenous Vein, Right S Lesser Saphenous Vein, Left T Foot Vein, Right V Foot Vein, Left Y Lower Vein	Ø Open 3 Percutaneous 4 Percutaneous Endoscopic	Z No Device	Z No Qualifier

Ø Medical and Surgical
6 Lower Veins
H Insertion Putting in a nonbiological appliance that monitors, assists, performs, or prevents a physiological function but does not physically take the place of a body part

Body Part Character 4	Approach Character 5	Device Character 6	Qualifier Character 7
Ø Inferior Vena Cava	Ø Open 3 Percutaneous	3 Infusion Device	T Via Umbilical Vein Z No Qualifier
Ø Inferior Vena Cava	Ø Open 3 Percutaneous	D Intraluminal Device	Z No Qualifier
Ø Inferior Vena Cava	4 Percutaneous Endoscopic	3 Infusion Device D Intraluminal Device	Z No Qualifier
1 Splenic Vein 2 Gastric Vein 3 Esophageal Vein 4 Hepatic Vein 5 Superior Mesenteric Vein 6 Inferior Mesenteric Vein 7 Colic Vein 8 Portal Vein 9 Renal Vein, Right B Renal Vein, Left C Common Iliac Vein, Right D Common Iliac Vein, Left F External Iliac Vein, Right G External Iliac Vein, Left H Hypogastric Vein, Right J Hypogastric Vein, Left M Femoral Vein, Right N Femoral Vein, Left P Greater Saphenous Vein, Right Q Greater Saphenous Vein, Left R Lesser Saphenous Vein, Right S Lesser Saphenous Vein, Left T Foot Vein, Right V Foot Vein, Left	Ø Open 3 Percutaneous 4 Percutaneous Endoscopic	3 Infusion Device D Intraluminal Device	Z No Qualifier
Y Lower Vein	Ø Open 3 Percutaneous 4 Percutaneous Endoscopic	2 Monitoring Device 3 Infusion Device D Intraluminal Device	Z No Qualifier

DRG_NONOR Ø6H[M,N]33Z
Non-OR Ø6HØ43Z
Non-OR Ø6HØ[Ø,3]3[T,Z]
Non-OR Ø6HY[Ø,3,4]3Z
Non-OR Ø6H[1,2,3,4,5,6,7,8,9,B,C,D,F,G,H,J,P,Q,R,S,T,V][Ø,3,4]3Z
Non-OR Ø6H[M,N][Ø,4]3Z
AHA: 2Ø13, 3Q, 18

No Procedure Combinations Specified
Combo-only Ø6H[M,N]33Z

Ø Medical and Surgical
6 Lower Veins
J Inspection Visually and/or manually exploring a body part

Body Part Character 4	Approach Character 5	Device Character 6	Qualifier Character 7
Y Lower Vein	Ø Open 3 Percutaneous 4 Percutaneous Endoscopic X External	Z No Device	Z No Qualifier

Non-OR Ø6JYXZZ

Ø Medical and Surgical
6 Lower Veins
L Occlusion Completely closing an orifice or the lumen of a tubular body part

Body Part Character 4	Approach Character 5	Device Character 6	Qualifier Character 7
Ø Inferior Vena Cava **1** Splenic Vein **2** Gastric Vein **3** Esophageal Vein **4** Hepatic Vein **5** Superior Mesenteric Vein **6** Inferior Mesenteric Vein **7** Colic Vein **8** Portal Vein **9** Renal Vein, Right **B** Renal Vein, Left **C** Common Iliac Vein, Right **D** Common Iliac Vein, Left **F** External Iliac Vein, Right **G** External Iliac Vein, Left **H** Hypogastric Vein, Right **J** Hypogastric Vein, Left **M** Femoral Vein, Right **N** Femoral Vein, Left **P** Greater Saphenous Vein, Right **Q** Greater Saphenous Vein, Left **R** Lesser Saphenous Vein, Right **S** Lesser Saphenous Vein, Left **T** Foot Vein, Right **V** Foot Vein, Left	**Ø** Open **3** Percutaneous **4** Percutaneous Endoscopic	**C** Extraluminal Device **D** Intraluminal Device **Z** No Device	**Z** No Qualifier
Y Lower Vein	**Ø** Open **3** Percutaneous **4** Percutaneous Endoscopic	**C** Extraluminal Device **D** Intraluminal Device **Z** No Device	**C** Hemorrhoidal Plexus **Z** No Qualifier

AHA: 2Ø13, 4Q, 112

Ø Medical and Surgical
6 Lower Veins
N Release Freeing a body part from an abnormal physical constraint

Body Part Character 4	Approach Character 5	Device Character 6	Qualifier Character 7
Ø Inferior Vena Cava **1** Splenic Vein **2** Gastric Vein **3** Esophageal Vein **4** Hepatic Vein **5** Superior Mesenteric Vein **6** Inferior Mesenteric Vein **7** Colic Vein **8** Portal Vein **9** Renal Vein, Right **B** Renal Vein, Left **C** Common Iliac Vein, Right **D** Common Iliac Vein, Left **F** External Iliac Vein, Right **G** External Iliac Vein, Left **H** Hypogastric Vein, Right **J** Hypogastric Vein, Left **M** Femoral Vein, Right **N** Femoral Vein, Left **P** Greater Saphenous Vein, Right **Q** Greater Saphenous Vein, Left **R** Lesser Saphenous Vein, Right **S** Lesser Saphenous Vein, Left **T** Foot Vein, Right **V** Foot Vein, Left **Y** Lower Vein	**Ø** Open **3** Percutaneous **4** Percutaneous Endoscopic	**Z** No Device	**Z** No Qualifier

Ø Medical and Surgical
6 Lower Veins
P Removal Taking out or off a device from a body part

Body Part Character 4	Approach Character 5	Device Character 6	Qualifier Character 7
Y Lower Vein	Ø Open 3 Percutaneous 4 Percutaneous Endoscopic	Ø Drainage Device 2 Monitoring Device 3 Infusion Device 7 Autologous Tissue Substitute C Extraluminal Device D Intraluminal Device J Synthetic Substitute K Nonautologous Tissue Substitute	Z No Qualifier
Y Lower Vein	X External	Ø Drainage Device 2 Monitoring Device 3 Infusion Device D Intraluminal Device	Z No Qualifier

Non-OR Ø6PYX[Ø,2,3,D]Z

Ø Medical and Surgical
6 Lower Veins
Q Repair Restoring, to the extent possible, a body part to its normal anatomic structure and function

Body Part Character 4	Approach Character 5	Device Character 6	Qualifier Character 7
Ø Inferior Vena Cava 1 Splenic Vein 2 Gastric Vein 3 Esophageal Vein 4 Hepatic Vein 5 Superior Mesenteric Vein 6 Inferior Mesenteric Vein 7 Colic Vein 8 Portal Vein 9 Renal Vein, Right B Renal Vein, Left C Common Iliac Vein, Right D Common Iliac Vein, Left F External Iliac Vein, Right G External Iliac Vein, Left H Hypogastric Vein, Right J Hypogastric Vein, Left M Femoral Vein, Right N Femoral Vein, Left P Greater Saphenous Vein, Right Q Greater Saphenous Vein, Left R Lesser Saphenous Vein, Right S Lesser Saphenous Vein, Left T Foot Vein, Right V Foot Vein, Left Y Lower Vein	Ø Open 3 Percutaneous 4 Percutaneous Endoscopic	Z No Device	Z No Qualifier

Ø **Medical and Surgical**
6 **Lower Veins**
R **Replacement** Putting in or on biological or synthetic material that physically takes the place and/or function of all or a portion of a body part

Body Part Character 4	Approach Character 5	Device Character 6	Qualifier Character 7
Ø Inferior Vena Cava 1 Splenic Vein 2 Gastric Vein 3 Esophageal Vein 4 Hepatic Vein 5 Superior Mesenteric Vein 6 Inferior Mesenteric Vein 7 Colic Vein 8 Portal Vein 9 Renal Vein, Right B Renal Vein, Left C Common Iliac Vein, Right D Common Iliac Vein, Left F External Iliac Vein, Right G External Iliac Vein, Left H Hypogastric Vein, Right J Hypogastric Vein, Left M Femoral Vein, Right N Femoral Vein, Left P Greater Saphenous Vein, Right Q Greater Saphenous Vein, Left R Lesser Saphenous Vein, Right S Lesser Saphenous Vein, Left T Foot Vein, Right V Foot Vein, Left Y Lower Vein	Ø Open 4 Percutaneous Endoscopic	7 Autologous Tissue Substitute J Synthetic Substitute K Nonautologous Tissue Substitute	Z No Qualifier

Ø **Medical and Surgical**
6 **Lower Veins**
S **Reposition** Moving to its normal location or other suitable location all or a portion of a body part

Body Part Character 4	Approach Character 5	Device Character 6	Qualifier Character 7
Ø Inferior Vena Cava 1 Splenic Vein 2 Gastric Vein 3 Esophageal Vein 4 Hepatic Vein 5 Superior Mesenteric Vein 6 Inferior Mesenteric Vein 7 Colic Vein 8 Portal Vein 9 Renal Vein, Right B Renal Vein, Left C Common Iliac Vein, Right D Common Iliac Vein, Left F External Iliac Vein, Right G External Iliac Vein, Left H Hypogastric Vein, Right J Hypogastric Vein, Left M Femoral Vein, Right N Femoral Vein, Left P Greater Saphenous Vein, Right Q Greater Saphenous Vein, Left R Lesser Saphenous Vein, Right S Lesser Saphenous Vein, Left T Foot Vein, Right V Foot Vein, Left Y Lower Vein	Ø Open 3 Percutaneous 4 Percutaneous Endoscopic	Z No Device	Z No Qualifier

0 Medical and Surgical
6 Lower Veins
U Supplement Putting in or on biological or synthetic material that physically reinforces and/or augments the function of a portion of a body part

Body Part Character 4	Approach Character 5	Device Character 6	Qualifier Character 7
0 Inferior Vena Cava	0 Open	7 Autologous Tissue Substitute	Z No Qualifier
1 Splenic Vein	3 Percutaneous	J Synthetic Substitute	
2 Gastric Vein	4 Percutaneous Endoscopic	K Nonautologous Tissue Substitute	
3 Esophageal Vein			
4 Hepatic Vein			
5 Superior Mesenteric Vein			
6 Inferior Mesenteric Vein			
7 Colic Vein			
8 Portal Vein			
9 Renal Vein, Right			
B Renal Vein, Left			
C Common Iliac Vein, Right			
D Common Iliac Vein, Left			
F External Iliac Vein, Right			
G External Iliac Vein, Left			
H Hypogastric Vein, Right			
J Hypogastric Vein, Left			
M Femoral Vein, Right			
N Femoral Vein, Left			
P Greater Saphenous Vein, Right			
Q Greater Saphenous Vein, Left			
R Lesser Saphenous Vein, Right			
S Lesser Saphenous Vein, Left			
T Foot Vein, Right			
V Foot Vein, Left			
Y Lower Vein			

0 Medical and Surgical
6 Lower Veins
V Restriction Partially closing an orifice or the lumen of a tubular body part

Body Part Character 4	Approach Character 5	Device Character 6	Qualifier Character 7
0 Inferior Vena Cava	0 Open	C Extraluminal Device	Z No Qualifier
1 Splenic Vein	3 Percutaneous	D Intraluminal Device	
2 Gastric Vein	4 Percutaneous Endoscopic	Z No Device	
3 Esophageal Vein			
4 Hepatic Vein			
5 Superior Mesenteric Vein			
6 Inferior Mesenteric Vein			
7 Colic Vein			
8 Portal Vein			
9 Renal Vein, Right			
B Renal Vein, Left			
C Common Iliac Vein, Right			
D Common Iliac Vein, Left			
F External Iliac Vein, Right			
G External Iliac Vein, Left			
H Hypogastric Vein, Right			
J Hypogastric Vein, Left			
M Femoral Vein, Right			
N Femoral Vein, Left			
P Greater Saphenous Vein, Right			
Q Greater Saphenous Vein, Left			
R Lesser Saphenous Vein, Right			
S Lesser Saphenous Vein, Left			
T Foot Vein, Right			
V Foot Vein, Left			
Y Lower Vein			

Ø Medical and Surgical
6 Lower Veins
W Revision Correcting, to the extent possible, a portion of a malfunctioning device or the position of a displaced device

Body Part Character 4	Approach Character 5	Device Character 6	Qualifier Character 7
Y Lower Vein	**Ø** Open **3** Percutaneous **4** Percutaneous Endoscopic **X** External	**Ø** Drainage Device **2** Monitoring Device **3** Infusion Device **7** Autologous Tissue Substitute **C** Extraluminal Device **D** Intraluminal Device **J** Synthetic Substitute **K** Nonautologous Tissue Substitute	**Z** No Qualifier

Non-OR Ø6WYX[Ø,2,3,7,C,D,J,K]Z

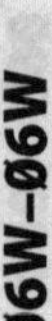

Lymphatic and Hemic Systems 072–07Y

0 Medical and Surgical
7 Lymphatic and Hemic Systems
2 Change Taking out or off a device from a body part and putting back an identical or similar device in or on the same body part without cutting or puncturing the skin or a mucous membrane

Body Part Character 4	Approach Character 5	Device Character 6	Qualifier Character 7
K Thoracic Duct L Cisterna Chyli M Thymus N Lymphatic P Spleen T Bone Marrow	X External	0 Drainage Device Y Other Device	Z No Qualifier

Non-OR For all body part, approach, device, and qualifier values

0 Medical and Surgical
7 Lymphatic and Hemic Systems
5 Destruction Physical eradication of all or a portion of a body part by the direct use of energy, force, or a destructive agent

Body Part Character 4	Approach Character 5	Device Character 6	Qualifier Character 7
0 Lymphatic, Head 1 Lymphatic, Right Neck 2 Lymphatic, Left Neck 3 Lymphatic, Right Upper Extremity 4 Lymphatic, Left Upper Extremity 5 Lymphatic, Right Axillary 6 Lymphatic, Left Axillary 7 Lymphatic, Thorax 8 Lymphatic, Internal Mammary, Right 9 Lymphatic, Internal Mammary, Left B Lymphatic, Mesenteric C Lymphatic, Pelvis D Lymphatic, Aortic F Lymphatic, Right Lower Extremity G Lymphatic, Left Lower Extremity H Lymphatic, Right Inguinal J Lymphatic, Left Inguinal K Thoracic Duct L Cisterna Chyli M Thymus P Spleen	0 Open 3 Percutaneous 4 Percutaneous Endoscopic	Z No Device	Z No Qualifier

Ø Medical and Surgical
7 Lymphatic and Hemic Systems
9 Drainage Taking or letting out fluids and/or gases from a body part

Body Part Character 4	Approach Character 5	Device Character 6	Qualifier Character 7
Ø Lymphatic, Head **1** Lymphatic, Right Neck **2** Lymphatic, Left Neck **3** Lymphatic, Right Upper Extremity **4** Lymphatic, Left Upper Extremity **5** Lymphatic, Right Axillary **6** Lymphatic, Left Axillary **7** Lymphatic, Thorax **8** Lymphatic, Internal Mammary, Right **9** Lymphatic, Internal Mammary, Left **B** Lymphatic, Mesenteric **C** Lymphatic, Pelvis **D** Lymphatic, Aortic **F** Lymphatic, Right Lower Extremity **G** Lymphatic, Left Lower Extremity **H** Lymphatic, Right Inguinal **J** Lymphatic, Left Inguinal **K** Thoracic Duct **L** Cisterna Chyli	**Ø** Open **3** Percutaneous **4** Percutaneous Endoscopic	**Ø** Drainage Device	**Z** No Qualifier
M Thymus **P** Spleen **T** Bone Marrow	**Ø** Open **3** Percutaneous **4** Percutaneous Endoscopic	**Ø** Drainage Device	**Z** No Qualifier
Ø Lymphatic, Head **1** Lymphatic, Right Neck **2** Lymphatic, Left Neck **3** Lymphatic, Right Upper Extremity **4** Lymphatic, Left Upper Extremity **5** Lymphatic, Right Axillary **6** Lymphatic, Left Axillary **7** Lymphatic, Thorax **8** Lymphatic, Internal Mammary, Right **9** Lymphatic, Internal Mammary, Left **B** Lymphatic, Mesenteric **C** Lymphatic, Pelvis **D** Lymphatic, Aortic **F** Lymphatic, Right Lower Extremity **G** Lymphatic, Left Lower Extremity **H** Lymphatic, Right Inguinal **J** Lymphatic, Left Inguinal **K** Thoracic Duct **L** Cisterna Chyli **M** Thymus **P** Spleen **T** Bone Marrow	**Ø** Open **3** Percutaneous **4** Percutaneous Endoscopic	**Z** No Device	**X** Diagnostic **Z** No Qualifier

Non-OR Ø79P[3,4]ØZ
Non-OR Ø79T[Ø,3,4]ØZ
Non-OR Ø79P[3,4]Z[X,Z]
Non-OR Ø79T[Ø,3,4]Z[X,Z]
AHA: 2Ø13, 4Q, 111

0 Medical and Surgical
7 Lymphatic and Hemic Systems
B Excision Cutting out or off, without replacement, a portion of a body part

Body Part Character 4	Approach Character 5	Device Character 6	Qualifier Character 7
0 Lymphatic, Head 1 Lymphatic, Right Neck 2 Lymphatic, Left Neck 3 Lymphatic, Right Upper Extremity 4 Lymphatic, Left Upper Extremity 5 Lymphatic, Right Axillary 6 Lymphatic, Left Axillary 7 Lymphatic, Thorax 8 Lymphatic, Internal Mammary, Right 9 Lymphatic, Internal Mammary, Left B Lymphatic, Mesenteric C Lymphatic, Pelvis D Lymphatic, Aortic F Lymphatic, Right Lower Extremity G Lymphatic, Left Lower Extremity H Lymphatic, Right Inguinal ⊞ J Lymphatic, Left Inguinal ⊞ K Thoracic Duct L Cisterna Chyli M Thymus P Spleen	0 Open 3 Percutaneous 4 Percutaneous Endoscopic	Z No Device	X Diagnostic Z No Qualifier

Non-OR 07BP[3,4]ZX
AHA: 2014, 1Q, 20, 26

See Appendix I for Procedure Combinations
⊞ 07B[H,J][0,4]ZZ

0 Medical and Surgical
7 Lymphatic and Hemic Systems
C Extirpation Taking or cutting out solid matter from a body part

Body Part Character 4	Approach Character 5	Device Character 6	Qualifier Character 7
0 Lymphatic, Head 1 Lymphatic, Right Neck 2 Lymphatic, Left Neck 3 Lymphatic, Right Upper Extremity 4 Lymphatic, Left Upper Extremity 5 Lymphatic, Right Axillary 6 Lymphatic, Left Axillary 7 Lymphatic, Thorax 8 Lymphatic, Internal Mammary, Right 9 Lymphatic, Internal Mammary, Left B Lymphatic, Mesenteric C Lymphatic, Pelvis D Lymphatic, Aortic F Lymphatic, Right Lower Extremity G Lymphatic, Left Lower Extremity H Lymphatic, Right Inguinal J Lymphatic, Left Inguinal K Thoracic Duct L Cisterna Chyli M Thymus P Spleen	0 Open 3 Percutaneous 4 Percutaneous Endoscopic	Z No Device	Z No Qualifier

Non-OR 07CP[3,4]ZZ

0 Medical and Surgical
7 Lymphatic and Hemic Systems
D Extraction Pulling or stripping out or off all or a portion of a body part by the use of force

Body Part Character 4	Approach Character 5	Device Character 6	Qualifier Character 7
Q Bone Marrow, Sternum R Bone Marrow, Iliac S Bone Marrow, Vertebral	0 Open 3 Percutaneous	Z No Device	X Diagnostic Z No Qualifier

Non-OR For all body part, approach, device, and qualifier values

0 Medical and Surgical
7 Lymphatic and Hemic Systems
H Insertion Putting in a nonbiological appliance that monitors, assists, performs, or prevents a physiological function but does not physically take the place of a body part

Body Part Character 4	Approach Character 5	Device Character 6	Qualifier Character 7
K Thoracic Duct L Cisterna Chyli M Thymus N Lymphatic P Spleen	0 Open 3 Percutaneous 4 Percutaneous Endoscopic	3 Infusion Device	Z No Qualifier

Non-OR For all body part, approach, device, and qualifier values

0 Medical and Surgical
7 Lymphatic and Hemic Systems
J Inspection Visually and/or manually exploring a body part

Body Part Character 4	Approach Character 5	Device Character 6	Qualifier Character 7
K Thoracic Duct L Cisterna Chyli M Thymus T Bone Marrow	0 Open 3 Percutaneous 4 Percutaneous Endoscopic	Z No Device	Z No Qualifier
N Lymphatic P Spleen	0 Open 3 Percutaneous 4 Percutaneous Endoscopic X External	Z No Device	Z No Qualifier

Non-OR 07JT[0,3,4]ZZ
Non-OR 07JNXZZ
Non-OR 07JP[3,4,X]ZZ

0 Medical and Surgical
7 Lymphatic and Hemic Systems
L Occlusion Completely closing an orifice or the lumen of a tubular body part

Body Part Character 4	Approach Character 5	Device Character 6	Qualifier Character 7
0 Lymphatic, Head 1 Lymphatic, Right Neck 2 Lymphatic, Left Neck 3 Lymphatic, Right Upper Extremity 4 Lymphatic, Left Upper Extremity 5 Lymphatic, Right Axillary 6 Lymphatic, Left Axillary 7 Lymphatic, Thorax 8 Lymphatic, Internal Mammary, Right 9 Lymphatic, Internal Mammary, Left B Lymphatic, Mesenteric C Lymphatic, Pelvis D Lymphatic, Aortic F Lymphatic, Right Lower Extremity G Lymphatic, Left Lower Extremity H Lymphatic, Right Inguinal J Lymphatic, Left Inguinal K Thoracic Duct L Cisterna Chyli	0 Open 3 Percutaneous 4 Percutaneous Endoscopic	C Extraluminal Device D Intraluminal Device Z No Device	Z No Qualifier

0 Medical and Surgical
7 Lymphatic and Hemic Systems
N Release Freeing a body part from an abnormal physical constraint

Body Part Character 4	Approach Character 5	Device Character 6	Qualifier Character 7
0 Lymphatic, Head 1 Lymphatic, Right Neck 2 Lymphatic, Left Neck 3 Lymphatic, Right Upper Extremity 4 Lymphatic, Left Upper Extremity 5 Lymphatic, Right Axillary 6 Lymphatic, Left Axillary 7 Lymphatic, Thorax 8 Lymphatic, Internal Mammary, Right 9 Lymphatic, Internal Mammary, Left B Lymphatic, Mesenteric C Lymphatic, Pelvis D Lymphatic, Aortic F Lymphatic, Right Lower Extremity G Lymphatic, Left Lower Extremity H Lymphatic, Right Inguinal J Lymphatic, Left Inguinal K Thoracic Duct L Cisterna Chyli M Thymus P Spleen	0 Open 3 Percutaneous 4 Percutaneous Endoscopic	Z No Device	Z No Qualifier

0 Medical and Surgical
7 Lymphatic and Hemic Systems
P Removal Taking out or off a device from a body part

Body Part Character 4	Approach Character 5	Device Character 6	Qualifier Character 7
K Thoracic Duct L Cisterna Chyli N Lymphatic	0 Open 3 Percutaneous 4 Percutaneous Endoscopic	0 Drainage Device 3 Infusion Device 7 Autologous Tissue Substitute C Extraluminal Device D Intraluminal Device J Synthetic Substitute K Nonautologous Tissue Substitute	Z No Qualifier
K Thoracic Duct L Cisterna Chyli N Lymphatic	X External	0 Drainage Device 3 Infusion Device D Intraluminal Device	Z No Qualifier
M Thymus P Spleen	0 Open 3 Percutaneous 4 Percutaneous Endoscopic X External	0 Drainage Device 3 Infusion Device	Z No Qualifier
T Bone Marrow	0 Open 3 Percutaneous 4 Percutaneous Endoscopic X External	0 Drainage Device	Z No Qualifier

Non-OR 07P[K,L,N]X[0,3,D]Z
Non-OR 07P[M,P]X[0,3]Z
Non-OR 07PT[0,3,4,X]0Z

Ø Medical and Surgical
7 Lymphatic and Hemic Systems
Q Repair Restoring, to the extent possible, a body part to its normal anatomic structure and function

Body Part Character 4	Approach Character 5	Device Character 6	Qualifier Character 7
Ø Lymphatic, Head **1** Lymphatic, Right Neck **2** Lymphatic, Left Neck **3** Lymphatic, Right Upper Extremity **4** Lymphatic, Left Upper Extremity **5** Lymphatic, Right Axillary **6** Lymphatic, Left Axillary **7** Lymphatic, Thorax **8** Lymphatic, Internal Mammary, Right **9** Lymphatic, Internal Mammary, Left **B** Lymphatic, Mesenteric **C** Lymphatic, Pelvis **D** Lymphatic, Aortic **F** Lymphatic, Right Lower Extremity **G** Lymphatic, Left Lower Extremity **H** Lymphatic, Right Inguinal **J** Lymphatic, Left Inguinal **K** Thoracic Duct **L** Cisterna Chyli **M** Thymus **P** Spleen	**Ø** Open **3** Percutaneous **4** Percutaneous Endoscopic	**Z** No Device	**Z** No Qualifier

Ø Medical and Surgical
7 Lymphatic and Hemic Systems
S Reposition Moving to its normal location or other suitable location all or a portion of a body part

Body Part Character 4	Approach Character 5	Device Character 6	Qualifier Character 7
M Thymus **P** Spleen	**Ø** Open	**Z** No Device	**Z** No Qualifier

Ø Medical and Surgical
7 Lymphatic and Hemic Systems
T Resection Cutting out or off, without replacement, all of a body part

Body Part Character 4	Approach Character 5	Device Character 6	Qualifier Character 7
Ø Lymphatic, Head **1** Lymphatic, Right Neck **2** Lymphatic, Left Neck **3** Lymphatic, Right Upper Extremity **4** Lymphatic, Left Upper Extremity **5** Lymphatic, Right Axillary ⊞ **6** Lymphatic, Left Axillary ⊞ **7** Lymphatic, Thorax ⊞ **8** Lymphatic, Internal Mammary, Right ⊞ **9** Lymphatic, Internal Mammary, Left ⊞ **B** Lymphatic, Mesenteric **C** Lymphatic, Pelvis **D** Lymphatic, Aortic **F** Lymphatic, Right Lower Extremity **G** Lymphatic, Left Lower Extremity **H** Lymphatic, Right Inguinal **J** Lymphatic, Left Inguinal **K** Thoracic Duct **L** Cisterna Chyli **M** Thymus **P** Spleen	**Ø** Open **4** Percutaneous Endoscopic	**Z** No Device	**Z** No Qualifier

See Appendix I for Procedure Combinations

⊞ Ø7T[5,6,7,8,9]ØZZ

0 Medical and Surgical
7 Lymphatic and Hemic Systems
U Supplement Putting in or on biological or synthetic material that physically reinforces and/or augments the function of a portion of a body part

Body Part Character 4	Approach Character 5	Device Character 6	Qualifier Character 7
0 Lymphatic, Head 1 Lymphatic, Right Neck 2 Lymphatic, Left Neck 3 Lymphatic, Right Upper Extremity 4 Lymphatic, Left Upper Extremity 5 Lymphatic, Right Axillary 6 Lymphatic, Left Axillary 7 Lymphatic, Thorax 8 Lymphatic, Internal Mammary, Right 9 Lymphatic, Internal Mammary, Left B Lymphatic, Mesenteric C Lymphatic, Pelvis D Lymphatic, Aortic F Lymphatic, Right Lower Extremity G Lymphatic, Left Lower Extremity H Lymphatic, Right Inguinal J Lymphatic, Left Inguinal K Thoracic Duct L Cisterna Chyli	0 Open 4 Percutaneous Endoscopic	7 Autologous Tissue Substitute J Synthetic Substitute K Nonautologous Tissue Substitute	Z No Qualifier

0 Medical and Surgical
7 Lymphatic and Hemic Systems
V Restriction Partially closing an orifice or the lumen of a tubular body part

Body Part Character 4	Approach Character 5	Device Character 6	Qualifier Character 7
0 Lymphatic, Head 1 Lymphatic, Right Neck 2 Lymphatic, Left Neck 3 Lymphatic, Right Upper Extremity 4 Lymphatic, Left Upper Extremity 5 Lymphatic, Right Axillary 6 Lymphatic, Left Axillary 7 Lymphatic, Thorax 8 Lymphatic, Internal Mammary, Right 9 Lymphatic, Internal Mammary, Left B Lymphatic, Mesenteric C Lymphatic, Pelvis D Lymphatic, Aortic F Lymphatic, Right Lower Extremity G Lymphatic, Left Lower Extremity H Lymphatic, Right Inguinal J Lymphatic, Left Inguinal K Thoracic Duct L Cisterna Chyli	0 Open 3 Percutaneous 4 Percutaneous Endoscopic	C Extraluminal Device D Intraluminal Device Z No Device	Z No Qualifier

0 Medical and Surgical
7 Lymphatic and Hemic Systems
W Revision Correcting, to the extent possible, a portion of a malfunctioning device or the position of a displaced device

Body Part Character 4	Approach Character 5	Device Character 6	Qualifier Character 7
K Thoracic Duct L Cisterna Chyli N Lymphatic	0 Open 3 Percutaneous 4 Percutaneous Endoscopic X External	0 Drainage Device 3 Infusion Device 7 Autologous Tissue Substitute C Extraluminal Device D Intraluminal Device J Synthetic Substitute K Nonautologous Tissue Substitute	Z No Qualifier
M Thymus P Spleen	0 Open 3 Percutaneous 4 Percutaneous Endoscopic X External	0 Drainage Device 3 Infusion Device	Z No Qualifier
T Bone Marrow	0 Open 3 Percutaneous 4 Percutaneous Endoscopic X External	0 Drainage Device	Z No Qualifier

Non-OR 07W[K,L,N]X[0,3,7,C,D,J,K]Z
Non-OR 07W[M,P]X[0,3]Z
Non-OR 07WT[0,3,4,X]0Z

Ø Medical and Surgical
7 Lymphatic and Hemic Systems
Y Transplantation Putting in or on all or a portion of a living body part taken from another individual or animal to physically take the place and/or function of all or a portion of a similar body part

Body Part Character 4	Approach Character 5	Device Character 6	Qualifier Character 7
M Thymus **P** Spleen	**Ø** Open	**Z** No Device	**Ø** Allogeneic **1** Syngeneic **2** Zooplastic

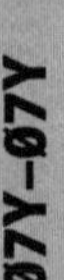

Eye 080–08X

0 Medical and Surgical
8 Eye
0 Alteration Modifying the anatomic structure of a body part without affecting the function of the body part

Body Part Character 4	Approach Character 5	Device Character 6	Qualifier Character 7
N Upper Eyelid, Right **P** Upper Eyelid, Left **Q** Lower Eyelid, Right **R** Lower Eyelid, Left	**0** Open **3** Percutaneous **X** External	**7** Autologous Tissue Substitute **J** Synthetic Substitute **K** Nonautologous Tissue Substitute **Z** No Device	**Z** No Qualifier

Non-OR For all body part, approach, device, and qualifier values

0 Medical and Surgical
8 Eye
1 Bypass Altering the route of passage of the contents of a tubular body part

Body Part Character 4	Approach Character 5	Device Character 6	Qualifier Character 7
2 Anterior Chamber, Right **3** Anterior Chamber, Left	**3** Percutaneous	**J** Synthetic Substitute **K** Nonautologous Tissue Substitute **Z** No Device	**4** Sclera
X Lacrimal Duct, Right **Y** Lacrimal Duct, Left	**0** Open **3** Percutaneous	**J** Synthetic Substitute **K** Nonautologous Tissue Substitute **Z** No Device	**3** Nasal Cavity

0 Medical and Surgical
8 Eye
2 Change Taking out or off a device from a body part and putting back an identical or similar device in or on the same body part without cutting or puncturing the skin or a mucous membrane

Body Part Character 4	Approach Character 5	Device Character 6	Qualifier Character 7
0 Eye, Right **1** Eye, Left	**X** External	**0** Drainage Device **Y** Other Device	**Z** No Qualifier

Non-OR For all body part, approach, device, and qualifier values

Ø Medical and Surgical
8 Eye
5 Destruction Physical eradication of all or a portion of a body part by the direct use of energy, force, or a destructive agent

Body Part Character 4	Approach Character 5	Device Character 6	Qualifier Character 7
Ø Eye, Right **1** Eye, Left **6** Sclera, Right **7** Sclera, Left **8** Cornea, Right **9** Cornea, Left **S** Conjunctiva, Right **T** Conjunctiva, Left	**X** External	**Z** No Device	**Z** No Qualifier
2 Anterior Chamber, Right **3** Anterior Chamber, Left **4** Vitreous, Right **5** Vitreous, Left **C** Iris, Right **D** Iris, Left **E** Retina, Right **F** Retina, Left **G** Retinal Vessel, Right **H** Retinal Vessel, Left **J** Lens, Right **K** Lens, Left	**3** Percutaneous	**Z** No Device	**Z** No Qualifier
A Choroid, Right **B** Choroid, Left **L** Extraocular Muscle, Right **M** Extraocular Muscle, Left **V** Lacrimal Gland, Right **W** Lacrimal Gland, Left	**Ø** Open **3** Percutaneous	**Z** No Device	**Z** No Qualifier
N Upper Eyelid, Right **P** Upper Eyelid, Left **Q** Lower Eyelid, Right **R** Lower Eyelid, Left	**Ø** Open **3** Percutaneous **X** External	**Z** No Device	**Z** No Qualifier
X Lacrimal Duct, Right **Y** Lacrimal Duct, Left	**Ø** Open **3** Percutaneous **7** Via Natural or Artificial Opening **8** Via Natural or Artificial Opening Endoscopic	**Z** No Device	**Z** No Qualifier

Ø Medical and Surgical
8 Eye
7 Dilation Expanding an orifice or the lumen of a tubular body part

Body Part Character 4	Approach Character 5	Device Character 6	Qualifier Character 7
X Lacrimal Duct, Right **Y** Lacrimal Duct, Left	**Ø** Open **3** Percutaneous **7** Via Natural or Artificial Opening **8** Via Natural or Artificial Opening Endoscopic	**D** Intraluminal Device **Z** No Device	**Z** No Qualifier

Ø Medical and Surgical
8 Eye
9 Drainage Taking or letting out fluids and/or gases from a body part

Body Part Character 4	Approach Character 5	Device Character 6	Qualifier Character 7
Ø Eye, Right **1** Eye, Left **6** Sclera, Right **7** Sclera, Left **8** Cornea, Right **9** Cornea, Left **S** Conjunctiva, Right **T** Conjunctiva, Left	**X** External	**Ø** Drainage Device	**Z** No Qualifier

Ø89 Continued on next page

Ø Medical and Surgical
8 Eye
9 Drainage Taking or letting out fluids and/or gases from a body part

Ø89 Continued

Body Part Character 4	Approach Character 5	Device Character 6	Qualifier Character 7
Ø Eye, Right **1** Eye, Left **6** Sclera, Right **7** Sclera, Left **8** Cornea, Right **9** Cornea, Left **S** Conjunctiva, Right **T** Conjunctiva, Left	**X** External	**Z** No Device	**X** Diagnostic **Z** No Qualifier
2 Anterior Chamber, Right **3** Anterior Chamber, Left **4** Vitreous, Right **5** Vitreous, Left **C** Iris, Right **D** Iris, Left **E** Retina, Right **F** Retina, Left **G** Retinal Vessel, Right **H** Retinal Vessel, Left **J** Lens, Right **K** Lens, Left	**3** Percutaneous	**Ø** Drainage Device	**Z** No Qualifier
2 Anterior Chamber, Right **3** Anterior Chamber, Left **4** Vitreous, Right **5** Vitreous, Left **C** Iris, Right **D** Iris, Left **E** Retina, Right **F** Retina, Left **G** Retinal Vessel, Right **H** Retinal Vessel, Left **J** Lens, Right **K** Lens, Left	**3** Percutaneous	**Z** No Device	**X** Diagnostic **Z** No Qualifier
A Choroid, Right **B** Choroid, Left **L** Extraocular Muscle, Right **M** Extraocular Muscle, Left **V** Lacrimal Gland, Right **W** Lacrimal Gland, Left	**Ø** Open **3** Percutaneous	**Ø** Drainage Device	**Z** No Qualifier
A Choroid, Right **B** Choroid, Left **L** Extraocular Muscle, Right **M** Extraocular Muscle, Left **V** Lacrimal Gland, Right **W** Lacrimal Gland, Left	**Ø** Open **3** Percutaneous	**Z** No Device	**X** Diagnostic **Z** No Qualifier
N Upper Eyelid, Right **P** Upper Eyelid, Left **Q** Lower Eyelid, Right **R** Lower Eyelid, Left	**Ø** Open **3** Percutaneous **X** External	**Ø** Drainage Device	**Z** No Qualifier
N Upper Eyelid, Right **P** Upper Eyelid, Left **Q** Lower Eyelid, Right **R** Lower Eyelid, Left	**Ø** Open **3** Percutaneous **X** External	**Z** No Device	**X** Diagnostic **Z** No Qualifier
X Lacrimal Duct, Right **Y** Lacrimal Duct, Left	**Ø** Open **3** Percutaneous **7** Via Natural or Artificial Opening **8** Via Natural or Artificial Opening Endoscopic	**Ø** Drainage Device	**Z** No Qualifier
X Lacrimal Duct, Right **Y** Lacrimal Duct, Left	**Ø** Open **3** Percutaneous **7** Via Natural or Artificial Opening **8** Via Natural or Artificial Opening Endoscopic	**Z** No Device	**X** Diagnostic **Z** No Qualifier

Non-OR Ø89[N,P,Q,R][Ø,3,X]ØZ
Non-OR Ø89[N,P,Q,R][Ø,3,X]ZZ

Ø Medical and Surgical
8 Eye
B Excision Cutting out or off, without replacement, a portion of a body part

Body Part Character 4	Approach Character 5	Device Character 6	Qualifier Character 7
Ø Eye, Right **1** Eye, Left **N** Upper Eyelid, Right **P** Upper Eyelid, Left **Q** Lower Eyelid, Right **R** Lower Eyelid, Left	**Ø** Open **3** Percutaneous **X** External	**Z** No Device	**X** Diagnostic **Z** No Qualifier
4 Vitreous, Right **5** Vitreous, Left **C** Iris, Right ⊞ **D** Iris, Left ⊞ **E** Retina, Right **F** Retina, Left **J** Lens, Right **K** Lens, Left	**3** Percutaneous	**Z** No Device	**X** Diagnostic **Z** No Qualifier
6 Sclera, Right ⊞ **7** Sclera, Left ⊞ **8** Cornea, Right **9** Cornea, Left **S** Conjunctiva, Right **T** Conjunctiva, Left	**X** External	**Z** No Device	**X** Diagnostic **Z** No Qualifier
A Choroid, Right **B** Choroid, Left **L** Extraocular Muscle, Right **M** Extraocular Muscle, Left **V** Lacrimal Gland, Right **W** Lacrimal Gland, Left	**Ø** Open **3** Percutaneous	**Z** No Device	**X** Diagnostic **Z** No Qualifier
X Lacrimal Duct, Right **Y** Lacrimal Duct, Left	**Ø** Open **3** Percutaneous **7** Via Natural or Artificial Opening **8** Via Natural or Artificial Opening Endoscopic	**Z** No Device	**X** Diagnostic **Z** No Qualifier

No Procedure Combinations Specified
⊞ Ø8B[C,D]3ZZ
⊞ Ø8B[6,7]XZZ

0 Medical and Surgical
8 Eye
C Extirpation Taking or cutting out solid matter from a body part

Body Part Character 4	Approach Character 5	Device Character 6	Qualifier Character 7
0 Eye, Right **1** Eye, Left **6** Sclera, Right **7** Sclera, Left **8** Cornea, Right **9** Cornea, Left **S** Conjunctiva, Right **T** Conjunctiva, Left	**X** External	**Z** No Device	**Z** No Qualifier
2 Anterior Chamber, Right **3** Anterior Chamber, Left **4** Vitreous, Right **5** Vitreous, Left **C** Iris, Right **D** Iris, Left **E** Retina, Right **F** Retina, Left **G** Retinal Vessel, Right **H** Retinal Vessel, Left **J** Lens, Right **K** Lens, Left	**3** Percutaneous **X** External	**Z** No Device	**Z** No Qualifier
A Choroid, Right **B** Choroid, Left **L** Extraocular Muscle, Right **M** Extraocular Muscle, Left **N** Upper Eyelid, Right **P** Upper Eyelid, Left **Q** Lower Eyelid, Right **R** Lower Eyelid, Left **V** Lacrimal Gland, Right **W** Lacrimal Gland, Left	**0** Open **3** Percutaneous **X** External	**Z** No Device	**Z** No Qualifier
X Lacrimal Duct, Right **Y** Lacrimal Duct, Left	**0** Open **3** Percutaneous **7** Via Natural or Artificial Opening **8** Via Natural or Artificial Opening Endoscopic	**Z** No Device	**Z** No Qualifier

Non-OR 08C[6,7]XZZ
Non-OR 08C[2,3]XZZ
Non-OR 08C[N,P,Q,R][0,3,X]ZZ

0 Medical and Surgical
8 Eye
D Extraction Pulling or stripping out or off all or a portion of a body part by the use of force

Body Part Character 4	Approach Character 5	Device Character 6	Qualifier Character 7
8 Cornea, Right **9** Cornea, Left	**X** External	**Z** No Device	**X** Diagnostic **Z** No Qualifier
J Lens, Right **K** Lens, Left	**3** Percutaneous	**Z** No Device	**Z** No Qualifier

0 Medical and Surgical
8 Eye
F Fragmentation Breaking solid matter in a body part into pieces

Body Part Character 4	Approach Character 5	Device Character 6	Qualifier Character 7
4 Vitreous, Right NC **5** Vitreous, Left NC	**3** Percutaneous **X** External	**Z** No Device	**Z** No Qualifier

Non-OR 08F[4,5]XZZ
NC 08F[4,5]XZZ

Ø Medical and Surgical
8 Eye
H Insertion Putting in a nonbiological appliance that monitors, assists, performs, or prevents a physiological function but does not physically take the place of a body part

Body Part Character 4	Approach Character 5	Device Character 6	Qualifier Character 7
Ø Eye, Right **1** Eye, Left	**Ø** Open	**5** Epiretinal Visual Prosthesis	**Z** No Qualifier
Ø Eye, Right **1** Eye, Left	**3** Percutaneous **X** External	**1** Radioactive Element **3** Infusion Device	**Z** No Qualifier

Ø Medical and Surgical
8 Eye
J Inspection Visually and/or manually exploring a body part

Body Part Character 4	Approach Character 5	Device Character 6	Qualifier Character 7
Ø Eye, Right **1** Eye, Left **J** Lens, Right **K** Lens, Left	**X** External	**Z** No Device	**Z** No Qualifier
L Extraocular Muscle, Right **M** Extraocular Muscle, Left	**Ø** Open **X** External	**Z** No Device	**Z** No Qualifier

Ø Medical and Surgical
8 Eye
L Occlusion Completely closing an orifice or the lumen of a tubular body part

Body Part Character 4	Approach Character 5	Device Character 6	Qualifier Character 7
X Lacrimal Duct, Right **Y** Lacrimal Duct, Left	**Ø** Open **3** Percutaneous	**C** Extraluminal Device **D** Intraluminal Device **Z** No Device	**Z** No Qualifier
X Lacrimal Duct, Right **Y** Lacrimal Duct, Left	**7** Via Natural or Artificial Opening **8** Via Natural or Artificial Opening Endoscopic	**D** Intraluminal Device **Z** No Device	**Z** No Qualifier

Ø Medical and Surgical
8 Eye
M Reattachment Putting back in or on all or a portion of a separated body part to its normal location or other suitable location

Body Part Character 4	Approach Character 5	Device Character 6	Qualifier Character 7
N Upper Eyelid, Right **P** Upper Eyelid, Left **Q** Lower Eyelid, Right **R** Lower Eyelid, Left	**X** External	**Z** No Device	**Z** No Qualifier

Ø **Medical and Surgical**
8 **Eye**
N **Release** Freeing a body part from an abnormal physical constraint

Body Part Character 4	Approach Character 5	Device Character 6	Qualifier Character 7
Ø Eye, Right **1** Eye, Left **6** Sclera, Right **7** Sclera, Left **8** Cornea, Right **9** Cornea, Left **S** Conjunctiva, Right **T** Conjunctiva, Left	**X** External	**Z** No Device	**Z** No Qualifier
2 Anterior Chamber, Right **3** Anterior Chamber, Left **4** Vitreous, Right **5** Vitreous, Left **C** Iris, Right **D** Iris, Left **E** Retina, Right **F** Retina, Left **G** Retinal Vessel, Right **H** Retinal Vessel, Left **J** Lens, Right **K** Lens, Left	**3** Percutaneous	**Z** No Device	**Z** No Qualifier
A Choroid, Right **B** Choroid, Left **L** Extraocular Muscle, Right **M** Extraocular Muscle, Left **V** Lacrimal Gland, Right **W** Lacrimal Gland, Left	**Ø** Open **3** Percutaneous	**Z** No Device	**Z** No Qualifier
N Upper Eyelid, Right **P** Upper Eyelid, Left **Q** Lower Eyelid, Right **R** Lower Eyelid, Left	**Ø** Open **3** Percutaneous **X** External	**Z** No Device	**Z** No Qualifier
X Lacrimal Duct, Right **Y** Lacrimal Duct, Left	**Ø** Open **3** Percutaneous **7** Via Natural or Artificial Opening **8** Via Natural or Artificial Opening Endoscopic	**Z** No Device	**Z** No Qualifier

Ø **Medical and Surgical**
8 **Eye**
P **Removal** Taking out or off a device from a body part

Body Part Character 4	Approach Character 5	Device Character 6	Qualifier Character 7
Ø Eye, Right **1** Eye, Left	**Ø** Open **3** Percutaneous **7** Via Natural or Artificial Opening **8** Via Natural or Artificial Opening Endoscopic **X** External	**Ø** Drainage Device **1** Radioactive Element **3** Infusion Device **7** Autologous Tissue Substitute **C** Extraluminal Device **D** Intraluminal Device **J** Synthetic Substitute **K** Nonautologous Tissue Substitute	**Z** No Qualifier
J Lens, Right **K** Lens, Left	**3** Percutaneous	**J** Synthetic Substitute	**Z** No Qualifier
L Extraocular Muscle, Right **M** Extraocular Muscle, Left	**Ø** Open **3** Percutaneous	**Ø** Drainage Device **7** Autologous Tissue Substitute **J** Synthetic Substitute **K** Nonautologous Tissue Substitute	**Z** No Qualifier

Non-OR Ø8PØX[Ø,3,C,D]Z
Non-OR Ø8P1X[Ø,1,3,C,D]Z

Ø Medical and Surgical
8 Eye
Q Repair Restoring, to the extent possible, a body part to its normal anatomic structure and function

Body Part Character 4	Approach Character 5	Device Character 6	Qualifier Character 7
Ø Eye, Right **1** Eye, Left **6** Sclera, Right **7** Sclera, Left **8** Cornea, Right NC **9** Cornea, Left NC **S** Conjunctiva, Right **T** Conjunctiva, Left	**X** External	**Z** No Device	**Z** No Qualifier
2 Anterior Chamber, Right **3** Anterior Chamber, Left **4** Vitreous, Right **5** Vitreous, Left **C** Iris, Right **D** Iris, Left **E** Retina, Right **F** Retina, Left **G** Retinal Vessel, Right **H** Retinal Vessel, Left **J** Lens, Right **K** Lens, Left	**3** Percutaneous	**Z** No Device	**Z** No Qualifier
A Choroid, Right **B** Choroid, Left **L** Extraocular Muscle, Right **M** Extraocular Muscle, Left **V** Lacrimal Gland, Right **W** Lacrimal Gland, Left	**Ø** Open **3** Percutaneous	**Z** No Device	**Z** No Qualifier
N Upper Eyelid, Right **P** Upper Eyelid, Left **Q** Lower Eyelid, Right **R** Lower Eyelid, Left	**Ø** Open **3** Percutaneous **X** External	**Z** No Device	**Z** No Qualifier
X Lacrimal Duct, Right **Y** Lacrimal Duct, Left	**Ø** Open **3** Percutaneous **7** Via Natural or Artificial Opening **8** Via Natural or Artificial Opening Endoscopic	**Z** No Device	**Z** No Qualifier

Non-OR Ø8Q[N,P,Q,R][Ø,3,X]ZZ
NC Ø8Q[8,9]XZZ

Ø Medical and Surgical
8 Eye
R Replacement Putting in or on biological or synthetic material that physically takes the place and/or function of all or a portion of a body part

Body Part Character 4	Approach Character 5	Device Character 6	Qualifier Character 7
Ø Eye, Right **1** Eye, Left **A** Choroid, Right **B** Choroid, Left	**Ø** Open **3** Percutaneous	**7** Autologous Tissue Substitute **J** Synthetic Substitute **K** Nonautologous Tissue Substitute	**Z** No Qualifier
4 Vitreous, Right **5** Vitreous, Left **C** Iris, Right **D** Iris, Left **G** Retinal Vessel, Right **H** Retinal Vessel, Left	**3** Percutaneous	**7** Autologous Tissue Substitute **J** Synthetic Substitute **K** Nonautologous Tissue Substitute	**Z** No Qualifier
6 Sclera, Right **7** Sclera, Left **S** Conjunctiva, Right **T** Conjunctiva, Left	**X** External	**7** Autologous Tissue Substitute **J** Synthetic Substitute **K** Nonautologous Tissue Substitute	**Z** No Qualifier
8 Cornea, Right **9** Cornea, Left	**3** Percutaneous **X** External	**7** Autologous Tissue Substitute **J** Synthetic Substitute **K** Nonautologous Tissue Substitute	**Z** No Qualifier
J Lens, Right **K** Lens, Left	**3** Percutaneous	**Ø** Synthetic Substitute, Intraocular Telescope **7** Autologous Tissue Substitute **J** Synthetic Substitute **K** Nonautologous Tissue Substitute	**Z** No Qualifier

Ø8R Continued on next page

Ø Medical and Surgical
8 Eye
R Replacement Putting in or on biological or synthetic material that physically takes the place and/or function of all or a portion of a body part

Ø8R Continued

Body Part Character 4	Approach Character 5	Device Character 6	Qualifier Character 7
N Upper Eyelid, Right P Upper Eyelid, Left Q Lower Eyelid, Right R Lower Eyelid, Left	Ø Open 3 Percutaneous X External	7 Autologous Tissue Substitute J Synthetic Substitute K Nonautologous Tissue Substitute	Z No Qualifier
X Lacrimal Duct, Right Y Lacrimal Duct, Left	Ø Open 3 Percutaneous 7 Via Natural or Artificial Opening 8 Via Natural or Artificial Opening Endoscopic	7 Autologous Tissue Substitute J Synthetic Substitute K Nonautologous Tissue Substitute	Z No Qualifier

Ø Medical and Surgical
8 Eye
S Reposition Moving to its normal location or other suitable location all or a portion of a body part

Body Part Character 4	Approach Character 5	Device Character 6	Qualifier Character 7
C Iris, Right D Iris, Left G Retinal Vessel, Right H Retinal Vessel, Left J Lens, Right K Lens, Left	3 Percutaneous	Z No Device	Z No Qualifier
L Extraocular Muscle, Right M Extraocular Muscle, Left V Lacrimal Gland, Right W Lacrimal Gland, Left	Ø Open 3 Percutaneous	Z No Device	Z No Qualifier
N Upper Eyelid, Right ⊞ P Upper Eyelid, Left ⊞ Q Lower Eyelid, Right ⊞ R Lower Eyelid, Left ⊞	Ø Open 3 Percutaneous X External	Z No Device	Z No Qualifier
X Lacrimal Duct, Right Y Lacrimal Duct, Left	Ø Open 3 Percutaneous 7 Via Natural or Artificial Opening 8 Via Natural or Artificial Opening Endoscopic	Z No Device	Z No Qualifier

No Procedure Combinations Specified
⊞ Ø8S[N,P,Q,R][Ø,3,X]ZZ

Ø Medical and Surgical
8 Eye
T Resection Cutting out or off, without replacement, all of a body part

Body Part Character 4	Approach Character 5	Device Character 6	Qualifier Character 7
Ø Eye, Right ⊞ 1 Eye, Left ⊞ 8 Cornea, Right 9 Cornea, Left	X External	Z No Device	Z No Qualifier
4 Vitreous, Right 5 Vitreous, Left C Iris, Right D Iris, Left J Lens, Right K Lens, Left	3 Percutaneous	Z No Device	Z No Qualifier
L Extraocular Muscle, Right M Extraocular Muscle, Left V Lacrimal Gland, Right W Lacrimal Gland, Left	Ø Open 3 Percutaneous	Z No Device	Z No Qualifier
N Upper Eyelid, Right P Upper Eyelid, Left Q Lower Eyelid, Right R Lower Eyelid, Left	Ø Open X External	Z No Device	Z No Qualifier
X Lacrimal Duct, Right Y Lacrimal Duct, Left	Ø Open 3 Percutaneous 7 Via Natural or Artificial Opening 8 Via Natural or Artificial Opening Endoscopic	Z No Device	Z No Qualifier

No Procedure Combinations Specified
⊞ Ø8T[Ø,1]XZZ

Ø Medical and Surgical
8 Eye
U Supplement Putting in or on biological or synthetic material that physically reinforces and/or augments the function of a portion of a body part

Body Part Character 4	Approach Character 5	Device Character 6	Qualifier Character 7
Ø Eye, Right **1** Eye, Left **C** Iris, Right **D** Iris, Left **E** Retina, Right **F** Retina, Left **G** Retinal Vessel, Right **H** Retinal Vessel, Left **L** Extraocular Muscle, Right **M** Extraocular Muscle, Left	**Ø** Open **3** Percutaneous	**7** Autologous Tissue Substitute **J** Synthetic Substitute **K** Nonautologous Tissue Substitute	**Z** No Qualifier
8 Cornea, Right NC **9** Cornea, Left NC **N** Upper Eyelid, Right **P** Upper Eyelid, Left **Q** Lower Eyelid, Right **R** Lower Eyelid, Left	**Ø** Open **3** Percutaneous **X** External	**7** Autologous Tissue Substitute **J** Synthetic Substitute **K** Nonautologous Tissue Substitute	**Z** No Qualifier
X Lacrimal Duct, Right **Y** Lacrimal Duct, Left	**Ø** Open **3** Percutaneous **7** Via Natural or Artificial Opening **8** Via Natural or Artificial Opening Endoscopic	**7** Autologous Tissue Substitute **J** Synthetic Substitute **K** Nonautologous Tissue Substitute	**Z** No Qualifier

NC Ø8U8[Ø,3,X]KZ
NC Ø8U9[Ø,3,X]KZ

Ø Medical and Surgical
8 Eye
V Restriction Partially closing an orifice or the lumen of a tubular body part

Body Part Character 4	Approach Character 5	Device Character 6	Qualifier Character 7
X Lacrimal Duct, Right **Y** Lacrimal Duct, Left	**Ø** Open **3** Percutaneous	**C** Extraluminal Device **D** Intraluminal Device **Z** No Device	**Z** No Qualifier
X Lacrimal Duct, Right **Y** Lacrimal Duct, Left	**7** Via Natural or Artificial Opening **8** Via Natural or Artificial Opening Endoscopic	**D** Intraluminal Device **Z** No Device	**Z** No Qualifier

Ø Medical and Surgical
8 Eye
W Revision Correcting, to the extent possible, a portion of a malfunctioning device or the position of a displaced device

Body Part Character 4	Approach Character 5	Device Character 6	Qualifier Character 7
Ø Eye, Right **1** Eye, Left	**Ø** Open **3** Percutaneous **7** Via Natural or Artificial Opening **8** Via Natural or Artificial Opening Endoscopic **X** External	**Ø** Drainage Device **3** Infusion Device **7** Autologous Tissue Substitute **C** Extraluminal Device **D** Intraluminal Device **J** Synthetic Substitute **K** Nonautologous Tissue Substitute	**Z** No Qualifier
J Lens, Right **K** Lens, Left	**3** Percutaneous **X** External	**J** Synthetic Substitute	**Z** No Qualifier
L Extraocular Muscle, Right **M** Extraocular Muscle, Left	**Ø** Open **3** Percutaneous	**Ø** Drainage Device **7** Autologous Tissue Substitute **J** Synthetic Substitute **K** Nonautologous Tissue Substitute	**Z** No Qualifier

Non-OR Ø8W[Ø,1]X[Ø,3,7,C,D,J,K]Z
Non-OR Ø8W[J,K]XJZ

Ø Medical and Surgical
8 Eye
X Transfer Moving, without taking out, all or a portion of a body part to another location to take over the function of all or a portion of a body part

Body Part Character 4	Approach Character 5	Device Character 6	Qualifier Character 7
L Extraocular Muscle, Right **M** Extraocular Muscle, Left	**Ø** Open **3** Percutaneous	**Z** No Device	**Z** No Qualifier

Ear, Nose, Sinus 090–09W

0 Medical and Surgical
9 Ear, Nose, Sinus
0 Alteration Modifying the anatomic structure of a body part without affecting the function of the body part

Body Part Character 4	Approach Character 5	Device Character 6	Qualifier Character 7
0 External Ear, Right 1 External Ear, Left 2 External Ear, Bilateral K Nose	0 Open 3 Percutaneous 4 Percutaneous Endoscopic X External	7 Autologous Tissue Substitute J Synthetic Substitute K Nonautologous Tissue Substitute Z No Device	Z No Qualifier

0 Medical and Surgical
9 Ear, Nose, Sinus
1 Bypass Altering the route of passage of the contents of a tubular body part

Body Part Character 4	Approach Character 5	Device Character 6	Qualifier Character 7
D Inner Ear, Right E Inner Ear, Left	0 Open	7 Autologous Tissue Substitute J Synthetic Substitute K Nonautologous Tissue Substitute Z No Device	0 Endolymphatic

0 Medical and Surgical
9 Ear, Nose, Sinus
2 Change Taking out or off a device from a body part and putting back an identical or similar device in or on the same body part without cutting or puncturing the skin or a mucous membrane

Body Part Character 4	Approach Character 5	Device Character 6	Qualifier Character 7
H Ear, Right J Ear, Left K Nose Y Sinus	X External	0 Drainage Device Y Other Device	Z No Qualifier

Non-OR For all body part, approach, device, and qualifier values

0 Medical and Surgical
9 Ear, Nose, Sinus
5 Destruction Physical eradication of all or a portion of a body part by the direct use of energy, force, or a destructive agent

Body Part Character 4	Approach Character 5	Device Character 6	Qualifier Character 7
0 External Ear, Right 1 External Ear, Left K Nose	0 Open 3 Percutaneous 4 Percutaneous Endoscopic X External	Z No Device	Z No Qualifier
3 External Auditory Canal, Right 4 External Auditory Canal, Left	0 Open 3 Percutaneous 4 Percutaneous Endoscopic 7 Via Natural or Artificial Opening 8 Via Natural or Artificial Opening Endoscopic X External	Z No Device	Z No Qualifier
5 Middle Ear, Right 6 Middle Ear, Left 9 Auditory Ossicle, Right A Auditory Ossicle, Left D Inner Ear, Right E Inner Ear, Left	0 Open	Z No Device	Z No Qualifier
7 Tympanic Membrane, Right 8 Tympanic Membrane, Left F Eustachian Tube, Right G Eustachian Tube, Left L Nasal Turbinate N Nasopharynx	0 Open 3 Percutaneous 4 Percutaneous Endoscopic 7 Via Natural or Artificial Opening 8 Via Natural or Artificial Opening Endoscopic	Z No Device	Z No Qualifier

095 Continued on next page

Non-OR 095[0,1,K][0,3,4,X]ZZ
Non-OR 095[3,4][0,3,4,7,8,X]ZZ
Non-OR 095[F,G][0,3,4,7,8]ZZ

Ø95 Continued

Ø Medical and Surgical
9 Ear, Nose, Sinus
5 Destruction Physical eradication of all or a portion of a body part by the direct use of energy, force, or a destructive agent

Body Part Character 4	Approach Character 5	Device Character 6	Qualifier Character 7
B Mastoid Sinus, Right **C** Mastoid Sinus, Left **M** Nasal Septum **P** Accessory Sinus **Q** Maxillary Sinus, Right **R** Maxillary Sinus, Left **S** Frontal Sinus, Right **T** Frontal Sinus, Left **U** Ethmoid Sinus, Right **V** Ethmoid Sinus, Left **W** Sphenoid Sinus, Right **X** Sphenoid Sinus, Left	**Ø** Open **3** Percutaneous **4** Percutaneous Endoscopic	**Z** No Device	**Z** No Qualifier

Non-OR Ø95M[Ø,3,4]ZZ

Ø Medical and Surgical
9 Ear, Nose, Sinus
7 Dilation Expanding an orifice or the lumen of a tubular body part

Body Part Character 4	Approach Character 5	Device Character 6	Qualifier Character 7
F Eustachian Tube, Right **G** Eustachian Tube, Left	**Ø** Open **7** Via Natural or Artificial Opening **8** Via Natural or Artificial Opening Endoscopic	**D** Intraluminal Device **Z** No Device	**Z** No Qualifier
F Eustachian Tube, Right **G** Eustachian Tube, Left	**3** Percutaneous **4** Percutaneous Endoscopic	**Z** No Device	**Z** No Qualifier

Non-OR For all body part, approach, device, and qualifier values

Ø Medical and Surgical
9 Ear, Nose, Sinus
8 Division Cutting into a body part without draining fluids and/or gases from the body part in order to separate or transect a body part

Body Part Character 4	Approach Character 5	Device Character 6	Qualifier Character 7
L Nasal Turbinate	**Ø** Open **3** Percutaneous **4** Percutaneous Endoscopic **7** Via Natural or Artificial Opening **8** Via Natural or Artificial Opening Endoscopic	**Z** No Device	**Z** No Qualifier

Ø Medical and Surgical
9 Ear, Nose, Sinus
9 Drainage Taking or letting out fluids and/or gases from a body part

Body Part Character 4	Approach Character 5	Device Character 6	Qualifier Character 7
Ø External Ear, Right **1** External Ear, Left **K** Nose	**Ø** Open **3** Percutaneous **4** Percutaneous Endoscopic **X** External	**Ø** Drainage Device	**Z** No Qualifier
Ø External Ear, Right **1** External Ear, Left **K** Nose	**Ø** Open **3** Percutaneous **4** Percutaneous Endoscopic **X** External	**Z** No Device	**X** Diagnostic **Z** No Qualifier
3 External Auditory Canal, Right **4** External Auditory Canal, Left	**Ø** Open **3** Percutaneous **4** Percutaneous Endoscopic **7** Via Natural or Artificial Opening **8** Via Natural or Artificial Opening Endoscopic **X** External	**Ø** Drainage Device	**Z** No Qualifier

Ø99 Continued on next page

Non-OR Ø99[Ø,1,K][Ø,3,4,X]ØZ
Non-OR Ø99[Ø,1,K][Ø,3,4,X]Z[X,Z]
Non-OR Ø99[3,4][Ø,3,4,7,8,X]ØZ

Ø Medical and Surgical
9 Ear, Nose, Sinus
9 Drainage Taking or letting out fluids and/or gases from a body part

Ø99 Continued

Body Part Character 4	Approach Character 5	Device Character 6	Qualifier Character 7
3 External Auditory Canal, Right 4 External Auditory Canal, Left	Ø Open 3 Percutaneous 4 Percutaneous Endoscopic 7 Via Natural or Artificial Opening 8 Via Natural or Artificial Opening Endoscopic X External	Z No Device	X Diagnostic Z No Qualifier
5 Middle Ear, Right 6 Middle Ear, Left 9 Auditory Ossicle, Right A Auditory Ossicle, Left D Inner Ear, Right E Inner Ear, Left	Ø Open	Ø Drainage Device	Z No Qualifier
5 Middle Ear, Right 6 Middle Ear, Left 9 Auditory Ossicle, Right A Auditory Ossicle, Left D Inner Ear, Right E Inner Ear, Left	Ø Open	Z No Device	X Diagnostic Z No Qualifier
7 Tympanic Membrane, Right 8 Tympanic Membrane, Left F Eustachian Tube, Right G Eustachian Tube, Left L Nasal Turbinate N Nasopharynx	Ø Open 3 Percutaneous 4 Percutaneous Endoscopic 7 Via Natural or Artificial Opening 8 Via Natural or Artificial Opening Endoscopic	Ø Drainage Device	Z No Qualifier
7 Tympanic Membrane, Right 8 Tympanic Membrane, Left F Eustachian Tube, Right G Eustachian Tube, Left L Nasal Turbinate N Nasopharynx	Ø Open 3 Percutaneous 4 Percutaneous Endoscopic 7 Via Natural or Artificial Opening 8 Via Natural or Artificial Opening Endoscopic	Z No Device	X Diagnostic Z No Qualifier
B Mastoid Sinus, Right C Mastoid Sinus, Left M Nasal Septum P Accessory Sinus Q Maxillary Sinus, Right R Maxillary Sinus, Left S Frontal Sinus, Right T Frontal Sinus, Left U Ethmoid Sinus, Right V Ethmoid Sinus, Left W Sphenoid Sinus, Right X Sphenoid Sinus, Left	Ø Open 3 Percutaneous 4 Percutaneous Endoscopic	Ø Drainage Device	Z No Qualifier
B Mastoid Sinus, Right C Mastoid Sinus, Left M Nasal Septum P Accessory Sinus Q Maxillary Sinus, Right R Maxillary Sinus, Left S Frontal Sinus, Right T Frontal Sinus, Left U Ethmoid Sinus, Right V Ethmoid Sinus, Left W Sphenoid Sinus, Right X Sphenoid Sinus, Left	Ø Open 3 Percutaneous 4 Percutaneous Endoscopic	Z No Device	X Diagnostic Z No Qualifier

Non-OR Ø99[3,4][Ø,3,4,7,8,X]Z[X,Z]
Non-OR Ø99[5,6]ØZZ
Non-OR Ø99[F,G,L][Ø,3,4,7,8]ØZ
Non-OR Ø99[7,8,F,G,L][Ø,3,4,7,8]ZZ
Non-OR Ø99[L,N][Ø,3,4,7,8]ZX
Non-OR Ø99M[Ø,3,4]ØZ
Non-OR Ø99[P,Q,R,S,T,U,V,W,X][3,4]ØZ
Non-OR Ø99M[Ø,3,4]Z[X,Z]
Non-OR Ø99[P,Q,R,S,T,U,V,W,X][3,4]Z[X,Z]

Ø Medical and Surgical
9 Ear, Nose, Sinus
B Excision Cutting out or off, without replacement, a portion of a body part

Body Part Character 4	Approach Character 5	Device Character 6	Qualifier Character 7
Ø External Ear, Right **1** External Ear, Left **K** Nose	**Ø** Open **3** Percutaneous **4** Percutaneous Endoscopic **X** External	**Z** No Device	**X** Diagnostic **Z** No Qualifier
3 External Auditory Canal, Right **4** External Auditory Canal, Left	**Ø** Open **3** Percutaneous **4** Percutaneous Endoscopic **7** Via Natural or Artificial Opening **8** Via Natural or Artificial Opening Endoscopic **X** External	**Z** No Device	**X** Diagnostic **Z** No Qualifier
5 Middle Ear, Right **6** Middle Ear, Left **9** Auditory Ossicle, Right **A** Auditory Ossicle, Left **D** Inner Ear, Right **E** Inner Ear, Left	**Ø** Open	**Z** No Device	**X** Diagnostic **Z** No Qualifier
7 Tympanic Membrane, Right **8** Tympanic Membrane, Left **F** Eustachian Tube, Right **G** Eustachian Tube, Left **L** Nasal Turbinate **N** Nasopharynx	**Ø** Open **3** Percutaneous **4** Percutaneous Endoscopic **7** Via Natural or Artificial Opening **8** Via Natural or Artificial Opening Endoscopic	**Z** No Device	**X** Diagnostic **Z** No Qualifier
B Mastoid Sinus, Right **C** Mastoid Sinus, Left **M** Nasal Septum **P** Accessory Sinus **Q** Maxillary Sinus, Right **R** Maxillary Sinus, Left **S** Frontal Sinus, Right **T** Frontal Sinus, Left **U** Ethmoid Sinus, Right **V** Ethmoid Sinus, Left **W** Sphenoid Sinus, Right **X** Sphenoid Sinus, Left	**Ø** Open **3** Percutaneous **4** Percutaneous Endoscopic	**Z** No Device	**X** Diagnostic **Z** No Qualifier

Non-OR Ø9B[Ø,1,K][Ø,3,4,X]Z[X,Z]
Non-OR Ø9B[3,4][Ø,3,4,7,8,X]Z[X,Z]
Non-OR Ø9B[F,G,L,N][Ø,3,4,7,8]ZX
Non-OR Ø9B[F,G][Ø,3,4,7,8]ZZ
Non-OR Ø9BM[Ø,3,4]ZX
Non-OR Ø9B[P,Q,R,S,T,U,V,W,X][3,4]ZX

0 Medical and Surgical
9 Ear, Nose, Sinus
C Extirpation Taking or cutting out solid matter from a body part

Body Part Character 4	Approach Character 5	Device Character 6	Qualifier Character 7
0 External Ear, Right 1 External Ear, Left K Nose	0 Open 3 Percutaneous 4 Percutaneous Endoscopic X External	Z No Device	Z No Qualifier
3 External Auditory Canal, Right 4 External Auditory Canal, Left	0 Open 3 Percutaneous 4 Percutaneous Endoscopic 7 Via Natural or Artificial Opening 8 Via Natural or Artificial Opening Endoscopic X External	Z No Device	Z No Qualifier
5 Middle Ear, Right 6 Middle Ear, Left 9 Auditory Ossicle, Right A Auditory Ossicle, Left D Inner Ear, Right E Inner Ear, Left	0 Open	Z No Device	Z No Qualifier
7 Tympanic Membrane, Right 8 Tympanic Membrane, Left F Eustachian Tube, Right G Eustachian Tube, Left L Nasal Turbinate N Nasopharynx	0 Open 3 Percutaneous 4 Percutaneous Endoscopic 7 Via Natural or Artificial Opening 8 Via Natural or Artificial Opening Endoscopic	Z No Device	Z No Qualifier
B Mastoid Sinus, Right C Mastoid Sinus, Left M Nasal Septum P Accessory Sinus Q Maxillary Sinus, Right R Maxillary Sinus, Left S Frontal Sinus, Right T Frontal Sinus, Left U Ethmoid Sinus, Right V Ethmoid Sinus, Left W Sphenoid Sinus, Right X Sphenoid Sinus, Left	0 Open 3 Percutaneous 4 Percutaneous Endoscopic	Z No Device	Z No Qualifier

Non-OR 09C[0,1,K][0,3,4,X]ZZ
Non-OR 09C[3,4][0,3,4,7,8,X]ZZ
Non-OR 09C[7,8,F,G,L][0,3,4,7,8]ZZ
Non-OR 09CM[0,3,4]ZZ

0 Medical and Surgical
9 Ear, Nose, Sinus
D Extraction Pulling or stripping out or off all or a portion of a body part by the use of force

Body Part Character 4	Approach Character 5	Device Character 6	Qualifier Character 7
7 Tympanic Membrane, Right 8 Tympanic Membrane, Left L Nasal Turbinate	0 Open 3 Percutaneous 4 Percutaneous Endoscopic 7 Via Natural or Artificial Opening 8 Via Natural or Artificial Opening Endoscopic	Z No Device	Z No Qualifier
9 Auditory Ossicle, Right A Auditory Ossicle, Left	0 Open	Z No Device	Z No Qualifier
B Mastoid Sinus, Right C Mastoid Sinus, Left M Nasal Septum P Accessory Sinus Q Maxillary Sinus, Right R Maxillary Sinus, Left S Frontal Sinus, Right T Frontal Sinus, Left U Ethmoid Sinus, Right V Ethmoid Sinus, Left W Sphenoid Sinus, Right X Sphenoid Sinus, Left	0 Open 3 Percutaneous 4 Percutaneous Endoscopic	Z No Device	Z No Qualifier

Ø Medical and Surgical
9 Ear, Nose, Sinus
H Insertion Putting in a nonbiological appliance that monitors, assists, performs, or prevents a physiological function but does not physically take the place of a body part

Body Part Character 4	Approach Character 5	Device Character 6	Qualifier Character 7
D Inner Ear, Right **E** Inner Ear, Left	**Ø** Open **3** Percutaneous **4** Percutaneous Endoscopic	**4** Hearing Device, Bone Conduction **5** Hearing Device, Single Channel Cochlear Prosthesis **6** Hearing Device, Multiple Channel Cochlear Prosthesis **S** Hearing Device	**Z** No Qualifier
N Nasopharynx	**7** Via Natural or Artificial Opening **8** Via Natural or Artificial Opening Endoscopic	**B** Intraluminal Device, Airway	**Z** No Qualifier

Non-OR Ø9HN[7,8]BZ

Ø Medical and Surgical
9 Ear, Nose, Sinus
J Inspection Visually and/or manually exploring a body part

Body Part Character 4	Approach Character 5	Device Character 6	Qualifier Character 7
7 Tympanic Membrane, Right **8** Tympanic Membrane, Left **H** Ear, Right **J** Ear, Left	**Ø** Open **3** Percutaneous **4** Percutaneous Endoscopic **7** Via Natural or Artificial Opening **8** Via Natural or Artificial Opening Endoscopic **X** External	**Z** No Device	**Z** No Qualifier
D Inner Ear, Right **E** Inner Ear, Left **K** Nose **Y** Sinus	**Ø** Open **3** Percutaneous **4** Percutaneous Endoscopic **X** External	**Z** No Device	**Z** No Qualifier

Non-OR Ø9J[7,8]8ZZ
Non-OR Ø9J[H,J][Ø,3,4,7,8,X]ZZ
Non-OR Ø9J[K,Y][Ø,3,4,X]ZZ

Ø Medical and Surgical
9 Ear, Nose, Sinus
M Reattachment Putting back in or on all or a portion of a separated body part to its normal location or other suitable location

Body Part Character 4	Approach Character 5	Device Character 6	Qualifier Character 7
Ø External Ear, Right **1** External Ear, Left **K** Nose	**X** External	**Z** No Device	**Z** No Qualifier

0 Medical and Surgical
9 Ear, Nose, Sinus
N Release Freeing a body part from an abnormal physical constraint

Body Part Character 4	Approach Character 5	Device Character 6	Qualifier Character 7
0 External Ear, Right 1 External Ear, Left K Nose	0 Open 3 Percutaneous 4 Percutaneous Endoscopic X External	Z No Device	Z No Qualifier
3 External Auditory Canal, Right 4 External Auditory Canal, Left	0 Open 3 Percutaneous 4 Percutaneous Endoscopic 7 Via Natural or Artificial Opening 8 Via Natural or Artificial Opening Endoscopic X External	Z No Device	Z No Qualifier
5 Middle Ear, Right 6 Middle Ear, Left 9 Auditory Ossicle, Right A Auditory Ossicle, Left D Inner Ear, Right E Inner Ear, Left	0 Open	Z No Device	Z No Qualifier
7 Tympanic Membrane, Right 8 Tympanic Membrane, Left F Eustachian Tube, Right G Eustachian Tube, Left L Nasal Turbinate N Nasopharynx	0 Open 3 Percutaneous 4 Percutaneous Endoscopic 7 Via Natural or Artificial Opening 8 Via Natural or Artificial Opening Endoscopic	Z No Device	Z No Qualifier
B Mastoid Sinus, Right C Mastoid Sinus, Left M Nasal Septum P Accessory Sinus Q Maxillary Sinus, Right R Maxillary Sinus, Left S Frontal Sinus, Right T Frontal Sinus, Left U Ethmoid Sinus, Right V Ethmoid Sinus, Left W Sphenoid Sinus, Right X Sphenoid Sinus, Left	0 Open 3 Percutaneous 4 Percutaneous Endoscopic	Z No Device	Z No Qualifier

Non-OR 09NK[0,3,4,X]ZZ
Non-OR 09N[F,G,L][0,3,4,7,8]ZZ
Non-OR 09NM[0,3,4]ZZ

0 Medical and Surgical
9 Ear, Nose, Sinus
P Removal Taking out or off a device from a body part

Body Part Character 4	Approach Character 5	Device Character 6	Qualifier Character 7
7 Tympanic Membrane, Right 8 Tympanic Membrane, Left	0 Open 7 Via Natural or Artificial Opening 8 Via Natural or Artificial Opening Endoscopic X External	0 Drainage Device	Z No Qualifier
D Inner Ear, Right E Inner Ear, Left	0 Open 7 Via Natural or Artificial Opening 8 Via Natural or Artificial Opening Endoscopic	S Hearing Device	Z No Qualifier
H Ear, Right J Ear, Left K Nose	0 Open 3 Percutaneous 4 Percutaneous Endoscopic 7 Via Natural or Artificial Opening 8 Via Natural or Artificial Opening Endoscopic X External	0 Drainage Device 7 Autologous Tissue Substitute D Intraluminal Device J Synthetic Substitute K Nonautologous Tissue Substitute	Z No Qualifier
Y Sinus	0 Open 3 Percutaneous 4 Percutaneous Endoscopic X External	0 Drainage Device	Z No Qualifier

Non-OR 09P[7,8][0,7,8,X]0Z
Non-OR 09P[H,J][3,4][0,J,K]Z
Non-OR 09P[H,J]X[0,7,D,J,K]Z
Non-OR 09P[H,J][7,8][0,D]Z
Non-OR 09PK[0,3,4,7,8,X][0,7,D,J,K]Z
Non-OR 09PYX0Z

Ø Medical and Surgical
9 Ear, Nose, Sinus
Q Repair Restoring, to the extent possible, a body part to its normal anatomic structure and function

Body Part Character 4	Approach Character 5	Device Character 6	Qualifier Character 7
Ø External Ear, Right **1** External Ear, Left **2** External Ear, Bilateral **K** Nose ⊞	**Ø** Open **3** Percutaneous **4** Percutaneous Endoscopic **X** External	**Z** No Device	**Z** No Qualifier
3 External Auditory Canal, Right **4** External Auditory Canal, Left **F** Eustachian Tube, Right **G** Eustachian Tube, Left	**Ø** Open **3** Percutaneous **4** Percutaneous Endoscopic **7** Via Natural or Artificial Opening **8** Via Natural or Artificial Opening Endoscopic **X** External	**Z** No Device	**Z** No Qualifier
5 Middle Ear, Right **6** Middle Ear, Left **9** Auditory Ossicle, Right **A** Auditory Ossicle, Left **D** Inner Ear, Right **E** Inner Ear, Left	**Ø** Open	**Z** No Device	**Z** No Qualifier
7 Tympanic Membrane, Right **8** Tympanic Membrane, Left **L** Nasal Turbinate **N** Nasopharynx	**Ø** Open **3** Percutaneous **4** Percutaneous Endoscopic **7** Via Natural or Artificial Opening **8** Via Natural or Artificial Opening Endoscopic	**Z** No Device	**Z** No Qualifier
B Mastoid Sinus, Right **C** Mastoid Sinus, Left **M** Nasal Septum **P** Accessory Sinus **Q** Maxillary Sinus, Right ⊞ **R** Maxillary Sinus, Left **S** Frontal Sinus, Right **T** Frontal Sinus, Left **U** Ethmoid Sinus, Right **V** Ethmoid Sinus, Left **W** Sphenoid Sinus, Right **X** Sphenoid Sinus, Left	**Ø** Open **3** Percutaneous **4** Percutaneous Endoscopic	**Z** No Device	**Z** No Qualifier

Non-OR Ø9Q[Ø,1,2]XZZ
Non-OR Ø9Q[3,4]XZZ
Non-OR Ø9Q[F,G][Ø,3,4,7,8,X]ZZ
AHA: 2Ø13, 4Q, 114

No Procedure Combinations Specified
⊞ Ø9QK[Ø,3,4]ZZ
⊞ Ø9QQ[Ø,3,4]ZZ

Ø Medical and Surgical
9 Ear, Nose, Sinus
R Replacement Putting in or on biological or synthetic material that physically takes the place and/or function of all or a portion of a body part

Body Part Character 4	Approach Character 5	Device Character 6	Qualifier Character 7
Ø External Ear, Right **1** External Ear, Left **2** External Ear, Bilateral **K** Nose	**Ø** Open **X** External	**7** Autologous Tissue Substitute **J** Synthetic Substitute **K** Nonautologous Tissue Substitute	**Z** No Qualifier
5 Middle Ear, Right **6** Middle Ear, Left **9** Auditory Ossicle, Right **A** Auditory Ossicle, Left **D** Inner Ear, Right **E** Inner Ear, Left	**Ø** Open	**7** Autologous Tissue Substitute **J** Synthetic Substitute **K** Nonautologous Tissue Substitute	**Z** No Qualifier
7 Tympanic Membrane, Right **8** Tympanic Membrane, Left **N** Nasopharynx	**Ø** Open **7** Via Natural or Artificial Opening **8** Via Natural or Artificial Opening Endoscopic	**7** Autologous Tissue Substitute **J** Synthetic Substitute **K** Nonautologous Tissue Substitute	**Z** No Qualifier
L Nasal Turbinate	**Ø** Open **3** Percutaneous **4** Percutaneous Endoscopic **7** Via Natural or Artificial Opening **8** Via Natural or Artificial Opening Endoscopic	**7** Autologous Tissue Substitute **J** Synthetic Substitute **K** Nonautologous Tissue Substitute	**Z** No Qualifier
M Nasal Septum	**Ø** Open **3** Percutaneous **4** Percutaneous Endoscopic	**7** Autologous Tissue Substitute **J** Synthetic Substitute **K** Nonautologous Tissue Substitute	**Z** No Qualifier

0 Medical and Surgical
9 Ear, Nose, Sinus
S Reposition Moving to its normal location or other suitable location all or a portion of a body part

Body Part Character 4	Approach Character 5	Device Character 6	Qualifier Character 7
0 External Ear, Right **1** External Ear, Left **2** External Ear, Bilateral **K** Nose	**0** Open **4** Percutaneous Endoscopic **X** External	**Z** No Device	**Z** No Qualifier
7 Tympanic Membrane, Right **8** Tympanic Membrane, Left **F** Eustachian Tube, Right **G** Eustachian Tube, Left **L** Nasal Turbinate	**0** Open **4** Percutaneous Endoscopic **7** Via Natural or Artificial Opening **8** Via Natural or Artificial Opening Endoscopic	**Z** No Device	**Z** No Qualifier
9 Auditory Ossicle, Right **A** Auditory Ossicle, Left **M** Nasal Septum	**0** Open **4** Percutaneous Endoscopic	**Z** No Device	**Z** No Qualifier

Non-OR 09S[F,G][0,4,7,8]ZZ

0 Medical and Surgical
9 Ear, Nose, Sinus
T Resection Cutting out or off, without replacement, all of a body part

Body Part Character 4	Approach Character 5	Device Character 6	Qualifier Character 7
0 External Ear, Right **1** External Ear, Left **K** Nose	**0** Open **4** Percutaneous Endoscopic **X** External	**Z** No Device	**Z** No Qualifier
5 Middle Ear, Right **6** Middle Ear, Left **9** Auditory Ossicle, Right **A** Auditory Ossicle, Left **D** Inner Ear, Right **E** Inner Ear, Left	**0** Open	**Z** No Device	**Z** No Qualifier
7 Tympanic Membrane, Right **8** Tympanic Membrane, Left **F** Eustachian Tube, Right **G** Eustachian Tube, Left **L** Nasal Turbinate **N** Nasopharynx	**0** Open **4** Percutaneous Endoscopic **7** Via Natural or Artificial Opening **8** Via Natural or Artificial Opening Endoscopic	**Z** No Device	**Z** No Qualifier
B Mastoid Sinus, Right **C** Mastoid Sinus, Left **M** Nasal Septum **P** Accessory Sinus **Q** Maxillary Sinus, Right **R** Maxillary Sinus, Left **S** Frontal Sinus, Right **T** Frontal Sinus, Left **U** Ethmoid Sinus, Right **V** Ethmoid Sinus, Left **W** Sphenoid Sinus, Right **X** Sphenoid Sinus, Left	**0** Open **4** Percutaneous Endoscopic	**Z** No Device	**Z** No Qualifier

Non-OR 09T[F,G][0,4,7,8]ZZ

Ø Medical and Surgical
9 Ear, Nose, Sinus
U Supplement Putting in or on biological or synthetic material that physically reinforces and/or augments the function of a portion of a body part

Body Part Character 4	Approach Character 5	Device Character 6	Qualifier Character 7
Ø External Ear, Right **1** External Ear, Left **2** External Ear, Bilateral **K** Nose	**Ø** Open **X** External	**7** Autologous Tissue Substitute **J** Synthetic Substitute **K** Nonautologous Tissue Substitute	**Z** No Qualifier
5 Middle Ear, Right **6** Middle Ear, Left **9** Auditory Ossicle, Right **A** Auditory Ossicle, Left **D** Inner Ear, Right **E** Inner Ear, Left	**Ø** Open	**7** Autologous Tissue Substitute **J** Synthetic Substitute **K** Nonautologous Tissue Substitute	**Z** No Qualifier
7 Tympanic Membrane, Right **8** Tympanic Membrane, Left **N** Nasopharynx	**Ø** Open **7** Via Natural or Artificial Opening **8** Via Natural or Artificial Opening Endoscopic	**7** Autologous Tissue Substitute **J** Synthetic Substitute **K** Nonautologous Tissue Substitute	**Z** No Qualifier
L Nasal Turbinate	**Ø** Open **3** Percutaneous **4** Percutaneous Endoscopic **7** Via Natural or Artificial Opening **8** Via Natural or Artificial Opening Endoscopic	**7** Autologous Tissue Substitute **J** Synthetic Substitute **K** Nonautologous Tissue Substitute	**Z** No Qualifier
M Nasal Septum	**Ø** Open **3** Percutaneous **4** Percutaneous Endoscopic	**7** Autologous Tissue Substitute **J** Synthetic Substitute **K** Nonautologous Tissue Substitute	**Z** No Qualifier

Ø Medical and Surgical
9 Ear, Nose, Sinus
W Revision Correcting, to the extent possible, a portion of a malfunctioning device or the position of a displaced device

Body Part Character 4	Approach Character 5	Device Character 6	Qualifier Character 7
7 Tympanic Membrane, Right **8** Tympanic Membrane, Left **9** Auditory Ossicle, Right **A** Auditory Ossicle, Left	**Ø** Open **7** Via Natural or Artificial Opening **8** Via Natural or Artificial Opening Endoscopic	**7** Autologous Tissue Substitute **J** Synthetic Substitute **K** Nonautologous Tissue Substitute	**Z** No Qualifier
D Inner Ear, Right **E** Inner Ear, Left	**Ø** Open **7** Via Natural or Artificial Opening **8** Via Natural or Artificial Opening Endoscopic	**S** Hearing Device	**Z** No Qualifier
H Ear, Right **J** Ear, Left **K** Nose	**Ø** Open **3** Percutaneous **4** Percutaneous Endoscopic **7** Via Natural or Artificial Opening **8** Via Natural or Artificial Opening Endoscopic **X** External	**Ø** Drainage Device **7** Autologous Tissue Substitute **D** Intraluminal Device **J** Synthetic Substitute **K** Nonautologous Tissue Substitute	**Z** No Qualifier
Y Sinus	**Ø** Open **3** Percutaneous **4** Percutaneous Endoscopic **X** External	**Ø** Drainage Device	**Z** No Qualifier

Non-OR Ø9W[H,J][3,4][J,K]Z
Non-OR Ø9WK[Ø,3,4,7,8,X][Ø,7,D,J,K]Z
Non-OR Ø9W[H,J][7,8]DZ
Non-OR Ø9W[H,J]X[Ø,7,D,J,K]Z
Non-OR Ø9WYXØZ

Respiratory System 0B1–0BY

0 Medical and Surgical
B Respiratory System
1 Bypass Altering the route of passage of the contents of a tubular body part

Body Part Character 4	Approach Character 5	Device Character 6	Qualifier Character 7
1 Trachea	0 Open	D Intraluminal Device	6 Esophagus
1 Trachea	0 Open 3 Percutaneous 4 Percutaneous Endoscopic	F Tracheostomy Device Z No Device	4 Cutaneous

DRG Non-OR 0B113[F,Z]4
Non-OR 0B110D6

0 Medical and Surgical
B Respiratory System
2 Change Taking out or off a device from a body part and putting back an identical or similar device in or on the same body part without cutting or puncturing the skin or a mucous membrane

Body Part Character 4	Approach Character 5	Device Character 6	Qualifier Character 7
0 Tracheobronchial Tree K Lung, Right L Lung, Left Q Pleura T Diaphragm	X External	0 Drainage Device Y Other Device	Z No Qualifier
1 Trachea	X External	0 Drainage Device E Intraluminal Device, Endotracheal Airway F Tracheostomy Device Y Other Device	Z No Qualifier

Non-OR For all body part, approach, device, and qualifier values

0 Medical and Surgical
B Respiratory System
5 Destruction Physical eradication of all or a portion of a body part by the direct use of energy, force, or a destructive agent

Body Part Character 4	Approach Character 5	Device Character 6	Qualifier Character 7
1 Trachea 2 Carina 3 Main Bronchus, Right 4 Upper Lobe Bronchus, Right 5 Middle Lobe Bronchus, Right 6 Lower Lobe Bronchus, Right 7 Main Bronchus, Left 8 Upper Lobe Bronchus, Left 9 Lingula Bronchus B Lower Lobe Bronchus, Left C Upper Lung Lobe, Right D Middle Lung Lobe, Right F Lower Lung Lobe, Right G Upper Lung Lobe, Left H Lung Lingula J Lower Lung Lobe, Left K Lung, Right L Lung, Left M Lungs, Bilateral	0 Open 3 Percutaneous 4 Percutaneous Endoscopic 7 Via Natural or Artificial Opening 8 Via Natural or Artificial Opening Endoscopic	Z No Device	Z No Qualifier
N Pleura, Right P Pleura, Left R Diaphragm, Right S Diaphragm, Left	0 Open 3 Percutaneous 4 Percutaneous Endoscopic	Z No Device	Z No Qualifier

Non-OR 0B5[3,4,5,6,7,8,9,B]4ZZ
Non-OR 0B5[C,D,F,G,H,J,K,L,M]8ZZ

Ø Medical and Surgical
B Respiratory System
7 Dilation Expanding an orifice or the lumen of a tubular body part

Body Part Character 4	Approach Character 5	Device Character 6	Qualifier Character 7
1 Trachea **2** Carina **3** Main Bronchus, Right **4** Upper Lobe Bronchus, Right **5** Middle Lobe Bronchus, Right **6** Lower Lobe Bronchus, Right **7** Main Bronchus, Left **8** Upper Lobe Bronchus, Left **9** Lingula Bronchus **B** Lower Lobe Bronchus, Left	**Ø** Open **3** Percutaneous **4** Percutaneous Endoscopic **7** Via Natural or Artificial Opening **8** Via Natural or Artificial Opening Endoscopic	**D** Intraluminal Device **Z** No Device	**Z** No Qualifier

Non-OR ØB7[3,4,5,6,7,8,9,B][Ø,3,4,7,8][D,Z]Z

Ø Medical and Surgical
B Respiratory System
9 Drainage Taking or letting out fluids and/or gases from a body part

Body Part Character 4	Approach Character 5	Device Character 6	Qualifier Character 7
1 Trachea **2** Carina **3** Main Bronchus, Right **4** Upper Lobe Bronchus, Right **5** Middle Lobe Bronchus, Right **6** Lower Lobe Bronchus, Right **7** Main Bronchus, Left **8** Upper Lobe Bronchus, Left **9** Lingula Bronchus **B** Lower Lobe Bronchus, Left **C** Upper Lung Lobe, Right **D** Middle Lung Lobe, Right **F** Lower Lung Lobe, Right **G** Upper Lung Lobe, Left **H** Lung Lingula **J** Lower Lung Lobe, Left **K** Lung, Right **L** Lung, Left **M** Lungs, Bilateral	**Ø** Open **3** Percutaneous **4** Percutaneous Endoscopic **7** Via Natural or Artificial Opening **8** Via Natural or Artificial Opening Endoscopic	**Ø** Drainage Device	**Z** No Qualifier
1 Trachea **2** Carina **3** Main Bronchus, Right **4** Upper Lobe Bronchus, Right **5** Middle Lobe Bronchus, Right **6** Lower Lobe Bronchus, Right **7** Main Bronchus, Left **8** Upper Lobe Bronchus, Left **9** Lingula Bronchus **B** Lower Lobe Bronchus, Left **C** Upper Lung Lobe, Right **D** Middle Lung Lobe, Right **F** Lower Lung Lobe, Right **G** Upper Lung Lobe, Left **H** Lung Lingula **J** Lower Lung Lobe, Left **K** Lung, Right **L** Lung, Left **M** Lungs, Bilateral	**Ø** Open **3** Percutaneous **4** Percutaneous Endoscopic **7** Via Natural or Artificial Opening **8** Via Natural or Artificial Opening Endoscopic	**Z** No Device	**X** Diagnostic **Z** No Qualifier
N Pleura, Right **P** Pleura, Left **R** Diaphragm, Right **S** Diaphragm, Left	**Ø** Open **3** Percutaneous **4** Percutaneous Endoscopic	**Ø** Drainage Device	**Z** No Qualifier
N Pleura, Right **P** Pleura, Left **R** Diaphragm, Right **S** Diaphragm, Left	**Ø** Open **3** Percutaneous **4** Percutaneous Endoscopic	**Z** No Device	**X** Diagnostic **Z** No Qualifier

Non-OR ØB9[1,2,3,4,5,6,7,8,9,B][3,4,7,8]ZX
Non-OR ØB9[C,D,F,G,H,J,K,L,M][3,4,7]ZX
Non-OR ØB9[N,P][Ø,3]ØZ
Non-OR ØB9[N,P][Ø,3,4]ZX

0 Medical and Surgical
B Respiratory System
B Excision Cutting out or off, without replacement, a portion of a body part

Body Part Character 4	Approach Character 5	Device Character 6	Qualifier Character 7
1 Trachea 2 Carina 3 Main Bronchus, Right 4 Upper Lobe Bronchus, Right 5 Middle Lobe Bronchus, Right 6 Lower Lobe Bronchus, Right 7 Main Bronchus, Left 8 Upper Lobe Bronchus, Left 9 Lingula Bronchus B Lower Lobe Bronchus, Left C Upper Lung Lobe, Right D Middle Lung Lobe, Right F Lower Lung Lobe, Right G Upper Lung Lobe, Left H Lung Lingula J Lower Lung Lobe, Left K Lung, Right L Lung, Left M Lungs, Bilateral	0 Open 3 Percutaneous 4 Percutaneous Endoscopic 7 Via Natural or Artificial Opening 8 Via Natural or Artificial Opening Endoscopic	Z No Device	X Diagnostic Z No Qualifier
N Pleura, Right P Pleura, Left R Diaphragm, Right S Diaphragm, Left	0 Open 3 Percutaneous 4 Percutaneous Endoscopic	Z No Device	X Diagnostic Z No Qualifier

Non-OR 0BB[1,2,3,4,5,6,7,8,9,B][3,4,7,8]ZX
Non-OR 0BB[3,4,5,6,7,8,9,B,M][4,8]ZZ
Non-OR 0BB[C,D,F,G,H,J,K,L,M]3ZX
Non-OR 0BB[C,D,F,G,H,J,K,L]8ZZ
Non-OR 0BB[N,P][0,3]ZX

AHA: 2014, 1Q, 20

0 Medical and Surgical
B Respiratory System
C Extirpation Taking or cutting out solid matter from a body part

Body Part Character 4	Approach Character 5	Device Character 6	Qualifier Character 7
1 Trachea 2 Carina 3 Main Bronchus, Right 4 Upper Lobe Bronchus, Right 5 Middle Lobe Bronchus, Right 6 Lower Lobe Bronchus, Right 7 Main Bronchus, Left 8 Upper Lobe Bronchus, Left 9 Lingula Bronchus B Lower Lobe Bronchus, Left C Upper Lung Lobe, Right D Middle Lung Lobe, Right F Lower Lung Lobe, Right G Upper Lung Lobe, Left H Lung Lingula J Lower Lung Lobe, Left K Lung, Right L Lung, Left M Lungs, Bilateral	0 Open 3 Percutaneous 4 Percutaneous Endoscopic 7 Via Natural or Artificial Opening 8 Via Natural or Artificial Opening Endoscopic	Z No Device	Z No Qualifier
N Pleura, Right P Pleura, Left R Diaphragm, Right S Diaphragm, Left	0 Open 3 Percutaneous 4 Percutaneous Endoscopic	Z No Device	Z No Qualifier

Non-OR 0BC[1,2,3,4,5,6,7,8,9,B][7,8]ZZ
Non-OR 0BC[N,P][0,3,4]ZZ

0 Medical and Surgical
B Respiratory System
D Extraction Pulling or stripping out or off all or a portion of a body part by the use of force

Body Part Character 4	Approach Character 5	Device Character 6	Qualifier Character 7
N Pleura, Right P Pleura, Left	0 Open 3 Percutaneous 4 Percutaneous Endoscopic	Z No Device	X Diagnostic Z No Qualifier

Ø Medical and Surgical
B Respiratory System
F Fragmentation Breaking solid matter in a body part into pieces

Body Part Character 4	Approach Character 5	Device Character 6	Qualifier Character 7
1 Trachea NC 2 Carina NC 3 Main Bronchus, Right NC 4 Upper Lobe Bronchus, Right NC 5 Middle Lobe Bronchus, Right NC 6 Lower Lobe Bronchus, Right NC 7 Main Bronchus, Left NC 8 Upper Lobe Bronchus, Left NC 9 Lingula Bronchus NC B Lower Lobe Bronchus, Left NC	Ø Open 3 Percutaneous 4 Percutaneous Endoscopic 7 Via Natural or Artificial Opening 8 Via Natural or Artificial Opening Endoscopic X External	Z No Device	Z No Qualifier

Non-OR ØBF[1,2,3,4,5,6,7,8,9,B]XZZ
NC ØBF[1,2,3,4,5,6,7,8,9,B]XZZ

Ø Medical and Surgical
B Respiratory System
H Insertion Putting in a nonbiological appliance that monitors, assists, performs, or prevents a physiological function but does not physically take the place of a body part

Body Part Character 4	Approach Character 5	Device Character 6	Qualifier Character 7
Ø Tracheobronchial Tree	Ø Open 3 Percutaneous 4 Percutaneous Endoscopic 7 Via Natural or Artificial Opening 8 Via Natural or Artificial Opening Endoscopic	1 Radioactive Element 2 Monitoring Device 3 Infusion Device D Intraluminal Device	Z No Qualifier
1 Trachea	Ø Open	2 Monitoring Device D Intraluminal Device	Z No Qualifier
1 Trachea	3 Percutaneous	D Intraluminal Device E Intraluminal Device, Endotracheal Airway	Z No Qualifier
1 Trachea	4 Percutaneous Endoscopic	D Intraluminal Device	Z No Qualifier
1 Trachea	7 Via Natural or Artificial Opening 8 Via Natural or Artificial Opening Endoscopic	2 Monitoring Device D Intraluminal Device E Intraluminal Device, Endotracheal Airway	Z No Qualifier
3 Main Bronchus, Right 4 Upper Lobe Bronchus, Right 5 Middle Lobe Bronchus, Right 6 Lower Lobe Bronchus, Right 7 Main Bronchus, Left 8 Upper Lobe Bronchus, Left 9 Lingula Bronchus B Lower Lobe Bronchus, Left	Ø Open 3 Percutaneous 4 Percutaneous Endoscopic 7 Via Natural or Artificial Opening 8 Via Natural or Artificial Opening Endoscopic	G Endobronchial Valve	Z No Qualifier
K Lung, Right L Lung, Left	Ø Open 3 Percutaneous 4 Percutaneous Endoscopic 7 Via Natural or Artificial Opening 8 Via Natural or Artificial Opening Endoscopic	1 Radioactive Element 2 Monitoring Device 3 Infusion Device	Z No Qualifier
R Diaphragm, Right S Diaphragm, Left	Ø Open 3 Percutaneous 4 Percutaneous Endoscopic	2 Monitoring Device M Diaphragmatic Pacemaker Lead	Z No Qualifier

Non-OR ØBHØ[7,8][2,3,D]Z
Non-OR ØBH13EZ
Non-OR ØBH1[7,8]EZ
Non-OR ØBH[3,4,5,6,7,8,9,B]8GZ

Ø Medical and Surgical
B Respiratory System
J Inspection Visually and/or manually exploring a body part

Body Part Character 4	Approach Character 5	Device Character 6	Qualifier Character 7
Ø Tracheobronchial Tree 1 Trachea K Lung, Right L Lung, Left Q Pleura T Diaphragm	Ø Open 3 Percutaneous 4 Percutaneous Endoscopic 7 Via Natural or Artificial Opening 8 Via Natural or Artificial Opening Endoscopic X External	Z No Device	Z No Qualifier

Non-OR ØBJ[Ø,K,L]8ZZ
Non-OR ØBJ1[3,4,7,8,X]ZZ
AHA: 2Ø14, 1Q, 2Ø

Ø Medical and Surgical
B Respiratory System
L Occlusion Completely closing an orifice or the lumen of a tubular body part

Body Part Character 4	Approach Character 5	Device Character 6	Qualifier Character 7
1 Trachea 2 Carina 3 Main Bronchus, Right 4 Upper Lobe Bronchus, Right 5 Middle Lobe Bronchus, Right 6 Lower Lobe Bronchus, Right 7 Main Bronchus, Left 8 Upper Lobe Bronchus, Left 9 Lingula Bronchus B Lower Lobe Bronchus, Left	Ø Open 3 Percutaneous 4 Percutaneous Endoscopic	C Extraluminal Device D Intraluminal Device Z No Device	Z No Qualifier
1 Trachea 2 Carina 3 Main Bronchus, Right 4 Upper Lobe Bronchus, Right 5 Middle Lobe Bronchus, Right 6 Lower Lobe Bronchus, Right 7 Main Bronchus, Left 8 Upper Lobe Bronchus, Left 9 Lingula Bronchus B Lower Lobe Bronchus, Left	7 Via Natural or Artificial Opening 8 Via Natural or Artificial Opening Endoscopic	D Intraluminal Device Z No Device	Z No Qualifier

Ø Medical and Surgical
B Respiratory System
M Reattachment Putting back in or on all or a portion of a separated body part to its normal location or other suitable location

Body Part Character 4	Approach Character 5	Device Character 6	Qualifier Character 7
1 Trachea 2 Carina 3 Main Bronchus, Right 4 Upper Lobe Bronchus, Right 5 Middle Lobe Bronchus, Right 6 Lower Lobe Bronchus, Right 7 Main Bronchus, Left 8 Upper Lobe Bronchus, Left 9 Lingula Bronchus B Lower Lobe Bronchus, Left C Upper Lung Lobe, Right D Middle Lung Lobe, Right F Lower Lung Lobe, Right G Upper Lung Lobe, Left H Lung Lingula J Lower Lung Lobe, Left K Lung, Right L Lung, Left R Diaphragm, Right S Diaphragm, Left	Ø Open	Z No Device	Z No Qualifier

Ø Medical and Surgical
B Respiratory System
N Release Freeing a body part from an abnormal physical constraint

Body Part Character 4	Approach Character 5	Device Character 6	Qualifier Character 7
1 Trachea 2 Carina 3 Main Bronchus, Right 4 Upper Lobe Bronchus, Right 5 Middle Lobe Bronchus, Right 6 Lower Lobe Bronchus, Right 7 Main Bronchus, Left 8 Upper Lobe Bronchus, Left 9 Lingula Bronchus B Lower Lobe Bronchus, Left C Upper Lung Lobe, Right D Middle Lung Lobe, Right F Lower Lung Lobe, Right G Upper Lung Lobe, Left H Lung Lingula J Lower Lung Lobe, Left K Lung, Right L Lung, Left M Lungs, Bilateral	Ø Open 3 Percutaneous 4 Percutaneous Endoscopic 7 Via Natural or Artificial Opening 8 Via Natural or Artificial Opening Endoscopic	Z No Device	Z No Qualifier
N Pleura, Right P Pleura, Left R Diaphragm, Right S Diaphragm, Left	Ø Open 3 Percutaneous 4 Percutaneous Endoscopic	Z No Device	Z No Qualifier

Ø Medical and Surgical
B Respiratory System
P Removal Taking out or off a device from a body part

Body Part Character 4	Approach Character 5	Device Character 6	Qualifier Character 7
Ø Tracheobronchial Tree	Ø Open 3 Percutaneous 4 Percutaneous Endoscopic 7 Via Natural or Artificial Opening 8 Via Natural or Artificial Opening Endoscopic	Ø Drainage Device 1 Radioactive Element 2 Monitoring Device 3 Infusion Device 7 Autologous Tissue Substitute C Extraluminal Device D Intraluminal Device J Synthetic Substitute K Nonautologous Tissue Substitute	Z No Qualifier
Ø Tracheobronchial Tree	X External	Ø Drainage Device 1 Radioactive Element 2 Monitoring Device 3 Infusion Device D Intraluminal Device	Z No Qualifier
1 Trachea	Ø Open 3 Percutaneous 4 Percutaneous Endoscopic 7 Via Natural or Artificial Opening 8 Via Natural or Artificial Opening Endoscopic	Ø Drainage Device 2 Monitoring Device 7 Autologous Tissue Substitute C Extraluminal Device D Intraluminal Device F Tracheostomy Device J Synthetic Substitute K Nonautologous Tissue Substitute	Z No Qualifier
1 Trachea	X External	Ø Drainage Device 2 Monitoring Device D Intraluminal Device F Tracheostomy Device	Z No Qualifier
K Lung, Right L Lung, Left	Ø Open 3 Percutaneous 4 Percutaneous Endoscopic 7 Via Natural or Artificial Opening 8 Via Natural or Artificial Opening Endoscopic X External	Ø Drainage Device 1 Radioactive Element 2 Monitoring Device 3 Infusion Device	Z No Qualifier

ØBP Continued on next page

Non-OR ØBPØX[Ø,1,2,3,D]Z
Non-OR ØBP1X[Ø,2,D,F]Z
Non-OR ØBP[K,L]X[Ø,1,2,3]Z

0 Medical and Surgical
B Respiratory System
P Removal Taking out or off a device from a body part

0BP Continued

Body Part Character 4	Approach Character 5	Device Character 6	Qualifier Character 7
Q Pleura	**0** Open **3** Percutaneous **4** Percutaneous Endoscopic **7** Via Natural or Artificial Opening **8** Via Natural or Artificial Opening Endoscopic **X** External	**0** Drainage Device **1** Radioactive Element **2** Monitoring Device	**Z** No Qualifier
T Diaphragm	**0** Open **3** Percutaneous **4** Percutaneous Endoscopic **7** Via Natural or Artificial Opening **8** Via Natural or Artificial Opening Endoscopic	**0** Drainage Device **2** Monitoring Device **7** Autologous Tissue Substitute **J** Synthetic Substitute **K** Nonautologous Tissue Substitute **M** Diaphragmatic Pacemaker Lead	**Z** No Qualifier
T Diaphragm	**X** External	**0** Drainage Device **2** Monitoring Device **M** Diaphragmatic Pacemaker Lead	**Z** No Qualifier

Non-OR 0BPQ[0,3,4,7,8,X][0,1,2]Z
Non-OR 0BPTX[0,2,M]Z

0 Medical and Surgical
B Respiratory System
Q Repair Restoring, to the extent possible, a body part to its normal anatomic structure and function

Body Part Character 4	Approach Character 5	Device Character 6	Qualifier Character 7
1 Trachea ⊞ **2** Carina **3** Main Bronchus, Right ⊞ **4** Upper Lobe Bronchus, Right ⊞ **5** Middle Lobe Bronchus, Right ⊞ **6** Lower Lobe Bronchus, Right ⊞ **7** Main Bronchus, Left ⊞ **8** Upper Lobe Bronchus, Left ⊞ **9** Lingula Bronchus ⊞ **B** Lower Lobe Bronchus, Left ⊞ **C** Upper Lung Lobe, Right **D** Middle Lung Lobe, Right **F** Lower Lung Lobe, Right **G** Upper Lung Lobe, Left **H** Lung Lingula **J** Lower Lung Lobe, Left **K** Lung, Right ⊞ **L** Lung, Left ⊞ **M** Lungs, Bilateral ⊞	**0** Open **3** Percutaneous **4** Percutaneous Endoscopic **7** Via Natural or Artificial Opening **8** Via Natural or Artificial Opening Endoscopic	**Z** No Device	**Z** No Qualifier
N Pleura, Right ⊞ **P** Pleura, Left ⊞ **R** Diaphragm, Right **S** Diaphragm, Left	**0** Open **3** Percutaneous **4** Percutaneous Endoscopic	**Z** No Device	**Z** No Qualifier

No Procedure Combinations Specified
⊞ 0BQ[1,3,4,5,6,7,8,9,B,K,L,M][0,3,4,7,8]ZZ
⊞ 0BQ[N,P][0,3,4]ZZ

Ø Medical and Surgical
B Respiratory System
S Reposition Moving to its normal location or other suitable location all or a portion of a body part

Body Part Character 4	Approach Character 5	Device Character 6	Qualifier Character 7
1 Trachea 2 Carina 3 Main Bronchus, Right 4 Upper Lobe Bronchus, Right 5 Middle Lobe Bronchus, Right 6 Lower Lobe Bronchus, Right 7 Main Bronchus, Left 8 Upper Lobe Bronchus, Left 9 Lingula Bronchus B Lower Lobe Bronchus, Left C Upper Lung Lobe, Right D Middle Lung Lobe, Right F Lower Lung Lobe, Right G Upper Lung Lobe, Left H Lung Lingula J Lower Lung Lobe, Left K Lung, Right L Lung, Left R Diaphragm, Right S Diaphragm, Left	Ø Open	Z No Device	Z No Qualifier

Ø Medical and Surgical
B Respiratory System
T Resection Cutting out or off, without replacement, all of a body part

Body Part Character 4	Approach Character 5	Device Character 6	Qualifier Character 7
1 Trachea 2 Carina 3 Main Bronchus, Right 4 Upper Lobe Bronchus, Right 5 Middle Lobe Bronchus, Right 6 Lower Lobe Bronchus, Right 7 Main Bronchus, Left 8 Upper Lobe Bronchus, Left 9 Lingula Bronchus B Lower Lobe Bronchus, Left C Upper Lung Lobe, Right D Middle Lung Lobe, Right F Lower Lung Lobe, Right G Upper Lung Lobe, Left H Lung Lingula J Lower Lung Lobe, Left K Lung, Right ⊞ L Lung, Left ⊞ M Lungs, Bilateral ⊞ R Diaphragm, Right S Diaphragm, Left	Ø Open 4 Percutaneous Endoscopic	Z No Device	Z No Qualifier

No Procedure Combinations Specified
⊞ ØBT[K,L,M]ØZZ

Ø Medical and Surgical
B Respiratory System
U Supplement Putting in or on biological or synthetic material that physically reinforces and/or augments the function of a portion of a body part

Body Part Character 4	Approach Character 5	Device Character 6	Qualifier Character 7
1 Trachea 2 Carina 3 Main Bronchus, Right 4 Upper Lobe Bronchus, Right 5 Middle Lobe Bronchus, Right 6 Lower Lobe Bronchus, Right 7 Main Bronchus, Left 8 Upper Lobe Bronchus, Left 9 Lingula Bronchus B Lower Lobe Bronchus, Left R Diaphragm, Right S Diaphragm, Left	Ø Open 4 Percutaneous Endoscopic	7 Autologous Tissue Substitute J Synthetic Substitute K Nonautologous Tissue Substitute	Z No Qualifier

0 Medical and Surgical
B Respiratory System
V Restriction Partially closing an orifice or the lumen of a tubular body part

Body Part Character 4	Approach Character 5	Device Character 6	Qualifier Character 7
1 Trachea **2** Carina **3** Main Bronchus, Right **4** Upper Lobe Bronchus, Right **5** Middle Lobe Bronchus, Right **6** Lower Lobe Bronchus, Right **7** Main Bronchus, Left **8** Upper Lobe Bronchus, Left **9** Lingula Bronchus **B** Lower Lobe Bronchus, Left	**0** Open **3** Percutaneous **4** Percutaneous Endoscopic	**C** Extraluminal Device **D** Intraluminal Device **Z** No Device	**Z** No Qualifier
1 Trachea **2** Carina **3** Main Bronchus, Right **4** Upper Lobe Bronchus, Right **5** Middle Lobe Bronchus, Right **6** Lower Lobe Bronchus, Right **7** Main Bronchus, Left **8** Upper Lobe Bronchus, Left **9** Lingula Bronchus **B** Lower Lobe Bronchus, Left	**7** Via Natural or Artificial Opening **8** Via Natural or Artificial Opening Endoscopic	**D** Intraluminal Device **Z** No Device	**Z** No Qualifier

0 Medical and Surgical
B Respiratory System
W Revision Correcting, to the extent possible, a portion of a malfunctioning device or the position of a displaced device

Body Part Character 4	Approach Character 5	Device Character 6	Qualifier Character 7
0 Tracheobronchial Tree	**0** Open **3** Percutaneous **4** Percutaneous Endoscopic **7** Via Natural or Artificial Opening **8** Via Natural or Artificial Opening Endoscopic **X** External	**0** Drainage Device **2** Monitoring Device **3** Infusion Device **7** Autologous Tissue Substitute **C** Extraluminal Device **D** Intraluminal Device **J** Synthetic Substitute **K** Nonautologous Tissue Substitute	**Z** No Qualifier
1 Trachea	**0** Open **3** Percutaneous **4** Percutaneous Endoscopic **7** Via Natural or Artificial Opening **8** Via Natural or Artificial Opening Endoscopic **X** External	**0** Drainage Device **2** Monitoring Device **7** Autologous Tissue Substitute **C** Extraluminal Device **D** Intraluminal Device **F** Tracheostomy Device **J** Synthetic Substitute **K** Nonautologous Tissue Substitute	**Z** No Qualifier
K Lung, Right **L** Lung, Left	**0** Open **3** Percutaneous **4** Percutaneous Endoscopic **7** Via Natural or Artificial Opening **8** Via Natural or Artificial Opening Endoscopic **X** External	**0** Drainage Device **2** Monitoring Device **3** Infusion Device	**Z** No Qualifier
Q Pleura	**0** Open **3** Percutaneous **4** Percutaneous Endoscopic **7** Via Natural or Artificial Opening **8** Via Natural or Artificial Opening Endoscopic **X** External	**0** Drainage Device **2** Monitoring Device	**Z** No Qualifier
T Diaphragm	**0** Open **3** Percutaneous **4** Percutaneous Endoscopic **7** Via Natural or Artificial Opening **8** Via Natural or Artificial Opening Endoscopic **X** External	**0** Drainage Device **2** Monitoring Device **7** Autologous Tissue Substitute **J** Synthetic Substitute **K** Nonautologous Tissue Substitute **M** Diaphragmatic Pacemaker Lead	**Z** No Qualifier

Non-OR 0BW0X[0,2,3,7,C,D,J,K]Z
Non-OR 0BW1X[0,2,7,C,D,F,J,K]Z
Non-OR 0BW[K,L]X[0,2,3]Z
Non-OR 0BWQ[0,3,4,7,8,X][0,2]Z
Non-OR 0BWTX[0,2,7,J,K,M]Z

Ø Medical and Surgical
B Respiratory System
Y Transplantation Putting in or on all or a portion of a living body part taken from another individual or animal to physically take the place and/or function of all or a portion of a similar body part

Body Part Character 4	Approach Character 5	Device Character 6	Qualifier Character 7
C Upper Lung Lobe, Right LC **D** Middle Lung Lobe, Right LC **F** Lower Lung Lobe, Right LC **G** Upper Lung Lobe, Left LC **H** Lung Lingula LC **J** Lower Lung Lobe, Left LC **K** Lung, Right LC **L** Lung, Left LC **M** Lungs, Bilateral LC	**Ø** Open	**Z** No Device	**Ø** Allogeneic **1** Syngeneic **2** Zooplastic

LC ØBY[C,D,F,G,H,J,K,L,M]ØZ[Ø,1,2]

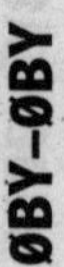

Mouth and Throat 0C0–0CX

0 Medical and Surgical
C Mouth and Throat
0 Alteration Modifying the anatomic structure of a body part without affecting the function of the body part

Body Part Character 4	Approach Character 5	Device Character 6	Qualifier Character 7
0 Upper Lip 1 Lower Lip	X External	7 Autologous Tissue Substitute J Synthetic Substitute K Nonautologous Tissue Substitute Z No Device	Z No Qualifier

0 Medical and Surgical
C Mouth and Throat
2 Change Taking out or off a device from a body part and putting back an identical or similar device in or on the same body part without cutting or puncturing the skin or a mucous membrane

Body Part Character 4	Approach Character 5	Device Character 6	Qualifier Character 7
A Salivary Gland S Larynx Y Mouth and Throat	X External	0 Drainage Device Y Other Device	Z No Qualifier

Non-OR For all body part, approach, device, and qualifier values

0 Medical and Surgical
C Mouth and Throat
5 Destruction Physical eradication of all or a portion of a body part by the direct use of energy, force, or a destructive agent

Body Part Character 4	Approach Character 5	Device Character 6	Qualifier Character 7
0 Upper Lip 1 Lower Lip 2 Hard Palate 3 Soft Palate 4 Buccal Mucosa 5 Upper Gingiva 6 Lower Gingiva 7 Tongue N Uvula P Tonsils Q Adenoids	0 Open 3 Percutaneous X External	Z No Device	Z No Qualifier
8 Parotid Gland, Right 9 Parotid Gland, Left B Parotid Duct, Right C Parotid Duct, Left D Sublingual Gland, Right F Sublingual Gland, Left G Submaxillary Gland, Right H Submaxillary Gland, Left J Minor Salivary Gland	0 Open 3 Percutaneous	Z No Device	Z No Qualifier
M Pharynx R Epiglottis S Larynx T Vocal Cord, Right V Vocal Cord, Left	0 Open 3 Percutaneous 4 Percutaneous Endoscopic 7 Via Natural or Artificial Opening 8 Via Natural or Artificial Opening Endoscopic	Z No Device	Z No Qualifier
W Upper Tooth X Lower Tooth	0 Open X External	Z No Device	0 Single 1 Multiple 2 All

Non-OR 0C5[5,6][0,3,X]ZZ
Non-OR 0C5[W,X][0,X]Z[0,1,2]

Ø Medical and Surgical
C Mouth and Throat
7 Dilation Expanding an orifice or the lumen of a tubular body part

Body Part Character 4	Approach Character 5	Device Character 6	Qualifier Character 7
B Parotid Duct, Right **C** Parotid Duct, Left	**Ø** Open **3** Percutaneous **7** Via Natural or Artificial Opening	**D** Intraluminal Device **Z** No Device	**Z** No Qualifier
M Pharynx	**7** Via Natural or Artificial Opening **8** Via Natural or Artificial Opening Endoscopic	**D** Intraluminal Device **Z** No Device	**Z** No Qualifier
S Larynx ⊞	**Ø** Open **3** Percutaneous **4** Percutaneous Endoscopic **7** Via Natural or Artificial Opening **8** Via Natural or Artificial Opening Endoscopic	**D** Intraluminal Device **Z** No Device	**Z** No Qualifier

Non-OR ØC7[B,C][Ø,3,7][D,Z]Z
Non-OR ØC7M[7,8][D,Z]Z

No Procedure Combinations Specified
⊞ ØC7S[Ø,3,4,7,8]DZ

Ø Medical and Surgical
C Mouth and Throat
9 Drainage Taking or letting out fluids and/or gases from a body part

Body Part Character 4	Approach Character 5	Device Character 6	Qualifier Character 7
Ø Upper Lip **1** Lower Lip **2** Hard Palate **3** Soft Palate **4** Buccal Mucosa **5** Upper Gingiva **6** Lower Gingiva **7** Tongue **N** Uvula **P** Tonsils **Q** Adenoids	**Ø** Open **3** Percutaneous **X** External	**Ø** Drainage Device	**Z** No Qualifier
Ø Upper Lip **1** Lower Lip **2** Hard Palate **3** Soft Palate **4** Buccal Mucosa **5** Upper Gingiva **6** Lower Gingiva **7** Tongue **N** Uvula **P** Tonsils **Q** Adenoids	**Ø** Open **3** Percutaneous **X** External	**Z** No Device	**X** Diagnostic **Z** No Qualifier
8 Parotid Gland, Right **9** Parotid Gland, Left **B** Parotid Duct, Right **C** Parotid Duct, Left **D** Sublingual Gland, Right **F** Sublingual Gland, Left **G** Submaxillary Gland, Right **H** Submaxillary Gland, Left **J** Minor Salivary Gland	**Ø** Open **3** Percutaneous	**Ø** Drainage Device	**Z** No Qualifier
8 Parotid Gland, Right **9** Parotid Gland, Left **B** Parotid Duct, Right **C** Parotid Duct, Left **D** Sublingual Gland, Right **F** Sublingual Gland, Left **G** Submaxillary Gland, Right **H** Submaxillary Gland, Left **J** Minor Salivary Gland	**Ø** Open **3** Percutaneous	**Z** No Device	**X** Diagnostic **Z** No Qualifier

ØC9 Continued on next page

Non-OR ØC9[5,6][Ø,3,X]ØZ
Non-OR ØC97[3,X]ZX
Non-OR ØC9[Ø,1,4,5,6][Ø,3,X]ZX
Non-OR ØC9[5,6][Ø,3,X]ZZ
Non-OR ØC9[8,9,B,C,D,F,G,H,J][Ø,3]ØZ
Non-OR ØC9[8,9,B,C,D,F,G,H,J]3ZX
Non-OR ØC9[8,9,B,C,D,F,G,H,J][Ø,3]ZZ

ØC9 Continued

Ø Medical and Surgical
C Mouth and Throat
9 Drainage Taking or letting out fluids and/or gases from a body part

Body Part Character 4	Approach Character 5	Device Character 6	Qualifier Character 7
M Pharynx R Epiglottis S Larynx T Vocal Cord, Right V Vocal Cord, Left	Ø Open 3 Percutaneous 4 Percutaneous Endoscopic 7 Via Natural or Artificial Opening 8 Via Natural or Artificial Opening Endoscopic	Ø Drainage Device	Z No Qualifier
M Pharynx R Epiglottis S Larynx T Vocal Cord, Right V Vocal Cord, Left	Ø Open 3 Percutaneous 4 Percutaneous Endoscopic 7 Via Natural or Artificial Opening 8 Via Natural or Artificial Opening Endoscopic	Z No Device	X Diagnostic Z No Qualifier
W Upper Tooth X Lower Tooth	Ø Open X External	Ø Drainage Device Z No Device	Ø Single 1 Multiple 2 All

Non-OR ØC9M[Ø,3,4,7,8]ZX
Non-OR ØC9[R,S,T,V][3,4,7,8]ZX
Non-OR ØC9[W,X][Ø,X][Ø,Z][Ø,1,2]

Ø Medical and Surgical
C Mouth and Throat
B Excision Cutting out or off, without replacement, a portion of a body part

Body Part Character 4	Approach Character 5	Device Character 6	Qualifier Character 7
Ø Upper Lip 1 Lower Lip 2 Hard Palate 3 Soft Palate 4 Buccal Mucosa 5 Upper Gingiva 6 Lower Gingiva 7 Tongue N Uvula P Tonsils Q Adenoids	Ø Open 3 Percutaneous X External	Z No Device	X Diagnostic Z No Qualifier
8 Parotid Gland, Right 9 Parotid Gland, Left B Parotid Duct, Right C Parotid Duct, Left D Sublingual Gland, Right F Sublingual Gland, Left G Submaxillary Gland, Right H Submaxillary Gland, Left J Minor Salivary Gland	Ø Open 3 Percutaneous	Z No Device	X Diagnostic Z No Qualifier
M Pharynx R Epiglottis S Larynx T Vocal Cord, Right V Vocal Cord, Left	Ø Open 3 Percutaneous 4 Percutaneous Endoscopic 7 Via Natural or Artificial Opening 8 Via Natural or Artificial Opening Endoscopic	Z No Device	X Diagnostic Z No Qualifier
W Upper Tooth X Lower Tooth	Ø Open X External	Z No Device	Ø Single 1 Multiple 2 All

Non-OR ØCB[Ø,1,4,5,6][Ø,3,X]ZX
Non-OR ØCB[5,6][Ø,3,X]ZZ
Non-OR ØCB7[3,X]ZX
Non-OR ØCB[8,9,B,C,D,F,G,H,J]3ZX
Non-OR ØCBM[Ø,3,4,7,8]ZX
Non-OR ØCB[R,S,T,V][3,4,7,8]ZX
Non-OR ØCB[W,X][Ø,X]Z[Ø,1,2]

Ø Medical and Surgical
C Mouth and Throat
C Extirpation Taking or cutting out solid matter from a body part

Body Part Character 4	Approach Character 5	Device Character 6	Qualifier Character 7
Ø Upper Lip **1** Lower Lip **2** Hard Palate **3** Soft Palate **4** Buccal Mucosa **5** Upper Gingiva **6** Lower Gingiva **7** Tongue **N** Uvula **P** Tonsils **Q** Adenoids	**Ø** Open **3** Percutaneous **X** External	**Z** No Device	**Z** No Qualifier
8 Parotid Gland, Right **9** Parotid Gland, Left **B** Parotid Duct, Right **C** Parotid Duct, Left **D** Sublingual Gland, Right **F** Sublingual Gland, Left **G** Submaxillary Gland, Right **H** Submaxillary Gland, Left **J** Minor Salivary Gland	**Ø** Open **3** Percutaneous	**Z** No Device	**Z** No Qualifier
M Pharynx **R** Epiglottis **S** Larynx **T** Vocal Cord, Right **V** Vocal Cord, Left	**Ø** Open **3** Percutaneous **4** Percutaneous Endoscopic **7** Via Natural or Artificial Opening **8** Via Natural or Artificial Opening Endoscopic	**Z** No Device	**Z** No Qualifier
W Upper Tooth **X** Lower Tooth	**Ø** Open **X** External	**Z** No Device	**Ø** Single **1** Multiple **2** All

Non-OR ØCC[Ø,1,2,3,4,7,N,P,Q]XZZ
Non-OR ØCC[5,6][Ø,3,X]ZZ
Non-OR ØCC[8,9,B,C,D,F,G,H,J][Ø,3]ZZ
Non-OR ØCC[M,S][7,8]ZZ
Non-OR ØCC[W,X][Ø,X]Z[Ø,1,2]

Ø Medical and Surgical
C Mouth and Throat
D Extraction Pulling or stripping out or off all or a portion of a body part by the use of force

Body Part Character 4	Approach Character 5	Device Character 6	Qualifier Character 7
T Vocal Cord, Right **V** Vocal Cord, Left	**Ø** Open **3** Percutaneous **4** Percutaneous Endoscopic **7** Via Natural or Artificial Opening **8** Via Natural or Artificial Opening Endoscopic	**Z** No Device	**Z** No Qualifier
W Upper Tooth **X** Lower Tooth	**X** External	**Z** No Device	**Ø** Single **1** Multiple **2** All

Non-OR ØCD[W,X]XZ[Ø,1,2]

Ø Medical and Surgical
C Mouth and Throat
F Fragmentation Breaking solid matter in a body part into pieces

Body Part Character 4	Approach Character 5	Device Character 6	Qualifier Character 7
B Parotid Duct, Right NC **C** Parotid Duct, Left NC	**Ø** Open **3** Percutaneous **7** Via Natural or Artificial Opening **X** External	**Z** No Device	**Z** No Qualifier

Non-OR For all body part, approach, device, and qualifier values
NC ØCF[B,C]XZZ

0 Medical and Surgical
C Mouth and Throat
H Insertion Putting in a nonbiological appliance that monitors, assists, performs, or prevents a physiological function but does not physically take the place of a body part

Body Part Character 4	Approach Character 5	Device Character 6	Qualifier Character 7
7 Tongue	0 Open 3 Percutaneous X External	1 Radioactive Element	Z No Qualifier
Y Mouth and Throat	7 Via Natural or Artificial Opening 8 Via Natural or Artificial Opening Endoscopic	B Intraluminal Device, Airway	Z No Qualifier

Non-OR 0CHY[7,8]BZ

0 Medical and Surgical
C Mouth and Throat
J Inspection Visually and/or manually exploring a body part

Body Part Character 4	Approach Character 5	Device Character 6	Qualifier Character 7
A Salivary Gland	0 Open 3 Percutaneous X External	Z No Device	Z No Qualifier
S Larynx Y Mouth and Throat	0 Open 3 Percutaneous 4 Percutaneous Endoscopic 7 Via Natural or Artificial Opening 8 Via Natural or Artificial Opening Endoscopic X External	Z No Device	Z No Qualifier

Non-OR 0CJA[0,3,X]ZZ
Non-OR 0CJ[S,Y][0,3,4,7,8,X]ZZ

0 Medical and Surgical
C Mouth and Throat
L Occlusion Completely closing an orifice or the lumen of a tubular body part

Body Part Character 4	Approach Character 5	Device Character 6	Qualifier Character 7
B Parotid Duct, Right C Parotid Duct, Left	0 Open 3 Percutaneous 4 Percutaneous Endoscopic	C Extraluminal Device D Intraluminal Device Z No Device	Z No Qualifier
B Parotid Duct, Right C Parotid Duct, Left	7 Via Natural or Artificial Opening 8 Via Natural or Artificial Opening Endoscopic	D Intraluminal Device Z No Device	Z No Qualifier

0 Medical and Surgical
C Mouth and Throat
M Reattachment Putting back in or on all or a portion of a separated body part to its normal location or other suitable location

Body Part Character 4	Approach Character 5	Device Character 6	Qualifier Character 7
0 Upper Lip 1 Lower Lip 3 Soft Palate 7 Tongue N Uvula	0 Open	Z No Device	Z No Qualifier
W Upper Tooth X Lower Tooth	0 Open X External	Z No Device	0 Single 1 Multiple 2 All

Non-OR 0CM[W,X][0,X]Z[0,1,2]

Ø Medical and Surgical
C Mouth and Throat
N Release Freeing a body part from an abnormal physical constraint

Body Part Character 4	Approach Character 5	Device Character 6	Qualifier Character 7
Ø Upper Lip 1 Lower Lip 2 Hard Palate 3 Soft Palate 4 Buccal Mucosa 5 Upper Gingiva 6 Lower Gingiva 7 Tongue N Uvula P Tonsils Q Adenoids	Ø Open 3 Percutaneous X External	Z No Device	Z No Qualifier
8 Parotid Gland, Right 9 Parotid Gland, Left B Parotid Duct, Right C Parotid Duct, Left D Sublingual Gland, Right F Sublingual Gland, Left G Submaxillary Gland, Right H Submaxillary Gland, Left J Minor Salivary Gland	Ø Open 3 Percutaneous	Z No Device	Z No Qualifier
W Upper Tooth X Lower Tooth	Ø Open X External	Z No Device	Ø Single 1 Multiple 2 All
M Pharynx R Epiglottis S Larynx T Vocal Cord, Right V Vocal Cord, Left	Ø Open 3 Percutaneous 4 Percutaneous Endoscopic 7 Via Natural or Artificial Opening 8 Via Natural or Artificial Opening Endoscopic	Z No Device	Z No Qualifier

Non-OR ØCN[Ø,1,5,6,7][Ø,3,X]ZZ
Non-OR ØCN[W,X][Ø,X]Z[Ø,1,2]

Ø Medical and Surgical
C Mouth and Throat
P Removal Taking out or off a device from a body part

Body Part Character 4	Approach Character 5	Device Character 6	Qualifier Character 7
A Salivary Gland	Ø Open 3 Percutaneous	Ø Drainage Device C Extraluminal Device	Z No Qualifier
S Larynx ⊞	Ø Open 3 Percutaneous 7 Via Natural or Artificial Opening 8 Via Natural or Artificial Opening Endoscopic X External	Ø Drainage Device 7 Autologous Tissue Substitute D Intraluminal Device J Synthetic Substitute K Nonautologous Tissue Substitute	Z No Qualifier
Y Mouth and Throat	Ø Open 3 Percutaneous 7 Via Natural or Artificial Opening 8 Via Natural or Artificial Opening Endoscopic X External	Ø Drainage Device 1 Radioactive Element 7 Autologous Tissue Substitute D Intraluminal Device J Synthetic Substitute K Nonautologous Tissue Substitute	Z No Qualifier

Non-OR ØCPA[Ø,3][Ø,C]Z
Non-OR ØCPSX[Ø,7,D,J,K]Z
Non-OR ØCPY[7,8][Ø,D]Z
Non-OR ØCPYX[Ø,1,7,D,J,K]Z

No Procedure Combinations Specified
⊞ ØCPS[Ø,3,7,8]DZ

Ø Medical and Surgical
C Mouth and Throat
Q Repair Restoring, to the extent possible, a body part to its normal anatomic structure and function

Body Part Character 4	Approach Character 5	Device Character 6	Qualifier Character 7
Ø Upper Lip ⊞ 1 Lower Lip ⊞ 2 Hard Palate 3 Soft Palate 4 Buccal Mucosa ⊞ 5 Upper Gingiva 6 Lower Gingiva 7 Tongue N Uvula P Tonsils Q Adenoids	Ø Open 3 Percutaneous X External	Z No Device	Z No Qualifier
8 Parotid Gland, Right 9 Parotid Gland, Left B Parotid Duct, Right C Parotid Duct, Left D Sublingual Gland, Right F Sublingual Gland, Left G Submaxillary Gland, Right H Submaxillary Gland, Left J Minor Salivary Gland	Ø Open 3 Percutaneous	Z No Device	Z No Qualifier
M Pharynx ⊞ R Epiglottis S Larynx T Vocal Cord, Right V Vocal Cord, Left	Ø Open 3 Percutaneous 4 Percutaneous Endoscopic 7 Via Natural or Artificial Opening 8 Via Natural or Artificial Opening Endoscopic	Z No Device	Z No Qualifier
W Upper Tooth X Lower Tooth	Ø Open X External	Z No Device	Ø Single 1 Multiple 2 All

Non-OR ØCQ[Ø,1]XZZ
Non-OR ØCQ[5,6][Ø,3,X]ZZ
Non-OR ØCQ[W,X][Ø,X]Z[Ø,1,2]

No Procedure Combinations Specified
⊞ ØCQ[Ø,1,4][Ø,3]ZZ
⊞ ØCQ4XZZ
⊞ ØCQM[Ø,3,4,7,8]ZZ

Ø Medical and Surgical
C Mouth and Throat
R Replacement Putting in or on biological or synthetic material that physically takes the place and/or function of all or a portion of a body part

Body Part Character 4	Approach Character 5	Device Character 6	Qualifier Character 7
Ø Upper Lip 1 Lower Lip 2 Hard Palate 3 Soft Palate 4 Buccal Mucosa 5 Upper Gingiva 6 Lower Gingiva 7 Tongue N Uvula	Ø Open 3 Percutaneous X External	7 Autologous Tissue Substitute J Synthetic Substitute K Nonautologous Tissue Substitute	Z No Qualifier
B Parotid Duct, Right C Parotid Duct, Left	Ø Open 3 Percutaneous	7 Autologous Tissue Substitute J Synthetic Substitute K Nonautologous Tissue Substitute	Z No Qualifier
M Pharynx R Epiglottis S Larynx ⊞ T Vocal Cord, Right V Vocal Cord, Left	Ø Open 7 Via Natural or Artificial Opening 8 Via Natural or Artificial Opening Endoscopic	7 Autologous Tissue Substitute J Synthetic Substitute K Nonautologous Tissue Substitute	Z No Qualifier
W Upper Tooth X Lower Tooth	Ø Open X External	7 Autologous Tissue Substitute J Synthetic Substitute K Nonautologous Tissue Substitute	Ø Single 1 Multiple 2 All

Non-OR ØCR[W,X][Ø,X][7,J,K][Ø,1,2]
AHA: 2014, 2Q, 5-6

No Procedure Combinations Specified
⊞ ØCRS[Ø,7,8]JZ

Ø Medical and Surgical
C Mouth and Throat
S Reposition Moving to its normal location or other suitable location all or a portion of a body part

Body Part Character 4	Approach Character 5	Device Character 6	Qualifier Character 7
Ø Upper Lip **1** Lower Lip **2** Hard Palate **3** Soft Palate **7** Tongue **N** Uvula	**Ø** Open **X** External	**Z** No Device	**Z** No Qualifier
B Parotid Duct, Right **C** Parotid Duct, Left	**Ø** Open **3** Percutaneous	**Z** No Device	**Z** No Qualifier
R Epiglottis **T** Vocal Cord, Right **V** Vocal Cord, Left	**Ø** Open **7** Via Natural or Artificial Opening **8** Via Natural or Artificial Opening Endoscopic	**Z** No Device	**Z** No Qualifier
W Upper Tooth **X** Lower Tooth	**Ø** Open **X** External	**5** External Fixation Device **Z** No Device	**Ø** Single **1** Multiple **2** All

Non-OR ØCS[W,X][Ø,X][5,Z][Ø,1,2]

Ø Medical and Surgical
C Mouth and Throat
T Resection Cutting out or off, without replacement, all of a body part

Body Part Character 4	Approach Character 5	Device Character 6	Qualifier Character 7
Ø Upper Lip **1** Lower Lip **2** Hard Palate **3** Soft Palate **7** Tongue **N** Uvula **P** Tonsils ⊞ **Q** Adenoids ⊞	**Ø** Open **X** External	**Z** No Device	**Z** No Qualifier
8 Parotid Gland, Right **9** Parotid Gland, Left **B** Parotid Duct, Right **C** Parotid Duct, Left **D** Sublingual Gland, Right **F** Sublingual Gland, Left **G** Submaxillary Gland, Right **H** Submaxillary Gland, Left **J** Minor Salivary Gland	**Ø** Open	**Z** No Device	**Z** No Qualifier
M Pharynx **R** Epiglottis **S** Larynx **T** Vocal Cord, Right **V** Vocal Cord, Left	**Ø** Open **4** Percutaneous Endoscopic **7** Via Natural or Artificial Opening **8** Via Natural or Artificial Opening Endoscopic	**Z** No Device	**Z** No Qualifier
W Upper Tooth **X** Lower Tooth	**Ø** Open	**Z** No Device	**Ø** Single **1** Multiple **2** All

Non-OR ØCT[W,X]ØZ[Ø,1,2]

No Procedure Combinations Specified
⊞ ØCT[P,Q][Ø,X]ZZ

0 Medical and Surgical
C Mouth and Throat
U Supplement Putting in or on biological or synthetic material that physically reinforces and/or augments the function of a portion of a body part

Body Part Character 4	Approach Character 5	Device Character 6	Qualifier Character 7
0 Upper Lip 1 Lower Lip 2 Hard Palate 3 Soft Palate 4 Buccal Mucosa 5 Upper Gingiva 6 Lower Gingiva 7 Tongue N Uvula	0 Open 3 Percutaneous X External	7 Autologous Tissue Substitute J Synthetic Substitute K Nonautologous Tissue Substitute	Z No Qualifier
M Pharynx R Epiglottis S Larynx ⊞ T Vocal Cord, Right V Vocal Cord, Left	0 Open 7 Via Natural or Artificial Opening 8 Via Natural or Artificial Opening Endoscopic	7 Autologous Tissue Substitute J Synthetic Substitute K Nonautologous Tissue Substitute	Z No Qualifier

Non-OR 0CU2[0,3]JZ

No Procedure Combinations Specified
⊞ 0CUS[0,7,8]JZ

0 Medical and Surgical
C Mouth and Throat
V Restriction Partially closing an orifice or the lumen of a tubular body part

Body Part Character 4	Approach Character 5	Device Character 6	Qualifier Character 7
B Parotid Duct, Right C Parotid Duct, Left	0 Open 3 Percutaneous	C Extraluminal Device D Intraluminal Device Z No Device	Z No Qualifier
B Parotid Duct, Right C Parotid Duct, Left	7 Via Natural or Artificial Opening 8 Via Natural or Artificial Opening Endoscopic	D Intraluminal Device Z No Device	Z No Qualifier

0 Medical and Surgical
C Mouth and Throat
W Revision Correcting, to the extent possible, a portion of a malfunctioning device or the position of a displaced device

Body Part Character 4	Approach Character 5	Device Character 6	Qualifier Character 7
A Salivary Gland	0 Open 3 Percutaneous X External	0 Drainage Device C Extraluminal Device	Z No Qualifier
S Larynx	0 Open 3 Percutaneous 7 Via Natural or Artificial Opening 8 Via Natural or Artificial Opening Endoscopic X External	0 Drainage Device 7 Autologous Tissue Substitute D Intraluminal Device J Synthetic Substitute K Nonautologous Tissue Substitute	Z No Qualifier
Y Mouth and Throat	0 Open 3 Percutaneous 7 Via Natural or Artificial Opening 8 Via Natural or Artificial Opening Endoscopic X External	0 Drainage Device 1 Radioactive Element 7 Autologous Tissue Substitute D Intraluminal Device J Synthetic Substitute K Nonautologous Tissue Substitute	Z No Qualifier

Non-OR 0CWA[0,3,X][0,C]Z
Non-OR 0CWSX[0,7,D,J,K]Z
Non-OR 0CWY07Z
Non-OR 0CWYX[0,1,7,D,J,K]Z

0 Medical and Surgical
C Mouth and Throat
X Transfer Moving, without taking out, all or a portion of a body part to another location to take over the function of all or a portion of a body part

Body Part Character 4	Approach Character 5	Device Character 6	Qualifier Character 7
0 Upper Lip 1 Lower Lip 3 Soft Palate 4 Buccal Mucosa 5 Upper Gingiva 6 Lower Gingiva 7 Tongue	0 Open X External	Z No Device	Z No Qualifier

Gastrointestinal System ØD1–ØDY

Ø Medical and Surgical
D Gastrointestinal System
1 Bypass Altering the route of passage of the contents of a tubular body part

Body Part Character 4	Approach Character 5	Device Character 6	Qualifier Character 7
1 Esophagus, Upper **2** Esophagus, Middle **3** Esophagus, Lower **5** Esophagus	**Ø** Open **4** Percutaneous Endoscopic **8** Via Natural or Artificial Opening Endoscopic	**7** Autologous Tissue Substitute **J** Synthetic Substitute **K** Nonautologous Tissue Substitute **Z** No Device	**4** Cutaneous **6** Stomach **9** Duodenum **A** Jejunum **B** Ileum
1 Esophagus, Upper **2** Esophagus, Middle **3** Esophagus, Lower **5** Esophagus **6** Stomach **9** Duodenum **A** Jejunum **B** Ileum **H** Cecum **K** Ascending Colon **L** Transverse Colon **M** Descending Colon **N** Sigmoid Colon	**3** Percutaneous	**J** Synthetic Substitute	**4** Cutaneous
6 Stomach ⊞ **9** Duodenum	**Ø** Open **4** Percutaneous Endoscopic **8** Via Natural or Artificial Opening Endoscopic	**7** Autologous Tissue Substitute **J** Synthetic Substitute **K** Nonautologous Tissue Substitute **Z** No Device	**4** Cutaneous **9** Duodenum **A** Jejunum **B** Ileum **L** Transverse Colon
A Jejunum	**Ø** Open **4** Percutaneous Endoscopic **8** Via Natural or Artificial Opening Endoscopic	**7** Autologous Tissue Substitute **J** Synthetic Substitute **K** Nonautologous Tissue Substitute **Z** No Device	**4** Cutaneous **A** Jejunum **B** Ileum **H** Cecum **K** Ascending Colon **L** Transverse Colon **M** Descending Colon **N** Sigmoid Colon **P** Rectum **Q** Anus
B Ileum	**Ø** Open **4** Percutaneous Endoscopic **8** Via Natural or Artificial Opening Endoscopic	**7** Autologous Tissue Substitute **J** Synthetic Substitute **K** Nonautologous Tissue Substitute **Z** No Device	**4** Cutaneous **B** Ileum **H** Cecum **K** Ascending Colon **L** Transverse Colon **M** Descending Colon **N** Sigmoid Colon **P** Rectum **Q** Anus
H Cecum	**Ø** Open **4** Percutaneous Endoscopic **8** Via Natural or Artificial Opening Endoscopic	**7** Autologous Tissue Substitute **J** Synthetic Substitute **K** Nonautologous Tissue Substitute **Z** No Device	**4** Cutaneous **H** Cecum **K** Ascending Colon **L** Transverse Colon **M** Descending Colon **N** Sigmoid Colon **P** Rectum
K Ascending Colon	**Ø** Open **4** Percutaneous Endoscopic **8** Via Natural or Artificial Opening Endoscopic	**7** Autologous Tissue Substitute **J** Synthetic Substitute **K** Nonautologous Tissue Substitute **Z** No Device	**4** Cutaneous **K** Ascending Colon **L** Transverse Colon **M** Descending Colon **N** Sigmoid Colon **P** Rectum

ØD1 Continued on next page

Non-OR ØD163J4
Non-OR ØD16[Ø,4,8][7,J,K,Z]4
HAC ØD16[Ø,4,8][7,J,K,Z][9,A,B,L] when reported with PDx E66.Ø1 and SDx K68.11 or K95.Ø1 or K95.81 or T81.4XXA

No Procedure Combinations Specified
⊞ ØD16Ø[7,J,K]A
⊞ ØD16ØZ[A,B]

ØD1 Continued

Ø Medical and Surgical
D Gastrointestinal System
1 Bypass Altering the route of passage of the contents of a tubular body part

Body Part Character 4	Approach Character 5	Device Character 6	Qualifier Character 7
L Transverse Colon	**Ø** Open **4** Percutaneous Endoscopic **8** Via Natural or Artificial Opening Endoscopic	**7** Autologous Tissue Substitute **J** Synthetic Substitute **K** Nonautologous Tissue Substitute **Z** No Device	**4** Cutaneous **L** Transverse Colon **M** Descending Colon **N** Sigmoid Colon **P** Rectum
M Descending Colon	**Ø** Open **4** Percutaneous Endoscopic **8** Via Natural or Artificial Opening Endoscopic	**7** Autologous Tissue Substitute **J** Synthetic Substitute **K** Nonautologous Tissue Substitute **Z** No Device	**4** Cutaneous **M** Descending Colon **N** Sigmoid Colon **P** Rectum
N Sigmoid Colon ⊞	**Ø** Open **4** Percutaneous Endoscopic **8** Via Natural or Artificial Opening Endoscopic	**7** Autologous Tissue Substitute **J** Synthetic Substitute **K** Nonautologous Tissue Substitute **Z** No Device	**4** Cutaneous **N** Sigmoid Colon **P** Rectum

No Procedure Combinations Specified
⊞ ØD1N[Ø,4]Z4

Ø Medical and Surgical
D Gastrointestinal System
2 Change Taking out or off a device from a body part and putting back an identical or similar device in or on the same body part without cutting or puncturing the skin or a mucous membrane

Body Part Character 4	Approach Character 5	Device Character 6	Qualifier Character 7
Ø Upper Intestinal Tract **D** Lower Intestinal Tract	**X** External	**Ø** Drainage Device **U** Feeding Device **Y** Other Device	**Z** No Qualifier
U Omentum **V** Mesentery **W** Peritoneum	**X** External	**Ø** Drainage Device **Y** Other Device	**Z** No Qualifier

Non-OR For all body part, approach, device, and qualifier values

Ø Medical and Surgical
D Gastrointestinal System
5 Destruction Physical eradication of all or a portion of a body part by the direct use of energy, force, or a destructive agent

Body Part Character 4	Approach Character 5	Device Character 6	Qualifier Character 7
1 Esophagus, Upper **2** Esophagus, Middle **3** Esophagus, Lower **4** Esophagogastric Junction **5** Esophagus **6** Stomach **7** Stomach, Pylorus **8** Small Intestine **9** Duodenum **A** Jejunum **B** Ileum **C** Ileocecal Valve **E** Large Intestine **F** Large Intestine, Right **G** Large Intestine, Left **H** Cecum **J** Appendix **K** Ascending Colon **L** Transverse Colon **M** Descending Colon **N** Sigmoid Colon **P** Rectum	**Ø** Open **3** Percutaneous **4** Percutaneous Endoscopic **7** Via Natural or Artificial Opening **8** Via Natural or Artificial Opening Endoscopic	**Z** No Device	**Z** No Qualifier

ØD5 Continued on next page

Non-OR ØD5[1,2,3,4,5,6,7,9,E,F,G,H,K,L,M,N][4,8]ZZ
Non-OR ØD5P[Ø,3,4,7,8]ZZ

ØD5 Continued

Ø Medical and Surgical
D Gastrointestinal System
5 Destruction Physical eradication of all or a portion of a body part by the direct use of energy, force, or a destructive agent

Body Part Character 4	Approach Character 5	Device Character 6	Qualifier Character 7
Q Anus	**Ø** Open **3** Percutaneous **4** Percutaneous Endoscopic **7** Via Natural or Artificial Opening **8** Via Natural or Artificial Opening Endoscopic **X** External	**Z** No Device	**Z** No Qualifier
R Anal Sphincter **S** Greater Omentum **T** Lesser Omentum **V** Mesentery **W** Peritoneum	**Ø** Open **3** Percutaneous **4** Percutaneous Endoscopic	**Z** No Device	**Z** No Qualifier

Non-OR ØD5Q[4,8]ZZ
Non-OR ØD5R4ZZ

Ø Medical and Surgical
D Gastrointestinal System
7 Dilation Expanding an orifice or the lumen of a tubular body part

Body Part Character 4	Approach Character 5	Device Character 6	Qualifier Character 7
1 Esophagus, Upper **2** Esophagus, Middle **3** Esophagus, Lower **4** Esophagogastric Junction **5** Esophagus **6** Stomach **7** Stomach, Pylorus **8** Small Intestine **9** Duodenum **A** Jejunum **B** Ileum **C** Ileocecal Valve **E** Large Intestine **F** Large Intestine, Right **G** Large Intestine, Left **H** Cecum **K** Ascending Colon **L** Transverse Colon **M** Descending Colon **N** Sigmoid Colon **P** Rectum **Q** Anus	**Ø** Open **3** Percutaneous **4** Percutaneous Endoscopic **7** Via Natural or Artificial Opening **8** Via Natural or Artificial Opening Endoscopic	**D** Intraluminal Device **Z** No Device	**Z** No Qualifier

Non-OR ØD7[1,2,3,4,5,8,9,A,B,C,E,F,G,H,K,L,M,N,P,Q][7,8][D,Z]Z
Non-OR ØD77[4,8]DZ
Non-OR ØD778ZZ
Non-OR ØD7[8,9,A,B,C,E,F,G,H,K,L,M,N][Ø,3,4]DZ

Ø Medical and Surgical
D Gastrointestinal System
8 Division Cutting into a body part without draining fluids and/or gases from the body part in order to separate or transect a body part

Body Part Character 4	Approach Character 5	Device Character 6	Qualifier Character 7
4 Esophagogastric Junction **7** Stomach, Pylorus	**Ø** Open **3** Percutaneous **4** Percutaneous Endoscopic **7** Via Natural or Artificial Opening **8** Via Natural or Artificial Opening Endoscopic	**Z** No Device	**Z** No Qualifier
R Anal Sphincter	**Ø** Open **3** Percutaneous	**Z** No Device	**Z** No Qualifier

Ø Medical and Surgical
D Gastrointestinal System
9 Drainage Taking or letting out fluids and/or gases from a body part

Body Part Character 4	Approach Character 5	Device Character 6	Qualifier Character 7
1 Esophagus, Upper 2 Esophagus, Middle 3 Esophagus, Lower 4 Esophagogastric Junction 5 Esophagus 6 Stomach 7 Stomach, Pylorus 8 Small Intestine 9 Duodenum A Jejunum B Ileum C Ileocecal Valve E Large Intestine F Large Intestine, Right G Large Intestine, Left H Cecum J Appendix K Ascending Colon L Transverse Colon M Descending Colon N Sigmoid Colon P Rectum	Ø Open 3 Percutaneous 4 Percutaneous Endoscopic 7 Via Natural or Artificial Opening 8 Via Natural or Artificial Opening Endoscopic	Ø Drainage Device	Z No Qualifier
1 Esophagus, Upper 2 Esophagus, Middle 3 Esophagus, Lower 4 Esophagogastric Junction 5 Esophagus 6 Stomach 7 Stomach, Pylorus 8 Small Intestine 9 Duodenum A Jejunum B Ileum C Ileocecal Valve E Large Intestine F Large Intestine, Right G Large Intestine, Left H Cecum J Appendix K Ascending Colon L Transverse Colon M Descending Colon N Sigmoid Colon P Rectum	Ø Open 3 Percutaneous 4 Percutaneous Endoscopic 7 Via Natural or Artificial Opening 8 Via Natural or Artificial Opening Endoscopic	Z No Device	X Diagnostic Z No Qualifier
Q Anus	Ø Open 3 Percutaneous 4 Percutaneous Endoscopic 7 Via Natural or Artificial Opening 8 Via Natural or Artificial Opening Endoscopic X External	Ø Drainage Device	Z No Qualifier
Q Anus	Ø Open 3 Percutaneous 4 Percutaneous Endoscopic 7 Via Natural or Artificial Opening 8 Via Natural or Artificial Opening Endoscopic X External	Z No Device	X Diagnostic Z No Qualifier
R Anal Sphincter S Greater Omentum T Lesser Omentum V Mesentery W Peritoneum	Ø Open 3 Percutaneous 4 Percutaneous Endoscopic	Ø Drainage Device	Z No Qualifier
R Anal Sphincter S Greater Omentum T Lesser Omentum V Mesentery W Peritoneum	Ø Open 3 Percutaneous 4 Percutaneous Endoscopic	Z No Device	X Diagnostic Z No Qualifier

Non-OR ØD9[6,7,8,9,A,B,E,F,G,H,K,L,M,N,P][7,8]ØZ
Non-OR ØD9[1,2,3,4,5,6,7,8,9,A,B,C,E,F,G,H,K,L,M,N,P][3,4,7,8]ZX
Non-OR ØD9Q[Ø,3,4,7,8,X]ZX
Non-OR ØD9[S,T,V,W][3,4]ØZ
Non-OR ØD9R[Ø,3,4]ZX
Non-OR ØD9[S,T,V,W][3,4]ZZ

Ø Medical and Surgical
D Gastrointestinal System
B Excision Cutting out or off, without replacement, a portion of a body part

Body Part Character 4	Approach Character 5	Device Character 6	Qualifier Character 7
1 Esophagus, Upper **2** Esophagus, Middle **3** Esophagus, Lower **4** Esophagogastric Junction **5** Esophagus **7** Stomach, Pylorus **8** Small Intestine ⊞ **9** Duodenum ⊞ **A** Jejunum **B** Ileum ⊞ **C** Ileocecal Valve **E** Large Intestine ⊞ **F** Large Intestine, Right **G** Large Intestine, Left **H** Cecum **J** Appendix **K** Ascending Colon **L** Transverse Colon **M** Descending Colon **N** Sigmoid Colon ⊞ **P** Rectum	**Ø** Open **3** Percutaneous **4** Percutaneous Endoscopic **7** Via Natural or Artificial Opening **8** Via Natural or Artificial Opening Endoscopic	**Z** No Device	**X** Diagnostic **Z** No Qualifier
6 Stomach	**Ø** Open **3** Percutaneous **4** Percutaneous Endoscopic **7** Via Natural or Artificial Opening **8** Via Natural or Artificial Opening Endoscopic	**Z** No Device	**3** Vertical **X** Diagnostic **Z** No Qualifier
Q Anus	**Ø** Open **3** Percutaneous **4** Percutaneous Endoscopic **7** Via Natural or Artificial Opening **8** Via Natural or Artificial Opening Endoscopic **X** External	**Z** No Device	**X** Diagnostic **Z** No Qualifier
R Anal Sphincter **S** Greater Omentum **T** Lesser Omentum **V** Mesentery **W** Peritoneum	**Ø** Open **3** Percutaneous **4** Percutaneous Endoscopic	**Z** No Device	**X** Diagnostic **Z** No Qualifier

Non-OR ØDB[1,2,3,4,5,7,8,9,A,B,C,E,F,G,H,K,L,M,N,P][3,4,7,8]ZX
Non-OR ØDB[1,2,3,5,7,9][4,8]ZZ
Non-OR ØDB[4,E,F,G,H,K,L,M,N,P]8ZZ
Non-OR ØDB6[3,4,7]ZX
Non-OR ØDB6[4,8]ZZ
Non-OR ØDBQ[Ø,3,4,7,8,X]ZX
Non-OR ØDBR[Ø,3,4]ZX
Non-OR ØDB[S,T,V,W][3,4]ZX

No Procedure Combinations Specified
⊞ ØDB[8,9,B,E,N]ØZZ

Ø Medical and Surgical
D Gastrointestinal System
C Extirpation Taking or cutting out solid matter from a body part

Body Part Character 4	Approach Character 5	Device Character 6	Qualifier Character 7
1 Esophagus, Upper 2 Esophagus, Middle 3 Esophagus, Lower 4 Esophagogastric Junction 5 Esophagus 6 Stomach 7 Stomach, Pylorus 8 Small Intestine 9 Duodenum A Jejunum B Ileum C Ileocecal Valve E Large Intestine F Large Intestine, Right G Large Intestine, Left H Cecum J Appendix K Ascending Colon L Transverse Colon M Descending Colon N Sigmoid Colon P Rectum	Ø Open 3 Percutaneous 4 Percutaneous Endoscopic 7 Via Natural or Artificial Opening 8 Via Natural or Artificial Opening Endoscopic	Z No Device	Z No Qualifier
Q Anus	Ø Open 3 Percutaneous 4 Percutaneous Endoscopic 7 Via Natural or Artificial Opening 8 Via Natural or Artificial Opening Endoscopic X External	Z No Device	Z No Qualifier
R Anal Sphincter S Greater Omentum T Lesser Omentum V Mesentery W Peritoneum	Ø Open 3 Percutaneous 4 Percutaneous Endoscopic	Z No Device	Z No Qualifier

Non-OR ØDC[1,2,3,4,5,6,7,8,9,A,B,C,E,F,G,H,K,L,M,N,P][7,8]ZZ
Non-OR ØDCQ[7,8,X]ZZ

Ø Medical and Surgical
D Gastrointestinal System
F Fragmentation Breaking solid matter in a body part into pieces

Body Part Character 4	Approach Character 5	Device Character 6	Qualifier Character 7
5 Esophagus NC 6 Stomach NC 8 Small Intestine NC 9 Duodenum NC A Jejunum NC B Ileum NC E Large Intestine NC F Large Intestine, Right NC G Large Intestine, Left NC H Cecum NC J Appendix NC K Ascending Colon NC L Transverse Colon NC M Descending Colon NC N Sigmoid Colon NC P Rectum NC Q Anus NC	Ø Open 3 Percutaneous 4 Percutaneous Endoscopic 7 Via Natural or Artificial Opening 8 Via Natural or Artificial Opening Endoscopic X External	Z No Device	Z No Qualifier

Non-OR ØDF[5,6,8,9,A,B,E,F,G,H,J,K,L,M,N,P,Q]XZZ
NC ØDF[5,6,8,9,A,B,E,F,G,H,J,K,L,M,N,P,Q]XZZ

Ø Medical and Surgical
D Gastrointestinal System
H Insertion Putting in a nonbiological appliance that monitors, assists, performs, or prevents a physiological function but does not physically take the place of a body part

Body Part Character 4	Approach Character 5	Device Character 6	Qualifier Character 7
5 Esophagus	**Ø** Open **3** Percutaneous **4** Percutaneous Endoscopic	**1** Radioactive Element **2** Monitoring Device **3** Infusion Device **D** Intraluminal Device **U** Feeding Device	**Z** No Qualifier
5 Esophagus	**7** Via Natural or Artificial Opening **8** Via Natural or Artificial Opening Endoscopic	**1** Radioactive Element **2** Monitoring Device **3** Infusion Device **B** Intraluminal Device, Airway **D** Intraluminal Device **U** Feeding Device	**Z** No Qualifier
6 Stomach ⊞	**Ø** Open **3** Percutaneous **4** Percutaneous Endoscopic	**2** Monitoring Device **3** Infusion Device **D** Intraluminal Device **M** Stimulator Lead **U** Feeding Device	**Z** No Qualifier
6 Stomach	**7** Via Natural or Artificial Opening **8** Via Natural or Artificial Opening Endoscopic	**2** Monitoring Device **3** Infusion Device **D** Intraluminal Device **U** Feeding Device	**Z** No Qualifier
8 Small Intestine **9** Duodenum **A** Jejunum **B** Ileum	**Ø** Open **3** Percutaneous **4** Percutaneous Endoscopic **7** Via Natural or Artificial Opening **8** Via Natural or Artificial Opening Endoscopic	**2** Monitoring Device **3** Infusion Device **D** Intraluminal Device **U** Feeding Device	**Z** No Qualifier
E Large Intestine	**Ø** Open **3** Percutaneous **4** Percutaneous Endoscopic **7** Via Natural or Artificial Opening **8** Via Natural or Artificial Opening Endoscopic	**D** Intraluminal Device	**Z** No Qualifier
P Rectum	**Ø** Open **3** Percutaneous **4** Percutaneous Endoscopic **7** Via Natural or Artificial Opening **8** Via Natural or Artificial Opening Endoscopic	**1** Radioactive Element **D** Intraluminal Device	**Z** No Qualifier
Q Anus	**Ø** Open **3** Percutaneous **4** Percutaneous Endoscopic	**D** Intraluminal Device **L** Artificial Sphincter	**Z** No Qualifier
Q Anus	**7** Via Natural or Artificial Opening **8** Via Natural or Artificial Opening Endoscopic	**D** Intraluminal Device	**Z** No Qualifier
R Anal Sphincter	**Ø** Open **3** Percutaneous **4** Percutaneous Endoscopic	**M** Stimulator Lead	**Z** No Qualifier

Non-OR ØDH5[Ø,3,4][D,U]Z
Non-OR ØDH5[7,8][B,D,U]Z
Non-OR ØDH6[3,4]UZ
Non-OR ØDH6[7,8]UZ
Non-OR ØDH[8,9,A,B][Ø,3,4,7,8][D,U]Z
Non-OR ØDHE[Ø,3,4,7,8]DZ
Non-OR ØDHP[Ø,3,4,7,8]DZ
AHA: 2Ø13, 4Q, 117

See Appendix I for Procedure Combinations
⊞ ØDH6[Ø,3,4]MZ

0 Medical and Surgical
D Gastrointestinal System
J Inspection Visually and/or manually exploring a body part

Body Part Character 4	Approach Character 5	Device Character 6	Qualifier Character 7
0 Upper Intestinal Tract 6 Stomach D Lower Intestinal Tract	0 Open 3 Percutaneous 4 Percutaneous Endoscopic 7 Via Natural or Artificial Opening 8 Via Natural or Artificial Opening Endoscopic X External	Z No Device	Z No Qualifier
U Omentum V Mesentery W Peritoneum	0 Open 3 Percutaneous 4 Percutaneous Endoscopic X External	Z No Device	Z No Qualifier

Non-OR 0DJ[0,6,D][3,7,8,X]ZZ
Non-OR 0DJ[U,V,W]XZZ

0 Medical and Surgical
D Gastrointestinal System
L Occlusion Completely closing an orifice or the lumen of a tubular body part

Body Part Character 4	Approach Character 5	Device Character 6	Qualifier Character 7
1 Esophagus, Upper 2 Esophagus, Middle 3 Esophagus, Lower 4 Esophagogastric Junction 5 Esophagus 6 Stomach 7 Stomach, Pylorus 8 Small Intestine 9 Duodenum A Jejunum B Ileum C Ileocecal Valve E Large Intestine F Large Intestine, Right G Large Intestine, Left H Cecum K Ascending Colon L Transverse Colon M Descending Colon N Sigmoid Colon P Rectum	0 Open 3 Percutaneous 4 Percutaneous Endoscopic	C Extraluminal Device D Intraluminal Device Z No Device	Z No Qualifier
1 Esophagus, Upper 2 Esophagus, Middle 3 Esophagus, Lower 4 Esophagogastric Junction 5 Esophagus 6 Stomach 7 Stomach, Pylorus 8 Small Intestine 9 Duodenum A Jejunum B Ileum C Ileocecal Valve E Large Intestine F Large Intestine, Right G Large Intestine, Left H Cecum K Ascending Colon L Transverse Colon M Descending Colon N Sigmoid Colon P Rectum Q Anus	7 Via Natural or Artificial Opening 8 Via Natural or Artificial Opening Endoscopic	D Intraluminal Device Z No Device	Z No Qualifier
Q Anus	0 Open 3 Percutaneous 4 Percutaneous Endoscopic X External	C Extraluminal Device D Intraluminal Device Z No Device	Z No Qualifier

Non-OR 0DL[1,2,3,4,5][0,3,4][C,D,Z]Z
Non-OR 0DL[1,2,3,4,5][7,8][D,Z]Z

Ø Medical and Surgical
D Gastrointestinal System
M Reattachment Putting back in or on all or a portion of a separated body part to its normal location or other suitable location

Body Part Character 4	Approach Character 5	Device Character 6	Qualifier Character 7
5 Esophagus 6 Stomach 8 Small Intestine 9 Duodenum A Jejunum B Ileum E Large Intestine F Large Intestine, Right G Large Intestine, Left H Cecum K Ascending Colon L Transverse Colon M Descending Colon N Sigmoid Colon P Rectum	Ø Open 4 Percutaneous Endoscopic	Z No Device	Z No Qualifier

Ø Medical and Surgical
D Gastrointestinal System
N Release Freeing a body part from an abnormal physical constraint

Body Part Character 4	Approach Character 5	Device Character 6	Qualifier Character 7
1 Esophagus, Upper 2 Esophagus, Middle 3 Esophagus, Lower 4 Esophagogastric Junction 5 Esophagus 6 Stomach 7 Stomach, Pylorus 8 Small Intestine 9 Duodenum A Jejunum B Ileum C Ileocecal Valve E Large Intestine F Large Intestine, Right G Large Intestine, Left H Cecum J Appendix K Ascending Colon L Transverse Colon M Descending Colon N Sigmoid Colon P Rectum	Ø Open 3 Percutaneous 4 Percutaneous Endoscopic 7 Via Natural or Artificial Opening 8 Via Natural or Artificial Opening Endoscopic	Z No Device	Z No Qualifier
Q Anus	Ø Open 3 Percutaneous 4 Percutaneous Endoscopic 7 Via Natural or Artificial Opening 8 Via Natural or Artificial Opening Endoscopic X External	Z No Device	Z No Qualifier
R Anal Sphincter S Greater Omentum T Lesser Omentum V Mesentery W Peritoneum	Ø Open 3 Percutaneous 4 Percutaneous Endoscopic	Z No Device	Z No Qualifier

Non-OR ØDN[8,9,A,B,E,F,G,H,K,L,M,N][7,8]ZZ

0 Medical and Surgical
D Gastrointestinal System
P Removal Taking out or off a device from a body part

Body Part Character 4	Approach Character 5	Device Character 6	Qualifier Character 7
0 Upper Intestinal Tract **6** Stomach **D** Lower Intestinal Tract	**X** External	**0** Drainage Device **2** Monitoring Device **3** Infusion Device **D** Intraluminal Device **U** Feeding Device	**Z** No Qualifier
0 Upper Intestinal Tract **D** Lower Intestinal Tract	**0** Open **3** Percutaneous **4** Percutaneous Endoscopic **7** Via Natural or Artificial Opening **8** Via Natural or Artificial Opening Endoscopic	**0** Drainage Device **2** Monitoring Device **3** Infusion Device **7** Autologous Tissue Substitute **C** Extraluminal Device **D** Intraluminal Device **J** Synthetic Substitute **K** Nonautologous Tissue Substitute **U** Feeding Device	**Z** No Qualifier
5 Esophagus	**0** Open **3** Percutaneous **4** Percutaneous Endoscopic	**1** Radioactive Element **2** Monitoring Device **3** Infusion Device **U** Feeding Device	**Z** No Qualifier
5 Esophagus	**7** Via Natural or Artificial Opening **8** Via Natural or Artificial Opening Endoscopic	**1** Radioactive Element **D** Intraluminal Device	**Z** No Qualifier
5 Esophagus	**X** External	**1** Radioactive Element **2** Monitoring Device **3** Infusion Device **D** Intraluminal Device **U** Feeding Device	**Z** No Qualifier
6 Stomach	**0** Open **3** Percutaneous **4** Percutaneous Endoscopic	**0** Drainage Device **2** Monitoring Device **3** Infusion Device **7** Autologous Tissue Substitute **C** Extraluminal Device **D** Intraluminal Device **J** Synthetic Substitute **K** Nonautologous Tissue Substitute **M** Stimulator Lead **U** Feeding Device	**Z** No Qualifier
6 Stomach	**7** Via Natural or Artificial Opening **8** Via Natural or Artificial Opening Endoscopic	**0** Drainage Device **2** Monitoring Device **3** Infusion Device **7** Autologous Tissue Substitute **C** Extraluminal Device **D** Intraluminal Device **J** Synthetic Substitute **K** Nonautologous Tissue Substitute **U** Feeding Device	**Z** No Qualifier
P Rectum	**0** Open **3** Percutaneous **4** Percutaneous Endoscopic **7** Via Natural or Artificial Opening **8** Via Natural or Artificial Opening Endoscopic **X** External	**1** Radioactive Element	**Z** No Qualifier
Q Anus	**0** Open **3** Percutaneous **4** Percutaneous Endoscopic **7** Via Natural or Artificial Opening **8** Via Natural or Artificial Opening Endoscopic	**L** Artificial Sphincter	**Z** No Qualifier
R Anal Sphincter	**0** Open **3** Percutaneous **4** Percutaneous Endoscopic	**M** Stimulator Lead	**Z** No Qualifier
U Omentum **V** Mesentery **W** Peritoneum	**0** Open **3** Percutaneous **4** Percutaneous Endoscopic	**0** Drainage Device **1** Radioactive Element **7** Autologous Tissue Substitute **J** Synthetic Substitute **K** Nonautologous Tissue Substitute	**Z** No Qualifier

Non-OR 0DP[0,6,D]X[0,2,3,D,U]Z
Non-OR 0DP5[7,8]1Z
Non-OR 0DP5X[1,2,3,D,U]Z
Non-OR 0DP6[7,8]DZ
Non-OR 0DPP[7,8,X]1Z

Ø Medical and Surgical
D Gastrointestinal System
Q Repair Restoring, to the extent possible, a body part to its normal anatomic structure and function

Body Part Character 4	Approach Character 5	Device Character 6	Qualifier Character 7
1 Esophagus, Upper 2 Esophagus, Middle 3 Esophagus, Lower 4 Esophagogastric Junction 5 Esophagus ⊞ 6 Stomach ⊞ 7 Stomach, Pylorus 8 Small Intestine ⊞ 9 Duodenum ⊞ A Jejunum ⊞ B Ileum ⊞ C Ileocecal Valve E Large Intestine ⊞ F Large Intestine, Right ⊞ G Large Intestine, Left ⊞ H Cecum ⊞ J Appendix ⊞ K Ascending Colon ⊞ L Transverse Colon ⊞ M Descending Colon ⊞ N Sigmoid Colon ⊞ P Rectum ⊞	Ø Open 3 Percutaneous 4 Percutaneous Endoscopic 7 Via Natural or Artificial Opening 8 Via Natural or Artificial Opening Endoscopic	Z No Device	Z No Qualifier
Q Anus ⊞	Ø Open 3 Percutaneous 4 Percutaneous Endoscopic 7 Via Natural or Artificial Opening 8 Via Natural or Artificial Opening Endoscopic X External	Z No Device	Z No Qualifier
R Anal Sphincter S Greater Omentum T Lesser Omentum V Mesentery W Peritoneum ⊞	Ø Open 3 Percutaneous 4 Percutaneous Endoscopic	Z No Device	Z No Qualifier

See Appendix I for Procedure Combinations
Combo-only ØDQ[F,G,L,M]ØZZ
⊞ ØDQ[8,9,A,B,E,F,G,H,K,L,M]ØZZ

No Procedure Combinations Specified
⊞ ØDQ[5,6,J,P,Q][Ø,3,4,7,8]ZZ
⊞ ØDQN[3,4,7,8]ZZ
⊞ ØDQW[Ø,3,4]ZZ

Ø Medical and Surgical
D Gastrointestinal System
R Replacement Putting in or on biological or synthetic material that physically takes the place and/or function of all or a portion of a body part

Body Part Character 4	Approach Character 5	Device Character 6	Qualifier Character 7
5 Esophagus	Ø Open 4 Percutaneous Endoscopic 7 Via Natural or Artificial Opening 8 Via Natural or Artificial Opening Endoscopic	7 Autologous Tissue Substitute J Synthetic Substitute K Nonautologous Tissue Substitute	Z No Qualifier
R Anal Sphincter S Greater Omentum T Lesser Omentum V Mesentery W Peritoneum	Ø Open 4 Percutaneous Endoscopic	7 Autologous Tissue Substitute J Synthetic Substitute K Nonautologous Tissue Substitute	Z No Qualifier

Ø Medical and Surgical
D Gastrointestinal System
S Reposition Moving to its normal location or other suitable location all or a portion of a body part

Body Part Character 4	Approach Character 5	Device Character 6	Qualifier Character 7
5 Esophagus 6 Stomach 9 Duodenum A Jejunum B Ileum H Cecum K Ascending Colon L Transverse Colon M Descending Colon N Sigmoid Colon P Rectum Q Anus	Ø Open 4 Percutaneous Endoscopic 7 Via Natural or Artificial Opening 8 Via Natural or Artificial Opening Endoscopic X External	Z No Device	Z No Qualifier

Non-OR ØDS[6,9,A,B,H,K,L,M,N,P]XZZ

Ø Medical and Surgical
D Gastrointestinal System
T Resection Cutting out or off, without replacement, all of a body part

Body Part Character 4	Approach Character 5	Device Character 6	Qualifier Character 7
1 Esophagus, Upper 2 Esophagus, Middle 3 Esophagus, Lower 4 Esophagogastric Junction 5 Esophagus 6 Stomach 7 Stomach, Pylorus 8 Small Intestine 9 Duodenum ⊞ A Jejunum B Ileum C Ileocecal Valve E Large Intestine F Large Intestine, Right G Large Intestine, Left H Cecum J Appendix K Ascending Colon L Transverse Colon M Descending Colon N Sigmoid Colon ⊞ P Rectum ⊞ Q Anus	Ø Open 4 Percutaneous Endoscopic 7 Via Natural or Artificial Opening 8 Via Natural or Artificial Opening Endoscopic	Z No Device	Z No Qualifier
R Anal Sphincter S Greater Omentum T Lesser Omentum	Ø Open 4 Percutaneous Endoscopic	Z No Device	Z No Qualifier

See Appendix I for Procedure Combinations
⊞ ØDT9ØZZ

No Procedure Combinations Specified
⊞ ØDTN[Ø,4]ZZ
⊞ ØDTP[Ø,4,7,8]ZZ

Ø Medical and Surgical
D Gastrointestinal System
U Supplement Putting in or on biological or synthetic material that physically reinforces and/or augments the function of a portion of a body part

Body Part Character 4	Approach Character 5	Device Character 6	Qualifier Character 7
1 Esophagus, Upper **2** Esophagus, Middle **3** Esophagus, Lower **4** Esophagogastric Junction **5** Esophagus **6** Stomach **7** Stomach, Pylorus **8** Small Intestine **9** Duodenum **A** Jejunum **B** Ileum **C** Ileocecal Valve **E** Large Intestine **F** Large Intestine, Right **G** Large Intestine, Left **H** Cecum **K** Ascending Colon **L** Transverse Colon **M** Descending Colon **N** Sigmoid Colon **P** Rectum	**Ø** Open **4** Percutaneous Endoscopic **7** Via Natural or Artificial Opening **8** Via Natural or Artificial Opening Endoscopic	**7** Autologous Tissue Substitute **J** Synthetic Substitute **K** Nonautologous Tissue Substitute	**Z** No Qualifier
Q Anus	**Ø** Open **4** Percutaneous Endoscopic **7** Via Natural or Artificial Opening **8** Via Natural or Artificial Opening Endoscopic **X** External	**7** Autologous Tissue Substitute **J** Synthetic Substitute **K** Nonautologous Tissue Substitute	**Z** No Qualifier
R Anal Sphincter **S** Greater Omentum **T** Lesser Omentum **V** Mesentery **W** Peritoneum	**Ø** Open **4** Percutaneous Endoscopic	**7** Autologous Tissue Substitute **J** Synthetic Substitute **K** Nonautologous Tissue Substitute	**Z** No Qualifier

Ø Medical and Surgical
D Gastrointestinal System
V Restriction Partially closing an orifice or the lumen of a tubular body part

Body Part Character 4	Approach Character 5	Device Character 6	Qualifier Character 7
1 Esophagus, Upper **2** Esophagus, Middle **3** Esophagus, Lower **4** Esophagogastric Junction **5** Esophagus **6** Stomach **7** Stomach, Pylorus **8** Small Intestine **9** Duodenum **A** Jejunum **B** Ileum **C** Ileocecal Valve **E** Large Intestine **F** Large Intestine, Right **G** Large Intestine, Left **H** Cecum **K** Ascending Colon **L** Transverse Colon **M** Descending Colon **N** Sigmoid Colon **P** Rectum	**Ø** Open **3** Percutaneous **4** Percutaneous Endoscopic	**C** Extraluminal Device **D** Intraluminal Device **Z** No Device	**Z** No Qualifier
1 Esophagus, Upper **2** Esophagus, Middle **3** Esophagus, Lower **4** Esophagogastric Junction **5** Esophagus **6** Stomach NC **7** Stomach, Pylorus **8** Small Intestine **9** Duodenum **A** Jejunum **B** Ileum **C** Ileocecal Valve **E** Large Intestine **F** Large Intestine, Right **G** Large Intestine, Left **H** Cecum **K** Ascending Colon **L** Transverse Colon **M** Descending Colon **N** Sigmoid Colon **P** Rectum **Q** Anus	**7** Via Natural or Artificial Opening **8** Via Natural or Artificial Opening Endoscopic	**D** Intraluminal Device **Z** No Device	**Z** No Qualifier
Q Anus	**Ø** Open **3** Percutaneous **4** Percutaneous Endoscopic **X** External	**C** Extraluminal Device **D** Intraluminal Device **Z** No Device	**Z** No Qualifier

Non-OR ØDV6[7,8]DZ
HAC ØDV64CZ when reported with PDx E66.Ø1 and SDx K68.11 or K95.Ø1 or K95.81 or T81.4XXA
NC ØDV6[7,8]DZ

Ø Medical and Surgical
D Gastrointestinal System
W Revision Correcting, to the extent possible, a portion of a malfunctioning device or the position of a displaced device

Body Part Character 4	Approach Character 5	Device Character 6	Qualifier Character 7
Ø Upper Intestinal Tract **D** Lower Intestinal Tract	**Ø** Open **3** Percutaneous **4** Percutaneous Endoscopic **7** Via Natural or Artificial Opening **8** Via Natural or Artificial Opening Endoscopic **X** External	**Ø** Drainage Device **2** Monitoring Device **3** Infusion Device **7** Autologous Tissue Substitute **C** Extraluminal Device **D** Intraluminal Device **J** Synthetic Substitute **K** Nonautologous Tissue Substitute **U** Feeding Device	**Z** No Qualifier
5 Esophagus	**7** Via Natural or Artificial Opening **8** Via Natural or Artificial Opening Endoscopic **X** External	**D** Intraluminal Device	**Z** No Qualifier
6 Stomach	**Ø** Open **3** Percutaneous **4** Percutaneous Endoscopic	**Ø** Drainage Device **2** Monitoring Device **3** Infusion Device **7** Autologous Tissue Substitute **C** Extraluminal Device **D** Intraluminal Device **J** Synthetic Substitute **K** Nonautologous Tissue Substitute **M** Stimulator Lead **U** Feeding Device	**Z** No Qualifier
6 Stomach	**7** Via Natural or Artificial Opening **8** Via Natural or Artificial Opening Endoscopic **X** External	**Ø** Drainage Device **2** Monitoring Device **3** Infusion Device **7** Autologous Tissue Substitute **C** Extraluminal Device **D** Intraluminal Device **J** Synthetic Substitute **K** Nonautologous Tissue Substitute **U** Feeding Device	**Z** No Qualifier
8 Small Intestine **E** Large Intestine	**Ø** Open **4** Percutaneous Endoscopic **7** Via Natural or Artificial Opening **8** Via Natural or Artificial Opening Endoscopic	**7** Autologous Tissue Substitute **J** Synthetic Substitute **K** Nonautologous Tissue Substitute	**Z** No Qualifier
Q Anus	**Ø** Open **3** Percutaneous **4** Percutaneous Endoscopic **7** Via Natural or Artificial Opening **8** Via Natural or Artificial Opening Endoscopic	**L** Artificial Sphincter	**Z** No Qualifier
R Anal Sphincter	**Ø** Open **3** Percutaneous **4** Percutaneous Endoscopic	**M** Stimulator Lead	**Z** No Qualifier
U Omentum **V** Mesentery **W** Peritoneum	**Ø** Open **3** Percutaneous **4** Percutaneous Endoscopic	**Ø** Drainage Device **7** Autologous Tissue Substitute **J** Synthetic Substitute **K** Nonautologous Tissue Substitute	**Z** No Qualifier

Non-OR ØDW[Ø,D]X[Ø,2,3,7,C,D,J,K,U]Z
Non-OR ØDW5XDZ
Non-OR ØDW6X[Ø,2,3,7,C,D,J,K,U]Z
Non-OR ØDW[U,V,W][Ø,3,4]ØZ

Ø Medical and Surgical
D Gastrointestinal System
X Transfer Moving, without taking out, all or a portion of a body part to another location to take over the function of all or a portion of a body part

Body Part Character 4	Approach Character 5	Device Character 6	Qualifier Character 7
6 Stomach **8** Small Intestine **E** Large Intestine	**Ø** Open **4** Percutaneous Endoscopic	**Z** No Device	**5** Esophagus

Ø Medical and Surgical
D Gastrointestinal System
Y Transplantation Putting in or on all or a portion of a living body part taken from another individual or animal to physically take the place and/or function of all or a portion of a similar body part

Body Part Character 4	Approach Character 5	Device Character 6	Qualifier Character 7
5 Esophagus 6 Stomach 8 Small Intestine LC E Large Intestine LC	Ø Open	Z No Device	Ø Allogeneic 1 Syngeneic 2 Zooplastic

Non-OR ØDY5ØZ[Ø,1,2]
LC ØDY[8,E]ØZ[Ø,1,2]

Hepatobiliary System and Pancreas

ØF1–ØF5

Hepatobiliary System and Pancreas ØF1–ØFY

Ø Medical and Surgical
F Hepatobiliary System and Pancreas
1 Bypass Altering the route of passage of the contents of a tubular body part

Body Part Character 4	Approach Character 5	Device Character 6	Qualifier Character 7
4 Gallbladder 5 Hepatic Duct, Right 6 Hepatic Duct, Left 8 Cystic Duct 9 Common Bile Duct ⊞	Ø Open 4 Percutaneous Endoscopic	D Intraluminal Device Z No Device	3 Duodenum 4 Stomach 5 Hepatic Duct, Right 6 Hepatic Duct, Left 7 Hepatic Duct, Caudate 8 Cystic Duct 9 Common Bile Duct B Small Intestine
D Pancreatic Duct F Pancreatic Duct, Accessory G Pancreas ⊞	Ø Open 4 Percutaneous Endoscopic	D Intraluminal Device Z No Device	3 Duodenum B Small Intestine C Large Intestine

No Procedure Combinations Specified
⊞ ØF19ØZ3
⊞ ØF1GØZC

Ø Medical and Surgical
F Hepatobiliary System and Pancreas
2 Change Taking out or off a device from a body part and putting back an identical or similar device in or on the same body part without cutting or puncturing the skin or a mucous membrane

Body Part Character 4	Approach Character 5	Device Character 6	Qualifier Character 7
Ø Liver 4 Gallbladder B Hepatobiliary Duct D Pancreatic Duct G Pancreas	X External	Ø Drainage Device Y Other Device	Z No Qualifier

Non-OR For all body part, approach, device, and qualifier values

Ø Medical and Surgical
F Hepatobiliary System and Pancreas
5 Destruction Physical eradication of all or a portion of a body part by the direct use of energy, force, or a destructive agent

Body Part Character 4	Approach Character 5	Device Character 6	Qualifier Character 7
Ø Liver 1 Liver, Right Lobe 2 Liver, Left Lobe 4 Gallbladder G Pancreas	Ø Open 3 Percutaneous 4 Percutaneous Endoscopic	Z No Device	Z No Qualifier
5 Hepatic Duct, Right 6 Hepatic Duct, Left 8 Cystic Duct 9 Common Bile Duct C Ampulla of Vater D Pancreatic Duct F Pancreatic Duct, Accessory	Ø Open 3 Percutaneous 4 Percutaneous Endoscopic 7 Via Natural or Artificial Opening 8 Via Natural or Artificial Opening Endoscopic	Z No Device	Z No Qualifier

Non-OR ØF5G4ZZ
Non-OR ØF5[5,6,8,9,C,D,F][4,8]ZZ

Ø Medical and Surgical
F Hepatobiliary System and Pancreas
7 Dilation Expanding an orifice or the lumen of a tubular body part

Body Part Character 4	Approach Character 5	Device Character 6	Qualifier Character 7
5 Hepatic Duct, Right 6 Hepatic Duct, Left 8 Cystic Duct 9 Common Bile Duct C Ampulla of Vater D Pancreatic Duct ⊞ F Pancreatic Duct, Accessory	Ø Open 3 Percutaneous 4 Percutaneous Endoscopic 7 Via Natural or Artificial Opening 8 Via Natural or Artificial Opening Endoscopic	D Intraluminal Device Z No Device	Z No Qualifier

DRG Non-OR ØF7[5,6,8,9,D][7,8]DZ
Non-OR ØF7D4[D,Z]Z
Non-OR ØF7[5,6,8,9,D]8ZZ
Non-OR ØF7[5,6,8,9][3,4][D,Z]Z
Non-OR ØF7C8[D,Z]Z
Non-OR ØF7F[4,8][D,Z]Z

See Appendix I for Procedure Combinations
Combo-only ØF7D8DZ
Combo-only ØF7[5,6,8,9][7,8]DZ
⊞ ØF7D7DZ

Ø Medical and Surgical
F Hepatobiliary System and Pancreas
8 Division Cutting into a body part without draining fluids and/or gases from the body part in order to separate or transect a body part

Body Part Character 4	Approach Character 5	Device Character 6	Qualifier Character 7
G Pancreas	Ø Open 3 Percutaneous 4 Percutaneous Endoscopic	Z No Device	Z No Qualifier

Ø Medical and Surgical
F Hepatobiliary System and Pancreas
9 Drainage Taking or letting out fluids and/or gases from a body part

Body Part Character 4	Approach Character 5	Device Character 6	Qualifier Character 7
Ø Liver 1 Liver, Right Lobe 2 Liver, Left Lobe 4 Gallbladder G Pancreas	Ø Open 3 Percutaneous 4 Percutaneous Endoscopic	Ø Drainage Device	Z No Qualifier
Ø Liver 1 Liver, Right Lobe 2 Liver, Left Lobe 4 Gallbladder G Pancreas	Ø Open 3 Percutaneous 4 Percutaneous Endoscopic	Z No Device	X Diagnostic Z No Qualifier
5 Hepatic Duct, Right 6 Hepatic Duct, Left 8 Cystic Duct 9 Common Bile Duct C Ampulla of Vater D Pancreatic Duct F Pancreatic Duct, Accessory	Ø Open 3 Percutaneous 4 Percutaneous Endoscopic 7 Via Natural or Artificial Opening 8 Via Natural or Artificial Opening Endoscopic	Ø Drainage Device	Z No Qualifier
5 Hepatic Duct, Right 6 Hepatic Duct, Left 8 Cystic Duct 9 Common Bile Duct C Ampulla of Vater D Pancreatic Duct F Pancreatic Duct, Accessory	Ø Open 3 Percutaneous 4 Percutaneous Endoscopic 7 Via Natural or Artificial Opening 8 Via Natural or Artificial Opening Endoscopic	Z No Device	X Diagnostic Z No Qualifier

Non-OR ØF9[Ø,1,2][3,4]ØZ
Non-OR ØF944ØZ
Non-OR ØF9[Ø,1,2,4,G][3,4]ZX
Non-OR ØF9[Ø,1,2,4][3,4]ZZ
Non-OR ØF9C[4,8]ØZ
Non-OR ØF9[9,D,F]8ØZ
Non-OR ØF9[5,6,8,9,C,D,F][3,4,7,8]ZX
Non-OR ØF99[3,4,7,8]ZZ
Non-OR ØF9C[4,8]ZZ

Ø Medical and Surgical
F Hepatobiliary System and Pancreas
B Excision Cutting out or off, without replacement, a portion of a body part

Body Part Character 4	Approach Character 5	Device Character 6	Qualifier Character 7
Ø Liver 1 Liver, Right Lobe 2 Liver, Left Lobe 4 Gallbladder G Pancreas	Ø Open 3 Percutaneous 4 Percutaneous Endoscopic	Z No Device	X Diagnostic Z No Qualifier
5 Hepatic Duct, Right 6 Hepatic Duct, Left 8 Cystic Duct 9 Common Bile Duct C Ampulla of Vater D Pancreatic Duct F Pancreatic Duct, Accessory	Ø Open 3 Percutaneous 4 Percutaneous Endoscopic 7 Via Natural or Artificial Opening 8 Via Natural or Artificial Opening Endoscopic	Z No Device	X Diagnostic Z No Qualifier

Non-OR ØFB[Ø,1,2]3ZX
Non-OR ØFB[4,G][3,4]ZX
Non-OR ØFB[5,6,8,9,C,D,F][3,4,7,8]ZX
Non-OR ØFB[5,6,8,9,C,D,F][4,8]ZZ

Ø Medical and Surgical
F Hepatobiliary System and Pancreas
C Extirpation Taking or cutting out solid matter from a body part

Body Part Character 4	Approach Character 5	Device Character 6	Qualifier Character 7
Ø Liver 1 Liver, Right Lobe 2 Liver, Left Lobe 4 Gallbladder G Pancreas	Ø Open 3 Percutaneous 4 Percutaneous Endoscopic	Z No Device	Z No Qualifier
5 Hepatic Duct, Right 6 Hepatic Duct, Left 8 Cystic Duct 9 Common Bile Duct C Ampulla of Vater D Pancreatic Duct F Pancreatic Duct, Accessory	Ø Open 3 Percutaneous 4 Percutaneous Endoscopic 7 Via Natural or Artificial Opening 8 Via Natural or Artificial Opening Endoscopic	Z No Device	Z No Qualifier

Non-OR ØFC[5,6,8,9][3,4,7,8]ZZ
Non-OR ØFCC[4,8]ZZ
Non-OR ØFC[D,F][3,4,8]ZZ

Ø Medical and Surgical
F Hepatobiliary System and Pancreas
F Fragmentation Breaking solid matter in a body part into pieces

Body Part Character 4	Approach Character 5	Device Character 6	Qualifier Character 7
4 Gallbladder NC 5 Hepatic Duct, Right NC 6 Hepatic Duct, Left NC 8 Cystic Duct NC 9 Common Bile Duct NC C Ampulla of Vater NC D Pancreatic Duct NC F Pancreatic Duct, Accessory NC	Ø Open 3 Percutaneous 4 Percutaneous Endoscopic 7 Via Natural or Artificial Opening 8 Via Natural or Artificial Opening Endoscopic X External	Z No Device	Z No Qualifier

Non-OR ØFF[4,5,6,8,9,C,][8,X]ZZ
Non-OR ØFF[D,F]XZZ
NC ØFF[4,5,6,8,9,C,D,F]XZZ

Ø Medical and Surgical
F Hepatobiliary System and Pancreas
H Insertion Putting in a nonbiological appliance that monitors, assists, performs, or prevents a physiological function but does not physically take the place of a body part

Body Part Character 4	Approach Character 5	Device Character 6	Qualifier Character 7
Ø Liver 1 Liver, Right Lobe 2 Liver, Left Lobe 4 Gallbladder G Pancreas	Ø Open 3 Percutaneous 4 Percutaneous Endoscopic	2 Monitoring Device 3 Infusion Device	Z No Qualifier
B Hepatobiliary Duct ⊞ D Pancreatic Duct	Ø Open 3 Percutaneous 4 Percutaneous Endoscopic 7 Via Natural or Artificial Opening 8 Via Natural or Artificial Opening Endoscopic	1 Radioactive Element 2 Monitoring Device 3 Infusion Device D Intraluminal Device	Z No Qualifier

Non-OR ØFH[Ø,1,2,4,G][Ø,3,4]3Z
Non-OR ØFH[B,D][Ø,3,7]3Z
Non-OR ØFH[B,D][4,8][3,D]Z

See Appendix I for Procedure Combinations
⊞ ØFHB[7,8]DZ

Ø Medical and Surgical
F Hepatobiliary System and Pancreas
J Inspection Visually and/or manually exploring a body part

Body Part Character 4	Approach Character 5	Device Character 6	Qualifier Character 7
Ø Liver 4 Gallbladder G Pancreas	Ø Open 3 Percutaneous 4 Percutaneous Endoscopic X External	Z No Device	Z No Qualifier
B Hepatobiliary Duct D Pancreatic Duct	Ø Open 3 Percutaneous 4 Percutaneous Endoscopic 7 Via Natural or Artificial Opening 8 Via Natural or Artificial Opening Endoscopic	Z No Device	Z No Qualifier

Non-OR ØFJ[Ø,4,G]XZZ

Ø Medical and Surgical
F Hepatobiliary System and Pancreas
L Occlusion Completely closing an orifice or the lumen of a tubular body part

Body Part Character 4	Approach Character 5	Device Character 6	Qualifier Character 7
5 Hepatic Duct, Right 6 Hepatic Duct, Left 8 Cystic Duct 9 Common Bile Duct C Ampulla of Vater D Pancreatic Duct F Pancreatic Duct, Accessory	Ø Open 3 Percutaneous 4 Percutaneous Endoscopic	C Extraluminal Device D Intraluminal Device Z No Device	Z No Qualifier
5 Hepatic Duct, Right 6 Hepatic Duct, Left 8 Cystic Duct 9 Common Bile Duct C Ampulla of Vater D Pancreatic Duct F Pancreatic Duct, Accessory	7 Via Natural or Artificial Opening 8 Via Natural or Artificial Opening Endoscopic	D Intraluminal Device Z No Device	Z No Qualifier

Non-OR ØFL[5,6,8,9][3,4][C,D,Z]Z
Non-OR ØFL[5,6,8,9][7,8][D,Z]Z

Ø Medical and Surgical
F Hepatobiliary System and Pancreas
M Reattachment Putting back in or on all or a portion of a separated body part to its normal location or other suitable location

Body Part Character 4	Approach Character 5	Device Character 6	Qualifier Character 7
Ø Liver 1 Liver, Right Lobe 2 Liver, Left Lobe 4 Gallbladder 5 Hepatic Duct, Right 6 Hepatic Duct, Left 8 Cystic Duct 9 Common Bile Duct C Ampulla of Vater D Pancreatic Duct F Pancreatic Duct, Accessory G Pancreas	Ø Open 4 Percutaneous Endoscopic	Z No Device	Z No Qualifier

Non-OR ØFM[4,5,6,8,9]4ZZ

Ø Medical and Surgical
F Hepatobiliary System and Pancreas
N Release Freeing a body part from an abnormal physical constraint

Body Part Character 4	Approach Character 5	Device Character 6	Qualifier Character 7
Ø Liver 1 Liver, Right Lobe 2 Liver, Left Lobe 4 Gallbladder G Pancreas	Ø Open 3 Percutaneous 4 Percutaneous Endoscopic	Z No Device	Z No Qualifier
5 Hepatic Duct, Right 6 Hepatic Duct, Left 8 Cystic Duct 9 Common Bile Duct C Ampulla of Vater D Pancreatic Duct F Pancreatic Duct, Accessory	Ø Open 3 Percutaneous 4 Percutaneous Endoscopic 7 Via Natural or Artificial Opening 8 Via Natural or Artificial Opening Endoscopic	Z No Device	Z No Qualifier

Ø Medical and Surgical
F Hepatobiliary System and Pancreas
P Removal Taking out or off a device from a body part

Body Part Character 4	Approach Character 5	Device Character 6	Qualifier Character 7
Ø Liver	Ø Open 3 Percutaneous 4 Percutaneous Endoscopic X External	Ø Drainage Device 2 Monitoring Device 3 Infusion Device	Z No Qualifier
4 Gallbladder G Pancreas	Ø Open 3 Percutaneous 4 Percutaneous Endoscopic X External	Ø Drainage Device 2 Monitoring Device 3 Infusion Device D Intraluminal Device	Z No Qualifier
B Hepatobiliary Duct ⊞ D Pancreatic Duct ⊞	Ø Open 3 Percutaneous 4 Percutaneous Endoscopic 7 Via Natural or Artificial Opening 8 Via Natural or Artificial Opening Endoscopic	Ø Drainage Device 1 Radioactive Element 2 Monitoring Device 3 Infusion Device 7 Autologous Tissue Substitute C Extraluminal Device D Intraluminal Device J Synthetic Substitute K Nonautologous Tissue Substitute	Z No Qualifier
B Hepatobiliary Duct D Pancreatic Duct	X External	Ø Drainage Device 1 Radioactive Element 2 Monitoring Device 3 Infusion Device D Intraluminal Device	Z No Qualifier

DRG Non-OR ØFP[B,D]XDZ
Non-OR ØFPØX[Ø,2,3]Z
Non-OR ØFP4X[Ø,2,3,D]Z
Non-OR ØFPGX[Ø,2,3]Z
Non-OR ØFP[B,D]X[Ø,1,2,3]Z

See Appendix I for Procedure Combinations
Combo-only ØFP[B,D]XDZ
⊞ ØFP[B,D][7,8]DZ

Ø Medical and Surgical
F Hepatobiliary System and Pancreas
Q Repair Restoring, to the extent possible, a body part to its normal anatomic structure and function

Body Part Character 4	Approach Character 5	Device Character 6	Qualifier Character 7
Ø Liver ⊞ 1 Liver, Right Lobe 2 Liver, Left Lobe 4 Gallbladder ⊞ G Pancreas	Ø Open 3 Percutaneous 4 Percutaneous Endoscopic	Z No Device	Z No Qualifier
5 Hepatic Duct, Right 6 Hepatic Duct, Left 8 Cystic Duct 9 Common Bile Duct C Ampulla of Vater D Pancreatic Duct F Pancreatic Duct, Accessory	Ø Open 3 Percutaneous 4 Percutaneous Endoscopic 7 Via Natural or Artificial Opening 8 Via Natural or Artificial Opening Endoscopic	Z No Device	Z No Qualifier

AHA: 2Ø13, 4Q, 1Ø9

No Procedure Combinations Specified
⊞ ØFQ[Ø,4][Ø,3,4]ZZ

Ø Medical and Surgical
F Hepatobiliary System and Pancreas
R Replacement Putting in or on biological or synthetic material that physically takes the place and/or function of all or a portion of a body part

Body Part Character 4	Approach Character 5	Device Character 6	Qualifier Character 7
5 Hepatic Duct, Right 6 Hepatic Duct, Left 8 Cystic Duct 9 Common Bile Duct C Ampulla of Vater D Pancreatic Duct F Pancreatic Duct, Accessory	Ø Open 4 Percutaneous Endoscopic	7 Autologous Tissue Substitute J Synthetic Substitute K Nonautologous Tissue Substitute	Z No Qualifier

Ø Medical and Surgical
F Hepatobiliary System and Pancreas
S Reposition Moving to its normal location or other suitable location all or a portion of a body part

Body Part Character 4	Approach Character 5	Device Character 6	Qualifier Character 7
Ø Liver 4 Gallbladder 5 Hepatic Duct, Right 6 Hepatic Duct, Left 8 Cystic Duct 9 Common Bile Duct C Ampulla of Vater D Pancreatic Duct F Pancreatic Duct, Accessory G Pancreas	Ø Open 4 Percutaneous Endoscopic	Z No Device	Z No Qualifier

Ø Medical and Surgical
F Hepatobiliary System and Pancreas
T Resection Cutting out or off, without replacement, all of a body part

Body Part Character 4	Approach Character 5	Device Character 6	Qualifier Character 7
Ø Liver 1 Liver, Right Lobe 2 Liver, Left Lobe 4 Gallbladder G Pancreas ⊞	Ø Open 4 Percutaneous Endoscopic	Z No Device	Z No Qualifier
5 Hepatic Duct, Right 6 Hepatic Duct, Left 8 Cystic Duct 9 Common Bile Duct C Ampulla of Vater D Pancreatic Duct F Pancreatic Duct, Accessory	Ø Open 4 Percutaneous Endoscopic 7 Via Natural or Artificial Opening 8 Via Natural or Artificial Opening Endoscopic	Z No Device	Z No Qualifier

Non-OR ØFT[D,F][4,8]ZZ
AHA: 2Ø13, 3Q, 22-23; 2Ø12, 4Q, 99

See Appendix I for Procedure Combinations
⊞ ØFTGØZZ

Ø Medical and Surgical
F Hepatobiliary System and Pancreas
U Supplement Putting in or on biological or synthetic material that physically reinforces and/or augments the function of a portion of a body part

Body Part Character 4	Approach Character 5	Device Character 6	Qualifier Character 7
5 Hepatic Duct, Right 6 Hepatic Duct, Left 8 Cystic Duct 9 Common Bile Duct C Ampulla of Vater D Pancreatic Duct F Pancreatic Duct, Accessory	Ø Open 3 Percutaneous 4 Percutaneous Endoscopic	7 Autologous Tissue Substitute J Synthetic Substitute K Nonautologous Tissue Substitute	Z No Qualifier

Ø Medical and Surgical
F Hepatobiliary System and Pancreas
V Restriction Partially closing an orifice or the lumen of a tubular body part

Body Part Character 4	Approach Character 5	Device Character 6	Qualifier Character 7
5 Hepatic Duct, Right 6 Hepatic Duct, Left 8 Cystic Duct 9 Common Bile Duct C Ampulla of Vater D Pancreatic Duct F Pancreatic Duct, Accessory	Ø Open 3 Percutaneous 4 Percutaneous Endoscopic	C Extraluminal Device D Intraluminal Device Z No Device	Z No Qualifier
5 Hepatic Duct, Right 6 Hepatic Duct, Left 8 Cystic Duct 9 Common Bile Duct C Ampulla of Vater D Pancreatic Duct F Pancreatic Duct, Accessory	7 Via Natural or Artificial Opening 8 Via Natural or Artificial Opening Endoscopic	D Intraluminal Device Z No Device	Z No Qualifier

Non-OR ØFV[5,6,8,9][3,4][C,D,Z]Z
Non-OR ØFV[5,6,8,9][7,8][D,Z]Z

Ø Medical and Surgical
F Hepatobiliary System and Pancreas
W Revision Correcting, to the extent possible, a portion of a malfunctioning device or the position of a displaced device

Body Part Character 4	Approach Character 5	Device Character 6	Qualifier Character 7
Ø Liver	Ø Open 3 Percutaneous 4 Percutaneous Endoscopic X External	Ø Drainage Device 2 Monitoring Device 3 Infusion Device	Z No Qualifier
4 Gallbladder G Pancreas	Ø Open 3 Percutaneous 4 Percutaneous Endoscopic X External	Ø Drainage Device 2 Monitoring Device 3 Infusion Device D Intraluminal Device	Z No Qualifier
B Hepatobiliary Duct D Pancreatic Duct	Ø Open 3 Percutaneous 4 Percutaneous Endoscopic 7 Via Natural or Artificial Opening 8 Via Natural or Artificial Opening Endoscopic X External	Ø Drainage Device 2 Monitoring Device 3 Infusion Device 7 Autologous Tissue Substitute C Extraluminal Device D Intraluminal Device J Synthetic Substitute K Nonautologous Tissue Substitute	Z No Qualifier

Non-OR ØFWØX[Ø,2,3]Z
Non-OR ØFW[4,G]X[Ø,2,3,D]Z
Non-OR ØFW[B,D]X[Ø,2,3,7,C,D,J,K]Z

Ø Medical and Surgical
F Hepatobiliary System and Pancreas
Y Transplantation Putting in or on all or a portion of a living body part taken from another individual or animal to physically take the place and/or function of all or a portion of a similar body part

Body Part Character 4	Approach Character 5	Device Character 6	Qualifier Character 7
Ø Liver LC G Pancreas ⊞ LC NC	Ø Open	Z No Device	Ø Allogeneic 1 Syngeneic 2 Zooplastic

LC ØFYØØZ[Ø,1,2]
LC ØFYGØZ[Ø,1]
NC ØFYGØZ2
NC ØFYGØZ[Ø,1] If reported alone without one of the following procedures ØTYØØZ[Ø,1,2], ØTY1ØZ[Ø,1,2] and without one of the following diagnoses E1Ø.1Ø-E1Ø.9, E89.1

See Appendix I for Procedure Combinations
⊞ ØFYGØZ[Ø,1,2]

AHA: 2Ø12, 4Q, 99

Endocrine System ØG2–ØGW

Ø Medical and Surgical
G Endocrine System
2 Change Taking out or off a device from a body part and putting back an identical or similar device in or on the same body part without cutting or puncturing the skin or a mucous membrane

Body Part Character 4	Approach Character 5	Device Character 6	Qualifier Character 7
Ø Pituitary Gland 1 Pineal Body 5 Adrenal Gland K Thyroid Gland R Parathyroid Gland S Endocrine Gland	X External	Ø Drainage Device Y Other Device	Z No Qualifier

Non-OR For all body part, approach, device, and qualifier values

Ø Medical and Surgical
G Endocrine System
5 Destruction Physical eradication of all or a portion of a body part by the direct use of energy, force, or a destructive agent

Body Part Character 4	Approach Character 5	Device Character 6	Qualifier Character 7
Ø Pituitary Gland 1 Pineal Body 2 Adrenal Gland, Left 3 Adrenal Gland, Right 4 Adrenal Glands, Bilateral 6 Carotid Body, Left 7 Carotid Body, Right 8 Carotid Bodies, Bilateral 9 Para-aortic Body B Coccygeal Glomus C Glomus Jugulare D Aortic Body F Paraganglion Extremity G Thyroid Gland Lobe, Left H Thyroid Gland Lobe, Right K Thyroid Gland L Superior Parathyroid Gland, Right M Superior Parathyroid Gland, Left N Inferior Parathyroid Gland, Right P Inferior Parathyroid Gland, Left Q Parathyroid Glands, Multiple R Parathyroid Gland	Ø Open 3 Percutaneous 4 Percutaneous Endoscopic	Z No Device	Z No Qualifier

Non-OR ØG5[6,7,8,9,B,C,D,F][Ø,3,4]ZZ

Ø Medical and Surgical
G Endocrine System
8 Division Cutting into a body part without draining fluids and/or gases from the body part in order to separate or transect a body part

Body Part Character 4	Approach Character 5	Device Character 6	Qualifier Character 7
Ø Pituitary Gland J Thyroid Gland Isthmus	Ø Open 3 Percutaneous 4 Percutaneous Endoscopic	Z No Device	Z No Qualifier

0 Medical and Surgical
G Endocrine System
9 Drainage Taking or letting out fluids and/or gases from a body part

Body Part Character 4	Approach Character 5	Device Character 6	Qualifier Character 7
0 Pituitary Gland **1** Pineal Body **2** Adrenal Gland, Left **3** Adrenal Gland, Right **4** Adrenal Glands, Bilateral **6** Carotid Body, Left **7** Carotid Body, Right **8** Carotid Bodies, Bilateral **9** Para-aortic Body **B** Coccygeal Glomus **C** Glomus Jugulare **D** Aortic Body **F** Paraganglion Extremity **G** Thyroid Gland Lobe, Left **H** Thyroid Gland Lobe, Right **K** Thyroid Gland **L** Superior Parathyroid Gland, Right **M** Superior Parathyroid Gland, Left **N** Inferior Parathyroid Gland, Right **P** Inferior Parathyroid Gland, Left **Q** Parathyroid Glands, Multiple **R** Parathyroid Gland	**0** Open **3** Percutaneous **4** Percutaneous Endoscopic	**0** Drainage Device	**Z** No Qualifier
0 Pituitary Gland **1** Pineal Body **2** Adrenal Gland, Left **3** Adrenal Gland, Right **4** Adrenal Glands, Bilateral **6** Carotid Body, Left **7** Carotid Body, Right **8** Carotid Bodies, Bilateral **9** Para-aortic Body **B** Coccygeal Glomus **C** Glomus Jugulare **D** Aortic Body **F** Paraganglion Extremity **G** Thyroid Gland Lobe, Left **H** Thyroid Gland Lobe, Right **K** Thyroid Gland **L** Superior Parathyroid Gland, Right **M** Superior Parathyroid Gland, Left **N** Inferior Parathyroid Gland, Right **P** Inferior Parathyroid Gland, Left **Q** Parathyroid Glands, Multiple **R** Parathyroid Gland	**0** Open **3** Percutaneous **4** Percutaneous Endoscopic	**Z** No Device	**X** Diagnostic **Z** No Qualifier

Non-OR 0G9[6,7,8,9,B,C,D,F][0,3,4]0Z
Non-OR 0G9[G,H,K,L,M,N,P,Q,R][3,4]0Z
Non-OR 0G9[2,3,4,G,H,K][3,4]ZX
Non-OR 0G9[6,7,8,9,B,C,D,F][0,3,4]Z[X,Z]
Non-OR 0G9[G,H,K,L,M,N,P,Q,R][3,4]ZZ

Ø Medical and Surgical
G Endocrine System
B Excision Cutting out or off, without replacement, a portion of a body part

Body Part Character 4	Approach Character 5	Device Character 6	Qualifier Character 7
Ø Pituitary Gland 1 Pineal Body 2 Adrenal Gland, Left 3 Adrenal Gland, Right 4 Adrenal Glands, Bilateral 6 Carotid Body, Left 7 Carotid Body, Right 8 Carotid Bodies, Bilateral 9 Para-aortic Body B Coccygeal Glomus C Glomus Jugulare D Aortic Body F Paraganglion Extremity G Thyroid Gland Lobe, Left H Thyroid Gland Lobe, Right L Superior Parathyroid Gland, Right M Superior Parathyroid Gland, Left N Inferior Parathyroid Gland, Right P Inferior Parathyroid Gland, Left Q Parathyroid Glands, Multiple R Parathyroid Gland	Ø Open 3 Percutaneous 4 Percutaneous Endoscopic	Z No Device	X Diagnostic Z No Qualifier

Non-OR ØGB[2,3,4,G,H][3,4]ZX
Non-OR ØGB[6,7,8,9,B,C,D,F][Ø,3,4]Z[X,Z]

Ø Medical and Surgical
G Endocrine System
C Extirpation Taking or cutting out solid matter from a body part

Body Part Character 4	Approach Character 5	Device Character 6	Qualifier Character 7
Ø Pituitary Gland 1 Pineal Body 2 Adrenal Gland, Left 3 Adrenal Gland, Right 4 Adrenal Glands, Bilateral 6 Carotid Body, Left 7 Carotid Body, Right 8 Carotid Bodies, Bilateral 9 Para-aortic Body B Coccygeal Glomus C Glomus Jugulare D Aortic Body F Paraganglion Extremity G Thyroid Gland Lobe, Left H Thyroid Gland Lobe, Right K Thyroid Gland L Superior Parathyroid Gland, Right M Superior Parathyroid Gland, Left N Inferior Parathyroid Gland, Right P Inferior Parathyroid Gland, Left Q Parathyroid Glands, Multiple R Parathyroid Gland	Ø Open 3 Percutaneous 4 Percutaneous Endoscopic	Z No Device	Z No Qualifier

Non-OR ØGC[6,7,8,9,B,C,D,F][Ø,3,4]ZZ

Ø Medical and Surgical
G Endocrine System
H Insertion Putting in a nonbiological appliance that monitors, assists, performs, or prevents a physiological function but does not physically take the place of a body part

Body Part Character 4	Approach Character 5	Device Character 6	Qualifier Character 7
S Endocrine Gland	Ø Open 3 Percutaneous 4 Percutaneous Endoscopic	2 Monitoring Device 3 Infusion Device	Z No Qualifier

0 Medical and Surgical
G Endocrine System
J Inspection Visually and/or manually exploring a body part

Body Part Character 4	Approach Character 5	Device Character 6	Qualifier Character 7
0 Pituitary Gland 1 Pineal Body 5 Adrenal Gland K Thyroid Gland R Parathyroid Gland S Endocrine Gland	0 Open 3 Percutaneous 4 Percutaneous Endoscopic	Z No Device	Z No Qualifier

0 Medical and Surgical
G Endocrine System
M Reattachment Putting back in or on all or a portion of a separated body part to its normal location or other suitable location

Body Part Character 4	Approach Character 5	Device Character 6	Qualifier Character 7
2 Adrenal Gland, Left 3 Adrenal Gland, Right G Thyroid Gland Lobe, Left H Thyroid Gland Lobe, Right L Superior Parathyroid Gland, Right M Superior Parathyroid Gland, Left N Inferior Parathyroid Gland, Right P Inferior Parathyroid Gland, Left Q Parathyroid Glands, Multiple R Parathyroid Gland	0 Open 4 Percutaneous Endoscopic	Z No Device	Z No Qualifier

0 Medical and Surgical
G Endocrine System
N Release Freeing a body part from an abnormal physical constraint

Body Part Character 4	Approach Character 5	Device Character 6	Qualifier Character 7
0 Pituitary Gland 1 Pineal Body 2 Adrenal Gland, Left 3 Adrenal Gland, Right 4 Adrenal Glands, Bilateral 6 Carotid Body, Left 7 Carotid Body, Right 8 Carotid Bodies, Bilateral 9 Para-aortic Body B Coccygeal Glomus C Glomus Jugulare D Aortic Body F Paraganglion Extremity G Thyroid Gland Lobe, Left H Thyroid Gland Lobe, Right K Thyroid Gland L Superior Parathyroid Gland, Right M Superior Parathyroid Gland, Left N Inferior Parathyroid Gland, Right P Inferior Parathyroid Gland, Left Q Parathyroid Glands, Multiple R Parathyroid Gland	0 Open 3 Percutaneous 4 Percutaneous Endoscopic	Z No Device	Z No Qualifier

Non-OR 0GN[6,7,8,9,B,C,D,F][0,3,4]ZZ

0 Medical and Surgical
G Endocrine System
P Removal Taking out or off a device from a body part

Body Part Character 4	Approach Character 5	Device Character 6	Qualifier Character 7
0 Pituitary Gland 1 Pineal Body 5 Adrenal Gland K Thyroid Gland R Parathyroid Gland	0 Open 3 Percutaneous 4 Percutaneous Endoscopic X External	0 Drainage Device	Z No Qualifier
S Endocrine Gland	0 Open 3 Percutaneous 4 Percutaneous Endoscopic X External	0 Drainage Device 2 Monitoring Device 3 Infusion Device	Z No Qualifier

Non-OR 0GP[0,1,5,K,R]X0Z
Non-OR 0GPS[0,3,4,X][0,2,3]Z

Ø Medical and Surgical
G Endocrine System
Q Repair Restoring, to the extent possible, a body part to its normal anatomic structure and function

Body Part Character 4	Approach Character 5	Device Character 6	Qualifier Character 7
Ø Pituitary Gland 1 Pineal Body 2 Adrenal Gland, Left 3 Adrenal Gland, Right 4 Adrenal Glands, Bilateral 6 Carotid Body, Left 7 Carotid Body, Right 8 Carotid Bodies, Bilateral 9 Para-aortic Body B Coccygeal Glomus C Glomus Jugulare D Aortic Body F Paraganglion Extremity G Thyroid Gland Lobe, Left H Thyroid Gland Lobe, Right J Thyroid Gland Isthmus K Thyroid Gland L Superior Parathyroid Gland, Right M Superior Parathyroid Gland, Left N Inferior Parathyroid Gland, Right P Inferior Parathyroid Gland, Left Q Parathyroid Glands, Multiple R Parathyroid Gland	Ø Open 3 Percutaneous 4 Percutaneous Endoscopic	Z No Device	Z No Qualifier

Non-OR ØGQ[6,7,8,9,B,C,D,F][Ø,3,4]ZZ

Ø Medical and Surgical
G Endocrine System
S Reposition Moving to its normal location or other suitable location all or a portion of a body part

Body Part Character 4	Approach Character 5	Device Character 6	Qualifier Character 7
2 Adrenal Gland, Left 3 Adrenal Gland, Right G Thyroid Gland Lobe, Left H Thyroid Gland Lobe, Right L Superior Parathyroid Gland, Right M Superior Parathyroid Gland, Left N Inferior Parathyroid Gland, Right P Inferior Parathyroid Gland, Left Q Parathyroid Glands, Multiple R Parathyroid Gland	Ø Open 4 Percutaneous Endoscopic	Z No Device	Z No Qualifier

Ø Medical and Surgical
G Endocrine System
T Resection Cutting out or off, without replacement, all of a body part

Body Part Character 4	Approach Character 5	Device Character 6	Qualifier Character 7
Ø Pituitary Gland 1 Pineal Body 2 Adrenal Gland, Left 3 Adrenal Gland, Right 4 Adrenal Glands, Bilateral 6 Carotid Body, Left 7 Carotid Body, Right 8 Carotid Bodies, Bilateral 9 Para-aortic Body B Coccygeal Glomus C Glomus Jugulare D Aortic Body F Paraganglion Extremity G Thyroid Gland Lobe, Left H Thyroid Gland Lobe, Right K Thyroid Gland L Superior Parathyroid Gland, Right M Superior Parathyroid Gland, Left N Inferior Parathyroid Gland, Right P Inferior Parathyroid Gland, Left Q Parathyroid Glands, Multiple R Parathyroid Gland	Ø Open 4 Percutaneous Endoscopic	Z No Device	Z No Qualifier

Non-OR ØGT[6,7,8,9,B,C,D,F][Ø,4]ZZ

Ø Medical and Surgical
G Endocrine System
W Revision Correcting, to the extent possible, a portion of a malfunctioning device or the position of a displaced device

Body Part Character 4	Approach Character 5	Device Character 6	Qualifier Character 7
Ø Pituitary Gland **1** Pineal Body **5** Adrenal Gland **K** Thyroid Gland **R** Parathyroid Gland	**Ø** Open **3** Percutaneous **4** Percutaneous Endoscopic **X** External	**Ø** Drainage Device	**Z** No Qualifier
S Endocrine Gland	**Ø** Open **3** Percutaneous **4** Percutaneous Endoscopic **X** External	**Ø** Drainage Device **2** Monitoring Device **3** Infusion Device	**Z** No Qualifier

Non-OR ØGW[Ø,1,5,K,R]XØZ
Non-OR ØGWS[Ø,3,4,X][Ø,2,3]Z

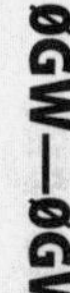

Skin and Breast ØHØ–ØHX

Ø Medical and Surgical
H Skin and Breast
Ø Alteration Modifying the anatomic structure of a body part without affecting the function of the body part

Body Part Character 4	Approach Character 5	Device Character 6	Qualifier Character 7
T Breast, Right U Breast, Left V Breast, Bilateral	Ø Open 3 Percutaneous X External	7 Autologous Tissue Substitute J Synthetic Substitute K Nonautologous Tissue Substitute Z No Device	Z No Qualifier

Ø Medical and Surgical
H Skin and Breast
2 Change Taking out or off a device from a body part and putting back an identical or similar device in or on the same body part without cutting or puncturing the skin or a mucous membrane

Body Part Character 4	Approach Character 5	Device Character 6	Qualifier Character 7
P Skin T Breast, Right U Breast, Left	X External	Ø Drainage Device Y Other Device	Z No Qualifier

Non-OR For all body part, approach, device, and qualifier values

Ø Medical and Surgical
H Skin and Breast
5 Destruction Physical eradication of all or a portion of a body part by the direct use of energy, force, or a destructive agent

Body Part Character 4	Approach Character 5	Device Character 6	Qualifier Character 7
Ø Skin, Scalp 1 Skin, Face 2 Skin, Right Ear 3 Skin, Left Ear 4 Skin, Neck 5 Skin, Chest 6 Skin, Back 7 Skin, Abdomen 8 Skin, Buttock 9 Skin, Perineum A Skin, Genitalia B Skin, Right Upper Arm C Skin, Left Upper Arm D Skin, Right Lower Arm E Skin, Left Lower Arm F Skin, Right Hand G Skin, Left Hand H Skin, Right Upper Leg J Skin, Left Upper Leg K Skin, Right Lower Leg L Skin, Left Lower Leg M Skin, Right Foot N Skin, Left Foot	X External	Z No Device	D Multiple Z No Qualifier
Q Finger Nail R Toe Nail	X External	Z No Device	Z No Qualifier
T Breast, Right U Breast, Left V Breast, Bilateral W Nipple, Right X Nipple, Left	Ø Open 3 Percutaneous 7 Via Natural or Artificial Opening 8 Via Natural or Artificial Opening Endoscopic X External	Z No Device	Z No Qualifier

DRG Non-OR ØH5[Ø,1,4,5,6,7,8,9,A,B,C,D,E,F,G,H,J,K,L,M,N]XZ[D,Z]
DRG Non-OR ØH5[Q,R]XZZ
Non-OR ØH5[2,3]XZ[D,Z]

Ø Medical and Surgical
H Skin and Breast
8 Division Cutting into a body part without draining fluids and/or gases from the body part in order to separate or transect a body part

Body Part Character 4	Approach Character 5	Device Character 6	Qualifier Character 7
Ø Skin, Scalp 1 Skin, Face 2 Skin, Right Ear 3 Skin, Left Ear 4 Skin, Neck 5 Skin, Chest 6 Skin, Back 7 Skin, Abdomen 8 Skin, Buttock 9 Skin, Perineum A Skin, Genitalia B Skin, Right Upper Arm C Skin, Left Upper Arm D Skin, Right Lower Arm E Skin, Left Lower Arm F Skin, Right Hand G Skin, Left Hand H Skin, Right Upper Leg J Skin, Left Upper Leg K Skin, Right Lower Leg L Skin, Left Lower Leg M Skin, Right Foot N Skin, Left Foot	X External	Z No Device	Z No Qualifier

Non-OR ØH8[2,3]XZZ

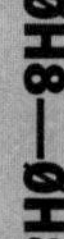

Ø Medical and Surgical
H Skin and Breast
9 Drainage Taking or letting out fluids and/or gases from a body part

Body Part Character 4	Approach Character 5	Device Character 6	Qualifier Character 7
Ø Skin, Scalp **1** Skin, Face **2** Skin, Right Ear **3** Skin, Left Ear **4** Skin, Neck **5** Skin, Chest **6** Skin, Back **7** Skin, Abdomen **8** Skin, Buttock **9** Skin, Perineum **A** Skin, Genitalia **B** Skin, Right Upper Arm **C** Skin, Left Upper Arm **D** Skin, Right Lower Arm **E** Skin, Left Lower Arm **F** Skin, Right Hand **G** Skin, Left Hand **H** Skin, Right Upper Leg **J** Skin, Left Upper Leg **K** Skin, Right Lower Leg **L** Skin, Left Lower Leg **M** Skin, Right Foot **N** Skin, Left Foot **Q** Finger Nail **R** Toe Nail	**X** External	**Ø** Drainage Device	**Z** No Qualifier
Ø Skin, Scalp **1** Skin, Face **2** Skin, Right Ear **3** Skin, Left Ear **4** Skin, Neck **5** Skin, Chest **6** Skin, Back **7** Skin, Abdomen **8** Skin, Buttock **9** Skin, Perineum **A** Skin, Genitalia **B** Skin, Right Upper Arm **C** Skin, Left Upper Arm **D** Skin, Right Lower Arm **E** Skin, Left Lower Arm **F** Skin, Right Hand **G** Skin, Left Hand **H** Skin, Right Upper Leg **J** Skin, Left Upper Leg **K** Skin, Right Lower Leg **L** Skin, Left Lower Leg **M** Skin, Right Foot **N** Skin, Left Foot **Q** Finger Nail **R** Toe Nail	**X** External	**Z** No Device	**X** Diagnostic **Z** No Qualifier
T Breast, Right **U** Breast, Left **V** Breast, Bilateral **W** Nipple, Right **X** Nipple, Left	**Ø** Open **3** Percutaneous **7** Via Natural or Artificial Opening **8** Via Natural or Artificial Opening Endoscopic **X** External	**Ø** Drainage Device	**Z** No Qualifier
T Breast, Right **U** Breast, Left **V** Breast, Bilateral **W** Nipple, Right **X** Nipple, Left	**Ø** Open **3** Percutaneous **7** Via Natural or Artificial Opening **8** Via Natural or Artificial Opening Endoscopic **X** External	**Z** No Device	**X** Diagnostic **Z** No Qualifier

Non-OR ØH9[Ø,1,2,3,4,5,6,7,8,A,B,C,D,E,F,G,H,J,K,L,M,N,Q,R]XØZ
Non-OR ØH9[Ø,1,2,3,4,5,6,7,8,9,A,B,C,D,E,F,G,H,J,K,L,M,N,Q,R]XZX
Non-OR ØH9[Ø,1,2,3,4,5,6,7,8,A,B,C,D,E,F,G,H,J,K,L,M,N,Q,R]XZZ
Non-OR ØH9[T,U,V,W,X][Ø,3,7,8,X]ØZ
Non-OR ØH9[T,U,V,W,X][3,7,8,X]ZX
Non-OR ØH9[T,U,V,W,X][Ø,3,7,8,X]ZZ

Ø Medical and Surgical
H Skin and Breast
B Excision Cutting out or off, without replacement, a portion of a body part

Body Part Character 4	Approach Character 5	Device Character 6	Qualifier Character 7
Ø Skin, Scalp **1** Skin, Face **2** Skin, Right Ear **3** Skin, Left Ear **4** Skin, Neck **5** Skin, Chest **6** Skin, Back **7** Skin, Abdomen **8** Skin, Buttock **9** Skin, Perineum **A** Skin, Genitalia **B** Skin, Right Upper Arm **C** Skin, Left Upper Arm **D** Skin, Right Lower Arm **E** Skin, Left Lower Arm **F** Skin, Right Hand **G** Skin, Left Hand **H** Skin, Right Upper Leg **J** Skin, Left Upper Leg **K** Skin, Right Lower Leg **L** Skin, Left Lower Leg **M** Skin, Right Foot **N** Skin, Left Foot **Q** Finger Nail **R** Toe Nail	**X** External	**Z** No Device	**X** Diagnostic **Z** No Qualifier
T Breast, Right **U** Breast, Left **V** Breast, Bilateral **W** Nipple, Right **X** Nipple, Left **Y** Supernumerary Breast	**Ø** Open **3** Percutaneous **7** Via Natural or Artificial Opening **8** Via Natural or Artificial Opening Endoscopic **X** External	**Z** No Device	**X** Diagnostic **Z** No Qualifier

DRG Non-OR ØHB9XZZ
Non-OR ØHB[Ø,1,2,3,4,5,6,7,8,9,A,B,C,D,E,F,G,H,J,K,L,M,N,Q,R]XZX
Non-OR ØHB[2,3,Q,R]XZZ
Non-OR ØHB[T,U,V,W,X,Y][3,7,8,X]ZX

Ø Medical and Surgical
H Skin and Breast
C Extirpation Taking or cutting out solid matter from a body part

Body Part Character 4	Approach Character 5	Device Character 6	Qualifier Character 7
Ø Skin, Scalp 1 Skin, Face 2 Skin, Right Ear 3 Skin, Left Ear 4 Skin, Neck 5 Skin, Chest 6 Skin, Back 7 Skin, Abdomen 8 Skin, Buttock 9 Skin, Perineum A Skin, Genitalia B Skin, Right Upper Arm C Skin, Left Upper Arm D Skin, Right Lower Arm E Skin, Left Lower Arm F Skin, Right Hand G Skin, Left Hand H Skin, Right Upper Leg J Skin, Left Upper Leg K Skin, Right Lower Leg L Skin, Left Lower Leg M Skin, Right Foot N Skin, Left Foot Q Finger Nail R Toe Nail	X External	Z No Device	Z No Qualifier
T Breast, Right U Breast, Left V Breast, Bilateral W Nipple, Right X Nipple, Left	Ø Open 3 Percutaneousv 7 Via Natural or Artificial Opening 8 Via Natural or Artificial Opening Endoscopic X External	Z No Device	Z No Qualifier

Non-OR For all body part, approach, device and qualifier values

Ø Medical and Surgical
H Skin and Breast
D Extraction Pulling or stripping out or off all or a portion of a body part by the use of force

Body Part Character 4	Approach Character 5	Device Character 6	Qualifier Character 7
Ø Skin, Scalp 1 Skin, Face 2 Skin, Right Ear 3 Skin, Left Ear 4 Skin, Neck 5 Skin, Chest 6 Skin, Back 7 Skin, Abdomen 8 Skin, Buttock 9 Skin, Perineum A Skin, Genitalia B Skin, Right Upper Arm C Skin, Left Upper Arm D Skin, Right Lower Arm E Skin, Left Lower Arm F Skin, Right Hand G Skin, Left Hand H Skin, Right Upper Leg J Skin, Left Upper Leg K Skin, Right Lower Leg L Skin, Left Lower Leg M Skin, Right Foot N Skin, Left Foot Q Finger Nail R Toe Nail S Hair	X External	Z No Device	Z No Qualifier

Non-OR For all body part, approach, device, and qualifier values

0 Medical and Surgical
H Skin and Breast
H Insertion Putting in a nonbiological appliance that monitors, assists, performs, or prevents a physiological function but does not physically take the place of a body part

Body Part Character 4	Approach Character 5	Device Character 6	Qualifier Character 7
T Breast, Right **U** Breast, Left **V** Breast, Bilateral **W** Nipple, Right **X** Nipple, Left	**0** Open **3** Percutaneous **7** Via Natural or Artificial Opening **8** Via Natural or Artificial Opening Endoscopic	**1** Radioactive Element **N** Tissue Expander	**Z** No Qualifier
T Breast, Right **U** Breast, Left **V** Breast, Bilateral **W** Nipple, Right **X** Nipple, Left	**X** External	**1** Radioactive Element	**Z** No Qualifier

AHA: 2014, 2Q, 12; 2013, 4Q, 107

0 Medical and Surgical
H Skin and Breast
J Inspection Visually and/or manually exploring a body part

Body Part Character 4	Approach Character 5	Device Character 6	Qualifier Character 7
P Skin **Q** Finger Nail **R** Toe Nail	**X** External	**Z** No Device	**Z** No Qualifier
T Breast, Right **U** Breast, Left	**0** Open **3** Percutaneous **7** Via Natural or Artificial Opening **8** Via Natural or Artificial Opening Endoscopic **X** External	**Z** No Device	**Z** No Qualifier

Non-OR For all body part, approach, device and qualifier values

0 Medical and Surgical
H Skin and Breast
M Reattachment Putting back in or on all or a portion of a separated body part to its normal location or other suitable location

Body Part Character 4	Approach Character 5	Device Character 6	Qualifier Character 7
0 Skin, Scalp **1** Skin, Face **2** Skin, Right Ear **3** Skin, Left Ear **4** Skin, Neck **5** Skin, Chest **6** Skin, Back **7** Skin, Abdomen **8** Skin, Buttock **9** Skin, Perineum **A** Skin, Genitalia **B** Skin, Right Upper Arm **C** Skin, Left Upper Arm **D** Skin, Right Lower Arm **E** Skin, Left Lower Arm **F** Skin, Right Hand **G** Skin, Left Hand **H** Skin, Right Upper Leg **J** Skin, Left Upper Leg **K** Skin, Right Lower Leg **L** Skin, Left Lower Leg **M** Skin, Right Foot **N** Skin, Left Foot **T** Breast, Right **U** Breast, Left **V** Breast, Bilateral **W** Nipple, Right **X** Nipple, Left	**X** External	**Z** No Device	**Z** No Qualifier

Non-OR 0HM0XZZ

Ø Medical and Surgical
H Skin and Breast
N Release Freeing a body part from an abnormal physical constraint

Body Part Character 4	Approach Character 5	Device Character 6	Qualifier Character 7
Ø Skin, Scalp 1 Skin, Face 2 Skin, Right Ear 3 Skin, Left Ear 4 Skin, Neck 5 Skin, Chest 6 Skin, Back 7 Skin, Abdomen 8 Skin, Buttock 9 Skin, Perineum A Skin, Genitalia B Skin, Right Upper Arm C Skin, Left Upper Arm D Skin, Right Lower Arm E Skin, Left Lower Arm F Skin, Right Hand G Skin, Left Hand H Skin, Right Upper Leg J Skin, Left Upper Leg K Skin, Right Lower Leg L Skin, Left Lower Leg M Skin, Right Foot N Skin, Left Foot Q Finger Nail R Toe Nail	X External	Z No Device	Z No Qualifier
T Breast, Right U Breast, Left V Breast, Bilateral W Nipple, Right X Nipple, Left	Ø Open 3 Percutaneous 7 Via Natural or Artificial Opening 8 Via Natural or Artificial Opening Endoscopic X External	Z No Device	Z No Qualifier

Ø Medical and Surgical
H Skin and Breast
P Removal Taking out or off a device from a body part

Body Part Character 4	Approach Character 5	Device Character 6	Qualifier Character 7
P Skin Q Finger Nail R Toe Nail	X External	Ø Drainage Device 7 Autologous Tissue Substitute J Synthetic Substitute K Nonautologous Tissue Substitute	Z No Qualifier
S Hair	X External	7 Autologous Tissue Substitute J Synthetic Substitute K Nonautologous Tissue Substitute	Z No Qualifier
T Breast, Right U Breast, Left	Ø Open 3 Percutaneous 7 Via Natural or Artificial Opening 8 Via Natural or Artificial Opening Endoscopic	Ø Drainage Device 1 Radioactive Element 7 Autologous Tissue Substitute J Synthetic Substitute K Nonautologous Tissue Substitute N Tissue Expander	Z No Qualifier
T Breast, Right U Breast, Left	X External	Ø Drainage Device 1 Radioactive Element 7 Autologous Tissue Substitute J Synthetic Substitute K Nonautologous Tissue Substitute	Z No Qualifier

Non-OR ØHP[P,Q,R]X[Ø,7,J,K]Z
Non-OR ØHPSX[7,J,K]Z
Non-OR ØHP[T,U][Ø,3][Ø,1,7,K]Z
Non-OR ØHP[T,U][7,8][Ø,1,7,J,K,N]Z
Non-OR ØHP[T,U]X[Ø,1,7,J,K]Z

Ø Medical and Surgical
H Skin and Breast
Q Repair Restoring, to the extent possible, a body part to its normal anatomic structure and function

Body Part Character 4	Approach Character 5	Device Character 6	Qualifier Character 7
Ø Skin, Scalp 1 Skin, Face 2 Skin, Right Ear 3 Skin, Left Ear 4 Skin, Neck 5 Skin, Chest 6 Skin, Back 7 Skin, Abdomen 8 Skin, Buttock 9 Skin, Perineum ⊞ A Skin, Genitalia B Skin, Right Upper Arm C Skin, Left Upper Arm D Skin, Right Lower Arm E Skin, Left Lower Arm F Skin, Right Hand G Skin, Left Hand H Skin, Right Upper Leg J Skin, Left Upper Leg K Skin, Right Lower Leg L Skin, Left Lower Leg M Skin, Right Foot N Skin, Left Foot Q Finger Nail R Toe Nail	X External	Z No Device	Z No Qualifier
T Breast, Right U Breast, Left V Breast, Bilateral W Nipple, Right X Nipple, Left Y Supernumerary Breast	Ø Open 3 Percutaneous 7 Via Natural or Artificial Opening 8 Via Natural or Artificial Opening Endoscopic X External	Z No Device	Z No Qualifier

DRG Non-OR ØHQ9XZZ
Non-OR ØHQ[Ø,1,2,3,4,5,6,7,8,A,B,C,D,E,F,G,H,J,K,L,M,N]XZZ
Non-OR ØHQ[T,U,V,Y]XZZ

No Procedure Combinations Specified
⊞ ØHQ9XZZ

Ø Medical and Surgical
H Skin and Breast
R Replacement Putting in or on biological or synthetic material that physically takes the place and/or function of all or a portion of a body part

Body Part Character 4	Approach Character 5	Device Character 6	Qualifier Character 7
Ø Skin, Scalp **1** Skin, Face **2** Skin, Right Ear **3** Skin, Left Ear **4** Skin, Neck **5** Skin, Chest **6** Skin, Back **7** Skin, Abdomen **8** Skin, Buttock **9** Skin, Perineum **A** Skin, Genitalia **B** Skin, Right Upper Arm **C** Skin, Left Upper Arm **D** Skin, Right Lower Arm **E** Skin, Left Lower Arm **F** Skin, Right Hand **G** Skin, Left Hand **H** Skin, Right Upper Leg **J** Skin, Left Upper Leg **K** Skin, Right Lower Leg **L** Skin, Left Lower Leg **M** Skin, Right Foot **N** Skin, Left Foot	**X** External	**7** Autologous Tissue Substitute **K** Nonautologous Tissue Substitute	**3** Full Thickness **4** Partial Thickness
Ø Skin, Scalp **1** Skin, Face **2** Skin, Right Ear **3** Skin, Left Ear **4** Skin, Neck **5** Skin, Chest **6** Skin, Back **7** Skin, Abdomen **8** Skin, Buttock **9** Skin, Perineum **A** Skin, Genitalia **B** Skin, Right Upper Arm **C** Skin, Left Upper Arm **D** Skin, Right Lower Arm **E** Skin, Left Lower Arm **F** Skin, Right Hand **G** Skin, Left Hand **H** Skin, Right Upper Leg **J** Skin, Left Upper Leg **K** Skin, Right Lower Leg **L** Skin, Left Lower Leg **M** Skin, Right Foot **N** Skin, Left Foot	**X** External	**J** Synthetic Substitute	**3** Full Thickness **4** Partial Thickness **Z** No Qualifier
Q Finger Nail **R** Toe Nail **S** Hair	**X** External	**7** Autologous Tissue Substitute **J** Synthetic Substitute **K** Nonautologous Tissue Substitute	**Z** No Qualifier
T Breast, Right **U** Breast, Left **V** Breast, Bilateral	**Ø** Open	**7** Autologous Tissue Substitute	**5** Latissimus Dorsi Myocutaneous Flap **6** Transverse Rectus Abdominis Myocutaneous Flap **7** Deep Inferior Epigastric Artery Perforator Flap **8** Superficial Inferior Epigastric Artery Flap **9** Gluteal Artery Perforator Flap **Z** No Qualifier
T Breast, Right **U** Breast, Left **V** Breast, Bilateral	**Ø** Open	**J** Synthetic Substitute **K** Nonautologous Tissue Substitute	**Z** No Qualifier
T Breast, Right ⊞ **U** Breast, Left ⊞ **V** Breast, Bilateral ⊞	**3** Percutaneous **X** External	**7** Autologous Tissue Substitute **J** Synthetic Substitute **K** Nonautologous Tissue Substitute	**Z** No Qualifier
W Nipple, Right **X** Nipple, Left	**Ø** Open **3** Percutaneous **X** External	**7** Autologous Tissue Substitute **J** Synthetic Substitute **K** Nonautologous Tissue Substitute	**Z** No Qualifier

Non-OR ØHRSX7Z

See Appendix I for Procedure Combinations
⊞ ØHR[T,U,V]37Z

Ø Medical and Surgical
H Skin and Breast
S Reposition Moving to its normal location or other suitable location all or a portion of a body part

Body Part Character 4	Approach Character 5	Device Character 6	Qualifier Character 7
S Hair W Nipple, Right X Nipple, Left	X External	Z No Device	Z No Qualifier
T Breast, Right U Breast, Left V Breast, Bilateral	Ø Open	Z No Device	Z No Qualifier

Non-OR ØHSSXZZ

Ø Medical and Surgical
H Skin and Breast
T Resection Cutting out or off, without replacement, all of a body part

Body Part Character 4	Approach Character 5	Device Character 6	Qualifier Character 7
Q Finger Nail R Toe Nail W Nipple, Right X Nipple, Left	X External	Z No Device	Z No Qualifier
T Breast, Right ⊞ U Breast, Left ⊞ V Breast, Bilateral ⊞ Y Supernumerary Breast	Ø Open	Z No Device	Z No Qualifier

Non-OR ØHT[Q,R]XZZ

See Appendix I for Procedure Combinations
⊞ ØHT[T,U,V]ØZZ

Ø Medical and Surgical
H Skin and Breast
U Supplement Putting in or on biological or synthetic material that physically reinforces and/or augments the function of a portion of a body part

Body Part Character 4	Approach Character 5	Device Character 6	Qualifier Character 7
T Breast, Right U Breast, Left V Breast, Bilateral W Nipple, Right X Nipple, Left	Ø Open 3 Percutaneous 7 Via Natural or Artificial Opening 8 Via Natural or Artificial Opening Endoscopic X External	7 Autologous Tissue Substitute J Synthetic Substitute K Nonautologous Tissue Substitute	Z No Qualifier

Ø Medical and Surgical
H Skin and Breast
W Revision Correcting, to the extent possible, a portion of a malfunctioning device or the position of a displaced device

Body Part Character 4	Approach Character 5	Device Character 6	Qualifier Character 7
P Skin Q Finger Nail R Toe Nail T Breast, Right U Breast, Left	X External	Ø Drainage Device 7 Autologous Tissue Substitute J Synthetic Substitute K Nonautologous Tissue Substitute	Z No Qualifier
S Hair	X External	7 Autologous Tissue Substitute J Synthetic Substitute K Nonautologous Tissue Substitute	Z No Qualifier
T Breast, Right U Breast, Left	Ø Open 3 Percutaneous 7 Via Natural or Artificial Opening 8 Via Natural or Artificial Opening Endoscopic	Ø Drainage Device 7 Autologous Tissue Substitute J Synthetic Substitute K Nonautologous Tissue Substitute N Tissue Expander	Z No Qualifier

Non-OR ØHW[P,Q,R,T,U]X[Ø,7,J,K]Z
Non-OR ØHWSX[7,J,K]Z
Non-OR ØHW[T,U][Ø,3][Ø,7,K,N]Z
Non-OR ØHW[T,U][7,8][Ø,7,J,K,N]Z

Ø Medical and Surgical
H Skin and Breast
X Transfer Moving, without taking out, all or a portion of a body part to another location to take over the function of all or a portion of a body part

Body Part Character 4	Approach Character 5	Device Character 6	Qualifier Character 7
Ø Skin, Scalp **1** Skin, Face **2** Skin, Right Ear **3** Skin, Left Ear **4** Skin, Neck **5** Skin, Chest **6** Skin, Back **7** Skin, Abdomen **8** Skin, Buttock **9** Skin, Perineum **A** Skin, Genitalia **B** Skin, Right Upper Arm **C** Skin, Left Upper Arm **D** Skin, Right Lower Arm **E** Skin, Left Lower Arm **F** Skin, Right Hand **G** Skin, Left Hand **H** Skin, Right Upper Leg **J** Skin, Left Upper Leg **K** Skin, Right Lower Leg **L** Skin, Left Lower Leg **M** Skin, Right Foot **N** Skin, Left Foot	**X** External	**Z** No Device	**Z** No Qualifier

Subcutaneous Tissue and Fascia 0J0–0JX

0 Medical and Surgical
J Subcutaneous Tissue and Fascia
0 Alteration Modifying the anatomic structure of a body part without affecting the function of the body part

Body Part Character 4	Approach Character 5	Device Character 6	Qualifier Character 7
1 Subcutaneous Tissue and Fascia, Face 4 Subcutaneous Tissue and Fascia, Anterior Neck 5 Subcutaneous Tissue and Fascia, Posterior Neck 6 Subcutaneous Tissue and Fascia, Chest 7 Subcutaneous Tissue and Fascia, Back 8 Subcutaneous Tissue and Fascia, Abdomen 9 Subcutaneous Tissue and Fascia, Buttock D Subcutaneous Tissue and Fascia, Right Upper Arm F Subcutaneous Tissue and Fascia, Left Upper Arm G Subcutaneous Tissue and Fascia, Right Lower Arm H Subcutaneous Tissue and Fascia, Left Lower Arm L Subcutaneous Tissue and Fascia, Right Upper Leg M Subcutaneous Tissue and Fascia, Left Upper Leg N Subcutaneous Tissue and Fascia, Right Lower Leg P Subcutaneous Tissue and Fascia, Left Lower Leg	0 Open 3 Percutaneous	Z No Device	Z No Qualifier

0 Medical and Surgical
J Subcutaneous Tissue and Fascia
2 Change Taking out or off a device from a body part and putting back an identical or similar device in or on the same body part without cutting or puncturing the skin or a mucous membrane

Body Part Character 4	Approach Character 5	Device Character 6	Qualifier Character 7
S Subcutaneous Tissue and Fascia, Head and Neck T Subcutaneous Tissue and Fascia, Trunk V Subcutaneous Tissue and Fascia, Upper Extremity W Subcutaneous Tissue and Fascia, Lower Extremity	X External	0 Drainage Device Y Other Device	Z No Qualifier

Non-OR For all body part, approach, device, and qualifier values

0 Medical and Surgical
J Subcutaneous Tissue and Fascia
5 Destruction Physical eradication of all or a portion of a body part by the direct use of energy, force, or a destructive agent

Body Part Character 4	Approach Character 5	Device Character 6	Qualifier Character 7
0 Subcutaneous Tissue and Fascia, Scalp 1 Subcutaneous Tissue and Fascia, Face 4 Subcutaneous Tissue and Fascia, Anterior Neck 5 Subcutaneous Tissue and Fascia, Posterior Neck 6 Subcutaneous Tissue and Fascia, Chest 7 Subcutaneous Tissue and Fascia, Back 8 Subcutaneous Tissue and Fascia, Abdomen 9 Subcutaneous Tissue and Fascia, Buttock B Subcutaneous Tissue and Fascia, Perineum C Subcutaneous Tissue and Fascia, Pelvic Region D Subcutaneous Tissue and Fascia, Right Upper Arm F Subcutaneous Tissue and Fascia, Left Upper Arm G Subcutaneous Tissue and Fascia, Right Lower Arm H Subcutaneous Tissue and Fascia, Left Lower Arm J Subcutaneous Tissue and Fascia, Right Hand K Subcutaneous Tissue and Fascia, Left Hand L Subcutaneous Tissue and Fascia, Right Upper Leg M Subcutaneous Tissue and Fascia, Left Upper Leg N Subcutaneous Tissue and Fascia, Right Lower Leg P Subcutaneous Tissue and Fascia, Left Lower Leg Q Subcutaneous Tissue and Fascia, Right Foot R Subcutaneous Tissue and Fascia, Left Foot	0 Open 3 Percutaneous	Z No Device	Z No Qualifier

DRG Non-OR For all body part, approach, device, and qualifier values

Ø Medical and Surgical
J Subcutaneous Tissue and Fascia
8 Division Cutting into a body part without draining fluids and/or gases from the body part in order to separate or transect a body part

Body Part Character 4	Approach Character 5	Device Character 6	Qualifier Character 7
Ø Subcutaneous Tissue and Fascia, Scalp 1 Subcutaneous Tissue and Fascia, Face 4 Subcutaneous Tissue and Fascia, Anterior Neck 5 Subcutaneous Tissue and Fascia, Posterior Neck 6 Subcutaneous Tissue and Fascia, Chest 7 Subcutaneous Tissue and Fascia, Back 8 Subcutaneous Tissue and Fascia, Abdomen 9 Subcutaneous Tissue and Fascia, Buttock B Subcutaneous Tissue and Fascia, Perineum C Subcutaneous Tissue and Fascia, Pelvic Region D Subcutaneous Tissue and Fascia, Right Upper Arm F Subcutaneous Tissue and Fascia, Left Upper Arm G Subcutaneous Tissue and Fascia, Right Lower Arm H Subcutaneous Tissue and Fascia, Left Lower Arm J Subcutaneous Tissue and Fascia, Right Hand K Subcutaneous Tissue and Fascia, Left Hand L Subcutaneous Tissue and Fascia, Right Upper Leg M Subcutaneous Tissue and Fascia, Left Upper Leg N Subcutaneous Tissue and Fascia, Right Lower Leg P Subcutaneous Tissue and Fascia, Left Lower Leg Q Subcutaneous Tissue and Fascia, Right Foot R Subcutaneous Tissue and Fascia, Left Foot S Subcutaneous Tissue and Fascia, Head and Neck T Subcutaneous Tissue and Fascia, Trunk V Subcutaneous Tissue and Fascia, Upper Extremity W Subcutaneous Tissue and Fascia, Lower Extremity	Ø Open 3 Percutaneous	Z No Device	Z No Qualifier

0 Medical and Surgical
J Subcutaneous Tissue and Fascia
9 Drainage Taking or letting out fluids and/or gases from a body part

Body Part Character 4	Approach Character 5	Device Character 6	Qualifier Character 7
0 Subcutaneous Tissue and Fascia, Scalp 1 Subcutaneous Tissue and Fascia, Face 4 Subcutaneous Tissue and Fascia, Anterior Neck 5 Subcutaneous Tissue and Fascia, Posterior Neck 6 Subcutaneous Tissue and Fascia, Chest 7 Subcutaneous Tissue and Fascia, Back 8 Subcutaneous Tissue and Fascia, Abdomen 9 Subcutaneous Tissue and Fascia, Buttock B Subcutaneous Tissue and Fascia, Perineum C Subcutaneous Tissue and Fascia, Pelvic Region D Subcutaneous Tissue and Fascia, Right Upper Arm F Subcutaneous Tissue and Fascia, Left Upper Arm G Subcutaneous Tissue and Fascia, Right Lower Arm H Subcutaneous Tissue and Fascia, Left Lower Arm J Subcutaneous Tissue and Fascia, Right Hand K Subcutaneous Tissue and Fascia, Left Hand L Subcutaneous Tissue and Fascia, Right Upper Leg M Subcutaneous Tissue and Fascia, Left Upper Leg N Subcutaneous Tissue and Fascia, Right Lower Leg P Subcutaneous Tissue and Fascia, Left Lower Leg Q Subcutaneous Tissue and Fascia, Right Foot R Subcutaneous Tissue and Fascia, Left Foot	0 Open 3 Percutaneous	0 Drainage Device	Z No Qualifier
0 Subcutaneous Tissue and Fascia, Scalp 1 Subcutaneous Tissue and Fascia, Face 4 Subcutaneous Tissue and Fascia, Anterior Neck 5 Subcutaneous Tissue and Fascia, Posterior Neck 6 Subcutaneous Tissue and Fascia, Chest 7 Subcutaneous Tissue and Fascia, Back 8 Subcutaneous Tissue and Fascia, Abdomen 9 Subcutaneous Tissue and Fascia, Buttock B Subcutaneous Tissue and Fascia, Perineum C Subcutaneous Tissue and Fascia, Pelvic Region D Subcutaneous Tissue and Fascia, Right Upper Arm F Subcutaneous Tissue and Fascia, Left Upper Arm G Subcutaneous Tissue and Fascia, Right Lower Arm H Subcutaneous Tissue and Fascia, Left Lower Arm J Subcutaneous Tissue and Fascia, Right Hand K Subcutaneous Tissue and Fascia, Left Hand L Subcutaneous Tissue and Fascia, Right Upper Leg M Subcutaneous Tissue and Fascia, Left Upper Leg N Subcutaneous Tissue and Fascia, Right Lower Leg P Subcutaneous Tissue and Fascia, Left Lower Leg Q Subcutaneous Tissue and Fascia, Right Foot R Subcutaneous Tissue and Fascia, Left Foot	0 Open 3 Percutaneous	Z No Device	X Diagnostic Z No Qualifier

DRG Non-OR 0J9[J,K]3ZZ
Non-OR 0J9[0,4,5,6,7,8,9,B,C,D,F,G,H,L,M,N,P,Q,R][0,3]0Z
Non-OR 0J9[0,1,4,5,6,7,8,9,B,C,D,F,G,H,J,K,L,M,N,P,Q,R][0,3]ZX
Non-OR 0J9[0,1,4,5,6,7,8,9,B,C,D,F,G,H,L,M,N,P,Q,R]3ZZ

Ø Medical and Surgical
J Subcutaneous Tissue and Fascia
B Excision Cutting out or off, without replacement, a portion of a body part

Body Part Character 4	Approach Character 5	Device Character 6	Qualifier Character 7
Ø Subcutaneous Tissue and Fascia, Scalp 1 Subcutaneous Tissue and Fascia, Face 4 Subcutaneous Tissue and Fascia, Anterior Neck 5 Subcutaneous Tissue and Fascia, Posterior Neck 6 Subcutaneous Tissue and Fascia, Chest 7 Subcutaneous Tissue and Fascia, Back 8 Subcutaneous Tissue and Fascia, Abdomen 9 Subcutaneous Tissue and Fascia, Buttock B Subcutaneous Tissue and Fascia, Perineum C Subcutaneous Tissue and Fascia, Pelvic Region D Subcutaneous Tissue and Fascia, Right Upper Arm F Subcutaneous Tissue and Fascia, Left Upper Arm G Subcutaneous Tissue and Fascia, Right Lower Arm H Subcutaneous Tissue and Fascia, Left Lower Arm J Subcutaneous Tissue and Fascia, Right Hand K Subcutaneous Tissue and Fascia, Left Hand L Subcutaneous Tissue and Fascia, Right Upper Leg ⊞ M Subcutaneous Tissue and Fascia, Left Upper Leg ⊞ N Subcutaneous Tissue and Fascia, Right Lower Leg P Subcutaneous Tissue and Fascia, Left Lower Leg Q Subcutaneous Tissue and Fascia, Right Foot R Subcutaneous Tissue and Fascia, Left Foot	Ø Open 3 Percutaneous	Z No Device	X Diagnostic Z No Qualifier

Non-OR ØJB[Ø,1,4,5,6,7,8,9,B,C,D,F,G,H,J,K,L,M,N,P,Q,R][Ø,3]ZX
Non-OR ØJB[Ø,4,5,6,7,8,9,B,C,D,F,G,H,L,M,N,P,Q,R]3ZZ

No Procedure Combinations Specified
⊞ ØJB[L,M]ØZZ

Ø Medical and Surgical
J Subcutaneous Tissue and Fascia
C Extirpation Taking or cutting out solid matter from a body part

Body Part Character 4	Approach Character 5	Device Character 6	Qualifier Character 7
Ø Subcutaneous Tissue and Fascia, Scalp 1 Subcutaneous Tissue and Fascia, Face 4 Subcutaneous Tissue and Fascia, Anterior Neck 5 Subcutaneous Tissue and Fascia, Posterior Neck 6 Subcutaneous Tissue and Fascia, Chest 7 Subcutaneous Tissue and Fascia, Back 8 Subcutaneous Tissue and Fascia, Abdomen 9 Subcutaneous Tissue and Fascia, Buttock B Subcutaneous Tissue and Fascia, Perineum C Subcutaneous Tissue and Fascia, Pelvic Region D Subcutaneous Tissue and Fascia, Right Upper Arm F Subcutaneous Tissue and Fascia, Left Upper Arm G Subcutaneous Tissue and Fascia, Right Lower Arm H Subcutaneous Tissue and Fascia, Left Lower Arm J Subcutaneous Tissue and Fascia, Right Hand K Subcutaneous Tissue and Fascia, Left Hand L Subcutaneous Tissue and Fascia, Right Upper Leg M Subcutaneous Tissue and Fascia, Left Upper Leg N Subcutaneous Tissue and Fascia, Right Lower Leg P Subcutaneous Tissue and Fascia, Left Lower Leg Q Subcutaneous Tissue and Fascia, Right Foot R Subcutaneous Tissue and Fascia, Left Foot	Ø Open 3 Percutaneous	Z No Device	Z No Qualifier

Non-OR For all body part, approach, device, and qualifier values

Ø Medical and Surgical
J Subcutaneous Tissue and Fascia
D Extraction Pulling or stripping out or off all or a portion of a body part by the use of force

Body Part Character 4	Approach Character 5	Device Character 6	Qualifier Character 7
Ø Subcutaneous Tissue and Fascia, Scalp 1 Subcutaneous Tissue and Fascia, Face 4 Subcutaneous Tissue and Fascia, Anterior Neck 5 Subcutaneous Tissue and Fascia, Posterior Neck 6 Subcutaneous Tissue and Fascia, Chest ⊞ 7 Subcutaneous Tissue and Fascia, Back ⊞ 8 Subcutaneous Tissue and Fascia, Abdomen ⊞ 9 Subcutaneous Tissue and Fascia, Buttock ⊞ B Subcutaneous Tissue and Fascia, Perineum C Subcutaneous Tissue and Fascia, Pelvic Region D Subcutaneous Tissue and Fascia, Right Upper Arm F Subcutaneous Tissue and Fascia, Left Upper Arm G Subcutaneous Tissue and Fascia, Right Lower Arm H Subcutaneous Tissue and Fascia, Left Lower Arm J Subcutaneous Tissue and Fascia, Right Hand K Subcutaneous Tissue and Fascia, Left Hand L Subcutaneous Tissue and Fascia, Right Upper Leg ⊞ M Subcutaneous Tissue and Fascia, Left Upper Leg ⊞ N Subcutaneous Tissue and Fascia, Right Lower Leg P Subcutaneous Tissue and Fascia, Left Lower Leg Q Subcutaneous Tissue and Fascia, Right Foot R Subcutaneous Tissue and Fascia, Left Foot	Ø Open 3 Percutaneous	Z No Device	Z No Qualifier

See Appendix I for Procedure Combinations
⊞ ØJD[6,7,8,9,L,M]3ZZ

Ø Medical and Surgical
J Subcutaneous Tissue and Fascia
H Insertion Putting in a nonbiological appliance that monitors, assists, performs, or prevents a physiological function but does not physically take the place of a body part

Body Part Character 4	Approach Character 5	Device Character 6	Qualifier Character 7
Ø Subcutaneous Tissue and Fascia, Scalp 1 Subcutaneous Tissue and Fascia, Face 4 Subcutaneous Tissue and Fascia, Anterior Neck 5 Subcutaneous Tissue and Fascia, Posterior Neck 9 Subcutaneous Tissue and Fascia, Buttock B Subcutaneous Tissue and Fascia, Perineum C Subcutaneous Tissue and Fascia, Pelvic Region J Subcutaneous Tissue and Fascia, Right Hand K Subcutaneous Tissue and Fascia, Left Hand Q Subcutaneous Tissue and Fascia, Right Foot R Subcutaneous Tissue and Fascia, Left Foot	Ø Open 3 Percutaneous	N Tissue Expander	Z No Qualifier

ØJH Continued on next page

Ø Medical and Surgical
J Subcutaneous Tissue and Fascia
H Insertion Putting in a nonbiological appliance that monitors, assists, performs, or prevents a physiological function but does not physically take the place of a body part

ØJH Continued

Body Part Character 4	Approach Character 5	Device Character 6	Qualifier Character 7
6 Subcutaneous Tissue and Fascia, Chest ⊞ **8** Subcutaneous Tissue and Fascia, Abdomen ⊞ NC	**Ø** Open **3** Percutaneous	**Ø** Monitoring Device, Hemodynamic **2** Monitoring Device **4** Pacemaker, Single Chamber **5** Pacemaker, Single Chamber Rate Responsive **6** Pacemaker, Dual Chamber **7** Cardiac Resynchronization Pacemaker Pulse Generator **8** Defibrillator Generator **9** Cardiac Resynchronization Defibrillator Pulse Generator **A** Contractility Modulation Device **B** Stimulator Generator, Single Array **C** Stimulator Generator, Single Array Rechargeable **D** Stimulator Generator, Multiple Array **E** Stimulator Generator, Multiple Array Rechargeable **H** Contraceptive Device **M** Stimulator Generator **N** Tissue Expander **P** Cardiac Rhythm Related Device **V** Infusion Device, Pump **W** Vascular Access Device, Reservoir **X** Vascular Access Device	**Z** No Qualifier
7 Subcutaneous Tissue and Fascia, Back ⊞ NC	**Ø** Open **3** Percutaneous	**B** Stimulator Generator, Single Array **C** Stimulator Generator, Single Array Rechargeable **D** Stimulator Generator, Multiple Array **E** Stimulator Generator, Multiple Array Rechargeable **M** Stimulator Generator **N** Tissue Expander **V** Infusion Device, Pump	**Z** No Qualifier
D Subcutaneous Tissue and Fascia, Right Upper Arm **F** Subcutaneous Tissue and Fascia, Left Upper Arm **G** Subcutaneous Tissue and Fascia, Right Lower Arm **H** Subcutaneous Tissue and Fascia, Left Lower Arm **L** Subcutaneous Tissue and Fascia, Right Upper Leg **M** Subcutaneous Tissue and Fascia, Left Upper Leg **N** Subcutaneous Tissue and Fascia, Right Lower Leg **P** Subcutaneous Tissue and Fascia, Left Lower Leg	**Ø** Open **3** Percutaneous	**H** Contraceptive Device **N** Tissue Expander **V** Infusion Pump **W** Reservoir **X** Vascular Access Device	**Z** No Qualifier
S Subcutaneous Tissue and Fascia, Head and Neck **V** Subcutaneous Tissue and Fascia, Upper Extremity **W** Subcutaneous Tissue and Fascia, Lower Extremity	**Ø** Open **3** Percutaneous	**1** Radioactive Element **3** Infusion Device	**Z** No Qualifier
T Subcutaneous Tissue and Fascia, Trunk	**Ø** Open **3** Percutaneous	**1** Radioactive Element **3** Infusion Device **V** Infusion Pump	**Z** No Qualifier

DRG Non-OR ØJH[6,8][Ø,3][2,4,5,6,H,W,X]Z
DRG Non-OR ØJH[D,F,G,H,L,M][Ø,3][W,X]
DRG Non-OR ØJHNØ[W,X]Z
DRG Non-OR ØJHN3[H,W,X]Z
DRG Non-OR ØJHP[Ø,3][H,W,X]Z
Non-OR ØJH[D,F,G,H,L,M][Ø,3][H,V]Z
Non-OR ØJHNØ[H,V]Z
Non-OR ØJHN3VZ
Non-OR ØJHP[Ø,3]VZ
Non-OR ØJH[S,V,W][Ø,3]3Z
Non-OR ØJHT[Ø,3]3Z

HAC ØJH[6,8][Ø,3][4,5,6,7,8,9,P]Z when reported with SDx K68.11 or T81.4XXA or T82.6XXA or T82.7XXA
HAC ØJH63XZ when reported with SDx J95.811
NC ØJH8[Ø,3]MZ
NC ØJH7[Ø,3]MZ

AHA: 2Ø13, 4Q, 116; 2Ø12, 4Q, 1Ø4

See Appendix I for Procedure Combinations

Combo-only ØJH[6,8][Ø,3][4,5,6]Z
⊞ ØJH[6,8][Ø,3][Ø,4,5,6,7,8,9,A,B,C,D,E,M,P]Z
⊞ ØJH7[Ø,3][B,C,D,E,M]Z

LC Limited Coverage NC Noncovered ⊞ Combination Member HAC associated procedure Combination Only DRG Non-OR Non-OR Revised Text in **GREEN**

Ø Medical and Surgical
J Subcutaneous Tissue and Fascia
J Inspection Visually and/or manually exploring a body part

Body Part Character 4	Approach Character 5	Device Character 6	Qualifier Character 7
S Subcutaneous Tissue and Fascia, Head and Neck **T** Subcutaneous Tissue and Fascia, Trunk **V** Subcutaneous Tissue and Fascia, Upper Extremity **W** Subcutaneous Tissue and Fascia, Lower Extremity	**Ø** Open **3** Percutaneous **X** External	**Z** No Device	**Z** No Qualifier

Non-OR For all body part, approach, device, and qualifier values

Ø Medical and Surgical
J Subcutaneous Tissue and Fascia
N Release Freeing a body part from an abnormal physical constraint

Body Part Character 4	Approach Character 5	Device Character 6	Qualifier Character 7
Ø Subcutaneous Tissue and Fascia, Scalp **1** Subcutaneous Tissue and Fascia, Face **4** Subcutaneous Tissue and Fascia, Anterior Neck **5** Subcutaneous Tissue and Fascia, Posterior Neck **6** Subcutaneous Tissue and Fascia, Chest **7** Subcutaneous Tissue and Fascia, Back **8** Subcutaneous Tissue and Fascia, Abdomen **9** Subcutaneous Tissue and Fascia, Buttock **B** Subcutaneous Tissue and Fascia, Perineum **C** Subcutaneous Tissue and Fascia, Pelvic Region **D** Subcutaneous Tissue and Fascia, Right Upper Arm **F** Subcutaneous Tissue and Fascia, Left Upper Arm **G** Subcutaneous Tissue and Fascia, Right Lower Arm **H** Subcutaneous Tissue and Fascia, Left Lower Arm **J** Subcutaneous Tissue and Fascia, Right Hand **K** Subcutaneous Tissue and Fascia, Left Hand **L** Subcutaneous Tissue and Fascia, Right Upper Leg **M** Subcutaneous Tissue and Fascia, Left Upper Leg **N** Subcutaneous Tissue and Fascia, Right Lower Leg **P** Subcutaneous Tissue and Fascia, Left Lower Leg **Q** Subcutaneous Tissue and Fascia, Right Foot **R** Subcutaneous Tissue and Fascia, Left Foot	**Ø** Open **3** Percutaneous **X** External	**Z** No Device	**Z** No Qualifier

Non-OR ØJN[Ø,1,4,5,6,7,8,9,B,C,D,F,G,H,J,K,L,M,N,P,Q,R]XZZ

Ø Medical and Surgical
J Subcutaneous Tissue and Fascia
P Removal Taking out or off a device from a body part

Body Part Character 4	Approach Character 5	Device Character 6	Qualifier Character 7
S Subcutaneous Tissue and Fascia, Head and Neck	**Ø** Open **3** Percutaneous	**Ø** Drainage Device **1** Radioactive Element **3** Infusion Device **7** Autologous Tissue Substitute **J** Synthetic Substitute **K** Nonautologous Tissue Substitute **N** Tissue Expander	**Z** No Qualifier
S Subcutaneous Tissue and Fascia, Head and Neck	**X** External	**Ø** Drainage Device **1** Radioactive Element **3** Infusion Device	**Z** No Qualifier
T Subcutaneous Tissue and Fascia, Trunk ⊞	**Ø** Open **3** Percutaneous	**Ø** Drainage Device **1** Radioactive Element **2** Monitoring Device **3** Infusion Device **7** Autologous Tissue Substitute **H** Contraceptive Device **J** Synthetic Substitute **K** Nonautologous Tissue Substitute **M** Stimulator Generator **N** Tissue Expander **P** Cardiac Rhythm Related Device **V** Infusion Pump **W** Reservoir **X** Vascular Access Device	**Z** No Qualifier
T Subcutaneous Tissue and Fascia, Trunk	**X** External	**Ø** Drainage Device **1** Radioactive Element **2** Monitoring Device **3** Infusion Device **H** Contraceptive Device **V** Infusion Pump **X** Vascular Access Device	**Z** No Qualifier
V Subcutaneous Tissue and Fascia, Upper Extremity **W** Subcutaneous Tissue and Fascia, Lower Extremity	**Ø** Open **3** Percutaneous	**Ø** Drainage Device **1** Radioactive Element **3** Infusion Device **7** Autologous Tissue Substitute **H** Contraceptive Device **J** Synthetic Substitute **K** Nonautologous Tissue Substitute **N** Tissue Expander **V** Infusion Pump **W** Reservoir **X** Vascular Access Device	**Z** No Qualifier
V Subcutaneous Tissue and Fascia, Upper Extremity **W** Subcutaneous Tissue and Fascia, Lower Extremity	**X** External	**Ø** Drainage Device **1** Radioactive Element **3** Infusion Device **H** Contraceptive Device **V** Infusion Pump **X** Vascular Access Device	**Z** No Qualifier

Non-OR ØJPS[Ø,3][Ø,1,3,7,J,K,N]Z
Non-OR ØJPSX[Ø,1,3]Z
Non-OR ØJPT[Ø,3][Ø,1,2,3,7,H,J,K,M,N,V,W,X]Z
Non-OR ØJPTX[Ø,1,2,3,H,V,X]Z
Non-OR ØJP[V,W][Ø,3][Ø,1,3,7,H,J,K,N,V,W,X]Z
Non-OR ØJP[V,W]X[Ø,1,3,H,V,X]Z
HAC ØJPT[Ø,3]PZ when reported with SDx K68.11 or T81.4XXA or T82.6XXA or T82.7XXA

AHA: 2Ø13, 4Q, 1Ø9; 2Ø12, 4Q, 1Ø4

See Appendix I for Procedure Combinations
⊞ ØJPT[Ø,3]PZ

0 Medical and Surgical
J Subcutaneous Tissue and Fascia
Q Repair Restoring, to the extent possible, a body part to its normal anatomic structure and function

Body Part Character 4	Approach Character 5	Device Character 6	Qualifier Character 7
0 Subcutaneous Tissue and Fascia, Scalp 1 Subcutaneous Tissue and Fascia, Face 4 Subcutaneous Tissue and Fascia, Anterior Neck 5 Subcutaneous Tissue and Fascia, Posterior Neck 6 Subcutaneous Tissue and Fascia, Chest 7 Subcutaneous Tissue and Fascia, Back 8 Subcutaneous Tissue and Fascia, Abdomen 9 Subcutaneous Tissue and Fascia, Buttock B Subcutaneous Tissue and Fascia, Perineum C Subcutaneous Tissue and Fascia, Pelvic Region D Subcutaneous Tissue and Fascia, Right Upper Arm F Subcutaneous Tissue and Fascia, Left Upper Arm G Subcutaneous Tissue and Fascia, Right Lower Arm H Subcutaneous Tissue and Fascia, Left Lower Arm J Subcutaneous Tissue and Fascia, Right Hand K Subcutaneous Tissue and Fascia, Left Hand L Subcutaneous Tissue and Fascia, Right Upper Leg M Subcutaneous Tissue and Fascia, Left Upper Leg N Subcutaneous Tissue and Fascia, Right Lower Leg P Subcutaneous Tissue and Fascia, Left Lower Leg Q Subcutaneous Tissue and Fascia, Right Foot R Subcutaneous Tissue and Fascia, Left Foot	0 Open 3 Percutaneous	Z No Device	Z No Qualifier

0 Medical and Surgical
J Subcutaneous Tissue and Fascia
R Replacement Putting in or on biological or synthetic material that physically takes the place and/or function of all or a portion of a body part

Body Part Character 4	Approach Character 5	Device Character 6	Qualifier Character 7
0 Subcutaneous Tissue and Fascia, Scalp 1 Subcutaneous Tissue and Fascia, Face 4 Subcutaneous Tissue and Fascia, Anterior Neck 5 Subcutaneous Tissue and Fascia, Posterior Neck 6 Subcutaneous Tissue and Fascia, Chest 7 Subcutaneous Tissue and Fascia, Back 8 Subcutaneous Tissue and Fascia, Abdomen 9 Subcutaneous Tissue and Fascia, Buttock B Subcutaneous Tissue and Fascia, Perineum C Subcutaneous Tissue and Fascia, Pelvic Region D Subcutaneous Tissue and Fascia, Right Upper Arm F Subcutaneous Tissue and Fascia, Left Upper Arm G Subcutaneous Tissue and Fascia, Right Lower Arm H Subcutaneous Tissue and Fascia, Left Lower Arm J Subcutaneous Tissue and Fascia, Right Hand K Subcutaneous Tissue and Fascia, Left Hand L Subcutaneous Tissue and Fascia, Right Upper Leg M Subcutaneous Tissue and Fascia, Left Upper Leg N Subcutaneous Tissue and Fascia, Right Lower Leg P Subcutaneous Tissue and Fascia, Left Lower Leg Q Subcutaneous Tissue and Fascia, Right Foot R Subcutaneous Tissue and Fascia, Left Foot	0 Open 3 Percutaneous	7 Autologous Tissue Substitute J Synthetic Substitute K Nonautologous Tissue Substitute	Z No Qualifier

Ø Medical and Surgical
J Subcutaneous Tissue and Fascia
U Supplement: Putting in or on biological or synthetic material that physically reinforces and/or augments the function of a portion of a body part

Body Part Character 4	Approach Character 5	Device Character 6	Qualifier Character 7
Ø Subcutaneous Tissue and Fascia, Scalp 1 Subcutaneous Tissue and Fascia, Face 4 Subcutaneous Tissue and Fascia, Anterior Neck 5 Subcutaneous Tissue and Fascia, Posterior Neck 6 Subcutaneous Tissue and Fascia, Chest 7 Subcutaneous Tissue and Fascia, Back 8 Subcutaneous Tissue and Fascia, Abdomen 9 Subcutaneous Tissue and Fascia, Buttock B Subcutaneous Tissue and Fascia, Perineum C Subcutaneous Tissue and Fascia, Pelvic Region D Subcutaneous Tissue and Fascia, Right Upper Arm F Subcutaneous Tissue and Fascia, Left Upper Arm G Subcutaneous Tissue and Fascia, Right Lower Arm H Subcutaneous Tissue and Fascia, Left Lower Arm J Subcutaneous Tissue and Fascia, Right Hand K Subcutaneous Tissue and Fascia, Left Hand L Subcutaneous Tissue and Fascia, Right Upper Leg M Subcutaneous Tissue and Fascia, Left Upper Leg N Subcutaneous Tissue and Fascia, Right Lower Leg P Subcutaneous Tissue and Fascia, Left Lower Leg Q Subcutaneous Tissue and Fascia, Right Foot R Subcutaneous Tissue and Fascia, Left Foot	Ø Open 3 Percutaneous	7 Autologous Tissue Substitute J Synthetic Substitute K Nonautologous Tissue Substitute	Z No Qualifier

Ø Medical and Surgical
J Subcutaneous Tissue and Fascia
W Revision Correcting, to the extent possible, a portion of a malfunctioning device or the position of a displaced device

Body Part Character 4	Approach Character 5	Device Character 6	Qualifier Character 7
S Subcutaneous Tissue and Fascia, Head and Neck	Ø Open 3 Percutaneous X External	Ø Drainage Device 3 Infusion Device 7 Autologous Tissue Substitute J Synthetic Substitute K Nonautologous Tissue Substitute N Tissue Expander	Z No Qualifier
T Subcutaneous Tissue and Fascia, Trunk	Ø Open 3 Percutaneous X External	Ø Drainage Device 2 Monitoring Device 3 Infusion Device 7 Autologous Tissue Substitute H Contraceptive Device J Synthetic Substitute K Nonautologous Tissue Substitute M Stimulator Generator N Tissue Expander P Cardiac Rhythm Related Device V Infusion Pump W Reservoir X Vascular Access Device	Z No Qualifier
V Subcutaneous Tissue and Fascia, Upper Extremity W Subcutaneous Tissue and Fascia, Lower Extremity	Ø Open 3 Percutaneous X External	Ø Drainage Device 3 Infusion Device 7 Autologous Tissue Substitute H Contraceptive Device J Synthetic Substitute K Nonautologous Tissue Substitute N Tissue Expander V Infusion Pump W Reservoir X Vascular Access Device	Z No Qualifier

DRG Non-OR ØJWS[Ø,3][Ø,3,7,J,K,N]Z
DRG Non-OR ØJWT[Ø,3][Ø,2,3,7,H,J,K,N,V,W,X]Z
DRG Non-OR ØJW[V,W][Ø,3][Ø,3,7,H,J,K,N,V,W,X]Z
Non-OR ØJWSX[Ø,3,7,J,K,N]Z
Non-OR ØJWTX[Ø,2,3,7,H,J,K,N,P,V,W,X]Z
Non-OR ØJW[V,W]X[Ø,3,7,H,J,K,N,V,W,X]Z
HAC ØJWT[Ø,3]PZ when reported with SDx K68.11 or T81.4XXA or T82.6XXA or T82.7XXA

AHA: 2Ø12, 4Q, 1Ø4

0 Medical and Surgical
J Subcutaneous Tissue and Fascia
X Transfer Moving, without taking out, all or a portion of a body part to another location to take over the function of all or a portion of a body part

Body Part Character 4	Approach Character 5	Device Character 6	Qualifier Character 7
0 Subcutaneous Tissue and Fascia, Scalp 1 Subcutaneous Tissue and Fascia, Face 4 Subcutaneous Tissue and Fascia, Anterior Neck 5 Subcutaneous Tissue and Fascia, Posterior Neck 6 Subcutaneous Tissue and Fascia, Chest 7 Subcutaneous Tissue and Fascia, Back 8 Subcutaneous Tissue and Fascia, Abdomen 9 Subcutaneous Tissue and Fascia, Buttock B Subcutaneous Tissue and Fascia, Perineum C Subcutaneous Tissue and Fascia, Pelvic Region D Subcutaneous Tissue and Fascia, Right Upper Arm F Subcutaneous Tissue and Fascia, Left Upper Arm G Subcutaneous Tissue and Fascia, Right Lower Arm H Subcutaneous Tissue and Fascia, Left Lower Arm J Subcutaneous Tissue and Fascia, Right Hand K Subcutaneous Tissue and Fascia, Left Hand L Subcutaneous Tissue and Fascia, Right Upper Leg M Subcutaneous Tissue and Fascia, Left Upper Leg N Subcutaneous Tissue and Fascia, Right Lower Leg P Subcutaneous Tissue and Fascia, Left Lower Leg Q Subcutaneous Tissue and Fascia, Right Foot R Subcutaneous Tissue and Fascia, Left Foot	0 Open 3 Percutaneous	Z No Device	B Skin and Subcutaneous Tissue C Skin, Subcutaneous Tissue and Fascia Z No Qualifier

AHA: 2013, 4Q, 109

Muscles ØK2–ØKX

Ø Medical and Surgical
K Muscles
2 Change Taking out or off a device from a body part and putting back an identical or similar device in or on the same body part without cutting or puncturing the skin or a mucous membrane

Body Part Character 4	Approach Character 5	Device Character 6	Qualifier Character 7
X Upper Muscle Y Lower Muscle	X External	Ø Drainage Device Y Other Device	Z No Qualifier

Non-OR For all body part, approach, device, and qualifier values

Ø Medical and Surgical
K Muscles
5 Destruction Physical eradication of all or a portion of a body part by the direct use of energy, force, or a destructive agent

Body Part Character 4	Approach Character 5	Device Character 6	Qualifier Character 7
Ø Head Muscle 1 Facial Muscle 2 Neck Muscle, Right 3 Neck Muscle, Left 4 Tongue, Palate, Pharynx Muscle 5 Shoulder Muscle, Right 6 Shoulder Muscle, Left 7 Upper Arm Muscle, Right 8 Upper Arm Muscle, Left 9 Lower Arm and Wrist Muscle, Right B Lower Arm and Wrist Muscle, Left C Hand Muscle, Right D Hand Muscle, Left F Trunk Muscle, Right G Trunk Muscle, Left H Thorax Muscle, Right J Thorax Muscle, Left K Abdomen Muscle, Right L Abdomen Muscle, Left M Perineum Muscle N Hip Muscle, Right P Hip Muscle, Left Q Upper Leg Muscle, Right R Upper Leg Muscle, Left S Lower Leg Muscle, Right T Lower Leg Muscle, Left V Foot Muscle, Right W Foot Muscle, Left	Ø Open 3 Percutaneous 4 Percutaneous Endoscopic	Z No Device	Z No Qualifier

Ø Medical and Surgical
K Muscles
8 Division Cutting into a body part without draining fluids and/or gases from the body part in order to separate or transect a body part

Body Part Character 4	Approach Character 5	Device Character 6	Qualifier Character 7
Ø Head Muscle 1 Facial Muscle 2 Neck Muscle, Right 3 Neck Muscle, Left 4 Tongue, Palate, Pharynx Muscle 5 Shoulder Muscle, Right 6 Shoulder Muscle, Left 7 Upper Arm Muscle, Right 8 Upper Arm Muscle, Left 9 Lower Arm and Wrist Muscle, Right B Lower Arm and Wrist Muscle, Left C Hand Muscle, Right D Hand Muscle, Left F Trunk Muscle, Right G Trunk Muscle, Left H Thorax Muscle, Right J Thorax Muscle, Left K Abdomen Muscle, Right L Abdomen Muscle, Left M Perineum Muscle N Hip Muscle, Right P Hip Muscle, Left Q Upper Leg Muscle, Right R Upper Leg Muscle, Left S Lower Leg Muscle, Right T Lower Leg Muscle, Left V Foot Muscle, Right W Foot Muscle, Left	Ø Open 3 Percutaneous 4 Percutaneous Endoscopic	Z No Device	Z No Qualifier

Ø Medical and Surgical
K Muscles
9 Drainage Taking or letting out fluids and/or gases from a body part

Body Part Character 4	Approach Character 5	Device Character 6	Qualifier Character 7
Ø Head Muscle 1 Facial Muscle 2 Neck Muscle, Right 3 Neck Muscle, Left 4 Tongue, Palate, Pharynx Muscle 5 Shoulder Muscle, Right 6 Shoulder Muscle, Left 7 Upper Arm Muscle, Right 8 Upper Arm Muscle, Left 9 Lower Arm and Wrist Muscle, Right B Lower Arm and Wrist Muscle, Left C Hand Muscle, Right D Hand Muscle, Left F Trunk Muscle, Right G Trunk Muscle, Left H Thorax Muscle, Right J Thorax Muscle, Left K Abdomen Muscle, Right L Abdomen Muscle, Left M Perineum Muscle N Hip Muscle, Right P Hip Muscle, Left Q Upper Leg Muscle, Right R Upper Leg Muscle, Left S Lower Leg Muscle, Right T Lower Leg Muscle, Left V Foot Muscle, Right W Foot Muscle, Left	Ø Open 3 Percutaneous 4 Percutaneous Endoscopic	Ø Drainage Device	Z No Qualifier

ØK9 Continued on next page

Ø Medical and Surgical
K Muscles
9 Drainage Taking or letting out fluids and/or gases from a body part

ØK9 Continued

Body Part Character 4	Approach Character 5	Device Character 6	Qualifier Character 7
Ø Head Muscle **1** Facial Muscle **2** Neck Muscle, Right **3** Neck Muscle, Left **4** Tongue, Palate, Pharynx Muscle **5** Shoulder Muscle, Right **6** Shoulder Muscle, Left **7** Upper Arm Muscle, Right **8** Upper Arm Muscle, Left **9** Lower Arm and Wrist Muscle, Right **B** Lower Arm and Wrist Muscle, Left **C** Hand Muscle, Right **D** Hand Muscle, Left **F** Trunk Muscle, Right **G** Trunk Muscle, Left **H** Thorax Muscle, Right **J** Thorax Muscle, Left **K** Abdomen Muscle, Right **L** Abdomen Muscle, Left **M** Perineum Muscle **N** Hip Muscle, Right **P** Hip Muscle, Left **Q** Upper Leg Muscle, Right **R** Upper Leg Muscle, Left **S** Lower Leg Muscle, Right **T** Lower Leg Muscle, Left **V** Foot Muscle, Right **W** Foot Muscle, Left	**Ø** Open **3** Percutaneous **4** Percutaneous Endoscopic	**Z** No Device	**X** Diagnostic **Z** No Qualifier

Non-OR ØK9[Ø,1,2,3,4,5,6,7,8,9,B,F,G,H,J,K,L,M,N,P,Q,R,S,T,V,W]3ZZ
Non-OR ØK9[C,D][3,4]ZZ

Ø Medical and Surgical
K Muscles
B Excision Cutting out or off, without replacement, a portion of a body part

Body Part Character 4	Approach Character 5	Device Character 6	Qualifier Character 7
Ø Head Muscle **1** Facial Muscle **2** Neck Muscle, Right **3** Neck Muscle, Left **4** Tongue, Palate, Pharynx Muscle **5** Shoulder Muscle, Right **6** Shoulder Muscle, Left **7** Upper Arm Muscle, Right **8** Upper Arm Muscle, Left **9** Lower Arm and Wrist Muscle, Right **B** Lower Arm and Wrist Muscle, Left **C** Hand Muscle, Right **D** Hand Muscle, Left **F** Trunk Muscle, Right **G** Trunk Muscle, Left **H** Thorax Muscle, Right **J** Thorax Muscle, Left **K** Abdomen Muscle, Right **L** Abdomen Muscle, Left **M** Perineum Muscle **N** Hip Muscle, Right **P** Hip Muscle, Left **Q** Upper Leg Muscle, Right **R** Upper Leg Muscle, Left **S** Lower Leg Muscle, Right **T** Lower Leg Muscle, Left **V** Foot Muscle, Right **W** Foot Muscle, Left	**Ø** Open **3** Percutaneous **4** Percutaneous Endoscopic	**Z** No Device	**X** Diagnostic **Z** No Qualifier

Ø Medical and Surgical
K Muscles
C Extirpation Taking or cutting out solid matter from a body part

Body Part Character 4	Approach Character 5	Device Character 6	Qualifier Character 7
Ø Head Muscle **1** Facial Muscle **2** Neck Muscle, Right **3** Neck Muscle, Left **4** Tongue, Palate, Pharynx Muscle **5** Shoulder Muscle, Right **6** Shoulder Muscle, Left **7** Upper Arm Muscle, Right **8** Upper Arm Muscle, Left **9** Lower Arm and Wrist Muscle, Right **B** Lower Arm and Wrist Muscle, Left **C** Hand Muscle, Right **D** Hand Muscle, Left **F** Trunk Muscle, Right **G** Trunk Muscle, Left **H** Thorax Muscle, Right **J** Thorax Muscle, Left **K** Abdomen Muscle, Right **L** Abdomen Muscle, Left **M** Perineum Muscle **N** Hip Muscle, Right **P** Hip Muscle, Left **Q** Upper Leg Muscle, Right **R** Upper Leg Muscle, Left **S** Lower Leg Muscle, Right **T** Lower Leg Muscle, Left **V** Foot Muscle, Right **W** Foot Muscle, Left	**Ø** Open **3** Percutaneous **4** Percutaneous Endoscopic	**Z** No Device	**Z** No Qualifier

Ø Medical and Surgical
K Muscles
H Insertion Putting in a nonbiological appliance that monitors, assists, performs, or prevents a physiological function but does not physically take the place of a body part

Body Part Character 4	Approach Character 5	Device Character 6	Qualifier Character 7
X Upper Muscle **Y** Lower Muscle	**Ø** Open **3** Percutaneous **4** Percutaneous Endoscopic	**M** Stimulator Lead	**Z** No Qualifier

Ø Medical and Surgical
K Muscles
J Inspection Visually and/or manually exploring a body part

Body Part Character 4	Approach Character 5	Device Character 6	Qualifier Character 7
X Upper Muscle **Y** Lower Muscle	**Ø** Open **3** Percutaneous **4** Percutaneous Endoscopic **X** External	**Z** No Device	**Z** No Qualifier

Non-OR ØKJ[X,Y]XZZ

Ø Medical and Surgical
K Muscles
M Reattachment Putting back in or on all or a portion of a separated body part to its normal location or other suitable location

Body Part Character 4	Approach Character 5	Device Character 6	Qualifier Character 7
Ø Head Muscle 1 Facial Muscle 2 Neck Muscle, Right 3 Neck Muscle, Left 4 Tongue, Palate, Pharynx Muscle 5 Shoulder Muscle, Right 6 Shoulder Muscle, Left 7 Upper Arm Muscle, Right 8 Upper Arm Muscle, Left 9 Lower Arm and Wrist Muscle, Right B Lower Arm and Wrist Muscle, Left C Hand Muscle, Right D Hand Muscle, Left F Trunk Muscle, Right G Trunk Muscle, Left H Thorax Muscle, Right J Thorax Muscle, Left K Abdomen Muscle, Right L Abdomen Muscle, Left M Perineum Muscle N Hip Muscle, Right P Hip Muscle, Left Q Upper Leg Muscle, Right R Upper Leg Muscle, Left S Lower Leg Muscle, Right T Lower Leg Muscle, Left V Foot Muscle, Right W Foot Muscle, Left	Ø Open 4 Percutaneous Endoscopic	Z No Device	Z No Qualifier

Ø Medical and Surgical
K Muscles
N Release Freeing a body part from an abnormal physical constraint

Body Part Character 4	Approach Character 5	Device Character 6	Qualifier Character 7
Ø Head Muscle 1 Facial Muscle 2 Neck Muscle, Right 3 Neck Muscle, Left 4 Tongue, Palate, Pharynx Muscle 5 Shoulder Muscle, Right 6 Shoulder Muscle, Left 7 Upper Arm Muscle, Right 8 Upper Arm Muscle, Left 9 Lower Arm and Wrist Muscle, Right B Lower Arm and Wrist Muscle, Left C Hand Muscle, Right D Hand Muscle, Left F Trunk Muscle, Right G Trunk Muscle, Left H Thorax Muscle, Right J Thorax Muscle, Left K Abdomen Muscle, Right L Abdomen Muscle, Left M Perineum Muscle N Hip Muscle, Right P Hip Muscle, Left Q Upper Leg Muscle, Right R Upper Leg Muscle, Left S Lower Leg Muscle, Right T Lower Leg Muscle, Left V Foot Muscle, Right W Foot Muscle, Left	Ø Open 3 Percutaneous 4 Percutaneous Endoscopic X External	Z No Device	Z No Qualifier

Non-OR ØKN[Ø,1,2,3,4,5,6,7,8,9,B,C,D,F,G,H,J,K,L,M,N,P,Q,R,S,T,V,W]XZZ

Ø Medical and Surgical
K Muscles
P Removal Taking out or off a device from a body part

Body Part Character 4	Approach Character 5	Device Character 6	Qualifier Character 7
X Upper Muscle **Y** Lower Muscle	**Ø** Open **3** Percutaneous **4** Percutaneous Endoscopic	**Ø** Drainage Device **7** Autologous Tissue Substitute **J** Synthetic Substitute **K** Nonautologous Tissue Substitute **M** Stimulator Lead	**Z** No Qualifier
X Upper Muscle **Y** Lower Muscle	**X** External	**Ø** Drainage Device **M** Stimulator Lead	**Z** No Qualifier

Non-OR ØKP[X,Y]X[Ø,M]Z

Ø Medical and Surgical
K Muscles
Q Repair Restoring, to the extent possible, a body part to its normal anatomic structure and function

Body Part Character 4	Approach Character 5	Device Character 6	Qualifier Character 7
Ø Head Muscle **1** Facial Muscle **2** Neck Muscle, Right **3** Neck Muscle, Left **4** Tongue, Palate, Pharynx Muscle **5** Shoulder Muscle, Right **6** Shoulder Muscle, Left **7** Upper Arm Muscle, Right **8** Upper Arm Muscle, Left **9** Lower Arm and Wrist Muscle, Right **B** Lower Arm and Wrist Muscle, Left **C** Hand Muscle, Right **D** Hand Muscle, Left **F** Trunk Muscle, Right **G** Trunk Muscle, Left **H** Thorax Muscle, Right **J** Thorax Muscle, Left **K** Abdomen Muscle, Right **L** Abdomen Muscle, Left **M** Perineum Muscle **N** Hip Muscle, Right **P** Hip Muscle, Left **Q** Upper Leg Muscle, Right **R** Upper Leg Muscle, Left **S** Lower Leg Muscle, Right **T** Lower Leg Muscle, Left **V** Foot Muscle, Right **W** Foot Muscle, Left	**Ø** Open **3** Percutaneous **4** Percutaneous Endoscopic	**Z** No Device	**Z** No Qualifier

AHA: 2Ø13, 4Q, 12Ø

Ø Medical and Surgical
K Muscles
S Reposition Moving to its normal location or other suitable location all or a portion of a body part

Body Part Character 4	Approach Character 5	Device Character 6	Qualifier Character 7
Ø Head Muscle **1** Facial Muscle **2** Neck Muscle, Right **3** Neck Muscle, Left **4** Tongue, Palate, Pharynx Muscle **5** Shoulder Muscle, Right **6** Shoulder Muscle, Left **7** Upper Arm Muscle, Right **8** Upper Arm Muscle, Left **9** Lower Arm and Wrist Muscle, Right **B** Lower Arm and Wrist Muscle, Left **C** Hand Muscle, Right **D** Hand Muscle, Left **F** Trunk Muscle, Right **G** Trunk Muscle, Left **H** Thorax Muscle, Right **J** Thorax Muscle, Left **K** Abdomen Muscle, Right **L** Abdomen Muscle, Left **M** Perineum Muscle **N** Hip Muscle, Right **P** Hip Muscle, Left **Q** Upper Leg Muscle, Right **R** Upper Leg Muscle, Left **S** Lower Leg Muscle, Right **T** Lower Leg Muscle, Left **V** Foot Muscle, Right **W** Foot Muscle, Left	**Ø** Open **4** Percutaneous Endoscopic	**Z** No Device	**Z** No Qualifier

Ø Medical and Surgical
K Muscles
T Resection Cutting out or off, without replacement, all of a body part

Body Part Character 4	Approach Character 5	Device Character 6	Qualifier Character 7
Ø Head Muscle **1** Facial Muscle **2** Neck Muscle, Right **3** Neck Muscle, Left **4** Tongue, Palate, Pharynx Muscle **5** Shoulder Muscle, Right **6** Shoulder Muscle, Left **7** Upper Arm Muscle, Right **8** Upper Arm Muscle, Left **9** Lower Arm and Wrist Muscle, Right **B** Lower Arm and Wrist Muscle, Left **C** Hand Muscle, Right **D** Hand Muscle, Left **F** Trunk Muscle, Right **G** Trunk Muscle, Left **H** Thorax Muscle, Right ⊞ **J** Thorax Muscle, Left ⊞ **K** Abdomen Muscle, Right **L** Abdomen Muscle, Left **M** Perineum Muscle **N** Hip Muscle, Right **P** Hip Muscle, Left **Q** Upper Leg Muscle, Right **R** Upper Leg Muscle, Left **S** Lower Leg Muscle, Right **T** Lower Leg Muscle, Left **V** Foot Muscle, Right **W** Foot Muscle, Left	**Ø** Open **4** Percutaneous Endoscopic	**Z** No Device	**Z** No Qualifier

See Appendix I for Procedure Combinations
⊞ ØKT[H,J]ØZZ

Ø Medical and Surgical
K Muscles
U Supplement Putting in or on biological or synthetic material that physically reinforces and/or augments the function of a portion of a body part

Body Part Character 4	Approach Character 5	Device Character 6	Qualifier Character 7
Ø Head Muscle **1** Facial Muscle **2** Neck Muscle, Right **3** Neck Muscle, Left **4** Tongue, Palate, Pharynx Muscle **5** Shoulder Muscle, Right **6** Shoulder Muscle, Left **7** Upper Arm Muscle, Right **8** Upper Arm Muscle, Left **9** Lower Arm and Wrist Muscle, Right **B** Lower Arm and Wrist Muscle, Left **C** Hand Muscle, Right **D** Hand Muscle, Left **F** Trunk Muscle, Right **G** Trunk Muscle, Left **H** Thorax Muscle, Right **J** Thorax Muscle, Left **K** Abdomen Muscle, Right **L** Abdomen Muscle, Left **M** Perineum Muscle **N** Hip Muscle, Right **P** Hip Muscle, Left **Q** Upper Leg Muscle, Right **R** Upper Leg Muscle, Left **S** Lower Leg Muscle, Right **T** Lower Leg Muscle, Left **V** Foot Muscle, Right **W** Foot Muscle, Left	**Ø** Open **4** Percutaneous Endoscopic	**7** Autologous Tissue Substitute **J** Synthetic Substitute **K** Nonautologous Tissue Substitute	**Z** No Qualifier

Ø Medical and Surgical
K Muscles
W Revision Correcting, to the extent possible, a portion of a malfunctioning device or the position of a displaced device

Body Part Character 4	Approach Character 5	Device Character 6	Qualifier Character 7
X Upper Muscle **Y** Lower Muscle	**Ø** Open **3** Percutaneous **4** Percutaneous Endoscopic **X** External	**Ø** Drainage Device **7** Autologous Tissue Substitute **J** Synthetic Substitute **K** Nonautologous Tissue Substitute **M** Stimulator Lead	**Z** No Qualifier

Non-OR ØKW[X,Y]X[Ø,7,J,K,M]Z

Ø Medical and Surgical
K Muscles
X Transfer Moving, without taking out, all or a portion of a body part to another location to take over the function of all or a portion of a body part

Body Part Character 4	Approach Character 5	Device Character 6	Qualifier Character 7
Ø Head Muscle 1 Facial Muscle ⊞ 2 Neck Muscle, Right 3 Neck Muscle, Left 4 Tongue, Palate, Pharynx Muscle 5 Shoulder Muscle, Right 6 Shoulder Muscle, Left 7 Upper Arm Muscle, Right 8 Upper Arm Muscle, Left 9 Lower Arm and Wrist Muscle, Right B Lower Arm and Wrist Muscle, Left C Hand Muscle, Right D Hand Muscle, Left F Trunk Muscle, Right G Trunk Muscle, Left H Thorax Muscle, Right J Thorax Muscle, Left M Perineum Muscle N Hip Muscle, Right P Hip Muscle, Left Q Upper Leg Muscle, Right R Upper Leg Muscle, Left S Lower Leg Muscle, Right ⊞ T Lower Leg Muscle, Left ⊞ V Foot Muscle, Right W Foot Muscle, Left	Ø Open 4 Percutaneous Endoscopic	Z No Device	Ø Skin 1 Subcutaneous Tissue 2 Skin and Subcutaneous Tissue Z No Qualifier
K Abdomen Muscle, Right L Abdomen Muscle, Left	Ø Open 4 Percutaneous Endoscopic	Z No Device	Ø Skin 1 Subcutaneous Tissue 2 Skin and Subcutaneous Tissue 6 Transverse Rectus Abdominis Myocutaneous Flap Z No Qualifier

No Procedure Combinations Specified
⊞ ØKX[1,S,T][Ø,4]ZZ

AHA: 2Ø14, 2Q, 1Ø-12

Tendons 0L2–0LX

0 Medical and Surgical
L Tendons
2 Change Taking out or off a device from a body part and putting back an identical or similar device in or on the same body part without cutting or puncturing the skin or a mucous membrane

Body Part Character 4	Approach Character 5	Device Character 6	Qualifier Character 7
X Upper Tendon Y Lower Tendon	X External	0 Drainage Device Y Other Device	Z No Qualifier

Non-OR For all body part, approach, device, and qualifier values

0 Medical and Surgical
L Tendons
5 Destruction Physical eradication of all or a portion of a body part by the direct use of energy, force, or a destructive agent

Body Part Character 4	Approach Character 5	Device Character 6	Qualifier Character 7
0 Head and Neck Tendon 1 Shoulder Tendon, Right 2 Shoulder Tendon, Left 3 Upper Arm Tendon, Right 4 Upper Arm Tendon, Left 5 Lower Arm and Wrist Tendon, Right 6 Lower Arm and Wrist Tendon, Left 7 Hand Tendon, Right 8 Hand Tendon, Left 9 Trunk Tendon, Right B Trunk Tendon, Left C Thorax Tendon, Right D Thorax Tendon, Left F Abdomen Tendon, Right G Abdomen Tendon, Left H Perineum Tendon J Hip Tendon, Right K Hip Tendon, Left L Upper Leg Tendon, Right M Upper Leg Tendon, Left N Lower Leg Tendon, Right P Lower Leg Tendon, Left Q Knee Tendon, Right R Knee Tendon, Left S Ankle Tendon, Right T Ankle Tendon, Left V Foot Tendon, Right W Foot Tendon, Left	0 Open 3 Percutaneous 4 Percutaneous Endoscopic	Z No Device	Z No Qualifier

Ø Medical and Surgical
L Tendons
8 Division Cutting into a body part without draining fluids and/or gases from the body part in order to separate or transect a body part

Body Part Character 4	Approach Character 5	Device Character 6	Qualifier Character 7
Ø Head and Neck Tendon 1 Shoulder Tendon, Right 2 Shoulder Tendon, Left 3 Upper Arm Tendon, Right 4 Upper Arm Tendon, Left 5 Lower Arm and Wrist Tendon, Right 6 Lower Arm and Wrist Tendon, Left 7 Hand Tendon, Right 8 Hand Tendon, Left 9 Trunk Tendon, Right B Trunk Tendon, Left C Thorax Tendon, Right D Thorax Tendon, Left F Abdomen Tendon, Right G Abdomen Tendon, Left H Perineum Tendon J Hip Tendon, Right K Hip Tendon, Left L Upper Leg Tendon, Right M Upper Leg Tendon, Left N Lower Leg Tendon, Right P Lower Leg Tendon, Left Q Knee Tendon, Right R Knee Tendon, Left S Ankle Tendon, Right T Ankle Tendon, Left V Foot Tendon, Right W Foot Tendon, Left	Ø Open 3 Percutaneous 4 Percutaneous Endoscopic	Z No Device	Z No Qualifier

Ø Medical and Surgical
L Tendons
9 Drainage Taking or letting out fluids and/or gases from a body part

Body Part Character 4	Approach Character 5	Device Character 6	Qualifier Character 7
Ø Head and Neck Tendon 1 Shoulder Tendon, Right 2 Shoulder Tendon, Left 3 Upper Arm Tendon, Right 4 Upper Arm Tendon, Left 5 Lower Arm and Wrist Tendon, Right 6 Lower Arm and Wrist Tendon, Left 7 Hand Tendon, Right 8 Hand Tendon, Left 9 Trunk Tendon, Right B Trunk Tendon, Left C Thorax Tendon, Right D Thorax Tendon, Left F Abdomen Tendon, Right G Abdomen Tendon, Left H Perineum Tendon J Hip Tendon, Right K Hip Tendon, Left L Upper Leg Tendon, Right M Upper Leg Tendon, Left N Lower Leg Tendon, Right P Lower Leg Tendon, Left Q Knee Tendon, Right R Knee Tendon, Left S Ankle Tendon, Right T Ankle Tendon, Left V Foot Tendon, Right W Foot Tendon, Left	Ø Open 3 Percutaneous 4 Percutaneous Endoscopic	Ø Drainage Device	Z No Qualifier

ØL9 Continued on next page

ØL9 Continued

Ø Medical and Surgical
L Tendons
9 Drainage Taking or letting out fluids and/or gases from a body part

Body Part Character 4	Approach Character 5	Device Character 6	Qualifier Character 7
Ø Head and Neck Tendon 1 Shoulder Tendon, Right 2 Shoulder Tendon, Left 3 Upper Arm Tendon, Right 4 Upper Arm Tendon, Left 5 Lower Arm and Wrist Tendon, Right 6 Lower Arm and Wrist Tendon, Left 7 Hand Tendon, Right 8 Hand Tendon, Left 9 Trunk Tendon, Right B Trunk Tendon, Left C Thorax Tendon, Right D Thorax Tendon, Left F Abdomen Tendon, Right G Abdomen Tendon, Left H Perineum Tendon J Hip Tendon, Right K Hip Tendon, Left L Upper Leg Tendon, Right M Upper Leg Tendon, Left N Lower Leg Tendon, Right P Lower Leg Tendon, Left Q Knee Tendon, Right R Knee Tendon, Left S Ankle Tendon, Right T Ankle Tendon, Left V Foot Tendon, Right W Foot Tendon, Left	Ø Open 3 Percutaneous 4 Percutaneous Endoscopic	Z No Device	X Diagnostic Z No Qualifier

Non-OR ØL9[7,8][3,4]ZZ

Ø Medical and Surgical
L Tendons
B Excision Cutting out or off, without replacement, a portion of a body part

Body Part Character 4	Approach Character 5	Device Character 6	Qualifier Character 7
Ø Head and Neck Tendon 1 Shoulder Tendon, Right 2 Shoulder Tendon, Left 3 Upper Arm Tendon, Right 4 Upper Arm Tendon, Left 5 Lower Arm and Wrist Tendon, Right 6 Lower Arm and Wrist Tendon, Left 7 Hand Tendon, Right 8 Hand Tendon, Left 9 Trunk Tendon, Right B Trunk Tendon, Left C Thorax Tendon, Right D Thorax Tendon, Left F Abdomen Tendon, Right G Abdomen Tendon, Left H Perineum Tendon J Hip Tendon, Right K Hip Tendon, Left L Upper Leg Tendon, Right M Upper Leg Tendon, Left N Lower Leg Tendon, Right P Lower Leg Tendon, Left Q Knee Tendon, Right R Knee Tendon, Left S Ankle Tendon, Right T Ankle Tendon, Left V Foot Tendon, Right W Foot Tendon, Left	Ø Open 3 Percutaneous 4 Percutaneous Endoscopic	Z No Device	X Diagnostic Z No Qualifier

Ø Medical and Surgical
L Tendons
C Extirpation Taking or cutting out solid matter from a body part

Body Part Character 4	Approach Character 5	Device Character 6	Qualifier Character 7
Ø Head and Neck Tendon 1 Shoulder Tendon, Right 2 Shoulder Tendon, Left 3 Upper Arm Tendon, Right 4 Upper Arm Tendon, Left 5 Lower Arm and Wrist Tendon, Right 6 Lower Arm and Wrist Tendon, Left 7 Hand Tendon, Right 8 Hand Tendon, Left 9 Trunk Tendon, Right B Trunk Tendon, Left C Thorax Tendon, Right D Thorax Tendon, Left F Abdomen Tendon, Right G Abdomen Tendon, Left H Perineum Tendon J Hip Tendon, Right K Hip Tendon, Left L Upper Leg Tendon, Right M Upper Leg Tendon, Left N Lower Leg Tendon, Right P Lower Leg Tendon, Left Q Knee Tendon, Right R Knee Tendon, Left S Ankle Tendon, Right T Ankle Tendon, Left V Foot Tendon, Right W Foot Tendon, Left	Ø Open 3 Percutaneous 4 Percutaneous Endoscopic	Z No Device	Z No Qualifier

Ø Medical and Surgical
L Tendons
J Inspection Visually and/or manually exploring a body part

Body Part Character 4	Approach Character 5	Device Character 6	Qualifier Character 7
X Upper Tendon Y Lower Tendon	Ø Open 3 Percutaneous 4 Percutaneous Endoscopic X External	Z No Device	Z No Qualifier

Non-OR ØLJ[X,Y]XZZ

Ø Medical and Surgical
L Tendons
M Reattachment Putting back in or on all or a portion of a separated body part to its normal location or other suitable location

Body Part Character 4	Approach Character 5	Device Character 6	Qualifier Character 7
Ø Head and Neck Tendon 1 Shoulder Tendon, Right 2 Shoulder Tendon, Left 3 Upper Arm Tendon, Right 4 Upper Arm Tendon, Left 5 Lower Arm and Wrist Tendon, Right 6 Lower Arm and Wrist Tendon, Left 7 Hand Tendon, Right 8 Hand Tendon, Left 9 Trunk Tendon, Right B Trunk Tendon, Left C Thorax Tendon, Right D Thorax Tendon, Left F Abdomen Tendon, Right G Abdomen Tendon, Left H Perineum Tendon J Hip Tendon, Right K Hip Tendon, Left L Upper Leg Tendon, Right M Upper Leg Tendon, Left N Lower Leg Tendon, Right P Lower Leg Tendon, Left Q Knee Tendon, Right R Knee Tendon, Left S Ankle Tendon, Right T Ankle Tendon, Left V Foot Tendon, Right W Foot Tendon, Left	Ø Open 4 Percutaneous Endoscopic	Z No Device	Z No Qualifier

Ø Medical and Surgical
L Tendons
N Release Freeing a body part from an abnormal physical constraint

Body Part Character 4	Approach Character 5	Device Character 6	Qualifier Character 7
Ø Head and Neck Tendon 1 Shoulder Tendon, Right 2 Shoulder Tendon, Left 3 Upper Arm Tendon, Right 4 Upper Arm Tendon, Left 5 Lower Arm and Wrist Tendon, Right 6 Lower Arm and Wrist Tendon, Left 7 Hand Tendon, Right 8 Hand Tendon, Left 9 Trunk Tendon, Right B Trunk Tendon, Left C Thorax Tendon, Right D Thorax Tendon, Left F Abdomen Tendon, Right G Abdomen Tendon, Left H Perineum Tendon J Hip Tendon, Right K Hip Tendon, Left L Upper Leg Tendon, Right M Upper Leg Tendon, Left N Lower Leg Tendon, Right P Lower Leg Tendon, Left Q Knee Tendon, Right R Knee Tendon, Left S Ankle Tendon, Right T Ankle Tendon, Left V Foot Tendon, Right W Foot Tendon, Left	Ø Open 3 Percutaneous 4 Percutaneous Endoscopic X External	Z No Device	Z No Qualifier

Non-OR ØLN[Ø,1,2,3,4,5,6,7,8,9,B,C,D,F,G,H,J,K,L,M,N,P,Q,R,S,T,V,W]XZZ

Ø Medical and Surgical
L Tendons
P Removal Taking out or off a device from a body part

Body Part Character 4	Approach Character 5	Device Character 6	Qualifier Character 7
X Upper Tendon **Y** Lower Tendon	**Ø** Open **3** Percutaneous **4** Percutaneous Endoscopic	**Ø** Drainage Device **7** Autologous Tissue Substitute **J** Synthetic Substitute **K** Nonautologous Tissue Substitute	**Z** No Qualifier
X Upper Tendon **Y** Lower Tendon	**X** External	**Ø** Drainage Device	**Z** No Qualifier

Non-OR ØLP[X,Y]XØZ

Ø Medical and Surgical
L Tendons
Q Repair Restoring, to the extent possible, a body part to its normal anatomic structure and function

Body Part Character 4	Approach Character 5	Device Character 6	Qualifier Character 7
Ø Head and Neck Tendon **1** Shoulder Tendon, Right **2** Shoulder Tendon, Left **3** Upper Arm Tendon, Right **4** Upper Arm Tendon, Left **5** Lower Arm and Wrist Tendon, Right **6** Lower Arm and Wrist Tendon, Left **7** Hand Tendon, Right **8** Hand Tendon, Left **9** Trunk Tendon, Right **B** Trunk Tendon, Left **C** Thorax Tendon, Right **D** Thorax Tendon, Left **F** Abdomen Tendon, Right **G** Abdomen Tendon, Left **H** Perineum Tendon **J** Hip Tendon, Right **K** Hip Tendon, Left **L** Upper Leg Tendon, Right **M** Upper Leg Tendon, Left **N** Lower Leg Tendon, Right **P** Lower Leg Tendon, Left **Q** Knee Tendon, Right **R** Knee Tendon, Left **S** Ankle Tendon, Right **T** Ankle Tendon, Left **V** Foot Tendon, Right **W** Foot Tendon, Left	**Ø** Open **3** Percutaneous **4** Percutaneous Endoscopic	**Z** No Device	**Z** No Qualifier

AHA: 2Ø13, 3Q, 2Ø

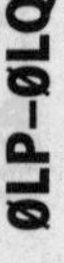

Ø Medical and Surgical
L Tendons
R Replacement Putting in or on biological or synthetic material that physically takes the place and/or function of all or a portion of a body part

Body Part Character 4	Approach Character 5	Device Character 6	Qualifier Character 7
Ø Head and Neck Tendon 1 Shoulder Tendon, Right 2 Shoulder Tendon, Left 3 Upper Arm Tendon, Right 4 Upper Arm Tendon, Left 5 Lower Arm and Wrist Tendon, Right 6 Lower Arm and Wrist Tendon, Left 7 Hand Tendon, Right 8 Hand Tendon, Left 9 Trunk Tendon, Right B Trunk Tendon, Left C Thorax Tendon, Right D Thorax Tendon, Left F Abdomen Tendon, Right G Abdomen Tendon, Left H Perineum Tendon J Hip Tendon, Right K Hip Tendon, Left L Upper Leg Tendon, Right M Upper Leg Tendon, Left N Lower Leg Tendon, Right P Lower Leg Tendon, Left Q Knee Tendon, Right R Knee Tendon, Left S Ankle Tendon, Right T Ankle Tendon, Left V Foot Tendon, Right W Foot Tendon, Left	Ø Open 4 Percutaneous Endoscopic	7 Autologous Tissue Substitute J Synthetic Substitute K Nonautologous Tissue Substitute	Z No Qualifier

Ø Medical and Surgical
L Tendons
S Reposition Moving to its normal location or other suitable location all or a portion of a body part

Body Part Character 4	Approach Character 5	Device Character 6	Qualifier Character 7
Ø Head and Neck Tendon 1 Shoulder Tendon, Right 2 Shoulder Tendon, Left 3 Upper Arm Tendon, Right 4 Upper Arm Tendon, Left 5 Lower Arm and Wrist Tendon, Right 6 Lower Arm and Wrist Tendon, Left 7 Hand Tendon, Right 8 Hand Tendon, Left 9 Trunk Tendon, Right B Trunk Tendon, Left C Thorax Tendon, Right D Thorax Tendon, Left F Abdomen Tendon, Right G Abdomen Tendon, Left H Perineum Tendon J Hip Tendon, Right K Hip Tendon, Left L Upper Leg Tendon, Right M Upper Leg Tendon, Left N Lower Leg Tendon, Right P Lower Leg Tendon, Left Q Knee Tendon, Right ⊞ R Knee Tendon, Left ⊞ S Ankle Tendon, Right T Ankle Tendon, Left V Foot Tendon, Right W Foot Tendon, Left	Ø Open 4 Percutaneous Endoscopic	Z No Device	Z No Qualifier

No Procedure Combinations Specified
⊞ ØLS[Q,R][Ø,4]ZZ

Ø Medical and Surgical
L Tendons
T Resection Cutting out or off, without replacement, all of a body part

Body Part Character 4	Approach Character 5	Device Character 6	Qualifier Character 7
Ø Head and Neck Tendon 1 Shoulder Tendon, Right 2 Shoulder Tendon, Left 3 Upper Arm Tendon, Right 4 Upper Arm Tendon, Left 5 Lower Arm and Wrist Tendon, Right 6 Lower Arm and Wrist Tendon, Left 7 Hand Tendon, Right 8 Hand Tendon, Left 9 Trunk Tendon, Right B Trunk Tendon, Left C Thorax Tendon, Right D Thorax Tendon, Left F Abdomen Tendon, Right G Abdomen Tendon, Left H Perineum Tendon J Hip Tendon, Right K Hip Tendon, Left L Upper Leg Tendon, Right M Upper Leg Tendon, Left N Lower Leg Tendon, Right P Lower Leg Tendon, Left Q Knee Tendon, Right R Knee Tendon, Left S Ankle Tendon, Right T Ankle Tendon, Left V Foot Tendon, Right W Foot Tendon, Left	Ø Open 4 Percutaneous Endoscopic	Z No Device	Z No Qualifier

Ø Medical and Surgical
L Tendons
U Supplement Putting in or on biological or synthetic material that physically reinforces and/or augments the function of a portion of a body part

Body Part Character 4	Approach Character 5	Device Character 6	Qualifier Character 7
Ø Head and Neck Tendon 1 Shoulder Tendon, Right 2 Shoulder Tendon, Left 3 Upper Arm Tendon, Right 4 Upper Arm Tendon, Left 5 Lower Arm and Wrist Tendon, Right 6 Lower Arm and Wrist Tendon, Left 7 Hand Tendon, Right 8 Hand Tendon, Left 9 Trunk Tendon, Right B Trunk Tendon, Left C Thorax Tendon, Right D Thorax Tendon, Left F Abdomen Tendon, Right G Abdomen Tendon, Left H Perineum Tendon J Hip Tendon, Right K Hip Tendon, Left L Upper Leg Tendon, Right M Upper Leg Tendon, Left N Lower Leg Tendon, Right P Lower Leg Tendon, Left Q Knee Tendon, Right R Knee Tendon, Left S Ankle Tendon, Right T Ankle Tendon, Left V Foot Tendon, Right W Foot Tendon, Left	Ø Open 4 Percutaneous Endoscopic	7 Autologous Tissue Substitute J Synthetic Substitute K Nonautologous Tissue Substitute	Z No Qualifier

Ø Medical and Surgical
L Tendons
W Revision Correcting, to the extent possible, a portion of a malfunctioning device or the position of a displaced device

Body Part Character 4	Approach Character 5	Device Character 6	Qualifier Character 7
X Upper Tendon **Y** Lower Tendon	**Ø** Open **3** Percutaneous **4** Percutaneous Endoscopic **X** External	**Ø** Drainage Device **7** Autologous Tissue Substitute **J** Synthetic Substitute **K** Nonautologous Tissue Substitute	**Z** No Qualifier

Non-OR ØLW[X,Y]X[Ø,7,J,K]Z

Ø Medical and Surgical
L Tendons
X Transfer Moving, without taking out, all or a portion of a body part to another location to take over the function of all or a portion of a body part

Body Part Character 4	Approach Character 5	Device Character 6	Qualifier Character 7
Ø Head and Neck Tendon **1** Shoulder Tendon, Right **2** Shoulder Tendon, Left **3** Upper Arm Tendon, Right **4** Upper Arm Tendon, Left **5** Lower Arm and Wrist Tendon, Right **6** Lower Arm and Wrist Tendon, Left **7** Hand Tendon, Right **8** Hand Tendon, Left **9** Trunk Tendon, Right **B** Trunk Tendon, Left **C** Thorax Tendon, Right **D** Thorax Tendon, Left **F** Abdomen Tendon, Right **G** Abdomen Tendon, Left **H** Perineum Tendon **J** Hip Tendon, Right **K** Hip Tendon, Left **L** Upper Leg Tendon, Right **M** Upper Leg Tendon, Left **N** Lower Leg Tendon, Right **P** Lower Leg Tendon, Left **Q** Knee Tendon, Right **R** Knee Tendon, Left **S** Ankle Tendon, Right **T** Ankle Tendon, Left **V** Foot Tendon, Right **W** Foot Tendon, Left	**Ø** Open **4** Percutaneous Endoscopic	**Z** No Device	**Z** No Qualifier

Bursae and Ligaments ØM2–ØMX

Ø Medical and Surgical
M Bursae and Ligaments
2 Change Taking out or off a device from a body part and putting back an identical or similar device in or on the same body part without cutting or puncturing the skin or a mucous membrane

Body Part Character 4	Approach Character 5	Device Character 6	Qualifier Character 7
X Upper Bursa and Ligament Y Lower Bursa and Ligament	X External	Ø Drainage Device Y Other Device	Z No Qualifier
Non-OR For all body part, approach, device, and qualifier values			

Ø Medical and Surgical
M Bursae and Ligaments
5 Destruction Physical eradication of all or a portion of a body part by the direct use of energy, force, or a destructive agent

Body Part Character 4	Approach Character 5	Device Character 6	Qualifier Character 7
Ø Head and Neck Bursa and Ligament 1 Shoulder Bursa and Ligament, Right 2 Shoulder Bursa and Ligament, Left 3 Elbow Bursa and Ligament, Right 4 Elbow Bursa and Ligament, Left 5 Wrist Bursa and Ligament, Right 6 Wrist Bursa and Ligament, Left 7 Hand Bursa and Ligament, Right 8 Hand Bursa and Ligament, Left 9 Upper Extremity Bursa and Ligament, Right B Upper Extremity Bursa and Ligament, Left C Trunk Bursa and Ligament, Right D Trunk Bursa and Ligament, Left F Thorax Bursa and Ligament, Right G Thorax Bursa and Ligament, Left H Abdomen Bursa and Ligament, Right J Abdomen Bursa and Ligament, Left K Perineum Bursa and Ligament L Hip Bursa and Ligament, Right M Hip Bursa and Ligament, Left N Knee Bursa and Ligament, Right P Knee Bursa and Ligament, Left Q Ankle Bursa and Ligament, Right R Ankle Bursa and Ligament, Left S Foot Bursa and Ligament, Right T Foot Bursa and Ligament, Left V Lower Extremity Bursa and Ligament, Right W Lower Extremity Bursa and Ligament, Left	Ø Open 3 Percutaneous 4 Percutaneous Endoscopic	Z No Device	Z No Qualifier

Ø Medical and Surgical
M Bursae and Ligaments
8 Division Cutting into a body part without draining fluids and/or gases from the body part in order to separate or transect a body part

Body Part Character 4	Approach Character 5	Device Character 6	Qualifier Character 7
Ø Head and Neck Bursa and Ligament 1 Shoulder Bursa and Ligament, Right 2 Shoulder Bursa and Ligament, Left 3 Elbow Bursa and Ligament, Right 4 Elbow Bursa and Ligament, Left 5 Wrist Bursa and Ligament, Right 6 Wrist Bursa and Ligament, Left 7 Hand Bursa and Ligament, Right 8 Hand Bursa and Ligament, Left 9 Upper Extremity Bursa and Ligament, Right B Upper Extremity Bursa and Ligament, Left C Trunk Bursa and Ligament, Right D Trunk Bursa and Ligament, Left F Thorax Bursa and Ligament, Right G Thorax Bursa and Ligament, Left H Abdomen Bursa and Ligament, Right J Abdomen Bursa and Ligament, Left K Perineum Bursa and Ligament L Hip Bursa and Ligament, Right M Hip Bursa and Ligament, Left N Knee Bursa and Ligament, Right P Knee Bursa and Ligament, Left Q Ankle Bursa and Ligament, Right R Ankle Bursa and Ligament, Left S Foot Bursa and Ligament, Right T Foot Bursa and Ligament, Left V Lower Extremity Bursa and Ligament, Right W Lower Extremity Bursa and Ligament, Left	Ø Open 3 Percutaneous 4 Percutaneous Endoscopic	Z No Device	Z No Qualifier

Non-OR ØM8[5,6][Ø,3,4]ZZ

Ø Medical and Surgical
M Bursae and Ligaments
9 Drainage Taking or letting out fluids and/or gases from a body part

Body Part Character 4	Approach Character 5	Device Character 6	Qualifier Character 7
Ø Head and Neck Bursa and Ligament 1 Shoulder Bursa and Ligament, Right 2 Shoulder Bursa and Ligament, Left 3 Elbow Bursa and Ligament, Right 4 Elbow Bursa and Ligament, Left 5 Wrist Bursa and Ligament, Right 6 Wrist Bursa and Ligament, Left 7 Hand Bursa and Ligament, Right 8 Hand Bursa and Ligament, Left 9 Upper Extremity Bursa and Ligament, Right B Upper Extremity Bursa and Ligament, Left C Trunk Bursa and Ligament, Right D Trunk Bursa and Ligament, Left F Thorax Bursa and Ligament, Right G Thorax Bursa and Ligament, Left H Abdomen Bursa and Ligament, Right J Abdomen Bursa and Ligament, Left K Perineum Bursa and Ligament L Hip Bursa and Ligament, Right M Hip Bursa and Ligament, Left N Knee Bursa and Ligament, Right P Knee Bursa and Ligament, Left Q Ankle Bursa and Ligament, Right R Ankle Bursa and Ligament, Left S Foot Bursa and Ligament, Right T Foot Bursa and Ligament, Left V Lower Extremity Bursa and Ligament, Right W Lower Extremity Bursa and Ligament, Left	Ø Open 3 Percutaneous 4 Percutaneous Endoscopic	Ø Drainage Device	Z No Qualifier

ØM9 Continued on next page

Non-OR ØM9[1,2,3,4,7,8,9,B,C,D,F,G,H,J,K,L,M,V,W][3,4]ØZ

ØM9 Continued

Ø Medical and Surgical
M Bursae and Ligaments
9 Drainage Taking or letting out fluids and/or gases from a body part

Body Part Character 4	Approach Character 5	Device Character 6	Qualifier Character 7
Ø Head and Neck Bursa and Ligament **1** Shoulder Bursa and Ligament, Right **2** Shoulder Bursa and Ligament, Left **3** Elbow Bursa and Ligament, Right **4** Elbow Bursa and Ligament, Left **5** Wrist Bursa and Ligament, Right **6** Wrist Bursa and Ligament, Left **7** Hand Bursa and Ligament, Right **8** Hand Bursa and Ligament, Left **9** Upper Extremity Bursa and Ligament, Right **B** Upper Extremity Bursa and Ligament, Left **C** Trunk Bursa and Ligament, Right **D** Trunk Bursa and Ligament, Left **F** Thorax Bursa and Ligament, Right **G** Thorax Bursa and Ligament, Left **H** Abdomen Bursa and Ligament, Right **J** Abdomen Bursa and Ligament, Left **K** Perineum Bursa and Ligament **L** Hip Bursa and Ligament, Right **M** Hip Bursa and Ligament, Left **N** Knee Bursa and Ligament, Right **P** Knee Bursa and Ligament, Left **Q** Ankle Bursa and Ligament, Right **R** Ankle Bursa and Ligament, Left **S** Foot Bursa and Ligament, Right **T** Foot Bursa and Ligament, Left **V** Lower Extremity Bursa and Ligament, Right **W** Lower Extremity Bursa and Ligament, Left	**Ø** Open **3** Percutaneous **4** Percutaneous Endoscopic	**Z** No Device	**X** Diagnostic **Z** No Qualifier

Non-OR ØM9[Ø,1,2,3,4,5,6,7,8,C,D,F,G,L,M,N,P,Q,R,S,T][Ø,3,4]ZX
Non-OR ØM9[Ø,5,6,7,8,9,B,C,D,F,G,H,J,K,N,P,Q,R,S,T,V,W][3,4]ZZ
Non-OR ØM9[1,2,3,4,L,M]3ZZ

Ø Medical and Surgical
M Bursae and Ligaments
B Excision Cutting out or off, without replacement, a portion of a body part

Body Part Character 4	Approach Character 5	Device Character 6	Qualifier Character 7
Ø Head and Neck Bursa and Ligament **1** Shoulder Bursa and Ligament, Right **2** Shoulder Bursa and Ligament, Left **3** Elbow Bursa and Ligament, Right **4** Elbow Bursa and Ligament, Left **5** Wrist Bursa and Ligament, Right **6** Wrist Bursa and Ligament, Left **7** Hand Bursa and Ligament, Right **8** Hand Bursa and Ligament, Left **9** Upper Extremity Bursa and Ligament, Right **B** Upper Extremity Bursa and Ligament, Left **C** Trunk Bursa and Ligament, Right **D** Trunk Bursa and Ligament, Left **F** Thorax Bursa and Ligament, Right **G** Thorax Bursa and Ligament, Left **H** Abdomen Bursa and Ligament, Right **J** Abdomen Bursa and Ligament, Left **K** Perineum Bursa and Ligament **L** Hip Bursa and Ligament, Right **M** Hip Bursa and Ligament, Left **N** Knee Bursa and Ligament, Right **P** Knee Bursa and Ligament, Left **Q** Ankle Bursa and Ligament, Right **R** Ankle Bursa and Ligament, Left **S** Foot Bursa and Ligament, Right **T** Foot Bursa and Ligament, Left **V** Lower Extremity Bursa and Ligament, Right **W** Lower Extremity Bursa and Ligament, Left	**Ø** Open **3** Percutaneous **4** Percutaneous Endoscopic	**Z** No Device	**X** Diagnostic **Z** No Qualifier

Non-OR ØMB[Ø,1,2,3,4,5,6,7,8,B,C,D,F,G,L,M,N,P,Q,R,S,T][Ø,3,4]ZX
Non-OR ØMB94ZX

Ø Medical and Surgical
M Bursae and Ligaments
C Extirpation Taking or cutting out solid matter from a body part

Body Part Character 4	Approach Character 5	Device Character 6	Qualifier Character 7
Ø Head and Neck Bursa and Ligament **1** Shoulder Bursa and Ligament, Right **2** Shoulder Bursa and Ligament, Left **3** Elbow Bursa and Ligament, Right **4** Elbow Bursa and Ligament, Left **5** Wrist Bursa and Ligament, Right **6** Wrist Bursa and Ligament, Left **7** Hand Bursa and Ligament, Right **8** Hand Bursa and Ligament, Left **9** Upper Extremity Bursa and Ligament, Right **B** Upper Extremity Bursa and Ligament, Left **C** Trunk Bursa and Ligament, Right **D** Trunk Bursa and Ligament, Left **F** Thorax Bursa and Ligament, Right **G** Thorax Bursa and Ligament, Left **H** Abdomen Bursa and Ligament, Right **J** Abdomen Bursa and Ligament, Left **K** Perineum Bursa and Ligament **L** Hip Bursa and Ligament, Right **M** Hip Bursa and Ligament, Left **N** Knee Bursa and Ligament, Right **P** Knee Bursa and Ligament, Left **Q** Ankle Bursa and Ligament, Right **R** Ankle Bursa and Ligament, Left **S** Foot Bursa and Ligament, Right **T** Foot Bursa and Ligament, Left **V** Lower Extremity Bursa and Ligament, Right **W** Lower Extremity Bursa and Ligament, Left	**Ø** Open **3** Percutaneous **4** Percutaneous Endoscopic	**Z** No Device	**Z** No Qualifier

Ø Medical and Surgical
M Bursae and Ligaments
D Extraction Pulling or stripping out or off all or a portion of a body part by the use of force

Body Part Character 4	Approach Character 5	Device Character 6	Qualifier Character 7
Ø Head and Neck Bursa and Ligament **1** Shoulder Bursa and Ligament, Right **2** Shoulder Bursa and Ligament, Left **3** Elbow Bursa and Ligament, Right **4** Elbow Bursa and Ligament, Left **5** Wrist Bursa and Ligament, Right **6** Wrist Bursa and Ligament, Left **7** Hand Bursa and Ligament, Right **8** Hand Bursa and Ligament, Left **9** Upper Extremity Bursa and Ligament, Right **B** Upper Extremity Bursa and Ligament, Left **C** Trunk Bursa and Ligament, Right **D** Trunk Bursa and Ligament, Left **F** Thorax Bursa and Ligament, Right **G** Thorax Bursa and Ligament, Left **H** Abdomen Bursa and Ligament, Right **J** Abdomen Bursa and Ligament, Left **K** Perineum Bursa and Ligament **L** Hip Bursa and Ligament, Right **M** Hip Bursa and Ligament, Left **N** Knee Bursa and Ligament, Right **P** Knee Bursa and Ligament, Left **Q** Ankle Bursa and Ligament, Right **R** Ankle Bursa and Ligament, Left **S** Foot Bursa and Ligament, Right **T** Foot Bursa and Ligament, Left **V** Lower Extremity Bursa and Ligament, Right **W** Lower Extremity Bursa and Ligament, Left	**Ø** Open **3** Percutaneous **4** Percutaneous Endoscopic	**Z** No Device	**Z** No Qualifier

Ø Medical and Surgical
M Bursae and Ligaments
J Inspection Visually and/or manually exploring a body part

Body Part Character 4	Approach Character 5	Device Character 6	Qualifier Character 7
X Upper Bursa and Ligament **Y** Lower Bursa and Ligament	**Ø** Open **3** Percutaneous **4** Percutaneous Endoscopic **X** External	**Z** No Device	**Z** No Qualifier

Non-OR ØMJ[X,Y]XZZ

Ø Medical and Surgical
M Bursae and Ligaments
M Reattachment Putting back in or on all or a portion of a separated body part to its normal location or other suitable location

Body Part Character 4	Approach Character 5	Device Character 6	Qualifier Character 7
Ø Head and Neck Bursa and Ligament **1** Shoulder Bursa and Ligament, Rightv **2** Shoulder Bursa and Ligament, Left **3** Elbow Bursa and Ligament, Right **4** Elbow Bursa and Ligament, Left **5** Wrist Bursa and Ligament, Right **6** Wrist Bursa and Ligament, Left **7** Hand Bursa and Ligament, Right **8** Hand Bursa and Ligament, Left **9** Upper Extremity Bursa and Ligament, Right **B** Upper Extremity Bursa and Ligament, Left **C** Trunk Bursa and Ligament, Right **D** Trunk Bursa and Ligament, Left **F** Thorax Bursa and Ligament, Right **G** Thorax Bursa and Ligament, Left **H** Abdomen Bursa and Ligament, Right **J** Abdomen Bursa and Ligament, Left **K** Perineum Bursa and Ligament **L** Hip Bursa and Ligament, Right **M** Hip Bursa and Ligament, Left **N** Knee Bursa and Ligament, Right **P** Knee Bursa and Ligament, Left **Q** Ankle Bursa and Ligament, Right **R** Ankle Bursa and Ligament, Left **S** Foot Bursa and Ligament, Right **T** Foot Bursa and Ligament, Left **V** Lower Extremity Bursa and Ligament, Right **W** Lower Extremity Bursa and Ligament, Left	**Ø** Open **4** Percutaneous Endoscopic	**Z** No Device	**Z** No Qualifier

AHA: 2Ø13, 3Q, 2Ø

0 Medical and Surgical
M Bursae and Ligaments
N Release Freeing a body part from an abnormal physical constraint

Body Part Character 4	Approach Character 5	Device Character 6	Qualifier Character 7
0 Head and Neck Bursa and Ligament 1 Shoulder Bursa and Ligament, Right 2 Shoulder Bursa and Ligament, Left 3 Elbow Bursa and Ligament, Right 4 Elbow Bursa and Ligament, Left 5 Wrist Bursa and Ligament, Right 6 Wrist Bursa and Ligament, Left 7 Hand Bursa and Ligament, Right 8 Hand Bursa and Ligament, Left 9 Upper Extremity Bursa and Ligament, Right B Upper Extremity Bursa and Ligament, Left C Trunk Bursa and Ligament, Right D Trunk Bursa and Ligament, Left F Thorax Bursa and Ligament, Right G Thorax Bursa and Ligament, Left H Abdomen Bursa and Ligament, Right J Abdomen Bursa and Ligament, Left K Perineum Bursa and Ligament L Hip Bursa and Ligament, Right M Hip Bursa and Ligament, Left N Knee Bursa and Ligament, Right P Knee Bursa and Ligament, Left Q Ankle Bursa and Ligament, Right R Ankle Bursa and Ligament, Left S Foot Bursa and Ligament, Right T Foot Bursa and Ligament, Left V Lower Extremity Bursa and Ligament, Right W Lower Extremity Bursa and Ligament, Left	0 Open 3 Percutaneous 4 Percutaneous Endoscopic X External	Z No Device	Z No Qualifier

0 Medical and Surgical
M Bursae and Ligaments
P Removal Taking out or off a device from a body part

Body Part Character 4	Approach Character 5	Device Character 6	Qualifier Character 7
X Upper Bursa and Ligament Y Lower Bursa and Ligament	0 Open 3 Percutaneous 4 Percutaneous Endoscopic	0 Drainage Device 7 Autologous Tissue Substitute J Synthetic Substitute K Nonautologous Tissue Substitute	Z No Qualifier
X Upper Bursa and Ligament Y Lower Bursa and Ligament	X External	0 Drainage Device	Z No Qualifier

Non-OR 0MP[X,Y]X0Z

Ø Medical and Surgical
M Bursae and Ligaments
Q Repair Restoring, to the extent possible, a body part to its normal anatomic structure and function

Body Part Character 4	Approach Character 5	Device Character 6	Qualifier Character 7
Ø Head and Neck Bursa and Ligament **1** Shoulder Bursa and Ligament, Right **2** Shoulder Bursa and Ligament, Left **3** Elbow Bursa and Ligament, Right **4** Elbow Bursa and Ligament, Left **5** Wrist Bursa and Ligament, Right **6** Wrist Bursa and Ligament, Left **7** Hand Bursa and Ligament, Right **8** Hand Bursa and Ligament, Left **9** Upper Extremity Bursa and Ligament, Right **B** Upper Extremity Bursa and Ligament, Left **C** Trunk Bursa and Ligament, Right **D** Trunk Bursa and Ligament, Left **F** Thorax Bursa and Ligament, Right **G** Thorax Bursa and Ligament, Left **H** Abdomen Bursa and Ligament, Right **J** Abdomen Bursa and Ligament, Left **K** Perineum Bursa and Ligament **L** Hip Bursa and Ligament, Right **M** Hip Bursa and Ligament, Left **N** Knee Bursa and Ligament, Right ⊞ **P** Knee Bursa and Ligament, Left ⊞ **Q** Ankle Bursa and Ligament, Right **R** Ankle Bursa and Ligament, Left **S** Foot Bursa and Ligament, Right ⊞ **T** Foot Bursa and Ligament, Left ⊞ **V** Lower Extremity Bursa and Ligament, Right **W** Lower Extremity Bursa and Ligament, Left	**Ø** Open **3** Percutaneous **4** Percutaneous Endoscopic	**Z** No Device	**Z** No Qualifier

No Procedure Combinations Specified
⊞ ØMQ[N,P,S,T][Ø,3,4]ZZ

Ø Medical and Surgical
M Bursae and Ligaments
S Reposition Moving to its normal location or other suitable location all or a portion of a body part

Body Part Character 4	Approach Character 5	Device Character 6	Qualifier Character 7
Ø Head and Neck Bursa and Ligament **1** Shoulder Bursa and Ligament, Right **2** Shoulder Bursa and Ligament, Left **3** Elbow Bursa and Ligament, Right **4** Elbow Bursa and Ligament, Left **5** Wrist Bursa and Ligament, Right **6** Wrist Bursa and Ligament, Left **7** Hand Bursa and Ligament, Right **8** Hand Bursa and Ligament, Left **9** Upper Extremity Bursa and Ligament, Right **B** Upper Extremity Bursa and Ligament, Left **C** Trunk Bursa and Ligament, Right **D** Trunk Bursa and Ligament, Left **F** Thorax Bursa and Ligament, Right **G** Thorax Bursa and Ligament, Left **H** Abdomen Bursa and Ligament, Right **J** Abdomen Bursa and Ligament, Left **K** Perineum Bursa and Ligament **L** Hip Bursa and Ligament, Right **M** Hip Bursa and Ligament, Left **N** Knee Bursa and Ligament, Right **P** Knee Bursa and Ligament, Left **Q** Ankle Bursa and Ligament, Right **R** Ankle Bursa and Ligament, Left **S** Foot Bursa and Ligament, Right **T** Foot Bursa and Ligament, Left **V** Lower Extremity Bursa and Ligament, Right **W** Lower Extremity Bursa and Ligament, Left	**Ø** Open **4** Percutaneous Endoscopic	**Z** No Device	**Z** No Qualifier

Ø Medical and Surgical
M Bursae and Ligaments
T Resection Cutting out or off, without replacement, all of a body part

Body Part Character 4	Approach Character 5	Device Character 6	Qualifier Character 7
Ø Head and Neck Bursa and Ligament 1 Shoulder Bursa and Ligament, Right 2 Shoulder Bursa and Ligament, Left 3 Elbow Bursa and Ligament, Right 4 Elbow Bursa and Ligament, Left 5 Wrist Bursa and Ligament, Right 6 Wrist Bursa and Ligament, Left 7 Hand Bursa and Ligament, Right 8 Hand Bursa and Ligament, Left 9 Upper Extremity Bursa and Ligament, Right B Upper Extremity Bursa and Ligament, Left C Trunk Bursa and Ligament, Right D Trunk Bursa and Ligament, Left F Thorax Bursa and Ligament, Right G Thorax Bursa and Ligament, Left H Abdomen Bursa and Ligament, Right J Abdomen Bursa and Ligament, Left K Perineum Bursa and Ligament L Hip Bursa and Ligament, Right M Hip Bursa and Ligament, Left N Knee Bursa and Ligament, Right P Knee Bursa and Ligament, Left Q Ankle Bursa and Ligament, Right R Ankle Bursa and Ligament, Left S Foot Bursa and Ligament, Right T Foot Bursa and Ligament, Left V Lower Extremity Bursa and Ligament, Right W Lower Extremity Bursa and Ligament, Left	Ø Open 4 Percutaneous Endoscopic	Z No Device	Z No Qualifier

Ø Medical and Surgical
M Bursae and Ligaments
U Supplement Putting in or on biological or synthetic material that physically reinforces and/or augments the function of a portion of a body part

Body Part Character 4	Approach Character 5	Device Character 6	Qualifier Character 7
Ø Head and Neck Bursa and Ligament 1 Shoulder Bursa and Ligament, Right 2 Shoulder Bursa and Ligament, Left 3 Elbow Bursa and Ligament, Right 4 Elbow Bursa and Ligament, Left 5 Wrist Bursa and Ligament, Right 6 Wrist Bursa and Ligament, Left 7 Hand Bursa and Ligament, Right 8 Hand Bursa and Ligament, Left 9 Upper Extremity Bursa and Ligament, Right B Upper Extremity Bursa and Ligament, Left C Trunk Bursa and Ligament, Right D Trunk Bursa and Ligament, Left F Thorax Bursa and Ligament, Right G Thorax Bursa and Ligament, Left H Abdomen Bursa and Ligament, Right J Abdomen Bursa and Ligament, Left K Perineum Bursa and Ligament L Hip Bursa and Ligament, Right M Hip Bursa and Ligament, Left N Knee Bursa and Ligament, Right P Knee Bursa and Ligament, Left Q Ankle Bursa and Ligament, Right R Ankle Bursa and Ligament, Left S Foot Bursa and Ligament, Right T Foot Bursa and Ligament, Left V Lower Extremity Bursa and Ligament, Right W Lower Extremity Bursa and Ligament, Left	Ø Open 4 Percutaneous Endoscopic	7 Autologous Tissue Substitute J Synthetic Substitute K Nonautologous Tissue Substitute	Z No Qualifier

Ø Medical and Surgical
M Bursae and Ligaments
W Revision Correcting, to the extent possible, a portion of a malfunctioning device or the position of a displaced device

Body Part Character 4	Approach Character 5	Device Character 6	Qualifier Character 7
X Upper Bursa and Ligament **Y** Lower Bursa and Ligament	**Ø** Open **3** Percutaneous **4** Percutaneous Endoscopic **X** External	**Ø** Drainage Device **7** Autologous Tissue Substitute **J** Synthetic Substitute **K** Nonautologous Tissue Substitute	**Z** No Qualifier

Non-OR ØMW[X,Y]X[Ø,7,J,K]Z

Ø Medical and Surgical
M Bursae and Ligaments
X Transfer Moving, without taking out, all or a portion of a body part to another location to take over the function of all or a portion of a body part

Body Part Character 4	Approach Character 5	Device Character 6	Qualifier Character 7
Ø Head and Neck Bursa and Ligament **1** Shoulder Bursa and Ligament, Right **2** Shoulder Bursa and Ligament, Left **3** Elbow Bursa and Ligament, Right **4** Elbow Bursa and Ligament, Left **5** Wrist Bursa and Ligament, Right **6** Wrist Bursa and Ligament, Left **7** Hand Bursa and Ligament, Right **8** Hand Bursa and Ligament, Left **9** Upper Extremity Bursa and Ligament, Right **B** Upper Extremity Bursa and Ligament, Left **C** Trunk Bursa and Ligament, Right **D** Trunk Bursa and Ligament, Left **F** Thorax Bursa and Ligament, Right **G** Thorax Bursa and Ligament, Left **H** Abdomen Bursa and Ligament, Right **J** Abdomen Bursa and Ligament, Left **K** Perineum Bursa and Ligament **L** Hip Bursa and Ligament, Right **M** Hip Bursa and Ligament, Left **N** Knee Bursa and Ligament, Right **P** Knee Bursa and Ligament, Left **Q** Ankle Bursa and Ligament, Right **R** Ankle Bursa and Ligament, Left **S** Foot Bursa and Ligament, Right **T** Foot Bursa and Ligament, Left **V** Lower Extremity Bursa and Ligament, Right **W** Lower Extremity Bursa and Ligament, Left	**Ø** Open **4** Percutaneous Endoscopic	**Z** No Device	**Z** No Qualifier

Head and Facial Bones 0N2–0NW

0 Medical and Surgical
N Head and Facial Bones
2 Change Taking out or off a device from a body part and putting back an identical or similar device in or on the same body part without cutting or puncturing the skin or a mucous membrane

Body Part Character 4	Approach Character 5	Device Character 6	Qualifier Character 7
0 Skull B Nasal Bone W Facial Bone	X External	0 Drainage Device Y Other Device	Z No Qualifier

Non-OR For all body part, approach, device, and qualifier values

0 Medical and Surgical
N Head and Facial Bones
5 Destruction Physical eradication of all or a portion of a body part by the direct use of energy, force, or a destructive agent

Body Part Character 4	Approach Character 5	Device Character 6	Qualifier Character 7
0 Skull 1 Frontal Bone, Right 2 Frontal Bone, Left 3 Parietal Bone, Right 4 Parietal Bone, Left 5 Temporal Bone, Right 6 Temporal Bone, Left 7 Occipital Bone, Right 8 Occipital Bone, Left B Nasal Bone C Sphenoid Bone, Right D Sphenoid Bone, Left F Ethmoid Bone, Right G Ethmoid Bone, Left H Lacrimal Bone, Right J Lacrimal Bone, Left K Palatine Bone, Right L Palatine Bone, Left M Zygomatic Bone, Right N Zygomatic Bone, Left P Orbit, Right Q Orbit, Left R Maxilla, Right S Maxilla, Left T Mandible, Right V Mandible, Left X Hyoid Bone	0 Open 3 Percutaneous 4 Percutaneous Endoscopic	Z No Device	Z No Qualifier

Ø Medical and Surgical
N Head and Facial Bones
8 Division Cutting into a body part without draining fluids and/or gases from the body part in order to separate or transect a body part

Body Part Character 4	Approach Character 5	Device Character 6	Qualifier Character 7
Ø Skull **1** Frontal Bone, Right **2** Frontal Bone, Left **3** Parietal Bone, Right **4** Parietal Bone, Left **5** Temporal Bone, Right **6** Temporal Bone, Left **7** Occipital Bone, Right **8** Occipital Bone, Left **B** Nasal Bone **C** Sphenoid Bone, Right **D** Sphenoid Bone, Left **F** Ethmoid Bone, Right **G** Ethmoid Bone, Left **H** Lacrimal Bone, Right **J** Lacrimal Bone, Left **K** Palatine Bone, Right **L** Palatine Bone, Left **M** Zygomatic Bone, Right **N** Zygomatic Bone, Left **P** Orbit, Right **Q** Orbit, Left **R** Maxilla, Right **S** Maxilla, Left **T** Mandible, Right **V** Mandible, Left **X** Hyoid Bone	**Ø** Open **3** Percutaneous **4** Percutaneous Endoscopic	**Z** No Device	**Z** No Qualifier

Non-OR ØN8B[Ø,3,4]ZZ

Ø Medical and Surgical
N Head and Facial Bones
9 Drainage Taking or letting out fluids and/or gases from a body part

Body Part Character 4	Approach Character 5	Device Character 6	Qualifier Character 7
Ø Skull 1 Frontal Bone, Right 2 Frontal Bone, Left 3 Parietal Bone, Right 4 Parietal Bone, Left 5 Temporal Bone, Right 6 Temporal Bone, Left 7 Occipital Bone, Right 8 Occipital Bone, Left B Nasal Bone C Sphenoid Bone, Right D Sphenoid Bone, Left F Ethmoid Bone, Right G Ethmoid Bone, Left H Lacrimal Bone, Right J Lacrimal Bone, Left K Palatine Bone, Right L Palatine Bone, Left M Zygomatic Bone, Right N Zygomatic Bone, Left P Orbit, Right Q Orbit, Left R Maxilla, Right S Maxilla, Left T Mandible, Right V Mandible, Left X Hyoid Bone	Ø Open 3 Percutaneous 4 Percutaneous Endoscopic	Ø Drainage Device	Z No Qualifier
Ø Skull 1 Frontal Bone, Right 2 Frontal Bone, Left 3 Parietal Bone, Right 4 Parietal Bone, Left 5 Temporal Bone, Right 6 Temporal Bone, Left 7 Occipital Bone, Right 8 Occipital Bone, Left B Nasal Bone C Sphenoid Bone, Right D Sphenoid Bone, Left F Ethmoid Bone, Right G Ethmoid Bone, Left H Lacrimal Bone, Right J Lacrimal Bone, Left K Palatine Bone, Right L Palatine Bone, Left M Zygomatic Bone, Right N Zygomatic Bone, Left P Orbit, Right Q Orbit, Left R Maxilla, Right S Maxilla, Left T Mandible, Right V Mandible, Left X Hyoid Bone	Ø Open 3 Percutaneous 4 Percutaneous Endoscopic	Z No Device	X Diagnostic Z No Qualifier

Non-OR ØN9[B,R,S,T,V][Ø,3,4]ØZ
Non-OR ØN9B[Ø,3,4]ZX
Non-OR ØN9[B,R,S,T,V][Ø,3,4]ZZ

Ø Medical and Surgical
N Head and Facial Bones
B Excision Cutting out or off, without replacement, a portion of a body part

Body Part Character 4	Approach Character 5	Device Character 6	Qualifier Character 7
Ø Skull **1** Frontal Bone, Right **2** Frontal Bone, Left **3** Parietal Bone, Right **4** Parietal Bone, Left **5** Temporal Bone, Right **6** Temporal Bone, Left **7** Occipital Bone, Right **8** Occipital Bone, Left **B** Nasal Bone **C** Sphenoid Bone, Right **D** Sphenoid Bone, Left **F** Ethmoid Bone, Right **G** Ethmoid Bone, Left **H** Lacrimal Bone, Right **J** Lacrimal Bone, Left **K** Palatine Bone, Right **L** Palatine Bone, Left **M** Zygomatic Bone, Right **N** Zygomatic Bone, Left **P** Orbit, Right ⊞ **Q** Orbit, Left ⊞ **R** Maxilla, Right ⊞ **S** Maxilla, Left ⊞ **T** Mandible, Right **V** Mandible, Left **X** Hyoid Bone	**Ø** Open **3** Percutaneous **4** Percutaneous Endoscopic	**Z** No Device	**X** Diagnostic **Z** No Qualifier

Non-OR ØNB[B,R,S,T,V][Ø,3,4]ZX

No Procedure Combinations Specified
⊞ ØNB[P,Q][Ø,3,4]ZZ
⊞ ØNB[R,S][Ø,4]ZZ

Ø Medical and Surgical
N Head and Facial Bones
C Extirpation Taking or cutting out solid matter from a body part

Body Part Character 4	Approach Character 5	Device Character 6	Qualifier Character 7
1 Frontal Bone, Right **2** Frontal Bone, Left **3** Parietal Bone, Right **4** Parietal Bone, Left **5** Temporal Bone, Right **6** Temporal Bone, Left **7** Occipital Bone, Right **8** Occipital Bone, Left **B** Nasal Bone **C** Sphenoid Bone, Right **D** Sphenoid Bone, Left **F** Ethmoid Bone, Right **G** Ethmoid Bone, Left **H** Lacrimal Bone, Right **J** Lacrimal Bone, Left **K** Palatine Bone, Right **L** Palatine Bone, Left **M** Zygomatic Bone, Right **N** Zygomatic Bone, Left **P** Orbit, Right **Q** Orbit, Left **R** Maxilla, Right **S** Maxilla, Left **T** Mandible, Right **V** Mandible, Left **X** Hyoid Bone	**Ø** Open **3** Percutaneous **4** Percutaneous Endoscopic	**Z** No Device	**Z** No Qualifier

Non-OR ØNC[B,R,S,T,V][Ø,3,4]ZZ

Ø Medical and Surgical
N Head and Facial Bones
H Insertion Putting in a nonbiological appliance that monitors, assists, performs, or prevents a physiological function but does not physically take the place of a body part

Body Part Character 4	Approach Character 5	Device Character 6	Qualifier Character 7
Ø Skull ⊞	**Ø** Open	**4** Internal Fixation Device **5** External Fixation Device **M** Bone Growth Stimulator **N** Neurostimulator Generator	**Z** No Qualifier
Ø Skull	**3** Percutaneous **4** Percutaneous Endoscopic	**4** Internal Fixation Device **5** External Fixation Device **M** Bone Growth Stimulator	**Z** No Qualifier
1 Frontal Bone, Right **2** Frontal Bone, Left **3** Parietal Bone, Right **4** Parietal Bone, Left **7** Occipital Bone, Right **8** Occipital Bone, Left **C** Sphenoid Bone, Right **D** Sphenoid Bone, Left **F** Ethmoid Bone, Right **G** Ethmoid Bone, Left **H** Lacrimal Bone, Right **J** Lacrimal Bone, Left **K** Palatine Bone, Right **L** Palatine Bone, Left **M** Zygomatic Bone, Right **N** Zygomatic Bone, Left **P** Orbit, Right **Q** Orbit, Left **X** Hyoid Bone	**Ø** Open **3** Percutaneous **4** Percutaneous Endoscopic	**4** Internal Fixation Device	**Z** No Qualifier
5 Temporal Bone, Right **6** Temporal Bone, Left	**Ø** Open **3** Percutaneous **4** Percutaneous Endoscopic	**4** Internal Fixation Device **S** Hearing Device	**Z** No Qualifier
B Nasal Bone	**Ø** Open **3** Percutaneous **4** Percutaneous Endoscopic	**4** Internal Fixation Device **M** Bone Growth Stimulator	**Z** No Qualifier
R Maxilla, Right **S** Maxilla, Left **T** Mandible, Right **V** Mandible, Left	**Ø** Open **3** Percutaneous **4** Percutaneous Endoscopic	**4** Internal Fixation Device **5** External Fixation Device	**Z** No Qualifier
W Facial Bone	**Ø** Open **3** Percutaneous **4** Percutaneous Endoscopic	**M** Bone Growth Stimulator	**Z** No Qualifier

Non-OR ØNHØØ5Z
Non-OR ØNHØ[3,4]5Z
Non-OR ØNHB[Ø,3,4][4,M]Z

See Appendix I for Procedure Combinations
⊞ ØNHØØNZ

Ø Medical and Surgical
N Head and Facial Bones
J Inspection Visually and/or manually exploring a body part

Body Part Character 4	Approach Character 5	Device Character 6	Qualifier Character 7
Ø Skull **B** Nasal Bone **W** Facial Bone	**Ø** Open **3** Percutaneous **4** Percutaneous Endoscopic **X** External	**Z** No Device	**Z** No Qualifier

Non-OR ØNJ[Ø,B,W]XZZ

Ø Medical and Surgical
N Head and Facial Bones
N Release Freeing a body part from an abnormal physical constraint

Body Part Character 4	Approach Character 5	Device Character 6	Qualifier Character 7
1 Frontal Bone, Right **2** Frontal Bone, Left **3** Parietal Bone, Right **4** Parietal Bone, Left **5** Temporal Bone, Right **6** Temporal Bone, Left **7** Occipital Bone, Right **8** Occipital Bone, Left **B** Nasal Bone **C** Sphenoid Bone, Right **D** Sphenoid Bone, Left **F** Ethmoid Bone, Right **G** Ethmoid Bone, Left **H** Lacrimal Bone, Right **J** Lacrimal Bone, Left **K** Palatine Bone, Right **L** Palatine Bone, Left **M** Zygomatic Bone, Right **N** Zygomatic Bone, Left **P** Orbit, Right **Q** Orbit, Left **R** Maxilla, Right **S** Maxilla, Left **T** Mandible, Right **V** Mandible, Left **X** Hyoid Bone	**Ø** Open **3** Percutaneous **4** Percutaneous Endoscopic	**Z** No Device	**Z** No Qualifier

Non-OR ØNNB[Ø,3,4]ZZ

Ø Medical and Surgical
N Head and Facial Bones
P Removal Taking out or off a device from a body part

Body Part Character 4	Approach Character 5	Device Character 6	Qualifier Character 7
Ø Skull	**Ø** Open	**Ø** Drainage Device **4** Internal Fixation Device **5** External Fixation Device **7** Autologous Tissue Substitute **J** Synthetic Substitute **K** Nonautologous Tissue Substitute **M** Bone Growth Stimulator **N** Neurostimulator Generator **S** Hearing Device	**Z** No Qualifier
Ø Skull	**3** Percutaneous **4** Percutaneous Endoscopic	**Ø** Drainage Device **4** Internal Fixation Device **5** External Fixation Device **7** Autologous Tissue Substitute **J** Synthetic Substitute **K** Nonautologous Tissue Substitute **M** Bone Growth Stimulator **S** Hearing Device	**Z** No Qualifier
Ø Skull	**X** External	**Ø** Drainage Device **4** Internal Fixation Device **5** External Fixation Device **M** Bone Growth Stimulator **S** Hearing Device	**Z** No Qualifier
B Nasal Bone **W** Facial Bone	**Ø** Open **3** Percutaneous **4** Percutaneous Endoscopic	**Ø** Drainage Device **4** Internal Fixation Device **7** Autologous Tissue Substitute **J** Synthetic Substitute **K** Nonautologous Tissue Substitute **M** Bone Growth Stimulator	**Z** No Qualifier
B Nasal Bone **W** Facial Bone	**X** External	**Ø** Drainage Device **4** Internal Fixation Device **M** Bone Growth Stimulator	**Z** No Qualifier

Non-OR ØNPØ[3,4]5Z
Non-OR ØNPØX[Ø,5]Z
Non-OR ØNPB[Ø,3,4][Ø,4,7,J,K,M]Z
Non-OR ØNPBX[Ø,4,M]Z
Non-OR ØNPWX[Ø,M]Z

Ø Medical and Surgical
N Head and Facial Bones
Q Repair Restoring, to the extent possible, a body part to its normal anatomic structure and function

Body Part Character 4	Approach Character 5	Device Character 6	Qualifier Character 7
Ø Skull **1** Frontal Bone, Right **2** Frontal Bone, Left **3** Parietal Bone, Right **4** Parietal Bone, Left **5** Temporal Bone, Right **6** Temporal Bone, Left **7** Occipital Bone, Right **8** Occipital Bone, Left **B** Nasal Bone **C** Sphenoid Bone, Right **D** Sphenoid Bone, Left **F** Ethmoid Bone, Right **G** Ethmoid Bone, Left **H** Lacrimal Bone, Right **J** Lacrimal Bone, Left **K** Palatine Bone, Right **L** Palatine Bone, Left **M** Zygomatic Bone, Right **N** Zygomatic Bone, Left **P** Orbit, Right **Q** Orbit, Left **R** Maxilla, Right **S** Maxilla, Left **T** Mandible, Right **V** Mandible, Left **X** Hyoid Bone	**Ø** Open **3** Percutaneous **4** Percutaneous Endoscopic **X** External	**Z** No Device	**Z** No Qualifier

Ø Medical and Surgical
N Head and Facial Bones
R Replacement Putting in or on biological or synthetic material that physically takes the place and/or function of all or a portion of a body part

Body Part Character 4	Approach Character 5	Device Character 6	Qualifier Character 7
Ø Skull **1** Frontal Bone, Right **2** Frontal Bone, Left **3** Parietal Bone, Right **4** Parietal Bone, Left **5** Temporal Bone, Right **6** Temporal Bone, Left **7** Occipital Bone, Right **8** Occipital Bone, Left **B** Nasal Bone **C** Sphenoid Bone, Right **D** Sphenoid Bone, Left **F** Ethmoid Bone, Right **G** Ethmoid Bone, Left **H** Lacrimal Bone, Right **J** Lacrimal Bone, Left **K** Palatine Bone, Right **L** Palatine Bone, Left **M** Zygomatic Bone, Right **N** Zygomatic Bone, Left **P** Orbit, Right **Q** Orbit, Left **R** Maxilla, Right **S** Maxilla, Left **T** Mandible, Right **V** Mandible, Left **X** Hyoid Bone	**Ø** Open **3** Percutaneous **4** Percutaneous Endoscopic	**7** Autologous Tissue Substitute **J** Synthetic Substitute **K** Nonautologous Tissue Substitute	**Z** No Qualifier

Ø Medical and Surgical
N Head and Facial Bones
S Reposition Moving to its normal location or other suitable location all or a portion of a body part

Body Part Character 4	Approach Character 5	Device Character 6	Qualifier Character 7
1 Frontal Bone, Right 2 Frontal Bone, Left 3 Parietal Bone, Right 4 Parietal Bone, Left 5 Temporal Bone, Right 6 Temporal Bone, Left 7 Occipital Bone, Right 8 Occipital Bone, Left B Nasal Bone C Sphenoid Bone, Right D Sphenoid Bone, Left F Ethmoid Bone, Right G Ethmoid Bone, Left H Lacrimal Bone, Right J Lacrimal Bone, Left K Palatine Bone, Right L Palatine Bone, Left M Zygomatic Bone, Right N Zygomatic Bone, Left P Orbit, Right Q Orbit, Left X Hyoid Bone	X External	Z No Device	Z No Qualifier
Ø Skull R Maxilla, Right S Maxilla, Left T Mandible, Right V Mandible, Left	Ø Open 3 Percutaneous 4 Percutaneous Endoscopic	4 Internal Fixation Device 5 External Fixation Device Z No Device	Z No Qualifier
Ø Skull R Maxilla, Right S Maxilla, Left T Mandible, Right V Mandible, Left	X External	Z No Device	Z No Qualifier
1 Frontal Bone, Right 2 Frontal Bone, Left 3 Parietal Bone, Right 4 Parietal Bone, Left 5 Temporal Bone, Right 6 Temporal Bone, Left 7 Occipital Bone, Right 8 Occipital Bone, Left B Nasal Bone C Sphenoid Bone, Right D Sphenoid Bone, Left F Ethmoid Bone, Right G Ethmoid Bone, Left H Lacrimal Bone, Right J Lacrimal Bone, Left K Palatine Bone, Right L Palatine Bone, Left M Zygomatic Bone, Right N Zygomatic Bone, Left P Orbit, Right Q Orbit, Left X Hyoid Bone	Ø Open 3 Percutaneous 4 Percutaneous Endoscopic	4 Internal Fixation Device Z No Device	Z No Qualifier

Non-OR ØNS[B,C,D,F,G,H,J,K,L,M,N,P,Q,X]XZZ
Non-OR ØNS[R,S,T,V][3,4][4,5,Z]Z
Non-OR ØNS[R,S,T,V]XZZ
Non-OR ØNS[B,C,D,F,G,H,J,K,L,M,N,P,Q,X][3,4][4,Z]Z
AHA: 2Ø13, 3Q, 24-25

0 Medical and Surgical
N Head and Facial Bones
T Resection Cutting out or off, without replacement, all of a body part

Body Part Character 4	Approach Character 5	Device Character 6	Qualifier Character 7
1 Frontal Bone, Right 2 Frontal Bone, Left 3 Parietal Bone, Right 4 Parietal Bone, Left 5 Temporal Bone, Right 6 Temporal Bone, Left 7 Occipital Bone, Right 8 Occipital Bone, Left B Nasal Bone C Sphenoid Bone, Right D Sphenoid Bone, Left F Ethmoid Bone, Right G Ethmoid Bone, Left H Lacrimal Bone, Right J Lacrimal Bone, Left K Palatine Bone, Right L Palatine Bone, Left M Zygomatic Bone, Right N Zygomatic Bone, Left P Orbit, Right Q Orbit, Left R Maxilla, Right S Maxilla, Left T Mandible, Right V Mandible, Left X Hyoid Bone	0 Open	Z No Device	Z No Qualifier

0 Medical and Surgical
N Head and Facial Bones
U Supplement Putting in or on biological or synthetic material that physically reinforces and/or augments the function of a portion of a body part

Body Part Character 4	Approach Character 5	Device Character 6	Qualifier Character 7
0 Skull 1 Frontal Bone, Right 2 Frontal Bone, Left 3 Parietal Bone, Right 4 Parietal Bone, Left 5 Temporal Bone, Right 6 Temporal Bone, Left 7 Occipital Bone, Right 8 Occipital Bone, Left B Nasal Bone C Sphenoid Bone, Right D Sphenoid Bone, Left F Ethmoid Bone, Right G Ethmoid Bone, Left H Lacrimal Bone, Right J Lacrimal Bone, Left K Palatine Bone, Right L Palatine Bone, Left M Zygomatic Bone, Right N Zygomatic Bone, Left P Orbit, Right Q Orbit, Left R Maxilla, Right S Maxilla, Left T Mandible, Right V Mandible, Left X Hyoid Bone	0 Open 3 Percutaneous 4 Percutaneous Endoscopic	7 Autologous Tissue Substitute J Synthetic Substitute K Nonautologous Tissue Substitute	Z No Qualifier

AHA: 2013, 3Q, 24

Ø Medical and Surgical
N Head and Facial Bones
W Revision Correcting, to the extent possible, a portion of a malfunctioning device or the position of a displaced device

Body Part Character 4	Approach Character 5	Device Character 6	Qualifier Character 7
Ø Skull	**Ø** Open	**Ø** Drainage Device **4** Internal Fixation Device **5** External Fixation Device **7** Autologous Tissue Substitute **J** Synthetic Substitute **K** Nonautologous Tissue Substitute **M** Bone Growth Stimulator **N** Neurostimulator Generator **S** Hearing Device	**Z** No Qualifier
Ø Skull	**3** Percutaneous **4** Percutaneous Endoscopic **X** External	**Ø** Drainage Device **4** Internal Fixation Device **5** External Fixation Device **7** Autologous Tissue Substitute **J** Synthetic Substitute **K** Nonautologous Tissue Substitute **M** Bone Growth Stimulator **S** Hearing Device	**Z** No Qualifier
B Nasal Bone **W** Facial Bone	**Ø** Open **3** Percutaneous **4** Percutaneous Endoscopic **X** External	**Ø** Drainage Device **4** Internal Fixation Device **7** Autologous Tissue Substitute **J** Synthetic Substitute **K** Nonautologous Tissue Substitute **M** Bone Growth Stimulator	**Z** No Qualifier

Non-OR ØNWØX[Ø,4,5,7,J,K,M,S]Z
Non-OR ØNWB[Ø,3,4,X][Ø,4,7,J,K,M]Z
Non-OR ØNWWX[Ø,4,7,J,K,M]Z

Upper Bones 0P2–0PW

0 Medical and Surgical
P Upper Bones
2 Change Taking out or off a device from a body part and putting back an identical or similar device in or on the same body part without cutting or puncturing the skin or a mucous membrane

Body Part Character 4	Approach Character 5	Device Character 6	Qualifier Character 7
Y Upper Bone	X External	0 Drainage Device Y Other Device	Z No Qualifier

Non-OR For all body part, approach, device, and qualifier values

0 Medical and Surgical
P Upper Bones
5 Destruction Physical eradication of all or a portion of a body part by the direct use of energy, force, or a destructive agent

Body Part Character 4	Approach Character 5	Device Character 6	Qualifier Character 7
0 Sternum 1 Rib, Right 2 Rib, Left 3 Cervical Vertebra 4 Thoracic Vertebra 5 Scapula, Right 6 Scapula, Left 7 Glenoid Cavity, Right 8 Glenoid Cavity, Left 9 Clavicle, Right B Clavicle, Left C Humeral Head, Right D Humeral Head, Left F Humeral Shaft, Right G Humeral Shaft, Left H Radius, Right J Radius, Left K Ulna, Right L Ulna, Left M Carpal, Right N Carpal, Left P Metacarpal, Right Q Metacarpal, Left R Thumb Phalanx, Right S Thumb Phalanx, Left T Finger Phalanx, Right V Finger Phalanx, Left	0 Open 3 Percutaneous 4 Percutaneous Endoscopic	Z No Device	Z No Qualifier

0 Medical and Surgical
P Upper Bones
8 Division Cutting into a body part without draining fluids and/or gases from the body part in order to separate or transect a body part

Body Part Character 4	Approach Character 5	Device Character 6	Qualifier Character 7
0 Sternum 1 Rib, Right 2 Rib, Left 3 Cervical Vertebra 4 Thoracic Vertebra 5 Scapula, Right 6 Scapula, Left 7 Glenoid Cavity, Right 8 Glenoid Cavity, Left 9 Clavicle, Right B Clavicle, Left C Humeral Head, Right D Humeral Head, Left F Humeral Shaft, Right ⊞ G Humeral Shaft, Left ⊞ H Radius, Right ⊞ J Radius, Left ⊞ K Ulna, Right ⊞ L Ulna, Left ⊞ M Carpal, Right ⊞ N Carpal, Left ⊞ P Metacarpal, Right ⊞ Q Metacarpal, Left ⊞ R Thumb Phalanx, Right S Thumb Phalanx, Left T Finger Phalanx, Right ⊞ V Finger Phalanx, Left ⊞	0 Open 3 Percutaneous 4 Percutaneous Endoscopic	Z No Device	Z No Qualifier

No Procedure Combinations Specified
⊞ 0P8[F,G,H,J,K,L,M,N,P,Q,T,V][0,3,4]ZZ

Ø Medical and Surgical
P Upper Bones
9 Drainage Taking or letting out fluids and/or gases from a body part

Body Part Character 4	Approach Character 5	Device Character 6	Qualifier Character 7
Ø Sternum **1** Rib, Right **2** Rib, Left **3** Cervical Vertebra **4** Thoracic Vertebra **5** Scapula, Right **6** Scapula, Left **7** Glenoid Cavity, Right **8** Glenoid Cavity, Left **9** Clavicle, Right **B** Clavicle, Left **C** Humeral Head, Right **D** Humeral Head, Left **F** Humeral Shaft, Right **G** Humeral Shaft, Left **H** Radius, Right **J** Radius, Left **K** Ulna, Right **L** Ulna, Left **M** Carpal, Right **N** Carpal, Left **P** Metacarpal, Right **Q** Metacarpal, Left **R** Thumb Phalanx, Right **S** Thumb Phalanx, Left **T** Finger Phalanx, Right **V** Finger Phalanx, Left	**Ø** Open **3** Percutaneous **4** Percutaneous Endoscopic	**Ø** Drainage Device	**Z** No Qualifier
Ø Sternum **1** Rib, Right **2** Rib, Left **3** Cervical Vertebra **4** Thoracic Vertebra **5** Scapula, Right **6** Scapula, Left **7** Glenoid Cavity, Right **8** Glenoid Cavity, Left **9** Clavicle, Right **B** Clavicle, Left **C** Humeral Head, Right **D** Humeral Head, Left **F** Humeral Shaft, Right **G** Humeral Shaft, Left **H** Radius, Right **J** Radius, Left **K** Ulna, Right **L** Ulna, Left **M** Carpal, Right **N** Carpal, Left **P** Metacarpal, Right **Q** Metacarpal, Left **R** Thumb Phalanx, Right **S** Thumb Phalanx, Left **T** Finger Phalanx, Right **V** Finger Phalanx, Left	**Ø** Open **3** Percutaneous **4** Percutaneous Endoscopic	**Z** No Device	**X** Diagnostic **Z** No Qualifier

Ø Medical and Surgical
P Upper Bones
B Excision Cutting out or off, without replacement, a portion of a body part

Body Part Character 4	Approach Character 5	Device Character 6	Qualifier Character 7
Ø Sternum 1 Rib, Right ⊞ 2 Rib, Left ⊞ 3 Cervical Vertebra 4 Thoracic Vertebra 5 Scapula, Right 6 Scapula, Left 7 Glenoid Cavity, Right 8 Glenoid Cavity, Left 9 Clavicle, Right B Clavicle, Left C Humeral Head, Right D Humeral Head, Left F Humeral Shaft, Right G Humeral Shaft, Left H Radius, Right J Radius, Left K Ulna, Right L Ulna, Left M Carpal, Right N Carpal, Left P Metacarpal, Right Q Metacarpal, Left R Thumb Phalanx, Right S Thumb Phalanx, Left T Finger Phalanx, Right V Finger Phalanx, Left	Ø Open 3 Percutaneous 4 Percutaneous Endoscopic	Z No Device	X Diagnostic Z No Qualifier

AHA: 2013, 4Q, 109; 2013, 3Q, 20; 2012, 4Q, 101

No Procedure Combinations Specified
⊞ ØPB[1,2]ØZZ

Ø Medical and Surgical
P Upper Bones
C Extirpation Taking or cutting out solid matter from a body part

Body Part Character 4	Approach Character 5	Device Character 6	Qualifier Character 7
Ø Sternum 1 Rib, Right 2 Rib, Left 3 Cervical Vertebra 4 Thoracic Vertebra 5 Scapula, Right 6 Scapula, Left 7 Glenoid Cavity, Right 8 Glenoid Cavity, Left 9 Clavicle, Right B Clavicle, Left C Humeral Head, Right D Humeral Head, Left F Humeral Shaft, Right G Humeral Shaft, Left H Radius, Right J Radius, Left K Ulna, Right L Ulna, Left M Carpal, Right N Carpal, Left P Metacarpal, Right Q Metacarpal, Left R Thumb Phalanx, Right S Thumb Phalanx, Left T Finger Phalanx, Right V Finger Phalanx, Left	Ø Open 3 Percutaneous 4 Percutaneous Endoscopic	Z No Device	Z No Qualifier

Ø Medical and Surgical
P Upper Bones
H Insertion Putting in a nonbiological appliance that monitors, assists, performs, or prevents a physiological function but does not physically take the place of a body part

Body Part Character 4	Approach Character 5	Device Character 6	Qualifier Character 7
Ø Sternum	**Ø** Open **3** Percutaneous **4** Percutaneous Endoscopic	**Ø** Internal Fixation Device, Rigid Plate **4** Internal Fixation Device	**Z** No Qualifier
1 Rib, Right **2** Rib, Left **3** Cervical Vertebra **4** Thoracic Vertebra **5** Scapula, Right **6** Scapula, Left **7** Glenoid Cavity, Right **8** Glenoid Cavity, Left **9** Clavicle, Right **B** Clavicle, Left	**Ø** Open **3** Percutaneous **4** Percutaneous Endoscopic	**4** Internal Fixation Device	**Z** No Qualifier
C Humeral Head, Right **D** Humeral Head, Left **F** Humeral Shaft, Right **G** Humeral Shaft, Left **H** Radius, Right **J** Radius, Left **K** Ulna, Right **L** Ulna, Left	**Ø** Open **3** Percutaneous **4** Percutaneous Endoscopic	**4** Internal Fixation Device **5** External Fixation Device **6** Internal Fixation Device, Intramedullary **8** External Fixation Device, Limb Lengthening **B** External Fixation Device, Monoplanar **C** External Fixation Device, Ring **D** External Fixation Device, Hybrid	**Z** No Qualifier
M Carpal, Right **N** Carpal, Left **P** Metacarpal, Right **Q** Metacarpal, Left **R** Thumb Phalanx, Right **S** Thumb Phalanx, Left **T** Finger Phalanx, Right **V** Finger Phalanx, Left	**Ø** Open **3** Percutaneous **4** Percutaneous Endoscopic	**4** Internal Fixation Device **5** External Fixation Device	**Z** No Qualifier
Y Upper Bone	**Ø** Open **3** Percutaneous **4** Percutaneous Endoscopic	**M** Bone Growth Stimulator	**Z** No Qualifier

Non-OR ØPH[C,D,F,G,H,J,K,L][Ø,3,4]8Z

Ø Medical and Surgical
P Upper Bones
J Inspection Visually and/or manually exploring a body part

Body Part Character 4	Approach Character 5	Device Character 6	Qualifier Character 7
Y Upper Bone	**Ø** Open **3** Percutaneous **4** Percutaneous Endoscopic **X** External	**Z** No Device	**Z** No Qualifier

Non-OR ØPJYXZZ

Ø Medical and Surgical
P Upper Bones
N Release Freeing a body part from an abnormal physical constraint

Body Part Character 4	Approach Character 5	Device Character 6	Qualifier Character 7
Ø Sternum **1** Rib, Right **2** Rib, Left **3** Cervical Vertebra **4** Thoracic Vertebra **5** Scapula, Right **6** Scapula, Left **7** Glenoid Cavity, Right **8** Glenoid Cavity, Left **9** Clavicle, Right **B** Clavicle, Left **C** Humeral Head, Right **D** Humeral Head, Left **F** Humeral Shaft, Right **G** Humeral Shaft, Left **H** Radius, Right **J** Radius, Left **K** Ulna, Right **L** Ulna, Left **M** Carpal, Right **N** Carpal, Left **P** Metacarpal, Right **Q** Metacarpal, Left **R** Thumb Phalanx, Right **S** Thumb Phalanx, Left **T** Finger Phalanx, Right **V** Finger Phalanx, Left	**Ø** Open **3** Percutaneous **4** Percutaneous Endoscopic	**Z** No Device	**Z** No Qualifier

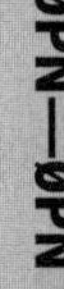

Ø Medical and Surgical
P Upper Bones
P Removal Taking out or off a device from a body part

Body Part Character 4	Approach Character 5	Device Character 6	Qualifier Character 7
Ø Sternum **1** Rib, Right **2** Rib, Left **3** Cervical Vertebra **4** Thoracic Vertebra **5** Scapula, Right **6** Scapula, Left **7** Glenoid Cavity, Right **8** Glenoid Cavity, Left **9** Clavicle, Right **B** Clavicle, Left	**Ø** Open **3** Percutaneous **4** Percutaneous Endoscopic	**4** Internal Fixation Device **7** Autologous Tissue Substitute **J** Synthetic Substitute **K** Nonautologous Tissue Substitute	**Z** No Qualifier
Ø Sternum **1** Rib, Right **2** Rib, Left **3** Cervical Vertebra **4** Thoracic Vertebra **5** Scapula, Right **6** Scapula, Left **7** Glenoid Cavity, Right **8** Glenoid Cavity, Left **9** Clavicle, Right **B** Clavicle, Left	**X** External	**4** Internal Fixation Device	**Z** No Qualifier
C Humeral Head, Right **D** Humeral Head, Left **F** Humeral Shaft, Right **G** Humeral Shaft, Left **H** Radius, Right **J** Radius, Left **K** Ulna, Right **L** Ulna, Left **M** Carpal, Right **N** Carpal, Left **P** Metacarpal, Right **Q** Metacarpal, Left **R** Thumb Phalanx, Right **S** Thumb Phalanx, Left **T** Finger Phalanx, Right **V** Finger Phalanx, Left	**Ø** Open **3** Percutaneous **4** Percutaneous Endoscopic	**4** Internal Fixation Device **5** External Fixation Device **7** Autologous Tissue Substitute **J** Synthetic Substitute **K** Nonautologous Tissue Substitute	**Z** No Qualifier
C Humeral Head, Right **D** Humeral Head, Left **F** Humeral Shaft, Right **G** Humeral Shaft, Left **H** Radius, Right **J** Radius, Left **K** Ulna, Right **L** Ulna, Left **M** Carpal, Right **N** Carpal, Left **P** Metacarpal, Right **Q** Metacarpal, Left **R** Thumb Phalanx, Right **S** Thumb Phalanx, Left **T** Finger Phalanx, Right **V** Finger Phalanx, Left	**X** External	**4** Internal Fixation Device **5** External Fixation Device	**Z** No Qualifier
Y Upper Bone	**Ø** Open **3** Percutaneous **4** Percutaneous Endoscopic **X** External	**Ø** Drainage Device **M** Bone Growth Stimulator	**Z** No Qualifier

Non-OR ØPP[Ø,1,2,3,4,5,6,7,8,9,B]X4Z
Non-OR ØPP[C,D,F,G,H,J,K,L,M,N,P,Q,R,S,T,V]X[4,5]Z
Non-OR ØPPYX[Ø,M]Z

Ø Medical and Surgical
P Upper Bones
Q Repair Restoring, to the extent possible, a body part to its normal anatomic structure and function

Body Part Character 4	Approach Character 5	Device Character 6	Qualifier Character 7
Ø Sternum **1** Rib, Right **2** Rib, Left **3** Cervical Vertebra **4** Thoracic Vertebra **5** Scapula, Right **6** Scapula, Left **7** Glenoid Cavity, Right **8** Glenoid Cavity, Left **9** Clavicle, Right **B** Clavicle, Left **C** Humeral Head, Right **D** Humeral Head, Left **F** Humeral Shaft, Right **G** Humeral Shaft, Left **H** Radius, Right **J** Radius, Left **K** Ulna, Right **L** Ulna, Left **M** Carpal, Right **N** Carpal, Left **P** Metacarpal, Right **Q** Metacarpal, Left **R** Thumb Phalanx, Right **S** Thumb Phalanx, Left **T** Finger Phalanx, Right **V** Finger Phalanx, Left	**Ø** Open **3** Percutaneous **4** Percutaneous Endoscopic **X** External	**Z** No Device	**Z** No Qualifier

Ø Medical and Surgical
P Upper Bones
R Replacement Putting in or on biological or synthetic material that physically takes the place and/or function of all or a portion of a body part

Body Part Character 4	Approach Character 5	Device Character 6	Qualifier Character 7
Ø Sternum **1** Rib, Right **2** Rib, Left **3** Cervical Vertebra **4** Thoracic Vertebra **5** Scapula, Right **6** Scapula, Left **7** Glenoid Cavity, Right **8** Glenoid Cavity, Left **9** Clavicle, Right **B** Clavicle, Left **C** Humeral Head, Right **D** Humeral Head, Left **F** Humeral Shaft, Right **G** Humeral Shaft, Left **H** Radius, Right **J** Radius, Left **K** Ulna, Right **L** Ulna, Left **M** Carpal, Right **N** Carpal, Left **P** Metacarpal, Right **Q** Metacarpal, Left **R** Thumb Phalanx, Right **S** Thumb Phalanx, Left **T** Finger Phalanx, Right **V** Finger Phalanx, Left	**Ø** Open **3** Percutaneous **4** Percutaneous Endoscopic	**7** Autologous Tissue Substitute **J** Synthetic Substitute **K** Nonautologous Tissue Substitute	**Z** No Qualifier

Non-OR ØPR[C,D]ØJZ

Ø Medical and Surgical
P Upper Bones
S Reposition Moving to its normal location or other suitable location all or a portion of a body part

Body Part Character 4	Approach Character 5	Device Character 6	Qualifier Character 7
Ø Sternum	Ø Open 3 Percutaneous 4 Percutaneous Endoscopic	Ø Internal Fixation Device, Rigid Plate 4 Internal Fixation Device Z No Device	Z No Qualifier
1 Rib, Right 2 Rib, Left 3 Cervical Vertebra ⊞ 4 Thoracic Vertebra ⊞ 5 Scapula, Right 6 Scapula, Left 7 Glenoid Cavity, Right 8 Glenoid Cavity, Left 9 Clavicle, Right B Clavicle, Left	Ø Open 3 Percutaneous 4 Percutaneous Endoscopic	4 Internal Fixation Device Z No Device	Z No Qualifier
Ø Sternum 1 Rib, Right 2 Rib, Left 3 Cervical Vertebra 4 Thoracic Vertebra 5 Scapula, Right 6 Scapula, Left 7 Glenoid Cavity, Right 8 Glenoid Cavity, Left 9 Clavicle, Right B Clavicle, Left	X External	Z No Device	Z No Qualifier
C Humeral Head, Right D Humeral Head, Left F Humeral Shaft, Right G Humeral Shaft, Left H Radius, Right J Radius, Left K Ulna, Right L Ulna, Left	Ø Open 3 Percutaneous 4 Percutaneous Endoscopic	4 Internal Fixation Device 5 External Fixation Device 6 Internal Fixation Device, Intramedullary B External Fixation Device, Monoplanar C External Fixation Device, Ring D External Fixation Device, Hybrid Z No Device	Z No Qualifier
C Humeral Head, Right D Humeral Head, Left F Humeral Shaft, Right G Humeral Shaft, Left H Radius, Right J Radius, Left K Ulna, Right L Ulna, Left	X External	Z No Device	Z No Qualifier
M Carpal, Right N Carpal, Left P Metacarpal, Right Q Metacarpal, Left R Thumb Phalanx, Right S Thumb Phalanx, Left T Finger Phalanx, Right V Finger Phalanx, Left	Ø Open 3 Percutaneous 4 Percutaneous Endoscopic	4 Internal Fixation Device 5 External Fixation Device Z No Device	Z No Qualifier
M Carpal, Right N Carpal, Left P Metacarpal, Right Q Metacarpal, Left R Thumb Phalanx, Right S Thumb Phalanx, Left T Finger Phalanx, Right V Finger Phalanx, Left	X External	Z No Device	Z No Qualifier

Non-OR ØPSØ[3,4]ZZ
Non-OR ØPS[1,2,5,6,7,8,9,B][3,4]ZZ
Non-OR ØPS[Ø,1,2,5,6,7,8,9,B]XZZ
Non-OR ØPS[C,D,F,G,H,J,K,L][3,4]ZZ
Non-OR ØPS[C,D,F,G,H,J,K,L]XZZ
Non-OR ØPS[M,N,P,Q,R,S,T,V][3,4]ZZ
Non-OR ØPS[M,N,P,Q,R,S,T,V]XZZ

See Appendix I for Procedure Combinations.
Combo_only ØPS[3,4]3ZZ
⊞ ØPS[3,4]3ZZ

0 Medical and Surgical
P Upper Bones
T Resection Cutting out or off, without replacement, all of a body part

Body Part Character 4	Approach Character 5	Device Character 6	Qualifier Character 7
0 Sternum **1** Rib, Right **2** Rib, Left **5** Scapula, Right **6** Scapula, Left **7** Glenoid Cavity, Right **8** Glenoid Cavity, Left **9** Clavicle, Right **B** Clavicle, Left **C** Humeral Head, Right ⊞ **D** Humeral Head, Left ⊞ **F** Humeral Shaft, Right ⊞ **G** Humeral Shaft, Left ⊞ **H** Radius, Right **J** Radius, Left **K** Ulna, Right **L** Ulna, Left **M** Carpal, Right **N** Carpal, Left **P** Metacarpal, Right **Q** Metacarpal, Left **R** Thumb Phalanx, Right **S** Thumb Phalanx, Left **T** Finger Phalanx, Right **V** Finger Phalanx, Left	**0** Open	**Z** No Device	**Z** No Qualifier

No Procedure Combinations Specified
⊞ 0PT[C,D,F,G]0ZZ

0 Medical and Surgical
P Upper Bones
U Supplement Putting in or on biological or synthetic material that physically reinforces and/or augments the function of a portion of a body part

Body Part Character 4	Approach Character 5	Device Character 6	Qualifier Character 7
0 Sternum **1** Rib, Right **2** Rib, Left **3** Cervical Vertebra ⊞ **4** Thoracic Vertebra ⊞ **5** Scapula, Right **6** Scapula, Left **7** Glenoid Cavity, Right **8** Glenoid Cavity, Left **9** Clavicle, Right **B** Clavicle, Left **C** Humeral Head, Right **D** Humeral Head, Left **F** Humeral Shaft, Right ⊞ **G** Humeral Shaft, Left ⊞ **H** Radius, Right ⊞ **J** Radius, Left ⊞ **K** Ulna, Right ⊞ **L** Ulna, Left ⊞ **M** Carpal, Right ⊞ **N** Carpal, Left ⊞ **P** Metacarpal, Right ⊞ **Q** Metacarpal, Left ⊞ **R** Thumb Phalanx, Right **S** Thumb Phalanx, Left **T** Finger Phalanx, Right ⊞ **V** Finger Phalanx, Left ⊞	**0** Open **3** Percutaneous **4** Percutaneous Endoscopic	**7** Autologous Tissue Substitute **J** Synthetic Substitute **K** Nonautologous Tissue Substitute	**Z** No Qualifier

AHA: 2013, 4Q, 109

See Appendix I for Procedure Combinations
⊞ 0PU[3,4]3JZ

No Procedure Combinations Specified
⊞ 0PU[F,G,H,J,K,L,M,N,P,Q,T,V][0,3,4][7,K]Z

Ø Medical and Surgical
P Upper Bones
W Revision Correcting, to the extent possible, a portion of a malfunctioning device or the position of a displaced device

Body Part Character 4	Approach Character 5	Device Character 6	Qualifier Character 7
Ø Sternum **1** Rib, Right **2** Rib, Left **3** Cervical Vertebra **4** Thoracic Vertebra **5** Scapula, Right **6** Scapula, Left **7** Glenoid Cavity, Right **8** Glenoid Cavity, Left **9** Clavicle, Right **B** Clavicle, Left	**Ø** Open **3** Percutaneous **4** Percutaneous Endoscopic **X** External	**4** Internal Fixation Device **7** Autologous Tissue Substitute **J** Synthetic Substitute **K** Nonautologous Tissue Substitute	**Z** No Qualifier
C Humeral Head, Right **D** Humeral Head, Left **F** Humeral Shaft, Right **G** Humeral Shaft, Left **H** Radius, Right **J** Radius, Left **K** Ulna, Right **L** Ulna, Left **M** Carpal, Right **N** Carpal, Left **P** Metacarpal, Right **Q** Metacarpal, Left **R** Thumb Phalanx, Right **S** Thumb Phalanx, Left **T** Finger Phalanx, Right **V** Finger Phalanx, Left	**Ø** Open **3** Percutaneous **4** Percutaneous Endoscopic **X** External	**4** Internal Fixation Device **5** External Fixation Device **7** Autologous Tissue Substitute **J** Synthetic Substitute **K** Nonautologous Tissue Substitute	**Z** No Qualifier
Y Upper Bone	**Ø** Open **3** Percutaneous **4** Percutaneous Endoscopic **X** External	**Ø** Drainage Device **M** Bone Growth Stimulator	**Z** No Qualifier

Non-OR ØPW[Ø,1,2,3,4,5,6,7,8,9,B]X[4,7,J,K]Z
Non-OR ØPW[C,D,F,G,H,J,K,L,M,N,P,Q,R,S,T,V]X[4,5,7,J,K]Z
Non-OR ØPWYX[Ø,M]Z

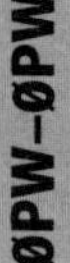

Lower Bones 0Q2–0QW

0 Medical and Surgical
Q Lower Bones
2 Change Taking out or off a device from a body part and putting back an identical or similar device in or on the same body part without cutting or puncturing the skin or a mucous membrane

Body Part Character 4	Approach Character 5	Device Character 6	Qualifier Character 7
Y Lower Bone	X External	0 Drainage Device Y Other Device	Z No Qualifier

Non-OR For all body part, approach, device, and qualifier values

0 Medical and Surgical
Q Lower Bones
5 Destruction Physical eradication of all or a portion of a body part by the direct use of energy, force, or a destructive agent

Body Part Character 4	Approach Character 5	Device Character 6	Qualifier Character 7
0 Lumbar Vertebra 1 Sacrum 2 Pelvic Bone, Right 3 Pelvic Bone, Left 4 Acetabulum, Right 5 Acetabulum, Left 6 Upper Femur, Right 7 Upper Femur, Left 8 Femoral Shaft, Right 9 Femoral Shaft, Left B Lower Femur, Right C Lower Femur, Left D Patella, Right F Patella, Left G Tibia, Right H Tibia, Left J Fibula, Right K Fibula, Left L Tarsal, Right M Tarsal, Left N Metatarsal, Right P Metatarsal, Left Q Toe Phalanx, Right R Toe Phalanx, Left S Coccyx	0 Open 3 Percutaneous 4 Percutaneous Endoscopic	Z No Device	Z No Qualifier

0 Medical and Surgical
Q Lower Bones
8 Division Cutting into a body part without draining fluids and/or gases from the body part in order to separate or transect a body part

Body Part Character 4	Approach Character 5	Device Character 6	Qualifier Character 7
0 Lumbar Vertebra 1 Sacrum 2 Pelvic Bone, Right 3 Pelvic Bone, Left 4 Acetabulum, Right 5 Acetabulum, Left 6 Upper Femur, Right 7 Upper Femur, Left 8 Femoral Shaft, Right ⊞ 9 Femoral Shaft, Left ⊞ B Lower Femur, Right C Lower Femur, Left D Patella, Right F Patella, Left G Tibia, Right ⊞ H Tibia, Left ⊞ J Fibula, Right ⊞ K Fibula, Left ⊞ L Tarsal, Right ⊞ M Tarsal, Left ⊞ N Metatarsal, Right ⊞ P Metatarsal, Left ⊞ Q Toe Phalanx, Right ⊞ R Toe Phalanx, Left ⊞ S Coccyx	0 Open 3 Percutaneous 4 Percutaneous Endoscopic	Z No Device	Z No Qualifier

No Procedure Combinations Specified
⊞ 0Q8[8,9,G,H,J,K,L,M,N,P,Q,R][0,3,4]ZZ

Ø Medical and Surgical
Q Lower Bones
9 Drainage Taking or letting out fluids and/or gases from a body part

Body Part Character 4	Approach Character 5	Device Character 6	Qualifier Character 7
Ø Lumbar Vertebra 1 Sacrum 2 Pelvic Bone, Right 3 Pelvic Bone, Left 4 Acetabulum, Right 5 Acetabulum, Left 6 Upper Femur, Right 7 Upper Femur, Left 8 Femoral Shaft, Right 9 Femoral Shaft, Left B Lower Femur, Right C Lower Femur, Left D Patella, Right F Patella, Left G Tibia, Right H Tibia, Left J Fibula, Right K Fibula, Left L Tarsal, Right M Tarsal, Left N Metatarsal, Right P Metatarsal, Left Q Toe Phalanx, Right R Toe Phalanx, Left S Coccyx	Ø Open 3 Percutaneous 4 Percutaneous Endoscopic	Ø Drainage Device	Z No Qualifier
Ø Lumbar Vertebra 1 Sacrum 2 Pelvic Bone, Right 3 Pelvic Bone, Left 4 Acetabulum, Right 5 Acetabulum, Left 6 Upper Femur, Right 7 Upper Femur, Left 8 Femoral Shaft, Right 9 Femoral Shaft, Left B Lower Femur, Right C Lower Femur, Left D Patella, Right F Patella, Left G Tibia, Right H Tibia, Left J Fibula, Right K Fibula, Left L Tarsal, Right M Tarsal, Left N Metatarsal, Right P Metatarsal, Left Q Toe Phalanx, Right R Toe Phalanx, Left S Coccyx	Ø Open 3 Percutaneous 4 Percutaneous Endoscopic	Z No Device	X Diagnostic Z No Qualifier

0 Medical and Surgical
Q Lower Bones
B Excision Cutting out or off, without replacement, a portion of a body part

Body Part Character 4	Approach Character 5	Device Character 6	Qualifier Character 7
0 Lumbar Vertebra **1** Sacrum **2** Pelvic Bone, Right **3** Pelvic Bone, Left **4** Acetabulum, Right **5** Acetabulum, Left **6** Upper Femur, Right **7** Upper Femur, Left **8** Femoral Shaft, Right **9** Femoral Shaft, Left **B** Lower Femur, Right **C** Lower Femur, Left **D** Patella, Right **F** Patella, Left **G** Tibia, Right **H** Tibia, Left **J** Fibula, Right **K** Fibula, Left **L** Tarsal, Right **M** Tarsal, Left **N** Metatarsal, Right ⊞ **P** Metatarsal, Left ⊞ **Q** Toe Phalanx, Right **R** Toe Phalanx, Left **S** Coccyx	**0** Open **3** Percutaneous **4** Percutaneous Endoscopic	**Z** No Device	**X** Diagnostic **Z** No Qualifier

AHA: 2014, 2Q, 6; 2013, 2Q, 39

No Procedure Combinations Specified
⊞ 0QB[N,P][0,3,4]ZZ

0 Medical and Surgical
Q Lower Bones
C Extirpation Taking or cutting out solid matter from a body part

Body Part Character 4	Approach Character 5	Device Character 6	Qualifier Character 7
0 Lumbar Vertebra **1** Sacrum **2** Pelvic Bone, Right **3** Pelvic Bone, Left **4** Acetabulum, Right **5** Acetabulum, Left **6** Upper Femur, Right **7** Upper Femur, Left **8** Femoral Shaft, Right **9** Femoral Shaft, Left **B** Lower Femur, Right **C** Lower Femur, Left **D** Patella, Right **F** Patella, Left **G** Tibia, Right **H** Tibia, Left **J** Fibula, Right **K** Fibula, Left **L** Tarsal, Right **M** Tarsal, Left **N** Metatarsal, Right **P** Metatarsal, Left **Q** Toe Phalanx, Right **R** Toe Phalanx, Left **S** Coccyx	**0** Open **3** Percutaneous **4** Percutaneous Endoscopic	**Z** No Device	**Z** No Qualifier

Ø Medical and Surgical
Q Lower Bones
H Insertion Putting in a nonbiological appliance that monitors, assists, performs, or prevents a physiological function but does not physically take the place of a body part

Body Part Character 4	Approach Character 5	Device Character 6	Qualifier Character 7
Ø Lumbar Vertebra **1** Sacrum **2** Pelvic Bone, Right **3** Pelvic Bone, Left **4** Acetabulum, Right **5** Acetabulum, Left **D** Patella, Right **F** Patella, Left **L** Tarsal, Right **M** Tarsal, Left **N** Metatarsal, Right **P** Metatarsal, Left **Q** Toe Phalanx, Right **R** Toe Phalanx, Left **S** Coccyx	**Ø** Open **3** Percutaneous **4** Percutaneous Endoscopic	**4** Internal Fixation Device **5** External Fixation Device	**Z** No Qualifier
6 Upper Femur, Right **7** Upper Femur, Left **8** Femoral Shaft, Right **9** Femoral Shaft, Left **B** Lower Femur, Right **C** Lower Femur, Left **G** Tibia, Right **H** Tibia, Left **J** Fibula, Right **K** Fibula, Left	**Ø** Open **3** Percutaneous **4** Percutaneous Endoscopic	**4** Internal Fixation Device **5** External Fixation Device **6** Internal Fixation Device, Intramedullary **8** External Fixation Device, Limb Lengthening **B** External Fixation Device, Monoplanar **C** External Fixation Device, Ring **D** External Fixation Device, Hybrid	**Z** No Qualifier
Y Lower Bone	**Ø** Open **3** Percutaneous **4** Percutaneous Endoscopic	**M** Bone Growth Stimulator	**Z** No Qualifier

Non-OR ØQH[6,7,8,9,B,C,G,H,J,K][Ø,3,4]8Z

Ø Medical and Surgical
Q Lower Bones
J Inspection Visually and/or manually exploring a body part

Body Part Character 4	Approach Character 5	Device Character 6	Qualifier Character 7
Y Lower Bone	**Ø** Open **3** Percutaneous **4** Percutaneous Endoscopic **X** External	**Z** No Device	**Z** No Qualifier

Non-OR ØQJYXZZ

Ø Medical and Surgical
Q Lower Bones
N Release Freeing a body part from an abnormal physical constraint

Body Part Character 4	Approach Character 5	Device Character 6	Qualifier Character 7
Ø Lumbar Vertebra **1** Sacrum **2** Pelvic Bone, Right **3** Pelvic Bone, Left **4** Acetabulum, Right **5** Acetabulum, Left **6** Upper Femur, Right **7** Upper Femur, Left **8** Femoral Shaft, Right **9** Femoral Shaft, Left **B** Lower Femur, Right **C** Lower Femur, Left **D** Patella, Right **F** Patella, Left **G** Tibia, Right **H** Tibia, Left **J** Fibula, Right **K** Fibula, Left **L** Tarsal, Right **M** Tarsal, Left **N** Metatarsal, Right **P** Metatarsal, Left **Q** Toe Phalanx, Right **R** Toe Phalanx, Left **S** Coccyx	**Ø** Open **3** Percutaneous **4** Percutaneous Endoscopic	**Z** No Device	**Z** No Qualifier

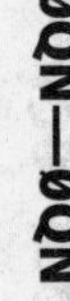

Ø Medical and Surgical
Q Lower Bones
P Removal Taking out or off a device from a body part

Body Part Character 4	Approach Character 5	Device Character 6	Qualifier Character 7
Ø Lumbar Vertebra **1** Sacrum **4** Acetabulum, Right **5** Acetabulum, Left **S** Coccyx	**Ø** Open **3** Percutaneous **4** Percutaneous Endoscopic	**4** Internal Fixation Device **7** Autologous Tissue Substitute **J** Synthetic Substitute **K** Nonautologous Tissue Substitute	**Z** No Qualifier
Ø Lumbar Vertebra **1** Sacrum **4** Acetabulum, Right **5** Acetabulum, Left **S** Coccyx	**X** External	**4** Internal Fixation Device	**Z** No Qualifier
2 Pelvic Bone, Right **3** Pelvic Bone, Left **6** Upper Femur, Right **7** Upper Femur, Left **8** Femoral Shaft, Right **9** Femoral Shaft, Left **B** Lower Femur, Right **C** Lower Femur, Left **D** Patella, Right **F** Patella, Left **G** Tibia, Right **H** Tibia, Left **J** Fibula, Right **K** Fibula, Left **L** Tarsal, Right **M** Tarsal, Left **N** Metatarsal, Right **P** Metatarsal, Left **Q** Toe Phalanx, Right **R** Toe Phalanx, Left	**X** External	**4** Internal Fixation Device **5** External Fixation Device	**Z** No Qualifier
2 Pelvic Bone, Right **3** Pelvic Bone, Left **6** Upper Femur, Right **7** Upper Femur, Left **8** Femoral Shaft, Right **9** Femoral Shaft, Left **B** Lower Femur, Right **C** Lower Femur, Left **D** Patella, Right ⊞ **F** Patella, Left ⊞ **G** Tibia, Right **H** Tibia, Left **J** Fibula, Right **K** Fibula, Left **L** Tarsal, Right **M** Tarsal, Left **N** Metatarsal, Right **P** Metatarsal, Left **Q** Toe Phalanx, Right **R** Toe Phalanx, Left	**Ø** Open **3** Percutaneous **4** Percutaneous Endoscopic	**4** Internal Fixation Device **5** External Fixation Device **7** Autologous Tissue Substitute **J** Synthetic Substitute **K** Nonautologous Tissue Substitute	**Z** No Qualifier
Y Lower Bone	**Ø** Open **3** Percutaneous **4** Percutaneous Endoscopic **X** External	**Ø** Drainage Device **M** Bone Growth Stimulator	**Z** No Qualifier

Non-OR ØQP[Ø,1,4,5,S]X4Z
Non-OR ØQP[2,3,6,7,8,9,B,C,D,F,G,H,J,K,L,M,N,P,Q,R]X[4,5]Z
Non-OR ØQPYX[Ø,M]Z

No Procedure Combinations Specified
⊞ ØQP[D,F][Ø,3,4]JZ

Ø Medical and Surgical
Q Lower Bones
Q Repair Restoring, to the extent possible, a body part to its normal anatomic structure and function

Body Part Character 4	Approach Character 5	Device Character 6	Qualifier Character 7
Ø Lumbar Vertebra 1 Sacrum 2 Pelvic Bone, Right 3 Pelvic Bone, Left 4 Acetabulum, Right 5 Acetabulum, Left 6 Upper Femur, Right 7 Upper Femur, Left 8 Femoral Shaft, Right 9 Femoral Shaft, Left B Lower Femur, Right C Lower Femur, Left D Patella, Right F Patella, Left G Tibia, Right H Tibia, Left J Fibula, Right K Fibula, Left L Tarsal, Right M Tarsal, Left N Metatarsal, Right P Metatarsal, Left Q Toe Phalanx, Right R Toe Phalanx, Left S Coccyx	Ø Open 3 Percutaneous 4 Percutaneous Endoscopic X External	Z No Device	Z No Qualifier

Ø Medical and Surgical
Q Lower Bones
R Replacement Putting in or on biological or synthetic material that physically takes the place and/or function of all or a portion of a body part

Body Part Character 4	Approach Character 5	Device Character 6	Qualifier Character 7
Ø Lumbar Vertebra 1 Sacrum 2 Pelvic Bone, Right 3 Pelvic Bone, Left 4 Acetabulum, Right 5 Acetabulum, Left 6 Upper Femur, Right 7 Upper Femur, Left 8 Femoral Shaft, Right ⊞ 9 Femoral Shaft, Left ⊞ B Lower Femur, Right C Lower Femur, Left D Patella, Right ⊞ F Patella, Left ⊞ G Tibia, Right ⊞ H Tibia, Left ⊞ J Fibula, Right ⊞ K Fibula, Left ⊞ L Tarsal, Right ⊞ M Tarsal, Left ⊞ N Metatarsal, Right ⊞ P Metatarsal, Left ⊞ Q Toe Phalanx, Right ⊞ R Toe Phalanx, Left ⊞ S Coccyx	Ø Open 3 Percutaneous 4 Percutaneous Endoscopic	7 Autologous Tissue Substitute J Synthetic Substitute K Nonautologous Tissue Substitute	Z No Qualifier

No Procedure Combinations Specified
⊞ ØQR[8,9,G,H,J,K,L,M,N,P,Q,R][Ø,3,4][7,K]Z
⊞ ØQR[D,F][Ø,3,4]JZ

Ø Medical and Surgical
Q Lower Bones
S Reposition Moving to its normal location or other suitable location all or a portion of a body part

Body Part Character 4	Approach Character 5	Device Character 6	Qualifier Character 7
Ø Lumbar Vertebra ⊞ **1** Sacrum ⊞ **4** Acetabulum, Right **5** Acetabulum, Left **S** Coccyx ⊞	**Ø** Open **3** Percutaneous **4** Percutaneous Endoscopic	**4** Internal Fixation Device **Z** No Device	**Z** No Qualifier
Ø Lumbar Vertebra **1** Sacrum **4** Acetabulum, Right **5** Acetabulum, Left **S** Coccyx	**X** External	**Z** No Device	**Z** No Qualifier
2 Pelvic Bone, Right **3** Pelvic Bone, Left **D** Patella, Right **F** Patella, Left **L** Tarsal, Right **M** Tarsal, Left **N** Metatarsal, Right **P** Metatarsal, Left **Q** Toe Phalanx, Right **R** Toe Phalanx, Left	**Ø** Open **3** Percutaneous **4** Percutaneous Endoscopic	**4** Internal Fixation Device **5** External Fixation Device **Z** No Device	**Z** No Qualifier
2 Pelvic Bone, Right **3** Pelvic Bone, Left **D** Patella, Right **F** Patella, Left **L** Tarsal, Right **M** Tarsal, Left **N** Metatarsal, Right **P** Metatarsal, Left **Q** Toe Phalanx, Right **R** Toe Phalanx, Left	**X** External	**Z** No Device	**Z** No Qualifier
6 Upper Femur, Right **7** Upper Femur, Left **8** Femoral Shaft, Right **9** Femoral Shaft, Left **B** Lower Femur, Right **C** Lower Femur, Left **G** Tibia, Right **H** Tibia, Left **J** Fibula, Right **K** Fibula, Left	**Ø** Open **3** Percutaneous **4** Percutaneous Endoscopic	**4** Internal Fixation Device **5** External Fixation Device **6** Internal Fixation Device, Intramedullary **B** External Fixation Device, Monoplanar **C** External Fixation Device, Ring **D** External Fixation Device, Hybrid **Z** No Device	**Z** No Qualifier
6 Upper Femur, Right **7** Upper Femur, Left **8** Femoral Shaft, Right **9** Femoral Shaft, Left **B** Lower Femur, Right **C** Lower Femur, Left **G** Tibia, Right **H** Tibia, Left **J** Fibula, Right **K** Fibula, Left	**X** External	**Z** No Device	**Z** No Qualifier

Non-OR ØQS[4,5][3,4]ZZ
Non-OR ØQS[4,5]XZZ
Non-OR ØQS[2,3,D,F,L,M,N,P,Q,R][3,4]ZZ
Non-OR ØQS[2,3,D,F,L,M,N,P,Q,R]XZZ
Non-OR ØQS[6,7,8,9,B,C,G,H,J,K][3,4]ZZ
Non-OR ØQS[6,7,8,9,B,C,G,H,J,K]XZZ

See Appendix I for Procedure Combinations
Combo-only ØQS[Ø,1]3ZZ
⊞ ØQS[Ø,1,S]3ZZ

0 Medical and Surgical
Q Lower Bones
T Resection Cutting out or off, without replacement, all of a body part

Body Part Character 4	Approach Character 5	Device Character 6	Qualifier Character 7
2 Pelvic Bone, Right 3 Pelvic Bone, Left 4 Acetabulum, Right 5 Acetabulum, Left 6 Upper Femur, Right ⊞ 7 Upper Femur, Left ⊞ 8 Femoral Shaft, Right ⊞ 9 Femoral Shaft, Left ⊞ B Lower Femur, Right ⊞ C Lower Femur, Left ⊞ D Patella, Right F Patella, Left G Tibia, Right H Tibia, Left J Fibula, Right K Fibula, Left L Tarsal, Right M Tarsal, Left N Metatarsal, Right P Metatarsal, Left Q Toe Phalanx, Right R Toe Phalanx, Left S Coccyx	0 Open	Z No Device	Z No Qualifier

No Procedure Combinations Specified
⊞ 0QT[6,7,8,9,B,C]0ZZ

0 Medical and Surgical
Q Lower Bones
U Supplement Putting in or on biological or synthetic material that physically reinforces and/or augments the function of a portion of a body part

Body Part Character 4	Approach Character 5	Device Character 6	Qualifier Character 7
0 Lumbar Vertebra ⊞ 1 Sacrum ⊞ 2 Pelvic Bone, Right 3 Pelvic Bone, Left 4 Acetabulum, Right 5 Acetabulum, Left 6 Upper Femur, Right 7 Upper Femur, Left 8 Femoral Shaft, Right ⊞ 9 Femoral Shaft, Left ⊞ B Lower Femur, Right C Lower Femur, Left D Patella, Right ⊞ F Patella, Left ⊞ G Tibia, Right ⊞ H Tibia, Left ⊞ J Fibula, Right ⊞ K Fibula, Left ⊞ L Tarsal, Right ⊞ M Tarsal, Left ⊞ N Metatarsal, Right ⊞ P Metatarsal, Left ⊞ Q Toe Phalanx, Right ⊞ R Toe Phalanx, Left ⊞ S Coccyx ⊞	0 Open 3 Percutaneous 4 Percutaneous Endoscopic	7 Autologous Tissue Substitute J Synthetic Substitute K Nonautologous Tissue Substitute	Z No Qualifier

AHA: 2014, 2Q, 12; 2013, 2Q, 35

See Appendix I for Procedure Combinations
⊞ 0QU[0,1,S]3JZ

No Procedure Combinations Specified
⊞ 0QU[8,9,G,H,J,K,L,M,N,P,Q,R][0,3,4][7,K]Z
⊞ 0QU[D,F][0,3,4]JZ

Ø Medical and Surgical
Q Lower Bones
W Revision Correcting, to the extent possible, a portion of a malfunctioning device or the position of a displaced device

Body Part Character 4	Approach Character 5	Device Character 6	Qualifier Character 7
Ø Lumbar Vertebra 1 Sacrum 4 Acetabulum, Right 5 Acetabulum, Left S Coccyx	Ø Open 3 Percutaneous 4 Percutaneous Endoscopic X External	4 Internal Fixation Device 7 Autologous Tissue Substitute J Synthetic Substitute K Nonautologous Tissue Substitute	Z No Qualifier
2 Pelvic Bone, Right 3 Pelvic Bone, Left 6 Upper Femur, Right 7 Upper Femur, Left 8 Femoral Shaft, Right 9 Femoral Shaft, Left B Lower Femur, Right C Lower Femur, Left D Patella, Right F Patella, Left G Tibia, Right H Tibia, Left J Fibula, Right K Fibula, Left L Tarsal, Right M Tarsal, Left N Metatarsal, Right P Metatarsal, Left Q Toe Phalanx, Right R Toe Phalanx, Left	Ø Open 3 Percutaneous 4 Percutaneous Endoscopic X External	4 Internal Fixation Device 5 External Fixation Device 7 Autologous Tissue Substitute J Synthetic Substitute K Nonautologous Tissue Substitute	Z No Qualifier
Y Lower Bone	Ø Open 3 Percutaneous 4 Percutaneous Endoscopic X External	Ø Drainage Device M Bone Growth Stimulator	Z No Qualifier

Non-OR ØQW[Ø,1,4,5,S]X[4,7,J,K]Z
Non-OR ØQW[2,3,6,7,8,9,B,C,D,F,G,H,J,K,L,M,N,P,Q,R]X[4,5,7,J,K]Z
Non-OR ØQWYX[Ø,M]Z

Upper Joints ØR2–ØRW

Ø Medical and Surgical
R Upper Joints
2 Change Taking out or off a device from a body part and putting back an identical or similar device in or on the same body part without cutting or puncturing the skin or a mucous membrane

Body Part Character 4	Approach Character 5	Device Character 6	Qualifier Character 7
Y Upper Joint	X External	Ø Drainage Device Y Other Device	Z No Qualifier

Non-OR For all body part, approach, device, and qualifier values

Ø Medical and Surgical
R Upper Joints
5 Destruction Physical eradication of all or a portion of a body part by the direct use of energy, force, or a destructive agent

Body Part Character 4	Approach Character 5	Device Character 6	Qualifier Character 7
Ø Occipital-cervical Joint 1 Cervical Vertebral Joint 3 Cervical Vertebral Disc 4 Cervicothoracic Vertebral Joint 5 Cervicothoracic Vertebral Disc 6 Thoracic Vertebral Joint 9 Thoracic Vertebral Disc A Thoracolumbar Vertebral Joint B Thoracolumbar Vertebral Disc C Temporomandibular Joint, Right D Temporomandibular Joint, Left E Sternoclavicular Joint, Right F Sternoclavicular Joint, Left G Acromioclavicular Joint, Right H Acromioclavicular Joint, Left J Shoulder Joint, Right K Shoulder Joint, Left L Elbow Joint, Right M Elbow Joint, Left N Wrist Joint, Right P Wrist Joint, Left Q Carpal Joint, Right R Carpal Joint, Left S Metacarpocarpal Joint, Right T Metacarpocarpal Joint, Left U Metacarpophalangeal Joint, Right V Metacarpophalangeal Joint, Left W Finger Phalangeal Joint, Right X Finger Phalangeal Joint, Left	Ø Open 3 Percutaneous 4 Percutaneous Endoscopic	Z No Device	Z No Qualifier

Non-OR ØR5[3,5,9,B][3,4]ZZ

Ø Medical and Surgical
R Upper Joints
9 Drainage Taking or letting out fluids and/or gases from a body part

Body Part Character 4	Approach Character 5	Device Character 6	Qualifier Character 7
Ø Occipital-cervical Joint **1** Cervical Vertebral Joint **3** Cervical Vertebral Disc **4** Cervicothoracic Vertebral Joint **5** Cervicothoracic Vertebral Disc **6** Thoracic Vertebral Joint **9** Thoracic Vertebral Disc **A** Thoracolumbar Vertebral Joint **B** Thoracolumbar Vertebral Disc **C** Temporomandibular Joint, Right **D** Temporomandibular Joint, Left **E** Sternoclavicular Joint, Right **F** Sternoclavicular Joint, Left **G** Acromioclavicular Joint, Right **H** Acromioclavicular Joint, Left **J** Shoulder Joint, Right **K** Shoulder Joint, Left **L** Elbow Joint, Right **M** Elbow Joint, Left **N** Wrist Joint, Right **P** Wrist Joint, Left **Q** Carpal Joint, Right **R** Carpal Joint, Left **S** Metacarpocarpal Joint, Right **T** Metacarpocarpal Joint, Left **U** Metacarpophalangeal Joint, Right **V** Metacarpophalangeal Joint, Left **W** Finger Phalangeal Joint, Right **X** Finger Phalangeal Joint, Left	**Ø** Open **3** Percutaneous **4** Percutaneous Endoscopic	**Ø** Drainage Device	**Z** No Qualifier
Ø Occipital-cervical Joint **1** Cervical Vertebral Joint **3** Cervical Vertebral Disc **4** Cervicothoracic Vertebral Joint **5** Cervicothoracic Vertebral Disc **6** Thoracic Vertebral Joint **9** Thoracic Vertebral Disc **A** Thoracolumbar Vertebral Joint **B** Thoracolumbar Vertebral Disc **C** Temporomandibular Joint, Right **D** Temporomandibular Joint, Left **E** Sternoclavicular Joint, Right **F** Sternoclavicular Joint, Left **G** Acromioclavicular Joint, Right **H** Acromioclavicular Joint, Left **J** Shoulder Joint, Right **K** Shoulder Joint, Left **L** Elbow Joint, Right **M** Elbow Joint, Left **N** Wrist Joint, Right **P** Wrist Joint, Left **Q** Carpal Joint, Right **R** Carpal Joint, Left **S** Metacarpocarpal Joint, Right **T** Metacarpocarpal Joint, Left **U** Metacarpophalangeal Joint, Right **V** Metacarpophalangeal Joint, Left **W** Finger Phalangeal Joint, Right **X** Finger Phalangeal Joint, Left	**Ø** Open **3** Percutaneous **4** Percutaneous Endoscopic	**Z** No Device	**X** Diagnostic **Z** No Qualifier

Non-OR ØR9[Ø,1,3,4,5,6,9,A,B,E,F,G,H,J,K,L,M,N,P,Q,R,S,T,U,V,W,X][3,4]ØZ
Non-OR ØR9[Ø,1,3,4,5,6,9,A,B,E,F,G,H,J,K,L,M,N,P,Q,R,S,T,U,V,W,X][Ø,3,4]ZX
Non-OR ØR9[Ø,1,3,4,5,6,9,A,B,E,F,G,H,J,K,L,M,N,P,Q,R,S,T,U,V,W,X][3,4]ZZ

Ø Medical and Surgical
R Upper Joints
B Excision Cutting out or off, without replacement, a portion of a body part

Body Part Character 4	Approach Character 5	Device Character 6	Qualifier Character 7
Ø Occipital-cervical Joint 1 Cervical Vertebral Joint 3 Cervical Vertebral Disc 4 Cervicothoracic Vertebral Joint 5 Cervicothoracic Vertebral Disc 6 Thoracic Vertebral Joint 9 Thoracic Vertebral Disc A Thoracolumbar Vertebral Joint B Thoracolumbar Vertebral Disc C Temporomandibular Joint, Right D Temporomandibular Joint, Left E Sternoclavicular Joint, Right F Sternoclavicular Joint, Left G Acromioclavicular Joint, Right H Acromioclavicular Joint, Left J Shoulder Joint, Right K Shoulder Joint, Left L Elbow Joint, Right M Elbow Joint, Left N Wrist Joint, Right P Wrist Joint, Left Q Carpal Joint, Right R Carpal Joint, Left S Metacarpocarpal Joint, Right T Metacarpocarpal Joint, Left U Metacarpophalangeal Joint, Right V Metacarpophalangeal Joint, Left W Finger Phalangeal Joint, Right X Finger Phalangeal Joint, Left	Ø Open 3 Percutaneous 4 Percutaneous Endoscopic	Z No Device	X Diagnostic Z No Qualifier

Non-OR ØRB[Ø,1,3,4,5,6,9,A,B,E,F,G,H,J,K,L,M,N,P,Q,R,S,T,U,V,W,X][Ø,3,4]ZX

Ø Medical and Surgical
R Upper Joints
C Extirpation Taking or cutting out solid matter from a body part

Body Part Character 4	Approach Character 5	Device Character 6	Qualifier Character 7
Ø Occipital-cervical Joint 1 Cervical Vertebral Joint 3 Cervical Vertebral Disc 4 Cervicothoracic Vertebral Joint 5 Cervicothoracic Vertebral Disc 6 Thoracic Vertebral Joint 9 Thoracic Vertebral Disc A Thoracolumbar Vertebral Joint B Thoracolumbar Vertebral Disc C Temporomandibular Joint, Right D Temporomandibular Joint, Left E Sternoclavicular Joint, Right F Sternoclavicular Joint, Left G Acromioclavicular Joint, Right H Acromioclavicular Joint, Left J Shoulder Joint, Right K Shoulder Joint, Left L Elbow Joint, Right M Elbow Joint, Left N Wrist Joint, Right P Wrist Joint, Left Q Carpal Joint, Right R Carpal Joint, Left S Metacarpocarpal Joint, Right T Metacarpocarpal Joint, Left U Metacarpophalangeal Joint, Right V Metacarpophalangeal Joint, Left W Finger Phalangeal Joint, Right X Finger Phalangeal Joint, Left	Ø Open 3 Percutaneous 4 Percutaneous Endoscopic	Z No Device	Z No Qualifier

Ø Medical and Surgical
R Upper Joints
G Fusion Joining together portions of an articular body part rendering the articular body part immobile

Body Part Character 4	Approach Character 5	Device Character 6	Qualifier Character 7
Ø Occipital-cervical Joint **1** Cervical Vertebral Joint **2** Cervical Vertebral Joints, 2 or more **4** Cervicothoracic Vertebral Joint **6** Thoracic Vertebral Joint **7** Thoracic Vertebral Joints, 2 to 7 ⊞ **8** Thoracic Vertebral Joints, 8 or more **A** Thoracolumbar Vertebral Joint	**Ø** Open **3** Percutaneous **4** Percutaneous Endoscopic	**7** Autologous Tissue Substitute **A** Interbody Fusion Device **J** Synthetic Substitute **K** Nonautologous Tissue Substitute **Z** No Device	**Ø** Anterior Approach, Anterior Column **1** Posterior Approach, Posterior Column **J** Posterior Approach, Anterior Column
C Temporomandibular Joint, Right **D** Temporomandibular Joint, Left **E** Sternoclavicular Joint, Right **F** Sternoclavicular Joint, Left **G** Acromioclavicular Joint, Right **H** Acromioclavicular Joint, Left **J** Shoulder Joint, Right **K** Shoulder Joint, Left	**Ø** Open **3** Percutaneous **4** Percutaneous Endoscopic	**4** Internal Fixation Device **7** Autologous Tissue Substitute **J** Synthetic Substitute **K** Nonautologous Tissue Substitute **Z** No Device	**Z** No Qualifier
L Elbow Joint, Right **M** Elbow Joint, Left **N** Wrist Joint, Right **P** Wrist Joint, Left **Q** Carpal Joint, Right **R** Carpal Joint, Left **S** Metacarpocarpal Joint, Right **T** Metacarpocarpal Joint, Left **U** Metacarpophalangeal Joint, Right **V** Metacarpophalangeal Joint, Left **W** Finger Phalangeal Joint, Right **X** Finger Phalangeal Joint, Left	**Ø** Open **3** Percutaneous **4** Percutaneous Endoscopic	**4** Internal Fixation Device **5** External Fixation Device **7** Autologous Tissue Substitute **J** Synthetic Substitute **K** Nonautologous Tissue Substitute **Z** No Device	**Z** No Qualifier

HAC ØRG[Ø,1,2,4,6,7,8,A][Ø,3,4][7,A,J,K,Z][Ø,1,J] when reported with SDx K68.11 or T81.4XXA or T81.6Ø-T84.7 with 7th character A

HAC ØRG[E,F,G,H,J,K][Ø,3,4][4,7,J,K,Z]Z when reported with SDx K68.11 or T81.4XXA or T81.6Ø-T84.7 with 7th character A

HAC ØRG[L,M][Ø,3,4][4,5,7,J,K,Z]Z when reported with SDx K68.11 or T81.4XXA or T81.6Ø-T84.7 with 7th character A

AHA: 2Ø14, 2Q, 7; 2Ø13, 1Q, 21, 29

See Appendix I for Procedure Combinations
⊞ ØRG7[Ø,3,4][7,A,J,K,Z][Ø,1,J]

0 Medical and Surgical
R Upper Joints
H Insertion Putting in a nonbiological appliance that monitors, assists, performs, or prevents a physiological function but does not physically take the place of a body part

Body Part Character 4	Approach Character 5	Device Character 6	Qualifier Character 7
0 Occipital-cervical Joint **1** Cervical Vertebral Joint **4** Cervicothoracic Vertebral Joint **6** Thoracic Vertebral Joint **A** Thoracolumbar Vertebral Joint	**0** Open **3** Percutaneous **4** Percutaneous Endoscopic	**3** Infusion Device **4** Internal Fixation Device **8** Spacer **B** Spinal Stabilization Device, Interspinous Process **C** Spinal Stabilization Device, Pedicle-Based **D** Spinal Stabilization Device, Facet Replacement	**Z** No Qualifier
3 Cervical Vertebral Disc **5** Cervicothoracic Vertebral Disc **9** Thoracic Vertebral Disc **B** Thoracolumbar Vertebral Disc	**0** Open **3** Percutaneous **4** Percutaneous Endoscopic	**3** Infusion Device	**Z** No Qualifier
C Temporomandibular Joint, Right **D** Temporomandibular Joint, Left **E** Sternoclavicular Joint, Right **F** Sternoclavicular Joint, Left **G** Acromioclavicular Joint, Right **H** Acromioclavicular Joint, Left **J** Shoulder Joint, Right **K** Shoulder Joint, Left	**0** Open **3** Percutaneous **4** Percutaneous Endoscopic	**3** Infusion Device **4** Internal Fixation Device **8** Spacer	**Z** No Qualifier
L Elbow Joint, Right **M** Elbow Joint, Left **N** Wrist Joint, Right **P** Wrist Joint, Left **Q** Carpal Joint, Right **R** Carpal Joint, Left **S** Metacarpocarpal Joint, Right **T** Metacarpocarpal Joint, Left **U** Metacarpophalangeal Joint, Right **V** Metacarpophalangeal Joint, Left **W** Finger Phalangeal Joint, Right **X** Finger Phalangeal Joint, Left	**0** Open **3** Percutaneous **4** Percutaneous Endoscopic	**3** Infusion Device **4** Internal Fixation Device **5** External Fixation Device **8** Spacer	**Z** No Qualifier

Non-OR 0RH[0,1,4,6,A][0,3,4][3,8]Z
Non-OR 0RH[3,5,9,B][0,3,4]3Z
Non-OR 0RH[E,F,G,H,J,K][0,3,4][3,8]Z
Non-OR 0RH[C,D][0,3,4]8Z
Non-OR 0RH[L,M,N,P,Q,R,S,T,U,V,W,X][0,3,4][3,8]Z

Ø Medical and Surgical
R Upper Joints
J Inspection Visually and/or manually exploring a body part

Body Part Character 4	Approach Character 5	Device Character 6	Qualifier Character 7
Ø Occipital-cervical Joint 1 Cervical Vertebral Joint 3 Cervical Vertebral Disc 4 Cervicothoracic Vertebral Joint 5 Cervicothoracic Vertebral Disc 6 Thoracic Vertebral Joint 9 Thoracic Vertebral Disc A Thoracolumbar Vertebral Joint B Thoracolumbar Vertebral Disc C Temporomandibular Joint, Right D Temporomandibular Joint, Left E Sternoclavicular Joint, Right F Sternoclavicular Joint, Left G Acromioclavicular Joint, Right H Acromioclavicular Joint, Left J Shoulder Joint, Right K Shoulder Joint, Left L Elbow Joint, Right M Elbow Joint, Left N Wrist Joint, Right P Wrist Joint, Left Q Carpal Joint, Right R Carpal Joint, Left S Metacarpocarpal Joint, Right T Metacarpocarpal Joint, Left U Metacarpophalangeal Joint, Right V Metacarpophalangeal Joint, Left W Finger Phalangeal Joint, Right X Finger Phalangeal Joint, Left	Ø Open 3 Percutaneous 4 Percutaneous Endoscopic X External	Z No Device	Z No Qualifier

Non-OR ØRJ[Ø,1,3,4,5,6,9,A,B,C,D,E,F,G,H,J,K,L,M,N,P,Q,R,S,T,U,V,W,X]XZZ

Ø Medical and Surgical
R Upper Joints
N Release Freeing a body part from an abnormal physical constraint

Body Part Character 4	Approach Character 5	Device Character 6	Qualifier Character 7
Ø Occipital-cervical Joint 1 Cervical Vertebral Joint 3 Cervical Vertebral Disc 4 Cervicothoracic Vertebral Joint 5 Cervicothoracic Vertebral Disc 6 Thoracic Vertebral Joint 9 Thoracic Vertebral Disc A Thoracolumbar Vertebral Joint B Thoracolumbar Vertebral Disc C Temporomandibular Joint, Right D Temporomandibular Joint, Left E Sternoclavicular Joint, Right F Sternoclavicular Joint, Left G Acromioclavicular Joint, Right H Acromioclavicular Joint, Left J Shoulder Joint, Right K Shoulder Joint, Left L Elbow Joint, Right M Elbow Joint, Left N Wrist Joint, Right P Wrist Joint, Left Q Carpal Joint, Right R Carpal Joint, Left S Metacarpocarpal Joint, Right T Metacarpocarpal Joint, Left U Metacarpophalangeal Joint, Right V Metacarpophalangeal Joint, Left W Finger Phalangeal Joint, Right X Finger Phalangeal Joint, Left	Ø Open 3 Percutaneous 4 Percutaneous Endoscopic X External	Z No Device	Z No Qualifier

Non-OR ØRN[Ø,1,3,4,5,6,9,A,B,C,D,E,F,G,H,J,K,L,M,N,P,Q,R,S,T,U,V,W,X]XZZ

Ø Medical and Surgical
R Upper Joints
P Removal Taking out or off a device from a body part

Body Part Character 4	Approach Character 5	Device Character 6	Qualifier Character 7
Ø Occipital-cervical Joint 1 Cervical Vertebral Joint 4 Cervicothoracic Vertebral Joint 6 Thoracic Vertebral Joint A Thoracolumbar Vertebral Joint C Temporomandibular Joint, Right D Temporomandibular Joint, Left E Sternoclavicular Joint, Right F Sternoclavicular Joint, Left G Acromioclavicular Joint, Right H Acromioclavicular Joint, Left J Shoulder Joint, Right K Shoulder Joint, Left	Ø Open 3 Percutaneous 4 Percutaneous Endoscopic	Ø Drainage Device 3 Infusion Device 4 Internal Fixation Device 7 Autologous Tissue Substitute 8 Spacer A Interbody Fusion Device J Synthetic Substitute K Nonautologous Tissue Substitute	Z No Qualifier
Ø Occipital-cervical Joint 1 Cervical Vertebral Joint 4 Cervicothoracic Vertebral Joint 6 Thoracic Vertebral Joint A Thoracolumbar Vertebral Joint C Temporomandibular Joint, Right D Temporomandibular Joint, Left E Sternoclavicular Joint, Right F Sternoclavicular Joint, Left G Acromioclavicular Joint, Right H Acromioclavicular Joint, Left J Shoulder Joint, Right K Shoulder Joint, Left	X External	Ø Drainage Device 3 Infusion Device 4 Internal Fixation Device	Z No Qualifier
3 Cervical Vertebral Disc 5 Cervicothoracic Vertebral Disc 9 Thoracic Vertebral Disc B Thoracolumbar Vertebral Disc	Ø Open 3 Percutaneous 4 Percutaneous Endoscopic	Ø Drainage Device 3 Infusion Device 7 Autologous Tissue Substitute J Synthetic Substitute K Nonautologous Tissue Substitute	Z No Qualifier
3 Cervical Vertebral Disc 5 Cervicothoracic Vertebral Disc 9 Thoracic Vertebral Disc B Thoracolumbar Vertebral Disc	X External	Ø Drainage Device 3 Infusion Device	Z No Qualifier
L Elbow Joint, Right M Elbow Joint, Left N Wrist Joint, Right P Wrist Joint, Left Q Carpal Joint, Right R Carpal Joint, Left S Metacarpocarpal Joint, Right T Metacarpocarpal Joint, Left U Metacarpophalangeal Joint, Right V Metacarpophalangeal Joint, Left W Finger Phalangeal Joint, Right X Finger Phalangeal Joint, Left	Ø Open 3 Percutaneous 4 Percutaneous Endoscopic	Ø Drainage Device 3 Infusion Device 4 Internal Fixation Device 5 External Fixation Device 7 Autologous Tissue Substitute 8 Spacer J Synthetic Substitute K Nonautologous Tissue Substitute	Z No Qualifier
L Elbow Joint, Right M Elbow Joint, Left N Wrist Joint, Right P Wrist Joint, Left Q Carpal Joint, Right R Carpal Joint, Left S Metacarpocarpal Joint, Right T Metacarpocarpal Joint, Left U Metacarpophalangeal Joint, Right V Metacarpophalangeal Joint, Left W Finger Phalangeal Joint, Right X Finger Phalangeal Joint, Left	X External	Ø Drainage Device 3 Infusion Device 4 Internal Fixation Device 5 External Fixation Device	Z No Qualifier

Non-OR ØRP[Ø,1,4,6,A,C,D,E,F,G,H,J,K][Ø,3,4]8Z
Non-OR ØRP[Ø,1,4,6,A,E,F,G,H,J,K]X[Ø,3,4]Z
Non-OR ØRP[C,D]X[Ø,3]Z
Non-OR ØRP[3,5,9,B]X[Ø,3]Z
Non-OR ØRP[L,M,N,P,Q,R,S,T,U,V,W,X][Ø,3,4]8Z
Non-OR ØRP[L,M,N,P,Q,R,S,T,U,V,W,X]X[Ø,3,4,5]Z

Ø Medical and Surgical
R Upper Joints
Q Repair Restoring, to the extent possible, a body part to its normal anatomic structure and function

Body Part Character 4	Approach Character 5	Device Character 6	Qualifier Character 7
Ø Occipital-cervical Joint 1 Cervical Vertebral Joint 3 Cervical Vertebral Disc 4 Cervicothoracic Vertebral Joint 5 Cervicothoracic Vertebral Disc 6 Thoracic Vertebral Joint 9 Thoracic Vertebral Disc A Thoracolumbar Vertebral Joint B Thoracolumbar Vertebral Disc C Temporomandibular Joint, Right D Temporomandibular Joint, Left E Sternoclavicular Joint, Right F Sternoclavicular Joint, Left G Acromioclavicular Joint, Right H Acromioclavicular Joint, Left J Shoulder Joint, Right K Shoulder Joint, Left L Elbow Joint, Right M Elbow Joint, Left N Wrist Joint, Right P Wrist Joint, Left Q Carpal Joint, Right R Carpal Joint, Left S Metacarpocarpal Joint, Right T Metacarpocarpal Joint, Left U Metacarpophalangeal Joint, Right V Metacarpophalangeal Joint, Left W Finger Phalangeal Joint, Right X Finger Phalangeal Joint, Left	Ø Open 3 Percutaneous 4 Percutaneous Endoscopic X External	Z No Device	Z No Qualifier

HAC ØRQ[E,F,G,H,J,K,L,M][Ø,3,4,X]ZZ when reported with SDx K68.11 or T81.4XXA or T81.6Ø-T84.7 with 7th character A
Non-OR ØRQ[C,D]XZZ

Ø Medical and Surgical
R Upper Joints
R Replacement Putting in or on biological or synthetic material that physically takes the place and/or function of all or a portion of a body part

Body Part Character 4	Approach Character 5	Device Character 6	Qualifier Character 7
Ø Occipital-cervical Joint 1 Cervical Vertebral Joint 3 Cervical Vertebral Disc 4 Cervicothoracic Vertebral Joint 5 Cervicothoracic Vertebral Disc 6 Thoracic Vertebral Joint 9 Thoracic Vertebral Disc A Thoracolumbar Vertebral Joint B Thoracolumbar Vertebral Disc C Temporomandibular Joint, Right D Temporomandibular Joint, Left E Sternoclavicular Joint, Right F Sternoclavicular Joint, Left G Acromioclavicular Joint, Right H Acromioclavicular Joint, Left L Elbow Joint, Right M Elbow Joint, Left N Wrist Joint, Right P Wrist Joint, Left Q Carpal Joint, Right R Carpal Joint, Left S Metacarpocarpal Joint, Right T Metacarpocarpal Joint, Left U Metacarpophalangeal Joint, Right V Metacarpophalangeal Joint, Left W Finger Phalangeal Joint, Right X Finger Phalangeal Joint, Left	Ø Open	7 Autologous Tissue Substitute J Synthetic Substitute K Nonautologous Tissue Substitute	Z No Qualifier
J Shoulder Joint, Right K Shoulder Joint, Left	Ø Open	Ø Synthetic Substitute, Reverse Ball and Socket 7 Autologous Tissue Substitute K Nonautologous Tissue Substitute	Z No Qualifier
J Shoulder Joint, Right K Shoulder Joint, Left	Ø Open	J Synthetic Substitute	6 Humeral Surface 7 Glenoid Surface Z No Qualifier

Ø Medical and Surgical
R Upper Joints
S Reposition Moving to its normal location or other suitable location all or a portion of a body part

Body Part Character 4	Approach Character 5	Device Character 6	Qualifier Character 7
Ø Occipital-cervical Joint 1 Cervical Vertebral Joint 4 Cervicothoracic Vertebral Joint 6 Thoracic Vertebral Joint A Thoracolumbar Vertebral Joint C Temporomandibular Joint, Right D Temporomandibular Joint, Left E Sternoclavicular Joint, Right F Sternoclavicular Joint, Left G Acromioclavicular Joint, Right H Acromioclavicular Joint, Left J Shoulder Joint, Right K Shoulder Joint, Left	Ø Open 3 Percutaneous 4 Percutaneous Endoscopic X External	4 Internal Fixation Device Z No Device	Z No Qualifier
L Elbow Joint, Right M Elbow Joint, Left N Wrist Joint, Right P Wrist Joint, Left Q Carpal Joint, Right R Carpal Joint, Left S Metacarpocarpal Joint, Right T Metacarpocarpal Joint, Left U Metacarpophalangeal Joint, Right V Metacarpophalangeal Joint, Left W Finger Phalangeal Joint, Right X Finger Phalangeal Joint, Left	Ø Open 3 Percutaneous 4 Percutaneous Endoscopic X External	4 Internal Fixation Device 5 External Fixation Device Z No Device	Z No Qualifier

Non-OR ØRS[Ø,1,4,6,A,C,D,E,F,G,H,J,K][3,4,X][4,Z]Z
Non-OR ØRS[L,M,N,P,Q,R,S,T,U,V,W,X][3,4,X][4,5,Z]Z
AHA: 2Ø13, 2Q, 39

Ø Medical and Surgical
R Upper Joints
T Resection Cutting out or off, without replacement, all of a body part

Body Part Character 4	Approach Character 5	Device Character 6	Qualifier Character 7
3 Cervical Vertebral Disc 4 Cervicothoracic Vertebral Joint 5 Cervicothoracic Vertebral Disc 9 Thoracic Vertebral Disc B Thoracolumbar Vertebral Disc C Temporomandibular Joint, Right D Temporomandibular Joint, Left E Sternoclavicular Joint, Right F Sternoclavicular Joint, Left G Acromioclavicular Joint, Right H Acromioclavicular Joint, Left J Shoulder Joint, Right K Shoulder Joint, Left L Elbow Joint, Right M Elbow Joint, Left N Wrist Joint, Right P Wrist Joint, Left Q Carpal Joint, Right R Carpal Joint, Left S Metacarpocarpal Joint, Right T Metacarpocarpal Joint, Left U Metacarpophalangeal Joint, Right V Metacarpophalangeal Joint, Left W Finger Phalangeal Joint, Right X Finger Phalangeal Joint, Left	Ø Open	Z No Device	Z No Qualifier

AHA: 2Ø14, 2Q, 7

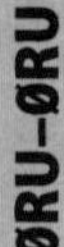

Ø Medical and Surgical
R Upper Joints
U Supplement Putting in or on biological or synthetic material that physically reinforces and/or augments the function of a portion of a body part

Body Part Character 4	Approach Character 5	Device Character 6	Qualifier Character 7
Ø Occipital-cervical Joint **1** Cervical Vertebral Joint **3** Cervical Vertebral Disc **4** Cervicothoracic Vertebral Joint **5** Cervicothoracic Vertebral Disc **6** Thoracic Vertebral Joint **9** Thoracic Vertebral Disc **A** Thoracolumbar Vertebral Joint **B** Thoracolumbar Vertebral Disc **C** Temporomandibular Joint, Right **D** Temporomandibular Joint, Left **E** Sternoclavicular Joint, Right **F** Sternoclavicular Joint, Left **G** Acromioclavicular Joint, Right **H** Acromioclavicular Joint, Left **J** Shoulder Joint, Right **K** Shoulder Joint, Left **L** Elbow Joint, Right **M** Elbow Joint, Left **N** Wrist Joint, Right **P** Wrist Joint, Left **Q** Carpal Joint, Right **R** Carpal Joint, Left **S** Metacarpocarpal Joint, Right **T** Metacarpocarpal Joint, Left **U** Metacarpophalangeal Joint, Right **V** Metacarpophalangeal Joint, Left **W** Finger Phalangeal **X** Finger Phalangeal Joint, Left	**Ø** Open **3** Percutaneous **4** Percutaneous Endoscopic	**7** Autologous Tissue Substitute **J** Synthetic Substitute **K** Nonautologous Tissue Substitute	**Z** No Qualifier

HAC ØRU[E,F,G,H,J,K,L,M][Ø,3,4][7,J,K]Z when reported with SDx K68.11 or T81.4XXA or T81.6Ø-T84.7 with 7th character A

Ø Medical and Surgical
R Upper Joints
W Revision Correcting, to the extent possible, a portion of a malfunctioning device or the position of a displaced device

Body Part Character 4	Approach Character 5	Device Character 6	Qualifier Character 7
Ø Occipital-cervical Joint 1 Cervical Vertebral Joint 4 Cervicothoracic Vertebral Joint 6 Thoracic Vertebral Joint A Thoracolumbar Vertebral Joint	Ø Open 3 Percutaneous 4 Percutaneous Endoscopic X External	Ø Drainage Device 3 Infusion Device 4 Internal Fixation Device 7 Autologous Tissue Substitute 8 Spacer A Interbody Fusion Device J Synthetic Substitute K Nonautologous Tissue Substitute	Z No Qualifier
3 Cervical Vertebral Disc 5 Cervicothoracic Vertebral Disc 9 Thoracic Vertebral Disc B Thoracolumbar Vertebral Disc	Ø Open 3 Percutaneous 4 Percutaneous Endoscopic X External	Ø Drainage Device 3 Infusion Device 7 Autologous Tissue Substitute J Synthetic Substitute K Nonautologous Tissue Substitute	Z No Qualifier
C Temporomandibular Joint, Right D Temporomandibular Joint, Left E Sternoclavicular Joint, Right F Sternoclavicular Joint, Left G Acromioclavicular Joint, Right H Acromioclavicular Joint, Left J Shoulder Joint, Right K Shoulder Joint, Left	Ø Open 3 Percutaneous 4 Percutaneous Endoscopic X External	Ø Drainage Device 3 Infusion Device 4 Internal Fixation Device 5 External Fixation Device 7 Autologous Tissue Substitute 8 Spacer J Synthetic Substitute K Nonautologous Tissue Substitute	Z No Qualifier
L Elbow Joint, Right M Elbow Joint, Left N Wrist Joint, Right P Wrist Joint, Left Q Carpal Joint, Right R Carpal Joint, Left S Metacarpocarpal Joint, Right T Metacarpocarpal Joint, Left U Metacarpophalangeal Joint, Right V Metacarpophalangeal Joint, Left W Finger Phalangeal Joint, Right X Finger Phalangeal Joint, Left	Ø Open 3 Percutaneous 4 Percutaneous Endoscopic X External	Ø Drainage Device 3 Infusion Device 4 Internal Fixation Device 5 External Fixation Device 7 Autologous Tissue Substitute 8 Spacer J Synthetic Substitute K Nonautologous Tissue Substitute	Z No Qualifier

Non-OR ØRW[Ø,1,4,6,A]X[Ø,3,4,7,8,A,J,K]Z
Non-OR ØRW[3,5,9,B]X[Ø,3,7,J,K]Z
Non-OR ØRW[C,D,E,F,G,H,J,K]X[Ø,3,4,5,7,8,J,K]Z
Non-OR ØRW[L,M,N,P,Q,R,S,T,U,V,W,X]X[Ø,3,4,5,7,8,J,K]Z

Lower Joints ØS2–ØSW

Ø Medical and Surgical
S Lower Joints
2 Change Taking out or off a device from a body part and putting back an identical or similar device in or on the same body part without cutting or puncturing the skin or a mucous membrane

Body Part Character 4	Approach Character 5	Device Character 6	Qualifier Character 7
Y Lower Joint	X External	Ø Drainage Device Y Other Device	Z No Qualifier

Non-OR For all body part, approach, device, and qualifier values

Ø Medical and Surgical
S Lower Joints
5 Destruction Physical eradication of all or a portion of a body part by the direct use of energy, force, or a destructive agent

Body Part Character 4	Approach Character 5	Device Character 6	Qualifier Character 7
Ø Lumbar Vertebral Joint 2 Lumbar Vertebral Disc 3 Lumbosacral Joint 4 Lumbosacral Disc 5 Sacrococcygeal Joint 6 Coccygeal Joint 7 Sacroiliac Joint, Right 8 Sacroiliac Joint, Left 9 Hip Joint, Right B Hip Joint, Left C Knee Joint, Right D Knee Joint, Left F Ankle Joint, Right G Ankle Joint, Left H Tarsal Joint, Right J Tarsal Joint, Left K Metatarsal-Tarsal Joint, Right L Metatarsal-Tarsal Joint, Left M Metatarsal-Phalangeal Joint, Right N Metatarsal-Phalangeal Joint, Left P Toe Phalangeal Joint, Right Q Toe Phalangeal Joint, Left	Ø Open 3 Percutaneous 4 Percutaneous Endoscopic	Z No Device	Z No Qualifier

Ø Medical and Surgical
S Lower Joints
9 Drainage Taking or letting out fluids and/or gases from a body part

Body Part Character 4	Approach Character 5	Device Character 6	Qualifier Character 7
Ø Lumbar Vertebral Joint 2 Lumbar Vertebral Disc 3 Lumbosacral Joint 4 Lumbosacral Disc 5 Sacrococcygeal Joint 6 Coccygeal Joint 7 Sacroiliac Joint, Right 8 Sacroiliac Joint, Left 9 Hip Joint, Right B Hip Joint, Left C Knee Joint, Right D Knee Joint, Left F Ankle Joint, Right G Ankle Joint, Left H Tarsal Joint, Right J Tarsal Joint, Left K Metatarsal-Tarsal Joint, Right L Metatarsal-Tarsal Joint, Left M Metatarsal-Phalangeal Joint, Right N Metatarsal-Phalangeal Joint, Left P Toe Phalangeal Joint, Right Q Toe Phalangeal Joint, Left	Ø Open 3 Percutaneous 4 Percutaneous Endoscopic	Ø Drainage Device	Z No Qualifier

ØS9 Continued on next page

Non-OR ØS9[Ø,2,3,4,5,6,7,8,9,B,C,D,F,G,H,J,K,L,M,N,P,Q][3,4]ØZ

0S9 Continued

0 Medical and Surgical
S Lower Joints
9 Drainage Taking or letting out fluids and/or gases from a body part

Body Part Character 4	Approach Character 5	Device Character 6	Qualifier Character 7
0 Lumbar Vertebral Joint 2 Lumbar Vertebral Disc 3 Lumbosacral Joint 4 Lumbosacral Disc 5 Sacrococcygeal Joint 6 Coccygeal Joint 7 Sacroiliac Joint, Right 8 Sacroiliac Joint, Left 9 Hip Joint, Right B Hip Joint, Left C Knee Joint, Right D Knee Joint, Left F Ankle Joint, Right G Ankle Joint, Left H Tarsal Joint, Right J Tarsal Joint, Left K Metatarsal-Tarsal Joint, Right L Metatarsal-Tarsal Joint, Left M Metatarsal-Phalangeal Joint, Right N Metatarsal-Phalangeal Joint, Left P Toe Phalangeal Joint, Right Q Toe Phalangeal Joint, Left	0 Open 3 Percutaneous 4 Percutaneous Endoscopic	Z No Device	X Diagnostic Z No Qualifier

Non-OR 0S9[0,2,3,4,5,6,7,8,9,B,C,D,F,G,H,J,K,L,M,N,P,Q][0,3,4]ZX
Non-OR 0S9[0,2,3,4,5,6,7,8,9,B,C,D,F,G,H,J,K,L,M,N,P,Q][3,4]ZZ

0 Medical and Surgical
S Lower Joints
B Excision Cutting out or off, without replacement, a portion of a body part

Body Part Character 4	Approach Character 5	Device Character 6	Qualifier Character 7
0 Lumbar Vertebral Joint 2 Lumbar Vertebral Disc 3 Lumbosacral Joint 4 Lumbosacral Disc 5 Sacrococcygeal Joint 6 Coccygeal Joint 7 Sacroiliac Joint, Right 8 Sacroiliac Joint, Left 9 Hip Joint, Right B Hip Joint, Left C Knee Joint, Right ⊞ D Knee Joint, Left ⊞ F Ankle Joint, Right G Ankle Joint, Left H Tarsal Joint, Right J Tarsal Joint, Left K Metatarsal-Tarsal Joint, Right L Metatarsal-Tarsal Joint, Left M Metatarsal-Phalangeal Joint, Right N Metatarsal-Phalangeal Joint, Left P Toe Phalangeal Joint, Right Q Toe Phalangeal Joint, Left	0 Open 3 Percutaneous 4 Percutaneous Endoscopic	Z No Device	X Diagnostic Z No Qualifier

Non-OR 0SB[0,2,3,4,5,6,7,8,9,B,C,D,F,G,H,J,K,L,M,N,P,Q][0,3,4]ZX
AHA: 2014, 2Q, 6

No Procedure Combinations Specified
⊞ 0SB[C,D][0,3,4]ZZ

Ø Medical and Surgical
S Lower Joints
C Extirpation Taking or cutting out solid matter from a body part

Body Part Character 4	Approach Character 5	Device Character 6	Qualifier Character 7
Ø Lumbar Vertebral Joint **2** Lumbar Vertebral Disc **3** Lumbosacral Joint **4** Lumbosacral Disc **5** Sacrococcygeal Joint **6** Coccygeal Joint **7** Sacroiliac Joint, Right **8** Sacroiliac Joint, Left **9** Hip Joint, Right **B** Hip Joint, Left **C** Knee Joint, Right **D** Knee Joint, Left **F** Ankle Joint, Right **G** Ankle Joint, Left **H** Tarsal Joint, Right **J** Tarsal Joint, Left **K** Metatarsal-Tarsal Joint, Right **L** Metatarsal-Tarsal Joint, Left **M** Metatarsal-Phalangeal Joint, Right **N** Metatarsal-Phalangeal Joint, Left **P** Toe Phalangeal Joint, Right **Q** Toe Phalangeal Joint, Left	**Ø** Open **3** Percutaneous **4** Percutaneous Endoscopic	**Z** No Device	**Z** No Qualifier

Ø Medical and Surgical
S Lower Joints
G Fusion Joining together portions of an articular body part rendering the articular body part immobile

Body Part Character 4	Approach Character 5	Device Character 6	Qualifier Character 7
Ø Lumbar Vertebral Joint **1** Lumbar Vertebral Joints, 2 or more ⊞ **3** Lumbosacral Joint	**Ø** Open **3** Percutaneous **4** Percutaneous Endoscopic	**7** Autologous Tissue Substitute **A** Interbody Fusion Device **J** Synthetic Substitute **K** Nonautologous Tissue Substitute **Z** No Device	**Ø** Anterior Approach, Anterior Column **1** Posterior Approach, Posterior Column **J** Posterior Approach, Anterior Column
5 Sacrococcygeal Joint **6** Coccygeal Joint **7** Sacroiliac Joint, Right **8** Sacroiliac Joint, Left	**Ø** Open **3** Percutaneous **4** Percutaneous Endoscopic	**4** Internal Fixation Device **7** Autologous Tissue Substitute **J** Synthetic Substitute **K** Nonautologous Tissue Substitute **Z** No Device	**Z** No Qualifier
9 Hip Joint, Right **B** Hip Joint, Left **C** Knee Joint, Right **D** Knee Joint, Left **F** Ankle Joint, Right **G** Ankle Joint, Left **H** Tarsal Joint, Right **J** Tarsal Joint, Left **K** Metatarsal-Tarsal Joint, Right **L** Metatarsal-Tarsal Joint, Left **M** Metatarsal-Phalangeal Joint, Right ⊞ **N** Metatarsal-Phalangeal Joint, Left ⊞ **P** Toe Phalangeal Joint, Right **Q** Toe Phalangeal Joint, Left	**Ø** Open **3** Percutaneous **4** Percutaneous Endoscopic	**4** Internal Fixation Device **5** External Fixation Device **7** Autologous Tissue Substitute **J** Synthetic Substitute **K** Nonautologous Tissue Substitute **Z** No Device	**Z** No Qualifier

HAC ØSG[Ø,1,3][Ø,3,4][7,A,J,K,Z][Ø,1,J] when reported with SDx K68.11 or T81.4XXA or T81.6Ø-T84.7 with 7th character A

HAC ØSG[7,8][Ø,3,4][4,7,J,K,Z]Z when reported with SDx K68.11 or T81.4XXA or T81.6Ø-T84.7 with 7th character A

AHA: 2Ø14, 2Q, 6; 2Ø13, 3Q, 25; 2Ø13, 2Q, 39; 2Ø13, 1Q, 21

See Appendix I for Procedure Combinations
⊞ ØSG1[Ø,3,4][7,A,J,K,Z][Ø,1,J]

No Procedure Combinations Specified
⊞ ØSG[M,N][Ø,3,4]ZZ

Lower Joints

Ø Medical and Surgical
S Lower Joints
H Insertion Putting in a nonbiological appliance that monitors, assists, performs, or prevents a physiological function but does not physically take the place of a body part

Body Part Character 4	Approach Character 5	Device Character 6	Qualifier Character 7
Ø Lumbar Vertebral Joint **3** Lumbosacral Joint	**Ø** Open **3** Percutaneous **4** Percutaneous Endoscopic	**3** Infusion Device **4** Internal Fixation Device **8** Spacer **B** Spinal Stabilization Device, Interspinous Process **C** Spinal Stabilization Device, Pedicle-Based **D** Spinal Stabilization Device, Facet Replacement	**Z** No Qualifier
2 Lumbar Vertebral Disc **4** Lumbosacral Disc	**Ø** Open **3** Percutaneous **4** Percutaneous Endoscopic	**3** Infusion Device **8** Spacer	**Z** No Qualifier
5 Sacrococcygeal Joint **6** Coccygeal Joint **7** Sacroiliac Joint, Right **8** Sacroiliac Joint, Left	**Ø** Open **3** Percutaneous **4** Percutaneous Endoscopic	**3** Infusion Device **4** Internal Fixation Device **8** Spacer	**Z** No Qualifier
9 Hip Joint, Right **B** Hip Joint, Left **C** Knee Joint, Right **D** Knee Joint, Left **F** Ankle Joint, Right **G** Ankle Joint, Left **H** Tarsal Joint, Right **J** Tarsal Joint, Left **K** Metatarsal-Tarsal Joint, Right **L** Metatarsal-Tarsal Joint, Left **M** Metatarsal-Phalangeal Joint, Right **N** Metatarsal-Phalangeal Joint, Left **P** Toe Phalangeal Joint, Right **Q** Toe Phalangeal Joint, Left	**Ø** Open **3** Percutaneous **4** Percutaneous Endoscopic	**3** Infusion Device **4** Internal Fixation Device **5** External Fixation Device **8** Spacer	**Z** No Qualifier

Non-OR ØSH[Ø,3][Ø,3,4][3,8]Z
Non-OR ØSH[2,4][Ø,3,4][3,8]Z
Non-OR ØSH[5,6,7,8][Ø,3,4][3,8]Z
Non-OR ØSH[9,B,C,D,F,G,H,J,K,L,M,N,P,Q][Ø,3,4][3,8]Z

Ø Medical and Surgical
S Lower Joints
J Inspection Visually and/or manually exploring a body part

Body Part Character 4	Approach Character 5	Device Character 6	Qualifier Character 7
Ø Lumbar Vertebral Joint **2** Lumbar Vertebral Disc **3** Lumbosacral Joint **4** Lumbosacral Disc **5** Sacrococcygeal Joint **6** Coccygeal Joint **7** Sacroiliac Joint, Right **8** Sacroiliac Joint, Left **9** Hip Joint, Right **B** Hip Joint, Left **C** Knee Joint, Right **D** Knee Joint, Left **F** Ankle Joint, Right **G** Ankle Joint, Left **H** Tarsal Joint, Right **J** Tarsal Joint, Left **K** Metatarsal-Tarsal Joint, Right **L** Metatarsal-Tarsal Joint, Left **M** Metatarsal-Phalangeal Joint, Right **N** Metatarsal-Phalangeal Joint, Left **P** Toe Phalangeal Joint, Right **Q** Toe Phalangeal Joint, Left	**Ø** Open **3** Percutaneous **4** Percutaneous Endoscopic **X** External	**Z** No Device	**Z** No Qualifier

Non-OR ØSJ[Ø,2,3,4,5,6,7,8,9,B,C,D,F,G,H,J,K,L,M,N,P,Q]XZZ

ØSH—ØSJ

Ø Medical and Surgical
S Lower Joints
N Release Freeing a body part from an abnormal physical constraint

Body Part Character 4	Approach Character 5	Device Character 6	Qualifier Character 7
Ø Lumbar Vertebral Joint 2 Lumbar Vertebral Disc 3 Lumbosacral Joint 4 Lumbosacral Disc 5 Sacrococcygeal Joint 6 Coccygeal Joint 7 Sacroiliac Joint, Right 8 Sacroiliac Joint, Left 9 Hip Joint, Right B Hip Joint, Left C Knee Joint, Right D Knee Joint, Left F Ankle Joint, Right G Ankle Joint, Left H Tarsal Joint, Right J Tarsal Joint, Left K Metatarsal-Tarsal Joint, Right L Metatarsal-Tarsal Joint, Left M Metatarsal-Phalangeal Joint, Right N Metatarsal-Phalangeal Joint, Left P Toe Phalangeal Joint, Right Q Toe Phalangeal Joint, Left	Ø Open 3 Percutaneous 4 Percutaneous Endoscopic X External	Z No Device	Z No Qualifier

Non-OR ØSN[Ø,2,3,4,5,6,7,8,9,B,C,D,F,G,H,J,K,L,M,N,P,Q]XZZ

Ø Medical and Surgical
S Lower Joints
P Removal Taking out or off a device from a body part

Body Part Character 4	Approach Character 5	Device Character 6	Qualifier Character 7
Ø Lumbar Vertebral Joint 3 Lumbosacral Joint	Ø Open 3 Percutaneous 4 Percutaneous Endoscopic	Ø Drainage Device 3 Infusion Device 4 Internal Fixation Device 7 Autologous Tissue Substitute 8 Spacer A Interbody Fusion Device J Synthetic Substitute K Nonautologous Tissue Substitute	Z No Qualifier
Ø Lumbar Vertebral Joint 3 Lumbosacral Joint	X External	Ø Drainage Device 3 Infusion Device 4 Internal Fixation Device	Z No Qualifier
5 Sacrococcygeal Joint 6 Coccygeal Joint 7 Sacroiliac Joint, Right 8 Sacroiliac Joint, Left	Ø Open 3 Percutaneous 4 Percutaneous Endoscopic	Ø Drainage Device 3 Infusion Device 4 Internal Fixation Device 7 Autologous Tissue Substitute 8 Spacer J Synthetic Substitute K Nonautologous Tissue Substitute	Z No Qualifier
5 Sacrococcygeal Joint 6 Coccygeal Joint 7 Sacroiliac Joint, Right 8 Sacroiliac Joint, Left	X External	Ø Drainage Device 3 Infusion Device 4 Internal Fixation Device	Z No Qualifier
2 Lumbar Vertebral Disc 4 Lumbosacral Disc	Ø Open 3 Percutaneous 4 Percutaneous Endoscopic	Ø Drainage Device 3 Infusion Device 7 Autologous Tissue Substitute J Synthetic Substitute K Nonautologous Tissue Substitute	Z No Qualifier
2 Lumbar Vertebral Disc 4 Lumbosacral Disc	X External	Ø Drainage Device 3 Infusion Device	Z No Qualifier

ØSP Continued on next page

Non-OR ØSP[Ø,3][Ø,3,4]8Z
Non-OR ØSP[Ø,3]X[Ø,3,4]Z
Non-OR ØSP[5,6,7,8][Ø,3,4]8Z
Non-OR ØSP[5,6,7,8]X[Ø,3,4]Z
Non-OR ØSP[2,4]X[Ø,3]Z
AHA: 2Ø13, 2Q, 39

ØSP Continued

Ø Medical and Surgical
S Lower Joints
P Removal Taking out or off a device from a body part

Body Part Character 4	Approach Character 5	Device Character 6	Qualifier Character 7
9 Hip Joint, Right ⊞ B Hip Joint, Left ⊞	Ø Open	Ø Drainage Device 3 Infusion Device 4 Internal Fixation Device 5 External Fixation Device 7 Autologous Tissue Substitute 8 Spacer 9 Liner B Resurfacing Device J Synthetic Substitute K Nonautologous Tissue Substitute	Z No Qualifier
9 Hip Joint, Right B Hip Joint, Left C Knee Joint, Right ⊞ D Knee Joint, Left ⊞	3 Percutaneous 4 Percutaneous Endoscopic	Ø Drainage Device 3 Infusion Device 4 Internal Fixation Device 5 External Fixation Device 7 Autologous Tissue Substitute 8 Spacer J Synthetic Substitute K Nonautologous Tissue Substitute	Z No Qualifier
9 Hip Joint, Right B Hip Joint, Left C Knee Joint, Right D Knee Joint, Left F Ankle Joint, Right G Ankle Joint, Left H Tarsal Joint, Right J Tarsal Joint, Left K Metatarsal-Tarsal Joint, Right L Metatarsal-Tarsal Joint, Left M Metatarsal-Phalangeal Joint, Right N Metatarsal-Phalangeal Joint, Left P Toe Phalangeal Joint, Right Q Toe Phalangeal Joint, Left	X External	Ø Drainage Device 3 Infusion Device 4 Internal Fixation Device 5 External Fixation Device	Z No Qualifier
C Knee Joint, Right ⊞ D Knee Joint, Left ⊞	Ø Open	Ø Drainage Device 3 Infusion Device 4 Internal Fixation Device 5 External Fixation Device 7 Autologous Tissue Substitute 8 Spacer 9 Liner J Synthetic Substitute K Nonautologous Tissue Substitute	Z No Qualifier
F Ankle Joint, Right G Ankle Joint, Left H Tarsal Joint, Right J Tarsal Joint, Left K Metatarsal-Tarsal Joint, Right L Metatarsal-Tarsal Joint, Left M Metatarsal-Phalangeal Joint, Right N Metatarsal-Phalangeal Joint, Left P Toe Phalangeal Joint, Right Q Toe Phalangeal Joint, Left	Ø Open 3 Percutaneous 4 Percutaneous Endoscopic	Ø Drainage Device 3 Infusion Device 4 Internal Fixation Device 5 External Fixation Device 7 Autologous Tissue Substitute 8 Spacer J Synthetic Substitute K Nonautologous Tissue Substitute	Z No Qualifier

Non-OR ØSP[9,B]Ø8Z
Non-OR ØSP[9,B,C,D][3,4]8Z
Non-OR ØSP[9,B,C,D,F,G,H,J,K,L,M,N,P,Q]X[Ø,3,4,5]Z
Non-OR ØSP[C,D]Ø8Z
Non-OR ØSP[F,G,H,J,K,L,M,N,P,Q][Ø,3,4]8Z
AHA: 2Ø13, 2Q, 39

See Appendix I for Procedure Combinations
⊞ ØSP[9,B]Ø[9,J]Z
⊞ ØSP[C,D]4JZ
⊞ ØSP[C,D]Ø[9,J]Z

DRAFT

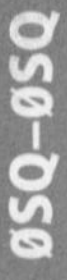

Ø Medical and Surgical
S Lower Joints
Q Repair Restoring, to the extent possible, a body part to its normal anatomic structure and function

Body Part Character 4	Approach Character 5	Device Character 6	Qualifier Character 7
Ø Lumbar Vertebral Joint **2** Lumbar Vertebral Disc **3** Lumbosacral Joint **4** Lumbosacral Disc **5** Sacrococcygeal Joint **6** Coccygeal Joint **7** Sacroiliac Joint, Right **8** Sacroiliac Joint, Left **9** Hip Joint, Right **B** Hip Joint, Left **C** Knee Joint, Right **D** Knee Joint, Left **F** Ankle Joint, Right **G** Ankle Joint, Left **H** Tarsal Joint, Right **J** Tarsal Joint, Left **K** Metatarsal-Tarsal Joint, Right **L** Metatarsal-Tarsal Joint, Left **M** Metatarsal-Phalangeal Joint, Right **N** Metatarsal-Phalangeal Joint, Left **P** Toe Phalangeal Joint, Right **Q** Toe Phalangeal Joint, Left	**Ø** Open **3** Percutaneous **4** Percutaneous Endoscopic **X** External	**Z** No Device	**Z** No Qualifier

Ø Medical and Surgical
S Lower Joints
R Replacement Putting in or on biological or synthetic material that physically takes the place and/or function of all or a portion of a body part

Body Part Character 4	Approach Character 5	Device Character 6	Qualifier Character 7
Ø Lumbar Vertebral Joint 2 Lumbar Vertebral Disc NC 3 Lumbosacral Joint 4 Lumbosacral Disc NC 5 Sacrococcygeal Joint 6 Coccygeal Joint 7 Sacroiliac Joint, Right 8 Sacroiliac Joint, Left H Tarsal Joint, Right J Tarsal Joint, Left K Metatarsal-Tarsal Joint, Right L Metatarsal-Tarsal Joint, Left M Metatarsal-Phalangeal Joint, Right N Metatarsal-Phalangeal Joint, Left P Toe Phalangeal Joint, Right Q Toe Phalangeal Joint, Left	Ø Open	7 Autologous Tissue Substitute J Synthetic Substitute K Nonautologous Tissue Substitute	Z No Qualifier
9 Hip Joint, Right ⊞ B Hip Joint, Left ⊞	Ø Open	1 Synthetic Substitute, Metal 2 Synthetic Substitute, Metal on Polyethylene 3 Synthetic Substitute, Ceramic 4 Synthetic Substitute, Ceramic on Polyethylene J Synthetic Substitute	9 Cemented A Uncemented Z No Qualifier
9 Hip Joint, Right B Hip Joint, Left	Ø Open	7 Autologous Tissue Substitute K Nonautologous Tissue Substitute	Z No Qualifier
A Hip Joint, Acetabular Surface, Right ⊞ E Hip Joint, Acetabular Surface, Left ⊞	Ø Open	Ø Synthetic Substitute, Polyethylene 1 Synthetic Substitute, Metal 3 Synthetic Substitute, Ceramic J Synthetic Substitute	9 Cemented A Uncemented Z No Qualifier
A Hip Joint, Acetabular Surface, Right E Hip Joint, Acetabular Surface, Left	Ø Open	7 Autologous Tissue Substitute K Nonautologous Tissue Substitute	Z No Qualifier
C Knee Joint, Right D Knee Joint, Left F Ankle Joint, Right G Ankle Joint, Left T Knee Joint, Femoral Surface, Right U Knee Joint, Femoral Surface, Left V Knee Joint, Tibial Surface, Right W Knee Joint, Tibial Surface, Left	Ø Open	7 Autologous Tissue Substitute K Nonautologous Tissue Substitute	Z No Qualifier
C Knee Joint, Right ⊞ D Knee Joint, Left ⊞ F Ankle Joint, Right G Ankle Joint, Left T Knee Joint, Femoral Surface, Right ⊞ U Knee Joint, Femoral Surface, Left ⊞ V Knee Joint, Tibial Surface, Right ⊞ W Knee Joint, Tibial Surface, Left ⊞	Ø Open	J Synthetic Substitute	9 Cemented A Uncemented Z No Qualifier
R Hip Joint, Femoral Surface, Right ⊞ S Hip Joint, Femoral Surface, Left ⊞	Ø Open	1 Synthetic Substitute, Metal 3 Synthetic Substitute, Ceramic J Synthetic Substitute	9 Cemented A Uncemented Z No Qualifier
R Hip Joint, Femoral Surface, Right S Hip Joint, Femoral Surface, Left	Ø Open	7 Autologous Tissue Substitute K Nonautologous Tissue Substitute	Z No Qualifier

HAC ØSR[9,B]Ø[1,2,3,4,J][9,A,Z] when reported with SDx from I26.Ø2-I26.Ø9, I26.92-I26.99, or I82.4Ø1-I82.4Z9

HAC ØSR[9,B]Ø[7,K]Z when reported with SDx from I26.Ø2-I26.Ø9, I26.92-I26.99, or I82.4Ø1-I82.4Z9

HAC ØSR[A,E]Ø[Ø,1,3,J][9,A,Z] when reported with SDx from I26.Ø2-I26.Ø9, I26.92-I26.99, or I82.4Ø1-I82.4Z9

HAC ØSR[A,E]Ø[7,K]Z when reported with SDx from I26.Ø2-I26.Ø9, I26.92-I26.99, or I82.4Ø1-I82.4Z9

HAC ØSR[C,D,T,U,V,W]Ø[7,K]Z when reported with SDx from I26.Ø2-I26.Ø9, I26.92-I26.99, or I82.4Ø1-I82.4Z9

HAC ØSR[C,D,T,U,V,W]ØJ[9,A,Z] when reported with SDx from I26.Ø2-I26.Ø9, I26.92-I26.99, or I82.4Ø1-I82.4Z9

HAC ØSR[R,S]Ø[1,3,J][9,A,Z] when reported with SDx from I26.Ø2-I26.Ø9, I26.92-I26.99, or I82.4Ø1-I82.4Z9

HAC ØSR[R,S]Ø[7,K]Z when reported with SDx from I26.Ø2-I26.Ø9, I26.92-I26.99, or I82.4Ø1-I82.4Z9

NC ØSR[2,4]ØJZ when beneficiary age is over 6Ø

See Appendix I for Procedure Combinations

⊞ ØSR[9,B]Ø[1,2,3,J][9,A,Z]
⊞ ØSR[A,E]Ø[Ø,1,3,J][9,A,Z]
⊞ ØSR[C,D]ØJZ[9,A,Z]
⊞ ØSR[T,U,V,W]ØJZ
⊞ ØSR[R,S]Ø[1,3,J][9,A,Z]

Ø Medical and Surgical
S Lower Joints
S Reposition Moving to its normal location or other suitable location all or a portion of a body part

Body Part Character 4	Approach Character 5	Device Character 6	Qualifier Character 7
Ø Lumbar Vertebral Joint **3** Lumbosacral Joint **5** Sacrococcygeal Joint **6** Coccygeal Joint **7** Sacroiliac Joint, Right **8** Sacroiliac Joint, Left	**Ø** Open **3** Percutaneous **4** Percutaneous Endoscopic **X** External	**4** Internal Fixation Device **Z** No Device	**Z** No Qualifier
9 Hip Joint, Right **B** Hip Joint, Left **C** Knee Joint, Right **D** Knee Joint, Left **F** Ankle Joint, Right **G** Ankle Joint, Left **H** Tarsal Joint, Right **J** Tarsal Joint, Left **K** Metatarsal-Tarsal Joint, Right **L** Metatarsal-Tarsal Joint, Left **M** Metatarsal-Phalangeal Joint, Right **N** Metatarsal-Phalangeal Joint, Left **P** Toe Phalangeal Joint, Right **Q** Toe Phalangeal Joint, Left	**Ø** Open **3** Percutaneous **4** Percutaneous Endoscopic **X** External	**4** Internal Fixation Device **5** External Fixation Device **Z** No Device	**Z** No Qualifier

Non-OR ØSS[Ø,3,5,6,7,8][3,4,X][4,Z]Z
Non-OR ØSS[9,B,C,D,F,G,H,J,K,L,M,N,P,Q][3,4,X][4,5,Z]Z

Ø Medical and Surgical
S Lower Joints
T Resection Cutting out or off, without replacement, all of a body part

Body Part Character 4	Approach Character 5	Device Character 6	Qualifier Character 7
2 Lumbar Vertebral Disc **4** Lumbosacral Disc **5** Sacrococcygeal Joint **6** Coccygeal Joint **7** Sacroiliac Joint, Right **8** Sacroiliac Joint, Left **9** Hip Joint, Right **B** Hip Joint, Left **C** Knee Joint, Right **D** Knee Joint, Left **F** Ankle Joint, Right **G** Ankle Joint, Left **H** Tarsal Joint, Right **J** Tarsal Joint, Left **K** Metatarsal-Tarsal Joint, Right **L** Metatarsal-Tarsal Joint, Left **M** Metatarsal-Phalangeal Joint, Right **N** Metatarsal-Phalangeal Joint, Left **P** Toe Phalangeal Joint, Right **Q** Toe Phalangeal Joint, Left	**Ø** Open	**Z** No Device	**Z** No Qualifier

0 Medical and Surgical
S Lower Joints
U Supplement Putting in or on biological or synthetic material that physically reinforces and/or augments the function of a portion of a body part

Body Part Character 4	Approach Character 5	Device Character 6	Qualifier Character 7
0 Lumbar Vertebral Joint 2 Lumbar Vertebral Disc 3 Lumbosacral Joint 4 Lumbosacral Disc 5 Sacrococcygeal Joint 6 Coccygeal Joint 7 Sacroiliac Joint, Right 8 Sacroiliac Joint, Left F Ankle Joint, Right G Ankle Joint, Left H Tarsal Joint, Right J Tarsal Joint, Left K Metatarsal-Tarsal Joint, Right L Metatarsal-Tarsal Joint, Left M Metatarsal-Phalangeal Joint, Right N Metatarsal-Phalangeal Joint, Left P Toe Phalangeal Joint, Right Q Toe Phalangeal Joint, Left	0 Open 3 Percutaneous 4 Percutaneous Endoscopic	7 Autologous Tissue Substitute J Synthetic Substitute K Nonautologous Tissue Substitute	Z No Qualifier
9 Hip Joint, Right ⊞ B Hip Joint, Left ⊞	0 Open	7 Autologous Tissue Substitute 9 Liner B Resurfacing Device J Synthetic Substitute K Nonautologous Tissue Substitute	Z No Qualifier
9 Hip Joint, Right B Hip Joint, Left	3 Percutaneous 4 Percutaneous Endoscopic	7 Autologous Tissue Substitute J Synthetic Substitute K Nonautologous Tissue Substitute	Z No Qualifier
A Hip Joint, Acetabular Surface, Right ⊞ E Hip Joint, Acetabular Surface, Left ⊞ R Hip Joint, Femoral Surface, Right ⊞ S Hip Joint, Femoral Surface, Left ⊞	0 Open	9 Liner B Resurfacing Device	Z No Qualifier
C Knee Joint, Right ⊞ D Knee Joint, Left ⊞	0 Open	7 Autologous Tissue Substitute J Synthetic Substitute K Nonautologous Tissue Substitute	Z No Qualifier
C Knee Joint, Right ⊞ D Knee Joint, Left ⊞	3 Percutaneous 4 Percutaneous Endoscopic	7 Autologous Tissue Substitute J Synthetic Substitute K Nonautologous Tissue Substitute	Z No Qualifier
C Knee Joint, Right ⊞ D Knee Joint, Left ⊞	0 Open	9 Liner	C Patellar Surface Z No Qualifier
T Knee Joint, Femoral Surface, Right ⊞ U Knee Joint, Femoral Surface, Left ⊞ V Knee Joint, Tibial Surface, Right ⊞ W Knee Joint, Tibial Surface, Left ⊞	0 Open	9 Liner	Z No Qualifier

HAC 0SU[9,B]0BZ when reported with SDx from I26.02-I26.09, I26.92-I26.99, or I82.401-I82.4Z9

HAC 0SU[A,E,R,S]0BZ when reported with SDx from I26.02-I26.09, I26.92-I26.99, or I82.401-I82.4Z9

See Appendix I for Procedure Combinations

⊞ 0SU[9,B]09Z
⊞ 0SU[A,E,R,S]09Z
⊞ 0SU[V,W]09Z

No Procedure Combinations Specified

⊞ 0SU[C,D]0JZ
⊞ 0SU[C,D]4JZ
⊞ 0SU[C,D]09C
⊞ 0SU[T,U]09Z

Ø Medical and Surgical
S Lower Joints
W Revision Correcting, to the extent possible, a portion of a malfunctioning device or the position of a displaced device

Body Part Character 4	Approach Character 5	Device Character 6	Qualifier Character 7
Ø Lumbar Vertebral Joint **3** Lumbosacral Joint	**Ø** Open **3** Percutaneous **4** Percutaneous Endoscopic **X** External	**Ø** Drainage Device **3** Infusion Device **4** Internal Fixation Device **7** Autologous Tissue Substitute **8** Spacer **A** Interbody Fusion Device **J** Synthetic Substitute **K** Nonautologous Tissue Substitute	**Z** No Qualifier
2 Lumbar Vertebral Disc **4** Lumbosacral Disc	**Ø** Open **3** Percutaneous **4** Percutaneous Endoscopic **X** External	**Ø** Drainage Device **3** Infusion Device **7** Autologous Tissue Substitute **J** Synthetic Substitute **K** Nonautologous Tissue Substitute	**Z** No Qualifier
5 Sacrococcygeal Joint **6** Coccygeal Joint **7** Sacroiliac Joint, Right **8** Sacroiliac Joint, Left	**Ø** Open **3** Percutaneous **4** Percutaneous Endoscopic **X** External	**Ø** Drainage Device **3** Infusion Device **4** Internal Fixation Device **7** Autologous Tissue Substitute **8** Spacer **J** Synthetic Substitute **K** Nonautologous Tissue Substitute	**Z** No Qualifier
9 Hip Joint, Right **B** Hip Joint, Left	**Ø** Open	**Ø** Drainage Device **3** Infusion Device **4** Internal Fixation Device **5** External Fixation Device **7** Autologous Tissue Substitute **8** Spacer **9** Liner **B** Resurfacing Device **J** Synthetic Substitute **K** Nonautologous Tissue Substitute	**Z** No Qualifier
9 Hip Joint, Right **B** Hip Joint, Left **C** Knee Joint, Right **D** Knee Joint, Left	**3** Percutaneous **4** Percutaneous Endoscopic **X** External	**Ø** Drainage Device **3** Infusion Device **4** Internal Fixation Device **5** External Fixation Device **7** Autologous Tissue Substitute **8** Spacer **J** Synthetic Substitute **K** Nonautologous Tissue Substitute	**Z** No Qualifier
C Knee Joint, Right **D** Knee Joint, Left	**Ø** Open	**Ø** Drainage Device **3** Infusion Device **4** Internal Fixation Device **5** External Fixation Device **7** Autologous Tissue Substitute **8** Spacer **9** Liner **J** Synthetic Substitute **K** Nonautologous Tissue Substitute	**Z** No Qualifier
F Ankle Joint, Right **G** Ankle Joint, Left **H** Tarsal Joint, Right **J** Tarsal Joint, Left **K** Metatarsal-Tarsal Joint, Right **L** Metatarsal-Tarsal Joint, Left **M** Metatarsal-Phalangeal Joint, Right **N** Metatarsal-Phalangeal Joint, Left **P** Toe Phalangeal Joint, Right **Q** Toe Phalangeal Joint, Left	**Ø** Open **3** Percutaneous **4** Percutaneous Endoscopic **X** External	**Ø** Drainage Device **3** Infusion Device **4** Internal Fixation Device **5** External Fixation Device **7** Autologous Tissue Substitute **8** Spacer **J** Synthetic Substitute **K** Nonautologous Tissue Substitute	**Z** No Qualifier

Non-OR ØSW[Ø,3]X[Ø,3,4,7,8,A,J,K]Z
Non-OR ØSW[2,4]X[Ø,3,7,J,K]Z
Non-OR ØSW[5,6,7,8]X[Ø,3,4,7,8,J,K]Z
Non-OR ØSW[9,B,C,D]X[Ø,3,4,5,7,8,J,K]Z
Non-OR ØSW[F,G,H,J,K,L,M,N,P,Q]X[Ø,3,4,5,7,8,J,K]Z

Urinary System ØT1–ØTY

Ø Medical and Surgical
T Urinary System
1 Bypass Altering the route of passage of the contents of a tubular body part

Body Part Character 4	Approach Character 5	Device Character 6	Qualifier Character 7
3 Kidney Pelvis, Right 4 Kidney Pelvis, Left	Ø Open 4 Percutaneous Endoscopic	7 Autologous Tissue Substitute J Synthetic Substitute K Nonautologous Tissue Substitute Z No Device	3 Kidney Pelvis, Right 4 Kidney Pelvis, Left 6 Ureter, Right 7 Ureter, Left 8 Colon 9 Colocutaneous A Ileum B Bladder C Ileocutaneous D Cutaneous
3 Kidney Pelvis, Right 4 Kidney Pelvis, Left 6 Ureter, Right 7 Ureter, Left 8 Ureters, Bilateral B Bladder	3 Percutaneous	J Synthetic Substitute	D Cutaneous
6 Ureter, Right 7 Ureter, Left 8 Ureters, Bilateral	Ø Open 4 Percutaneous Endoscopic	7 Autologous Tissue Substitute J Synthetic Substitute K Nonautologous Tissue Substitute Z No Device	6 Ureter, Right 7 Ureter, Left 8 Colon 9 Colocutaneous A Ileum B Bladder C Ileocutaneous D Cutaneous
B Bladder	Ø Open 4 Percutaneous Endoscopic	7 Autologous Tissue Substitute J Synthetic Substitute K Nonautologous Tissue Substitute Z No Device	9 Colocutaneous C Ileocutaneous D Cutaneous

Ø Medical and Surgical
T Urinary System
2 Change Taking out or off a device from a body part and putting back an identical or similar device in or on the same body part without cutting or puncturing the skin or a mucous membrane

Body Part Character 4	Approach Character 5	Device Character 6	Qualifier Character 7
5 Kidney 9 Ureter B Bladder D Urethra	X External	Ø Drainage Device Y Other Device	Z No Qualifier

Non-OR For all body part, approach, device, and qualifier values

Ø Medical and Surgical
T Urinary System
5 Destruction Physical eradication of all or a portion of a body part by the direct use of energy, force, or a destructive agent

Body Part Character 4	Approach Character 5	Device Character 6	Qualifier Character 7
Ø Kidney, Right 1 Kidney, Left 3 Kidney Pelvis, Right 4 Kidney Pelvis, Left 6 Ureter, Right 7 Ureter, Left B Bladder C Bladder Neck	Ø Open 3 Percutaneous 4 Percutaneous Endoscopic 7 Via Natural or Artificial Opening 8 Via Natural or Artificial Opening Endoscopic	Z No Device	Z No Qualifier
D Urethra	Ø Open 3 Percutaneous 4 Percutaneous Endoscopic 7 Via Natural or Artificial Opening 8 Via Natural or Artificial Opening Endoscopic X External	Z No Device	Z No Qualifier

Non-OR ØT5D[Ø,3,4,7,8,X]ZZ

Ø Medical and Surgical
T Urinary System
7 Dilation Expanding an orifice or the lumen of a tubular body part

Body Part Character 4	Approach Character 5	Device Character 6	Qualifier Character 7
3 Kidney Pelvis, Right **4** Kidney Pelvis, Left **6** Ureter, Right **7** Ureter, Left **8** Ureters, Bilateral **B** Bladder **C** Bladder Neck **D** Urethra	**Ø** Open **3** Percutaneous **4** Percutaneous Endoscopic **7** Via Natural or Artificial Opening **8** Via Natural or Artificial Opening Endoscopic	**D** Intraluminal Device **Z** No Device	**Z** No Qualifier

Non-OR ØT7[6,7][Ø,3,4,7,8]DZ
Non-OR ØT7[8,D][Ø,3,4]DZ
Non-OR ØT7[8,D][7,8][D,Z]Z
Non-OR ØT7C[Ø,3,4,7,8][D,Z]Z
AHA: 2Ø13, 4Q, 123

Ø Medical and Surgical
T Urinary System
8 Division Cutting into a body part without draining fluids and/or gases from the body part in order to separate or transect a body part

Body Part Character 4	Approach Character 5	Device Character 6	Qualifier Character 7
2 Kidneys, Bilateral **C** Bladder Neck	**Ø** Open **3** Percutaneous **4** Percutaneous Endoscopic	**Z** No Device	**Z** No Qualifier

Ø Medical and Surgical
T Urinary System
9 Drainage Taking or letting out fluids and/or gases from a body part

Body Part Character 4	Approach Character 5	Device Character 6	Qualifier Character 7
Ø Kidney, Right **1** Kidney, Left **3** Kidney Pelvis, Right **4** Kidney Pelvis, Left **6** Ureter, Right **7** Ureter, Left **8** Ureters, Bilateral **B** Bladder **C** Bladder Neck	**Ø** Open **3** Percutaneous **4** Percutaneous Endoscopic **7** Via Natural or Artificial Opening **8** Via Natural or Artificial Opening Endoscopic	**Ø** Drainage Device	**Z** No Qualifier
Ø Kidney, Right **1** Kidney, Left **3** Kidney Pelvis, Right **4** Kidney Pelvis, Left **6** Ureter, Right **7** Ureter, Left **8** Ureters, Bilateral **B** Bladder **C** Bladder Neck	**Ø** Open **3** Percutaneous **4** Percutaneous Endoscopic **7** Via Natural or Artificial Opening **8** Via Natural or Artificial Opening Endoscopic	**Z** No Device	**X** Diagnostic **Z** No Qualifier
D Urethra	**Ø** Open **3** Percutaneous **4** Percutaneous Endoscopic **7** Via Natural or Artificial Opening **8** Via Natural or Artificial Opening Endoscopic **X** External	**Ø** Drainage Device	**Z** No Qualifier
D Urethra	**Ø** Open **3** Percutaneous **4** Percutaneous Endoscopic **7** Via Natural or Artificial Opening **8** Via Natural or Artificial Opening Endoscopic **X** External	**Z** No Device	**X** Diagnostic **Z** No Qualifier

Non-OR ØT9[6,7,8][Ø,3,4,7,8]ØZ
Non-OR ØT9[B,C][3,4,7,8]ØZ
Non-OR ØT9[Ø,1,3,4,6,7,8][3,4,7,8]ZX
Non-OR ØT9[Ø,1,3,4][3,4]ZZ
Non-OR ØT9[B,C][3,4,7,8]ZZ
Non-OR ØT9D[Ø,3,4,7,8,X]ZX

0 Medical and Surgical
T Urinary System
B Excision Cutting out or off, without replacement, a portion of a body part

Body Part Character 4	Approach Character 5	Device Character 6	Qualifier Character 7
0 Kidney, Right 1 Kidney, Left 3 Kidney Pelvis, Right 4 Kidney Pelvis, Left 6 Ureter, Right 7 Ureter, Left B Bladder C Bladder Neck	0 Open 3 Percutaneous 4 Percutaneous Endoscopic 7 Via Natural or Artificial Opening 8 Via Natural or Artificial Opening Endoscopic	Z No Device	X Diagnostic Z No Qualifier
D Urethra	0 Open 3 Percutaneous 4 Percutaneous Endoscopic 7 Via Natural or Artificial Opening 8 Via Natural or Artificial Opening Endoscopic X External	Z No Device	X Diagnostic Z No Qualifier

Non-OR 0TB[0,1,3,4,6,7][3,4,7,8]ZX
Non-OR 0TBD[0,3,4,7,8,X]ZX
AHA: 2014, 2Q, 8

0 Medical and Surgical
T Urinary System
C Extirpation Taking or cutting out solid matter from a body part

Body Part Character 4	Approach Character 5	Device Character 6	Qualifier Character 7
0 Kidney, Right 1 Kidney, Left 3 Kidney Pelvis, Right 4 Kidney Pelvis, Left 6 Ureter, Right 7 Ureter, Left B Bladder C Bladder Neck	0 Open 3 Percutaneous 4 Percutaneous Endoscopic 7 Via Natural or Artificial Opening 8 Via Natural or Artificial Opening Endoscopic	Z No Device	Z No Qualifier
D Urethra	0 Open 3 Percutaneous 4 Percutaneous Endoscopic 7 Via Natural or Artificial Opening 8 Via Natural or Artificial Opening Endoscopic X External	Z No Device	Z No Qualifier

Non-OR 0TC[B,C][7,8]ZZ
Non-OR 0TCD[7,8,X]ZZ
AHA: 2013, 4Q, 122

0 Medical and Surgical
T Urinary System
D Extraction Pulling or stripping out or off all or a portion of a body part by the use of force

Body Part Character 4	Approach Character 5	Device Character 6	Qualifier Character 7
0 Kidney, Right 1 Kidney, Left	0 Open 3 Percutaneous 4 Percutaneous Endoscopic	Z No Device	Z No Qualifier

0 Medical and Surgical
T Urinary System
F Fragmentation Breaking solid matter in a body part into pieces

Body Part Character 4	Approach Character 5	Device Character 6	Qualifier Character 7
3 Kidney Pelvis, Right 4 Kidney Pelvis, Left 6 Ureter, Right 7 Ureter, Left B Bladder C Bladder Neck D Urethra NC	0 Open 3 Percutaneous 4 Percutaneous Endoscopic 7 Via Natural or Artificial Opening 8 Via Natural or Artificial Opening Endoscopic X External	Z No Device	Z No Qualifier

DRG Non-OR 0TF[3,4,6,7,B,C]XZZ
Non-OR 0TF[3,4][0,7,8]ZZ
Non-OR 0TF[6,7,B,C][0,3,4,7,8]ZZ
Non-OR 0TFD[0,3,4,7,8,X]ZZ
NC 0TFDXZZ
AHA: 2013, 4Q, 122

Ø Medical and Surgical
T Urinary System
H Insertion Putting in a nonbiological appliance that monitors, assists, performs, or prevents a physiological function but does not physically take the place of a body part

Body Part Character 4	Approach Character 5	Device Character 6	Qualifier Character 7
5 Kidney	**Ø** Open **3** Percutaneous **4** Percutaneous Endoscopic **7** Via Natural or Artificial Opening **8** Via Natural or Artificial Opening Endoscopic	**2** Monitoring Device **3** Infusion Device	**Z** No Qualifier
9 Ureter ⊞	**Ø** Open **3** Percutaneous **4** Percutaneous Endoscopic **7** Via Natural or Artificial Opening **8** Via Natural or Artificial Opening Endoscopic	**2** Monitoring Device **3** Infusion Device **M** Stimulator Lead	**Z** No Qualifier
B Bladder ⊞ NC	**Ø** Open **3** Percutaneous **4** Percutaneous Endoscopic **7** Via Natural or Artificial Opening **8** Via Natural or Artificial Opening Endoscopic	**2** Monitoring Device **3** Infusion Device **L** Artificial Sphincter **M** Stimulator Lead	**Z** No Qualifier
C Bladder Neck	**Ø** Open **3** Percutaneous **4** Percutaneous Endoscopic **7** Via Natural or Artificial Opening **8** Via Natural or Artificial Opening Endoscopic	**L** Artificial Sphincter	**Z** No Qualifier
D Urethra	**Ø** Open **3** Percutaneous **4** Percutaneous Endoscopic **7** Via Natural or Artificial Opening **8** Via Natural or Artificial Opening Endoscopic **X** External	**2** Monitoring Device **3** Infusion Device **L** Artificial Sphincter	**Z** No Qualifier

Non-OR ØTH5[Ø,3,4,7,8]3Z
Non-OR ØTH9[Ø,3,4,7,8]3Z
Non-OR ØTHB[Ø,3,4,7,8]3Z
Non-OR ØTHD[Ø,3,4,7,8,X]3Z
NC ØTHB[Ø,3,4,7,8]MZ

No Procedure Combinations Specified
⊞ ØTH[9,B][Ø,3,4,7,8]MZ

Ø Medical and Surgical
T Urinary System
J Inspection Visually and/or manually exploring a body part

Body Part Character 4	Approach Character 5	Device Character 6	Qualifier Character 7
5 Kidney **9** Ureter **B** Bladder **D** Urethra	**Ø** Open **3** Percutaneous **4** Percutaneous Endoscopic **7** Via Natural or Artificial Opening **8** Via Natural or Artificial Opening Endoscopic **X** External	**Z** No Device	**Z** No Qualifier

Non-OR ØTJ[5,9][4,8,X]ZZ
Non-OR ØTJB[8,X]ZZ
Non-OR ØTJD[3,4,7,8,X]ZZ

Ø Medical and Surgical
T Urinary System
L Occlusion Completely closing an orifice or the lumen of a tubular body part

Body Part Character 4	Approach Character 5	Device Character 6	Qualifier Character 7
3 Kidney Pelvis, Right **4** Kidney Pelvis, Left **6** Ureter, Right **7** Ureter, Left **B** Bladder **C** Bladder Neck	**Ø** Open **3** Percutaneous **4** Percutaneous Endoscopic	**C** Extraluminal Device **D** Intraluminal Device **Z** No Device	**Z** No Qualifier
3 Kidney Pelvis, Right **4** Kidney Pelvis, Left **6** Ureter, Right **7** Ureter, Left **B** Bladder **C** Bladder Neck **D** Urethra	**7** Via Natural or Artificial Opening **8** Via Natural or Artificial Opening Endoscopic	**D** Intraluminal Device **Z** No Device	**Z** No Qualifier
D Urethra	**Ø** Open **3** Percutaneous **4** Percutaneous Endoscopic **X** External	**C** Extraluminal Device **D** Intraluminal Device **Z** No Device	**Z** No Qualifier

Ø Medical and Surgical
T Urinary System
M Reattachment Putting back in or on all or a portion of a separated body part to its normal location or other suitable location

Body Part Character 4	Approach Character 5	Device Character 6	Qualifier Character 7
Ø Kidney, Right **1** Kidney, Left **2** Kidneys, Bilateral **3** Kidney Pelvis, Right **4** Kidney Pelvis, Left **6** Ureter, Right **7** Ureter, Left **8** Ureters, Bilateral **B** Bladder **C** Bladder Neck **D** Urethra	**Ø** Open **4** Percutaneous Endoscopic	**Z** No Device	**Z** No Qualifier

Ø Medical and Surgical
T Urinary System
N Release Freeing a body part from an abnormal physical constraint

Body Part Character 4	Approach Character 5	Device Character 6	Qualifier Character 7
Ø Kidney, Right **1** Kidney, Left **3** Kidney Pelvis, Right **4** Kidney Pelvis, Left **6** Ureter, Right **7** Ureter, Left **B** Bladder **C** Bladder Neck	**Ø** Open **3** Percutaneous **4** Percutaneous Endoscopic **7** Via Natural or Artificial Opening **8** Via Natural or Artificial Opening Endoscopic	**Z** No Device	**Z** No Qualifier
D Urethra	**Ø** Open **3** Percutaneous **4** Percutaneous Endoscopic **7** Via Natural or Artificial Opening **8** Via Natural or Artificial Opening Endoscopic **X** External	**Z** No Device	**Z** No Qualifier

Ø Medical and Surgical
T Urinary System
P Removal Taking out or off a device from a body part

Body Part Character 4	Approach Character 5	Device Character 6	Qualifier Character 7
5 Kidney	Ø Open 3 Percutaneous 4 Percutaneous Endoscopic 7 Via Natural or Artificial Opening 8 Via Natural or Artificial Opening Endoscopic	Ø Drainage Device 2 Monitoring Device 3 Infusion Device 7 Autologous Tissue Substitute C Extraluminal Device D Intraluminal Device J Synthetic Substitute K Nonautologous Tissue Substitute	Z No Qualifier
5 Kidney	X External	Ø Drainage Device 2 Monitoring Device 3 Infusion Device D Intraluminal Device	Z No Qualifier
9 Ureter ⊞	Ø Open 3 Percutaneous 4 Percutaneous Endoscopic 7 Via Natural or Artificial Opening 8 Via Natural or Artificial Opening Endoscopic	Ø Drainage Device 2 Monitoring Device 3 Infusion Device 7 Autologous Tissue Substitute C Extraluminal Device D Intraluminal Device J Synthetic Substitute K Nonautologous Tissue Substitute M Stimulator Lead	Z No Qualifier
9 Ureter	X External	Ø Drainage Device 2 Monitoring Device 3 Infusion Device D Intraluminal Device M Stimulator Lead	Z No Qualifier
B Bladder ⊞ NC	Ø Open 3 Percutaneous 4 Percutaneous Endoscopic 7 Via Natural or Artificial Opening 8 Via Natural or Artificial Opening Endoscopic	Ø Drainage Device 2 Monitoring Device 3 Infusion Device 7 Autologous Tissue Substitute C Extraluminal Device D Intraluminal Device J Synthetic Substitute K Nonautologous Tissue Substitute L Artificial Sphincter M Stimulator Lead	Z No Qualifier
B Bladder	X External	Ø Drainage Device 2 Monitoring Device 3 Infusion Device D Intraluminal Device L Artificial Sphincter M Stimulator Lead	Z No Qualifier
D Urethra	Ø Open 3 Percutaneous 4 Percutaneous Endoscopic 7 Via Natural or Artificial Opening 8 Via Natural or Artificial Opening Endoscopic	Ø Drainage Device 2 Monitoring Device 3 Infusion Device 7 Autologous Tissue Substitute C Extraluminal Device D Intraluminal Device J Synthetic Substitute K Nonautologous Tissue Substitute L Artificial Sphincter	Z No Qualifier
D Urethra	X External	Ø Drainage Device 2 Monitoring Device 3 Infusion Device D Intraluminal Device L Artificial Sphincter	Z No Qualifier

Non-OR ØTP5X[Ø,2,3,D]Z
Non-OR ØTP9X[Ø,2,3,D]Z
Non-OR ØTPBX[Ø,2,3,D,L]Z
Non-OR ØTPDX[Ø,2,3,D]Z
NC ØTPB[Ø,3,4,7,8]MZ

No Procedure Combinations Specified
⊞ ØTP[9,B][Ø,3,4,7,8]MZ

0 Medical and Surgical
T Urinary System
Q Repair Restoring, to the extent possible, a body part to its normal anatomic structure and function

Body Part Character 4	Approach Character 5	Device Character 6	Qualifier Character 7
0 Kidney, Right ⊞ 1 Kidney, Left ⊞ 3 Kidney Pelvis, Right ⊞ 4 Kidney Pelvis, Left ⊞ 6 Ureter, Right ⊞ 7 Ureter, Left ⊞ B Bladder ⊞ C Bladder Neck	0 Open 3 Percutaneous 4 Percutaneous Endoscopic 7 Via Natural or Artificial Opening 8 Via Natural or Artificial Opening Endoscopic	Z No Device	Z No Qualifier
D Urethra ⊞	0 Open 3 Percutaneous 4 Percutaneous Endoscopic 7 Via Natural or Artificial Opening 8 Via Natural or Artificial Opening Endoscopic X External	Z No Device	Z No Qualifier

Non-OR 0TQC[0,3,4,7,8]ZZ

See Appendix I for Procedure Combinations
⊞ 0TQB[0,3,4]ZZ

No Procedure Combinations Specified
⊞ 0TQ[0,1,3,4,6,7,D][0,3,4]ZZ

0 Medical and Surgical
T Urinary System
R Replacement Putting in or on biological or synthetic material that physically takes the place and/or function of all or a portion of a body part

Body Part Character 4	Approach Character 5	Device Character 6	Qualifier Character 7
3 Kidney Pelvis, Right 4 Kidney Pelvis, Left 6 Ureter, Right 7 Ureter, Left B Bladder ⊞ C Bladder Neck	0 Open 4 Percutaneous Endoscopic 7 Via Natural or Artificial Opening 8 Via Natural or Artificial Opening Endoscopic	7 Autologous Tissue Substitute J Synthetic Substitute K Nonautologous Tissue Substitute	Z No Qualifier
D Urethra	0 Open 4 Percutaneous Endoscopic 7 Via Natural or Artificial Opening 8 Via Natural or Artificial Opening Endoscopic X External	7 Autologous Tissue Substitute J Synthetic Substitute K Nonautologous Tissue Substitute	Z No Qualifier

No Procedure Combinations Specified
⊞ 0TRB07Z

0 Medical and Surgical
T Urinary System
S Reposition Moving to its normal location or other suitable location all or a portion of a body part

Body Part Character 4	Approach Character 5	Device Character 6	Qualifier Character 7
0 Kidney, Right 1 Kidney, Left 2 Kidneys, Bilateral 3 Kidney Pelvis, Right 4 Kidney Pelvis, Left 6 Ureter, Right 7 Ureter, Left 8 Ureters, Bilateral B Bladder C Bladder Neck D Urethra	0 Open 4 Percutaneous Endoscopic	Z No Device	Z No Qualifier

Ø Medical and Surgical
T Urinary System
T Resection Cutting out or off, without replacement, all of a body part

Body Part Character 4	Approach Character 5	Device Character 6	Qualifier Character 7
Ø Kidney, Right **1** Kidney, Left **2** Kidneys, Bilateral	**Ø** Open **4** Percutaneous Endoscopic	**Z** No Device	**Z** No Qualifier
3 Kidney Pelvis, Right **4** Kidney Pelvis, Left **6** Ureter, Right **7** Ureter, Left **B** Bladder ⊞ **C** Bladder Neck **D** Urethra	**Ø** Open **4** Percutaneous Endoscopic **7** Via Natural or Artificial Opening **8** Via Natural or Artificial Opening Endoscopic	**Z** No Device	**Z** No Qualifier

Non-OR ØTTD[4,7,8]ZZ

See Appendix I for Procedure Combinations
Combo-only ØTTDØZZ
⊞ ØTTBØZZ

No Procedure Combinations Specified
⊞ ØTTB[4,7,8]ZZ

Ø Medical and Surgical
T Urinary System
U Supplement Putting in or on biological or synthetic material that physically reinforces and/or augments the function of a portion of a body part

Body Part Character 4	Approach Character 5	Device Character 6	Qualifier Character 7
3 Kidney Pelvis, Right **4** Kidney Pelvis, Left **6** Ureter, Right **7** Ureter, Left **B** Bladder **C** Bladder Neck	**Ø** Open **4** Percutaneous Endoscopic **7** Via Natural or Artificial Opening **8** Via Natural or Artificial Opening Endoscopic	**7** Autologous Tissue Substitute **J** Synthetic Substitute **K** Nonautologous Tissue Substitute	**Z** No Qualifier
D Urethra	**Ø** Open **4** Percutaneous Endoscopic **7** Via Natural or Artificial Opening **8** Via Natural or Artificial Opening Endoscopic **X** External	**7** Autologous Tissue Substitute **J** Synthetic Substitute **K** Nonautologous Tissue Substitute	**Z** No Qualifier

Ø Medical and Surgical
T Urinary System
V Restriction Partially closing an orifice or the lumen of a tubular body part

Body Part Character 4	Approach Character 5	Device Character 6	Qualifier Character 7
3 Kidney Pelvis, Right **4** Kidney Pelvis, Left **6** Ureter, Right **7** Ureter, Left **B** Bladder **C** Bladder Neck **D** Urethra	**Ø** Open **3** Percutaneous **4** Percutaneous Endoscopic	**C** Extraluminal Device **D** Intraluminal Device **Z** No Device	**Z** No Qualifier
3 Kidney Pelvis, Right **4** Kidney Pelvis, Left **6** Ureter, Right **7** Ureter, Left **B** Bladder **C** Bladder Neck **D** Urethra	**7** Via Natural or Artificial Opening **8** Via Natural or Artificial Opening Endoscopic	**D** Intraluminal Device **Z** No Device	**Z** No Qualifier
D Urethra	**X** External	**Z** No Device	**Z** No Qualifier

0 Medical and Surgical
T Urinary System
W Revision Correcting, to the extent possible, a portion of a malfunctioning device or the position of a displaced device

Body Part Character 4	Approach Character 5	Device Character 6	Qualifier Character 7
5 Kidney	0 Open 3 Percutaneous 4 Percutaneous Endoscopic 7 Via Natural or Artificial Opening 8 Via Natural or Artificial Opening Endoscopic X External	0 Drainage Device 2 Monitoring Device 3 Infusion Device 7 Autologous Tissue Substitute C Extraluminal Device D Intraluminal Device J Synthetic Substitute K Nonautologous Tissue Substitute	Z No Qualifier
9 Ureter	0 Open 3 Percutaneous 4 Percutaneous Endoscopic 7 Via Natural or Artificial Opening 8 Via Natural or Artificial Opening Endoscopic X External	0 Drainage Device 2 Monitoring Device 3 Infusion Device 7 Autologous Tissue Substitute C Extraluminal Device D Intraluminal Device J Synthetic Substitute K Nonautologous Tissue Substitute M Stimulator Lead	Z No Qualifier
B Bladder	0 Open 3 Percutaneous 4 Percutaneous Endoscopic 7 Via Natural or Artificial Opening 8 Via Natural or Artificial Opening Endoscopic X External	0 Drainage Device 2 Monitoring Device 3 Infusion Device 7 Autologous Tissue Substitute C Extraluminal Device D Intraluminal Device J Synthetic Substitute K Nonautologous Tissue Substitute L Artificial Sphincter M Stimulator Lead	Z No Qualifier
D Urethra	0 Open 3 Percutaneous 4 Percutaneous Endoscopic 7 Via Natural or Artificial Opening 8 Via Natural or Artificial Opening Endoscopic X External	0 Drainage Device 2 Monitoring Device 3 Infusion Device 7 Autologous Tissue Substitute C Extraluminal Device D Intraluminal Device J Synthetic Substitute K Nonautologous Tissue Substitute L Artificial Sphincter	Z No Qualifier

Non-OR 0TW5X[0,2,3,7,C,D,J,K]Z
Non-OR 0TW9X[0,2,3,7,C,D,J,K,M]Z
Non-OR 0TWBX[0,2,3,7,C,D,J,K,L,M]Z
Non-OR 0TWDX[0,2,3,7,C,D,J,K,L]Z

0 Medical and Surgical
T Urinary System
Y Transplantation Putting in or on all or a portion of a living body part taken from another individual or animal to physically take the place and/or function of all or a portion of a similar body part

Body Part Character 4	Approach Character 5	Device Character 6	Qualifier Character 7
0 Kidney, Right ⊞ LC 1 Kidney, Left ⊞ LC	0 Open	Z No Device	0 Allogeneic 1 Syngeneic 2 Zooplastic

LC 0TY[0,1]0Z[0,1,2]

See Appendix I for Procedure Combinations
⊞ 0TY[0,1]0Z[0,1,2]

Female Reproductive System ØU1–ØUY

Ø Medical and Surgical
U Female Reproductive System
1 Bypass Altering the route of passage of the contents of a tubular body part

Body Part Character 4	Approach Character 5	Device Character 6	Qualifier Character 7
5 Fallopian Tube, Right ♀ 6 Fallopian Tube, Left ♀	Ø Open 4 Percutaneous Endoscopic	7 Autologous Tissue Substitute J Synthetic Substitute K Nonautologous Tissue Substitute Z No Device	5 Fallopian Tube, Right 6 Fallopian Tube, Left 9 Uterus

Ø Medical and Surgical
U Female Reproductive System
2 Change Taking out or off a device from a body part and putting back an identical or similar device in or on the same body part without cutting or puncturing the skin or a mucous membrane

Body Part Character 4	Approach Character 5	Device Character 6	Qualifier Character 7
3 Ovary ♀ 8 Fallopian Tube ♀ M Vulva ♀	X External	Ø Drainage Device Y Other Device	Z No Qualifier
D Uterus and Cervix ♀	X External	Ø Drainage Device H Contraceptive Device Y Other Device	Z No Qualifier
H Vagina and Cul-de-sac ♀	X External	Ø Drainage Device G Pessary Y Other Device	Z No Qualifier

Non-OR For all body part, approach, device, and qualifier values

Ø Medical and Surgical
U Female Reproductive System
5 Destruction Physical eradication of all or a portion of a body part by the direct use of energy, force, or a destructive agent

Body Part Character 4	Approach Character 5	Device Character 6	Qualifier Character 7
Ø Ovary, Right ♀ 1 Ovary, Left ♀ 2 Ovaries, Bilateral ♀ 4 Uterine Supporting Structure ♀	Ø Open 3 Percutaneous 4 Percutaneous Endoscopic	Z No Device	Z No Qualifier
5 Fallopian Tube, Right ♀ 6 Fallopian Tube, Left ♀ 7 Fallopian Tubes, Bilateral NC ♀ 9 Uterus ♀ B Endometrium ♀ C Cervix ♀ F Cul-de-sac ♀	Ø Open 3 Percutaneous 4 Percutaneous Endoscopic 7 Via Natural or Artificial Opening 8 Via Natural or Artificial Opening Endoscopic	Z No Device	Z No Qualifier
G Vagina ♀ K Hymen ♀	Ø Open 3 Percutaneous 4 Percutaneous Endoscopic 7 Via Natural or Artificial Opening 8 Via Natural or Artificial Opening Endoscopic X External	Z No Device	Z No Qualifier
J Clitoris ♀ L Vestibular Gland ♀ M Vulva ♀	Ø Open X External	Z No Device	Z No Qualifier

NC ØU57[Ø,3,4,7,8]ZZ

0 Medical and Surgical
U Female Reproductive System
7 Dilation Expanding an orifice or lumen of a tabular body part

Body Part Character 4	Approach Character 5	Device Character 6	Qualifier Character 7
5 Fallopian Tube, Right ♀ 6 Fallopian Tube, Left ♀ 7 Fallopian Tubes, Bilateral ♀ 9 Uterus ♀ C Cervix ♀ G Vagina ♀	0 Open 3 Percutaneous 4 Percutaneous Endoscopic 7 Via Natural or Artificial Opening 8 Via Natural or Artificial Opening Endoscopic	D Intraluminal Device Z No Device	Z No Qualifier
K Hymen ♀	0 Open 3 Percutaneous 4 Percutaneous Endoscopic 7 Via Natural or Artificial Opening 8 Via Natural or Artificial Opening Endoscopic X External	D Intraluminal Device Z No Device	Z No Qualifier

Non-OR 0U7C[0,3,4,7,8][D,Z]Z
Non-OR 0U7G[7,8][D,Z]Z

0 Medical and Surgical
U Female Reproductive System
8 Division Cutting into a body part without draining fluids and/or gases from the body part in order to separate or transect a body part

Body Part Character 4	Approach Character 5	Device Character 6	Qualifier Character 7
0 Ovary, Right ♀ 1 Ovary, Left ♀ 2 Ovaries, Bilateral ♀ 4 Uterine Supporting Structure ♀	0 Open 3 Percutaneous 4 Percutaneous Endoscopic	Z No Device	Z No Qualifier
K Hymen ♀	7 Via Natural or Artificial Opening 8 Via Natural or Artificial Opening Endoscopic X External	Z No Device	Z No Qualifier

Non-OR 0U8K[7,8,X]ZZ

0 Medical and Surgical
U Female Reproductive System
9 Drainage Taking or letting out fluids and/or gases from a body part

Body Part Character 4	Approach Character 5	Device Character 6	Qualifier Character 7
0 Ovary, Right ♀ 1 Ovary, Left ♀ 2 Ovaries, Bilateral ♀	X External	Z No Device	Z No Qualifier
0 Ovary, Right ♀ 1 Ovary, Left ♀ 2 Ovaries, Bilateral ♀ 4 Uterine Supporting Structure ♀	0 Open 3 Percutaneous 4 Percutaneous Endoscopic	0 Drainage Device	Z No Qualifier
0 Ovary, Right ♀ 1 Ovary, Left ♀ 2 Ovaries, Bilateral ♀ 4 Uterine Supporting Structure ♀	0 Open 3 Percutaneous 4 Percutaneous Endoscopic	Z No Device	X Diagnostic Z No Qualifier
5 Fallopian Tube, Right ♀ 6 Fallopian Tube, Left ♀ 7 Fallopian Tubes, Bilateral ♀ 9 Uterus ♀ C Cervix ♀ F Cul-de-sac ♀	0 Open 3 Percutaneous 4 Percutaneous Endoscopic 7 Via Natural or Artificial Opening 8 Via Natural or Artificial Opening Endoscopic	0 Drainage Device	Z No Qualifier
5 Fallopian Tube, Right ♀ 6 Fallopian Tube, Left ♀ 7 Fallopian Tubes, Bilateral ♀ 9 Uterus ♀ C Cervix ♀ F Cul-de-sac ♀	0 Open 3 Percutaneous 4 Percutaneous Endoscopic 7 Via Natural or Artificial Opening 8 Via Natural or Artificial Opening Endoscopic	Z No Device	X Diagnostic Z No Qualifier

0U9 Continued on next page

Non-OR 0U9F[3,4]0Z
Non-OR 0U9[5,6,7][3,4,7,8]ZZ
Non-OR 0U9F[3,4]ZZ

Ø Medical and Surgical
U Female Reproductive System
9 Drainage Taking or letting out fluids and/or gases from a body part

ØU9 Continued

Body Part Character 4	Approach Character 5	Device Character 6	Qualifier Character 7
G Vagina ♀ K Hymen ♀	Ø Open 3 Percutaneous 4 Percutaneous Endoscopic 7 Via Natural or Artificial Opening 8 Via Natural or Artificial Opening Endoscopic X External	Ø Drainage Device	Z No Qualifier
G Vagina ♀ K Hymen ♀	Ø Open 3 Percutaneous 4 Percutaneous Endoscopic 7 Via Natural or Artificial Opening 8 Via Natural or Artificial Opening Endoscopic X External	Z No Device	X Diagnostic Z No Qualifier
J Clitoris ♀ L Vestibular Gland ♀ M Vulva ♀	Ø Open X External	Ø Drainage Device	Z No Qualifier
J Clitoris ♀ L Vestibular Gland ♀ M Vulva ♀	Ø Open X External	Z No Device	X Diagnostic Z No Qualifier

Non-OR ØU9K[Ø,3,4,7,8,X]ØZ
Non-OR ØU9K[Ø,3,4,7,8,X]ZZ
Non-OR ØU9L [Ø,X]ØZ
Non-OR ØU9L [Ø,X]ZZ

Ø Medical and Surgical
U Female Reproductive System
B Excision Cutting out or off, without replacement, a portion of a body part

Body Part Character 4	Approach Character 5	Device Character 6	Qualifier Character 7
Ø Ovary, Right ♀ 1 Ovary, Left ♀ 2 Ovaries, Bilateral ♀ 4 Uterine Supporting Structure ♀ 5 Fallopian Tube, Right ♀ 6 Fallopian Tube, Left ♀ 7 Fallopian Tubes, Bilateral ♀ 9 Uterus ♀ C Cervix ♀ F Cul-de-sac ♀	Ø Open 3 Percutaneous 4 Percutaneous Endoscopic 7 Via Natural or Artificial Opening 8 Via Natural or Artificial Opening Endoscopic	Z No Device	X Diagnostic Z No Qualifier
G Vagina ♀ K Hymen ♀	Ø Open 3 Percutaneous 4 Percutaneous Endoscopic 7 Via Natural or Artificial Opening 8 Via Natural or Artificial Opening Endoscopic X External	Z No Device	X Diagnostic Z No Qualifier
J Clitoris ♀ L Vestibular Gland ♀ M Vulva ♀	Ø Open X External	Z No Device	X Diagnostic Z No Qualifier

0 Medical and Surgical
U Female Reproductive System
C Extirpation Taking or cutting out solid matter from a body part

Body Part Character 4	Approach Character 5	Device Character 6	Qualifier Character 7
0 Ovary, Right ♀ 1 Ovary, Left ♀ 2 Ovaries, Bilateral ♀ 4 Uterine Supporting Structure ♀	0 Open 3 Percutaneous 4 Percutaneous Endoscopic	Z No Device	Z No Qualifier
5 Fallopian Tube, Right ♀ 6 Fallopian Tube, Left ♀ 7 Fallopian Tubes, Bilateral ♀ 9 Uterus ♀ B Endometrium ♀ C Cervix ♀ F Cul-de-sac ♀	0 Open 3 Percutaneous 4 Percutaneous Endoscopic 7 Via Natural or Artificial Opening 8 Via Natural or Artificial Opening Endoscopic	Z No Device	Z No Qualifier
G Vagina ♀ K Hymen ♀	0 Open 3 Percutaneous 4 Percutaneous Endoscopic 7 Via Natural or Artificial Opening 8 Via Natural or Artificial Opening Endoscopic X External	Z No Device	Z No Qualifier
J Clitoris ♀ L Vestibular Gland ♀ M Vulva ♀	0 Open X External	Z No Device	Z No Qualifier

Non-OR 0UC9[7,8]ZZ
Non-OR 0UCG[7,8,X]ZZ
Non-OR 0UCK[0,3,4,7,8,X]ZZ
Non-OR 0UCMXZZ
AHA: 2013, 2Q, 38

0 Medical and Surgical
U Female Reproductive System
D Extraction Pulling or stripping out or off all or a portion of a body part by the use of force

Body Part Character 4	Approach Character 5	Device Character 6	Qualifier Character 7
B Endometrium ♀	7 Via Natural or Artificial Opening 8 Via Natural or Artificial Opening Endoscopic	Z No Device	X Diagnostic Z No Qualifier
N Ova ♀	0 Open 3 Percutaneous 4 Percutaneous Endoscopic	Z No Device	Z No Qualifier

0 Medical and Surgical
U Female Reproductive System
F Fragmentation Breaking solid matter in a body part into pieces

Body Part Character 4	Approach Character 5	Device Character 6	Qualifier Character 7
5 Fallopian Tube, Right NC ♀ 6 Fallopian Tube, Left NC ♀ 7 Fallopian Tubes, Bilateral NC ♀ 9 Uterus NC ♀	0 Open 3 Percutaneous 4 Percutaneous Endoscopic 7 Via Natural or Artificial Opening 8 Via Natural or Artificial Opening Endoscopic X External	Z No Device	Z No Qualifier

Non-OR 0UF[5,6,7,9]XZZ
NC 0UF[5,6,7,9]XZZ

Ø Medical and Surgical
U Female Reproductive System
H Insertion Putting in a nonbiological appliance that monitors, assists, performs, or prevents a physiological function but does not physically take the place of a body part

Body Part Character 4	Approach Character 5	Device Character 6	Qualifier Character 7
3 Ovary ♀	**Ø** Open **3** Percutaneous **4** Percutaneous Endoscopic	**3** Infusion Device	**Z** No Qualifier
8 Fallopian Tube ♀ **D** Uterus and Cervix ♀ **H** Vagina and Cul-de-sac ♀	**Ø** Open **3** Percutaneous **4** Percutaneous Endoscopic **7** Via Natural or Artificial Opening **8** Via Natural or Artificial Opening Endoscopic	**3** Infusion Device	**Z** No Qualifier
9 Uterus ♀ **C** Cervix ♀	**7** Via Natural or Artificial Opening **8** Via Natural or Artificial Opening Endoscopic	**H** Contraceptive Device	**Z** No Qualifier
C Cervix ♀	**Ø** Open **3** Percutaneous **4** Percutaneous Endoscopic **7** Via Natural or Artificial Opening **8** Via Natural or Artificial Opening Endoscopic	**1** Radioactive Element	**Z** No Qualifier
F Cul-de-sac ♀	**7** Via Natural or Artificial Opening **8** Via Natural or Artificial Opening Endoscopic	**G** Intraluminal Device, Pessary	**Z** No Qualifier
G Vagina ♀	**Ø** Open **3** Percutaneous **4** Percutaneous Endoscopic **X** External	**1** Radioactive Element	**Z** No Qualifier
G Vagina ♀	**7** Via Natural or Artificial Opening **8** Via Natural or Artificial Opening Endoscopic	**1** Radioactive Element **G** Intraluminal Device, Pessary	**Z** No Qualifier

Non-OR ØUH3[Ø,3,4]3Z
Non-OR ØUH[8,D][Ø,3,4,7,8]3Z
Non-OR ØUH[9,C][7,8]HZ
Non-OR ØUHF[7,8]GZ
Non-OR ØUHG[7,8]GZ

AHA: 2Ø13, 2Q, 34

Ø Medical and Surgical
U Female Reproductive System
J Inspection Visually and/or manually exploring a body part

Body Part Character 4	Approach Character 5	Device Character 6	Qualifier Character 7
3 Ovary ♀	**Ø** Open **3** Percutaneous **4** Percutaneous Endoscopic **X** External	**Z** No Device	**Z** No Qualifier
8 Fallopian Tube ♀ **D** Uterus and Cervix ♀ **H** Vagina and Cul-de-sac ♀	**Ø** Open **3** Percutaneous **4** Percutaneous Endoscopic **7** Via Natural or Artificial Opening **8** Via Natural or Artificial Opening Endoscopic **X** External	**Z** No Device	**Z** No Qualifier
M Vulva ♀	**Ø** Open **X** External	**Z** No Device	**Z** No Qualifier

Non-OR ØUJ3XZZ
Non-OR ØUJ8XZZ
Non-OR ØUJD[7,8,X]ZZ
Non-OR ØUJH[8,X]ZZ
Non-OR ØUJMXZZ

0 Medical and Surgical
U Female Reproductive System
L Occlusion Completely closing an orifice or the lumen of a tubular body part

Body Part Character 4	Approach Character 5	Device Character 6	Qualifier Character 7
5 Fallopian Tube, Right ♀ 6 Fallopian Tube, Left ♀ 7 Fallopian Tubes, Bilateral NC ♀	0 Open 3 Percutaneous 4 Percutaneous Endoscopic	C Extraluminal Device D Intraluminal Device Z No Device	Z No Qualifier
5 Fallopian Tube, Right ♀ 6 Fallopian Tube, Left ♀ 7 Fallopian Tubes, Bilateral NC ♀ F Cul-de-sac ♀ G Vagina ♀	7 Via Natural or Artificial Opening 8 Via Natural or Artificial Opening Endoscopic	D Intraluminal Device Z No Device	Z No Qualifier

NC 0UL7[0,3,4][C,D,Z]Z
NC 0UL7[7,8][D,Z]Z

0 Medical and Surgical
U Female Reproductive System
M Reattachment Putting back in or on all or a portion of a separated body part to its normal location or other suitable location

Body Part Character 4	Approach Character 5	Device Character 6	Qualifier Character 7
0 Ovary, Right ♀ 1 Ovary, Left ♀ 2 Ovaries, Bilateral ♀ 4 Uterine Supporting Structure ♀ 5 Fallopian Tube, Right ♀ 6 Fallopian Tube, Left ♀ 7 Fallopian Tubes, Bilateral ♀ 9 Uterus ♀ C Cervix ♀ F Cul-de-sac ♀ G Vagina ♀ K Hymen ♀	0 Open 4 Percutaneous Endoscopic	Z No Device	Z No Qualifier
J Clitoris ♀ M Vulva ♀	X External	Z No Device	Z No Qualifier
K Hymen ♀	0 Open 4 Percutaneous Endoscopic X External	Z No Device	Z No Qualifier

0 Medical and Surgical
U Female Reproductive System
N Release Freeing a body part from an abnormal physical constraint

Body Part Character 4	Approach Character 5	Device Character 6	Qualifier Character 7
0 Ovary, Right ♀ 1 Ovary, Left ♀ 2 Ovaries, Bilateral ♀ 4 Uterine Supporting Structure ♀	0 Open 3 Percutaneous 4 Percutaneous Endoscopic	Z No Device	Z No Qualifier
5 Fallopian Tube, Right ♀ 6 Fallopian Tube, Left ♀ 7 Fallopian Tubes, Bilateral ♀ 9 Uterus ♀ C Cervix ♀ F Cul-de-sac ♀	0 Open 3 Percutaneous 4 Percutaneous Endoscopic 7 Via Natural or Artificial Opening 8 Via Natural or Artificial Opening Endoscopic	Z No Device	Z No Qualifier
G Vagina ♀ K Hymen ♀	0 Open 3 Percutaneous 4 Percutaneous Endoscopic 7 Via Natural or Artificial Opening 8 Via Natural or Artificial Opening Endoscopic X External	Z No Device	Z No Qualifier
J Clitoris ♀ L Vestibular Gland ♀ M Vulva ♀	0 Open X External	Z No Device	Z No Qualifier

Ø Medical and Surgical
U Female Reproductive System
P Removal Taking out or off a device from a body part

Body Part Character 4	Approach Character 5	Device Character 6	Qualifier Character 7
3 Ovary ♀	**Ø** Open **3** Percutaneous **4** Percutaneous Endoscopic **X** External	**Ø** Drainage Device **3** Infusion Device	**Z** No Qualifier
8 Fallopian Tube ♀	**Ø** Open **3** Percutaneous **4** Percutaneous Endoscopic **7** Via Natural or Artificial Opening **8** Via Natural or Artificial Opening Endoscopic	**Ø** Drainage Device **3** Infusion Device **7** Autologous Tissue Substitute **C** Extraluminal Device **D** Intraluminal Device **J** Synthetic Substitute **K** Nonautologous Tissue Substitute	**Z** No Qualifier
8 Fallopian Tube ♀	**X** External	**Ø** Drainage Device **3** Infusion Device **D** Intraluminal Device	**Z** No Qualifier
D Uterus and Cervix ♀	**Ø** Open **3** Percutaneous **4** Percutaneous Endoscopic **7** Via Natural or Artificial Opening **8** Via Natural or Artificial Opening Endoscopic	**Ø** Drainage Device **1** Radioactive Element **3** Infusion Device **7** Autologous Tissue Substitute **C** Extraluminal Device **D** Intraluminal Device **H** Contraceptive Device **J** Synthetic Substitute **K** Nonautologous Tissue Substitute	**Z** No Qualifier
D Uterus and Cervix ♀	**X** External	**Ø** Drainage Device **3** Infusion Device **D** Intraluminal Device **H** Contraceptive Device	**Z** No Qualifier
H Vagina and Cul-de-sac ♀	**Ø** Open **3** Percutaneous **4** Percutaneous Endoscopic **7** Via Natural or Artificial Opening **8** Via Natural or Artificial Opening Endoscopic	**Ø** Drainage Device **1** Radioactive Element **3** Infusion Device **7** Autologous Tissue Substitute **D** Intraluminal Device **J** Synthetic Substitute **K** Nonautologous Tissue Substitute	**Z** No Qualifier
H Vagina and Cul-de-sac ♀	**X** External	**Ø** Drainage Device **1** Radioactive Element **3** Infusion Device **D** Intraluminal Device	**Z** No Qualifier
M Vulva ♀	**Ø** Open	**Ø** Drainage Device **7** Autologous Tissue Substitute **J** Synthetic Substitute **K** Nonautologous Tissue Substitute	**Z** No Qualifier
M Vulva ♀	**X** External	**Ø** Drainage Device	**Z** No Qualifier

Non-OR ØUP3X[Ø,3]Z
Non-OR ØUP8X[Ø,3,D]Z
Non-OR ØUPD[3,4]CZ
Non-OR ØUPD[7,8][C,H]Z
Non-OR ØUPDX[Ø,3,D,H]Z
Non-OR ØUPHX[Ø,1,3,D]Z
Non-OR ØUPMXØZ

Ø Medical and Surgical
U Female Reproductive System
Q Repair Restoring, to the extent possible, a body part to its normal anatomic structure and function

Body Part Character 4	Approach Character 5	Device Character 6	Qualifier Character 7
Ø Ovary, Right ⊞♀ **1** Ovary, Left ⊞♀ **2** Ovaries, Bilateral ⊞♀ **4** Uterine Supporting Structure ♀	**Ø** Open **3** Percutaneous **4** Percutaneous Endoscopic	**Z** No Device	**Z** No Qualifier
5 Fallopian Tube, Right ⊞♀ **6** Fallopian Tube, Left ⊞♀ **7** Fallopian Tubes, Bilateral ⊞♀ **9** Uterus ♀ **C** Cervix ♀ **F** Cul-de-sac ♀	**Ø** Open **3** Percutaneous **4** Percutaneous Endoscopic **7** Via Natural or Artificial Opening **8** Via Natural or Artificial Opening Endoscopic	**Z** No Device	**Z** No Qualifier
G Vagina ♀ **K** Hymen ♀	**Ø** Open **3** Percutaneous **4** Percutaneous Endoscopic **7** Via Natural or Artificial Opening **8** Via Natural or Artificial Opening Endoscopic **X** External	**Z** No Device	**Z** No Qualifier
J Clitoris ♀ **L** Vestibular Gland ♀ **M** Vulva ⊞♀	**Ø** Open **X** External	**Z** No Device	**Z** No Qualifier

DRG Non-OR ØUQG[7,8,X]ZZ
DRG Non-OR ØUQM[Ø,X]ZZ
AHA: 2Ø13, 4Q, 12Ø

No Procedure Combinations Specified
⊞ ØUQ[Ø,1,2,5,6,7][Ø,3,4]ZZ
⊞ ØUQM[Ø,X]ZZ

Ø Medical and Surgical
U Female Reproductive System
S Reposition Moving to its normal location or other suitable location all or a portion of a body part

Body Part Character 4	Approach Character 5	Device Character 6	Qualifier Character 7
Ø Ovary, Right ♀ **1** Ovary, Left ♀ **2** Ovaries, Bilateral ♀ **4** Uterine Supporting Structure ♀ **5** Fallopian Tube, Right ♀ **6** Fallopian Tube, Left ♀ **7** Fallopian Tubes, Bilateral ♀ **C** Cervix ♀ **F** Cul-de-sac ♀	**Ø** Open **4** Percutaneous Endoscopic	**Z** No Device	**Z** No Qualifier
9 Uterus ♀ **G** Vagina ♀	**Ø** Open **4** Percutaneous Endoscopic **X** External	**Z** No Device	**Z** No Qualifier

Non-OR ØUS9XZZ

Ø Medical and Surgical
U Female Reproductive System
T Resection Cutting out or off, without replacement, all of a body part

Body Part Character 4	Approach Character 5	Device Character 6	Qualifier Character 7
Ø Ovary, Right ⊞♀ **1** Ovary, Left ⊞♀ **2** Ovaries, Bilateral ⊞♀ **5** Fallopian Tube, Right ⊞♀ **6** Fallopian Tube, Left ⊞♀ **7** Fallopian Tubes, Bilateral ⊞♀ **9** Uterus ⊞♀	**Ø** Open **4** Percutaneous Endoscopic **7** Via Natural or Artificial Opening **8** Via Natural or Artificial Opening Endoscopic **F** Via Natural or Artificial Opening With Percutaneous Endoscopic Assistance	**Z** No Device	**Z** No Qualifier
4 Uterine Supporting Structure ⊞♀ **C** Cervix ⊞♀ **F** Cul-de-sac ♀ **G** Vagina ⊞♀ **K** Hymen ♀	**Ø** Open **4** Percutaneous Endoscopic **7** Via Natural or Artificial Opening **8** Via Natural or Artificial Opening Endoscopic	**Z** No Device	**Z** No Qualifier
J Clitoris ♀ **L** Vestibular Gland ♀ **M** Vulva ⊞♀	**Ø** Open **X** External	**Z** No Device	**Z** No Qualifier
K Hymen ♀	**Ø** Open **4** Percutaneous Endoscopic **7** Via Natural or Artificial Opening **8** Via Natural or Artificial Opening Endoscopic **X** External	**Z** No Device	**Z** No Device

AHA: 2Ø13, 3Q, 28; 2Ø13, 1Q, 24

See Appendix I for Procedure Combinations
⊞ ØUT[2,7][Ø,4]ZZ
⊞ ØUT4[Ø,4,7,8]ZZ
⊞ ØUT9[Ø,4,7,8,F]ZZ
⊞ ØUTC[Ø,4,7,8]ZZ
⊞ ØUTGØZZ
⊞ ØUTM[Ø,X]ZZ

No Procedure Combinations Specified
⊞ ØUT[Ø,1,5,6][Ø,4]ZZ

Ø Medical and Surgical
U Female Reproductive System
U Supplement Putting in or on biological or synthetic material that physically reinforces and/or augments the function of a portion of a body part

Body Part Character 4	Approach Character 5	Device Character 6	Qualifier Character 7
4 Uterine Supporting Structure ♀	**Ø** Open **4** Percutaneous Endoscopic	**7** Autologous Tissue Substitute **J** Synthetic Substitute **K** Nonautologous Tissue Substitute	**Z** No Qualifier
5 Fallopian Tube, Right ♀ **6** Fallopian Tube, Left ♀ **7** Fallopian Tubes, Bilateral ♀ **F** Cul-de-sac ♀	**Ø** Open **4** Percutaneous Endoscopic **7** Via Natural or Artificial Opening **8** Via Natural or Artificial Opening Endoscopic	**7** Autologous Tissue Substitute **J** Synthetic Substitute **K** Nonautologous Tissue Substitute	**Z** No Qualifier
G Vagina ♀ **K** Hymen ♀	**Ø** Open **4** Percutaneous Endoscopic **7** Via Natural or Artificial Opening **8** Via Natural or Artificial Opening Endoscopic **X** External	**7** Autologous Tissue Substitute **J** Synthetic Substitute **K** Nonautologous Tissue Substitute	**Z** No Qualifier
J Clitoris ♀ **M** Vulva ♀	**Ø** Open **X** External	**7** Autologous Tissue Substitute **J** Synthetic Substitute **K** Nonautologous Tissue Substitute	**Z** No Qualifier

Ø Medical and Surgical
U Female Reproductive System
V Restriction Partially closing an orifice or the lumen of a tubular body part

Body Part Character 4	Approach Character 5	Device Character 6	Qualifier Character 7
C Cervix ♀	**Ø** Open **3** Percutaneous **4** Percutaneous Endoscopic	**C** Extraluminal Device **D** Intraluminal Device **Z** No Device	**Z** No Qualifier
C Cervix ♀	**7** Via Natural or Artificial Opening **8** Via Natural or Artificial Opening Endoscopic	**D** Intraluminal Device **Z** No Device	**Z** No Qualifier

0 Medical and Surgical
U Female Reproductive System
W Revision Correcting, to the extent possible, a portion of a malfunctioning device or the position of a displaced device

Body Part Character 4	Approach Character 5	Device Character 6	Qualifier Character 7
3 Ovary ♀	0 Open 3 Percutaneous 4 Percutaneous Endoscopic X External	0 Drainage Device 3 Infusion Device	Z No Qualifier
8 Fallopian Tube ♀	0 Open 3 Percutaneous 4 Percutaneous Endoscopic 7 Via Natural or Artificial Opening 8 Via Natural or Artificial Opening Endoscopic X External	0 Drainage Device 3 Infusion Device 7 Autologous Tissue Substitute C Extraluminal Device D Intraluminal Device J Synthetic Substitute K Nonautologous Tissue Substitute	Z No Qualifier
D Uterus and Cervix ♀	0 Open 3 Percutaneous 4 Percutaneous Endoscopic 7 Via Natural or Artificial Opening 8 Via Natural or Artificial Opening Endoscopic X External	0 Drainage Device 1 Radioactive Element 3 Infusion Device 7 Autologous Tissue Substitute C Extraluminal Device D Intraluminal Device H Contraceptive Device J Synthetic Substitute K Nonautologous Tissue Substitute	Z No Qualifier
H Vagina and Cul-de-sac ♀	0 Open 3 Percutaneous 4 Percutaneous Endoscopic 7 Via Natural or Artificial Opening 8 Via Natural or Artificial Opening Endoscopic X External	0 Drainage Device 1 Radioactive Element 3 Infusion Device 7 Autologous Tissue Substitute D Intraluminal Device J Synthetic Substitute K Nonautologous Tissue Substitute	Z No Qualifier
M Vulva ♀	0 Open X External	0 Drainage Device 7 Autologous Tissue Substitute J Synthetic Substitute K Nonautologous Tissue Substitute	Z No Qualifier

Non-OR 0UW3X[0,3]Z
Non-OR 0UW8X[0,3,7,C,D,J,K]Z
Non-OR 0UWDX[0,3,7,C,D,H,J,K]Z
Non-OR 0UWHX[0,3,7,C,D,J,K]Z
Non-OR 0UWMX[0,7,J,K]Z

0 Medical and Surgical
U Female Reproductive System
Y Transplantation Putting in or on all or a portion of a living body part taken from another individual or animal to physically take the place and/or function of all or a portion of a similar body part

Body Part Character 4	Approach Character 5	Device Character 6	Qualifier Character 7
0 Ovary, Right ♀ 1 Ovary, Left ♀	0 Open	Z No Device	0 Allogeneic 1 Syngeneic 2 Zooplastic

Male Reproductive System ØV1–ØVW

Ø Medical and Surgical
V Male Reproductive System
1 Bypass Altering the route of passage of the contents of a tubular body part

Body Part Character 4	Approach Character 5	Device Character 6	Qualifier Character 7
N Vas Deferens, Right ♂ **P** Vas Deferens, Left ♂ **Q** Vas Deferens, Bilateral ♂	**Ø** Open **4** Percutaneous Endoscopic	**7** Autologous Tissue Substitute **J** Synthetic Substitute **K** Nonautologous Tissue Substitute **Z** No Device	**J** Epididymis, Right **K** Epididymis, Left **N** Vas Deferens, Right **P** Vas Deferens, Left

Ø Medical and Surgical
V Male Reproductive System
2 Change Taking out or off a device from a body part and putting back an identical or similar device in or on the same body part without cutting or puncturing the skin or a mucous membrane

Body Part Character 4	Approach Character 5	Device Character 6	Qualifier Character 7
4 Prostate and Seminal Vesicles ♂ **8** Scrotum and Tunica Vaginalis ♂ **D** Testis ♂ **M** Epididymis and Spermatic Cord ♂ **R** Vas Deferens ♂ **S** Penis ♂	**X** External	**Ø** Drainage Device **Y** Other Device	**Z** No Qualifier

Non-OR For all body part, approach, device, and qualifier values

Ø Medical and Surgical
V Male Reproductive System
5 Destruction Physical eradication of all or a portion of a body part by the direct use of energy, force, or a destructive agent

Body Part Character 4	Approach Character 5	Device Character 6	Qualifier Character 7
Ø Prostate ♂	**Ø** Open **3** Percutaneous **4** Percutaneous Endoscopic **7** Via Natural or Artificial Opening **8** Via Natural or Artificial Opening Endoscopic	**Z** No Device	**Z** No Qualifier
1 Seminal Vesicle, Right ♂ **2** Seminal Vesicle, Left ♂ **3** Seminal Vesicles, Bilateral ♂ **6** Tunica Vaginalis, Right ♂ **7** Tunica Vaginalis, Left ♂ **9** Testis, Right ♂ **B** Testis, Left ♂ **C** Testes, Bilateral ♂ **F** Spermatic Cord, Right ♂ **G** Spermatic Cord, Left ♂ **H** Spermatic Cords, Bilateral ♂ **J** Epididymis, Right ♂ **K** Epididymis, Left ♂ **L** Epididymis, Bilateral ♂ **N** Vas Deferens, Right NC ♂ **P** Vas Deferens, Left NC ♂ **Q** Vas Deferens, Bilateral NC ♂	**Ø** Open **3** Percutaneous **4** Percutaneous Endoscopic	**Z** No Device	**Z** No Qualifier
5 Scrotum ♂ **S** Penis ♂ **T** Prepuce ♂	**Ø** Open **3** Percutaneous **4** Percutaneous Endoscopic **X** External	**Z** No Device	**Z** No Qualifier

Non-OR ØV5[N,P,Q][Ø,3,4]ZZ
Non-OR ØV55[Ø,3,4,X]ZZ
NC ØV5[N,P,Q][Ø,3,4]ZZ

0 Medical and Surgical
V Male Reproductive System
7 Dilation Expanding an orifice or the lumen of a tubular body part

Body Part Character 4	Approach Character 5	Device Character 6	Qualifier Character 7
N Vas Deferens, Right ♂ **P** Vas Deferens, Left ♂ **Q** Vas Deferens, Bilateral ♂	**0** Open **3** Percutaneous **4** Percutaneous Endoscopic	**D** Intraluminal Device **Z** No Device	**Z** No Qualifier

0 Medical and Surgical
V Male Reproductive System
9 Drainage Taking or letting out fluids and/or gases from a body part

Body Part Character 4	Approach Character 5	Device Character 6	Qualifier Character 7
0 Prostate ♂	**0** Open **3** Percutaneous **4** Percutaneous Endoscopic **7** Via Natural or Artificial Opening **8** Via Natural or Artificial Opening Endoscopic	**0** Drainage Device	**Z** No Qualifier
0 Prostate ♂	**0** Open **3** Percutaneous **4** Percutaneous Endoscopic **7** Via Natural or Artificial Opening **8** Via Natural or Artificial Opening Endoscopic	**Z** No Device	**X** Diagnostic **Z** No Qualifier
1 Seminal Vesicle, Right ♂ **2** Seminal Vesicle, Left ♂ **3** Seminal Vesicles, Bilateral ♂ **6** Tunica Vaginalis, Right ♂ **7** Tunica Vaginalis, Left ♂ **9** Testis, Right ♂ **B** Testis, Left ♂ **C** Testes, Bilateral ♂ **F** Spermatic Cord, Right ♂ **G** Spermatic Cord, Left ♂ **H** Spermatic Cords, Bilateral ♂ **J** Epididymis, Right ♂ **K** Epididymis, Left ♂ **L** Epididymis, Bilateral ♂ **N** Vas Deferens, Right ♂ **P** Vas Deferens, Left ♂ **Q** Vas Deferens, Bilateral ♂	**0** Open **3** Percutaneous **4** Percutaneous Endoscopic	**0** Drainage Device	**Z** No Qualifier
1 Seminal Vesicle, Right ♂ **2** Seminal Vesicle, Left ♂ **3** Seminal Vesicles, Bilateral ♂ **6** Tunica Vaginalis, Right ♂ **7** Tunica Vaginalis, Left ♂ **9** Testis, Right ♂ **B** Testis, Left ♂ **C** Testes, Bilateral ♂ **F** Spermatic Cord, Right ♂ **G** Spermatic Cord, Left ♂ **H** Spermatic Cords, Bilateral ♂ **J** Epididymis, Right ♂ **K** Epididymis, Left ♂ **L** Epididymis, Bilateral ♂ **N** Vas Deferens, Right ♂ **P** Vas Deferens, Left ♂ **Q** Vas Deferens, Bilateral ♂	**0** Open **3** Percutaneous **4** Percutaneous Endoscopic	**Z** No Device	**X** Diagnostic **Z** No Qualifier
5 Scrotum ♂ **S** Penis ♂ **T** Prepuce ♂	**0** Open **3** Percutaneous **4** Percutaneous Endoscopic **X** External	**0** Drainage Device	**Z** No Qualifier
5 Scrotum ♂ **S** Penis ♂ **T** Prepuce ♂	**0** Open **3** Percutaneous **4** Percutaneous Endoscopic **X** External	**Z** No Device	**X** Diagnostic **Z** No Qualifier

Non-OR 0V90[3,4]0Z
Non-OR 0V90[3,4]ZZ
Non-OR 0V90[3,4,7,8]ZX
Non-OR 0V9[1,2,3,9,B,C][3,4]0Z
Non-OR 0V9[6,7,F,G,H,N,P,Q][0,3,4]0Z
Non-OR 0V9[1,2,3,9,B,C][3,4]Z[X,Z]
Non-OR 0V9[6,7,F,G,H,J,K,L,N,P,Q][0,3,4]ZX
Non-OR 0V9[6,7,F,G,H,N,P,Q][0,3,4]ZZ
Non-OR 0V95[0,3,4,X]0Z
Non-OR 0V95[0,3,4,X]Z[X,Z]

Ø Medical and Surgical
V Male Reproductive System
B Excision Cutting out or off, without replacement, a portion of a body part

Body Part Character 4	Approach Character 5	Device Character 6	Qualifier Character 7
Ø Prostate ♂	Ø Open 3 Percutaneous 4 Percutaneous Endoscopic 7 Via Natural or Artificial Opening 8 Via Natural or Artificial Opening Endoscopic	Z No Device	X Diagnostic Z No Qualifier
1 Seminal Vesicle, Right ♂ 2 Seminal Vesicle, Left ♂ 3 Seminal Vesicles, Bilateral ♂ 6 Tunica Vaginalis, Right ♂ 7 Tunica Vaginalis, Left ♂ 9 Testis, Right ♂ B Testis, Left ♂ C Testes, Bilateral ♂ F Spermatic Cord, Right ♂ G Spermatic Cord, Left ♂ H Spermatic Cords, Bilateral ♂ J Epididymis, Right ♂ K Epididymis, Left ♂ L Epididymis, Bilateral ♂ N Vas Deferens, Right NC ♂ P Vas Deferens, Left NC ♂ Q Vas Deferens, Bilateral NC ♂	Ø Open 3 Percutaneous 4 Percutaneous Endoscopic	Z No Device	X Diagnostic Z No Qualifier
5 Scrotum ♂ S Penis ♂ T Prepuce ♂	Ø Open 3 Percutaneous 4 Percutaneous Endoscopic X External	Z No Device	X Diagnostic Z No Qualifier

Non-OR ØVBØ[3,4,7,8]ZX
Non-OR ØVB[1,2,3,9,B,C][3,4]ZX
Non-OR ØVB[6,7,F,G,H,J,K,L][Ø,3,4]ZX
Non-OR ØVB[N,P,Q][Ø,3,4]Z[X,Z]
Non-OR ØVB5[Ø,3,4,X]Z[X,Z]
NC ØVB[N,P,Q][Ø,3,4]ZZ

Ø Medical and Surgical
V Male Reproductive System
C Extirpation Taking or cutting out solid matter from a body part

Body Part Character 4	Approach Character 5	Device Character 6	Qualifier Character 7
Ø Prostate ♂	Ø Open 3 Percutaneous 4 Percutaneous Endoscopic 7 Via Natural or Artificial Opening 8 Via Natural or Artificial Opening Endoscopic	Z No Device	Z No Qualifier
1 Seminal Vesicle, Right ♂ 2 Seminal Vesicle, Left ♂ 3 Seminal Vesicles, Bilateral ♂ 6 Tunica Vaginalis, Right ♂ 7 Tunica Vaginalis, Left ♂ 9 Testis, Right ♂ B Testis, Left ♂ C Testes, Bilateral ♂ F Spermatic Cord, Right ♂ G Spermatic Cord, Left ♂ H Spermatic Cords, Bilateral ♂ J Epididymis, Right ♂ K Epididymis, Left ♂ L Epididymis, Bilateral ♂ N Vas Deferens, Right ♂ P Vas Deferens, Left ♂ Q Vas Deferens, Bilateral ♂	Ø Open 3 Percutaneous 4 Percutaneous Endoscopic	Z No Device	Z No Qualifier
5 Scrotum ♂ S Penis ♂ T Prepuce ♂	Ø Open 3 Percutaneous 4 Percutaneous Endoscopic X External	Z No Device	Z No Qualifier

Non-OR ØVC[6,7,N,P,Q][Ø,3,4]ZZ
Non-OR ØVC5[Ø,3,4,X]ZZ
Non-OR ØVCSXZZ

Ø Medical and Surgical
V Male Reproductive System
H Insertion Putting in a nonbiological appliance that monitors, assists, performs, or prevents a physiological function but does not physically take the place of a body part

Body Part Character 4	Approach Character 5	Device Character 6	Qualifier Character 7
Ø Prostate ♂	**Ø** Open **3** Percutaneous **4** Percutaneous Endoscopic **7** Via Natural or Artificial Opening **8** Via Natural or Artificial Opening Endoscopic	**1** Radioactive Element	**Z** No Qualifier
4 Prostate and Seminal Vesicles ♂ **8** Scrotum and Tunica Vaginalis ♂ **D** Testis ♂ **M** Epididymis and Spermatic Cord ♂ **R** Vas Deferens ♂	**Ø** Open **3** Percutaneous **4** Percutaneous Endoscopic **7** Via Natural or Artificial Opening **8** Via Natural or Artificial Opening Endoscopic	**3** Infusion Device	**Z** No Qualifier
S Penis ♂	**Ø** Open **3** Percutaneous **4** Percutaneous Endoscopic **X** External	**3** Infusion Device	**Z** No Qualifier

Non-OR ØVH[4,8,D,M,R][Ø,3,4,7,8]3Z
Non-OR ØVHS[Ø,3,4,X]3Z

Ø Medical and Surgical
V Male Reproductive System
J Inspection Visually and/or manually exploring a body part

Body Part Character 4	Approach Character 5	Device Character 6	Qualifier Character 7
4 Prostate and Seminal Vesicles ♂ **8** Scrotum and Tunica Vaginalis ♂ **D** Testis ♂ **M** Epididymis and Spermatic Cord ♂ **R** Vas Deferens ♂ **S** Penis ♂	**Ø** Open **3** Percutaneous **4** Percutaneous Endoscopic **X** External	**Z** No Device	**Z** No Qualifier

Non-OR ØVJ[4,D,M,R]XZZ
Non-OR ØVJ[8,S][Ø,3,4,X]ZZ

Ø Medical and Surgical
V Male Reproductive System
L Occlusion Completely closing an orifice or the lumen of a tubular body part

Body Part Character 4	Approach Character 5	Device Character 6	Qualifier Character 7
F Spermatic Cord, Right NC ♂ **G** Spermatic Cord, Left NC ♂ **H** Spermatic Cords, Bilateral NC ♂ **N** Vas Deferens, Right NC ♂ **P** Vas Deferens, Left NC ♂ **Q** Vas Deferens, Bilateral NC ♂	**Ø** Open **3** Percutaneous **4** Percutaneous Endoscopic	**C** Extraluminal Device **D** Intraluminal Device **Z** No Device	**Z** No Qualifier

Non-OR ØVL[F,G,H][Ø,3,4][C,D,Z]Z
Non-OR ØVL[N,P,Q][Ø,3,4][C,Z]Z
NC ØVL[F,G,H][Ø,3,4][C,D,Z]Z
NC ØVL[N,P,Q][Ø,3,4][C,Z]Z

Ø Medical and Surgical
V Male Reproductive System
M Reattachment Putting back in or on all or a portion of a separated body part to its normal location or other suitable location

Body Part Character 4	Approach Character 5	Device Character 6	Qualifier Character 7
5 Scrotum ♂ **S** Penis ♂	**X** External	**Z** No Device	**Z** No Qualifier
6 Tunica Vaginalis, Right ♂ **7** Tunica Vaginalis, Left ♂ **9** Testis, Right ♂ **B** Testis, Left ♂ **C** Testes, Bilateral ♂ **F** Spermatic Cord, Right ♂ **G** Spermatic Cord, Left ♂ **H** Spermatic Cords, Bilateral ♂	**Ø** Open **4** Percutaneous Endoscopic	**Z** No Device	**Z** No Qualifier

Ø Medical and Surgical
V Male Reproductive System
N Release Freeing a body part from an abnormal physical constraint

Body Part Character 4	Approach Character 5	Device Character 6	Qualifier Character 7
Ø Prostate ♂	**Ø** Open **3** Percutaneous **4** Percutaneous Endoscopic **7** Via Natural or Artificial Opening **8** Via Natural or Artificial Opening Endoscopic	**Z** No Device	**Z** No Qualifier
1 Seminal Vesicle, Right ♂ **2** Seminal Vesicle, Left ♂ **3** Seminal Vesicles, Bilateral ♂ **6** Tunica Vaginalis, Right ♂ **7** Tunica Vaginalis, Left ♂ **9** Testis, Right ♂ **B** Testis, Left ♂ **C** Testes, Bilateral ♂ **F** Spermatic Cord, Right ♂ **G** Spermatic Cord, Left ♂ **H** Spermatic Cords, Bilateral ♂ **J** Epididymis, Right ♂ **K** Epididymis, Left ♂ **L** Epididymis, Bilateral ♂ **N** Vas Deferens, Right ♂ **P** Vas Deferens, Left ♂ **Q** Vas Deferens, Bilateral ♂	**Ø** Open **3** Percutaneous **4** Percutaneous Endoscopic	**Z** No Device	**Z** No Qualifier
5 Scrotum ♂ **S** Penis ♂ **T** Prepuce ♂	**Ø** Open **3** Percutaneous **4** Percutaneous Endoscopic **X** External	**Z** No Device	**Z** No Qualifier

Non-OR ØVN[9,B,C][Ø,3,4]ZZ
Non-OR ØVNT[Ø,3,4,X]ZZ

Ø Medical and Surgical
V Male Reproductive System
P Removal Taking out or off a device from a body part

Body Part Character 4	Approach Character 5	Device Character 6	Qualifier Character 7
4 Prostate and Seminal Vesicles ♂	**Ø** Open **3** Percutaneous **4** Percutaneous Endoscopic **7** Via Natural or Artificial Opening **8** Via Natural or Artificial Opening Endoscopic	**Ø** Drainage Device **1** Radioactive Element **3** Infusion Device **7** Autologous Tissue Substitute **J** Synthetic Substitute **K** Nonautologous Tissue Substitute	**Z** No Qualifier
4 Prostate and Seminal Vesicles ♂	**X** External	**Ø** Drainage Device **1** Radioactive Element **3** Infusion Device	**Z** No Qualifier
8 Scrotum and Tunica Vaginalis ♂ **D** Testis ♂ **M** Epididymis and Spermatic Cord ♂ **S** Penis ♂	**X** External	**Ø** Drainage Device **3** Infusion Device	**Z** No Qualifier
8 Scrotum and Tunica Vaginalis ♂ **D** Testis ♂ **S** Penis ♂	**Ø** Open **3** Percutaneous **4** Percutaneous Endoscopic **7** Via Natural or Artificial Opening **8** Via Natural or Artificial Opening Endoscopic	**Ø** Drainage Device **3** Infusion Device **7** Autologous Tissue Substitute **J** Synthetic Substitute **K** Nonautologous Tissue Substitute	**Z** No Qualifier
M Epididymis and Spermatic Cord ♂	**Ø** Open **3** Percutaneous **4** Percutaneous Endoscopic **7** Via Natural or Artificial Opening **8** Via Natural or Artificial Opening Endoscopic	**Ø** Drainage Device **3** Infusion Device **7** Autologous Tissue Substitute **C** Extraluminal Device **J** Synthetic Substitute **K** Nonautologous Tissue Substitute	**Z** No Qualifier

ØVP Continued on next page

Non-OR ØVP4X[Ø,1,3]Z
Non-OR ØVP[8,D,M,S]X[Ø,3]Z
Non-OR ØVP8[Ø,3,4,7,8][Ø,3,7,J,K]Z

ØVP Continued

Ø Medical and Surgical
V Male Reproductive System
P Removal Taking out or off a device from a body part

Body Part Character 4	Approach Character 5	Device Character 6	Qualifier Character 7
R Vas Deferens ♂	Ø Open 3 Percutaneous 4 Percutaneous Endoscopic 7 Via Natural or Artificial Opening 8 Via Natural or Artificial Opening Endoscopic	Ø Drainage Device 3 Infusion Device 7 Autologous Tissue Substitute C Extraluminal Device D Intraluminal Device J Synthetic Substitute K Nonautologous Tissue Substitute	Z No Qualifier
R Vas Deferens ♂	X External	Ø Drainage Device 3 Infusion Device D Intraluminal Device	Z No Qualifier

Non-OR ØVPR[Ø,3,4,7,8][Ø,3,7,C,J,K]Z
Non-OR ØVPRX[Ø,3,D]Z

Ø Medical and Surgical
V Male Reproductive System
Q Repair Restoring, to the extent possible, a body part to its normal anatomic structure and function

Body Part Character 4	Approach Character 5	Device Character 6	Qualifier Character 7
Ø Prostate ♂	Ø Open 3 Percutaneous 4 Percutaneous Endoscopic 7 Via Natural or Artificial Opening 8 Via Natural or Artificial Opening Endoscopic	Z No Device	Z No Qualifier
1 Seminal Vesicle, Right ♂ 2 Seminal Vesicle, Left ♂ 3 Seminal Vesicles, Bilateral ♂ 6 Tunica Vaginalis, Right ♂ 7 Tunica Vaginalis, Left ♂ 9 Testis, Right ♂ B Testis, Left ♂ C Testes, Bilateral ♂ F Spermatic Cord, Right ♂ G Spermatic Cord, Left ♂ H Spermatic Cords, Bilateral ♂ J Epididymis, Right ♂ K Epididymis, Left ♂ L Epididymis, Bilateral ♂ N Vas Deferens, Right ♂ P Vas Deferens, Left ♂ Q Vas Deferens, Bilateral ♂	Ø Open 3 Percutaneous 4 Percutaneous Endoscopic	Z No Device	Z No Qualifier
5 Scrotum ♂ S Penis ♂ T Prepuce ♂	Ø Open 3 Percutaneous 4 Percutaneous Endoscopic X External	Z No Device	Z No Qualifier

Non-OR ØVQ[6,7][Ø,3,4]ZZ
Non-OR ØVQ5[Ø,3,4,X]ZZ

Ø Medical and Surgical
V Male Reproductive System
R Replacement Putting in or on biological or synthetic material that physically takes the place and/or function of all or a portion of a body part

Body Part Character 4	Approach Character 5	Device Character 6	Qualifier Character 7
9 Testis, Right ♂ B Testis, Left ♂ C Testes, Bilateral ♂	Ø Open	J Synthetic Substitute	Z No Qualifier

Ø Medical and Surgical
V Male Reproductive System
S Reposition Moving to its normal location or other suitable location all or a portion of a body part

Body Part Character 4	Approach Character 5	Device Character 6	Qualifier Character 7
9 Testis, Right ♂ B Testis, Left ♂ C Testes, Bilateral ♂ F Spermatic Cord, Right ♂ G Spermatic Cord, Left ♂ H Spermatic Cords, Bilateral ♂	Ø Open 3 Percutaneous 4 Percutaneous Endoscopic	Z No Device	Z No Qualifier

Ø Medical and Surgical
V Male Reproductive System
T Resection Cutting out or off, without replacement, all of a body part

Body Part Character 4	Approach Character 5	Device Character 6	Qualifier Character 7
Ø Prostate ⊞♂	Ø Open 4 Percutaneous Endoscopic 7 Via Natural or Artificial Opening 8 Via Natural or Artificial Opening Endoscopic	Z No Device	Z No Qualifier
1 Seminal Vesicle, Right ♂ 2 Seminal Vesicle, Left ♂ 3 Seminal Vesicles, Bilateral ⊞♂ 6 Tunica Vaginalis, Right ♂ 7 Tunica Vaginalis, Left ♂ 9 Testis, Right ♂ B Testis, Left ♂ C Testes, Bilateral ♂ F Spermatic Cord, Right ♂ G Spermatic Cord, Left ♂ H Spermatic Cords, Bilateral ♂ J Epididymis, Right ♂ K Epididymis, Left ♂ L Epididymis, Bilateral ♂ N Vas Deferens, Right NC♂ P Vas Deferens, Left NC♂ Q Vas Deferens, Bilateral NC♂	Ø Open 4 Percutaneous Endoscopic	Z No Device	Z No Qualifier
5 Scrotum ♂ S Penis ♂ T Prepuce ♂	Ø Open 4 Percutaneous Endoscopic X External	Z No Device	Z No Qualifier

Non-OR ØVT[N,P,Q][Ø,4]ZZ
Non-OR ØVT[5,T][Ø,4,X]ZZ
NC ØVT[N,P,Q][Ø,4]ZZ

See Appendix I for Procedure Combinations
⊞ ØVTØ[Ø,4,7,8]ZZ
⊞ ØVT3[Ø,4]ZZ

Ø Medical and Surgical
V Male Reproductive System
U Supplement Putting in or on biological or synthetic material that physically reinforces and/or augments the function of a portion of a body part

Body Part Character 4	Approach Character 5	Device Character 6	Qualifier Character 7
1 Seminal Vesicle, Right ♂ **2** Seminal Vesicle, Left ♂ **3** Seminal Vesicles, Bilateral ♂ **6** Tunica Vaginalis, Right ♂ **7** Tunica Vaginalis, Left ♂ **F** Spermatic Cord, Right ♂ **G** Spermatic Cord, Left ♂ **H** Spermatic Cords, Bilateral ♂ **J** Epididymis, Right ♂ **K** Epididymis, Left ♂ **L** Epididymis, Bilateral ♂ **N** Vas Deferens, Right ♂ **P** Vas Deferens, Left ♂ **Q** Vas Deferens, Bilateral ♂	**Ø** Open **4** Percutaneous Endoscopic	**7** Autologous Tissue Substitute **J** Synthetic Substitute **K** Nonautologous Tissue Substitute	**Z** No Qualifier
5 Scrotum ♂ **S** Penis ♂ **T** Prepuce ♂	**Ø** Open **4** Percutaneous Endoscopic **X** External	**7** Autologous Tissue Substitute **J** Synthetic Substitute **K** Nonautologous Tissue Substitute	**Z** No Qualifier
9 Testis, Right ♂ **B** Testis, Left ♂ **C** Testes, Bilateral ♂	**Ø** Open	**7** Autologous Tissue Substitute **J** Synthetic Substitute **K** Nonautologous Tissue Substitute	**Z** No Qualifier

Non-OR ØVUSX[7,J,K]Z

Ø Medical and Surgical
V Male Reproductive System
W Revision Correcting, to the extent possible, a portion of a malfunctioning device or the position of a displaced device

Body Part Character 4	Approach Character 5	Device Character 6	Qualifier Character 7
4 Prostate and Seminal Vesicles ♂ **8** Scrotum and Tunica Vaginalis ♂ **D** Testis ♂ **S** Penis ♂	**Ø** Open **3** Percutaneous **4** Percutaneous Endoscopic **7** Via Natural or Artificial Opening **8** Via Natural or Artificial Opening Endoscopic **X** External	**Ø** Drainage Device **3** Infusion Device **7** Autologous Tissue Substitute **J** Synthetic Substitute **K** Nonautologous Tissue Substitute	**Z** No Qualifier
M Epididymis and Spermatic Cord ♂	**Ø** Open **3** Percutaneous **4** Percutaneous Endoscopic **7** Via Natural or Artificial Opening **8** Via Natural or Artificial Opening Endoscopic **X** External	**Ø** Drainage Device **3** Infusion Device **7** Autologous Tissue Substitute **C** Extraluminal Device **J** Synthetic Substitute **K** Nonautologous Tissue Substitute	**Z** No Qualifier
R Vas Deferens ♂	**Ø** Open **3** Percutaneous **4** Percutaneous Endoscopic **7** Via Natural or Artificial Opening **8** Via Natural or Artificial Opening Endoscopic **X** External	**Ø** Drainage Device **3** Infusion Device **7** Autologous Tissue Substitute **C** Extraluminal Device **D** Intraluminal Device **J** Synthetic Substitute **K** Nonautologous Tissue Substitute	**Z** No Qualifier

Non-OR ØVW8[Ø,3,4,7,8,X][Ø,3,7,J,K]Z
Non-OR ØVW[4,D,S]X[Ø,3,7,J,K]Z
Non-OR ØVWMX[Ø,3,7,C,J,K]Z
Non-OR ØVWR[Ø,3,4,7,8,X][Ø,3,7,C,D,J,K]Z

Anatomical Regions, General ØWØ–ØWW

Ø Medical and Surgical
W Anatomical Regions, General
Ø Alteration Modifying the anatomic structure of a body part without affecting the function of the body part

Body Part Character 4	Approach Character 5	Device Character 6	Qualifier Character 7
Ø Head **2** Face **4** Upper Jaw **5** Lower Jaw **6** Neck **8** Chest Wall **F** Abdominal Wall **K** Upper Back **L** Lower Back **M** Perineum, Male ♂ **N** Perineum, Female ♀	**Ø** Open **3** Percutaneous **4** Percutaneous Endoscopic	**7** Autologous Tissue Substitute **J** Synthetic Substitute **K** Nonautologous Tissue Substitute **Z** No Device	**Z** No Qualifier

Ø Medical and Surgical
W Anatomical Regions, General
1 Bypass Altering the route of passage of the contents of a tubular body part

Body Part Character 4	Approach Character 5	Device Character 6	Qualifier Character 7
1 Cranial Cavity	**Ø** Open	**J** Synthetic Substitute	**9** Pleural Cavity, Right **B** Pleural Cavity, Left **G** Peritoneal Cavity **J** Pelvic Cavity
9 Pleural Cavity, Right **B** Pleural Cavity, Left **G** Peritoneal Cavity **J** Pelvic Cavity ♀	**Ø** Open **4** Percutaneous Endoscopic	**J** Synthetic Substitute	**4** Cutaneous **9** Pleural Cavity, Right **B** Pleural Cavity, Left **G** Peritoneal Cavity **J** Pelvic Cavity **Y** Lower Vein
9 Pleural Cavity, Right **B** Pleural Cavity, Left **G** Peritoneal Cavity **J** Pelvic Cavity ♀	**3** Percutaneous	**J** Synthetic Substitute	**4** Cutaneous

Non-OR ØW1[9,B,G][Ø,4]JG
Non-OR ØW1[9,B,J][Ø,4]J[4,Y]
Non-OR ØW1G[Ø,4]J[9,B,J]
Non-OR ØW1[9,B,J]3J4
AHA: 2013, 4Q, 126-127

Ø Medical and Surgical
W Anatomical Regions, General
2 Change Taking out or off a device from a body part and putting back an identical or similar device in or on the same body part without cutting or puncturing the skin or a mucous membrane

Body Part Character 4	Approach Character 5	Device Character 6	Qualifier Character 7
Ø Head **1** Cranial Cavity **2** Face **4** Upper Jaw **5** Lower Jaw **6** Neck **8** Chest Wall **9** Pleural Cavity, Right **B** Pleural Cavity, Left **C** Mediastinum **D** Pericardial Cavity **F** Abdominal Wall **G** Peritoneal Cavity **H** Retroperitoneum **J** Pelvic Cavity **K** Upper Back **L** Lower Back **M** Perineum, Male **N** Perineum, Female	**X** External	**Ø** Drainage Device **Y** Other Device	**Z** No Qualifier

Non-OR For all body part, approach, device, and qualifier values

Ø Medical and Surgical
W Anatomical Regions, General
3 Control Stopping, or attempting to stop, postprocedural bleeding

Body Part Character 4	Approach Character 5	Device Character 6	Qualifier Character 7
Ø Head 1 Cranial Cavity 2 Face 4 Upper Jaw 5 Lower Jaw 6 Neck 8 Chest Wall 9 Pleural Cavity, Right B Pleural Cavity, Left C Mediastinum D Pericardial Cavity F Abdominal Wall G Peritoneal Cavity H Retroperitoneum J Pelvic Cavity K Upper Back L Lower Back M Perineum, Male ♂ N Perineum, Female ♀	Ø Open 3 Percutaneous 4 Percutaneous Endoscopic	Z No Device	Z No Qualifier
3 Oral Cavity and Throat	Ø Open 3 Percutaneous 4 Percutaneous Endoscopic 7 Via Natural or Artificial Opening 8 Via Natural or Artificial Opening Endoscopic X External	Z No Device	Z No Qualifier
P Gastrointestinal Tract Q Respiratory Tract R Genitourinary Tract	Ø Open 3 Percutaneous 4 Percutaneous Endoscopic 7 Via Natural or Artificial Opening 8 Via Natural or Artificial Opening Endoscopic	Z No Device	Z No Qualifier

Non-OR ØW3GØZZ
Non-OR ØW3P8ZZ

Ø Medical and Surgical
W Anatomical Regions, General
4 Creation Making a new genital structure that does not take over the function of a body part

Body Part Character 4	Approach Character 5	Device Character 6	Qualifier Character 7
M Perineum, Male NC ♂	Ø Open	7 Autologous Tissue Substitute J Synthetic Substitute K Nonautologous Tissue Substitute Z No Device	Ø Vagina
N Perineum, Female NC ♀	Ø Open	7 Autologous Tissue Substitute J Synthetic Substitute K Nonautologous Tissue Substitute Z No Device	1 Penis

NC ØW4MØ[7,J,K,Z]Ø
NC ØW4NØ[7,J,K,Z]1

Ø Medical and Surgical
W Anatomical Regions, General
8 Division Cutting into a body part without draining fluids and/or gases from the body part in order to separate or transect a body part

Body Part Character 4	Approach Character 5	Device Character 6	Qualifier Character 7
N Perineum, Female ♀	X External	Z No Device	Z No Qualifier

Non-OR ØW8NXZZ

Ø Medical and Surgical
W Anatomical Regions, General
9 Drainage Taking or letting out fluids and/or gases from a body part

Body Part Character 4	Approach Character 5	Device Character 6	Qualifier Character 7
Ø Head 1 Cranial Cavity 2 Face 3 Oral Cavity and Throat 4 Upper Jaw 5 Lower Jaw 6 Neck 8 Chest Wall 9 Pleural Cavity, Right B Pleural Cavity, Left C Mediastinum D Pericardial Cavity F Abdominal Wall G Peritoneal Cavity H Retroperitoneum J Pelvic Cavity K Upper Back L Lower Back M Perineum, Male ♂ N Perineum, Female ♀	Ø Open 3 Percutaneous 4 Percutaneous Endoscopic	Ø Drainage Device	Z No Qualifier
Ø Head 1 Cranial Cavity 2 Face 3 Oral Cavity and Throat 4 Upper Jaw 5 Lower Jaw 6 Neck 8 Chest Wall 9 Pleural Cavity, Right B Pleural Cavity, Left C Mediastinum D Pericardial Cavity F Abdominal Wall G Peritoneal Cavity H Retroperitoneum J Pelvic Cavity K Upper Back L Lower Back M Perineum, Male ♂ N Perineum, Female ♀	Ø Open 3 Percutaneous 4 Percutaneous Endoscopic	Z No Device	X Diagnostic Z No Qualifier

Non-OR ØW9[Ø,8,9,B,K,L,M][Ø,3,4]ØZ
Non-OR ØW9[1,D,F,G][3,4]ØZ
Non-OR ØW9J3ØZ
Non-OR ØW9[Ø,2,3,4,5,6,8,9,B,K,L,M,N][Ø,3,4]ZX
Non-OR ØW9[Ø,8,9,B,K,L,M][Ø,3,4]ZZ
Non-OR ØW9[1,C,D][3,4]ZX
Non-OR ØW9[1,D,F,G][3,4]ZZ
Non-OR ØW9J3ZZ

Ø Medical and Surgical
W Anatomical Regions, General
B Excision Cutting out or off, without replacement, a portion of a body part

Body Part Character 4	Approach Character 5	Device Character 6	Qualifier Character 7
Ø Head 2 Face 4 Upper Jaw 5 Lower Jaw 8 Chest Wall K Upper Back L Lower Back M Perineum, Male ♂ N Perineum, Female ♀	Ø Open 3 Percutaneous 4 Percutaneous Endoscopic X External	Z No Device	X Diagnostic Z No Qualifier
6 Neck C Mediastinum F Abdominal Wall H Retroperitoneum	Ø Open 3 Percutaneous 4 Percutaneous Endoscopic	Z No Device	X Diagnostic Z No Qualifier
6 Neck F Abdominal Wall	X External	Z No Device	2 Stoma X Diagnostic Z No Qualifier

Non-OR ØWB[Ø,2,4,5,8,K,L,M][Ø,3,4,X]ZX
Non-OR ØWB6[Ø,3,4]ZX
Non-OR ØWB[C,H][3,4]ZX
Non-OR ØWB6XZX

AHA: 2Ø13, 4Q, 119

Ø Medical and Surgical
W Anatomical Regions, General
C Extirpation Taking or cutting out solid matter from a body part

Body Part Character 4	Approach Character 5	Device Character 6	Qualifier Character 7
1 Cranial Cavity 3 Oral Cavity and Throat 9 Pleural Cavity, Right B Pleural Cavity, Left C Mediastinum D Pericardial Cavity G Peritoneal Cavity J Pelvic Cavity	Ø Open 3 Percutaneous 4 Percutaneous Endoscopic X External	Z No Device	Z No Qualifier
P Gastrointestinal Tract Q Respiratory Tract R Genitourinary Tract	Ø Open 3 Percutaneous 4 Percutaneous Endoscopic 7 Via Natural or Artificial Opening 8 Via Natural or Artificial Opening Endoscopic X External	Z No Device	Z No Qualifier

Non-OR ØWC[1,3]XZZ
Non-OR ØWC[9,B][Ø,3,4,X]ZZ
Non-OR ØWC[C,D,G,J]XZZ
Non-OR ØWCP[7,8,X]ZZ
Non-OR ØWCQ[Ø,3,4,X]ZZ
Non-OR ØWCR[7,8,X]ZZ

Ø Medical and Surgical
W Anatomical Regions, General
F Fragmentation Breaking solid matter in a body part into pieces

Body Part Character 4	Approach Character 5	Device Character 6	Qualifier Character 7
1 Cranial Cavity NC 3 Oral Cavity and Throat NC 9 Pleural Cavity, Right NC B Pleural Cavity, Left NC C Mediastinum NC D Pericardial Cavity G Peritoneal Cavity NC J Pelvic Cavity NC	Ø Open 3 Percutaneous 4 Percutaneous Endoscopic X External	Z No Device	Z No Qualifier
P Gastrointestinal Tract NC Q Respiratory Tract NC R Genitourinary Tract	Ø Open 3 Percutaneous 4 Percutaneous Endoscopic 7 Via Natural or Artificial Opening 8 Via Natural or Artificial Opening Endoscopic X External	Z No Device	Z No Qualifier

DRG Non-OR ØWFRXZZ
Non-OR ØWF[1,3,9,B,C,G]XZZ
Non-OR ØWFJ[Ø,3,4,X]ZZ
Non-OR ØWFP[Ø,3,4,7,8,X]ZZ
Non-OR ØWFQXZZ
Non-OR ØWFR[Ø,3,4,7,8]ZZ
NC ØWF[1,3,9,B,C,G,J]XZZ
NC ØWF[P,Q]XZZ

Ø Medical and Surgical
W Anatomical Regions, General
H Insertion Putting in a nonbiological appliance that monitors, assists, performs, or prevents a physiological function but does not physically take the place of a body part

Body Part Character 4	Approach Character 5	Device Character 6	Qualifier Character 7
Ø Head **1** Cranial Cavity **2** Face **3** Oral Cavity and Throat **4** Upper Jaw **5** Lower Jaw **6** Neck **8** Chest Wall **9** Pleural Cavity, Right **B** Pleural Cavity, Left **C** Mediastinum **D** Pericardial Cavity **F** Abdominal Wall **G** Peritoneal Cavity **H** Retroperitoneum **J** Pelvic Cavity **K** Upper Back **L** Lower Back **M** Perineum, Male **N** Perineum, Female ♀	**Ø** Open **3** Percutaneous **4** Percutaneous Endoscopic	**1** Radioactive Element **3** Infusion Device **Y** Other Device	**Z** No Qualifier
P Gastrointestinal Tract **Q** Respiratory Tract **R** Genitourinary Tract	**Ø** Open **3** Percutaneous **4** Percutaneous Endoscopic **7** Via Natural or Artificial Opening **8** Via Natural or Artificial Opening Endoscopic	**1** Radioactive Element **3** Infusion Device **Y** Other Device	**Z** No Qualifier

DRG Non-OR ØWH[Ø,2,4,5,6,K,L,M][Ø,3,4][3,Y]Z
Non-OR ØWH1[Ø,3,4]3Z
Non-OR ØWH[8,9,B][Ø,3,4][3,Y]Z
Non-OR ØWHPØYZ
Non-OR ØWHP[3,4,7,8][3,Y]Z
Non-OR ØWHQ[Ø,7,8][3,Y]Z
Non-OR ØWHR[Ø,3,4,7,8][3,Y]Z

Ø Medical and Surgical
W Anatomical Regions, General
J Inspection Visually and/or manually exploring a body part

Body Part Character 4	Approach Character 5	Device Character 6	Qualifier Character 7
Ø Head **2** Face **3** Oral Cavity and Throat **4** Upper Jaw **5** Lower Jaw **6** Neck **8** Chest Wall **F** Abdominal Wall **K** Upper Back **L** Lower Back **M** Perineum, Male ♂ **N** Perineum, Female ♀	**Ø** Open **3** Percutaneous **4** Percutaneous Endoscopic **X** External	**Z** No Device	**Z** No Qualifier
1 Cranial Cavity **9** Pleural Cavity, Right **B** Pleural Cavity, Left **C** Mediastinum **D** Pericardial Cavity **G** Peritoneal Cavity **H** Retroperitoneum **J** Pelvic Cavity	**Ø** Open **3** Percutaneous **4** Percutaneous Endoscopic	**Z** No Device	**Z** No Qualifier
P Gastrointestinal Tract **Q** Respiratory Tract **R** Genitourinary Tract	**Ø** Open **3** Percutaneous **4** Percutaneous Endoscopic **7** Via Natural or Artificial Opening **8** Via Natural or Artificial Opening Endoscopic	**Z** No Device	**Z** No Qualifier

DRG Non-OR ØWJ[Ø,2,4,5,K,L]ØZZ
DRG Non-OR ØWJM[Ø,4]ZZ
AHA: 2Ø13, 2Q, 36
Non-OR ØWJ[Ø,2,4,5,K,L][3,4,X]ZZ
Non-OR ØWJ3[Ø,3,4,X]ZZ
Non-OR ØWJ[6,8,F,N]XZZ
Non-OR ØWJM[3,X]ZZ
Non-OR ØWJD[Ø,3]ZZ

Ø Medical and Surgical
W Anatomical Regions, General
M Reattachment Putting back in or on all or a portion of a separated body part to its normal location or other suitable location

Body Part Character 4	Approach Character 5	Device Character 6	Qualifier Character 7
2 Face **4** Upper Jaw **5** Lower Jaw **6** Neck **8** Chest Wall **F** Abdominal Wall **K** Upper Back **L** Lower Back **M** Perineum, Male ♂ **N** Perineum, Female ♀	**Ø** Open	**Z** No Device	**Z** No Qualifier

Ø Medical and Surgical
W Anatomical Regions, General
P Removal Taking out or off a device from a body part

Body Part Character 4	Approach Character 5	Device Character 6	Qualifier Character 7
Ø Head **2** Face **4** Upper Jaw **5** Lower Jaw **6** Neck **8** Chest Wall **C** Mediastinum **F** Abdominal Wall **K** Upper Back **L** Lower Back **M** Perineum, Male ♂ **N** Perineum, Female ♀	**Ø** Open **3** Percutaneous **4** Percutaneous Endoscopic **X** External	**Ø** Drainage Device **1** Radioactive Element **3** Infusion Device **7** Autologous Tissue Substitute **J** Synthetic Substitute **K** Nonautologous Tissue Substitute **Y** Other Device	**Z** No Qualifier
1 Cranial Cavity **9** Pleural Cavity, Right **B** Pleural Cavity, Left **D** Pericardial Cavity **G** Peritoneal Cavity **H** Retroperitoneum **J** Pelvic Cavity	**X** External	**Ø** Drainage Device **1** Radioactive Element **3** Infusion Device	**Z** No Qualifier
1 Cranial Cavity **9** Pleural Cavity, Right **B** Pleural Cavity, Left **G** Peritoneal Cavity **J** Pelvic Cavity	**Ø** Open **3** Percutaneous **4** Percutaneous Endoscopic	**Ø** Drainage Device **1** Radioactive Element **3** Infusion Device **J** Synthetic Substitute **Y** Other Device	**Z** No Qualifier
D Pericardial Cavity **H** Retroperitoneum	**Ø** Open **3** Percutaneous **4** Percutaneous Endoscopic	**Ø** Drainage Device **1** Radioactive Element **3** Infusion Device **Y** Other Device	**Z** No Qualifier
P Gastrointestinal Tract **Q** Respiratory Tract **R** Genitourinary Tract	**Ø** Open **3** Percutaneous **4** Percutaneous Endoscopic **7** Via Natural or Artificial Opening **8** Via Natural or Artificial Opening Endoscopic **X** External	**1** Radioactive Element **3** Infusion Device **Y** Other Device	**Z** No Qualifier

Non-OR ØWP[Ø,2,4,5,6,8,K,L][Ø,3,4,X][Ø,1,3,7,J,K,Y]Z
Non-OR ØWPM[Ø,3,4][Ø,1,3,J,Y]Z
Non-OR ØWPMX[Ø,1,3,Y]Z
Non-OR ØWP[C,F,N]X[Ø,1,3,7,J,K,Y]Z
Non-OR ØWP[1,9,B,D,G,H,J]X[Ø,1,3]Z
Non-OR ØWP1[Ø,3,4]3Z
Non-OR ØWP[9,B,J][Ø,3,4][Ø,1,3,J,Y]Z
Non-OR ØWPP[3,4,7,8,X][1,3,Y]Z
Non-OR ØWPQ8[3,Y]Z
Non-OR ØWPQ[Ø,X][1,3,Y]Z
Non-OR ØWPR[Ø,3,4,7,8,X][1,3,Y]Z

Ø Medical and Surgical
W Anatomical Regions, General
Q Repair Restoring, to the extent possible, a body part to its normal anatomic structure and function

Body Part Character 4	Approach Character 5	Device Character 6	Qualifier Character 7
Ø Head **2** Face **4** Upper Jaw **5** Lower Jaw **8** Chest Wall ⊞ **K** Upper Back **L** Lower Back **M** Perineum, Male **N** Perineum, Female ⊞♀	**Ø** Open **3** Percutaneous **4** Percutaneous Endoscopic **X** External	**Z** No Device	**Z** No Qualifier
6 Neck **C** Mediastinum ⊞ **F** Abdominal Wall	**Ø** Open **3** Percutaneous **4** Percutaneous Endoscopic	**Z** No Device	**Z** No Qualifier
6 Neck **F** Abdominal Wall ⊞	**X** External	**Z** No Device	**2** Stoma **Z** No Qualifier

Non-OR ØWQNXZZ

See Appendix I for Procedure Combinations
⊞ ØWQFXZ[2,Z]

No Procedure Combinations Specified
⊞ ØWQ[8,N][Ø,3,4]ZZ
⊞ ØWQC[Ø,3,4]ZZ

Ø Medical and Surgical
W Anatomical Regions, General
U Supplement Putting in or on biological or synthetic material that physically reinforces and/or augments the function of a portion of a body part

Body Part Character 4	Approach Character 5	Device Character 6	Qualifier Character 7
Ø Head **2** Face **4** Upper Jaw **5** Lower Jaw **6** Neck **8** Chest Wall **C** Mediastinum **F** Abdominal Wall **K** Upper Back **L** Lower Back **M** Perineum, Male ♂ **N** Perineum, Female ♀	**Ø** Open **4** Percutaneous Endoscopic	**7** Autologous Tissue Substitute **J** Synthetic Substitute **K** Nonautologous Tissue Substitute	**Z** No Qualifier

AHA: 2Ø12, 4Q, 1Ø1

Ø Medical and Surgical
W Anatomical Regions, General
W Revision Correcting, to the extent possible, a portion of a malfunctioning device or the position of a displaced device

Body Part Character 4	Approach Character 5	Device Character 6	Qualifier Character 7
Ø Head 2 Face 4 Upper Jaw 5 Lower Jaw 6 Neck 8 Chest Wall C Mediastinum F Abdominal Wall K Upper Back L Lower Back M Perineum, Male ♂ N Perineum, Female ♀	Ø Open 3 Percutaneous 4 Percutaneous Endoscopic X External	Ø Drainage Device 1 Radioactive Element 3 Infusion Device 7 Autologous Tissue Substitute J Synthetic Substitute K Nonautologous Tissue Substitute Y Other Device	Z No Qualifier
1 Cranial Cavity 9 Pleural Cavity, Right B Pleural Cavity, Left G Peritoneal Cavity J Pelvic Cavity	Ø Open 3 Percutaneous 4 Percutaneous Endoscopic X External	Ø Drainage Device 1 Radioactive Element 3 Infusion Device J Synthetic Substitute Y Other Device	Z No Qualifier
D Pericardial Cavity H Retroperitoneum	Ø Open 3 Percutaneous 4 Percutaneous Endoscopic X External	Ø Drainage Device 1 Radioactive Element 3 Infusion Device Y Other Device	Z No Qualifier
P Gastrointestinal Tract Q Respiratory Tract R Genitourinary Tract	Ø Open 3 Percutaneous 4 Percutaneous Endoscopic 7 Via Natural or Artificial Opening 8 Via Natural or Artificial Opening Endoscopic X External	1 Radioactive Element 3 Infusion Device Y Other Device	Z No Qualifier

DRG Non-OR ØWW[Ø,2,4,5,6,K,L][Ø,3,4][Ø,1,3,7,J,K,Y]Z
DRG Non-OR ØWWM[Ø,3,4][Ø,1,3,J,Y]Z
Non-OR ØWW[Ø,2,4,5,6,C,F,K,L,M,N]X[Ø,1,3,7,J,K,Y]Z
Non-OR ØWW8[Ø,3,4,X][Ø,1,3,7,J,K,Y]Z
Non-OR ØWW[1,G,J]X[Ø,1,3,J,Y]Z
Non-OR ØWW[9,B][Ø,3,4,X][Ø,1,3,J,Y]Z
Non-OR ØWW[D,H]X[Ø,1,3,Y]Z
Non-OR ØWWP[3,4,7,8,X][1,3,Y]Z
Non-OR ØWWQ[Ø,X][1,3,Y]Z
Non-OR ØWWR[Ø,3,4,7,8,X][1,3,Y]Z

Anatomical Regions, Upper Extremities ØXØ–ØXX

Ø Medical and Surgical
X Anatomical Regions, Upper Extremities
Ø Alteration Modifying the anatomic structure of a body part without affecting the function of the body part

Body Part Character 4	Approach Character 5	Device Character 6	Qualifier Character 7
2 Shoulder Region, Right **3** Shoulder Region, Left **4** Axilla, Right **5** Axilla, Left **6** Upper Extremity, Right **7** Upper Extremity, Left **8** Upper Arm, Right **9** Upper Arm, Left **B** Elbow Region, Right **C** Elbow Region, Left **D** Lower Arm, Right **F** Lower Arm, Left **G** Wrist Region, Right **H** Wrist Region, Left	**Ø** Open **3** Percutaneous **4** Percutaneous Endoscopic	**7** Autologous Tissue Substitute **J** Synthetic Substitute **K** Nonautologous Tissue Substitute **Z** No Device	**Z** No Qualifier

Ø Medical and Surgical
X Anatomical Regions, Upper Extremities
2 Change Taking out or off a device from a body part and putting back an identical or similar device in or on the same body part without cutting or puncturing the skin or a mucous membrane

Body Part Character 4	Approach Character 5	Device Character 6	Qualifier Character 7
6 Upper Extremity, Right **7** Upper Extremity, Left	**X** External	**Ø** Drainage Device **Y** Other Device	**Z** No Qualifier

Non-OR For all body part, approach, device, and qualifier values

Ø Medical and Surgical
X Anatomical Regions, Upper Extremities
3 Control Stopping, or attempting to stop, postprocedural bleeding

Body Part Character 4	Approach Character 5	Device Character 6	Qualifier Character 7
2 Shoulder Region, Right **3** Shoulder Region, Left **4** Axilla, Right **5** Axilla, Left **6** Upper Extremity, Right **7** Upper Extremity, Left **8** Upper Arm, Right **9** Upper Arm, Left **B** Elbow Region, Right **C** Elbow Region, Left **D** Lower Arm, Right **F** Lower Arm, Left **G** Wrist Region, Right **H** Wrist Region, Left **J** Hand, Right **K** Hand, Left	**Ø** Open **3** Percutaneous **4** Percutaneous Endoscopic	**Z** No Device	**Z** No Qualifier

Ø Medical and Surgical
X Anatomical Regions, Upper Extremities
6 Detachment Cutting off all or a portion of the upper or lower extremities

Body Part Character 4	Approach Character 5	Device Character 6	Qualifier Character 7
Ø Forequarter, Right **1** Forequarter, Left **2** Shoulder Region, Right **3** Shoulder Region, Left **B** Elbow Region, Right **C** Elbow Region, Left	**Ø** Open	**Z** No Device	**Z** No Qualifier
8 Upper Arm, Right **9** Upper Arm, Left **D** Lower Arm, Right **F** Lower Arm, Left	**Ø** Open	**Z** No Device	**1** High **2** Mid **3** Low

ØX6 Continued on next page

ØX6 Continued

Ø Medical and Surgical
X Anatomical Regions, Upper Extremities
6 Detachment Cutting off all or a portion of the upper or lower extremities

Body Part Character 4	Approach Character 5	Device Character 6	Qualifier Character 7
J Hand, Right K Hand, Left	Ø Open	Z No Device	Ø Complete 4 Complete 1st Ray 5 Complete 2nd Ray 6 Complete 3rd Ray 7 Complete 4th Ray 8 Complete 5th Ray 9 Partial 1st Ray B Partial 2nd Ray C Partial 3rd Ray D Partial 4th Ray F Partial 5th Ray
L Thumb, Right M Thumb, Left N Index Finger, Right P Index Finger, Left Q Middle Finger, Right R Middle Finger, Left S Ring Finger, Right T Ring Finger, Left V Little Finger, Right W Little Finger, Left	Ø Open	Z No Device	Ø Complete 1 High 2 Mid 3 Low

Ø Medical and Surgical
X Anatomical Regions, Upper Extremities
9 Drainage Taking or letting out fluids and/or gases from a body part

Body Part Character 4	Approach Character 5	Device Character 6	Qualifier Character 7
2 Shoulder Region, Right 3 Shoulder Region, Left 4 Axilla, Right 5 Axilla, Left 6 Upper Extremity, Right 7 Upper Extremity, Left 8 Upper Arm, Right 9 Upper Arm, Left B Elbow Region, Right C Elbow Region, Left D Lower Arm, Right F Lower Arm, Left G Wrist Region, Right H Wrist Region, Left J Hand, Right K Hand, Left	Ø Open 3 Percutaneous 4 Percutaneous Endoscopic	Ø Drainage Device	Z No Qualifier
2 Shoulder Region, Right 3 Shoulder Region, Left 4 Axilla, Right 5 Axilla, Left 6 Upper Extremity, Right 7 Upper Extremity, Left 8 Upper Arm, Right 9 Upper Arm, Left B Elbow Region, Right C Elbow Region, Left D Lower Arm, Right F Lower Arm, Left G Wrist Region, Right H Wrist Region, Left J Hand, Right K Hand, Left	Ø Open 3 Percutaneous 4 Percutaneous Endoscopic	Z No Device	X Diagnostic Z No Qualifier

Non-OR For all body part, approach, device, and qualifier values

Ø Medical and Surgical
X Anatomical Regions, Upper Extremities
B Excision Cutting out or off, without replacement, a portion of a body part

Body Part Character 4	Approach Character 5	Device Character 6	Qualifier Character 7
2 Shoulder Region, Right 3 Shoulder Region, Left 4 Axilla, Right 5 Axilla, Left 6 Upper Extremity, Right 7 Upper Extremity, Left 8 Upper Arm, Right 9 Upper Arm, Left B Elbow Region, Right C Elbow Region, Left D Lower Arm, Right F Lower Arm, Left G Wrist Region, Right H Wrist Region, Left J Hand, Right K Hand, Left	Ø Open 3 Percutaneous 4 Percutaneous Endoscopic	Z No Device	X Diagnostic Z No Qualifier

Non-OR ØXB[2,3,4,5,6,7,8,9,B,C,D,F,G,H,J,K][Ø,3,4]ZX

Ø Medical and Surgical
X Anatomical Regions, Upper Extremities
H Insertion Putting in a nonbiological appliance that monitors, assists, performs, or prevents a physiological function but does not physically take the place of a body part

Body Part Character 4	Approach Character 5	Device Character 6	Qualifier Character 7
2 Shoulder Region, Right 3 Shoulder Region, Left 4 Axilla, Right 5 Axilla, Left 6 Upper Extremity, Right 7 Upper Extremity, Left 8 Upper Arm, Right 9 Upper Arm, Left B Elbow Region, Right C Elbow Region, Left D Lower Arm, Right F Lower Arm, Left G Wrist Region, Right H Wrist Region, Left J Hand, Right K Hand, Left	Ø Open 3 Percutaneous 4 Percutaneous Endoscopic	1 Radioactive Element 3 Infusion Device Y Other Device	Z No Qualifier

DRG Non-OR ØXH[2,3,4,5,6,7,8,9,B,C,D,F,G,H,J,K][Ø,3,4][3,Y]Z

Ø Medical and Surgical
X Anatomical Regions, Upper Extremities
J Inspection Visually and/or manually exploring a body part

Body Part Character 4	Approach Character 5	Device Character 6	Qualifier Character 7
2 Shoulder Region, Right 3 Shoulder Region, Left 4 Axilla, Right 5 Axilla, Left 6 Upper Extremity, Right 7 Upper Extremity, Left 8 Upper Arm, Right 9 Upper Arm, Left B Elbow Region, Right C Elbow Region, Left D Lower Arm, Right F Lower Arm, Left G Wrist Region, Right H Wrist Region, Left J Hand, Right K Hand, Left	Ø Open 3 Percutaneous 4 Percutaneous Endoscopic X External	Z No Device	Z No Qualifier

DRG Non-OR ØXJ[2,3,4,5,6,7,8,9,B,C,D,F,G,H,J,K]ØZZ
Non-OR ØXJ[2,3,4,5,6,7,8,9,B,C,D,F,G,H][3,4,X]ZZ
Non-OR ØXJ[J,K]XZZ

Ø Medical and Surgical
X Anatomical Regions, Upper Extremities
M Reattachment Putting back in or on all or a portion of a separated body part to its normal location or other suitable location

Body Part Character 4	Approach Character 5	Device Character 6	Qualifier Character 7
Ø Forequarter, Right 1 Forequarter, Left 2 Shoulder Region, Right 3 Shoulder Region, Left 4 Axilla, Right 5 Axilla, Left 6 Upper Extremity, Right 7 Upper Extremity, Left 8 Upper Arm, Right 9 Upper Arm, Left B Elbow Region, Right C Elbow Region, Left D Lower Arm, Right F Lower Arm, Left G Wrist Region, Right H Wrist Region, Left J Hand, Right K Hand, Left L Thumb, Right M Thumb, Left N Index Finger, Right P Index Finger, Left Q Middle Finger, Right R Middle Finger, Left S Ring Finger, Right T Ring Finger, Left V Little Finger, Right W Little Finger, Left	Ø Open	Z No Device	Z No Qualifier

Ø Medical and Surgical
X Anatomical Regions, Upper Extremities
P Removal Taking out or off a device from a body part

Body Part Character 4	Approach Character 5	Device Character 6	Qualifier Character 7
6 Upper Extremity, Right 7 Upper Extremity, Left	Ø Open 3 Percutaneous 4 Percutaneous Endoscopic X External	Ø Drainage Device 1 Radioactive Element 3 Infusion Device 7 Autologous Tissue Substitute J Synthetic Substitute K Nonautologous Tissue Substitute Y Other Device	Z No Qualifier

Non-OR For all body part, approach, device, and qualifier values

Ø Medical and Surgical
X Anatomical Regions, Upper Extremities
Q Repair Restoring, to the extent possible, a body part to its normal anatomic structure and function

Body Part Character 4	Approach Character 5	Device Character 6	Qualifier Character 7
2 Shoulder Region, Right **3** Shoulder Region, Left **4** Axilla, Right **5** Axilla, Left **6** Upper Extremity, Right **7** Upper Extremity, Left **8** Upper Arm, Right **9** Upper Arm, Left **B** Elbow Region, Right **C** Elbow Region, Left **D** Lower Arm, Right **F** Lower Arm, Left **G** Wrist Region, Right **H** Wrist Region, Left **J** Hand, Right **K** Hand, Left **L** Thumb, Right **M** Thumb, Left **N** Index Finger, Right **P** Index Finger, Left **Q** Middle Finger, Right **R** Middle Finger, Left **S** Ring Finger, Right **T** Ring Finger, Left **V** Little Finger, Right **W** Little Finger, Left	**Ø** Open **3** Percutaneous **4** Percutaneous Endoscopic **X** External	**Z** No Device	**Z** No Qualifier

Ø Medical and Surgical
X Anatomical Regions, Upper Extremities
R Replacement Putting in or on biological or synthetic material that physically takes the place and/or function of all or a portion of a body part

Body Part Character 4	Approach Character 5	Device Character 6	Qualifier Character 7
L Thumb, Right **M** Thumb, Left	**Ø** Open **4** Percutaneous Endoscopic	**7** Autologous Tissue Substitute	**N** Toe, Right **P** Toe, Left

Ø Medical and Surgical
X Anatomical Regions, Upper Extremities
U Supplement Putting in or on biological or synthetic material that physically reinforces and/or augments the function of a portion of a body part

Body Part Character 4	Approach Character 5	Device Character 6	Qualifier Character 7
2 Shoulder Region, Right **3** Shoulder Region, Left **4** Axilla, Right **5** Axilla, Left **6** Upper Extremity, Right **7** Upper Extremity, Left **8** Upper Arm, Right **9** Upper Arm, Left **B** Elbow Region, Right **C** Elbow Region, Left **D** Lower Arm, Right **F** Lower Arm, Left **G** Wrist Region, Right **H** Wrist Region, Left **J** Hand, Right **K** Hand, Left **L** Thumb, Right **M** Thumb, Left **N** Index Finger, Right **P** Index Finger, Left **Q** Middle Finger, Right **R** Middle Finger, Left **S** Ring Finger, Right **T** Ring Finger, Left **V** Little Finger, Right **W** Little Finger, Left	**Ø** Open **4** Percutaneous Endoscopic	**7** Autologous Tissue Substitute **J** Synthetic Substitute **K** Nonautologous Tissue Substitute	**Z** No Qualifier

Ø Medical and Surgical
X Anatomical Regions, Upper Extremities
W Revision Correcting, to the extent possible, a portion of a malfunctioning device or the position of a displaced device

Body Part Character 4	Approach Character 5	Device Character 6	Qualifier Character 7
6 Upper Extremity, Right **7** Upper Extremity, Left	**Ø** Open **3** Percutaneous **4** Percutaneous Endoscopic **X** External	**Ø** Drainage Device **3** Infusion Device **7** Autologous Tissue Substitute **J** Synthetic Substitute **K** Nonautologous Tissue Substitute **Y** Other Device	**Z** No Qualifier

DRG Non-OR ØXW[6,7][Ø,3,4][Ø,3,7,J,K,Y]Z
Non-OR ØXW[6,7]X[Ø,3,7,J,K,Y]Z

Ø Medical and Surgical
X Anatomical Regions, Upper Extremities
X Transfer Moving, without taking out, all or a portion of a body part to another location to take over the function of all or a portion of a body part

Body Part Character 4	Approach Character 5	Device Character 6	Qualifier Character 7
N Index Finger, Right	**Ø** Open	**Z** No Device	**L** Thumb, Right
P Index Finger, Left	**Ø** Open	**Z** No Device	**M** Thumb, Left

Anatomical Regions, Lower Extremities ØYØ–ØYW

Ø Medical and Surgical
Y Anatomical Regions, Lower Extremities
Ø Alteration Modifying the anatomic structure of a body part without affecting the function of the body part

Body Part Character 4	Approach Character 5	Device Character 6	Qualifier Character 7
Ø Buttock, Right 1 Buttock, Left 9 Lower Extremity, Right B Lower Extremity, Left C Upper Leg, Right D Upper Leg, Left F Knee Region, Right G Knee Region, Left H Lower Leg, Right J Lower Leg, Left K Ankle Region, Right L Ankle Region, Left	Ø Open 3 Percutaneous 4 Percutaneous Endoscopic	7 Autologous Tissue Substitute J Synthetic Substitute K Nonautologous Tissue Substitute Z No Device	Z No Qualifier

Ø Medical and Surgical
Y Anatomical Regions, Lower Extremities
2 Change Taking out or off a device from a body part and putting back an identical or similar device in or on the same body part without cutting or puncturing the skin or a mucous membrane

Body Part Character 4	Approach Character 5	Device Character 6	Qualifier Character 7
9 Lower Extremity, Right B Lower Extremity, Left	X External	Ø Drainage Device Y Other Device	Z No Qualifier

Non-OR For all body part, approach, device, and qualifier values

Ø Medical and Surgical
Y Anatomical Regions, Lower Extremities
3 Control Stopping, or attempting to stop, postprocedural bleeding

Body Part Character 4	Approach Character 5	Device Character 6	Qualifier Character 7
Ø Buttock, Right 1 Buttock, Left 5 Inguinal Region, Right 6 Inguinal Region, Left 7 Femoral Region, Right 8 Femoral Region, Left 9 Lower Extremity, Right B Lower Extremity, Left C Upper Leg, Right D Upper Leg, Left F Knee Region, Right G Knee Region, Left H Lower Leg, Right J Lower Leg, Left K Ankle Region, Right L Ankle Region, Left M Foot, Right N Foot, Left	Ø Open 3 Percutaneous 4 Percutaneous Endoscopic	Z No Device	Z No Qualifier

Ø Medical and Surgical
Y Anatomical Regions, Lower Extremities
6 Detachment Cutting off all or a portion of the upper or lower extremities

Body Part Character 4	Approach Character 5	Device Character 6	Qualifier Character 7
2 Hindquarter, Right 3 Hindquarter, Left 4 Hindquarter, Bilateral 7 Femoral Region, Right 8 Femoral Region, Left F Knee Region, Right G Knee Region, Left	Ø Open	Z No Device	Z No Qualifier
C Upper Leg, Right D Upper Leg, Left H Lower Leg, Right J Lower Leg, Left	Ø Open	Z No Device	1 High 2 Mid 3 Low

ØY6 Continued on next page

0Y6 Continued

0 Medical and Surgical
Y Anatomical Regions, Lower Extremities
6 Detachment Cutting off all or a portion of the upper or lower extremities

Body Part Character 4	Approach Character 5	Device Character 6	Qualifier Character 7
M Foot, Right **N** Foot, Left	**0** Open	**Z** No Device	**0** Complete **4** Complete 1st Ray **5** Complete 2nd Ray **6** Complete 3rd Ray **7** Complete 4th Ray **8** Complete 5th Ray **9** Partial 1st Ray **B** Partial 2nd Ray **C** Partial 3rd Ray **D** Partial 4th Ray **F** Partial 5th Ray
P 1st Toe, Right **Q** 1st Toe, Left **R** 2nd Toe, Right **S** 2nd Toe, Left **T** 3rd Toe, Right **U** 3rd Toe, Left **V** 4th Toe, Right **W** 4th Toe, Left **X** 5th Toe, Right **Y** 5th Toe, Left	**0** Open	**Z** No Device	**0** Complete **1** High **2** Mid **3** Low

0 Medical and Surgical
Y Anatomical Regions, Lower Extremities
9 Drainage Taking or letting out fluids and/or gases from a body part

Body Part Character 4	Approach Character 5	Device Character 6	Qualifier Character 7
0 Buttock, Right **1** Buttock, Left **5** Inguinal Region, Right **6** Inguinal Region, Left **7** Femoral Region, Right **8** Femoral Region, Left **9** Lower Extremity, Right **B** Lower Extremity, Left **C** Upper Leg, Right **D** Upper Leg, Left **F** Knee Region, Right **G** Knee Region, Left **H** Lower Leg, Right **J** Lower Leg, Left **K** Ankle Region, Right **L** Ankle Region, Left **M** Foot, Right **N** Foot, Left	**0** Open **3** Percutaneous **4** Percutaneous Endoscopic	**0** Drainage Device	**Z** No Qualifier
0 Buttock, Right **1** Buttock, Left **5** Inguinal Region, Right **6** Inguinal Region, Left **7** Femoral Region, Right **8** Femoral Region, Left **9** Lower Extremity, Right **B** Lower Extremity, Left **C** Upper Leg, Right **D** Upper Leg, Left **F** Knee Region, Right **G** Knee Region, Left **H** Lower Leg, Right **J** Lower Leg, Left **K** Ankle Region, Right **L** Ankle Region, Left **M** Foot, Right **N** Foot, Left	**0** Open **3** Percutaneous **4** Percutaneous Endoscopic	**Z** No Device	**X** Diagnostic **Z** No Qualifier

Non-OR 0Y9[0,1,7,8,9,B,C,D,F,G,H,J,K,L,M,N][0,3,4]0Z
Non-OR 0Y9[0,1,7,8,9,B,C,D,F,G,H,J,K,L,M,N][0,3,4]Z[X,Z]

Ø Medical and Surgical
Y Anatomical Regions, Lower Extremities
B Excision Cutting out or off, without replacement, a portion of a body part

Body Part Character 4	Approach Character 5	Device Character 6	Qualifier Character 7
Ø Buttock, Right 1 Buttock, Left 5 Inguinal Region, Right 6 Inguinal Region, Left 7 Femoral Region, Right 8 Femoral Region, Left 9 Lower Extremity, Right B Lower Extremity, Left C Upper Leg, Right D Upper Leg, Left F Knee Region, Right G Knee Region, Left H Lower Leg, Right J Lower Leg, Left K Ankle Region, Right L Ankle Region, Left M Foot, Right N Foot, Left	Ø Open 3 Percutaneous 4 Percutaneous Endoscopic	Z No Device	X Diagnostic Z No Qualifier

Non-OR ØYB[Ø,1,9,B,C,D,F,G,H,J,K,L,M,N][Ø,3,4]ZX

Ø Medical and Surgical
Y Anatomical Regions, Lower Extremities
H Insertion Putting in a nonbiological appliance that monitors, assists, performs, or prevents a physiological function but does not physically take the place of a body part

Body Part Character 4	Approach Character 5	Device Character 6	Qualifier Character 7
Ø Buttock, Right 1 Buttock, Left 5 Inguinal Region, Right 6 Inguinal Region, Left 7 Femoral Region, Right 8 Femoral Region, Left 9 Lower Extremity, Right B Lower Extremity, Left C Upper Leg, Right D Upper Leg, Left F Knee Region, Right G Knee Region, Left H Lower Leg, Right J Lower Leg, Left K Ankle Region, Right L Ankle Region, Left M Foot, Right N Foot, Left	Ø Open 3 Percutaneous 4 Percutaneous Endoscopic	1 Radioactive Element 3 Infusion Device Y Other Device	Z No Qualifier

DRG Non-OR ØYH[Ø,1,5,6,7,8,9,B,C,D,F,G,H,J,K,L,M,N][Ø,3,4][3,Y]Z

Ø Medical and Surgical
Y Anatomical Regions, Lower Extremities
J Inspection Visually and/or manually exploring a body part

Body Part Character 4	Approach Character 5	Device Character 6	Qualifier Character 7
Ø Buttock, Right 1 Buttock, Left 5 Inguinal Region, Right 6 Inguinal Region, Left 7 Femoral Region, Right 8 Femoral Region, Left 9 Lower Extremity, Right A Inguinal Region, Bilateral B Lower Extremity, Left C Upper Leg, Right D Upper Leg, Left E Femoral Region, Bilateral F Knee Region, Right G Knee Region, Left H Lower Leg, Right J Lower Leg, Left K Ankle Region, Right L Ankle Region, Left M Foot, Right N Foot, Left	Ø Open 3 Percutaneous 4 Percutaneous Endoscopic X External	Z No Device	Z No Qualifier

DRG Non-OR ØYJ[Ø,1,8,9,B,C,D,E,F,G,H,J,K,L,M,N]ØZZ
Non-OR ØYJ[Ø,1,9,B,C,D,F,G,H,J,K,L,M,N][3,4,X]ZZ
Non-OR ØYJ[5,6,7,8,A,E]XZZ

Ø Medical and Surgical
Y Anatomical Regions, Lower Extremities
M Reattachment Putting back in or on all or a portion of a separated body part to its normal location or other suitable location

Body Part Character 4	Approach Character 5	Device Character 6	Qualifier Character 7
Ø Buttock, Right 1 Buttock, Left 2 Hindquarter, Right 3 Hindquarter, Left 4 Hindquarter, Bilateral 5 Inguinal Region, Right 6 Inguinal Region, Left 7 Femoral Region, Right 8 Femoral Region, Left 9 Lower Extremity, Right B Lower Extremity, Left C Upper Leg, Right D Upper Leg, Left F Knee Region, Right G Knee Region, Left H Lower Leg, Right J Lower Leg, Left K Ankle Region, Right L Ankle Region, Left M Foot, Right N Foot, Left P 1st Toe, Right Q 1st Toe, Left R 2nd Toe, Right S 2nd Toe, Left T 3rd Toe, Right U 3rd Toe, Left V 4th Toe, Right W 4th Toe, Left X 5th Toe, Right Y 5th Toe, Left	Ø Open	Z No Device	Z No Qualifier

Ø Medical and Surgical
Y Anatomical Regions, Lower Extremities
P Removal Taking out or off a device from a body part

Body Part Character 4	Approach Character 5	Device Character 6	Qualifier Character 7
9 Lower Extremity, Right B Lower Extremity, Left	Ø Open 3 Percutaneous 4 Percutaneous Endoscopic X External	Ø Drainage Device 1 Radioactive Element 3 Infusion Device 7 Autologous Tissue Substitute J Synthetic Substitute K Nonautologous Tissue Substitute Y Other Device	Z No Qualifier

Non-OR For all body part, approach, device, and qualifier values

Ø Medical and Surgical
Y Anatomical Regions, Lower Extremities
Q Repair Restoring, to the extent possible, a body part to its normal anatomic structure and function

Body Part Character 4	Approach Character 5	Device Character 6	Qualifier Character 7
Ø Buttock, Right 1 Buttock, Left 5 Inguinal Region, Right 6 Inguinal Region, Left 7 Femoral Region, Right 8 Femoral Region, Left 9 Lower Extremity, Right A Inguinal Region, Bilateral B Lower Extremity, Left C Upper Leg, Right D Upper Leg, Left E Femoral Region, Bilateral F Knee Region, Right G Knee Region, Left H Lower Leg, Right J Lower Leg, Left K Ankle Region, Right L Ankle Region, Left M Foot, Right N Foot, Left P 1st Toe, Right Q 1st Toe, Left R 2nd Toe, Right S 2nd Toe, Left T 3rd Toe, Right U 3rd Toe, Left V 4th Toe, Right W 4th Toe, Left X 5th Toe, Right Y 5th Toe, Left	Ø Open 3 Percutaneous 4 Percutaneous Endoscopic X External	Z No Device	Z No Qualifier

Non-OR ØYQ[5,6,7,8,A,E]XZZ

Ø Medical and Surgical
Y Anatomical Regions, Lower Extremities
U Supplement Putting in or on biological or synthetic material that physically reinforces and/or augments the function of a portion of a body part

Body Part Character 4	Approach Character 5	Device Character 6	Qualifier Character 7
Ø Buttock, Right **1** Buttock, Left **5** Inguinal Region, Right **6** Inguinal Region, Left **7** Femoral Region, Right **8** Femoral Region, Left **9** Lower Extremity, Right **A** Inguinal Region, Bilateral **B** Lower Extremity, Left **C** Upper Leg, Right **D** Upper Leg, Left **E** Femoral Region, Bilateral **F** Knee Region, Right **G** Knee Region, Left **H** Lower Leg, Right **J** Lower Leg, Left **K** Ankle Region, Right **L** Ankle Region, Left **M** Foot, Right **N** Foot, Left **P** 1st Toe, Right **Q** 1st Toe, Left **R** 2nd Toe, Right **S** 2nd Toe, Left **T** 3rd Toe, Right **U** 3rd Toe, Left **V** 4th Toe, Right **W** 4th Toe, Left **X** 5th Toe, Right **Y** 5th Toe, Left	**Ø** Open **4** Percutaneous Endoscopic	**7** Autologous Tissue Substitute **J** Synthetic Substitute **K** Nonautologous Tissue Substitute	**Z** No Qualifier

Ø Medical and Surgical
Y Anatomical Regions, Lower Extremities
W Revision Correcting, to the extent possible, a portion of a malfunctioning device or the position of a displaced device

Body Part Character 4	Approach Character 5	Device Character 6	Qualifier Character 7
9 Lower Extremity, Right **B** Lower Extremity, Left	**Ø** Open **3** Percutaneous **4** Percutaneous Endoscopic **X** External	**Ø** Drainage Device **3** Infusion Device **7** Autologous Tissue Substitute **J** Synthetic Substitute **K** Nonautologous Tissue Substitute **Y** Other Device	**Z** No Qualifier

DRG Non-OR ØYW[9,B][Ø,3,4][Ø,3,7,J,K,Y]Z
Non-OR ØYW[9,B]X[Ø,3,7,J,K,Y]Z

Obstetrics 1Ø2–1ØY

1 Obstetrics
Ø Pregnancy
2 Change Taking out or off a device from a body part and putting back an identical or similar device in or on the same body part without cutting or puncturing the skin or a mucous membrane

Body Part Character 4	Approach Character 5	Device Character 6	Qualifier Character 7
Ø Products of Conception ♀	7 Via Natural or Artificial Opening	3 Monitoring Electrode Y Other Device	Z No Qualifier

Non-OR For all body part, approach, device, and qualifier values

1 Obstetrics
Ø Pregnancy
9 Drainage Taking or letting out fluids and/or gases from a body part

Body Part Character 4	Approach Character 5	Device Character 6	Qualifier Character 7
Ø Products of Conception ♀	Ø Open 3 Percutaneous 4 Percutaneous Endoscopic 7 Via Natural or Artificial Opening 8 Via Natural or Artificial Opening Endoscopic	Z No Device	9 Fetal Blood A Fetal Cerebrospinal Fluid B Fetal Fluid, Other C Amniotic Fluid, Therapeutic D Fluid, Other U Amniotic Fluid, Diagnostic

Non-OR For all body part, approach, device, and qualifier values
AHA: 2Ø14, 2Q, 9

1 Obstetrics
Ø Pregnancy
A Abortion Artificially terminating a pregnancy

Body Part Character 4	Approach Character 5	Device Character 6	Qualifier Character 7
Ø Products of Conception ♀	Ø Open 3 Percutaneous 4 Percutaneous Endoscopic 8 Via Natural or Artificial Opening Endoscopic	Z No Device	Z No Qualifier
Ø Products of Conception ♀	7 Via Natural or Artificial Opening	Z No Device	6 Vacuum W Laminaria X Abortifacient Z No Qualifier

DRG Non-OR 1ØAØ7Z6
Non-OR 1ØAØ7Z[W,X]

1 Obstetrics
Ø Pregnancy
D Extraction Pulling or stripping out or off all or a portion of a body part

Body Part Character 4	Approach Character 5	Device Character 6	Qualifier Character 7
Ø Products of Conception ♀	Ø Open	Z No Device	Ø Classical 1 Low Cervical 2 Extraperitoneal
Ø Products of Conception ⊞♀	7 Via Natural or Artificial Opening	Z No Device	3 Low Forceps 4 Mid Forceps 5 High Forceps 6 Vacuum 7 Internal Version 8 Other
1 Products of Conception, Retained ♀ 2 Products of Conception, Ectopic ♀	7 Via Natural or Artificial Opening 8 Via Natural or Artificial Opening Endoscopic	Z No Device	Z No Qualifier

DRG Non-OR 1ØDØ7Z[3,4,5,6,7,8]
No Procedure Combinations Specified
⊞ 1ØDØ7Z[3,4,5,6]

1 Obstetrics
0 Pregnancy
E Delivery Assisting the passage of the products of conception from the genital canal

Body Part Character 4	Approach Character 5	Device Character 6	Qualifier Character 7
0 Products of Conception ⊞♀	X External	Z No Device	Z No Qualifier

DRG Non-OR 10E0XZZ
AHA: 2014, 2Q, 9

No Procedure Combinations Specified
⊞ 10E0XZZ

1 Obstetrics
0 Pregnancy
H Insertion Putting in a nonbiological appliance that monitors, assists, performs, or prevents a physiological function but does not physically take the place of a body part

Body Part Character 4	Approach Character 5	Device Character 6	Qualifier Character 7
0 Products of Conception ♀	0 Open 7 Via Natural or Artificial Opening	3 Monitoring Electrode Y Other Device	Z No Qualifier

Non-OR 10H07[3,Y]Z
AHA: 2013, 2Q, 36

1 Obstetrics
0 Pregnancy
J Inspection Visually and/or manually exploring a body part

Body Part Character 4	Approach Character 5	Device Character 6	Qualifier Character 7
0 Products of Conception ♀ 1 Products of Conception, Retained ♀ 2 Products of Conception, Ectopic ♀	0 Open 3 Percutaneous 4 Percutaneous Endoscopic 7 Via Natural or Artificial Opening 8 Via Natural or Artificial Opening Endoscopic X External	Z No Device	Z No Qualifier

Non-OR For all body part, approach, device, and qualifier values

1 Obstetrics
0 Pregnancy
P Removal Taking out or off a device from a body part, region or orifice

Body Part Character 4	Approach Character 5	Device Character 6	Qualifier Character 7
0 Products of Conception ♀	0 Open 7 Via Natural or Artificial Opening	3 Monitoring Electrode Y Other Device	Z No Qualifier

1 Obstetrics
0 Pregnancy
Q Repair Restoring, to the extent possible, a body part to its normal anatomic structure and function

Body Part Character 4	Approach Character 5	Device Character 6	Qualifier Character 7
0 Products of Conception ♀	0 Open 3 Percutaneous 4 Percutaneous Endoscopic 7 Via Natural or Artificial Opening 8 Via Natural or Artificial Opening Endoscopic	Y Other Device Z No Device	E Nervous System F Cardiovascular System G Lymphatics and Hemic H Eye J Ear, Nose and Sinus K Respiratory System L Mouth and Throat M Gastrointestinal System N Hepatobiliary and Pancreas P Endocrine System Q Skin R Musculoskeletal System S Urinary System T Female Reproductive System V Male Reproductive System Y Other Body System

Non-OR For all body part, approach, device, and qualifier values

1 Obstetrics
Ø Pregnancy
S Reposition Moving to its normal location or other suitable location all or a portion of a body part

Body Part Character 4	Approach Character 5	Device Character 6	Qualifier Character 7
Ø Products of Conception ♀	**7** Via Natural or Artificial Opening **X** External	**Z** No Device	**Z** No Qualifier
2 Products of Conception, Ectopic ♀	**Ø** Open **3** Percutaneous **4** Percutaneous Endoscopic **7** Via Natural or Artificial Opening **8** Via Natural or Artificial Opening Endoscopic	**Z** No Device	**Z** No Qualifier

DRG Non-OR 1ØSØ7ZZ
Non-OR 1ØSØXZZ

1 Obstetrics
Ø Pregnancy
T Resection Cutting out or off, without replacement, all of a body part

Body Part Character 4	Approach Character 5	Device Character 6	Qualifier Character 7
2 Products of Conception, Ectopic ♀	**Ø** Open **3** Percutaneous **4** Percutaneous Endoscopic **7** Via Natural or Artificial Opening **8** Via Natural or Artificial Opening Endoscopic	**Z** No Device	**Z** No Qualifier

1 Obstetrics
Ø Pregnancy
Y Transplantation Putting in or on all or a portion of a living body part taken from another individual or animal to physically take the place and/or function of all or a portion of a similar body part

Body Part Character 4	Approach Character 5	Device Character 6	Qualifier Character 7
Ø Products of Conception ♀	**3** Percutaneous **4** Percutaneous Endoscopic **7** Via Natural or Artificial Opening	**Z** No Device	**E** Nervous System **F** Cardiovascular System **G** Lymphatics and Hemic **H** Eye **J** Ear, Nose and Sinus **K** Respiratory System **L** Mouth and Throat **M** Gastrointestinal System **N** Hepatobiliary and Pancreas **P** Endocrine System **Q** Skin **R** Musculoskeletal System **S** Urinary System **T** Female Reproductive System **V** Male Reproductive System **Y** Other Body System

Non-OR For all body part, approach, device, and qualifier values

Placement—Anatomical Regions 2W0–2W6

2 Placement
W Anatomical Regions
0 Change Taking out or off a device from a body part and putting back an identical or similar device in or on the same body part without cutting or puncturing the skin or a mucous membrane

Body Region Character 4	Approach Character 5	Device Character 6	Qualifier Character 7
0 Head **1** Face **2** Neck **3** Abdominal Wall **4** Chest Wall **5** Back **6** Inguinal Region, Right **7** Inguinal Region, Left **8** Upper Extremity, Right **9** Upper Extremity, Left **A** Upper Arm, Right **B** Upper Arm, Left **C** Lower Arm, Right **D** Lower Arm, Left **E** Hand, Right **F** Hand, Left **G** Thumb, Right **H** Thumb, Left **J** Finger, Right **K** Finger, Left **L** Lower Extremity, Right **M** Lower Extremity, Left **N** Upper Leg, Right **P** Upper Leg, Left **Q** Lower Leg, Right **R** Lower Leg, Left **S** Foot, Right **T** Foot, Left **U** Toe, Right **V** Toe, Left	**X** External	**0** Traction Apparatus **1** Splint **2** Cast **3** Brace **4** Bandage **5** Packing Material **6** Pressure Dressing **7** Intermittent Pressure Device **Y** Other Device	**Z** No Qualifier
1 Face	**X** External	**0** Traction Apparatus **1** Splint **2** Cast **3** Brace **4** Bandage **5** Packing Material **6** Pressure Dressing **7** Intermittent Pressure Device **9** Wire **Y** Other Device	**Z** No Qualifier

2 Placement
W Anatomical Regions
1 Compression Putting pressure on a body region

Body Region Character 4	Approach Character 5	Device Character 6	Qualifier Character 7
Ø Head **1** Face **2** Neck **3** Abdominal Wall **4** Chest Wall **5** Back **6** Inguinal Region, Right **7** Inguinal Region, Left **8** Upper Extremity, Right **9** Upper Extremity, Left **A** Upper Arm, Right **B** Upper Arm, Left **C** Lower Arm, Right **D** Lower Arm, Left **E** Hand, Right **F** Hand, Left **G** Thumb, Right **H** Thumb, Left **J** Finger, Right **K** Finger, Left **L** Lower Extremity, Right **M** Lower Extremity, Left **N** Upper Leg, Right **P** Upper Leg, Left **Q** Lower Leg, Right **R** Lower Leg, Left **S** Foot, Right **T** Foot, Left **U** Toe, Right **V** Toe, Left	**X** External	**6** Pressure Dressing **7** Intermittent Pressure Device	**Z** No Qualifier

2 Placement
W Anatomical Regions
2 Dressing Putting material on a body region for protection

Body Region Character 4	Approach Character 5	Device Character 6	Qualifier Character 7
Ø Head **1** Face **2** Neck **3** Abdominal Wall **4** Chest Wall **5** Back **6** Inguinal Region, Right **7** Inguinal Region, Left **8** Upper Extremity, Right **9** Upper Extremity, Left **A** Upper Arm, Right **B** Upper Arm, Left **C** Lower Arm, Right **D** Lower Arm, Left **E** Hand, Right **F** Hand, Left **G** Thumb, Right **H** Thumb, Left **J** Finger, Right **K** Finger, Left **L** Lower Extremity, Right **M** Lower Extremity, Left **N** Upper Leg, Right **P** Upper Leg, Left **Q** Lower Leg, Right **R** Lower Leg, Left **S** Foot, Right **T** Foot, Left **U** Toe, Right **V** Toe, Left	**X** External	**4** Bandage	**Z** No Qualifier

2 Placement
W Anatomical Regions
3 Immobilization Limiting or preventing motion of a body region

Body Region Character 4	Approach Character 5	Device Character 6	Qualifier Character 7
0 Head **2** Neck **3** Abdominal Wall **4** Chest Wall **5** Back **6** Inguinal Region, Right **7** Inguinal Region, Left **8** Upper Extremity, Right **9** Upper Extremity, Left **A** Upper Arm, Right **B** Upper Arm, Left **C** Lower Arm, Right **D** Lower Arm, Left **E** Hand, Right **F** Hand, Left **G** Thumb, Right **H** Thumb, Left **J** Finger, Right **K** Finger, Left **L** Lower Extremity, Right **M** Lower Extremity, Left **N** Upper Leg, Right **P** Upper Leg, Left **Q** Lower Leg, Right **R** Lower Leg, Left **S** Foot, Right **T** Foot, Left **U** Toe, Right **V** Toe, Left	**X** External	**1** Splint **2** Cast **3** Brace **Y** Other Device	**Z** No Qualifier
1 Face	**X** External	**1** Splint **2** Cast **3** Brace **9** Wire **Y** Other Device	**Z** No Qualifier

2 Placement
W Anatomical Regions
4 Packing Putting material in a body region or orifice

Body Region Character 4	Approach Character 5	Device Character 6	Qualifier Character 7
0 Head **1** Face **2** Neck **3** Abdominal Wall **4** Chest Wall **5** Back **6** Inguinal Region, Right **7** Inguinal Region, Left **8** Upper Extremity, Right **9** Upper Extremity, Left **A** Upper Arm, Right **B** Upper Arm, Left **C** Lower Arm, Right **D** Lower Arm, Left **E** Hand, Right **F** Hand, Left **G** Thumb, Right **H** Thumb, Left **J** Finger, Right **K** Finger, Left **L** Lower Extremity, Right **M** Lower Extremity, Left **N** Upper Leg, Right **P** Upper Leg, Left **Q** Lower Leg, Right **R** Lower Leg, Left **S** Foot, Right **T** Foot, Left **U** Toe, Right **V** Toe, Left	**X** External	**5** Packing Material	**Z** No Qualifier

2 Placement
W Anatomical Regions
5 Removal Taking out or off a device from a body part

Body Region Character 4	Approach Character 5	Device Character 6	Qualifier Character 7
Ø Head 2 Neck 3 Abdominal Wall 4 Chest Wall 5 Back 6 Inguinal Region, Right 7 Inguinal Region, Left 8 Upper Extremity, Right 9 Upper Extremity, Left A Upper Arm, Right B Upper Arm, Left C Lower Arm, Right D Lower Arm, Left E Hand, Right F Hand, Left G Thumb, Right H Thumb, Left J Finger, Right K Finger, Left L Lower Extremity, Right M Lower Extremity, Left N Upper Leg, Right P Upper Leg, Left Q Lower Leg, Right R Lower Leg, Left S Foot, Right T Foot, Left U Toe, Right V Toe, Left	X External	Ø Traction Apparatus 1 Splint 2 Cast 3 Brace 4 Bandage 5 Packing Material 6 Pressure Dressing 7 Intermittent Pressure Device Y Other Device	Z No Qualifier
1 Face	X External	Ø Traction Apparatus 1 Splint 2 Cast 3 Brace 4 Bandage 5 Packing Material 6 Pressure Dressing 7 Intermittent Pressure Device 9 Wire Y Other Device	Z No Qualifier

2 Placement
W Anatomical Regions
6 Traction Exerting a pulling force on a body region in a distal direction

Body Region Character 4	Approach Character 5	Device Character 6	Qualifier Character 7
0 Head **1** Face **2** Neck **3** Abdominal Wall **4** Chest Wall **5** Back **6** Inguinal Region, Right **7** Inguinal Region, Left **8** Upper Extremity, Right **9** Upper Extremity, Left **A** Upper Arm, Right **B** Upper Arm, Left **C** Lower Arm, Right **D** Lower Arm, Left **E** Hand, Right **F** Hand, Left **G** Thumb, Right **H** Thumb, Left **J** Finger, Right **K** Finger, Left **L** Lower Extremity, Right **M** Lower Extremity, Left **N** Upper Leg, Right **P** Upper Leg, Left **Q** Lower Leg, Right **R** Lower Leg, Left **S** Foot, Right **T** Foot, Left **U** Toe, Right **V** Toe, Left	**X** External	**0** Traction Apparatus **Z** No Device	**Z** No Qualifier

AHA: 2013, 2Q, 39

Placement—Anatomical Orifices 2YØ–2Y5

2 Placement
Y Anatomical Orifices
Ø Change Taking out or off a device from a body part and putting back an identical or similar device in or on the same body part without cutting or puncturing the skin or a mucous membrane

Body Region Character 4	Approach Character 5	Device Character 6	Qualifier Character 7
Ø Mouth and Pharynx **1** Nasal **2** Ear **3** Anorectal **4** Female Genital Tract ♀ **5** Urethra	**X** External	**5** Packing Material	**Z** No Qualifier

2 Placement
Y Anatomical Orifices
4 Packing Putting material in a body region or orifice

Body Region Character 4	Approach Character 5	Device Character 6	Qualifier Character 7
Ø Mouth and Pharynx **1** Nasal **2** Ear **3** Anorectal **4** Female Genital Tract ♀ **5** Urethra	**X** External	**5** Packing Material	**Z** No Qualifier

2 Placement
Y Anatomical Orifices
5 Removal Taking out or off a device from a body part

Body Region Character 4	Approach Character 5	Device Character 6	Qualifier Character 7
Ø Mouth and Pharynx **1** Nasal **2** Ear **3** Anorectal **4** Female Genital Tract ♀ **5** Urethra	**X** External	**5** Packing Material	**Z** No Qualifier

Administration 302–3E1

3 Administration
0 Circulatory
2 Transfusion Putting in blood or blood products

Body System/Region Character 4	Approach Character 5	Substance Character 6	Qualifier Character 7
3 Peripheral Vein NC 4 Central Vein NC	0 Open 3 Percutaneous	A Stem Cells, Embryonic	Z No Qualifier
3 Peripheral Vein NC 4 Central Vein NC 5 Peripheral Artery NC 6 Central Artery NC	0 Open 3 Percutaneous	G Bone Marrow H Whole Blood J Serum Albumin K Frozen Plasma L Fresh Plasma M Plasma Cryoprecipitate N Red Blood Cells P Frozen Red Cells Q White Cells R Platelets S Globulin T Fibrinogen V Antihemophilic Factors W Factor IX X Stem Cells, Cord Blood Y Stem Cells, Hematopoietic	0 Autologous 1 Nonautologous
7 Products of Conception, Circulatory ♀	3 Percutaneous 7 Via Natural or Artificial Opening	H Whole Blood J Serum Albumin K Frozen Plasma L Fresh Plasma M Plasma Cryoprecipitate N Red Blood Cells P Frozen Red Cells Q White Cells R Platelets S Globulin T Fibrinogen V Antihemophilic Factors W Factor IX	1 Nonautologous
8 Vein	0 Open 3 Percutaneous	B 4-Factor Prothrombin Complex Concentrate	1 Nonautologous

NC 3023[0,3]AZ Only when reported with PDx or SDx of C91.00, C92.00, C92.10, C92.11, C92.40, C92.50, C92.60, C92.A0, C93.00, C94.00, C95.00
NC 3024[0,3]AZ Only when reported with PDx or SDx of C91.00, C92.00, C92.10, C92.11, C92.40, C92.50, C92.60, C92.A0, C93.00, C94.00, C95.00
NC 302[3,4,5,6][0,3][G,Y]0 Only when reported with PDx or SDx of C91.00, C92.00, C92.10, C92.11, C92.40, C92.50, C92.60, C92.A0, C93.00, C94.00, C95.00
NC 302[3,4,5,6][0,3][G,Y]1 Only when reported with PDx or SDx of C90.00 or C90.01

3 Administration
C Indwelling Device
1 Irrigation Putting in or on a cleansing substance

Body System/Region Character 4	Approach Character 5	Substance Character 6	Qualifier Character 7
Z None	X External	8 Irrigating Substance	Z No Qualifier

3 Administration
E Physiological Systems and Anatomical Regions
Ø Introduction Putting in or on a therapeutic, diagnostic, nutritional, physiological, or prophylactic substance except blood or blood products

Body System/Region Character 4	Approach Character 5	Substance Character 6	Qualifier Character 7
Ø Skin and Mucous Membranes	**X** External	**Ø** Antineoplastic	**5** Other Antineoplastic **M** Monoclonal Antibody
Ø Skin and Mucous Membranes	**X** External	**2** Anti-infective	**8** Oxazolidinones **9** Other Anti-infective
Ø Skin and Mucous Membranes	**X** External	**3** Anti-inflammatory **4** Serum, Toxoid and Vaccine **B** Local Anesthetic **K** Other Diagnostic Substance **M** Pigment **N** Analgesics, Hypnotics, Sedatives **T** Destructive Agent	**Z** No Qualifier
Ø Skin and Mucous Membranes	**X** External	**G** Other Therapeutic Substance	**C** Other Substance
1 Subcutaneous Tissue	**Ø** Open	**2** Anti-infective	**A** Anti-infective Envelope
1 Subcutaneous Tissue	**3** Percutaneous	**V** Hormone	**G** Insulin **J** Other Hormone
1 Subcutaneous Tissue	**3** Percutaneous	**2** Anti-infective	**8** Oxazolidinones **9** Other Anti-infective **A** Anti-infective Envelope
1 Subcutaneous Tissue **2** Muscle	**3** Percutaneous	**3** Anti-inflammatory **4** Serum, Toxoid and Vaccine **6** Nutritional Substance **7** Electrolytic and Water Balance Substance **B** Local Anesthetic **H** Radioactive Substance **K** Other Diagnostic Substance **N** Analgesics, Hypnotics, Sedatives **T** Destructive Agent	**Z** No Qualifier
1 Subcutaneous Tissue **2** Muscle **A** Bone Marrow **F** Respiratory Tract **L** Pleural Cavity **M** Peritoneal Cavity **Q** Cranial Cavity and Brain **R** Spinal Canal **S** Epidural Space **T** Peripheral Nerves and Plexi **W** Lymphatics **X** Cranial Nerves **Y** Pericardial Cavity	**3** Percutaneous	**G** Other Therapeutic Substance	**C** Other Substance
1 Subcutaneous Tissue **2** Muscle **A** Bone Marrow **V** Bones **W** Lymphatics	**3** Percutaneous	**Ø** Antineoplastic	**5** Other Antineoplastic **M** Monoclonal Antibody
2 Muscle **F** Respiratory Tract **L** Pleural Cavity **M** Peritoneal Cavity **Q** Cranial Cavity and Brain **R** Spinal Canal **S** Epidural Space **U** Joints **V** Bones **W** Lymphatics **Y** Pericardial Cavity	**3** Percutaneous	**2** Anti-infective	**8** Oxazolidinones **9** Other Anti-infective
3 Peripheral Vein	**Ø** Open **3** Percutaneous	**U** Pancreatic Islet Cells	**Ø** Autologous **1** Nonautologous

3EØ Continued on next page

DRG Non-OR 3EØ3[Ø,3]U[Ø,1]

AHA: 2Ø14, 2Q, 8, 1Ø; 2Ø13, 1Q, 27

3E0 Continued

3 Administration
E Physiological Systems and Anatomical Regions
0 Introduction Putting in or on a therapeutic, diagnostic, nutritional, physiological, or prophylactic substance except blood or blood products

Body System/Region Character 4	Approach Character 5	Substance Character 6	Qualifier Character 7
3 Peripheral Vein 4 Central Vein 5 Peripheral Artery 6 Central Artery	0 Open 3 Percutaneous	0 Antineoplastic	2 High-dose Interleukin-2 3 Low-dose Interleukin-2 5 Other Antineoplastic M Monoclonal Antibody P Clofarabine
3 Peripheral Vein 4 Central Vein 5 Peripheral Artery 6 Central Artery	0 Open 3 Percutaneous	2 Anti-infective	8 Oxazolidinones 9 Other Anti-infective
3 Peripheral Vein 4 Central Vein 5 Peripheral Artery 6 Central Artery	0 Open 3 Percutaneous	3 Anti-inflammatory 4 Serum, Toxoid and Vaccine 6 Nutritional Substance 7 Electrolytic and Water Balance Substance F Intracirculatory Anesthetic H Radioactive Substance K Other Diagnostic Substance N Analgesics, Hypnotics, Sedatives P Platelet Inhibitor R Antiarrhythmic T Destructive Agent X Vasopressor	Z No Qualifier
5 Peripheral Artery 6 Central Artery	0 Open 3 Percutaneous	G Other Therapeutic Substance	C Other Substance N Blood Brain Barrier Disruption
3 Peripheral Vein 4 Central Vein 5 Peripheral Artery 6 Central Artery	0 Open 3 Percutaneous	V Hormone	G Insulin H Human B-type Natriuretic Peptide J Other Hormone
3 Peripheral Vein 4 Central Vein	0 Open	G Other Therapeutic Substance	C Other Substance N Blood Brain Barrier Disruption Q Glucarpidase
3 Peripheral Vein 4 Central Vein	3 Percutaneous Substance	G Other Therapeutic Substance	C Other Substance N Blood Brain Barrier Disruption Q Glucarpidase
3 Peripheral Vein 4 Central Vein 5 Peripheral Artery 6 Central Artery	0 Open 3 Percutaneous	W Immunotherapeutic	K Immunostimulator L Immunosuppressive
3 Peripheral Vein 4 Central Vein 5 Peripheral Artery 6 Central Artery 7 Coronary Artery 8 Heart	0 Open 3 Percutaneous	1 Thrombolytic	6 Recombinant Human-activated Protein C 7 Other Thrombolytic
7 Coronary Artery 8 Heart	0 Open 3 Percutaneous	G Other Therapeutic Substance	C Other Substance
7 Coronary Artery 8 Heart	0 Open 3 Percutaneous	K Other Diagnostic Substance P Platelet Inhibitor	Z No Qualifier
9 Nose	3 Percutaneous 7 Via Natural or Artificial Opening X External	0 Antineoplastic	5 Other Antineoplastic M Monoclonal Antibody
9 Nose	3 Percutaneous 7 Via Natural or Artificial Opening X External	3 Anti-inflammatory 4 Serum, Toxoid and Vaccine B Local Anesthetic H Radioactive Substance K Other Diagnostic Substance N Analgesics, Hypnotics, Sedatives T Destructive Agent	Z No Qualifier

3E0 Continued on next page

DRG Non-OR 3E0[3,4,5,6][0,3]02
DRG Non-OR 3E0[3,4,5,6,8][0,3]17
AHA: 2014, 2Q, 8, 10; 2013, 1Q, 27

3 Administration
E Physiological Systems and Anatomical Regions
Ø Introduction Putting in or on a therapeutic, diagnostic, nutritional, physiological, or prophylactic substance except blood or blood products

3EØ Continued

Body System/Region Character 4	Approach Character 5	Substance Character 6	Qualifier Character 7
9 Nose **B** Ear **C** Eye **D** Mouth and Pharynx	**3** Percutaneous **7** Via Natural or Artificial Opening **X** External	**2** Anti-infective	**8** Oxazolidinones **9** Other Anti-infective
9 Nose **B** Ear **C** Eye **D** Mouth and Pharynx	**3** Percutaneous **7** Via Natural or Artificial Opening **X** External	**G** Other Therapeutic Substance	**C** Other Substance
B Ear	**3** Percutaneous **7** Via Natural or Artificial Opening **X** External	**3** Anti-inflammatory **B** Local Anesthetic **H** Radioactive Substance **K** Other Diagnostic Substance **N** Analgesics, Hypnotics, Sedatives **T** Destructive Agent	**Z** No Qualifier
B Ear **C** Eye **D** Mouth and Pharynx	**3** Percutaneous **7** Via Natural or Artificial Opening **X** External	**Ø** Antineoplastic	**4** Liquid Brachytherapy Radioisotope **5** Other Antineoplastic **M** Monoclonal Antibody
C Eye	**3** Percutaneous **7** Via Natural or Artificial Opening **X** External	**3** Anti-inflammatory **B** Local Anesthetic **H** Radioactive Substance **K** Other Diagnostic Substance **M** Pigment **N** Analgesics, Hypnotics, Sedatives **T** Destructive Agent	**Z** No Qualifier
C Eye	**3** Percutaneous **7** Via Natural or Artificial Opening **X** External	**S** Gas	**F** Other Gas
D Mouth and Pharynx	**3** Percutaneous **7** Via Natural or Artificial Opening **X** External	**3** Anti-inflammatory **4** Serum, Toxoid and Vaccine **6** Nutritional Substance **7** Electrolytic and Water Balance Substance **B** Local Anesthetic **H** Radioactive Substance **K** Other Diagnostic Substance **N** Analgesics, Hypnotics, Sedatives **R** Antiarrhythmic **T** Destructive Agent	**Z** No Qualifier
E Products of Conception ♀ **F** Respiratory Tract **G** Upper GI **H** Lower GI **J** Biliary and Pancreatic Tract **K** Genitourinary Tract **N** Male Reproductive ♂ **P** Female Reproductive ♀	**3** Percutaneous **7** Via Natural or Artificial Opening **8** Via Natural or Artificial Opening Endoscopic	**Ø** Antineoplastic	**4** Liquid Brachytherapy Radioisotope **5** Other Antineoplastic **M** Monoclonal Antibody
E Products of Conception ♀ **F** Respiratory Tract **G** Upper GI **H** Lower GI **J** Biliary and Pancreatic Tract **K** Genitourinary Tract **N** Male Reproductive ♂ **P** Female Reproductive ♀	**3** Percutaneous **7** Via Natural or Artificial Opening **8** Via Natural or Artificial Opening Endoscopic	**2** Anti-infective	**8** Oxazolidinones **9** Other Anti-infective
E Products of Conception ♀ **F** Respiratory Tract **G** Upper GI **H** Lower GI **J** Biliary and Pancreatic Tract **K** Genitourinary Tract **N** Male Reproductive ♂ **P** Female Reproductive ♀	**3** Percutaneous **7** Via Natural or Artificial Opening **8** Via Natural or Artificial Opening Endoscopic	**G** Other Therapeutic Substance	**C** Other Substance

3EØ Continued on next page

AHA: 2Ø14, 2Q, 8, 1Ø; 2Ø13, 1Q, 27

3 Administration
E Physiological Systems and Anatomical Regions
0 Introduction Putting in or on a therapeutic, diagnostic, nutritional, physiological, or prophylactic substance except blood or blood products

3E0 Continued

Body System/Region Character 4	Approach Character 5	Substance Character 6	Qualifier Character 7
E Products of Conception ♀ **G** Upper GI **H** Lower GI **J** Biliary and Pancreatic Tract **K** Genitourinary Tract **N** Male Reproductive ♂	**3** Percutaneous **7** Via Natural or Artificial Opening **8** Via Natural or Artificial Opening Endoscopic	**3** Anti-inflammatory **6** Nutritional Substance **7** Electrolytic and Water Balance Substance **B** Local Anesthetic **H** Radioactive Substance **K** Other Diagnostic Substance **N** Analgesics, Hypnotics, Sedatives **T** Destructive Agent	**Z** No Qualifier
E Products of Conception ♀ **G** Upper GI **H** Lower GI **J** Biliary and Pancreatic Tract **K** Genitourinary Tract **N** Male Reproductive ♂ **P** Female Reproductive ♀	**3** Percutaneous **7** Via Natural or Artificial Opening **8** Via Natural or Artificial Opening Endoscopic	**S** Gas	**F** Other Gas
F Respiratory Tract	**3** Percutaneous **7** Via Natural or Artificial Opening **8** Via Natural or Artificial Opening Endoscopic	**S** Gas	**D** Nitric Oxide **F** Other Gas
F Respiratory Tract	**7** Via Natural or Artificial Opening **8** Via Natural or Artificial Opening Endoscopic	**3** Anti-inflammatory **6** Nutritional Substance **7** Electrolytic and Water Balance Substance **B** Local Anesthetic **D** Inhalation Anesthetic **H** Radioactive Substance **K** Other Diagnostic Substance **N** Analgesics, Hypnotics, Sedatives **T** Destructive Agent	**Z** No Qualifier
F Respiratory Tract **L** Pleural Cavity **M** Peritoneal Cavity **W** Lymphatics **Y** Pericardial Cavity	**3** Percutaneous	**3** Anti-inflammatory **6** Nutritional Substance **7** Electrolytic and Water Balance Substance **B** Local Anesthetic **H** Radioactive Substance **K** Other Diagnostic Substance **N** Analgesics, Hypnotics, Sedatives **T** Destructive Agent	**Z** No Qualifier
J Biliary and Pancreatic Tract	**3** Percutaneous **7** Via Natural or Artificial Opening **8** Via Natural or Artificial Opening Endoscopic	**U** Pancreatic Islet Cells	**0** Autologous **1** Nonautologous
L Pleural Cavity **M** Peritoneal Cavity **P** Female Reproductive ♀	**0** Open	**5** Adhesion Barrier	**Z** No Qualifier
L Pleural Cavity **M** Peritoneal Cavity **Q** Cranial Cavity and Brain **R** Spinal Canal **S** Epidural Space **Y** Pericardial Cavity	**3** Percutaneous **7** Via Natural or Artificial Opening	**S** Gas	**F** Other Gas
L Pleural Cavity **M** Peritoneal Cavity **Q** Cranial Cavity and Brain **Y** Pericardial Cavity	**3** Percutaneous **7** Via Natural or Artificial Opening	**0** Antineoplastic	**4** Liquid Brachytherapy Radioisotope **5** Other Antineoplastic **M** Monoclonal Antibody

3E0 Continued on next page

DRG Non-OR 3E0J[3,7,8]U[0,1]
DRG Non-OR 3E0Q[3,7]05
AHA: 2014, 2Q, 8, 10; 2013, 1Q, 27

3 Administration
E Physiological Systems and Anatomical Regions
Ø Introduction Putting in or on a therapeutic, diagnostic, nutritional, physiological, or prophylactic substance except blood or blood products

3EØ Continued

Body System/Region Character 4	Approach Character 5	Substance Character 6	Qualifier Character 7
P Female Reproductive ♀	3 Percutaneous 7 Via Natural or Artificial Opening	3 Anti-inflammatory 6 Nutritional Substance 7 Electrolytic and Water Balance Substance B Local Anesthetic H Radioactive Substance K Other Diagnostic Substance L Sperm N Analgesics, Hypnotics, Sedatives T Destructive Agent	Z No Qualifier
P Female Reproductive ♀	3 Percutaneous 7 Via Natural or Artificial Opening	Q Fertilized Ovum	Ø Autologous 1 Nonautologous
P Female Reproductive ♀	8 Via Natural or Artificial Opening Endoscopic	3 Anti-inflammatory 6 Nutritional Substance 7 Electrolytic and Water Balance Substance B Local Anesthetic H Radioactive Substance K Other Diagnostic Substance N Analgesics, Hypnotics, Sedatives T Destructive Agent	Z No Qualifier
Q Cranial Cavity and Brain	3 Percutaneous	3 Anti-inflammatory 6 Nutritional Substance 7 Electrolytic and Water Balance Substance A Stem Cells, Embryonic B Local Anesthetic H Radioactive Substance K Other Diagnostic Substance N Analgesics, Hypnotics, Sedatives T Destructive Agent	Z No Qualifier
Q Cranial Cavity and Brain R Spinal Canal	Ø Open	A Stem Cells, Embryonic	Z No Qualifier
Q Cranial Cavity and Brain R Spinal Canal	Ø Open 3 Percutaneous	E Stem Cells, Somatic	Ø Autologous 1 Nonautologous
R Spinal Canal	3 Percutaneous	3 Anti-inflammatory 6 Nutritional Substance 7 Electrolytic and Water Balance Substance A Stem Cells, Embryonic B Local Anesthetic C Regional Anesthetic H Radioactive Substance K Other Diagnostic Substance N Analgesics, Hypnotics, Sedatives T Destructive Agent	Z No Qualifier
R Spinal Canal S Epidural Space	3 Percutaneous	Ø Antineoplastic	2 High-dose Interleukin-2 3 Low-dose Interleukin-2 4 Liquid Brachytherapy Radioisotope 5 Other Antineoplastic M Monoclonal Antibody
S Epidural Space	3 Percutaneous	3 Anti-inflammatory 6 Nutritional Substance 7 Electrolytic and Water Balance Substance B Local Anesthetic C Regional Anesthetic H Radioactive Substance K Other Diagnostic Substance N Analgesics, Hypnotics, Sedatives T Destructive Agent	Z No Qualifier
T Peripheral Nerves and Plexi X Cranial Nerves	3 Percutaneous	3 Anti-inflammatory B Local Anesthetic C Regional Anesthetic T Destructive Agent	Z No Qualifier

3EØ Continued on next page

DRG Non-OR 3EØ[R,S]3Ø2
AHA: 2Ø14, 2Q, 8, 1Ø; 2Ø13, 1Q, 27

3EØ Continued

3 Administration
E Physiological Systems and Anatomical Regions
Ø Introduction Putting in or on a therapeutic, diagnostic, nutritional, physiological, or prophylactic substance except blood or blood products

Body System/Region Character 4	Approach Character 5	Substance Character 6	Qualifier Character 7
U Joints V Bones	Ø Open	G Other Therapeutic Substance	B Recombinant Bone Morphogenetic Protein
U Joints	Ø Open	2 Anti-infective	8 Oxazolidinones 9 Other Anti-infective
U Joints	3 Percutaneous	Ø Antineoplastic	4 Liquid Brachytherapy Radioisotope 5 Other Antineoplastic M Monoclonal Antibody
U Joints	3 Percutaneous	2 Anti-infective	8 Oxazolidinones 9 Other Anti-infective
U Joints	3 Percutaneous	S Gas	F Other Gas
U Joints V Bones	3 Percutaneous	3 Anti-inflammatory 6 Nutritional Substance 7 Electrolytic and Water Balance Substance B Local Anesthetic H Radioactive Substance K Other Diagnostic Substance N Analgesics, Hypnotics, Sedatives T Destructive Agent	Z No Qualifier
V Bones	3 Percutaneous	Ø Antineoplastic	5 Other Antineoplastic M Monoclonal Antibody
V Bones	3 Percutaneous	2 Anti-infective	8 Oxazolidinones 9 Other Anti-infective
U Joints V Bones	3 Percutaneous	G Other Therapeutic Substance	B Recombinant Bone Morphogenetic Protein C Other Substance

AHA: 2Ø14, 2Q, 8, 1Ø; 2Ø13, 1Q, 27

3 Administration
E Physiological Systems and Anatomical Regions
1 Irrigation Putting in or on a cleansing substance

Body System/Region Character 4	Approach Character 5	Substance Character 6	Qualifier Character 7
Ø Skin and Mucous Membranes C Eye	3 Percutaneous X External	8 Irrigating Substance	X Diagnostic Z No Qualifier
9 Nose B Ear F Respiratory Tract G Upper GI H Lower GI J Biliary and Pancreatic Tract K Genitourinary Tract N Male Reproductive ♂ P Female Reproductive ♀	3 Percutaneous 7 Via Natural or Artificial Opening 8 Via Natural or Artificial Opening Endoscopic	8 Irrigating Substance	X Diagnostic Z No Qualifier
L Pleural Cavity M Peritoneal Cavity Q Cranial Cavity and Brain R Spinal Canal S Epidural Space U Joints Y Pericardial Cavity	3 Percutaneous	8 Irrigating Substance	X Diagnostic Z No Qualifier
M Peritoneal Cavity	3 Percutaneous	9 Dialysate	Z No Qualifier

Measurement and Monitoring 4AØ–4BØ

4 Measurement and Monitoring
A Physiological Systems
Ø Measurement Determining the level of a physiological or physical function at a point in time

Body System Character 4	Approach Character 5	Function/Device Character 6	Qualifier Character 7
Ø Central Nervous	**Ø** Open	**2** Conductivity **4** Electrical Activity **B** Pressure	**Z** No Qualifier
Ø Central Nervous	**3** Percutaneous	**4** Electrical Activity	**Z** No Qualifier
Ø Central Nervous	**3** Percutaneous **7** Via Natural or Artificial Opening	**B** Pressure **K** Temperature **R** Saturation	**D** Intracranial
Ø Central Nervous	**X** External	**2** Conductivity **4** Electrical Activity	**Z** No Qualifier
1 Peripheral Nervous	**Ø** Open **3** Percutaneous **X** External	**2** Conductivity	**9** Sensory **B** Motor
1 Peripheral Nervous	**Ø** Open **3** Percutaneous **X** External	**4** Electrical Activity	**Z** No Qualifier
2 Cardiac	**Ø** Open **3** Percutaneous	**N** Sampling and Pressure	**6** Right Heart **7** Left Heart **8** Bilateral
2 Cardiac	**Ø** Open **3** Percutaneous	**4** Electrical Activity **9** Output **C** Rate **F** Rhythm **H** Sound **P** Action Currents	**Z** No Qualifier
2 Cardiac	**X** External	**9** Output **C** Rate **F** Rhythm **H** Sound **P** Action Currents	**Z** No Qualifier
2 Cardiac	**X** External	**M** Total Activity	**4** Stress
2 Cardiac ⊞	**X** External	**4** Electrical Activity	**A** Guidance **Z** No Qualifier
3 Arterial	**Ø** Open **3** Percutaneous	**5** Flow **J** Pulse	**1** Peripheral **3** Pulmonary **C** Coronary
3 Arterial	**Ø** Open **3** Percutaneous	**B** Pressure	**1** Peripheral **3** Pulmonary **C** Coronary **F** Other Thoracic
3 Arterial	**Ø** Open **3** Percutaneous	**H** Sound **R** Saturation	**1** Peripheral
3 Arterial	**X** External	**5** Flow **B** Pressure **H** Sound **J** Pulse **R** Saturation	**1** Peripheral
4 Venous	**Ø** Open **3** Percutaneous	**5** Flow **B** Pressure **J** Pulse	**Ø** Central **1** Peripheral **2** Portal **3** Pulmonary
4 Venous	**Ø** Open **3** Percutaneous	**R** Saturation	**1** Peripheral
4 Venous	**X** External	**5** Flow **B** Pressure **J** Pulse **R** Saturation	**1** Peripheral
5 Circulatory	**X** External	**L** Volume	**Z** No Qualifier

4AØ Continued on next page

DRG Non-OR	4AØ2[Ø,3]N[6,7,8]	**No Procedure Combinations Specified**	
DRG Non-OR	4AØ23FZ	**Combo-only**	4AØ2X4A
DRG Non-OR	4AØ2X4A	⊞	4AØ2X4A

4A0 Continued

4 Measurement and Monitoring
A Physiological Systems
0 Measurement Determining the level of a physiological or physical function at a point in time

Body System Character 4	Approach Character 5	Function/Device Character 6	Qualifier Character 7
6 Lymphatic	**0** Open **3** Percutaneous	**5** Flow **B** Pressure	**Z** No Qualifier
7 Visual	**X** External	**0** Acuity **7** Mobility **B** Pressure	**Z** No Qualifier
8 Olfactory	**X** External	**0** Acuity	**Z** No Qualifier
9 Respiratory	**7** Via Natural or Artificial Opening **8** Via Natural or Artificial Opening Endoscopic **X** External	**1** Capacity **5** Flow **C** Rate **D** Resistance **L** Volume **M** Total Activity	**Z** No Qualifier
B Gastrointestinal	**7** Via Natural or Artificial Opening **8** Via Natural or Artificial Opening Endoscopic	**8** Motility **B** Pressure **G** Secretion	**Z** No Qualifier
C Biliary	**3** Percutaneous **4** Percutaneous Endoscopic **7** Via Natural or Artificial Opening **8** Via Natural or Artificial Opening Endoscopic	**5** Flow **B** Pressure	**Z** No Qualifier
D Urinary	**7** Via Natural or Artificial Opening	**3** Contractility **5** Flow **B** Pressure **D** Resistance **L** Volume	**Z** No Qualifier
F Musculoskeletal	**3** Percutaneous **X** External	**3** Contractility	**Z** No Qualifier
H Products of Conception, Cardiac ♀	**7** Via Natural or Artificial Opening **8** Via Natural or Artificial Opening Endoscopic **X** External	**4** Electrical Activity **C** Rate **F** Rhythm **H** Sound	**Z** No Qualifier
J Products of Conception, Nervous ♀	**7** Via Natural or Artificial Opening **8** Via Natural or Artificial Opening Endoscopic **X** External	**2** Conductivity **4** Electrical Activity **B** Pressure	**Z** No Qualifier
Z None	**7** Via Natural or Artificial Opening	**6** Metabolism **K** Temperature	**Z** No Qualifier
Z None	**X** External	**6** Metabolism **K** Temperature **Q** Sleep	**Z** No Qualifier

4 Measurement and Monitoring
A Physiological Systems
1 Monitoring Determining the level of a physiological or physical function repetitively over a period of time

Body System Character 4	Approach Character 5	Function/Device Character 6	Qualifier Character 7
0 Central Nervous	**0** Open	**2** Conductivity **B** Pressure	**Z** No Qualifier
0 Central Nervous	**0** Open **X** External	**4** Electrical Activity	**G** Intraoperative **Z** No Qualifier
0 Central Nervous	**3** Percutaneous **7** Via Natural or Artificial Opening	**B** Pressure **K** Temperature **R** Saturation	**D** Intracranial
0 Central Nervous	**3** Percutaneous	**4** Electrical Activity	**G** Intraoperative **Z** No Qualifier
0 Central Nervous	**X** External	**2** Conductivity	**Z** No Qualifier
1 Peripheral Nervous	**0** Open **3** Percutaneous **X** External	**2** Conductivity	**9** Sensory **B** Motor
1 Peripheral Nervous	**0** Open **3** Percutaneous **X** External	**4** Electrical Activity	**G** Intraoperative **Z** No Qualifier

4A1 Continued on next page

4A1 Continued

4 Measurement and Monitoring
A Physiological Systems
1 Monitoring Determining the level of a physiological or physical function repetitively over a period of time

Body System Character 4	Approach Character 5	Function/Device Character 6	Qualifier Character 7
2 Cardiac	0 Open 3 Percutaneous	4 Electrical Activity 9 Output C Rate F Rhythm H Sound	Z No Qualifier
2 Cardiac	X External	4 Electrical Activity	5 Ambulatory Z No Qualifier
2 Cardiac	X External	9 Output C Rate F Rhythm H Sound	Z No Qualifier
2 Cardiac	X External	M Total Activity	4 Stress
3 Arterial	0 Open 3 Percutaneous	5 Flow B Pressure J Pulse	1 Peripheral 3 Pulmonary C Coronary
3 Arterial	0 Open 3 Percutaneous	H Sound R Saturation	1 Peripheral
3 Arterial	X External	5 Flow B Pressure H Sound J Pulse R Saturation	1 Peripheral
4 Venous	0 Open 3 Percutaneous	5 Flow B Pressure J Pulse	0 Central 1 Peripheral 2 Portal 3 Pulmonary
4 Venous	0 Open 3 Percutaneous	R Saturation	0 Central 2 Portal 3 Pulmonary
4 Venous	X External	5 Flow B Pressure J Pulse	1 Peripheral
6 Lymphatic	0 Open 3 Percutaneous	5 Flow B Pressure	Z No Qualifier
9 Respiratory	7 Via Natural or Artificial Opening X External	1 Capacity 5 Flow C Rate D Resistance L Volume	Z No Qualifier
B Gastrointestinal	7 Via Natural or Artificial Opening 8 Via Natural or Artificial Opening Endoscopic	8 Motility B Pressure G Secretion	Z No Qualifier
D Urinary	7 Via Natural or Artificial Opening	3 Contractility 5 Flow B Pressure D Resistance L Volume	Z No Qualifier
H Products of Conception, Cardiac ♀	7 Via Natural or Artificial Opening 8 Via Natural or Artificial Opening Endoscopic X External	4 Electrical Activity C Rate F Rhythm H Sound	Z No Qualifier
J Products of Conception, Nervous ♀	7 Via Natural or Artificial Opening 8 Via Natural or Artificial Opening Endoscopic X External	2 Conductivity 4 Electrical Activity B Pressure	Z No Qualifier
Z None	7 Via Natural or Artificial Opening	K Temperature	Z No Qualifier
Z None	X External	K Temperature Q Sleep	Z No Qualifier

4 Measurement and Monitoring
B Physiological Devices
0 Measurement Determining the level of a physiological or physical function at a point in time

Body System Character 4	Approach Character 5	Function/Device Character 6	Qualifier Character 7
0 Central Nervous **1** Peripheral Nervous **F** Musculoskeletal	**X** External	**V** Stimulator	**Z** No Qualifier
2 Cardiac	**X** External	**S** Pacemaker **T** Defibrillator	**Z** No Qualifier
9 Respiratory	**X** External	**S** Pacemaker	**Z** No Qualifier

Extracorporeal Assistance and Performance 5AØ–5A2

5 Extracorporeal Assistance and Performance
A Physiological Systems
Ø Assistance Taking over a portion of a physiological function by extracorporeal means

Body System Character 4	Duration Character 5	Function Character 6	Qualifier Character 7
2 Cardiac	1 Intermittent 2 Continuous	1 Output	Ø Balloon Pump 5 Pulsatile Compression 6 Other Pump D Impeller Pump
5 Circulatory	1 Intermittent 2 Continuous	2 Oxygenation	1 Hyperbaric C Supersaturated
9 Respiratory	3 Less than 24 Consecutive Hours 4 24-96 Consecutive Hours 5 Greater than 96 Consecutive Hours	5 Ventilation	7 Continuous Positive Airway Pressure 8 Intermittent Positive Airway Pressure 9 Continuous Negative Airway Pressure B Intermittent Negative Airway Pressure Z No Qualifier

AHA: 2Ø13, 3Q, 18

5 Extracorporeal Assistance and Performance
A Physiological Systems
1 Performance Completely taking over a physiological function by extracorporeal means

Body System Character 4	Duration Character 5	Function Character 6	Qualifier Character 7
2 Cardiac	Ø Single	1 Output	2 Manual
2 Cardiac	1 Intermittent	3 Pacing	Z No Qualifier
2 Cardiac	2 Continuous	1 Output 3 Pacing	Z No Qualifier
5 Circulatory	2 Continuous	2 Oxygenation	3 Membrane
9 Respiratory	Ø Single	5 Ventilation	4 Nonmechanical
9 Respiratory	3 Less than 24 Consecutive Hours 4 24-96 Consecutive Hours 5 Greater than 96 Consecutive Hours	5 Ventilation	Z No Qualifier
C Biliary D Urinary	Ø Single 6 Multiple	Ø Filtration	Z No Qualifier

DRG Non-OR 5A19[3,4,5]5Z
Note: For code 5A1955Z, length of stay must be >= 4 days.
AHA: 2Ø14, 1Q, 1Ø; 2Ø13, 3Q, 18

5 Extracorporeal Assistance and Performance
A Physiological Systems
2 Restoration Returning, or attempting to return, a physiological function to its original state by extracorporeal means.

Body System Character 4	Duration Character 5	Function Character 6	Qualifier Character 7
2 Cardiac	Ø Single	4 Rhythm	Z No Qualifier

Extracorporeal Therapies 6A0–6A9

6 Extracorporeal Therapies
A Physiological Systems
0 Atmospheric Control Extracorporeal control of atmospheric pressure and composition

Body System Character 4	Duration Character 5	Qualifier Character 6	Qualifier Character 7
Z None	0 Single 1 Multiple	Z No Qualifier	Z No Qualifier

6 Extracorporeal Therapies
A Physiological Systems
1 Decompression Extracorporeal elimination of undissolved gas from body fluids

Body System Character 4	Duration Character 5	Qualifier Character 6	Qualifier Character 7
5 Circulatory	0 Single 1 Multiple	Z No Qualifier	Z No Qualifier

6 Extracorporeal Therapies
A Physiological Systems
2 Electromagnetic Therapy Extracorporeal treatment by electromagnetic rays

Body System Character 4	Duration Character 5	Qualifier Character 6	Qualifier Character 7
1 Urinary 2 Central Nervous	0 Single 1 Multiple	Z No Qualifier	Z No Qualifier

6 Extracorporeal Therapies
A Physiological Systems
3 Hyperthermia Extracorporeal raising of body temperature

Body System Character 4	Duration Character 5	Qualifier Character 6	Qualifier Character 7
Z None	0 Single 1 Multiple	Z No Qualifier	Z No Qualifier

6 Extracorporeal Therapies
A Physiological Systems
4 Hypothermia Extracorporeal lowering of body temperature

Body System Character 4	Duration Character 5	Qualifier Character 6	Qualifier Character 7
Z None	0 Single 1 Multiple	Z No Qualifier	Z No Qualifier

6 Extracorporeal Therapies
A Physiological Systems
5 Pheresis Extracorporeal separation of blood products

Body System Character 4	Duration Character 5	Qualifier Character 6	Qualifier Character 7
5 Circulatory	0 Single 1 Multiple	Z No Qualifier	0 Erythrocytes 1 Leukocytes 2 Platelets 3 Plasma T Stem Cells, Cord Blood V Stem Cells, Hematopoietic

6 Extracorporeal Therapies
A Physiological Systems
6 Phototherapy Extracorporeal treatment by light rays

Body System Character 4	Duration Character 5	Qualifier Character 6	Qualifier Character 7
0 Skin 5 Circulatory	0 Single 1 Multiple	Z No Qualifier	Z No Qualifier

6 Extracorporeal Therapies
A Physiological Systems
7 Ultrasound Therapy Extracorporeal treatment by ultrasound

Body System Character 4	Duration Character 5	Qualifier Character 6	Qualifier Character 7
5 Circulatory	Ø Single 1 Multiple	Z No Qualifier	4 Head and Neck Vessels 5 Heart 6 Peripheral Vessels 7 Other Vessels Z No Qualifier

6 Extracorporeal Therapies
A Physiological Systems
8 Ultraviolet Light Therapy Extracorporeal treatment by ultraviolet light

Body System Character 4	Duration Character 5	Qualifier Character 6	Qualifier Character 7
Ø Skin	Ø Single 1 Multiple	Z No Qualifier	Z No Qualifier

6 Extracorporeal Therapies
A Physiological Systems
9 Shock Wave Therapy Extracorporeal treatment by shock waves

Body System Character 4	Duration Character 5	Qualifier Character 6	Qualifier Character 7
3 Musculoskeletal	Ø Single 1 Multiple	Z No Qualifier	Z No Qualifier

Osteopathic 7WØ

7 Osteopathic
W Anatomical Regions
Ø Treatment Manual treatment to eliminate or alleviate somatic dysfunction and related disorders

Body Region Character 4	Approach Character 5	Method Character 6	Qualifier Character 7
Ø Head	**X** External	**Ø** Articulatory-Raising	**Z** None
1 Cervical		**1** Fascial Release	
2 Thoracic		**2** General Mobilization	
3 Lumbar		**3** High Velocity-Low Amplitude	
4 Sacrum		**4** Indirect	
5 Pelvis		**5** Low Velocity-High Amplitude	
6 Lower Extremities		**6** Lymphatic Pump	
7 Upper Extremities		**7** Muscle Energy-Isometric	
8 Rib Cage		**8** Muscle Energy-Isotonic	
9 Abdomen		**9** Other Method	

Other Procedures 8CØ–8EØ

8 Other Procedures
C Indwelling Device
Ø Other Procedures Methodologies which attempt to remediate or cure a disorder or disease

Body Region Character 4	Approach Character 5	Method Character 6	Qualifier Character 7
1 Nervous System	**X** External	**6** Collection	**J** Cerebrospinal Fluid **L** Other Fluid
2 Circulatory System	**X** External	**6** Collection	**K** Blood **L** Other Fluid

8 Other Procedures
E Physiological Systems and Anatomical Regions
Ø Other Procedures Methodologies which attempt to remediate or cure a disorder or disease

Body Region Character 4	Approach Character 5	Method Character 6	Qualifier Character 7
1 Nervous System **K** Musculoskeletal System **U** Female Reproductive System ♀	**X** External	**Y** Other Method	**7** Examination
2 Circulatory System	**3** Percutaneous	**D** Near Infrared Spectroscopy	**Z** No Qualifier
9 Head and Neck Region **W** Trunk Region	**Ø** Open **3** Percutaneous **4** Percutaneous Endoscopic **7** Via Natural or Artificial Opening **8** Via Natural or Artificial Opening Endoscopic **X** External	**C** Robotic Assisted Procedure	**Z** No Qualifier
9 Head and Neck Region **W** Trunk Region **X** Upper Extremity **Y** Lower Extremity	**X** External	**B** Computer Assisted Procedure	**F** With Fluoroscopy **G** With Computerized Tomography **H** With Magnetic Resonance Imaging **Z** No Qualifier
9 Head and Neck Region **W** Trunk Region **X** Upper Extremity **Y** Lower Extremity	**X** External	**Y** Other Method	**8** Suture Removal
H Integumentary System and Breast	**3** Percutaneous	**Ø** Acupuncture	**Ø** Anesthesia **Z** No Qualifier
H Integumentary System and Breast ♀	**X** External	**6** Collection	**2** Breast Milk
H Integumentary System and Breast	**X** External	**Y** Other Method	**9** Piercing
K Musculoskeletal System	**X** External	**1** Therapeutic Massage	**Z** No Qualifier
V Male Reproductive System ♂	**X** External	**1** Therapeutic Massage	**C** Prostate **D** Rectum
V Male Reproductive System ♂	**X** External	**6** Collection	**3** Sperm
X Upper Extremity **Y** Lower Extremity	**Ø** Open **3** Percutaneous **4** Percutaneous Endoscopic **X** External	**C** Robotic Assisted Procedure	**Z** No Qualifier
Z None	**X** External	**Y** Other Method	**1** In Vitro Fertilization **4** Yoga Therapy **5** Meditation **6** Isolation

Chiropractic 9WB

9 Chiropractic
W Anatomical Regions
B Manipulation Manual procedure that involves a directed thrust to move a joint past the physiological range of motion, without exceeding the anatomical limit

Body Region Character 4	Approach Character 5	Method Character 6	Qualifier Character 7
0 Head **1** Cervical **2** Thoracic **3** Lumbar **4** Sacrum **5** Pelvis **6** Lower Extremities **7** Upper Extremities **8** Rib Cage **9** Abdomen	**X** External	**B** Non-Manual **C** Indirect Visceral **D** Extra-Articular **F** Direct Visceral **G** Long Lever Specific Contact **H** Short Lever Specific Contact **J** Long and Short Lever Specific Contact **K** Mechanically Assisted **L** Other Method	**Z** None

Imaging BØØ–BY4

B Imaging
Ø Central Nervous System
Ø Plain Radiography Planar display of an image developed from the capture of external ionizing radiation on photographic or photoconductive plate

Body Part Character 4	Contrast Character 5	Qualifier Character 6	Qualifier Character 7
B Spinal Cord	Ø High Osmolar 1 Low Osmolar Y Other Contrast Z None	Z None	Z None

B Imaging
Ø Central Nervous System
1 Fluoroscopy Single plane or bi-plane real time display of an image developed from the capture of external ionizing radioation on a fluorescent screen. The image may also be stored by either digital or analog means

Body Part Character 4	Contrast Character 5	Qualifier Character 6	Qualifier Character 7
B Spinal Cord	Ø High Osmolar 1 Low Osmolar Y Other Contrast Z None	Z None	Z None

B Imaging
Ø Central Nervous System
2 Computerized Tomography (CT Scan) Computer reformatted digital display of multiplanar images developed from the capture of multiple exposures of external ionizing radiation

Body Part Character 4	Contrast Character 5	Qualifier Character 6	Qualifier Character 7
Ø Brain 7 Cisterna 8 Cerebral Ventricle(s) 9 Sella Turcica/Pituitary Gland B Spinal Cord	Ø High Osmolar 1 Low Osmolar Y Other Contrast	Ø Unenhanced and Enhanced Z None	Z None
Ø Brain 7 Cisterna 8 Cerebral Ventricle(s) 9 Sella Turcica/Pituitary Gland B Spinal Cord	Z None	Z None	Z None

B Imaging
Ø Central Nervous System
3 Magnetic Resonance Imaging (MRI) Computer reformatted digital display of multiplanar images developed from the capture of radio-frequency signals emitted by nuclei in a body site excited within a magnetic field

Body Part Character 4	Contrast Character 5	Qualifier Character 6	Qualifier Character 7
Ø Brain 9 Sella Turcica/Pituitary Gland B Spinal Cord C Acoustic Nerves	Y Other Contrast	Ø Unenhanced and Enhanced Z None	Z None
Ø Brain 9 Sella Turcica/Pituitary Gland B Spinal Cord C Acoustic Nerves	Z None	Z None	Z None

B Imaging
Ø Central Nervous System
4 Ultrasonography Real time display of images of anatomy or flow information developed from the capture of relected and attenuated high frequency sound waves

Body Part Character 4	Contrast Character 5	Qualifier Character 6	Qualifier Character 7
Ø Brain B Spinal Cord	Z None	Z None	Z None

B Imaging
2 Heart
0 Plain Radiography Planar display of an image developed from the capture of external ionizing radiation on photographic or photoconductive plate

Body Part Character 4	Contrast Character 5	Qualifier Character 6	Qualifier Character 7
0 Coronary Artery, Single 1 Coronary Arteries, Multiple 2 Coronary Artery Bypass Graft, Single 3 Coronary Artery Bypass Grafts, Multiple 4 Heart, Right 5 Heart, Left 6 Heart, Right and Left 7 Internal Mammary Bypass Graft, Right 8 Internal Mammary Bypass Graft, Left F Bypass Graft, Other	0 High Osmolar 1 Low Osmolar Y Other Contrast	Z None	Z None

DRG Non-OR For all body part, approach, device, and qualifier values

B Imaging
2 Heart
1 Fluoroscopy Single plane or bi-plane real time display of an image developed from the capture of external ionizing radioation on a fluorescent screen. The image may also be stored by either digital or analog means

Body Part Character 4	Contrast Character 5	Qualifier Character 6	Qualifier Character 7
0 Coronary Artery, Single 1 Coronary Arteries, Multiple 2 Coronary Artery Bypass Graft, Single 3 Coronary Artery Bypass Grafts, Multiple	0 High Osmolar 1 Low Osmolar Y Other Contrast	1 Laser	0 Intraoperative
0 Coronary Artery, Single 1 Coronary Arteries, Multiple 2 Coronary Artery Bypass Graft, Single 3 Coronary Artery Bypass Grafts, Multiple 4 Heart, Right 5 Heart, Left 6 Heart, Right and Left 7 Internal Mammary Bypass Graft, Right 8 Internal Mammary Bypass Graft, Left F Bypass Graft, Other	0 High Osmolar 1 Low Osmolar Y Other Contrast	Z None	Z None

DRG Non-OR All body part values, all contrast values, with qualifier values of NONE

B Imaging
2 Heart
2 Computerized Tomography (CT Scan) Computer reformatted digital display of multiplanar images developed from the capture of multiple exposures of external ionizing radiation

Body Part Character 4	Contrast Character 5	Qualifier Character 6	Qualifier Character 7
1 Coronary Arteries, Multiple 3 Coronary Artery Bypass Grafts, Multiple 6 Heart, Right and Left	0 High Osmolar 1 Low Osmolar Y Other Contrast	0 Unenhanced and Enhanced Z None	Z None
1 Coronary Arteries, Multiple 3 Coronary Artery Bypass Grafts, Multiple 6 Heart, Right and Left	Z None	2 Intravascular Optical Coherence Z None	Z None

B Imaging
2 Heart
3 Magnetic Resonance Imaging (MRI) Computer reformatted digital display of multiplanar images developed from the capture of radio-frequency signals emitted by nuclei in a body site excited within a magnetic field

Body Part Character 4	Contrast Character 5	Qualifier Character 6	Qualifier Character 7
1 Coronary Arteries, Multiple 3 Coronary Artery Bypass Grafts, Multiple 6 Heart, Right and Left	Y Other Contrast	Ø Unenhanced and Enhanced Z None	Z None
1 Coronary Arteries, Multiple 3 Coronary Artery Bypass Grafts, Multiple 6 Heart, Right and Left	Z None	Z None	Z None

B Imaging
2 Heart
4 Ultrasonography Real time display of images of anatomy or flow information developed from the capture of relected and attenuated high frequency sound waves

Body Part Character 4	Contrast Character 5	Qualifier Character 6	Qualifier Character 7
Ø Coronary Artery, Single 1 Coronary Arteries, Multiple 4 Heart, Right 5 Heart, Left 6 Heart, Right and Left B Heart with Aorta C Pericardium D Pediatric Heart	Y Other Contrast	Z None	Z None
Ø Coronary Artery, Single 1 Coronary Arteries, Multiple 4 Heart, Right 5 Heart, Left 6 Heart, Right and Left B Heart with Aorta C Pericardium D Pediatric Heart	Z None	Z None	3 Intravascular 4 Transesophageal Z None

B Imaging
3 Upper Arteries
Ø Plain Radiography Planar display of an image developed from the capture of external ionizing radiation on photographic or photoconductive plate

Body Part Character 4	Contrast Character 5	Qualifier Character 6	Qualifier Character 7
Ø Thoracic Aorta 1 Brachiocephalic-Subclavian Artery, Right 2 Subclavian Artery, Left 3 Common Carotid Artery, Right 4 Common Carotid Artery, Left 5 Common Carotid Arteries, Bilateral 6 Internal Carotid Artery, Right 7 Internal Carotid Artery, Left 8 Internal Carotid Arteries, Bilateral 9 External Carotid Artery, Right B External Carotid Artery, Left C External Carotid Arteries, Bilateral D Vertebral Artery, Right F Vertebral Artery, Left G Vertebral Arteries, Bilateral H Upper Extremity Arteries, Right J Upper Extremity Arteries, Left K Upper Extremity Arteries, Bilateral L Intercostal and Bronchial Arteries M Spinal Arteries N Upper Arteries, Other P Thoraco-Abdominal Aorta Q Cervico-Cerebral Arch R Intracranial Arteries S Pulmonary Artery, Right T Pulmonary Artery, Left	Ø High Osmolar 1 Low Osmolar Y Other Contrast Z None	Z None	Z None

B Imaging
3 Upper Arteries
1 Fluoroscopy Fluoroscopy: Single plane or bi-plane real time display of an image developed from the capture of external ionizing radiation on a fluorescent screen. The image may also be stored by either digital or analog means

Body Part Character 4	Contrast Character 5	Qualifier Character 6	Qualifier Character 7
0 Thoracic Aorta 1 Brachiocephalic-Subclavian Artery, Right 2 Subclavian Artery, Left 3 Common Carotid Artery, Right 4 Common Carotid Artery, Left 5 Common Carotid Arteries, Bilateral 6 Internal Carotid Artery, Right 7 Internal Carotid Artery, Left 8 Internal Carotid Arteries, Bilateral 9 External Carotid Artery, Right B External Carotid Artery, Left C External Carotid Arteries, Bilateral D Vertebral Artery, Right F Vertebral Artery, Left G Vertebral Arteries, Bilateral H Upper Extremity Arteries, Right J Upper Extremity Arteries, Left K Upper Extremity Arteries, Bilateral L Intercostal and Bronchial Arteries M Spinal Arteries N Upper Arteries, Other P Thoraco-Abdominal Aorta Q Cervico-Cerebral Arch R Intracranial Arteries S Pulmonary Artery, Right T Pulmonary Artery, Left	0 High Osmolar 1 Low Osmolar Y Other Contrast	1 Laser	0 Intraoperative
0 Thoracic Aorta 1 Brachiocephalic-Subclavian Artery, Right 2 Subclavian Artery, Left 3 Common Carotid Artery, Right 4 Common Carotid Artery, Left 5 Common Carotid Arteries, Bilateral 6 Internal Carotid Artery, Right 7 Internal Carotid Artery, Left 8 Internal Carotid Arteries, Bilateral 9 External Carotid Artery, Right B External Carotid Artery, Left C External Carotid Arteries, Bilateral D Vertebral Artery, Right F Vertebral Artery, Left G Vertebral Arteries, Bilateral H Upper Extremity Arteries, Right J Upper Extremity Arteries, Left K Upper Extremity Arteries, Bilateral L Intercostal and Bronchial Arteries M Spinal Arteries N Upper Arteries, Other P Thoraco-Abdominal Aorta Q Cervico-Cerebral Arch R Intracranial Arteries S Pulmonary Artery, Right T Pulmonary Artery, Left	0 High Osmolar 1 Low Osmolar Y Other Contrast	Z None	Z None

B31 Continued on next page

B Imaging
3 Upper Arteries
1 Fluoroscopy Fluoroscopy: Single plane or bi-plane real time display of an image developed from the capture of external ionizing radiation on a fluorescent screen. The image may also be stored by either digital or analog means

B31 Continued

Body Part Character 4	Contrast Character 5	Qualifier Character 6	Qualifier Character 7
Ø Thoracic Aorta **1** Brachiocephalic-Subclavian Artery, Right **2** Subclavian Artery, Left **3** Common Carotid Artery, Right **4** Common Carotid Artery, Left **5** Common Carotid Arteries, Bilateral **6** Internal Carotid Artery, Right **7** Internal Carotid Artery, Left **8** Internal Carotid Arteries, Bilateral **9** External Carotid Artery, Right **B** External Carotid Artery, Left **C** External Carotid Arteries, Bilateral **D** Vertebral Artery, Right **F** Vertebral Artery, Left **G** Vertebral Arteries, Bilateral **H** Upper Extremity Arteries, Right **J** Upper Extremity Arteries, Left **K** Upper Extremity Arteries, Bilateral **L** Intercostal and Bronchial Arteries **M** Spinal Arteries **N** Upper Arteries, Other **P** Thoraco-Abdominal Aorta **Q** Cervico-Cerebral Arch **R** Intracranial Arteries **S** Pulmonary Artery, Right **T** Pulmonary Artery, Left	**Z** None	**Z** None	**Z** None

B Imaging
3 Upper Arteries
2 Computerized Tomography (CT Scan) Computer reformatted digital display of multiplanar images developed from the capture of multiple exposures of external ionizing radiation

Body Part Character 4	Contrast Character 5	Qualifier Character 6	Qualifier Character 7
Ø Thoracic Aorta **5** Common Carotid Arteries, Bilateral **8** Internal Carotid Arteries, Bilateral **G** Vertebral Arteries, Bilateral **R** Intracranial Arteries **S** Pulmonary Artery, Right **T** Pulmonary Artery, Left	**Ø** High Osmolar **1** Low Osmolar **Y** Other Contrast	**Z** None	**Z** None
Ø Thoracic Aorta **5** Common Carotid Arteries, Bilateral **8** Internal Carotid Arteries, Bilateral **G** Vertebral Arteries, Bilateral **R** Intracranial Arteries **S** Pulmonary Artery, Right **T** Pulmonary Artery, Left	**Z** None	**2** Intravascular Optical Coherence **Z** None	**Z** None

B Imaging
3 Upper Arteries
3 Magnetic Resonance Imaging (MRI) Computer reformatted digital display of multiplanar images developed from the capture of radio-frequency signals emitted by nuclei in a body site excited within a magnetic field

Body Part Character 4	Contrast Character 5	Qualifier Character 6	Qualifier Character 7
0 Thoracic Aorta **5** Common Carotid Arteries, Bilateral **8** Internal Carotid Arteries, Bilateral **G** Vertebral Arteries, Bilateral **H** Upper Extremity Arteries, Right **J** Upper Extremity Arteries, Left **K** Upper Extremity Arteries, Bilateral **M** Spinal Arteries **Q** Cervico-Cerebral Arch **R** Intracranial Arteries	**Y** Other Contrast	**0** Unenhanced and Enhanced **Z** None	**Z** None
0 Thoracic Aorta **5** Common Carotid Arteries, Bilateral **8** Internal Carotid Arteries, Bilateral **G** Vertebral Arteries, Bilateral **H** Upper Extremity Arteries, Right **J** Upper Extremity Arteries, Left **K** Upper Extremity Arteries, Bilateral **M** Spinal Arteries **Q** Cervico-Cerebral Arch **R** Intracranial Arteries	**Z** None	**Z** None	**Z** None

B Imaging
3 Upper Arteries
4 Ultrasonography Real time display of images of anatomy or flow information developed from the capture of relected and attenuated high frequency sound waves

Body Part Character 4	Contrast Character 5	Qualifier Character 6	Qualifier Character 7
0 Thoracic Aorta **1** Brachiocephalic-Subclavian Artery, Right **2** Subclavian Artery, Left **3** Common Carotid Artery, Right **4** Common Carotid Artery, Left **5** Common Carotid Arteries, Bilateral **6** Internal Carotid Artery, Right **7** Internal Carotid Artery, Left **8** Internal Carotid Arteries, Bilateral **H** Upper Extremity Arteries, Right **J** Upper Extremity Arteries, Left **K** Upper Extremity Arteries, Bilateral **R** Intracranial Arteries **S** Pulmonary Artery, Right **T** Pulmonary Artery, Left **V** Ophthalmic Arteries	**Z** None	**Z** None	**3** Intravascular **Z** None

B Imaging
4 Lower Arteries
0 Plain Radiography Planar display of an image developed from the capture of external ionizing radiation on photographic or photoconductive plate

Body Part Character 4	Contrast Character 5	Qualifier Character 6	Qualifier Character 7
0 Abdominal Aorta **2** Hepatic Artery **3** Splenic Arteries **4** Superior Mesenteric Artery **5** Inferior Mesenteric Artery **6** Renal Artery, Right **7** Renal Artery, Left **8** Renal Arteries, Bilateral **9** Lumbar Arteries **B** Intra-Abdominal Arteries, Other **C** Pelvic Arteries **D** Aorta and Bilateral Lower Extremity Arteries **F** Lower Extremity Arteries, Right **G** Lower Extremity Arteries, Left **J** Lower Arteries, Other **M** Renal Artery Transplant	**0** High Osmolar **1** Low Osmolar **Y** Other Contrast	**Z** None	**Z** None

B Imaging
4 Lower Arteries
1 Fluoroscopy Single plane or bi-plane real time display of an image developed from the capture of external ionizing radiation on a fluorescent screen. The image may also be stored by either digital or analog means

Body Part Character 4	Contrast Character 5	Qualifier Character 6	Qualifier Character 7
0 Abdominal Aorta **2** Hepatic Artery **3** Splenic Arteries **4** Superior Mesenteric Artery **5** Inferior Mesenteric Artery **6** Renal Artery, Right **7** Renal Artery, Left **8** Renal Arteries, Bilateral **9** Lumbar Arteries **B** Intra-Abdominal Arteries, Other **C** Pelvic Arteries **D** Aorta and Bilateral Lower Extremity Arteries **F** Lower Extremity Arteries, Right **G** Lower Extremity Arteries, Left **J** Lower Arteries, Other	**0** High Osmolar **1** Low Osmolar **Y** Other Contrast	**1** Laser	**0** Intraoperative
0 Abdominal Aorta **2** Hepatic Artery **3** Splenic Arteries **4** Superior Mesenteric Artery **5** Inferior Mesenteric Artery **6** Renal Artery, Right **7** Renal Artery, Left **8** Renal Arteries, Bilateral **9** Lumbar Arteries **B** Intra-Abdominal Arteries, Other **C** Pelvic Arteries **D** Aorta and Bilateral Lower Extremity Arteries **F** Lower Extremity Arteries, Right **G** Lower Extremity Arteries, Left **J** Lower Arteries, Other	**0** High Osmolar **1** Low Osmolar **Y** Other Contrast	**Z** None	**Z** None
0 Abdominal Aorta **2** Hepatic Artery **3** Splenic Arteries **4** Superior Mesenteric Artery **5** Inferior Mesenteric Artery **6** Renal Artery, Right **7** Renal Artery, Left **8** Renal Arteries, Bilateral **9** Lumbar Arteries **B** Intra-Abdominal Arteries, Other **C** Pelvic Arteries **D** Aorta and Bilateral Lower Extremity Arteries **F** Lower Extremity Arteries, Right **G** Lower Extremity Arteries, Left **J** Lower Arteries, Other	**Z** None	**Z** None	**Z** None

B Imaging
4 Lower Arteries
2 Computerized Tomography (CT Scan) Computer reformatted digital display of multiplanar images developed from the capture of multiple exposures of external ionizing radiation

Body Part Character 4	Contrast Character 5	Qualifier Character 6	Qualifier Character 7
Ø Abdominal Aorta **1** Celiac Artery **4** Superior Mesenteric Artery **8** Renal Arteries, Bilateral **C** Pelvic Arteries **F** Lower Extremity Arteries, Right **G** Lower Extremity Arteries, Left **H** Lower Extremity Arteries, Bilateral **M** Renal Artery Transplant	**Ø** High Osmolar **1** Low Osmolar **Y** Other Contrast	**Z** None	**Z** None
Ø Abdominal Aorta **1** Celiac Artery **4** Superior Mesenteric Artery **8** Renal Arteries, Bilateral **C** Pelvic Arteries **F** Lower Extremity Arteries, Right **G** Lower Extremity Arteries, Left **H** Lower Extremity Arteries, Bilateral **M** Renal Artery Transplant	**Z** None	**2** Intravascular Optical Coherence **Z** None	**Z** None

B Imaging
4 Lower Arteries
3 Magnetic Resonance Imaging (MRI) Computer reformatted digital display of multiplanar images developed from the capture of radio-frequency signals emitted by nuclei in a body site excited within a magnetic field

Body Part Character 4	Contrast Character 5	Qualifier Character 6	Qualifier Character 7
Ø Abdominal Aorta **1** Celiac Artery **4** Superior Mesenteric Artery **8** Renal Arteries, Bilateral **C** Pelvic Arteries **F** Lower Extremity Arteries, Right **G** Lower Extremity Arteries, Left **H** Lower Extremity Arteries, Bilateral	**Y** Other Contrast	**Ø** Unenhanced and Enhanced **Z** None	**Z** None
Ø Abdominal Aorta **1** Celiac Artery **4** Superior Mesenteric Artery **8** Renal Arteries, Bilateral **C** Pelvic Arteries **F** Lower Extremity Arteries, Right **G** Lower Extremity Arteries, Left **H** Lower Extremity Arteries, Bilateral	**Z** None	**Z** None	**Z** None

B Imaging
4 Lower Arteries
4 Ultrasonography Real time display of images of anatomy or flow information developed from the capture of relected and attenuated high frequency sound waves

Body Part Character 4	Contrast Character 5	Qualifier Character 6	Qualifier Character 7
Ø Abdominal Aorta **4** Superior Mesenteric Artery **5** Inferior Mesenteric Artery **6** Renal Artery, Right **7** Renal Artery, Left **8** Renal Arteries, Bilateral **B** Intra-Abdominal Arteries, Other **F** Lower Extremity Arteries, Right **G** Lower Extremity Arteries, Left **H** Lower Extremity Arteries, Bilateral **K** Celiac and Mesenteric Arteries **L** Femoral Artery **N** Penile Arteries	**Z** None	**Z** None	**3** Intravascular **Z** None

B Imaging
5 Veins
0 Plain Radiography Planar display of an image developed from the capture of external ionizing radiation on photographic or photoconductive plate

Body Part Character 4	Contrast Character 5	Qualifier Character 6	Qualifier Character 7
0 Epidural Veins 1 Cerebral and Cerebellar Veins 2 Intracranial Sinuses 3 Jugular Veins, Right 4 Jugular Veins, Left 5 Jugular Veins, Bilateral 6 Subclavian Vein, Right 7 Subclavian Vein, Left 8 Superior Vena Cava 9 Inferior Vena Cava B Lower Extremity Veins, Right C Lower Extremity Veins, Left D Lower Extremity Veins, Bilateral F Pelvic (Iliac) Veins, Right G Pelvic (Iliac) Veins, Left H Pelvic (Iliac) Veins, Bilateral J Renal Vein, Right K Renal Vein, Left L Renal Veins, Bilateral M Upper Extremity Veins, Right N Upper Extremity Veins, Left P Upper Extremity Veins, Bilateral Q Pulmonary Vein, Right R Pulmonary Vein, Left S Pulmonary Veins, Bilateral T Portal and Splanchnic Veins V Veins, Other W Dialysis Shunt/Fistula	0 High Osmolar 1 Low Osmolar Y Other Contrast	Z None	Z None

B Imaging
5 Veins
1 Fluoroscopy Single plane or bi-plane real time display of an image developed from the capture of external ionizing radioation on a fluorescent screen. The image may also be stored by either digital or analog means

Body Part Character 4	Contrast Character 5	Qualifier Character 6	Qualifier Character 7
0 Epidural Veins 1 Cerebral and Cerebellar Veins 2 Intracranial Sinuses 3 Jugular Veins, Right ⊞ 4 Jugular Veins, Left ⊞ 5 Jugular Veins, Bilateral ⊞ 6 Subclavian Vein, Right ⊞ 7 Subclavian Vein, Left ⊞ 8 Superior Vena Cava 9 Inferior Vena Cava B Lower Extremity Veins, Right ⊞ C Lower Extremity Veins, Left ⊞ D Lower Extremity Veins, Bilateral ⊞ F Pelvic (Iliac) Veins, Right G Pelvic (Iliac) Veins, Left H Pelvic (Iliac) Veins, Bilateral J Renal Vein, Right K Renal Vein, Left L Renal Veins, Bilateral M Upper Extremity Veins, Right N Upper Extremity Veins, Left P Upper Extremity Veins, Bilateral Q Pulmonary Vein, Right R Pulmonary Vein, Left S Pulmonary Veins, Bilateral T Portal and Splanchnic Veins V Veins, Other W Dialysis Shunt/Fistula	0 High Osmolar 1 Low Osmolar Y Other Contrast Z None	Z None	A Guidance Z None

DRG Non-OR B51[3,4,5,6,7,B,C,D][0,1,Y,Z]ZA

No Procedure Combinations Specified
Combo-only B51[3,4,5,6,7,B,C,D][0,1,Y,Z]ZA
⊞ B51[3,4,5,6,7,B,C,D][0,1,Y,Z]ZA

B Imaging
5 Veins
2 Computerized Tomography (CT Scan) Computer reformatted digital display of multiplanar images developed from the capture of multiple exposures of external ionizing radiation

Body Part Character 4	Contrast Character 5	Qualifier Character 6	Qualifier Character 7
2 Intracranial Sinuses **8** Superior Vena Cava **9** Inferior Vena Cava **F** Pelvic (Iliac) Veins, Right **G** Pelvic (Iliac) Veins, Left **H** Pelvic (Iliac) Veins, Bilateral **J** Renal Vein, Right **K** Renal Vein, Left **L** Renal Veins, Bilateral **Q** Pulmonary Vein, Right **R** Pulmonary Vein, Left **S** Pulmonary Veins, Bilateral **T** Portal and Splanchnic Veins	**0** High Osmolar **1** Low Osmolar **Y** Other Contrast	**0** Unenhanced and Enhanced **Z** None	**Z** None
2 Intracranial Sinuses **8** Superior Vena Cava **9** Inferior Vena Cava **F** Pelvic (Iliac) Veins, Right **G** Pelvic (Iliac) Veins, Left **H** Pelvic (Iliac) Veins, Bilateral **J** Renal Vein, Right **K** Renal Vein, Left **L** Renal Veins, Bilateral **Q** Pulmonary Vein, Right **R** Pulmonary Vein, Left **S** Pulmonary Veins, Bilateral **T** Portal and Splanchnic Veins	**Z** None	**2** Intravascular Optical Coherence **Z** None	**Z** None

B Imaging
5 Veins
3 Magnetic Resonance Imaging (MRI) Computer reformatted digital display of multiplanar images developed from the capture of radio-frequency signals emitted by nuclei in a body site excited within a magnetic field

Body Part Character 4	Contrast Character 5	Qualifier Character 6	Qualifier Character 7
1 Cerebral and Cerebellar Veins **2** Intracranial Sinuses **5** Jugular Veins, Bilateral **8** Superior Vena Cava **9** Inferior Vena Cava **B** Lower Extremity Veins, Right **C** Lower Extremity Veins, Left **D** Lower Extremity Veins, Bilateral **H** Pelvic (Iliac) Veins, Bilateral **L** Renal Veins, Bilateral **M** Upper Extremity Veins, Right **N** Upper Extremity Veins, Left **P** Upper Extremity Veins, Bilateral **S** Pulmonary Veins, Bilateral **T** Portal and Splanchnic Veins **V** Veins, Other	**Y** Other Contrast	**0** Unenhanced and Enhanced **Z** None	**Z** None
1 Cerebral and Cerebellar Veins **2** Intracranial Sinuses **5** Jugular Veins, Bilateral **8** Superior Vena Cava **9** Inferior Vena Cava **B** Lower Extremity Veins, Right **C** Lower Extremity Veins, Left **D** Lower Extremity Veins, Bilateral **H** Pelvic (Iliac) Veins, Bilateral **L** Renal Veins, Bilateral **M** Upper Extremity Veins, Right **N** Upper Extremity Veins, Left **P** Upper Extremity Veins, Bilateral **S** Pulmonary Veins, Bilateral **T** Portal and Splanchnic Veins **V** Veins, Other	**Z** None	**Z** None	**Z** None

B Imaging
5 Veins
4 Ultrasonography Real time display of images of anatomy or flow information developed from the capture of relected and attenuated high frequency sound waves

Body Part Character 4	Contrast Character 5	Qualifier Character 6	Qualifier Character 7
3 Jugular Veins, Right ⊞ **4** Jugular Veins, Left ⊞ **6** Subclavian Vein, Right ⊞ **7** Subclavian Vein, Left ⊞ **8** Superior Vena Cava **9** Inferior Vena Cava **B** Lower Extremity Veins, Right ⊞ **C** Lower Extremity Veins, Left ⊞ **D** Lower Extremity Veins, Bilateral ⊞ **J** Renal Vein, Right **K** Renal Vein, Left **L** Renal Veins, Bilateral **M** Upper Extremity Veins, Right **N** Upper Extremity Veins, Left **P** Upper Extremity Veins, Bilateral **T** Portal and Splanchnic Veins	**Z** None	**Z** None	**3** Intravascular **A** Guidance **Z** None

DRG Non-OR B54[3,4,6,7,B,C,D]ZZA **No Procedure Combinations Specified**
Combo-only B54[3,4,6,7,B,C,D]ZZA
⊞ B54[3,4,6,7,B,C,D]ZZA

B Imaging
7 Lymphatic System
Ø Plain Radiography Planar display of an image developed from the capture of external ionizing radiation on photographic or photoconductive plate

Body Part Character 4	Contrast Character 5	Qualifier Character 6	Qualifier Character 7
Ø Abdominal/Retroperitoneal Lymphatics, Unilateral **1** Abdominal/Retroperitoneal Lymphatics, Bilateral **4** Lymphatics, Head and Neck **5** Upper Extremity Lymphatics, Right **6** Upper Extremity Lymphatics, Left **7** Upper Extremity Lymphatics, Bilateral **8** Lower Extremity Lymphatics, Right **9** Lower Extremity Lymphatics, Left **B** Lower Extremity Lymphatics, Bilateral **C** Lymphatics, Pelvic	**Ø** High Osmolar **1** Low Osmolar **Y** Other Contrast	**Z** None	**Z** None

B Imaging
8 Eye
Ø Plain Radiography Planar display of an image developed from the capture of external ionizing radiation on photographic or photoconductive plate

Body Part Character 4	Contrast Character 5	Qualifier Character 6	Qualifier Character 7
Ø Lacrimal Duct, Right **1** Lacrimal Duct, Left **2** Lacrimal Ducts, Bilateral	**Ø** High Osmolar **1** Low Osmolar **Y** Other Contrast	**Z** None	**Z** None
3 Optic Foramina, Right **4** Optic Foramina, Left **5** Eye, Right **6** Eye, Left **7** Eyes, Bilateral	**Z** None	**Z** None	**Z** None

B Imaging
8 Eye
2 Computerized Tomography (CT Scan) Computer reformatted digital display of multiplanar images developed from the capture of multiple exposures of external ionizing radiation

Body Part Character 4	Contrast Character 5	Qualifier Character 6	Qualifier Character 7
5 Eye, Right **6** Eye, Left **7** Eyes, Bilateral	**Ø** High Osmolar **1** Low Osmolar **Y** Other Contrast	**Ø** Unenhanced and Enhanced **Z** None	**Z** None
5 Eye, Right **6** Eye, Left **7** Eyes, Bilateral	**Z** None	**Z** None	**Z** None

B Imaging
8 Eye
3 Magnetic Resonance Imaging (MRI) Computer reformatted digital display of multiplanar images developed from the capture of radio-frequency signals emitted by nuclei in a body site excited within a magnetic field

Body Part Character 4	Contrast Character 5	Qualifier Character 6	Qualifier Character 7
5 Eye, Right 6 Eye, Left 7 Eyes, Bilateral	Y Other Contrast	Ø Unenhanced and Enhanced Z None	Z None
5 Eye, Right 6 Eye, Left 7 Eyes, Bilateral	Z None	Z None	Z None

B Imaging
8 Eye
4 Ultrasonography Real time display of images of anatomy or flow information developed from the capture of relected and attenuated high frequency sound waves

Body Part Character 4	Contrast Character 5	Qualifier Character 6	Qualifier Character 7
5 Eye, Right 6 Eye, Left 7 Eyes, Bilateral	Z None	Z None	Z None

B Imaging
9 Ear, Nose, Mouth and Throat
Ø Plain Radiography Planar display of an image developed from the capture of external ionizing radiation on photographic or photoconductive plate

Body Part Character 4	Contrast Character 5	Qualifier Character 6	Qualifier Character 7
2 Paranasal Sinuses F Nasopharynx/Oropharynx H Mastoids	Z None	Z None	Z None
4 Parotid Gland, Right 5 Parotid Gland, Left 6 Parotid Glands, Bilateral 7 Submandibular Gland, Right 8 Submandibular Gland, Left 9 Submandibular Glands, Bilateral B Salivary Gland, Right C Salivary Gland, Left D Salivary Glands, Bilateral	Ø High Osmolar 1 Low Osmolar Y Other Contrast	Z None	Z None

B Imaging
9 Ear, Nose, Mouth and Throat
1 Fluoroscopy Single plane or bi-plane real time display of an image developed from the capture of external ionizing radioation on a fluorescent screen. The image may also be stored by either digital or analog means

Body Part Character 4	Contrast Character 5	Qualifier Character 6	Qualifier Character 7
G Pharynx and Epiglottis J Larynx	Y Other Contrast Z None	Z None	Z None

B Imaging
9 Ear, Nose, Mouth and Throat
2 Computerized Tomography (CT Scan) Computer reformatted digital display of multiplanar images developed from the capture of multiple exposures of external ionizing radiation

Body Part Character 4	Contrast Character 5	Qualifier Character 6	Qualifier Character 7
Ø Ear 2 Paranasal Sinuses 6 Parotid Glands, Bilateral 9 Submandibular Glands, Bilateral D Salivary Glands, Bilateral F Nasopharynx/Oropharynx J Larynx	Ø High Osmolar 1 Low Osmolar Y Other Contrast	Ø Unenhanced and Enhanced Z None	Z None
Ø Ear 2 Paranasal Sinuses 6 Parotid Glands, Bilateral 9 Submandibular Glands, Bilateral D Salivary Glands, Bilateral F Nasopharynx/Oropharynx J Larynx	Z None	Z None	Z None

B Imaging
9 Ear, Nose, Mouth and Throat
3 Magnetic Resonance Imaging (MRI) Computer reformatted digital display of multiplanar images developed from the capture of radio-frequency signals emitted by nuclei in a body site excited within a magnetic field

Body Part Character 4	Contrast Character 5	Qualifier Character 6	Qualifier Character 7
Ø Ear **2** Paranasal Sinuses **6** Parotid Glands, Bilateral **9** Submandibular Glands, Bilateral **D** Salivary Glands, Bilateral **F** Nasopharynx/Oropharynx **J** Larynx	**Y** Other Contrast	**Ø** Unenhanced and Enhanced **Z** None	**Z** None
Ø Ear **2** Paranasal Sinuses **6** Parotid Glands, Bilateral **9** Submandibular Glands, Bilateral **D** Salivary Glands, Bilateral **F** Nasopharynx/Oropharynx **J** Larynx	**Z** None	**Z** None	**Z** None

B Imaging
B Respiratory System
Ø Plain Radiography Planar display of an image developed from the capture of external ionizing radiation on photographic or photoconductive plate

Body Part Character 4	Contrast Character 5	Qualifier Character 6	Qualifier Character 7
7 Tracheobronchial Tree, Right **8** Tracheobronchial Tree, Left **9** Tracheobronchial Trees, Bilateral	**Y** Other Contrast	**Z** None	**Z** None
D Upper Airways	**Z** None	**Z** None	**Z** None

B Imaging
B Respiratory System
1 Fluoroscopy Single plane or bi-plane real time display of an image developed from the capture of external ionizing radioation on a fluorescent screen. The image may also be stored by either digital or analog means

Body Part Character 4	Contrast Character 5	Qualifier Character 6	Qualifier Character 7
2 Lung, Right **3** Lung, Left **4** Lungs, Bilateral **6** Diaphragm **C** Mediastinum **D** Upper Airways	**Z** None	**Z** None	**Z** None
7 Tracheobronchial Tree, Right **8** Tracheobronchial Tree, Left **9** Tracheobronchial Trees, Bilateral	**Y** Other Contrast	**Z** None	**Z** None

B Imaging
B Respiratory System
2 Computerized Tomography (CT Scan) Computer reformatted digital display of multiplanar images developed from the capture of multiple exposures of external ionizing radiation

Body Part Character 4	Contrast Character 5	Qualifier Character 6	Qualifier Character 7
4 Lungs, Bilateral **7** Tracheobronchial Tree, Right **8** Tracheobronchial Tree, Left **9** Tracheobronchial Trees, Bilateral **F** Trachea/Airways	**Ø** High Osmolar **1** Low Osmolar **Y** Other Contrast	**Ø** Unenhanced and Enhanced **Z** None	**Z** None
4 Lungs, Bilateral **7** Tracheobronchial Tree, Right **8** Tracheobronchial Tree, Left **9** Tracheobronchial Trees, Bilateral **F** Trachea/Airways	**Z** None	**Z** None	**Z** None

B Imaging
B Respiratory System
3 Magnetic Resonance Imaging (MRI) Computer reformatted digital display of multiplanar images developed from the capture of radio-frequency signals emitted by nuclei in a body site excited within a magnetic field

Body Part Character 4	Contrast Character 5	Qualifier Character 6	Qualifier Character 7
G Lung Apices	Y Other Contrast	Ø Unenhanced and Enhanced Z None	Z None
G Lung Apices	Z None	Z None	Z None

B Imaging
B Respiratory System
4 Ultrasonography Real time display of images of anatomy or flow information developed from the capture of relected and attenuated high frequency sound waves

Body Part Character 4	Contrast Character 5	Qualifier Character 6	Qualifier Character 7
B Pleura C Mediastinum	Z None	Z None	Z None

B Imaging
D Gastrointestinal System
1 Fluoroscopy Single plane or bi-plane real time display of an image developed from the capture of external ionizing radioation on a fluorescent screen. The image may also be stored by either digital or analog means

Body Part Character 4	Contrast Character 5	Qualifier Character 6	Qualifier Character 7
1 Esophagus 2 Stomach 3 Small Bowel 4 Colon 5 Upper GI 6 Upper GI and Small Bowel 9 Duodenum B Mouth/Oropharynx	Y Other Contrast Z None	Z None	Z None

B Imaging
D Gastrointestinal System
2 Computerized Tomography (CT Scan) Computer reformatted digital display of multiplanar images developed from the capture of multiple exposures of external ionizing radiation

Body Part Character 4	Contrast Character 5	Qualifier Character 6	Qualifier Character 7
4 Colon	Ø High Osmolar 1 Low Osmolar Y Other Contrast	Ø Unenhanced and Enhanced Z None	Z None
4 Colon	Z None	Z None	Z None

B Imaging
D Gastrointestinal System
4 Ultrasonography Real time display of images of anatomy or flow information developed from the capture of relected and attenuated high frequency sound waves

Body Part Character 4	Contrast Character 5	Qualifier Character 6	Qualifier Character 7
1 Esophagus 2 Stomach 7 Gastrointestinal Tract 8 Appendix 9 Duodenum C Rectum	Z None	Z None	Z None

B Imaging
F Hepatobiliary System and Pancreas
Ø Plain Radiography Planar display of an image developed from the capture of external ionizing radiation on photographic or photoconductive plate

Body Part Character 4	Contrast Character 5	Qualifier Character 6	Qualifier Character 7
Ø Bile Ducts 3 Gallbladder and Bile Ducts C Hepatobiliary System, All	Ø High Osmolar 1 Low Osmolar Y Other Contrast	Z None	Z None

B Imaging
F Hepatobiliary System and Pancreas
1 Fluoroscopy Single plane or bi-plane real time display of an image developed from the capture of external ionizing radioation on a fluorescent screen. The image may also be stored by either digital or analog means

Body Part Character 4	Contrast Character 5	Qualifier Character 6	Qualifier Character 7
Ø Bile Ducts 1 Biliary and Pancreatic Ducts 2 Gallbladder 3 Gallbladder and Bile Ducts 4 Gallbladder, Bile Ducts and Pancreatic Ducts 8 Pancreatic Ducts	Ø High Osmolar 1 Low Osmolar Y Other Contrast	Z None	Z None

B Imaging
F Hepatobiliary System and Pancreas
2 Computerized Tomography (CT Scan) Computer reformatted digital display of multiplanar images developed from the capture of multiple exposures of external ionizing radiation

Body Part Character 4	Contrast Character 5	Qualifier Character 6	Qualifier Character 7
5 Liver 6 Liver and Spleen 7 Pancreas C Hepatobiliary System, All	Ø High Osmolar 1 Low Osmolar Y Other Contrast	Ø Unenhanced and Enhanced Z None	Z None
5 Liver 6 Liver and Spleen 7 Pancreas C Hepatobiliary System, All	Z None	Z None	Z None

B Imaging
F Hepatobiliary System and Pancreas
3 Magnetic Resonance Imaging (MRI) Computer reformatted digital display of multiplanar images developed from the capture of radio-frequency signals emitted by nuclei in a body site excited within a magnetic field

Body Part Character 4	Contrast Character 5	Qualifier Character 6	Qualifier Character 7
5 Liver 6 Liver and Spleen 7 Pancreas	Y Other Contrast	Ø Unenhanced and Enhanced Z None	Z None
5 Liver 6 Liver and Spleen 7 Pancreas	Z None	Z None	Z None

B Imaging
F Hepatobiliary System and Pancreas
4 Ultrasonography Real time display of images of anatomy or flow information developed from the capture of relected and attenuated high frequency sound waves

Body Part Character 4	Contrast Character 5	Qualifier Character 6	Qualifier Character 7
Ø Bile Ducts 2 Gallbladder 3 Gallbladder and Bile Ducts 5 Liver 6 Liver and Spleen 7 Pancreas C Hepatobiliary System, All	Z None	Z None	Z None

B Imaging
G Endocrine System
2 Computerized Tomography (CT Scan) Computer reformatted digital display of multiplanar images developed from the capture of multiple exposures of external ionizing radiation

Body Part Character 4	Contrast Character 5	Qualifier Character 6	Qualifier Character 7
2 Adrenal Glands, Bilateral 3 Parathyroid Glands 4 Thyroid Gland	Ø High Osmolar 1 Low Osmolar Y Other Contrast	Ø Unenhanced and Enhanced Z None	Z None
2 Adrenal Glands, Bilateral 3 Parathyroid Glands 4 Thyroid Gland	Z None	Z None	Z None

B Imaging
G Endocrine System
3 Magnetic Resonance Imaging (MRI) Computer reformatted digital display of multiplanar images developed from the capture of radio-frequency signals emitted by nuclei in a body site excited within a magnetic field

Body Part Character 4	Contrast Character 5	Qualifier Character 6	Qualifier Character 7
2 Adrenal Glands, Bilateral 3 Parathyroid Glands 4 Thyroid Gland	Y Other Contrast	0 Unenhanced and Enhanced Z None	Z None
2 Adrenal Glands, Bilateral 3 Parathyroid Glands 4 Thyroid Gland	Z None	Z None	Z None

B Imaging
G Endocrine System
4 Ultrasonography Real time display of images of anatomy or flow information developed from the capture of relected and attenuated high frequency sound waves

Body Part Character 4	Contrast Character 5	Qualifier Character 6	Qualifier Character 7
0 Adrenal Gland, Right 1 Adrenal Gland, Left 2 Adrenal Glands, Bilateral 3 Parathyroid Glands 4 Thyroid Gland	Z None	Z None	Z None

B Imaging
H Skin, Subcutaneous Tissue and Breast
0 Plain Radiography Planar display of an image developed from the capture of external ionizing radiation on photographic or photoconductive plate

Body Part Character 4	Contrast Character 5	Qualifier Character 6	Qualifier Character 7
0 Breast, Right 1 Breast, Left 2 Breasts, Bilateral	Z None	Z None	Z None
3 Single Mammary Duct, Right 4 Single Mammary Duct, Left 5 Multiple Mammary Ducts, Right 6 Multiple Mammary Ducts, Left	0 High Osmolar 1 Low Osmolar Y Other Contrast Z None	Z None	Z None

B Imaging
H Skin, Subcutaneous Tissue and Breast
3 Magnetic Resonance Imaging (MRI) Computer reformatted digital display of multiplanar images developed from the capture of radio-frequency signals emitted by nuclei in a body site excited within a magnetic field

Body Part Character 4	Contrast Character 5	Qualifier Character 6	Qualifier Character 7
0 Breast, Right 1 Breast, Left 2 Breasts, Bilateral D Subcutaneous Tissue, Head/Neck F Subcutaneous Tissue, Upper Extremity G Subcutaneous Tissue, Thorax H Subcutaneous Tissue, Abdomen and Pelvis J Subcutaneous Tissue, Lower Extremity	Y Other Contrast	0 Unenhanced and Enhanced Z None	Z None
0 Breast, Right 1 Breast, Left 2 Breasts, Bilateral D Subcutaneous Tissue, Head/Neck F Subcutaneous Tissue, Upper Extremity G Subcutaneous Tissue, Thorax H Subcutaneous Tissue, Abdomen and Pelvis J Subcutaneous Tissue, Lower Extremity	Z None	Z None	Z None

B Imaging
H Skin, Subcutaneous Tissue and Breast
4 Ultrasonography Real time display of images of anatomy or flow information developed from the capture of relected and attenuated high frequency sound waves

Body Part Character 4	Contrast Character 5	Qualifier Character 6	Qualifier Character 7
Ø Breast, Right 1 Breast, Left 2 Breasts, Bilateral 7 Extremity, Upper 8 Extremity, Lower 9 Abdominal Wall B Chest Wall C Head and Neck	Z None	Z None	Z None

B Imaging
L Connective Tissue
3 Magnetic Resonance Imaging (MRI) Computer reformatted digital display of multiplanar images developed from the capture of radio-frequency signals emitted by nuclei in a body site excited within a magnetic field

Body Part Character 4	Contrast Character 5	Qualifier Character 6	Qualifier Character 7
Ø Connective Tissue, Upper Extremity 1 Connective Tissue, Lower Extremity 2 Tendons, Upper Extremity 3 Tendons, Lower Extremity	Y Other Contrast	Ø Unenhanced and Enhanced Z None	Z None
Ø Connective Tissue, Upper Extremity 1 Connective Tissue, Lower Extremity 2 Tendons, Upper Extremity 3 Tendons, Lower Extremity	Z None	Z None	Z None

B Imaging
L Connective Tissue
4 Ultrasonography Real time display of images of anatomy or flow information developed from the capture of relected and attenuated high frequency sound waves

Body Part Character 4	Contrast Character 5	Qualifier Character 6	Qualifier Character 7
Ø Connective Tissue, Upper Extremity 1 Connective Tissue, Lower Extremity 2 Tendons, Upper Extremity 3 Tendons, Lower Extremity	Z None	Z None	Z None

B Imaging
N Skull and Facial Bones
Ø Plain Radiography Planar display of an image developed from the capture of external ionizing radiation on photographic or photoconductive plate

Body Part Character 4	Contrast Character 5	Qualifier Character 6	Qualifier Character 7
Ø Skull 1 Orbit, Right 2 Orbit, Left 3 Orbits, Bilateral 4 Nasal Bones 5 Facial Bones 6 Mandible B Zygomatic Arch, Right C Zygomatic Arch, Left D Zygomatic Arches, Bilateral G Tooth, Single H Teeth, Multiple J Teeth, All	Z None	Z None	Z None
7 Temporomandibular Joint, Right 8 Temporomandibular Joint, Left 9 Temporomandibular Joints, Bilateral	Ø High Osmolar 1 Low Osmolar Y Other Contrast Z None	Z None	Z None

B Imaging
N Skull and Facial Bones
1 Fluoroscopy Single plane or bi-plane real time display of an image developed from the capture of external ionizing radioation on a fluorescent screen. The image may also be stored by either digital or analog means

Body Part Character 4	Contrast Character 5	Qualifier Character 6	Qualifier Character 7
7 Temporomandibular Joint, Right 8 Temporomandibular Joint, Left 9 Temporomandibular Joints, Bilateral	0 High Osmolar 1 Low Osmolar Y Other Contrast Z None	Z None	Z None

B Imaging
N Skull and Facial Bones
2 Computerized Tomography (CT Scan) Computer reformatted digital display of multiplanar images developed from the capture of multiple exposures of external ionizing radiation

Body Part Character 4	Contrast Character 5	Qualifier Character 6	Qualifier Character 7
0 Skull 3 Orbits, Bilateral 5 Facial Bones 6 Mandible 9 Temporomandibular Joints, Bilateral F Temporal Bones	0 High Osmolar 1 Low Osmolar Y Other Contrast Z None	Z None	Z None

B Imaging
N Skull and Facial Bones
3 Magnetic Resonance Imaging (MRI) Computer reformatted digital display of multiplanar images developed from the capture of radio-frequency signals emitted by nuclei in a body site excited within a magnetic field

Body Part Character 4	Contrast Character 5	Qualifier Character 6	Qualifier Character 7
9 Temporomandibular Joints, Bilateral	Y Other Contrast Z None	Z None	Z None

B Imaging
P Non-Axial Upper Bones
0 Plain Radiography Planar display of an image developed from the capture of external ionizing radiation on photographic or photoconductive plate

Body Part Character 4	Contrast Character 5	Qualifier Character 6	Qualifier Character 7
0 Sternoclavicular Joint, Right 1 Sternoclavicular Joint, Left 2 Sternoclavicular Joints, Bilateral 3 Acromioclavicular Joints, Bilateral 4 Clavicle, Right 5 Clavicle, Left 6 Scapula, Right 7 Scapula, Left A Humerus, Right B Humerus, Left E Upper Arm, Right F Upper Arm, Left J Forearm, Right K Forearm, Left N Hand, Right P Hand, Left R Finger(s), Right S Finger(s), Left X Ribs, Right Y Ribs, Left	Z None	Z None	Z None
8 Shoulder, Right 9 Shoulder, Left C Hand/Finger Joint, Right D Hand/Finger Joint, Left G Elbow, Right H Elbow, Left L Wrist, Right M Wrist, Left	0 High Osmolar 1 Low Osmolar Y Other Contrast Z None	Z None	Z None

B Imaging
P Non-Axial Upper Bones
1 Fluoroscopy Single plane or bi-plane real time display of an image developed from the capture of external ionizing radioation on a fluorescent screen. The image may also be stored by either digital or analog means

Body Part Character 4	Contrast Character 5	Qualifier Character 6	Qualifier Character 7
Ø Sternoclavicular Joint, Right **1** Sternoclavicular Joint, Left **2** Sternoclavicular Joints, Bilateral **3** Acromioclavicular Joints, Bilateral **4** Clavicle, Right **5** Clavicle, Left **6** Scapula, Right **7** Scapula, Left **A** Humerus, Right **B** Humerus, Left **E** Upper Arm, Right **F** Upper Arm, Left **J** Forearm, Right **K** Forearm, Left **N** Hand, Right **P** Hand, Left **R** Finger(s), Right **S** Finger(s), Left **X** Ribs, Right **Y** Ribs, Left	**Z** None	**Z** None	**Z** None
8 Shoulder, Right **9** Shoulder, Left **L** Wrist, Right **M** Wrist, Left	**Ø** High Osmolar **1** Low Osmolar **Y** Other Contrast **Z** None	**Z** None	**Z** None
C Hand/Finger Joint, Right **D** Hand/Finger Joint, Left **G** Elbow, Right **H** Elbow, Left	**Ø** High Osmolar **1** Low Osmolar **Y** Other Contrast	**Z** None	**Z** None

B Imaging
P Non-Axial Upper Bones
2 Computerized Tomography (CT Scan) Computer reformatted digital display of multiplanar images developed from the capture of multiple exposures of external ionizing radiation

Body Part Character 4	Contrast Character 5	Qualifier Character 6	Qualifier Character 7
Ø Sternoclavicular Joint, Right **1** Sternoclavicular Joint, Left **W** Thorax	**Ø** High Osmolar **1** Low Osmolar **Y** Other Contrast	**Z** None	**Z** None
2 Sternoclavicular Joints, Bilateral **3** Acromioclavicular Joints, Bilateral **4** Clavicle, Right **5** Clavicle, Left **6** Scapula, Right **7** Scapula, Left **8** Shoulder, Right **9** Shoulder, Left **A** Humerus, Right **B** Humerus, Left **E** Upper Arm, Right **F** Upper Arm, Left **G** Elbow, Right **H** Elbow, Left **J** Forearm, Right **K** Forearm, Left **L** Wrist, Right **M** Wrist, Left **N** Hand, Right **P** Hand, Left **Q** Hands and Wrists, Bilateral **R** Finger(s), Right **S** Finger(s), Left **T** Upper Extremity, Right **U** Upper Extremity, Left **V** Upper Extremities, Bilateral **X** Ribs, Right **Y** Ribs, Left	**Ø** High Osmolar **1** Low Osmolar **Y** Other Contrast **Z** None	**Z** None	**Z** None
C Hand/Finger Joint, Right **D** Hand/Finger Joint, Left	**Z** None	**Z** None	**Z** None

B Imaging
P Non-Axial Upper Bones
3 Magnetic Resonance Imaging (MRI) Computer reformatted digital display of multiplanar images developed from the capture of radio-frequency signals emitted by nuclei in a body site excited within a magnetic field

Body Part Character 4	Contrast Character 5	Qualifier Character 6	Qualifier Character 7
8 Shoulder, Right **9** Shoulder, Left **C** Hand/Finger Joint, Right **D** Hand/Finger Joint, Left **E** Upper Arm, Right **F** Upper Arm, Left **G** Elbow, Right **H** Elbow, Left **J** Forearm, Right **K** Forearm, Left **L** Wrist, Right **M** Wrist, Left	**Y** Other Contrast	**0** Unenhanced and Enhanced **Z** None	**Z** None
8 Shoulder, Right **9** Shoulder, Left **C** Hand/Finger Joint, Right **D** Hand/Finger Joint, Left **E** Upper Arm, Right **F** Upper Arm, Left **G** Elbow, Right **H** Elbow, Left **J** Forearm, Right **K** Forearm, Left **L** Wrist, Right **M** Wrist, Left	**Z** None	**Z** None	**Z** None

B Imaging
P Non-Axial Upper Bones
4 Ultrasonography Real time display of images of anatomy or flow information developed from the capture of relected and attenuated high frequency sound waves

Body Part Character 4	Contrast Character 5	Qualifier Character 6	Qualifier Character 7
8 Shoulder, Right **9** Shoulder, Left **G** Elbow, Right **H** Elbow, Left **L** Wrist, Right **M** Wrist, Left **N** Hand, Right **P** Hand, Left	**Z** None	**Z** None	**1** Densitometry **Z** None

B Imaging
Q Non-Axial Lower Bones
0 Plain Radiography Planar display of an image developed from the capture of external ionizing radiation on photographic or photoconductive plate

Body Part Character 4	Contrast Character 5	Qualifier Character 6	Qualifier Character 7
0 Hip, Right **1** Hip, Left **3** Femur, Right **4** Femur, Left	**Z** None	**Z** None	**1** Densitometry **Z** None
0 Hip, Right **1** Hip, Left **X** Foot/Toe Joint, Right **Y** Foot/Toe Joint, Left	**0** High Osmolar **1** Low Osmolar **Y** Other Contrast	**Z** None	**Z** None
7 Knee, Right **8** Knee, Left **G** Ankle, Right **H** Ankle, Left	**0** High Osmolar **1** Low Osmolar **Y** Other Contrast **Z** None	**Z** None	**Z** None
D Lower Leg, Right **F** Lower Leg, Left **J** Calcaneus, Right **K** Calcaneus, Left **L** Foot, Right **M** Foot, Left **P** Toe(s), Right **Q** Toe(s), Left **V** Patella, Right **W** Patella, Left	**Z** None	**Z** None	**Z** None

B Imaging
Q Non-Axial Lower Bones
1 Fluoroscopy Single plane or bi-plane real time display of an image developed from the capture of external ionizing radioation on a fluorescent screen. The image may also be stored by either digital or analog means

Body Part Character 4	Contrast Character 5	Qualifier Character 6	Qualifier Character 7
0 Hip, Right **1** Hip, Left **7** Knee, Right **8** Knee, Left **G** Ankle, Right **H** Ankle, Left **X** Foot/Toe Joint, Right **Y** Foot/Toe Joint, Left	**0** High Osmolar **1** Low Osmolar **Y** Other Contrast **Z** None	**Z** None	**Z** None
3 Femur, Right **4** Femur, Left **D** Lower Leg, Right **F** Lower Leg, Left **J** Calcaneus, Right **K** Calcaneus, Left **L** Foot, Right **M** Foot, Left **P** Toe(s), Right **Q** Toe(s), Left **V** Patella, Right **W** Patella, Left	**Z** None	**Z** None	**Z** None

B Imaging
Q Non-Axial Lower Bones
2 Computerized Tomography (CT Scan) Computer reformatted digital display of multiplanar images developed from the capture of multiple exposures of external ionizing radiation

Body Part Character 4	Contrast Character 5	Qualifier Character 6	Qualifier Character 7
0 Hip, Right **1** Hip, Left **3** Femur, Right **4** Femur, Left **7** Knee, Right **8** Knee, Left **D** Lower Leg, Right **F** Lower Leg, Left **G** Ankle, Right **H** Ankle, Left **J** Calcaneus, Right **K** Calcaneus, Left **L** Foot, Right **M** Foot, Left **P** Toe(s), Right **Q** Toe(s), Left **R** Lower Extremity, Right **S** Lower Extremity, Left **V** Patella, Right **W** Patella, Left **X** Foot/Toe Joint, Right **Y** Foot/Toe Joint, Left	**0** High Osmolar **1** Low Osmolar **Y** Other Contrast **Z** None	**Z** None	**Z** None
B Tibia/Fibula, Right **C** Tibia/Fibula, Left	**0** High Osmolar **1** Low Osmolar **Y** Other Contrast	**Z** None	**Z** None

B Imaging
Q Non-Axial Lower Bones
3 Magnetic Resonance Imaging (MRI) Computer reformatted digital display of multiplanar images developed from the capture of radio-frequency signals emitted by nuclei in a body site excited within a magnetic field

Body Part Character 4	Contrast Character 5	Qualifier Character 6	Qualifier Character 7
0 Hip, Right **1** Hip, Left **3** Femur, Right **4** Femur, Left **7** Knee, Right **8** Knee, Left **D** Lower Leg, Right **F** Lower Leg, Left **G** Ankle, Right **H** Ankle, Left **J** Calcaneus, Right **K** Calcaneus, Left **L** Foot, Right **M** Foot, Left **P** Toe(s), Right **Q** Toe(s), Left **V** Patella, Right **W** Patella, Left	**Y** Other Contrast	**0** Unenhanced and Enhanced **Z** None	**Z** None
0 Hip, Right **1** Hip, Left **3** Femur, Right **4** Femur, Left **7** Knee, Right **8** Knee, Left **D** Lower Leg, Right **F** Lower Leg, Left **G** Ankle, Right **H** Ankle, Left **J** Calcaneus, Right **K** Calcaneus, Left **L** Foot, Right **M** Foot, Left **P** Toe(s), Right **Q** Toe(s), Left **V** Patella, Right **W** Patella, Left	**Z** None	**Z** None	**Z** None

B Imaging
Q Non-Axial Lower Bones
4 Ultrasonography Real time display of images of anatomy or flow information developed from the capture of relected and attenuated high frequency sound waves

Body Part Character 4	Contrast Character 5	Qualifier Character 6	Qualifier Character 7
0 Hip, Right **1** Hip, Left **2** Hips, Bilateral **7** Knee, Right **8** Knee, Left **9** Knees, Bilateral	**Z** None	**Z** None	**Z** None

B Imaging
R Axial Skeleton, Except Skull and Facial Bones
Ø Plain Radiography Planar display of an image developed from the capture of external ionizing radiation on photographic or photoconductive plate

Body Part Character 4	Contrast Character 5	Qualifier Character 6	Qualifier Character 7
Ø Cervical Spine **7** Thoracic Spine **9** Lumbar Spine **G** Whole Spine	**Z** None	**Z** None	**1** Densitometry **Z** None
1 Cervical Disc(s) **2** Thoracic Disc(s) **3** Lumbar Disc(s) **4** Cervical Facet Joint(s) **5** Thoracic Facet Joint(s) **6** Lumbar Facet Joint(s) **D** Sacroiliac Joints	**Ø** High Osmolar **1** Low Osmolar **Y** Other Contrast **Z** None	**Z** None	**Z** None
8 Thoracolumbar Joint **B** Lumbosacral Joint **C** Pelvis **F** Sacrum and Coccyx **H** Sternum	**Z** None	**Z** None	**Z** None

B Imaging
R Axial Skeleton, Except Skull and Facial Bones
1 Fluoroscopy Single plane or bi-plane real time display of an image developed from the capture of external ionizing radioation on a fluorescent screen. The image may also be stored by either digital or analog means

Body Part Character 4	Contrast Character 5	Qualifier Character 6	Qualifier Character 7
Ø Cervical Spine **1** Cervical Disc(s) **2** Thoracic Disc(s) **3** Lumbar Disc(s) **4** Cervical Facet Joint(s) **5** Thoracic Facet Joint(s) **6** Lumbar Facet Joint(s) **7** Thoracic Spine **8** Thoracolumbar Joint **9** Lumbar Spine **B** Lumbosacral Joint **C** Pelvis **D** Sacroiliac Joints **F** Sacrum and Coccyx **G** Whole Spine **H** Sternum	**Ø** High Osmolar **1** Low Osmolar **Y** Other Contrast **Z** None	**Z** None	**Z** None

B Imaging
R Axial Skeleton, Except Skull and Facial Bones
2 Computerized Tomography (CT Scan) Computer reformatted digital display of multiplanar images developed from the capture of multiple exposures of external ionizing radiation

Body Part Character 4	Contrast Character 5	Qualifier Character 6	Qualifier Character 7
Ø Cervical Spine **7** Thoracic Spine **9** Lumbar Spine **C** Pelvis **D** Sacroiliac Joints **F** Sacrum and Coccyx	**Ø** High Osmolar **1** Low Osmolar **Y** Other Contrast **Z** None	**Z** None	**Z** None

B Imaging
R Axial Skeleton, Except Skull and Facial Bones
3 Magnetic Resonance Imaging (MRI) Computer reformatted digital display of multiplanar images developed from the capture of radio-frequency signals emitted by nuclei in a body site excited within a magnetic field

Body Part Character 4	Contrast Character 5	Qualifier Character 6	Qualifier Character 7
0 Cervical Spine **1** Cervical Disc(s) **2** Thoracic Disc(s) **3** Lumbar Disc(s) **7** Thoracic Spine **9** Lumbar Spine **C** Pelvis **F** Sacrum and Coccyx	**Y** Other Contrast	**0** Unenhanced and Enhanced **Z** None	**Z** None
0 Cervical Spine **1** Cervical Disc(s) **2** Thoracic Disc(s) **3** Lumbar Disc(s) **7** Thoracic Spine **9** Lumbar Spine **C** Pelvis **F** Sacrum and Coccyx	**Z** None	**Z** None	**Z** None

B Imaging
R Axial Skeleton, Except Skull and Facial Bones
4 Ultrasonography Real time display of images of anatomy or flow information developed from the capture of relected and attenuated high frequency sound waves

Body Part Character 4	Contrast Character 5	Qualifier Character 6	Qualifier Character 7
0 Cervical Spine **7** Thoracic Spine **9** Lumbar Spine **F** Sacrum and Coccyx	**Z** None	**Z** None	**Z** None

B Imaging
T Urinary System
0 Plain Radiography Planar display of an image developed from the capture of external ionizing radiation on photographic or photoconductive plate

Body Part Character 4	Contrast Character 5	Qualifier Character 6	Qualifier Character 7
0 Bladder **1** Kidney, Right **2** Kidney, Left **3** Kidneys, Bilateral **4** Kidneys, Ureters and Bladder **5** Urethra **6** Ureter, Right **7** Ureter, Left **8** Ureters, Bilateral **B** Bladder and Urethra **C** Ileal Diversion Loop	**0** High Osmolar **1** Low Osmolar **Y** Other Contrast **Z** None	**Z** None	**Z** None

B Imaging
T Urinary System
1 Fluoroscopy Single plane or bi-plane real time display of an image developed from the capture of external ionizing radioation on a fluorescent screen. The image may also be stored by either digital or analog means

Body Part Character 4	Contrast Character 5	Qualifier Character 6	Qualifier Character 7
0 Bladder **1** Kidney, Right **2** Kidney, Left **3** Kidneys, Bilateral **4** Kidneys, Ureters and Bladder **5** Urethra **6** Ureter, Right **7** Ureter, Left **B** Bladder and Urethra **C** Ileal Diversion Loop **D** Kidney, Ureter and Bladder, Right **F** Kidney, Ureter and Bladder, Left **G** Ileal Loop, Ureters and Kidneys	**0** High Osmolar **1** Low Osmolar **Y** Other Contrast **Z** None	**Z** None	**Z** None

B Imaging
T Urinary System
2 Computerized Tomography (CT Scan) Computer reformatted digital display of multiplanar images developed from the capture of multiple exposures of external ionizing radiation

Body Part Character 4	Contrast Character 5	Qualifier Character 6	Qualifier Character 7
Ø Bladder 1 Kidney, Right 2 Kidney, Left 3 Kidneys, Bilateral 9 Kidney Transplant	Ø High Osmolar 1 Low Osmolar Y Other Contrast	Ø Unenhanced and Enhanced Z None	Z None
Ø Bladder 1 Kidney, Right 2 Kidney, Left 3 Kidneys, Bilateral 9 Kidney Transplant	Z None	Z None	Z None

B Imaging
T Urinary System
3 Magnetic Resonance Imaging (MRI) Computer reformatted digital display of multiplanar images developed from the capture of radio-frequency signals emitted by nuclei in a body site excited within a magnetic field

Body Part Character 4	Contrast Character 5	Qualifier Character 6	Qualifier Character 7
Ø Bladder 1 Kidney, Right 2 Kidney, Left 3 Kidneys, Bilateral 9 Kidney Transplant	Y Other Contrast	Ø Unenhanced and Enhanced Z None	Z None
Ø Bladder 1 Kidney, Right 2 Kidney, Left 3 Kidneys, Bilateral 9 Kidney Transplant	Z None	Z None	Z None

B Imaging
T Urinary System
4 Ultrasonography Real time display of images of anatomy or flow information developed from the capture of relected and attenuated high frequency sound waves

Body Part Character 4	Contrast Character 5	Qualifier Character 6	Qualifier Character 7
Ø Bladder 1 Kidney, Right 2 Kidney, Left 3 Kidneys, Bilateral 5 Urethra 6 Ureter, Right 7 Ureter, Left 8 Ureters, Bilateral 9 Kidney Transplant J Kidneys and Bladder	Z None	Z None	Z None

B Imaging
U Female Reproductive System
Ø Plain Radiography Planar display of an image developed from the capture of external ionizing radiation on photographic or photoconductive plate

Body Part Character 4	Contrast Character 5	Qualifier Character 6	Qualifier Character 7
Ø Fallopian Tube, Right ♀ 1 Fallopian Tube, Left ♀ 2 Fallopian Tubes, Bilateral ♀ 6 Uterus ♀ 8 Uterus and Fallopian Tubes ♀ 9 Vagina ♀	Ø High Osmolar 1 Low Osmolar Y Other Contrast	Z None	Z None

B Imaging
U Female Reproductive System
1 Fluoroscopy Single plane or bi-plane real time display of an image developed from the capture of external ionizing radioation on a fluorescent screen. The image may also be stored by either digital or analog means

Body Part Character 4	Contrast Character 5	Qualifier Character 6	Qualifier Character 7
0 Fallopian Tube, Right ♀ **1** Fallopian Tube, Left ♀ **2** Fallopian Tubes, Bilateral ♀ **6** Uterus ♀ **8** Uterus and Fallopian Tubes ♀ **9** Vagina ♀	**0** High Osmolar **1** Low Osmolar **Y** Other Contrast **Z** None	**Z** None	**Z** None

B Imaging
U Female Reproductive System
3 Magnetic Resonance Imaging (MRI) Computer reformatted digital display of multiplanar images developed from the capture of radio-frequency signals emitted by nuclei in a body site excited within a magnetic field

Body Part Character 4	Contrast Character 5	Qualifier Character 6	Qualifier Character 7
3 Ovary, Right ♀ **4** Ovary, Left ♀ **5** Ovaries, Bilateral ♀ **6** Uterus ♀ **9** Vagina ♀ **B** Pregnant Uterus ♀ **C** Uterus and Ovaries ♀	**Y** Other Contrast	**0** Unenhanced and Enhanced **Z** None	**Z** None
3 Ovary, Right ♀ **4** Ovary, Left ♀ **5** Ovaries, Bilateral ♀ **6** Uterus ♀ **9** Vagina ♀ **B** Pregnant Uterus ♀ **C** Uterus and Ovaries ♀	**Z** None	**Z** None	**Z** None

B Imaging
U Female Reproductive System
4 Ultrasonography Real time display of images of anatomy or flow information developed from the capture of relected and attenuated high frequency sound waves

Body Part Character 4	Contrast Character 5	Qualifier Character 6	Qualifier Character 7
0 Fallopian Tube, Right ♀ **1** Fallopian Tube, Left ♀ **2** Fallopian Tubes, Bilateral ♀ **3** Ovary, Right ♀ **4** Ovary, Left ♀ **5** Ovaries, Bilateral ♀ **6** Uterus ♀ **C** Uterus and Ovaries ♀	**Y** Other Contrast **Z** None	**Z** None	**Z** None

B Imaging
V Male Reproductive System
0 Plain Radiography Planar display of an image developed from the capture of external ionizing radiation on photographic or photoconductive plate

Body Part Character 4	Contrast Character 5	Qualifier Character 6	Qualifier Character 7
0 Corpora Cavernosa ♂ **1** Epididymis, Right ♂ **2** Epididymis, Left ♂ **3** Prostate ♂ **5** Testicle, Right ♂ **6** Testicle, Left ♂ **8** Vasa Vasorum ♂	**0** High Osmolar **1** Low Osmolar **Y** Other Contrast	**Z** None	**Z** None

B Imaging
V Male Reproductive System
1 Fluoroscopy Single plane or bi-plane real time display of an image developed from the capture of external ionizing radioation on a fluorescent screen. The image may also be stored by either digital or analog means

Body Part Character 4	Contrast Character 5	Qualifier Character 6	Qualifier Character 7
0 Corpora Cavernosa ♂ **8** Vasa Vasorum ♂	**0** High Osmolar **1** Low Osmolar **Y** Other Contrast **Z** None	**Z** None	**Z** None

B Imaging
V Male Reproductive System
2 Computerized Tomography (CT Scan) Computer reformatted digital display of multiplanar images developed from the capture of multiple exposures of external ionizing radiation

Body Part Character 4	Contrast Character 5	Qualifier Character 6	Qualifier Character 7
3 Prostate ♂	**0** High Osmolar **1** Low Osmolar **Y** Other Contrast	**0** Unenhanced and Enhanced **Z** None	**Z** None
3 Prostate ♂	**Z** None	**Z** None	**Z** None

B Imaging
V Male Reproductive System
3 Magnetic Resonance Imaging (MRI) Computer reformatted digital display of multiplanar images developed from the capture of radio-frequency signals emitted by nuclei in a body site excited within a magnetic field

Body Part Character 4	Contrast Character 5	Qualifier Character 6	Qualifier Character 7
0 Corpora Cavernosa ♂ **3** Prostate ♂ **4** Scrotum ♂ **5** Testicle, Right ♂ **6** Testicle, Left ♂ **7** Testicles, Bilateral ♂	**Y** Other Contrast	**0** Unenhanced and Enhanced **Z** None	**Z** None
0 Corpora Cavernosa ♂ **3** Prostate ♂ **4** Scrotum ♂ **5** Testicle, Right ♂ **6** Testicle, Left ♂ **7** Testicles, Bilateral ♂	**Z** None	**Z** None	**Z** None

B Imaging
V Male Reproductive System
4 Ultrasonography Real time display of images of anatomy or flow information developed from the capture of relected and attenuated high frequency sound waves

Body Part Character 4	Contrast Character 5	Qualifier Character 6	Qualifier Character 7
4 Scrotum ♂ **9** Prostate and Seminal Vesicles ♂ **B** Penis ♂	**Z** None	**Z** None	**Z** None

B Imaging
W Anatomical Regions
0 Plain Radiography Planar display of an image developed from the capture of external ionizing radiation on photographic or photoconductive plate

Body Part Character 4	Contrast Character 5	Qualifier Character 6	Qualifier Character 7
0 Abdomen **1** Abdomen and Pelvis **3** Chest **B** Long Bones, All **C** Lower Extremity **J** Upper Extremity **K** Whole Body **L** Whole Skeleton **M** Whole Body, Infant	**Z** None	**Z** None	**Z** None

B Imaging
W Anatomical Regions
1 Fluoroscopy Single plane or bi-plane real time display of an image developed from the capture of external ionizing radioation on a fluorescent screen. The image may also be stored by either digital or analog means

Body Part Character 4	Contrast Character 5	Qualifier Character 6	Qualifier Character 7
1 Abdomen and Pelvis **9** Head and Neck **C** Lower Extremity **J** Upper Extremity	**0** High Osmolar **1** Low Osmolar **Y** Other Contrast **Z** None	**Z** None	**Z** None

B Imaging
W Anatomical Regions
2 Computerized Tomography (CT Scan) Computer reformatted digital display of multiplanar images developed from the capture of multiple exposures of external ionizing radiation

Body Part Character 4	Contrast Character 5	Qualifier Character 6	Qualifier Character 7
Ø Abdomen **1** Abdomen and Pelvis **4** Chest and Abdomen **5** Chest, Abdomen and Pelvis **8** Head **9** Head and Neck **F** Neck **G** Pelvic Region	**Ø** High Osmolar **1** Low Osmolar **Y** Other Contrast	**Ø** Unenhanced and Enhanced **Z** None	**Z** None
Ø Abdomen **1** Abdomen and Pelvis **4** Chest and Abdomen **5** Chest, Abdomen and Pelvis **8** Head **9** Head and Neck **F** Neck **G** Pelvic Region	**Z** None	**Z** None	**Z** None

B Imaging
W Anatomical Regions
3 Magnetic Resonance Imaging (MRI) Computer reformatted digital display of multiplanar images developed from the capture of radio-frequency signals emitted by nuclei in a body site excited within a magnetic field

Body Part Character 4	Contrast Character 5	Qualifier Character 6	Qualifier Character 7
Ø Abdomen **3** Chest **8** Head **F** Neck **G** Pelvic Region **H** Retroperitoneum **P** Brachial Plexus	**Y** Other Contrast	**Ø** Unenhanced and Enhanced **Z** None	**Z** None
Ø Abdomen **8** Head **F** Neck **G** Pelvic Region **H** Retroperitoneum **P** Brachial Plexus	**Z** None	**Z** None	**Z** None

B Imaging
W Anatomical Regions
4 Ultrasonography Real time display of images of anatomy or flow information developed from the capture of relected and attenuated high frequency sound waves

Body Part Character 4	Contrast Character 5	Qualifier Character 6	Qualifier Character 7
Ø Abdomen **1** Abdomen and Pelvis **F** Neck **G** Pelvic Region	**Z** None	**Z** None	**Z** None

B Imaging
Y Fetus and Obstetrical
3 Magnetic Resonance Imaging (MRI) Computer reformatted digital display of multiplanar images developed from the capture of radio-frequency signals emitted by nuclei in a body site excited within a magnetic field

Body Part Character 4	Contrast Character 5	Qualifier Character 6	Qualifier Character 7
0 Fetal Head ♀ **1** Fetal Heart ♀ **2** Fetal Thorax ♀ **3** Fetal Abdomen ♀ **4** Fetal Spine ♀ **5** Fetal Extremities ♀ **6** Whole Fetus ♀	**Y** Other Contrast	**0** Unenhanced and Enhanced **Z** None	**Z** None
0 Fetal Head ♀ **1** Fetal Heart ♀ **2** Fetal Thorax ♀ **3** Fetal Abdomen ♀ **4** Fetal Spine ♀ **5** Fetal Extremities ♀ **6** Whole Fetus ♀	**Z** None	**Z** None	**Z** None

B Imaging
Y Fetus and Obstetrical
4 Ultrasonography Real time display of images of anatomy or flow information developed from the capture of relected and attenuated high frequency sound waves

Body Part Character 4	Contrast Character 5	Qualifier Character 6	Qualifier Character 7
7 Fetal Umbilical Cord ♀ **8** Placenta ♀ **9** First Trimester, Single Fetus ♀ **B** First Trimester, Multiple Gestation ♀ **C** Second Trimester, Single Fetus ♀ **D** Second Trimester, Multiple Gestation ♀ **F** Third Trimester, Single Fetus ♀ **G** Third Trimester, Multiple Gestation ♀	**Z** None	**Z** None	**Z** None

Nuclear Medicine C01–CW7

C Nuclear Medicine
0 Central Nervous System
1 Planar Nuclear Medicine Imaging Introduction of radioactive materials into the body for single plane display of images developed from the capture of radioactive emissions

Body Part Character 4	Radionuclide Character 5	Qualifier Character 6	Qualifier Character 7
0 Brain	1 Technetium 99m (Tc-99m) Y Other Radionuclide	Z None	Z None
5 Cerebrospinal Fluid	D Indium 111 (In-111) Y Other Radionuclide	Z None	Z None
Y Central Nervous System	Y Other Radionuclide	Z None	Z None

C Nuclear Medicine
0 Central Nervous System
2 Tomographic (Tomo) Nuclear Medicine Imaging Introduction of radioactive materials into the body for three dimensional display of images developed from the capture of radioactive emissions

Body Part Character 4	Radionuclide Character 5	Qualifier Character 6	Qualifier Character 7
0 Brain	1 Technetium 99m (Tc-99m) F Iodine 123 (I-123) S Thallium 201 (Tl-201) Y Other Radionuclide	Z None	Z None
5 Cerebrospinal Fluid	D Indium 111 (In-111) Y Other Radionuclide	Z None	Z None
Y Central Nervous System	Y Other Radionuclide	Z None	Z None

C Nuclear Medicine
0 Central Nervous System
3 Positron Emission Tomographic (PET) Imaging Introduction of radioactive materials into the body for three dimensional display of images developed from the simultaneous capture, 180 degrees apart, of radioactive emissions

Body Part Character 4	Radionuclide Character 5	Qualifier Character 6	Qualifier Character 7
0 Brain	B Carbon 11 (C-11) K Fluorine 18 (F-18) M Oxygen 15 (O-15) Y Other Radionuclide	Z None	Z None
Y Central Nervous System	Y Other Radionuclide	Z None	Z None

C Nuclear Medicine
0 Central Nervous System
5 Nonimaging Nuclear Medicine Probe Introduction of radioactive materials into the body for the study of distribution and fate of certain substances by the detection of radioactive emissions; or, alternatively, measurement of absorption of radioactive emissions from an external source

Body Part Character 4	Radionuclide Character 5	Qualifier Character 6	Qualifier Character 7
0 Brain	V Xenon 133 (Xe-133) Y Other Radionuclide	Z None	Z None
Y Central Nervous System	Y Other Radionuclide	Z None	Z None

C Nuclear Medicine
2 Heart
1 Planar Nuclear Medicine Imaging Introduction of radioactive materials into the body for single plane display of images developed from the capture of radioactive emissions

Body Part Character 4	Radionuclide Character 5	Qualifier Character 6	Qualifier Character 7
6 Heart, Right and Left	1 Technetium 99m (Tc-99m) Y Other Radionuclide	Z None	Z None
G Myocardium	1 Technetium 99m (Tc-99m) D Indium 111 (In-111) S Thallium 201 (Tl-201) Y Other Radionuclide Z None	Z None	Z None
Y Heart	Y Other Radionuclide	Z None	Z None

C Nuclear Medicine
2 Heart
2 Tomographic (Tomo) Nuclear Medicine Imaging Introduction of radioactive materials into the body for three dimensional display of images developed from the capture of radioactive emissions

Body Part Character 4	Radionuclide Character 5	Qualifier Character 6	Qualifier Character 7
6 Heart, Right and Left	**1** Technetium 99m (Tc-99m) **Y** Other Radionuclide	**Z** None	**Z** None
G Myocardium	**1** Technetium 99m (Tc-99m) **D** Indium 111 (In-111) **K** Fluorine 18 (F-18) **S** Thallium 201 (Tl-201) **Y** Other Radionuclide **Z** None	**Z** None	**Z** None
Y Heart	**Y** Other Radionuclide	**Z** None	**Z** None

C Nuclear Medicine
2 Heart
3 Positron Emission Tomographic (PET) Imaging Introduction of radioactive materials into the body for three dimensional display of images developed from the simultaneous capture, 180 degrees apart, of radioactive emissions

Body Part Character 4	Radionuclide Character 5	Qualifier Character 6	Qualifier Character 7
G Myocardium	**K** Fluorine 18 (F-18) **M** Oxygen 15 (O-15) **Q** Rubidium 82 (Rb-82) **R** Nitrogen 13 (N-13) **Y** Other Radionuclide	**Z** None	**Z** None
Y Heart	**Y** Other Radionuclide	**Z** None	**Z** None

C Nuclear Medicine
2 Heart
5 Nonimaging Nuclear Medicine Probe Introduction of radioactive materials into the body for the study of distribution and fate of certain substances by the detection of radioactive emissions; or, alternatively, measurement of absorption of radioactive emissions from an external source

Body Part Character 4	Radionuclide Character 5	Qualifier Character 6	Qualifier Character 7
6 Heart, Right and Left	**1** Technetium 99m (Tc-99m) **Y** Other Radionuclide	**Z** None	**Z** None
Y Heart	**Y** Other Radionuclide	**Z** None	**Z** None

C Nuclear Medicine
5 Veins
1 Planar Nuclear Medicine Imaging Introduction of radioactive materials into the body for single plane display of images developed from the capture of radioactive emissions

Body Part Character 4	Radionuclide Character 5	Qualifier Character 6	Qualifier Character 7
B Lower Extremity Veins, Right **C** Lower Extremity Veins, Left **D** Lower Extremity Veins, Bilateral **N** Upper Extremity Veins, Right **P** Upper Extremity Veins, Left **Q** Upper Extremity Veins, Bilateral **R** Central Veins	**1** Technetium 99m (Tc-99m) **Y** Other Radionuclide	**Z** None	**Z** None
Y Veins	**Y** Other Radionuclide	**Z** None	**Z** None

C Nuclear Medicine
7 Lymphatic and Hematologic System
1 Planar Nuclear Medicine Imaging Introduction of radioactive materials into the body for single plane display of images developed from the capture of radioactive emissions

Body Part Character 4	Radionuclide Character 5	Qualifier Character 6	Qualifier Character 7
0 Bone Marrow	**1** Technetium 99m (Tc-99m) **D** Indium 111 (In-111) **Y** Other Radionuclide	**Z** None	**Z** None
2 Spleen **5** Lymphatics, Head and Neck **D** Lymphatics, Pelvic **J** Lymphatics, Head **K** Lymphatics, Neck **L** Lymphatics, Upper Chest **M** Lymphatics, Trunk **N** Lymphatics, Upper Extremity **P** Lymphatics, Lower Extremity	**1** Technetium 99m (Tc-99m) **Y** Other Radionuclide	**Z** None	**Z** None
3 Blood	**D** Indium 111 (In-111) **Y** Other Radionuclide	**Z** None	**Z** None
Y Lymphatic and Hematologic System	**Y** Other Radionuclide	**Z** None	**Z** None

C Nuclear Medicine
7 Lymphatic and Hematologic System
2 Tomographic (Tomo) Nuclear Medicine Imaging Introduction of radioactive materials into the body for three dimensional display of images developed from the capture of radioactive emissions

Body Part Character 4	Radionuclide Character 5	Qualifier Character 6	Qualifier Character 7
2 Spleen	**1** Technetium 99m (Tc-99m) **Y** Other Radionuclide	**Z** None	**Z** None
Y Lymphatic and Hematologic System	**Y** Other Radionuclide	**Z** None	**Z** None

C Nuclear Medicine
7 Lymphatic and Hematologic System
5 Nonimaging Nuclear Medicine Probe Introduction of radioactive materials into the body for the study of distribution and fate of certain substances by the detection of radioactive emissions; or, alternatively, measurement of absorption of radioactive emissions from an external source

Body Part Character 4	Radionuclide Character 5	Qualifier Character 6	Qualifier Character 7
5 Lymphatics, Head and Neck **D** Lymphatics, Pelvic **J** Lymphatics, Head **K** Lymphatics, Neck **L** Lymphatics, Upper Chest **M** Lymphatics, Trunk **N** Lymphatics, Upper Extremity **P** Lymphatics, Lower Extremity	**1** Technetium 99m (Tc-99m) **Y** Other Radionuclide	**Z** None	**Z** None
Y Lymphatic and Hematologic System	**Y** Other Radionuclide	**Z** None	**Z** None

C Nuclear Medicine
7 Lymphatic and Hematologic System
6 Nonimaging Nuclear Medicine Assay Introduction of radioactive materials into the body for the study of body fluids and blood elements, by the detection of radioactive emissions

Body Part Character 4	Radionuclide Character 5	Qualifier Character 6	Qualifier Character 7
3 Blood	**1** Technetium 99m (Tc-99m) **7** Cobalt 58 (Co-58) **C** Cobalt 57 (Co-57) **D** Indium 111 (In-111) **H** Iodine 125 (I-125) **W** Chromium (Cr-51) **Y** Other Radionuclide	**Z** None	**Z** None
Y Lymphatic and Hematologic System	**Y** Other Radionuclide	**Z** None	**Z** None

C Nuclear Medicine
8 Eye
1 Planar Nuclear Medicine Imaging Introduction of radioactive materials into the body for single plane display of images developed from the capture of radioactive emissions

Body Part Character 4	Radionuclide Character 5	Qualifier Character 6	Qualifier Character 7
9 Lacrimal Ducts, Bilateral	1 Technetium 99m (Tc-99m) Y Other Radionuclide	Z None	Z None
Y Eye	Y Other Radionuclide	Z None	Z None

C Nuclear Medicine
9 Ear, Nose, Mouth and Throat
1 Planar Nuclear Medicine Imaging Introduction of radioactive materials into the body for single plane display of images developed from the capture of radioactive emissions

Body Part Character 4	Radionuclide Character 5	Qualifier Character 6	Qualifier Character 7
B Salivary Glands, Bilateral	1 Technetium 99m (Tc-99m) Y Other Radionuclide	Z None	Z None
Y Ear, Nose, Mouth and Throat	Y Other Radionuclide	Z None	Z None

C Nuclear Medicine
B Respiratory System
1 Planar Nuclear Medicine Imaging Introduction of radioactive materials into the body for single plane display of images developed from the capture of radioactive emissions

Body Part Character 4	Radionuclide Character 5	Qualifier Character 6	Qualifier Character 7
2 Lungs and Bronchi	1 Technetium 99m (Tc-99m) 9 Krypton (Kr-81m) T Xenon 127 (Xe-127) V Xenon 133 (Xe-133) Y Other Radionuclide	Z None	Z None
Y Respiratory System	Y Other Radionuclide	Z None	Z None

C Nuclear Medicine
B Respiratory System
2 Tomographic (Tomo) Nuclear Medicine Imaging Introduction of radioactive materials into the body for three dimensional display of images developed from the capture of radioactive emissions

Body Part Character 4	Radionuclide Character 5	Qualifier Character 6	Qualifier Character 7
2 Lungs and Bronchi	1 Technetium 99m (Tc-99m) 9 Krypton (Kr-81m) Y Other Radionuclide	Z None	Z None
Y Respiratory System	Y Other Radionuclide	Z None	Z None

C Nuclear Medicine
B Respiratory System
3 Positron Emission Tomographic (PET) Imaging Introduction of radioactive materials into the body for three dimensional display of images developed from the simultaneous capture, 180 degrees apart, of radioactive emissions

Body Part Character 4	Radionuclide Character 5	Qualifier Character 6	Qualifier Character 7
2 Lungs and Bronchi	K Fluorine 18 (F-18) Y Other Radionuclide	Z None	Z None
Y Respiratory System	Y Other Radionuclide	Z None	Z None

C Nuclear Medicine
D Gastrointestinal System
1 Planar Nuclear Medicine Imaging Introduction of radioactive materials into the body for single plane display of images developed from the capture of radioactive emissions

Body Part Character 4	Radionuclide Character 5	Qualifier Character 6	Qualifier Character 7
5 Upper Gastrointestinal Tract 7 Gastrointestinal Tract	1 Technetium 99m (Tc-99m) D Indium 111 (In-111) Y Other Radionuclide	Z None	Z None
Y Digestive System	Y Other Radionuclide	Z None	Z None

C Nuclear Medicine
D Gastrointestinal System
2 Tomographic (Tomo) Nuclear Medicine Imaging Introduction of radioactive materials into the body for three dimensional display of images developed from the capture of radioactive emissions

Body Part Character 4	Radionuclide Character 5	Qualifier Character 6	Qualifier Character 7
7 Gastrointestinal Tract	**1** Technetium 99m (Tc-99m) **D** Indium 111 (In-111) **Y** Other Radionuclide	**Z** None	**Z** None
Y Digestive System	**Y** Other Radionuclide	**Z** None	**Z** None

C Nuclear Medicine
F Hepatobiliary System and Pancreas
1 Planar Nuclear Medicine Imaging Introduction of radioactive materials into the body for single plane display of images developed from the capture of radioactive emissions

Body Part Character 4	Radionuclide Character 5	Qualifier Character 6	Qualifier Character 7
4 Gallbladder **5** Liver **6** Liver and Spleen **C** Hepatobiliary System, All	**1** Technetium 99m (Tc-99m) **Y** Other Radionuclide	**Z** None	**Z** None
Y Hepatobiliary System and Pancreas	**Y** Other Radionuclide	**Z** None	**Z** None

C Nuclear Medicine
F Hepatobiliary System and Pancreas
2 Tomographic (Tomo) Nuclear Medicine Imaging Introduction of radioactive materials into the body for three dimensional display of images developed from the capture of radioactive emissions

Body Part Character 4	Radionuclide Character 5	Qualifier Character 6	Qualifier Character 7
4 Gallbladder **5** Liver **6** Liver and Spleen	**1** Technetium 99m (Tc-99m) **Y** Other Radionuclide	**Z** None	**Z** None
Y Hepatobiliary System and Pancreas	**Y** Other Radionuclide	**Z** None	**Z** None

C Nuclear Medicine
G Endocrine System
1 Planar Nuclear Medicine Imaging Introduction of radioactive materials into the body for single plane display of images developed from the capture of radioactive emissions

Body Part Character 4	Radionuclide Character 5	Qualifier Character 6	Qualifier Character 7
1 Parathyroid Glands	**1** Technetium 99m (Tc-99m) **S** Thallium 201 (Tl-201) **Y** Other Radionuclide	**Z** None	**Z** None
2 Thyroid Gland	**1** Technetium 99m (Tc-99m) **F** Iodine 123 (I-123) **G** Iodine 131 (I-131) **Y** Other Radionuclide	**Z** None	**Z** None
4 Adrenal Glands, Bilateral	**G** Iodine 131 (I-131) **Y** Other Radionuclide	**Z** None	**Z** None
Y Endocrine System	**Y** Other Radionuclide	**Z** None	**Z** None

C Nuclear Medicine
G Endocrine System
2 Tomographic (Tomo) Nuclear Medicine Imaging Introduction of radioactive materials into the body for three dimensional display of images developed from the capture of radioactive emissions

Body Part Character 4	Radionuclide Character 5	Qualifier Character 6	Qualifier Character 7
1 Parathyroid Glands	**1** Technetium 99m (Tc-99m) **S** Thallium 201 (Tl-201) **Y** Other Radionuclide	**Z** None	**Z** None
Y Endocrine System	**Y** Other Radionuclide	**Z** None	**Z** None

C Nuclear Medicine
G Endocrine System
4 Nonimaging Nuclear Medicine Uptake Introduction of radioactive materials into the body for measurements of organ function, from the detection of radioactive emmissions

Body Part Character 4	Radionuclide Character 5	Qualifier Character 6	Qualifier Character 7
2 Thyroid Gland	1 Technetium 99m (Tc-99m) F Iodine 123 (I-123) G Iodine 131 (I-131) Y Other Radionuclide	Z None	Z None
Y Endocrine System	Y Other Radionuclide	Z None	Z None

C Nuclear Medicine
H Skin, Subcutaneous Tissue and Breast
1 Planar Nuclear Medicine Imaging Introduction of radioactive materials into the body for single plane display of images developed from the capture of radioactive emissions

Body Part Character 4	Radionuclide Character 5	Qualifier Character 6	Qualifier Character 7
Ø Breast, Right 1 Breast, Left 2 Breasts, Bilateral	1 Technetium 99m (Tc-99m) S Thallium 2Ø1 (Tl-2Ø1) Y Other Radionuclide	Z None	Z None
Y Skin, Subcutaneous Tissue and Breast	Y Other Radionuclide	Z None	Z None

C Nuclear Medicine
H Skin, Subcutaneous Tissue and Breast
2 Tomographic (Tomo) Nuclear Medicine Imaging Introduction of radioactive materials into the body for three dimensional display of images developed from the capture of radioactive emissions

Body Part Character 4	Radionuclide Character 5	Qualifier Character 6	Qualifier Character 7
Ø Breast, Right 1 Breast, Left 2 Breasts, Bilateral	1 Technetium 99m (Tc-99m) S Thallium 2Ø1 (Tl-2Ø1) Y Other Radionuclide	Z None	Z None
Y Skin, Subcutaneous Tissue and Breast	Y Other Radionuclide	Z None	Z None

C Nuclear Medicine
P Musculoskeletal System
1 Planar Nuclear Medicine Imaging Introduction of radioactive materials into the body for single plane display of images developed from the capture of radioactive emissions

Body Part Character 4	Radionuclide Character 5	Qualifier Character 6	Qualifier Character 7
1 Skull 4 Thorax 5 Spine 6 Pelvis 7 Spine and Pelvis 8 Upper Extremity, Right 9 Upper Extremity, Left B Upper Extremities, Bilateral C Lower Extremity, Right D Lower Extremity, Left F Lower Extremities, Bilateral Z Musculoskeletal System, All	1 Technetium 99m (Tc-99m) Y Other Radionuclide	Z None	Z None
Y Musculoskeletal System, Other	Y Other Radionuclide	Z None	Z None

C Nuclear Medicine
P Musculoskeletal System
2 Tomographic (Tomo) Nuclear Medicine Imaging Introduction of radioactive materials into the body for three dimensional display of images developed from the capture of radioactive emissions

Body Part Character 4	Radionuclide Character 5	Qualifier Character 6	Qualifier Character 7
1 Skull **2** Cervical Spine **3** Skull and Cervical Spine **4** Thorax **6** Pelvis **7** Spine and Pelvis **8** Upper Extremity, Right **9** Upper Extremity, Left **B** Upper Extremities, Bilateral **C** Lower Extremity, Right **D** Lower Extremity, Left **F** Lower Extremities, Bilateral **G** Thoracic Spine **H** Lumbar Spine **J** Thoracolumbar Spine	**1** Technetium 99m (Tc-99m) **Y** Other Radionuclide	**Z** None	**Z** None
Y Musculoskeletal System, Other	**Y** Other Radionuclide	**Z** None	**Z** None

C Nuclear Medicine
P Musculoskeletal System
5 Nonimaging Nuclear Medicine Probe Introduction of radioactive materials into the body for the study of distribution and fate of certain substances by the detection of radioactive emissions; or, alternatively, measurement of absorption of radioactive emissions from an external source

Body Part Character 4	Radionuclide Character 5	Qualifier Character 6	Qualifier Character 7
5 Spine **N** Upper Extremities **P** Lower Extremities	**Z** None	**Z** None	**Z** None
Y Musculoskeletal System, Other	**Y** Other Radionuclide	**Z** None	**Z** None

C Nuclear Medicine
T Urinary System
1 Planar Nuclear Medicine Imaging Introduction of radioactive materials into the body for single plane display of images developed from the capture of radioactive emissions

Body Part Character 4	Radionuclide Character 5	Qualifier Character 6	Qualifier Character 7
3 Kidneys, Ureters and Bladder	**1** Technetium 99m (Tc-99m) **F** Iodine 123 (I-123) **G** Iodine 131 (I-131) **Y** Other Radionuclide	**Z** None	**Z** None
H Bladder and Ureters	**1** Technetium 99m (Tc-99m) **Y** Other Radionuclide	**Z** None	**Z** None
Y Urinary System	**Y** Other Radionuclide	**Z** None	**Z** None

C Nuclear Medicine
T Urinary System
2 Tomographic (Tomo) Nuclear Medicine Imaging Introduction of radioactive materials into the body for three dimensional display of images developed from the capture of radioactive emissions

Body Part Character 4	Radionuclide Character 5	Qualifier Character 6	Qualifier Character 7
3 Kidneys, Ureters and Bladder	**1** Technetium 99m (Tc-99m) **Y** Other Radionuclide	**Z** None	**Z** None
Y Urinary System	**Y** Other Radionuclide	**Z** None	**Z** None

C Nuclear Medicine
T Urinary System
6 Nonimaging Nuclear Medicine Assay Introduction of radioactive materials into the body for the study of body fluids and blood elements, by the detection of radioactive emissions

Body Part Character 4	Radionuclide Character 5	Qualifier Character 6	Qualifier Character 7
3 Kidneys, Ureters and Bladder	**1** Technetium 99m (Tc-99m) **F** Iodine 123 (I-123) **G** Iodine 131 (I-131) **H** Iodine 125 (I-125) **Y** Other Radionuclide	**Z** None	**Z** None
Y Urinary System	**Y** Other Radionuclide	**Z** None	**Z** None

C Nuclear Medicine
V Male Reproductive System
1 Planar Nuclear Medicine Imaging Introduction of radioactive materials into the body for single plane display of images developed from the capture of radioactive emissions

Body Part Character 4	Radionuclide Character 5	Qualifier Character 6	Qualifier Character 7
9 Testicles, Bilateral	**1** Technetium 99m (Tc-99m) **Y** Other Radionuclide	**Z** None	**Z** None
Y Male Reproductive System	**Y** Other Radionuclide	**Z** None	**Z** None

C Nuclear Medicine
W Anatomical Regions
1 Planar Nuclear Medicine Imaging Introduction of radioactive materials into the body for single plane display of images developed from the capture of radioactive emissions

Body Part Character 4	Radionuclide Character 5	Qualifier Character 6	Qualifier Character 7
Ø Abdomen **1** Abdomen and Pelvis **4** Chest and Abdomen **6** Chest and Neck **B** Head and Neck **D** Lower Extremity **J** Pelvic Region **M** Upper Extremity **N** Whole Body	**1** Technetium 99m (Tc-99m) **D** Indium 111 (In-111) **F** Iodine 123 (I-123) **G** Iodine 131 (I-131) **L** Gallium 67 (Ga-67) **S** Thallium 2Ø1 (Tl-2Ø1) **Y** Other Radionuclide	**Z** None	**Z** None
3 Chest	**1** Technetium 99m (Tc-99m) **D** Indium 111 (In-111) **F** Iodine 123 (I-123) **G** Iodine 131 (I-131) **K** Fluorine 18 (F-18) **L** Gallium 67 (Ga-67) **S** Thallium 2Ø1 (Tl-2Ø1) **Y** Other Radionuclide	**Z** None	**Z** None
Y Anatomical Regions, Multiple	**Y** Other Radionuclide	**Z** None	**Z** None
Z Anatomical Region, Other	**Z** None	**Z** None	**Z** None

C Nuclear Medicine
W Anatomical Regions
2 Tomographic (Tomo) Nuclear Medicine Imaging Introduction of radioactive materials into the body for three dimensional display of images developed from the capture of radioactive emissions

Body Part Character 4	Radionuclide Character 5	Qualifier Character 6	Qualifier Character 7
Ø Abdomen **1** Abdomen and Pelvis **3** Chest **4** Chest and Abdomen **6** Chest and Neck **B** Head and Neck **D** Lower Extremity **J** Pelvic Region **M** Upper Extremity	**1** Technetium 99m (Tc-99m) **D** Indium 111 (In-111) **F** Iodine 123 (I-123) **G** Iodine 131 (I-131) **K** Fluorine 18 (F-18) **L** Gallium 67 (Ga-67) **S** Thallium 2Ø1 (Tl-2Ø1) **Y** Other Radionuclide	**Z** None	**Z** None
Y Anatomical Regions, Multiple	**Y** Other Radionuclide	**Z** None	**Z** None

C Nuclear Medicine
W Anatomical Regions
3 Positron Emission Tomographic (PET) Imaging Introduction of radioactive materials into the body for three dimensional display of images developed from the simultaneous capture, 18Ø degrees apart, of radioactive emissions

Body Part Character 4	Radionuclide Character 5	Qualifier Character 6	Qualifier Character 7
N Whole Body	**Y** Other Radionuclide	**Z** None	**Z** None

C Nuclear Medicine
W Anatomical Regions
5 Nonimaging Nuclear Medicine Probe Introduction of radioactive materials into the body for the study of distribution and fate of certain substances by the detection of radioactive emissions; or, alternatively, measurement of absorption of radioactive emissions from an external source

Body Part Character 4	Radionuclide Character 5	Qualifier Character 6	Qualifier Character 7
Ø Abdomen 1 Abdomen and Pelvis 3 Chest 4 Chest and Abdomen 6 Chest and Neck B Head and Neck D Lower Extremity J Pelvic Region M Upper Extremity	1 Technetium 99m (Tc-99m) D Indium 111 (In-111) Y Other Radionuclide	Z None	Z None

C Nuclear Medicine
W Anatomical Regions
7 Systemic Nuclear Medicine Therapy Introduction of radioactive materials into the body for treatment

Body Part Character 4	Radionuclide Character 5	Qualifier Character 6	Qualifier Character 7
Ø Abdomen 3 Chest	N Phosphorus 32 (P-32) Y Other Radionuclide	Z None	Z None
G Thyroid	G Iodine 131 (I-131) Y Other Radionuclide	Z None	Z None
N Whole Body	8 Samarium 153 (Sm-153) G Iodine 131 (I-131) N Phosphorus 32 (P-32) P Strontium 89 (Sr-89) Y Other Radionuclide	Z None	Z None
Y Anatomical Regions, Multiple	Y Other Radionuclide	Z None	Z None

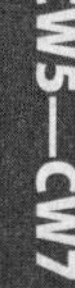

Radiation Therapy DØØ–DWY

D Radiation Therapy
Ø Central and Peripheral Nervous System
Ø Beam Radiation

Treatment Site Character 4	Modal. Qualifier Character 5	Isotope Character 6	Qualifier Character 7
Ø Brain 1 Brain Stem 6 Spinal Cord 7 Peripheral Nerve	Ø Photons <1 MeV 1 Photons 1-1Ø MeV 2 Photons >1Ø MeV 4 Heavy Particles (Protons, Ions) 5 Neutrons 6 Neutron Capture	Z None	Z None
Ø Brain 1 Brain Stem 6 Spinal Cord 7 Peripheral Nerve	3 Electrons	Z None	Ø Intraoperative Z None

D Radiation Therapy
Ø Central and Peripheral Nervous System
1 Brachytherapy

Treatment Site Character 4	Modal. Qualifier Character 5	Isotope Character 6	Qualifier Character 7
Ø Brain 1 Brain Stem 6 Spinal Cord 7 Peripheral Nerve	9 High Dose Rate (HDR) B Low Dose Rate (LDR)	7 Cesium 137 (Cs-137) 8 Iridium 192 (Ir-192) 9 Iodine 125 (I-125) B Palladium 1Ø3 (Pd-1Ø3) C Californium 252 (Cf-252) Y Other Isotope	Z None

D Radiation Therapy
Ø Central and Peripheral Nervous System
2 Stereotactic Radiosurgery

Treatment Site Character 4	Modal. Qualifier Character 5	Isotope Character 6	Qualifier Character 7
Ø Brain 1 Brain Stem 6 Spinal Cord 7 Peripheral Nerve	D Stereotactic Other Photon Radiosurgery H Stereotactic Particulate Radiosurgery J Stereotactic Gamma Beam Radiosurgery	Z None	Z None

DRG Non-OR For all body part, approach, device, and qualifier values

D Radiation Therapy
Ø Central and Peripheral Nervous System
Y Other Radiation

Treatment Site Character 4	Modal. Qualifier Character 5	Isotope Character 6	Qualifier Character 7
Ø Brain 1 Brain Stem 6 Spinal Cord 7 Peripheral Nerve	7 Contact Radiation 8 Hyperthermia F Plaque Radiation K Laser Interstitial Thermal Therapy	Z None	Z None

D Radiation Therapy
7 Lymphatic and Hematologic System
Ø Beam Radiation

Treatment Site Character 4	Modal. Qualifier Character 5	Isotope Character 6	Qualifier Character 7
Ø Bone Marrow 1 Thymus 2 Spleen 3 Lymphatics, Neck 4 Lymphatics, Axillary 5 Lymphatics, Thorax 6 Lymphatics, Abdomen 7 Lymphatics, Pelvis 8 Lymphatics, Inguinal	Ø Photons <1 MeV 1 Photons 1- 1Ø MeV 2 Photons >1Ø MeV 4 Heavy Particles (Protons, Ions) 5 Neutrons 6 Neutron Capture	Z None	Z None
Ø Bone Marrow 1 Thymus 2 Spleen 3 Lymphatics, Neck 4 Lymphatics, Axillary 5 Lymphatics, Thorax 6 Lymphatics, Abdomen 7 Lymphatics, Pelvis 8 Lymphatics, Inguinal	3 Electrons	Z None	Ø Intraoperative Z None

D Radiation Therapy
7 Lymphatic and Hematologic System
1 Brachytherapy

Treatment Site Character 4	Modal. Qualifier Character 5	Isotope Character 6	Qualifier Character 7
Ø Bone Marrow 1 Thymus 2 Spleen 3 Lymphatics, Neck 4 Lymphatics, Axillary 5 Lymphatics, Thorax 6 Lymphatics, Abdomen 7 Lymphatics, Pelvis 8 Lymphatics, Inguinal	9 High Dose Rate (HDR) B Low Dose Rate (LDR)	7 Cesium 137 (Cs-137) 8 Iridium 192 (Ir-192) 9 Iodine 125 (I-125) B Palladium 1Ø3 (Pd-1Ø3) C Californium 252 (Cf-252) Y Other Isotope	Z None

D Radiation Therapy
7 Lymphatic and Hematologic System
2 Stereotactic Radiosurgery

Treatment Site Character 4	Modal. Qualifier Character 5	Isotope Character 6	Qualifier Character 7
Ø Bone Marrow 1 Thymus 2 Spleen 3 Lymphatics, Neck 4 Lymphatics, Axillary 5 Lymphatics, Thorax 6 Lymphatics, Abdomen 7 Lymphatics, Pelvis 8 Lymphatics, Inguinal	D Stereotactic Other Photon Radiosurgery H Stereotactic Particulate Radiosurgery J Stereotactic Gamma Beam Radiosurgery	Z None	Z None

DRG Non-OR For all body part, approach, device, and qualifier values

D Radiation Therapy
7 Lymphatic and Hematologic System
Y Other Radiation

Treatment Site Character 4	Modal. Qualifier Character 5	Isotope Character 6	Qualifier Character 7
Ø Bone Marrow 1 Thymus 2 Spleen 3 Lymphatics, Neck 4 Lymphatics, Axillary 5 Lymphatics, Thorax 6 Lymphatics, Abdomen 7 Lymphatics, Pelvis 8 Lymphatics, Inguinal	8 Hyperthermia F Plaque Radiation	Z None	Z None

D Radiation Therapy
8 Eye
Ø Beam Radiation

Treatment Site Character 4	Modal. Qualifier Character 5	Isotope Character 6	Qualifier Character 7
Ø Eye	**Ø** Photons <1 MeV **1** Photons 1- 1Ø MeV **2** Photons >1Ø MeV **4** Heavy Particles (Protons, Ions) **5** Neutrons **6** Neutron Capture	**Z** None	**Z** None
Ø Eye	**3** Electrons	**Z** None	**Ø** Intraoperative **Z** None

D Radiation Therapy
8 Eye
1 Brachytherapy

Treatment Site Character 4	Modal. Qualifier Character 5	Isotope Character 6	Qualifier Character 7
Ø Eye	**9** High Dose Rate (HDR) **B** Low Dose Rate (LDR)	**7** Cesium 137 (Cs-137) **8** Iridium 192 (Ir-192) **9** Iodine 125 (I-125) **B** Palladium 1Ø3 (Pd-1Ø3) **C** Californium 252 (Cf-252) **Y** Other Isotope	**Z** None

D Radiation Therapy
8 Eye
2 Stereotactic Radiosurgery

Treatment Site Character 4	Modal. Qualifier Character 5	Isotope Character 6	Qualifier Character 7
Ø Eye	**D** Stereotactic Other Photon Radiosurgery **H** Stereotactic Particulate Radiosurgery **J** Stereotactic Gamma Beam Radiosurgery	**Z** None	**Z** None

DRG Non-OR For all body part, approach, device, and qualifier values

D Radiation Therapy
8 Eye
Y Other Radiation

Treatment Site Character 4	Modal. Qualifier Character 5	Isotope Character 6	Qualifier Character 7
Ø Eye	**7** Contact Radiation **8** Hyperthermia **F** Plaque Radiation	**Z** None	**Z** None

D Radiation Therapy
9 Ear, Nose, Mouth and Throat
0 Beam Radiation

Treatment Site Character 4	Modal. Qualifier Character 5	Isotope Character 6	Qualifier Character 7
0 Ear 1 Nose 3 Hypopharynx 4 Mouth 5 Tongue 6 Salivary Glands 7 Sinuses 8 Hard Palate 9 Soft Palate B Larynx D Nasopharynx F Oropharynx	0 Photons <1 MeV 1 Photons 1- 10 MeV 2 Photons >10 MeV 4 Heavy Particles (Protons, Ions) 5 Neutrons 6 Neutron Capture	Z None	Z None
0 Ear 1 Nose 3 Hypopharynx 4 Mouth 5 Tongue 6 Salivary Glands 7 Sinuses 8 Hard Palate 9 Soft Palate B Larynx D Nasopharynx F Oropharynx	3 Electrons	Z None	0 Intraoperative Z None

D Radiation Therapy
9 Ear, Nose, Mouth and Throat
1 Brachytherapy

Treatment Site Character 4	Modal. Qualifier Character 5	Isotope Character 6	Qualifier Character 7
0 Ear 1 Nose 3 Hypopharynx 4 Mouth 5 Tongue 6 Salivary Glands 7 Sinuses 8 Hard Palate 9 Soft Palate B Larynx D Nasopharynx F Oropharynx	9 High Dose Rate (HDR) B Low Dose Rate (LDR)	7 Cesium 137 (Cs-137) 8 Iridium 192 (Ir-192) 9 Iodine 125 (I-125) B Palladium 103 (Pd-103) C Californium 252 (Cf-252) Y Other Isotope	Z None

D Radiation Therapy
9 Ear, Nose, Mouth and Throat
2 Stereotactic Radiosurgery

Treatment Site Character 4	Modal. Qualifier Character 5	Isotope Character 6	Qualifier Character 7
0 Ear 1 Nose 4 Mouth 5 Tongue 6 Salivary Glands 7 Sinuses 8 Hard Palate 9 Soft Palate B Larynx C Pharynx D Nasopharynx	D Stereotactic Other Photon Radiosurgery H Stereotactic Particulate Radiosurgery J Stereotactic Gamma Beam Radiosurgery	Z None	Z None

DRG Non-OR For all body part, approach, device, and qualifier values

D Radiation Therapy
9 Ear, Nose, Mouth and Throat
Y Other Radiation

Treatment Site Character 4	Modal. Qualifier Character 5	Isotope Character 6	Qualifier Character 7
0 Ear 1 Nose 5 Tongue 6 Salivary Glands 7 Sinuses 8 Hard Palate 9 Soft Palate	7 Contact Radiation 8 Hyperthermia F Plaque Radiation	Z None	Z None
3 Hypopharynx F Oropharynx	7 Contact Radiation 8 Hyperthermia	Z None	Z None
4 Mouth B Larynx D Nasopharynx	7 Contact Radiation 8 Hyperthermia C Intraoperative Radiation Therapy (IORT) F Plaque Radiation	Z None	Z None
C Pharynx	C Intraoperative Radiation Therapy (IORT) F Plaque Radiation	Z None	Z None

D Radiation Therapy
B Respiratory System
0 Beam Radiation

Treatment Site Character 4	Modal. Qualifier Character 5	Isotope Character 6	Qualifier Character 7
0 Trachea 1 Bronchus 2 Lung 5 Pleura 6 Mediastinum 7 Chest Wall 8 Diaphragm	0 Photons <1 MeV 1 Photons 1-10 MeV 2 Photons >10 MeV 4 Heavy Particles (Protons, Ions) 5 Neutrons 6 Neutron Capture	Z None	Z None
0 Trachea 1 Bronchus 2 Lung 5 Pleura 6 Mediastinum 7 Chest Wall 8 Diaphragm	3 Electrons	Z None	0 Intraoperative Z None

D Radiation Therapy
B Respiratory System
1 Brachytherapy

Treatment Site Character 4	Modal. Qualifier Character 5	Isotope Character 6	Qualifier Character 7
0 Trachea 1 Bronchus 2 Lung 5 Pleura 6 Mediastinum 7 Chest Wall 8 Diaphragm	9 High Dose Rate (HDR) B Low Dose Rate (LDR)	7 Cesium 137 (Cs-137) 8 Iridium 192 (Ir-192) 9 Iodine 125 (I-125) B Palladium 103 (Pd-103) C Californium 252 (Cf-252) Y Other Isotope	Z None

D Radiation Therapy
B Respiratory System
2 Stereotactic Radiosurgery

Treatment Site Character 4	Modal. Qualifier Character 5	Isotope Character 6	Qualifier Character 7
0 Trachea 1 Bronchus 2 Lung 5 Pleura 6 Mediastinum 7 Chest Wall 8 Diaphragm	D Stereotactic Other Photon Radiosurgery H Stereotactic Particulate Radiosurgery J Stereotactic Gamma Beam Radiosurgery	Z None	Z None

DRG Non-OR For all body part, approach, device, and qualifier values

D Radiation Therapy
B Respiratory System
Y Other Radiation

Treatment Site Character 4	Modal. Qualifier Character 5	Isotope Character 6	Qualifier Character 7
0 Trachea 1 Bronchus 2 Lung 5 Pleura 6 Mediastinum 7 Chest Wall 8 Diaphragm	7 Contact Radiation 8 Hyperthermia F Plaque Radiation K Laser Interstitial Thermal Therapy	Z None	Z None

D Radiation Therapy
D Gastrointestinal System
0 Beam Radiation

Treatment Site Character 4	Modal. Qualifier Character 5	Isotope Character 6	Qualifier Character 7
0 Esophagus 1 Stomach 2 Duodenum 3 Jejunum 4 Ileum 5 Colon 7 Rectum	0 Photons <1 MeV 1 Photons 1- 10 MeV 2 Photons >10 MeV 4 Heavy Particles (Protons, Ions) 5 Neutrons 6 Neutron Capture	Z None	Z None
0 Esophagus 1 Stomach 2 Duodenum 3 Jejunum 4 Ileum 5 Colon 7 Rectum	3 Electrons	Z None	0 Intraoperative Z None

D Radiation Therapy
D Gastrointestinal System
1 Brachytherapy

Treatment Site Character 4	Modal. Qualifier Character 5	Isotope Character 6	Qualifier Character 7
0 Esophagus 1 Stomach 2 Duodenum 3 Jejunum 4 Ileum 5 Colon 7 Rectum	9 High Dose Rate (HDR) B Low Dose Rate (LDR)	7 Cesium 137 (Cs-137) 8 Iridium 192 (Ir-192) 9 Iodine 125 (I-125) B Palladium 103 (Pd-103) C Californium 252 (Cf-252) Y Other Isotope	Z None

D Radiation Therapy
D Gastrointestinal System
2 Stereotactic Radiosurgery

Treatment Site Character 4	Modal. Qualifier Character 5	Isotope Character 6	Qualifier Character 7
0 Esophagus 1 Stomach 2 Duodenum 3 Jejunum 4 Ileum 5 Colon 7 Rectum	D Stereotactic Other Photon Radiosurgery H Stereotactic Particulate Radiosurgery J Stereotactic Gamma Beam Radiosurgery	Z None	Z None

DRG Non-OR For all body part, approach, device, and qualifier values

D Radiation therapy
D Gastrointestinal System
Y Other Radiation

Treatment Site Character 4	Modal. Qualifier Character 5	Isotope Character 6	Qualifier Character 7
Ø Esophagus	7 Contact Radiation 8 Hyperthermia F Plaque Radiation K Laser Interstitial Thermal Therapy	Z None	Z None
1 Stomach 2 Duodenum 3 Jejunum 4 Ileum 5 Colon 7 Rectum	7 Contact Radiation 8 Hyperthermia C Intraoperative Radiation Therapy (IORT) F Plaque Radiation K Laser Interstitial Thermal Therapy	Z None	Z None
8 Anus	C Intraoperative Radiation Therapy (IORT) F Plaque Radiation K Laser Interstitial Thermal Therapy	Z None	Z None

D Radiation Therapy
F Hepatobiliary System and Pancreas
Ø Beam Radiation

Treatment Site Character 4	Modal. Qualifier Character 5	Isotope Character 6	Qualifier Character 7
Ø Liver 1 Gallbladder 2 Bile Ducts 3 Pancreas	Ø Photons <1 MeV 1 Photons 1-1Ø MeV 2 Photons >1Ø MeV 4 Heavy Particles (Protons, Ions) 5 Neutrons 6 Neutron Capture	Z None	Z None
Ø Liver 1 Gallbladder 2 Bile Ducts 3 Pancreas	3 Electrons	Z None	Ø Intraoperative Z None

D Radiation Therapy
F Hepatobiliary System and Pancreas
1 Brachytherapy

Treatment Site Character 4	Modal. Qualifier Character 5	Isotope Character 6	Qualifier Character 7
Ø Liver 1 Gallbladder 2 Bile Ducts 3 Pancreas	9 High Dose Rate (HDR) B Low Dose Rate (LDR)	7 Cesium 137 (Cs-137) 8 Iridium 192 (Ir-192) 9 Iodine 125 (I-125) B Palladium 1Ø3 (Pd-1Ø3) C Californium 252 (Cf-252) Y Other Isotope	Z None

D Radiation Therapy
F Hepatobiliary System and Pancreas
2 Stereotactic Radiosurgery

Treatment Site Character 4	Modal. Qualifier Character 5	Isotope Character 6	Qualifier Character 7
Ø Liver 1 Gallbladder 2 Bile Ducts 3 Pancreas	D Stereotactic Other Photon Radiosurgery H Stereotactic Particulate Radiosurgery J Stereotactic Gamma Beam Radiosurgery	Z None	Z None

DRG Non-OR For all body part, approach, device, and qualifier values

D Radiation Therapy
F Hepatobiliary System and Pancreas
Y Other Radiation

Treatment Site Character 4	Modal. Qualifier Character 5	Isotope Character 6	Qualifier Character 7
Ø Liver 1 Gallbladder 2 Bile Ducts 3 Pancreas	7 Contact Radiation 8 Hyperthermia C Intraoperative Radiation Therapy (IORT) F Plaque Radiation K Laser Interstitial Thermal Therapy	Z None	Z None

D Radiation Therapy
G Endocrine System
0 Beam Radiation

Treatment Site Character 4	Modal. Qualifier Character 5	Isotope Character 6	Qualifier Character 7
0 Pituitary Gland **1** Pineal Body **2** Adrenal Glands **4** Parathyroid Glands **5** Thyroid	**0** Photons <1 MeV **1** Photons 1-10 MeV **2** Photons >10 MeV **5** Neutrons **6** Neutron Capture	**Z** None	**Z** None
0 Pituitary Gland **1** Pineal Body **2** Adrenal Glands **4** Parathyroid Glands **5** Thyroid	**3** Electrons	**Z** None	**0** Intraoperative **Z** None

D Radiation Therapy
G Endocrine System
1 Brachytherapy

Treatment Site Character 4	Modal. Qualifier Character 5	Isotope Character 6	Qualifier Character 7
0 Pituitary Gland **1** Pineal Body **2** Adrenal Glands **4** Parathyroid Glands **5** Thyroid	**9** High Dose Rate (HDR) **B** Low Dose Rate (LDR)	**7** Cesium 137 (Cs-137) **8** Iridium 192 (Ir-192) **9** Iodine 125 (I-125) **B** Palladium 103 (Pd-103) **C** Californium 252 (Cf-252) **Y** Other Isotope	**Z** None

D Radiation Therapy
G Endocrine System
2 Stereotactic Radiosurgery

Treatment Site Character 4	Modal. Qualifier Character 5	Isotope Character 6	Qualifier Character 7
0 Pituitary Gland **1** Pineal Body **2** Adrenal Glands **4** Parathyroid Glands **5** Thyroid	**D** Stereotactic Other Photon Radiosurgery **H** Stereotactic Particulate Radiosurgery **J** Stereotactic Gamma Beam Radiosurgery	**Z** None	**Z** None

DRG Non-OR For all body part, approach, device, and qualifier values

D Radiation therapy
G Endocrine System
Y Other Radiation

Treatment Site Character 4	Modal. Qualifier Character 5	Isotope Character 6	Qualifier Character 7
0 Pituitary Gland **1** Pineal Body **2** Adrenal Glands **4** Parathyroid Glands **5** Thyroid	**7** Contact Radiation **8** Hyperthermia **F** Plaque Radiation **K** Laser Interstitial Thermal Therapy	**Z** None	**Z** None

D Radiation Therapy
H Skin
0 Beam Radiation

Treatment Site Character 4	Modal. Qualifier Character 5	Isotope Character 6	Qualifier Character 7
2 Skin, Face **3** Skin, Neck **4** Skin, Arm **6** Skin, Chest **7** Skin, Back **8** Skin, Abdomen **9** Skin, Buttock **B** Skin, Leg	**0** Photons <1 MeV **1** Photons 1-10 MeV **2** Photons >10 MeV **4** Heavy Particles (Protons, Ions) **5** Neutrons **6** Neutron Capture	**Z** None	**Z** None
2 Skin, Face **3** Skin, Neck **4** Skin, Arm **6** Skin, Chest **7** Skin, Back **8** Skin, Abdomen **9** Skin, Buttock **B** Skin, Leg	**3** Electrons	**Z** None	**0** Intraoperative **Z** None

D Radiation Therapy
H Skin
Y Other Radiation

Treatment Site Character 4	Modal. Qualifier Character 5	Isotope Character 6	Qualifier Character 7
2 Skin, Face 3 Skin, Neck 4 Skin, Arm 6 Skin, Chest 7 Skin, Back 8 Skin, Abdomen 9 Skin, Buttock B Skin, Leg	7 Contact Radiation 8 Hyperthermia F Plaque Radiation	Z None	Z None
5 Skin, Hand C Skin, Foot	F Plaque Radiation	Z None	Z None

D Radiation Therapy
M Breast
Ø Beam Radiation

Treatment Site Character 4	Modal. Qualifier Character 5	Isotope Character 6	Qualifier Character 7
Ø Breast, Left 1 Breast, Right	Ø Photons <1 MeV 1 Photons 1-1Ø MeV 2 Photons >1Ø MeV 4 Heavy Particles (Protons, Ions) 5 Neutrons 6 Neutron Capture	Z None	Z None
Ø Breast, Left 1 Breast, Right	3 Electrons	Z None	Ø Intraoperative Z None

D Radiation Therapy
M Breast
1 Brachytherapy

Treatment Site Character 4	Modal. Qualifier Character 5	Isotope Character 6	Qualifier Character 7
Ø Breast, Left 1 Breast, Right	9 High Dose Rate (HDR) B Low Dose Rate (LDR)	7 Cesium 137 (Cs-137) 8 Iridium 192 (Ir-192) 9 Iodine 125 (I-125) B Palladium 1Ø3 (Pd-1Ø3) C Californium 252 (Cf-252) Y Other Isotope	Z None

D Radiation Therapy
M Breast
2 Stereotactic Radiosurgery

Treatment Site Character 4	Modal. Qualifier Character 5	Isotope Character 6	Qualifier Character 7
Ø Breast, Left 1 Breast, Right	D Stereotactic Other Photon Radiosurgery H Stereotactic Particulate Radiosurgery J Stereotactic Gamma Beam Radiosurgery	Z None	Z None

DRG Non-OR For all body part, approach, device, and qualifier values

D Radiation Therapy
M Breast
Y Other Radiation

Treatment Site Character 4	Modal. Qualifier Character 5	Isotope Character 6	Qualifier Character 7
Ø Breast, Left 1 Breast, Right	7 Contact Radiation 8 Hyperthermia F Plaque Radiation K Laser Interstitial Thermal Therapy	Z None	Z None

D Radiation Therapy
P Musculoskeletal System
0 Beam Radiation

Treatment Site Character 4	Modal. Qualifier Character 5	Isotope Character 6	Qualifier Character 7
0 Skull 2 Maxilla 3 Mandible 4 Sternum 5 Rib(s) 6 Humerus 7 Radius/Ulna 8 Pelvic Bones 9 Femur B Tibia/Fibula C Other Bone	0 Photons <1 MeV 1 Photons 1-10 MeV 2 Photons >10 MeV 4 Heavy Particles (Protons, Ions) 5 Neutrons 6 Neutron Capture	Z None	Z None
0 Skull 2 Maxilla 3 Mandible 4 Sternum 5 Rib(s) 6 Humerus 7 Radius/Ulna 8 Pelvic Bones 9 Femur B Tibia/Fibula C Other Bone	3 Electrons	Z None	0 Intraoperative Z None

D Radiation Therapy
P Musculoskeletal System
Y Other Radiation

Treatment Site Character 4	Modal. Qualifier Character 5	Isotope Character 6	Qualifier Character 7
0 Skull 2 Maxilla 3 Mandible 4 Sternum 5 Rib(s) 6 Humerus 7 Radius/Ulna 8 Pelvic Bones 9 Femur B Tibia/Fibula C Other Bone	7 Contact Radiation 8 Hyperthermia F Plaque Radiation	Z None	Z None

D Radiation Therapy
T Urinary System
0 Beam Radiation

Treatment Site Character 4	Modal. Qualifier Character 5	Isotope Character 6	Qualifier Character 7
0 Kidney 1 Ureter 2 Bladder 3 Urethra	0 Photons <1 MeV 1 Photons 1-10 MeV 2 Photons >10 MeV 4 Heavy Particles (Protons, Ions) 5 Neutrons 6 Neutron Capture	Z None	Z None
0 Kidney 1 Ureter 2 Bladder 3 Urethra	3 Electrons	Z None	0 Intraoperative Z None

D Radiation Therapy
T Urinary System
1 Brachytherapy

Treatment Site Character 4	Modal. Qualifier Character 5	Isotope Character 6	Qualifier Character 7
0 Kidney 1 Ureter 2 Bladder 3 Urethra	9 High Dose Rate (HDR) B Low Dose Rate (LDR)	7 Cesium 137 (Cs-137) 8 Iridium 192 (Ir-192) 9 Iodine 125 (I-125) B Palladium 103 (Pd-103) C Californium 252 (Cf-252) Y Other Isotope	Z None

Radiation Therapy DP0—DT1

D Radiation Therapy
T Urinary System
2 Stereotactic Radiosurgery

Treatment Site Character 4	Modal. Qualifier Character 5	Isotope Character 6	Qualifier Character 7
Ø Kidney 1 Ureter 2 Bladder 3 Urethra	D Stereotactic Other Photon Radiosurgery H Stereotactic Particulate Radiosurgery J Stereotactic Gamma Beam Radiosurgery	Z None	Z None

DRG Non-OR For all body part, approach, device, and qualifier values

D Radiation Therapy
T Urinary System
Y Other Radiation

Treatment Site Character 4	Modal. Qualifier Character 5	Isotope Character 6	Qualifier Character 7
Ø Kidney 1 Ureter 2 Bladder 3 Urethra	7 Contact Radiation 8 Hyperthermia C Intraoperative Radiation Therapy (IORT) F Plaque Radiation	Z None	Z None

D Radiation Therapy
U Female Reproductive System
Ø Beam Radiation

Treatment Site Character 4	Modal. Qualifier Character 5	Isotope Character 6	Qualifier Character 7
Ø Ovary ♀ 1 Cervix ♀ 2 Uterus ♀	Ø Photons <1 MeV 1 Photons 1 - 1Ø MeV 2 Photons >1Ø MeV 4 Heavy Particles (Protons, Ions) 5 Neutrons 6 Neutron Capture	Z None	Z None
Ø Ovary ♀ 1 Cervix ♀ 2 Uterus ♀	3 Electrons	Z None	Ø Intraoperative Z None

D Radiation Therapy
U Female Reproductive System
1 Brachytherapy

Treatment Site Character 4	Modal. Qualifier Character 5	Isotope Character 6	Qualifier Character 7
Ø Ovary ♀ 1 Cervix ♀ 2 Uterus ♀	9 High Dose Rate (HDR) B Low Dose Rate (LDR)	7 Cesium 137 (Cs-137) 8 Iridium 192 (Ir-192) 9 Iodine 125 (I-125) B Palladium 1Ø3 (Pd-1Ø3) C Californium 252 (Cf-252) Y Other Isotope	Z None

D Radiation Therapy
U Female Reproductive System
2 Stereotactic Radiosurgery

Treatment Site Character 4	Modal. Qualifier Character 5	Isotope Character 6	Qualifier Character 7
Ø Ovary ♀ 1 Cervix ♀ 2 Uterus ♀	D Stereotactic Other Photon Radiosurgery H Stereotactic Particulate Radiosurgery J Stereotactic Gamma Beam Radiosurgery	Z None	Z None

DRG Non-OR For all body part, approach, device, and qualifier values

D Radiation Therapy
U Female Reproductive System
Y Other Radiation

Treatment Site Character 4	Modal. Qualifier Character 5	Isotope Character 6	Qualifier Character 7
Ø Ovary ♀ 1 Cervix ♀ 2 Uterus ♀	7 Contact Radiation 8 Hyperthermia C Intraoperative Radiation Therapy (IORT) F Plaque Radiation	Z None	Z None

D Radiation Therapy
V Male Reproductive System
Ø Beam Radiation

Treatment Site Character 4	Modal. Qualifier Character 5	Isotope Character 6	Qualifier Character 7
Ø Prostate ♂ 1 Testis ♂	Ø Photons <1 MeV 1 Photons 1- 1Ø MeV 2 Photons >1Ø MeV 4 Heavy Particles (Protons, Ions) 5 Neutrons 6 Neutron Capture	Z None	Z None
Ø Prostate ♂ 1 Testis ♂	3 Electrons	Z None	Ø Intraoperative Z None

D Radiation Therapy
V Male Reproductive System
1 Brachytherapy

Treatment Site Character 4	Modal. Qualifier Character 5	Isotope Character 6	Qualifier Character 7
Ø Prostate ♂ 1 Testis ♂	9 High Dose Rate (HDR) B Low Dose Rate (LDR)	7 Cesium 137 (Cs-137) 8 Iridium 192 (Ir-192) 9 Iodine 125 (I-125) B Palladium 1Ø3 (Pd-1Ø3) C Californium 252 (Cf-252) Y Other Isotope	Z None

D Radiation Therapy
V Male Reproductive System
2 Stereotactic Radiosurgery

Treatment Site Character 4	Modal. Qualifier Character 5	Isotope Character 6	Qualifier Character 7
Ø Prostate ♂ 1 Testis ♂	D Stereotactic Other Photon Radiosurgery H Stereotactic Particulate Radiosurgery J Stereotactic Gamma Beam Radiosurgery	Z None	Z None

DRG Non-OR For all body part, approach, device, and qualifier values

D Radiation Therapy
V Male Reproductive System
Y Other Radiation

Treatment Site Character 4	Modal. Qualifier Character 5	Isotope Character 6	Qualifier Character 7
Ø Prostate ♂	7 Contact Radiation 8 Hyperthermia C Intraoperative Radiation Therapy (IORT) F Plaque Radiation K Laser Interstitial Thermal Therapy	Z None	Z None
1 Testis ♂	7 Contact Radiation 8 Hyperthermia F Plaque Radiation	Z None	Z None

D Radiation Therapy
W Anatomical Regions
Ø Beam Radiation

Treatment Site Character 4	Modal. Qualifier Character 5	Isotope Character 6	Qualifier Character 7
1 Head and Neck 2 Chest 3 Abdomen 4 Hemibody 5 Whole Body 6 Pelvic Region	Ø Photons <1 MeV 1 Photons 1-1Ø MeV 2 Photons >1Ø MeV 4 Heavy Particles (Protons, Ions) 5 Neutrons 6 Neutron Capture	Z None	Z None
1 Head and Neck 2 Chest 3 Abdomen 4 Hemibody 5 Whole Body 6 Pelvic Region	3 Electrons	Z None	Ø Intraoperative Z None

D Radiation Therapy
W Anatomical Regions
1 Brachytherapy

Treatment Site Character 4	Modal. Qualifier Character 5	Isotope Character 6	Qualifier Character 7
1 Head and Neck 2 Chest 3 Abdomen 6 Pelvic Region	9 High Dose Rate (HDR) B Low Dose Rate (LDR)	7 Cesium 137 (Cs-137) 8 Iridium 192 (Ir-192) 9 Iodine 125 (I-125) B Palladium 1Ø3 (Pd-1Ø3) C Californium 252 (Cf-252) Y Other Isotope	Z None

D Radiation Therapy
W Anatomical Regions
2 Stereotactic Radiosurgery

Treatment Site Character 4	Modal. Qualifier Character 5	Isotope Character 6	Qualifier Character 7
1 Head and Neck 2 Chest 3 Abdomen 6 Pelvic Region	D Stereotactic Other Photon Radiosurgery H Stereotactic Particulate Radiosurgery J Stereotactic Gamma Beam Radiosurgery	Z None	Z None

DRG Non-OR For all body part, approach, device, and qualifier values

D Radiation Therapy
W Anatomical Regions
Y Other Radiation

Treatment Site Character 4	Modal. Qualifier Character 5	Isotope Character 6	Qualifier Character 7
1 Head and Neck 2 Chest 3 Abdomen 4 Hemibody 5 Whole Body 6 Pelvic Region	7 Contact Radiation 8 Hyperthermia F Plaque Radiation	Z None	Z None
5 Whole Body	G Isotope Administration	D Iodine 131 (I-131) F Phosphorus 32 (P-32) G Strontium 89 (Sr-89) H Strontium 9Ø (Sr-9Ø) Y Other Isotope	Z None

Physical Rehabilitation and Diagnostic Audiology F00–F15

F Physical Rehabilitation and Diagnostic Audiology
0 Rehabilitation
0 Speech Assessment Measurement of speech and related functions

Body System/Region Character 4	Type Qualifier Character 5	Equipment Character 6	Qualifier Character 7
3 Neurological System - Whole Body	G Communicative/Cognitive Integration Skills	K Audiovisual M Augmentative / Alternative Communication P Computer Y Other Equipment Z None	Z None
Z None	0 Filtered Speech 3 Staggered Spondaic Word Q Performance Intensity Phonetically Balanced Speech Discrimination R Brief Tone Stimuli S Distorted Speech T Dichotic Stimuli V Temporal Ordering of Stimuli W Masking Patterns	1 Audiometer 2 Sound Field / Booth K Audiovisual Z None	Z None
Z None	1 Speech Threshold 2 Speech/Word Recognition	1 Audiometer 2 Sound Field / Booth 9 Cochlear Implant K Audiovisual Z None	Z None
Z None	4 Sensorineural Acuity Level	1 Audiometer 2 Sound Field / Booth Z None	Z None
Z None	5 Synthetic Sentence Identification	1 Audiometer 2 Sound Field / Booth 9 Cochlear Implant K Audiovisual	Z None
Z None	6 Speech and/or Language Screening 7 Nonspoken Language 8 Receptive/Expressive Language C Aphasia G Communicative/Cognitive Integration Skills L Augmentative/Alternative Communication System	K Audiovisual M Augmentative / Alternative Communication P Computer Y Other Equipment Z None	Z None
Z None	9 Articulation/Phonology	K Audiovisual P Computer Q Speech Analysis Y Other Equipment Z None	Z None
Z None	B Motor Speech	K Audiovisual N Biosensory Feedback P Computer Q Speech Analysis T Aerodynamic Function Y Other Equipment Z None	Z None
Z None	D Fluency	K Audiovisual N Biosensory Feedback P Computer Q Speech Analysis S Voice Analysis T Aerodynamic Function Y Other Equipment Z None	Z None

F00 Continued on next page

DRG Non-OR All body system/region, type qualifier, equipment, and qualifier values

FØØ Continued

F Physical Rehabilitation and Diagnostic Audiology
Ø Rehabilitation
Ø Speech Assessment Measurement of speech and related functions

Body System/Region Character 4	Type Qualifier Character 5	Equipment Character 6	Qualifier Character 7
Z None	F Voice	K Audiovisual N Biosensory Feedback P Computer S Voice Analysis T Aerodynamic Function Y Other Equipment Z None	Z None
Z None	H Bedside Swallowing and Oral Function P Oral Peripheral Mechanism	Y Other Equipment Z None	Z None
Z None	J Instrumental Swallowing and Oral Function	T Aerodynamic Function W Swallowing Y Other Equipment	Z None
Z None	K Orofacial Myofunctional	K Audiovisual P Computer Y Other Equipment Z None	Z None
Z None	M Voice Prosthetic	K Audiovisual P Computer S Voice Analysis V Speech Prosthesis Y Other Equipment Z None	Z None
Z None	N Non-invasive Instrumental Status	N Biosensory Feedback P Computer Q Speech Analysis S Voice Analysis T Aerodynamic Function Y Other Equipment	Z None
Z None	X Other Specified Central Auditory Processing	Z None	Z None

DRG Non-OR All body system/region, type qualifier, equipment, and qualifier values

F Physical Rehabilitation and Diagnostic Audiology
Ø Rehabilitation
1 Motor and/or Nerve Function Assessment Measurement of motor, nerve, and related functions

Body System/Region Character 4	Type Qualifier Character 5	Equipment Character 6	Qualifier Character 7
Ø Neurological System - Head and Neck 1 Neurological System - Upper Back/ Upper Extremity 2 Neurological System - Lower Back/ Lower Extremity 3 Neurological System - Whole Body	1 Integumentary Integrity 3 Coordination/Dexterity 4 Motor Function G Reflex Integrity	Z None	Z None
Ø Neurological System - Head and Neck 1 Neurological System - Upper Back/ Upper Extremity 2 Neurological System - Lower Back/ Lower Extremity 3 Neurological System - Whole Body D Integumentary System - Head and Neck F Integumentary System - Upper Back/ Upper Extremity G Integumentary System - Lower Back/ Lower Extremity H Integumentary System - Whole Body J Musculoskeletal System - Head and Neck K Musculoskeletal System - Upper Back/ Upper Extremity L Musculoskeletal System - Lower Back/ Lower Extremity M Musculoskeletal System - Whole Body	5 Range of Motion and Joint Integrity 6 Sensory Awareness/Processing/ Integrity	Y Other Equipment Z None	Z None

FØ1 Continued on next page

DRG Non-OR All body system/region, type qualifier, equipment, and qualifier values

F Physical Rehabilitation and Diagnostic Audiology ***F01 Continued***
0 Rehabilitation
1 Motor and/or Nerve Function Assessment Measurement of motor, nerve, and related functions

Body System/Region Character 4	Type Qualifier Character 5	Equipment Character 6	Qualifier Character 7
0 Neurological System - Head and Neck **1** Neurological System - Upper Back/ Upper Extremity **2** Neurological System - Lower Back/ Lower Extremity **3** Neurological System - Whole Body **D** Integumentary System - Head and Neck **F** Integumentary System - Upper Back/ Upper Extremity **G** Integumentary System - Lower Back/ Lower Extremity **H** Integumentary System - Whole Body **J** Musculoskeletal System - Head and Neck **K** Musculoskeletal System - Upper Back/ Upper Extremity **L** Musculoskeletal System - Lower Back/ Lower Extremity **M** Musculoskeletal System - Whole Body **N** Genitourinary System	**0** Muscle Performance	**E** Orthosis **F** Assistive, Adaptive, Supportive or Protective **U** Prosthesis **Y** Other Equipment **Z** None	**Z** None
D Integumentary System - Head and Neck **F** Integumentary System - Upper Back/ Upper Extremity **G** Integumentary System - Lower Back/ Lower Extremity **H** Integumentary System - Whole Body **J** Musculoskeletal System - Head and Neck **K** Musculoskeletal System - Upper Back/ Upper Extremity **L** Musculoskeletal System - Lower Back/ Lower Extremity **M** Musculoskeletal System - Whole Body	**1** Integumentary Integrity	**Z** None	**Z** None
Z None	**2** Visual Motor Integration	**K** Audiovisual **M** Augmentative / Alternative Communication **N** Biosensory Feedback **P** Computer **Q** Speech Analysis **S** Voice Analysis **Y** Other Equipment **Z** None	**Z** None
Z None	**7** Facial Nerve Function	**7** Electrophysiologic	**Z** None
Z None	**9** Somatosensory Evoked Potentials	**J** Somatosensory	**Z** None
Z None	**B** Bed Mobility **C** Transfer **F** Wheelchair Mobility	**E** Orthosis **F** Assistive, Adaptive, Supportive or Protective **U** Prosthesis **Z** None	**Z** None
Z None	**D** Gait and/or Balance	**E** Orthosis **F** Assistive, Adaptive, Supportive or Protective **U** Prosthesis **Y** Other Equipment **Z** None	**Z** None

DRG Non-OR All body system/region, type qualifier, equipment, and qualifier values

F Physical Rehabilitation and Diagnostic Audiology
Ø Rehabilitation
2 Activities of Daily Living Assessment Measurement of functional level for activities of daily living

Body System/Region Character 4	Type Qualifier Character 5	Equipment Character 6	Qualifier Character 7
Ø Neurological System - Head and Neck	**9** Cranial Nerve Integrity **D** Neuromotor Development	**Y** Other Equipment **Z** None	**Z** None
1 Neurological System - Upper Back/ Upper Extremity **2** Neurological System - Lower Back/ Lower Extremity **3** Neurological System - Whole Body	**D** Neuromotor Development	**Y** Other Equipment **Z** None	**Z** None
4 Circulatory System - Head and Neck **5** Circulatory System - Upper Back/Upper Extremity **6** Circulatory System - Lower Back/Lower Extremity **7** Circulatory System - Whole Body **8** Respiratory System - Head and Neck **9** Respiratory System - Upper Back/ Upper Extremity **B** Respiratory System - Lower Back/ Lower Extremity **C** Respiratory System - Whole Body	**G** Ventilation, Respiration and Circulation	**C** Mechanical **G** Aerobic Endurance and Conditioning **Y** Other Equipment **Z** None	**Z** None
7 Circulatory System - Whole Body **C** Respiratory System - Whole Body	**7** Aerobic Capacity and Endurance	**E** Orthosis **G** Aerobic Endurance and Conditioning **U** Prosthesis **Y** Other Equipment **Z** None	**Z** None
Z None	**Ø** Bathing/Showering **1** Dressing **3** Grooming/Personal Hygiene **4** Home Management	**E** Orthosis **F** Assistive, Adaptive, Supportive or Protective **U** Prosthesis **Z** None	**Z** None
Z None	**2** Feeding/Eating **8** Anthropometric Characteristics **F** Pain	**Y** Other Equipment **Z** None	**Z** None
Z None	**5** Perceptual Processing	**K** Audiovisual **M** Augmentative / Alternative Communication **N** Biosensory Feedback **P** Computer **Q** Speech Analysis **S** Voice Analysis **Y** Other Equipment **Z** None	**Z** None
Z None	**6** Psychosocial Skills	**Z** None	**Z** None
Z None	**B** Environmental, Home and Work Barriers **C** Ergonomics and Body Mechanics	**E** Orthosis **F** Assistive, Adaptive, Supportive or Protective **U** Prosthesis **Y** Other Equipment **Z** None	**Z** None
Z None	**H** Vocational Activities and Functional Community or Work Reintegration Skills	**E** Orthosis **F** Assistive, Adaptive, Supportive or Protective **G** Aerobic Endurance and Conditioning **U** Prosthesis **Y** Other Equipment **Z** None	**Z** None

DRG Non-OR All body system/region, type qualifier, equipment, and qualifier values

F Physical Rehabilitation and Diagnostic Audiology
0 Rehabilitation
6 Speech Treatment Application of techniques to improve, augment, or compensate for speech and related functional impairment

Body System/Region Character 4	Type Qualifier Character 5	Equipment Character 6	Qualifier Character 7
3 Neurological System - Whole Body	6 Communicative/Cognitive Integration Skills	K Audiovisual M Augmentative / Alternative Communication P Computer Y Other Equipment Z None	Z None
Z None	0 Nonspoken Language 3 Aphasia 6 Communicative/Cognitive Integration Skills	K Audiovisual M Augmentative / Alternative Communication P Computer Y Other Equipment Z None	Z None
Z None	1 Speech-Language Pathology and Related Disorders Counseling 2 Speech-Language Pathology and Related Disorders Prevention	K Audiovisual Z None	Z None
Z None	4 Articulation/Phonology	K Audiovisual P Computer Q Speech Analysis T Aerodynamic Function Y Other Equipment Z None	Z None
Z None	5 Aural Rehabilitation	K Audiovisual L Assistive Listening M Augmentative / Alternative Communication N Biosensory Feedback P Computer Q Speech Analysis S Voice Analysis Y Other Equipment Z None	Z None
Z None	7 Fluency	4 Electroacoustic Immitance / Acoustic Reflex K Audiovisual N Biosensory Feedback Q Speech Analysis S Voice Analysis T Aerodynamic Function Y Other Equipment Z None	Z None
Z None	8 Motor Speech	K Audiovisual N Biosensory Feedback P Computer Q Speech Analysis S Voice Analysis T Aerodynamic Function Y Other Equipment Z None	Z None
Z None	9 Orofacial Myofunctional	K Audiovisual P Computer Y Other Equipment Z None	Z None
Z None	B Receptive/Expressive Language	K Audiovisual L Assistive Listening M Augmentative / Alternative Communication P Computer Y Other Equipment Z None	Z None

F06 Continued on next page

DRG Non-OR All body system/region, type qualifier, equipment, and qualifier values

F06 Continued

F Physical Rehabilitation and Diagnostic Audiology
0 Rehabilitation
6 Speech Treatment Application of techniques to improve, augment, or compensate for speech and related functional impairment

Body System/Region Character 4	Type Qualifier Character 5	Equipment Character 6	Qualifier Character 7
Z None	**C** Voice	**K** Audiovisual **N** Biosensory Feedback **P** Computer **S** Voice Analysis **T** Aerodynamic Function **V** Speech Prosthesis **Y** Other Equipment **Z** None	**Z** None
Z None	**D** Swallowing Dysfunction	**M** Augmentative / Alternative Communication **T** Aerodynamic Function **V** Speech Prosthesis **Y** Other Equipment **Z** None	**Z** None

DRG Non-OR All body system/region, type qualifier, equipment, and qualifier values

F Physical Rehabilitation and Diagnostic Audiology
0 Rehabilitation
7 Motor Treatment Exercise or activities to increase or facilitate motor function

Body System/Region Character 4	Type Qualifier Character 5	Equipment Character 6	Qualifier Character 7
0 Neurological System - Head and Neck **1** Neurological System - Upper Back/Upper Extremity **2** Neurological System - Lower Back/Lower Extremity **3** Neurological System - Whole Body **4** Circulatory System - Head and Neck **5** Circulatory System - Upper Back/Upper Extremity **6** Circulatory System - Lower Back/Lower Extremity **7** Circulatory System - Whole Body **8** Respiratory System - Head and Neck **9** Respiratory System - Upper Back/Upper Extremity **B** Respiratory System - Lower Back/Lower Extremity **C** Respiratory System - Whole Body **D** Integumentary System - Head and Neck **F** Integumentary System - Upper Back/Upper Extremity **G** Integumentary System - Lower Back/Lower Extremity **H** Integumentary System - Whole Body **J** Musculoskeletal System - Head and Neck **K** Musculoskeletal System - Upper Back/ Upper Extremity **L** Musculoskeletal System - Lower Back/ Lower Extremity **M** Musculoskeletal System - Whole Body **N** Genitourinary System	**6** Therapeutic Exercise	**B** Physical Agents **C** Mechanical **D** Electrotherapeutic **E** Orthosis **F** Assistive, Adaptive, Supportive or Protective **G** Aerobic Endurance and Conditioning **H** Mechanical or Electromechanical **U** Prosthesis **Y** Other Equipment **Z** None	**Z** None

F07 Continued on next page

DRG Non-OR All body system/region, type qualifier, equipment, and qualifier values

F Physical Rehabilitation and Diagnostic Audiology
Ø Rehabilitation
7 Motor Treatment Exercise or activities to increase or facilitate motor function

FØ7 Continued

Body System/Region Character 4	Type Qualifier Character 5	Equipment Character 6	Qualifier Character 7
Ø Neurological System - Head and Neck **1** Neurological System - Upper Back/Upper Extremity **2** Neurological System - Lower Back/Lower Extremity **3** Neurological System - Whole Body **D** Integumentary System - Head and Neck **F** Integumentary System - Upper Back/Upper Extremity **G** Integumentary System - Lower Back/Lower Extremity **H** Integumentary System - Whole Body **J** Musculoskeletal System - Head and Neck **K** Musculoskeletal System - Upper Back/ Upper Extremity **L** Musculoskeletal System - Lower Back/ Lower Extremity **M** Musculoskeletal System - Whole Body	**Ø** Range of Motion and Joint Mobility **1** Muscle Performance **2** Coordination/Dexterity **3** Motor Function	**E** Orthosis **F** Assistive, Adaptive, Supportive or Protective **U** Prosthesis **Y** Other Equipment **Z** None	**Z** None
Ø Neurological System - Head and Neck **1** Neurological System - Upper Back/Upper Extremity **2** Neurological System - Lower Back/Lower Extremity **3** Neurological System - Whole Body **D** Integumentary System - Head and Neck **F** Integumentary System - Upper Back/Upper Extremity **G** Integumentary System - Lower Back/Lower Extremity **H** Integumentary System - Whole Body **J** Musculoskeletal System - Head and Neck **K** Musculoskeletal System - Upper Back/ Upper Extremity **L** Musculoskeletal System - Lower Back/ Lower Extremity **M** Musculoskeletal System - Whole Body	**7** Manual Therapy Techniques	**Z** None	**Z** None
N Genitourinary System	**1** Muscle Performance	**E** Orthosis **F** Assistive, Adaptive, Supportive or Protective **U** Prosthesis **Y** Other Equipment **Z** None	**Z** None
Z None	**4** Wheelchair Mobility	**D** Electrotherapeutic **E** Orthosis **F** Assistive, Adaptive, Supportive or Protective **U** Prosthesis **Y** Other Equipment **Z** None	**Z** None
Z None	**5** Bed Mobility	**C** Mechanical **E** Orthosis **F** Assistive, Adaptive, Supportive or Protective **U** Prosthesis **Y** Other Equipment **Z** None	**Z** None
Z None	**8** Transfer Training	**C** Mechanical **D** Electrotherapeutic **E** Orthosis **F** Assistive, Adaptive, Supportive or Protective **U** Prosthesis **Y** Other Equipment **Z** None	**Z** None

DRG Non-OR All body system/region, type qualifier, equipment, and qualifier values

F Physical Rehabilitation and Diagnostic Audiology
Ø Rehabilitation
7 Motor Treatment Exercise or activities to increase or facilitate motor function

FØ7 Continued

Body System/Region Character 4	Type Qualifier Character 5	Equipment Character 6	Qualifier Character 7
Z None	**9** Gait Training/Functional Ambulation	**C** Mechanical **D** Electrotherapeutic **E** Orthosis **F** Assistive, Adaptive, Supportive or Protective **G** Aerobic Endurance and Conditioning **U** Prosthesis **Y** Other Equipment **Z** None	**Z** None

DRG Non-OR All body system/region, type qualifier, equipment, and qualifier values

F Physical Rehabilitation and Diagnostic Audiology
Ø Rehabilitation
8 Activities of Daily Living Treatment Exercise or activities to facilitate functional competence for activities of daily living

Body System/Region Character 4	Type Qualifier Character 5	Equipment Character 6	Qualifier Character 7
D Integumentary System - Head and Neck **F** Integumentary System - Upper Back/Upper Extremity **G** Integumentary System - Lower Back/Lower Extremity **H** Integumentary System - Whole Body **J** Musculoskeletal System - Head and Neck **K** Musculoskeletal System - Upper Back/Upper Extremity **L** Musculoskeletal System - Lower Back/Lower Extremity **M** Musculoskeletal System - Whole Body	**5** Wound Management	**B** Physical Agents **C** Mechanical **D** Electrotherapeutic **E** Orthosis **F** Assistive, Adaptive, Supportive or Protective **U** Prosthesis **Y** Other Equipment **Z** None	**Z** None
Z None	**Ø** Bathing/Showering Techniques **1** Dressing Techniques **2** Grooming/Personal Hygiene	**E** Orthosis **F** Assistive, Adaptive, Supportive or Protective **U** Prosthesis **Y** Other Equipment **Z** None	**Z** None
Z None	**3** Feeding/Eating	**C** Mechanical **D** Electrotherapeutic **E** Orthosis **F** Assistive, Adaptive, Supportive or Protective **U** Prosthesis **Y** Other Equipment **Z** None	**Z** None
Z None	**4** Home Management	**D** Electrotherapeutic **E** Orthosis **F** Assistive, Adaptive, Supportive or Protective **U** Prosthesis **Y** Other Equipment **Z** None	**Z** None
Z None	**6** Psychosocial Skills	**Z** None	**Z** None
Z None	**7** Vocational Activities and Functional Community or Work Reintegration Skills	**B** Physical Agents **C** Mechanical **D** Electrotherapeutic **E** Orthosis **F** Assistive, Adaptive, Supportive or Protective **G** Aerobic Endurance and Conditioning **U** Prosthesis **Y** Other Equipment **Z** None	**Z** None

DRG Non-OR All body system/region, type qualifier, equipment, and qualifier values

F Physical Rehabilitation and Diagnostic Audiology
Ø Rehabilitation
9 Hearing Treatment Application of techniques to improve, augment, or compensate for hearing and related functional impairment

Body System/Region Character 4	Type Qualifier Character 5	Equipment Character 6	Qualifier Character 7
Z None	Ø Hearing and Related Disorders Counseling 1 Hearing and Related Disorders Prevention	K Audiovisual Z None	Z None
Z None	2 Auditory Processing	K Audiovisual L Assistive Listening P Computer Y Other Equipment Z None	Z None
Z None	3 Cerumen Management	X Cerumen Management Z None	Z None

DRG Non-OR All body system/region, type qualifier, equipment, and qualifier values

F Physical Rehabilitation and Diagnostic Audiology
Ø Rehabilitation
B Cochlear Implant Treatment Application of techniques to improve the communication abilities of individuals with cochlear implant

Body System/Region Character 4	Type Qualifier Character 5	Equipment Character 6	Qualifier Character 7
Z None	Ø Cochlear Implant Rehabilitation	1 Audiometer 2 Sound Field / Booth 9 Cochlear Implant K Audiovisual P Computer Y Other Equipment	Z None

DRG Non-OR All body system/region, type qualifier, equipment, and qualifier values

F Physical Rehabilitation and Diagnostic Audiology
Ø Rehabilitation
C Vestibular Treatment Application of techniques to improve, augment, or compensate for vestibular and related functional impairment

Body System/Region Character 4	Type Qualifier Character 5	Equipment Character 6	Qualifier Character 7
3 Neurological System - Whole Body H Integumentary System - Whole Body M Musculoskeletal System - Whole Body	3 Postural Control	E Orthosis F Assistive, Adaptive, Supportive or Protective U Prosthesis Y Other Equipment Z None	Z None
Z None	Ø Vestibular	8 Vestibular / Balance Z None	Z None
Z None	1 Perceptual Processing 2 Visual Motor Integration	K Audiovisual L Assistive Listening N Biosensory Feedback P Computer Q Speech Analysis S Voice Analysis T Aerodynamic Function Y Other Equipment Z None	Z None

DRG Non-OR All body system/region, type qualifier, equipment, and qualifier values

F Physical Rehabilitation and Diagnostic Audiology
Ø Rehabilitation
D Device Fitting Fitting of a device designed to facilitate or support achievement of a higher level of function

Body System/Region Character 4	Type Qualifier Character 5	Equipment Character 6	Qualifier Character 7
Z None	**Ø** Tinnitus Masker	**5** Hearing Aid Selection / Fitting / Test **Z** None	**Z** None
Z None	**1** Monaural Hearing Aid **2** Binaural Hearing Aid **5** Assistive Listening Device	**1** Audiometer **2** Sound Field / Booth **5** Hearing Aid Selection / Fitting / Test **K** Audiovisual **L** Assistive Listening **Z** None	**Z** None
Z None	**3** Augmentative/Alternative Communication System	**M** Augmentative / Alternative Communication	**Z** None
Z None	**4** Voice Prosthetic	**S** Voice Analysis **V** Speech Prosthesis	**Z** None
Z None	**6** Dynamic Orthosis **7** Static Orthosis **8** Prosthesis **9** Assistive, Adaptive,Supportive or Protective Devices	**E** Orthosis **F** Assistive, Adaptive, Supportive or Protective **U** Prosthesis **Z** None	**Z** None

DRG Non-OR FØDZØ[5,Z]Z
DRG Non-OR FØDZ[1, 2,5][1,2,5, K,L,Z]Z
DRG Non-OR FØDZ3MZ
DRG Non-OR FØDZ4[S,V]Z
DRG Non-OR FØDZ[6,7][E,F,U,Z]Z
DRG Non-OR FØDZ8[E,F,U]Z

F Physical Rehabilitation and Diagnostic Audiology
Ø Rehabilitation
F Caregiver Training Training in activities to support patient's optimal level of function

Body System/Region Character 4	Type Qualifier Character 5	Equipment Character 6	Qualifier Character 7
Z None	**Ø** Bathing/Showering Technique **1** Dressing **2** Feeding and Eating **3** Grooming/Personal Hygiene **4** Bed Mobility **5** Transfer **6** Wheelchair Mobility **7** Therapeutic Exercise **8** Airway Clearance Techniques **9** Wound Management **B** Vocational Activities and Functional Community or Work Reintegration Skills **C** Gait Training/Functional Ambulation **D** Application, Proper Use and Care of Assistive, Adaptive, Supportive or Protective Devices **F** Application, Proper Use and Care of Orthoses **G** Application, Proper Use and Care of Prosthesis **H** Home Management	**E** Orthosis **F** Assistive, Adaptive, Supportive or Protective **U** Prosthesis **Z** None	**Z** None
Z None	**J** Communication Skills	**K** Audiovisual **L** Assistive Listening **M** Augmentative / Alternative Communication **P** Computer **Z** None	**Z** None

DRG Non-OR All body system/region, type qualifier, equipment, and qualifier values

F Physical Rehabilitation and Diagnostic Audiology
1 Diagnostic Audiology
3 Hearing Assessment Measurement of hearing and related functions

Body System/Region Character 4	Type Qualifier Character 5	Equipment Character 6	Qualifier Character 7
Z None	**0** Hearing Screening	**0** Occupational Hearing **1** Audiometer **2** Sound Field / Booth **3** Tympanometer **8** Vestibular / Balance **9** Cochlear Implant **Z** None	**Z** None
Z None	**1** Pure Tone Audiometry, Air **2** Pure Tone Audiometry, Air and Bone	**0** Occupational Hearing **1** Audiometer **2** Sound Field / Booth **Z** None	**Z** None
Z None	**3** Bekesy Audiometry **6** Visual Reinforcement Audiometry **9** Short Increment Sensitivity Index **B** Stenger **C** Pure Tone Stenger	**1** Audiometer **2** Sound Field / Booth **Z** None	**Z** None
Z None	**4** Conditioned Play Audiometry **5** Select Picture Audiometry	**1** Audiometer **2** Sound Field / Booth **K** Audiovisual **Z** None	**Z** None
Z None	**7** Alternate Binaural or Monaural Loudness Balance	**1** Audiometer **K** Audiovisual **Z** None	**Z** None
Z None	**8** Tone Decay **D** Tympanometry **F** Eustachian Tube Function **G** Acoustic Reflex Patterns **H** Acoustic Reflex Threshold **J** Acoustic Reflex Decay	**3** Tympanometer **4** Electroacoustic Immitance / Acoustic Reflex **Z** None	**Z** None
Z None	**K** Electrocochleography **L** Auditory Evoked Potentials	**7** Electrophysiologic **Z** None	**Z** None
Z None	**M** Evoked Otoacoustic Emissions, Screening **N** Evoked Otoacoustic Emissions, Diagnostic	**6** Otoacoustic Emission (OAE) **Z** None	**Z** None
Z None	**P** Aural Rehabilitation Status	**1** Audiometer **2** Sound Field / Booth **4** Electroacoustic Immitance / Acoustic Reflex **9** Cochlear Implant **K** Audiovisual **L** Assistive Listening **P** Computer **Z** None	**Z** None
Z None	**Q** Auditory Processing	**K** Audiovisual **P** Computer **Y** Other Equipment **Z** None	**Z** None

F Physical Rehabilitation and Diagnostic Audiology
1 Diagnostic Audiology
4 Hearing Aid Assessment Measurement of the appropriateness and/or effectiveness of a hearing device

Body System/Region Character 4	Type Qualifier Character 5	Equipment Character 6	Qualifier Character 7
Z None	**0** Cochlear Implant	**1** Audiometer **2** Sound Field / Booth **3** Tympanometer **4** Electroacoustic Immitance / Acoustic Reflex **5** Hearing Aid Selection / Fitting / Test **7** Electrophysiologic **9** Cochlear Implant **K** Audiovisual **L** Assistive Listening **P** Computer **Y** Other Equipment **Z** None	**Z** None
Z None	**1** Ear Canal Probe Microphone **6** Binaural Electroacoustic Hearing Aid Check **8** Monaural Electroacoustic Hearing Aid Check	**5** Hearing Aid Selection / Fitting / Test **Z** None	**Z** None
Z None	**2** Monaural Hearing Aid **3** Binaural Hearing Aid	**1** Audiometer **2** Sound Field / Booth **3** Tympanometer **4** Electroacoustic Immitance / Acoustic Reflex **5** Hearing Aid Selection / Fitting / Test **K** Audiovisual **L** Assistive Listening **P** Computer **Z** None	**Z** None
Z None	**4** Assistive Listening System/Device Selection	**1** Audiometer **2** Sound Field / Booth **3** Tympanometer **4** Electroacoustic Immitance / Acoustic Reflex **K** Audiovisual **L** Assistive Listening **Z** None	**Z** None
Z None	**5** Sensory Aids	**1** Audiometer **2** Sound Field / Booth **3** Tympanometer **4** Electroacoustic Immitance / Acoustic Reflex **5** Hearing Aid Selection / Fitting / Test **K** Audiovisual **L** Assistive Listening **Z** None	**Z** None
Z None	**7** Ear Protector Attentuation	**0** Occupational Hearing **Z** None	**Z** None

F Physical Rehabilitation and Diagnostic Audiology
1 Diagnostic Audiology
5 Vestibular Assessment Measurement of the vestibular system and related functions

Body System/Region Character 4	Type Qualifier Character 5	Equipment Character 6	Qualifier Character 7
Z None	**0** Bithermal, Binaural Caloric Irrigation **1** Bithermal, Monaural Caloric Irrigation **2** Unithermal Binaural Screen **3** Oscillating Tracking **4** Sinusoidal Vertical Axis Rotational **5** Dix-Hallpike Dynamic **6** Computerized Dynamic Posturography	**8** Vestibular / Balance **Z** None	**Z** None
Z None	**7** Tinnitus Masker	**5** Hearing Aid Selection / Fitting / Test **Z** None	**Z** None

Mental Health GZ1–GZJ

G Mental Health
Z None
1 Psychological Tests The administration and interpretation of standardized psychological tests and measurement instruments for the assessment of psychological function

Type Qualifier Character 4	Qualifier Character 5	Qualifier Character 6	Qualifier Character 7
0 Developmental 1 Personality and Behavioral 2 Intellectual and Psychoeducational 3 Neuropsychological 4 Neurobehavioral and Cognitive Status	Z None	Z None	Z None

G Mental Health
Z None
2 Crisis Intervention Treatment of a traumatized, acutely disturbed or distressed individual for the purpose of short-term stabilization

Type Qualifier Character 4	Qualifier Character 5	Qualifier Character 6	Qualifier Character 7
Z None	Z None	Z None	Z None

G Mental Health
Z None
3 Medication Management Monitoring and adjusting the use of medications for the treatment of a mental health disorder

Type Qualifier Character 4	Qualifier Character 5	Qualifier Character 6	Qualifier Character 7
Z None	Z None	Z None	Z None

G Mental Health
Z None
5 Individual Psychotherapy Treatment of an individual with a mental health disorder by behavioral, cognitive, psychoanalytic, psychodynamic or psychophysiological means to improve functioning or well-being

Type Qualifier Character 4	Qualifier Character 5	Qualifier Character 6	Qualifier Character 7
0 Interactive 1 Behavioral 2 Cognitive 3 Interpersonal 4 Psychoanalysis 5 Psychodynamic 6 Supportive 8 Cognitive-Behavioral 9 Psychophysiological	Z None	Z None	Z None

G Mental Health
Z None
6 Counseling The application of psychological methods to treat an individual with normal developmental issues and psychological problems in order to increase function, improve well-being, alleviate distress, maladjustment or resolve crises

Type Qualifier Character 4	Qualifier Character 5	Qualifier Character 6	Qualifier Character 7
0 Educational 1 Vocational 3 Other Counseling	Z None	Z None	Z None

G Mental Health
Z None
7 Family Psychotherapy Treatment that includes one or more family members of an individual with a mental health disorder by behavioral, cognitive, psychoanalytic, psychodynamic or psychophysiological means to improve functioning or well-being

Type Qualifier Character 4	Qualifier Character 5	Qualifier Character 6	Qualifier Character 7
2 Other Family Psychotherapy	Z None	Z None	Z None

G Mental Health
Z None
B Electroconvulsive Therapy The application of controlled electrical voltages to treat a mental health disorder

Type Qualifier Character 4	Qualifier Character 5	Qualifier Character 6	Qualifier Character 7
0 Unilateral-Single Seizure 1 Unilateral-Multiple Seizure 2 Bilateral-Single Seizure 3 Bilateral-Multiple Seizure 4 Other Electroconvulsive Therapy	Z None	Z None	Z None

G Mental Health
Z None
C Biofeedback Provision of information from the monitoring and regulating of physiological processes in conjunction with cognitive-behavioral techniques to improve patient functioning or well-being

Type Qualifier Character 4	Qualifier Character 5	Qualifier Character 6	Qualifier Character 7
9 Other Biofeedback	Z None	Z None	Z None

G Mental Health
Z None
F Hypnosis Induction of a state of heightened suggestibility by auditory, visual and tactile techniques to elicit an emotional or behavioral response

Type Qualifier Character 4	Qualifier Character 5	Qualifier Character 6	Qualifier Character 7
Z None	Z None	Z None	Z None

G Mental Health
Z None
G Narcosynthesis Administration of intravenous barbiturates in order to release suppressed or repressed thoughts

Type Qualifier Character 4	Qualifier Character 5	Qualifier Character 6	Qualifier Character 7
Z None	Z None	Z None	Z None

G Mental Health
Z None
H Group Psychotherapy Treatment of two or more individuals with a mental health disorder by behavioral, cognitive, psychoanalytic, psychodynamic or psychophysiological means to improve functioning or well-being

Type Qualifier Character 4	Qualifier Character 5	Qualifier Character 6	Qualifier Character 7
Z None	Z None	Z None	Z None

G Mental Health
Z None
J Light Therapy Application of specialized light treatments to improve functioning or well-being

Type Qualifier Character 4	Qualifier Character 5	Qualifier Character 6	Qualifier Character 7
Z None	Z None	Z None	Z None

Substance Abuse Treatment HZ2–HZ9

H Substance Abuse Treatment
Z None
2 Detoxification Services Detoxification from alcohol and/or drugs

Type Qualifier Character 4	Qualifier Character 5	Qualifier Character 6	Qualifier Character 7
Z None ⊞	Z None	Z None	Z None

DRG Non-OR HZ2ZZZZ

See Appendix I for Procedure Combinations
Combo-only HZ2ZZZZ
⊞ HZ2ZZZZ

H Substance Abuse Treatment
Z None
3 Individual Counseling The application of psychological methods to treat an individual with addictive behavior

Type Qualifier Character 4	Qualifier Character 5	Qualifier Character 6	Qualifier Character 7
0 Cognitive ⊞	Z None	Z None	Z None
1 Behavioral ⊞			
2 Cognitive-Behavioral ⊞			
3 12-Step ⊞			
4 Interpersonal ⊞			
5 Vocational ⊞			
6 Psychoeducation ⊞			
7 Motivational Enhancement ⊞			
8 Confrontational ⊞			
9 Continuing Care ⊞			
B Spiritual ⊞			
C Pre/Post-Test Infectious Disease			

See Appendix I for Procedure Combinations
⊞ HZ3[0,1,2,3,4,5,6,7,8,9,B]ZZZ

H Substance Abuse Treatment
Z None
4 Group Counseling The application of psychological methods to treat two or more individuals with addictive behavior

Type Qualifier Character 4	Qualifier Character 5	Qualifier Character 6	Qualifier Character 7
0 Cognitive ⊞	Z None	Z None	Z None
1 Behavioral ⊞			
2 Cognitive-Behavioral ⊞			
3 12-Step ⊞			
4 Interpersonal ⊞			
5 Vocational ⊞			
6 Psychoeducation ⊞			
7 Motivational Enhancement ⊞			
8 Confrontational ⊞			
9 Continuing Care ⊞			
B Spiritual ⊞			
C Pre/Post-Test Infectious Disease			

See Appendix I for Procedure Combinations
⊞ HZ4[0,1,2,3,4,5,6,7,8,9,B]ZZZ

H Substance Abuse Treatment
Z None
5 Individual Psychotherapy Treatment of an individual with addictive behavior by behavioral, cognitive, psychoanalytic, psychodynamic or psychophysiological means

Type Qualifier Character 4	Qualifier Character 5	Qualifier Character 6	Qualifier Character 7
Ø Cognitive 1 Behavioral 2 Cognitive-Behavioral 3 12-Step 4 Interpersonal 5 Interactive 6 Psychoeducation 7 Motivational Enhancement 8 Confrontational 9 Supportive B Psychoanalysis C Psychodynamic D Psychophysiological	Z None	Z None	Z None

DRG Non-OR For all type qualifier and qualifier values

H Substance Abuse Treatment
Z None
6 Family Counseling The application of psychological methods that includes one or more family members to treat an individual with addictive behavior

Type Qualifier Character 4	Qualifier Character 5	Qualifier Character 6	Qualifier Character 7
3 Other Family Counseling	Z None	Z None	Z None

DRG Non-OR For all type qualifier and qualifier values

H Substance Abuse Treatment
Z None
8 Medication Management Monitoring or adjusting the use of replacement medications for the treatment of addiction

Type Qualifier Character 4	Qualifier Character 5	Qualifier Character 6	Qualifier Character 7
Ø Nicotine Replacement 1 Methadone Maintenance 2 Levo-alpha-acetyl-methadol (LAAM) 3 Antabuse 4 Naltrexone 5 Naloxone 6 Clonidine 7 Bupropion 8 Psychiatric Medication 9 Other Replacement Medication	Z None	Z None	Z None

DRG Non-OR For all type qualifier and qualifier values

H Substance Abuse Treatment
Z None
9 Pharmacotherapy The use of replacement medications for the treatment of addiction

Type Qualifier Character 4	Qualifier Character 5	Qualifier Character 6	Qualifier Character 7
Ø Nicotine Replacement 1 Methadone Maintenance 2 Levo-alpha-acetyl-methadol (LAAM) 3 Antabuse 4 Naltrexone 5 Naloxone 6 Clonidine 7 Bupropion 8 Psychiatric Medication 9 Other Replacement Medication	Z None	Z None	Z None

DRG Non-OR For all type qualifier and qualifier values

Appendix A: Root Operations Definitions

Ø	Medical and Surgical		
Ø	Alteration	Definition:	Modifying the natural anatomic structure of a body part without affecting the function of the body part
		Explanation:	Principal purpose is to improve appearance
		Examples:	Face lift, breast augmentation
1	Bypass	Definition:	Altering the route of passage of the contents of a tubular body part
		Explanation:	Rerouting contents of a body part to a downstream area of the normal route, to a similar route and body part, or to an abnormal route and dissimilar body part. Includes one or more anastomoses, with or without the use of a device
		Examples:	Coronary artery bypass, colostomy formation
2	Change	Definition:	Taking out or off a device from a body part and putting back an identical or similar device in or on the same body part without cutting or puncturing the skin or a mucous membrane
		Explanation:	All CHANGE procedures are coded using the approach EXTERNAL
		Example:	Urinary catheter change, gastrostomy tube change
3	Control	Definition:	Stopping, or attempting to stop, postprocedural bleeding
		Explanation:	The site of the bleeding is coded as an anatomical region and not to a specific body part.
		Examples:	Control of post-prostatectomy hemorrhage, control of post-tonsillectomy hemorrhage
4	Creation	Definition:	Making a new genital structure that does not take over the function of a body part
		Explanation:	Used only for sex change operations
		Examples:	Creation of vagina in a male, creation of penis in a female
5	Destruction	Definition:	Physical eradication of all or a portion of a body part by the direct use of energy, force, or a destructive agent
		Explanation:	None of the body part is physically taken out.
		Examples:	Fulguration of rectal polyp, cautery of skin lesion
6	Detachment	Definition:	Cutting off all or part of the upper or lower extremities
		Explanation:	The body part value is the site of the detachment, with a qualifier if applicable to further specify the level where the extremity was detached
		Examples:	Below knee amputation, disarticulation of shoulder
7	Dilation	Definition:	Expanding an orifice or the lumen of a tubular body part
		Explanation:	The orifice can be a natural orifice or an artificially created orifice. Accomplished by stretching a tubular body part using intraluminal pressure or by cutting part of the orifice or wall of the tubular body part.
		Examples:	Percutaneous transluminal angioplasty, pyloromyotomy
8	Division	Definition:	Cutting into a body part without draining fluids and/or gases from the body part in order to separate or transect a body part
		Explanation:	All or a portion of the body part is separated into two or more portions.
		Examples:	Spinal cordotomy, osteotomy
9	Drainage	Definition:	Taking or letting out fluids and/or gases from a body part
		Explanation:	The qualifier *diagnostic* is used to identify drainage procedures that are biopsies.
		Examples:	Thoracentesis, incision and drainage
B	Excision	Definition:	Cutting out or off, without replacement, a portion of a body part
		Explanation:	The qualifier *diagnostic* is used to identify excision procedures that are biopsies.
		Examples:	Partial nephrectomy, liver biopsy
C	Extirpation	Definition:	Taking or cutting out solid matter from a body part
		Explanation:	The solid matter may be an abnormal byproduct of a biological function or a foreign body; it may be imbedded in a body part or in the lumen of a tubular body part. The solid matter may or may not have been previously broken into pieces.
		Examples:	Thrombectomy, choledocholithotomy, endarterectomy

Continued on next page

Ø Medical and Surgical

Continued from previous page

D	Extraction	Definition:	Pulling or stripping out or off all or a portion of a body part by the use of force
		Explanation:	The qualifier DIAGNOSTIC is used to identify extractions that are biopsies.
		Examples:	Dilation and curettage, vein stripping
F	Fragmentation	Definition:	Breaking solid matter in a body part into pieces
		Explanation:	Physical force (e.g., manual, ultrasonic) applied directly or indirectly through intervening body parts are used to break the solid matter into pieces. The solid matter may be an abnormal byproduct of a biological function or a foreign body. The pieces of solid matter are not taken out, but are eliminated or absorbed through normal biological functions.
		Examples:	Extracorporeal shockwave lithotripsy, transurethral lithotripsy
G	Fusion	Definition:	Joining together portions of an articular body part, rendering the articular body part immobile
		Explanation:	The body part is joined together by fixation device, bone graft, or other means.
		Examples:	Spinal fusion, ankle arthrodesis
H	Insertion	Definition:	Putting in a nonbiological appliance that monitors, assists, performs, or prevents a physiological function but does not physically take the place of a body part
		Explanation:	None
		Examples:	Insertion of radioactive implant, insertion of central venous catheter
J	Inspection	Definition:	Visually and/or manually exploring a body part
		Explanation:	Visual exploration may be performed with or without optical instrumentation. Manual exploration may be performed directly or through intervening body layers.
		Examples:	Diagnostic arthroscopy, exploratory laparotomy
K	Map	Definition:	Locating the route of passage of electrical impulses and/or locating functional areas in a body part
		Explanation:	Applicable only to the cardiac conduction mechanism and the central nervous system
		Examples:	Cardiac mapping, cortical mapping
L	Occlusion	Definition:	Completely closing an orifice or lumen of a tubular body part
		Explanation:	The orifice can be a natural orifice or an artificially created orifice.
		Examples:	Fallopian tube ligation, ligation of inferior vena cava
M	Reattachment	Definition:	Putting back in or on all or a portion of a separated body part to its normal location or other suitable location
		Explanation:	Vascular circulation and nervous pathways may or may not be reestablished.
		Examples:	Reattachment of hand, reattachment of avulsed kidney
N	Release	Definition:	Freeing a body part from an abnormal physical constraint by cutting or by use of force
		Explanation:	Some of the restraining tissue may be taken out but none of the body part is taken out.
		Examples:	Adhesiolysis, carpal tunnel release
P	Removal	Definition:	Taking out or off a device from a body part
		Explanation:	If a device is taken out and a similar device put in without cutting or puncturing the skin or mucous membrane, the procedure is coded to the root operation CHANGE. Otherwise, the procedure for taking out the device is coded to the root operation REMOVAL, and the procedure for putting in the new device is coded to the root operation performed.
		Examples:	Drainage tube removal, cardiac pacemaker removal
Q	Repair	Definition:	Restoring, to the extent possible, a body part to its normal anatomic structure and function
		Explanation:	Used only when the method to accomplish the repair is not one of the other root operations
		Examples:	Colostomy takedown, herniorrhaphy, suture of laceration
R	Replacement	Definition:	Putting in or on a biological or synthetic material that physically takes the place and/or function of all or a portion of a body part
		Explanation:	The body part may have been taken out or replaced, or may be taken out, physically eradicated, or rendered nonfunctional during the REPLACEMENT procedure. A REMOVAL procedure is coded for taking out the device used in a previous replacement procedure
		Examples:	Total hip replacement, free skin graft
S	Reposition	Definition:	Moving to its normal location or other suitable location all or a portion of a body part
		Explanation:	The body part is moved to a new location from an abnormal location, or from a normal location where it is not functioning correctly. The body part may or may not be cut out or off to be moved to the new location.
		Examples:	Reposition of undescended testicle, fracture reduction

Continued on next page

Ø	Medical and Surgical		*Continued from previous page*
T	Resection	Definition:	Cutting out or off, without replacement, all of a body part
		Explanation:	None
		Examples:	Total nephrectomy, total lobectomy of lung
V	Restriction	Definition:	Partially closing an orifice or the lumen of a tubular body part
		Explanation:	The orifice can be a natural orifice or an artificially created orifice.
		Examples:	Esophagogastric fundoplication, cervical cerclage
W	Revision	Definition:	Correcting, to the extent possible, a portion of a malfunctioning device or the position of a displaced device
		Explanation:	Revision can include correcting a malfunctioning or displaced device by taking out or putting in components of the device such as a screw or pin.
		Examples:	Adjustment of position of pacemaker lead, recementing of hip prosthesis
U	Supplement	Definition:	Putting in or on biological or synthetic material that physically reinforces and/or augments the function of a portion of a body part
		Explanation:	The biological material is non-living, or is living and from the same individual. The body part may have been previously replaced, and the SUPPLEMENT procedure is performed to physically reinforce and/or augment the function of the replaced body part
		Examples:	Herniorrhaphy using mesh, free nerve graft, mitral valve ring annuloplasty, put a new acetabular liner in a previous hip replacement
X	Transfer	Definition:	Moving, without taking out, all or a portion of a body part to another location to take over the function of all or a portion of a body part
		Explanation:	The body part transferred remains connected to its vascular and nervous supply.
		Examples:	Tendon transfer, skin pedicle flap transfer
Y	Transplantation	Definition:	Putting in or on all or a portion of a living body part taken from another individual or animal to physically take the place and/or function of all or a portion of a similar body part
		Explanation:	The native body part may or may not be taken out, and the transplanted body part may take over all or a portion of its function.
		Examples:	Kidney transplant, heart transplant

Root Operation Definitions for Other Sections

1	Obstetrics		
A	Abortion	Definition:	Artificially terminating a pregnancy
		Explanation:	Subdivided according to whether an additional device such as a laminaria or abortifacient is used, or whether the abortion was performed by mechanical means
		Examples:	Transvaginal abortion using vacuum aspiration technique
E	Delivery	Definition:	Assisting the passage of the products of conception from the genital canal
		Explanation:	Applies only to manually-assisted, vaginal delivery
		Examples:	Manually-assisted delivery

2	Placement		
Ø	Change	Definition:	Taking out or off a device from a body region and putting back an identical or similar device in or on the same body region without cutting or puncturing the skin or a mucous membrane
		Explanation:	Procedures performed without making an incision or a puncture.
		Examples:	Change of vaginal packing
1	Compression	Definition:	Putting pressure on a body region
		Explanation:	Procedures performed without making an incision or a puncture
		Examples:	Placement of pressure dressing on abdominal wall
2	Dressing	Definition:	Putting material on a body region for protection
		Explanation:	Procedures performed without making an incision or a puncture
		Examples:	Application of sterile dressing to head wound

Continued on next page

2 Placement

Continued from previous page

3	Immobilization	Definition:	Limiting or preventing motion of a body region
		Explanation:	Procedures to fit a device, such as splints and braces, as described in FØDZ6EZ and FØDZ7EZ, apply only to the rehabilitation setting.
		Examples:	Placement of splint on left finger
4	Packing	Definition:	Putting material in a body region or orifice
		Explanation:	Procedures performed without making an incision or a puncture
		Examples:	Placement of nasal packing
5	Removal	Definition:	Taking out or off a device from a body region
		Explanation:	Procedures performed without making an incision or a puncture
		Examples:	Removal of stereotactic head frame
6	Traction	Definition:	Exerting a pulling force on a body region in a distal direction
		Explanation:	Traction in this section includes only the task performed using a mechanical traction apparatus.
		Examples:	Lumbar traction using motorized split-traction table

3 Administration

Ø	Introduction	Definition:	Putting in or on a therapeutic, diagnostic, nutritional, physiological, or prophylactic substance except blood or blood products
		Explanation:	All other substances administered, such as antineoplastic substance
		Examples:	Nerve block injection to median nerve
1	Irrigation	Definition:	Putting in or on a cleansing substance
		Explanation:	Substance given is a cleansing substance or dialysate
		Examples:	Flushing of eye
2	Transfusion	Definition:	Putting in blood or blood products
		Explanation:	Substance given is a blood product or a stem cell substance
		Examples:	Transfusion of cell saver red cells into central venous line

4 Measurement and Monitoring

Ø	Measurement	Definition:	Determining the level of a physiological or physical function at a point in time
		Explanation:	A single temperature reading is considered measurement.
		Examples:	External electrocardiogram(EKG), single reading
1	Monitoring	Definition:	Determining the level of a physiological or physical function repetitively over a period of time
		Explanation:	Temperature taken every half hour for 8 hours is considered monitoring
		Examples:	Urinary pressure monitoring

5 Extracorporeal Assistance and Performance

Ø	Assistance	Definition:	Taking over a portion of a physiological function by extracorporeal means
		Explanation:	Procedures that support a physiological function but do not take complete control of it, such as intra-aortic balloon pump to support cardiac output and hyperbaric oxygen treatment
		Examples:	Hyperbaric oxygenation of wound
1	Performance	Definition:	Completely taking over a physiological function by extracorporeal means
		Explanation:	Procedures in which complete control is exercised over a physiological function, such as total mechanical ventilation, cardiac pacing, and cardiopulmonary bypass
		Examples:	Cardiopulmonary bypass in conjunction with CABG
2	Restoration	Definition:	Returning, or attempting to return, a physiological function to its original state by extracorporeal means
		Explanation:	Only external cardioversion and defibrillation procedures. Failed cardioversion procedures are also included in the definition of restoration, and are coded the same as successful procedures
		Examples:	Attempted cardiac defibrillation, unsuccessful

6 Extracorporeal Therapies

0	Atmospheric Control	Definition:	Extracorporeal control of atmospheric pressure and composition
		Explanation:	None
		Examples:	Antigen-free air conditioning, series treatment
1	Decompression	Definition:	Extracorporeal elimination of undissolved gas from body fluids
		Explanation:	A single type of procedure—treatment for decompression sickness (the bends) in a hyperbaric chamber
		Examples:	Hyperbaric decompression treatment, single
2	Electromagnetic Therapy	Definition:	Extracorporeal treatment by electromagnetic rays
		Explanation:	None
		Examples:	TMS (transcranial magnetic stimulation), series treatment
3	Hyperthermia	Definition:	Extracorporeal raising of body temperature
		Explanation:	To treat temperature imbalance, and as an adjunct radiation treatment for cancer. When performed to treat temperature imbalance, the procedure is coded to this section. When performed for cancer treatment, whole-body hyperthermia is classified as a modality qualifier in section D, "Radiation Therapy."
		Examples:	None
4	Hypothermia	Definition:	Extracorporeal lowering of body temperature
		Explanation:	None
		Examples:	Whole body hypothermia treatment for temperature imbalances, series
5	Pheresis	Definition:	Extracorporeal separation of blood products
		Explanation:	Used in medical practice for two main purposes: to treat diseases where too much of a blood component is produced, such as leukemia, or to remove a blood product such as platelets from a donor, for transfusion into a patient who needs them
		Examples:	Therapeutic leukopheresis, single treatment
6	Phototherapy	Definition:	Extracorporeal treatment by light rays
		Explanation:	Phototherapy to the circulatory system means exposing the blood to light rays outside the body, using a machine that recirculates the blood and returns it to the body after phototherapy.
		Examples:	Phototherapy of circulatory system, series treatment
7	Ultrasound Therapy	Definition:	Extracorporeal treatment by ultrasound
		Explanation:	None
		Examples:	Therapeutic ultrasound of peripheral vessels, single treatment
8	Ultraviolet Light Therapy	Definition:	Extracorporeal treatment by ultraviolet light
		Explanation:	None
		Examples:	Ultraviolet light phototherapy, series treatment
9	Shock Wave Therapy	Definition:	Extracorporeal treatment by shockwaves
		Explanation:	None
		Examples:	Shockwave therapy of plantar fascia, single treatment

7 Osteopathic

0	Treatment	Definition:	Manual treatment to eliminate or alleviate somatic dysfunction and related disorders
		Explanation:	None
		Examples:	Fascial release of abdomen, osteopathic treatment

8 Other Procedures

0	Other Procedures	Definition:	Methodologies that attempt to remediate or cure a disorder or disease
		Explanation:	For nontraditional, whole-body therapies including acupuncture and meditation
		Examples:	Acupuncture

9	Chiropractic		
B	Manipulation	Definition:	Manual procedure that involves a directed thrust to move a joint past the physiological range of motion, without exceeding the anatomical limit
		Explanation:	None
		Examples:	Chiropractic treatment of cervical spine, short lever specific contact

Note: Sections B-H (Imaging through Substance Abuse Treatment) do not include root operations. Character 3 position represents type of procedure, therefore those definitions are not included in this appendix. See appendix E for definitions of the type (character 3) or type qualifiers (character 5) that provide details of the procedures performed.

Appendix B: Comparison of Medical and Surgical Root Operations

Note: the character associated with each operation appears in parentheses after its title.

Procedures That Take Out Some or All of a Body Part

Operation	Action	Target	Clarification	Example
Excision (B)	Cutting out or off	Some of a body part	Without replacing body part	Breast lumpectomy
Resection (T)	Cutting out or off	All of a body part	Without replacing body part	Total nephrectomy
Extraction (D)	Pulling out or off	All or a portion of a body part	Without replacing body part	Suction D&C
Destruction (5)	Eradicating	All or a portion of a body part	Without taking out or replacing body part	Rectal polyp fulguration
Detachment (6)	Cutting out/off	Extremity only, any level	Without replacing extremity	Below knee amputation

Procedures That Put in/Put Back or Move Some/All of a Body Part

Operation	Action	Target	Clarification	Example
Transplantation (Y)	Putting in	All or a portion of a living body part from other individual or animal	Physically takes the place and/or function of all or a portion of a body part	Heart transplant, kidney transplant
Reattachment (M)	Putting back in or on	All or a portion of a separated body part	Put in its normal or other suitable location. The vascular circulation and nervous pathways may or may not be reestablished.	Finger reattachment
Reposition (S)	Moving	All or a portion of a body part	Moving to its normal or other suitable location. Body part may or may not be cut out or off	Reposition undescended testicle
Transfer (X)	Moving to function for a similar body part	All or a portion of a body part	Without taking out body part; assumes function of similar body part and remains connected to its vascular and nervous supply	Tendon transfer, skin transfer flap

Procedures That Take Out or Eliminate Solid Matter, Fluids, or Gases From a Body Part

Operation	Action	Target	Clarification	Example
Drainage (9)	Taking or letting out	Fluids and/or gases from a body part	Without taking out any of the body part. The qualifier DIAGNOSTIC is used to identify drainage procedures that are biopsies.	Incision and drainage
Extirpation (C)	Taking or cutting out	Solid matter in a body part	Without taking out any of the body part. The solid matter may be an abnormal byproduct of a biological function or a foreign body; it may be imbedded in a body part or in the lumen of a tubular body part. The solid matter may or may not have been previously broken into pieces.	Thrombectomy
Fragmentation (F)	Breaking down	Solid matter into pieces within a body part	The physical force (e.g., manual, ultrasonic) is applied directly or indirectly, without taking out any of the body part or any solid matter. The solid matter may be an abnormal byproduct of a biological function or a foreign body. The pieces of solid matter are not taken out.	Lithotripsy

Procedures That Involve Only Examination of Body Parts and Regions

Operation	Action	Target	Clarification	Example
Inspection (J)	Visual and/or manual exploration	Some or all of a body part	Performed with or without optical instrumentation, directly or through body layers	Diagnostic arthroscopy, diagnostic cystoscopy
Map (K)	Locating	Route of passage of electrical impulses or functional areas in a body part	Applicable only to cardiac conduction mechanism and central nervous system	Cardiac mapping

Procedures That Alter the Diameter/Route of a Tubular Body Part

Operation	Action	Target	Clarification	Example
Bypass (1)	Altering the route of passage	Contents of tubular body part	May include use of living tissue, nonliving biological material or synthetic material which does not take the place of the body part. Includes one or more anastomoses, with or without the use of a device.	Gastrojejunal bypass, coronary artery bypass (CABG)
Dilation (7)	Expanding	Orifice or lumen of tubular body part	By application of intraluminal pressure or by cutting the wall of the orifice	Percutaneous transluminal angioplasty
Occlusion (L)	Completely closing	Orifice or lumen of tubular body part	Orifice may be natural or artificially created	Fallopian tube ligation
Restriction (V)	Partially closing	Orifice or lumen of tubular body part	Orifice may be natural or artificially created	Cervical cerclage, gastroesophageal fundoplication

Procedures That Always Involve Devices

Operation	Action	Target	Clarification	Example
Insertion (H)	Putting in non-biological device	Device in or on a body part	Putting in a non-biological device that monitors, performs, assists, or prevents a physical function, does not physically take the place of a body part	Pacemaker insertion, central line insertion
Replacement (R)	Putting in or on	Biological or synthetic material; living tissue taken from same individual	Physically takes the place of all or a portion of a body part. A REMOVAL procedure is assigned for taking out the device used in a previous replacement procedure.	Total hip replacement
Supplement (U)	Putting in or on	Device that reinforces or augments a body part	Biological material is nonliving or living and from the same individual	Herniorrhaphy using mesh
Removal (P)	Taking a device out or off	Device from a body part	If a new device is inserted via an incision or puncture, that procedure is coded separately	Cardiac pacemaker removal, central line removal
Change (2)	Taking a device out or off and putting back an indentical or similar device	Identical or similar device in or on a body part	Without cutting or puncturing skin or mucous membrane; all *change* procedures are coded using the *External* approach	Drainage tube change
Revision (W)	Correcting	Malfunctioning or displaced device in or on a body part	To the extent possible	Hip prosthesis adjustment, revision of pacemaker lead

Procedures Involving Cutting or Separation Only

Operation	Action	Target	Clarification	Example
Division (8)	Cutting into/Separating	A body part	Without taking out any of the body part or draining fluids and/or gases. All or a portion of the body part is separated into two or more portions.	Osteotomy, neurotomy
Release (N)	Freeing, by cutting or by the use of force	A body part	Eliminating abnormal constraint without taking out any of the body part. Some of the restraining tissue may be taken out, but none of the body part is taken out.	Peritoneal adhesiolysis

Procedures That Define Other Repairs

Operation	Action	Target	Clarification	Example
Control (3)	Stopping or attempting to stop	Postprocedural bleeding	Limited to anatomic regions not specific body parts	Control of postprostatectomy bleeding
Repair (Q)	Restoring	A body part to its natural anatomic structure and function	To the extent possible	Hernia repair, suture laceration

Procedures That Define Objectives

Operation	Action	Target	Clarification	Example
Alteration (Ø)	Modifying	Natural anatomical structure of a body part	Without affecting function of body part, performed for cosmetic purposes	Face lift
Creation (4)	Making	New genital structure	Does not physically take the place of a body part, used only for sex change operations	Artificial vagina creation
Fusion (G)	Unification and immobilization	Joint or articular body part	Stabilization of damaged joints by graft and/or fixation	Spinal fusion

Appendix C: Body Part Key

Anatomical Term	PCS Description
Abdominal aortic plexus	Abdominal Sympathetic Nerve
Abdominal esophagus	Esophagus, Lower
Abductor hallucis muscle	Foot Muscle, Right
	Foot Muscle, Left
Accessory cephalic vein	Cephalic Vein, Right
	Cephalic Vein, Left
Accessory obturator nerve	Lumbar Plexus
Accessory phrenic nerve	Phrenic nerve
Accessory spleen	Spleen
Acetabulofemoral joint	Hip Joint, Left
	Hip Joint, Right
Achilles tendon	Lower Leg Tendon, Right
	Lower Leg Tendon, Left
Acromioclavicular ligament	Shoulder Bursa and Ligament, Right
	Shoulder Bursa and Ligament, Left
Acromion (process)	Scapula, Left
	Scapula, Right
Adductor brevis muscle	Upper Leg Muscle, Right
	Upper Leg Muscle, Left
Adductor hallucis muscle	Foot Muscle, Right
	Foot Muscle, Left
Adductor longus muscle	Upper Leg Muscle, Right
	Upper Leg Muscle, Left
Adductor magnus muscle	Upper Leg Muscle, Right
	Upper Leg Muscle, Left
Adenohypophysis	Pituitary Gland
Alar ligament of axis	Head and Neck Bursa and Ligament
Alveolar process of mandible	Mandible, Left
	Mandible, Right
Alveolar process of maxilla	Maxilla, Left
	Maxilla, Right
Anal orifice	Anus
Anatomical snuffbox	Lower Arm and Wrist Tendon, Right
	Lower Arm and Wrist Tendon, Left
Angular artery	Face Artery
Angular vein	Face Vein, Left
	Face Vein, Right
Annular ligament	Elbow Bursa and Ligament, Right
	Elbow Bursa and Ligament, Left
Anorectal junction	Rectum
Ansa cervicalis	Cervical Plexus
Antebrachial fascia	Subcutaneous Tissue and Fascia, Right Lower Arm
	Subcutaneous Tissue and Fascia, Left Lower Arm
Anterior (pectoral) lymph node	Lymphatic, Left Axillary
	Lymphatic, Right Axillary

Anatomical Term	PCS Description
Anterior cerebral artery	Intracranial Artery
Anterior cerebral vein	Intracranial Vein
Anterior choroidal artery	Intracranial Artery
Anterior circumflex humeral artery	Axillary Artery, Right
	Axillary Artery, Left
Anterior communicating artery	Intracranial Artery
Anterior cruciate ligament (ACL)	Knee Bursa and Ligament, Right
	Knee Bursa and Ligament, Left
Anterior crural nerve	Femoral Nerve
Anterior facial vein	Face Vein, Left
	Face Vein, Right
Anterior intercostal artery	Internal Mammary Artery, Right
	Internal Mammary Artery, Left
Anterior interosseous nerve	Median Nerve
Anterior lateral malleolar artery	Anterior Tibial Artery, Right
	Anterior Tibial Artery, Left
Anterior lingual gland	Minor Salivary Gland
Anterior medial malleolar artery	Anterior Tibial Artery, Right
	Anterior Tibial Artery, Left
Anterior spinal artery	Vertebral Artery, Right
	Vertebral Artery, Left
Anterior tibial recurrent artery	Anterior Tibial Artery, Right
	Anterior Tibial Artery, Left
Anterior ulnar recurrent artery	Ulnar Artery, Right
	Ulnar Artery, Left
Anterior vagal trunk	Vagus Nerve
Anterior vertebral muscle	Neck Muscle, Right
	Neck Muscle, Left
Antihelix	External Ear, Right
	External Ear, Left
	External Ear, Bilateral
Antitragus	External Ear, Right
	External Ear, Left
	External Ear, Bilateral
Antrum of Highmore	Maxillary Sinus, Right
	Maxillary Sinus, Left
Aortic annulus	Aortic Valve
Aortic arch	Thoracic Aorta
Aortic intercostal artery	Thoracic Aorta
Apical (subclavicular) lymph node	Lymphatic, Left Axillary
	Lymphatic, Right Axillary
Apneustic center	Pons
Aqueduct of Sylvius	Cerebral Ventricle
Aqueous humour	Anterior Chamber, Right
	Anterior Chamber, Left

Anatomical Term	PCS Description
Arachnoid mater	Cerebral Meninges
	Spinal Meninges
Arcuate artery	Foot Artery, Right
	Foot Artery, Right
Areola	Nipple, Left
	Nipple, Right
Arterial canal (duct)	Pulmonary Artery, Left
Aryepiglottic fold	Larynx
Arytenoid cartilage	Larynx
Arytenoid muscle	Neck Muscle, Right
	Neck Muscle, Left
Ascending aorta	Thoracic Aorta
Ascending palatine artery	Face Artery
Ascending pharyngeal artery	External Carotid Artery, Right
	External Carotid Artery, Left
Atlantoaxial joint	Cervical Vertebral Joint
Atrioventricular node	Conduction Mechanism
Atrium dextrum cordis	Atrium, Right
Atrium pulmonale	Atrium, Left
Auditory tube	Eustachian Tube, Right
	Eustachian Tube, Left
Auerbach's (myenteric) plexus	Abdominal Sympathetic Nerve
Auricle	External Ear, Right
	External Ear, Left
	External Ear, Bilateral
Auricularis muscle	Head Muscle
Axillary fascia	Subcutaneous Tissue and Fascia, Right Upper Arm
	Subcutaneous Tissue and Fascia, Left Upper Arm
Axillary nerve	Brachial Plexus
Bartholin's (greater vestibular) gland	Vestibular Gland
Basal (internal) cerebral vein	Intracranial Vein
Basal nuclei	Basal Ganglia
Basilar artery	Intracranial Artery
Basis pontis	Pons
Biceps brachii muscle	Upper Arm Muscle, Right
	Upper Arm Muscle, Left
Biceps femoris muscle	Upper Leg Muscle, Right
	Upper Leg Muscle, Left
Bicipital aponeurosis	Subcutaneous Tissue and Fascia, Right Lower Arm
	Subcutaneous Tissue and Fascia, Left Lower Arm
Bicuspid valve	Mitral Valve
Body of femur	Femoral Shaft, Right
	Femoral Shaft, Left
Body of fibula	Fibula, Left
	Fibula, Right

Anatomical Term	PCS Description
Bony labyrinth	Inner Ear, Left
	Inner Ear, Right
Bony orbit	Orbit, Left
	Orbit, Right
Bony vestibule	Inner Ear, Left
	Inner Ear, Right
Botallo's duct	Pulmonary Artery, Left
Brachial (lateral) lymph node	Lymphatic, Left Axillary
	Lymphatic, Right Axillary
Brachialis muscle	Upper Arm Muscle, Right
	Upper Arm Muscle, Left
Brachiocephalic artery or trunk	Innominate Artery
	Innominate Artery
Brachiocephalic vein	Innominate Vein, Right
	Innominate Vein, Left
Brachioradialis muscle	Lower Arm and Wrist Muscle, Right
	Lower Arm and Wrist Muscle, Left
Broad ligament	Uterine Supporting Structure
Bronchial artery	Thoracic Aorta
Buccal gland	Buccal Mucosa
Buccinator lymph node	Lymphatic, Head
Buccinator muscle	Facial Muscle
Bulbospongiosus muscle	Perineum Muscle
Bulbourethral (Cowper's) gland	Urethra
Bundle of His	Conduction Mechanism
Bundle of Kent	Conduction Mechanism
Calcaneocuboid ligament	Foot Bursa and Ligament, Right
	Foot Bursa and Ligament, Left
Calcaneocuboid joint	Tarsal Joint, Right
	Tarsal Joint, Left
Calcaneofibular ligament	Ankle Bursa and Ligament, Right
	Ankle Bursa and Ligament, Left
Calcaneus	Tarsal, Left
	Tarsal, Right
Capitate bone	Carpal, Left
	Carpal, Right
Cardia	Esophagogastric Junction
Cardiac plexus	Thoracic Sympathetic Nerve
Cardioesophageal junction	Esophagogastric Junction
Caroticotympanic artery	Internal Carotid Artery, Right
	Internal Carotid Artery, Left
Carotid glomus	Carotid Bodies, Bilateral
	Carotid Body, Right
	Carotid Body, Left
Carotid sinus nerve	Glossopharyngeal Nerve
Carotid sinus	Internal Carotid Artery, Right
	Internal Carotid Artery, Left
Carpometacarpal (CMC) joint	Metacarpocarpal Joint, Right
	Metacarpocarpal Joint, Left

Anatomical Term	PCS Description
Carpometacarpal ligament	Hand Bursa and Ligament, Right
	Hand Bursa and Ligament, Left
Cauda equina	Lumbar Spinal Cord
Cavernous plexus	Head and Neck Sympathetic Nerve
Celiac ganglion	Abdominal Sympathetic Nerve
Celiac (solar) plexus	Abdominal Sympathetic Nerve
Celiac lymph node	Lymphatic, Aortic
Celiac trunk	Celiac Artery
Central axillary lymph node	Lymphatic, Left Axillary
	Lymphatic, Right Axillary
Cerebral aqueduct (Sylvius)	Cerebral Ventricle
Cerebrum	Brain
Cervical esophagus	Esophagus, Upper
Cervical facet joint	Cervical Vertebral Joints, 2 or more
	Cervical Vertebral Joint
Cervical ganglion	Head and Neck Sympathetic Nerve
Cervical intertransverse ligament	Head and Neck Bursa and Ligament
Cervical interspinous ligament	Head and Neck Bursa and Ligament
Cervical ligamentum flavum	Head and Neck Bursa and Ligament
Cervical lymph node	Lymphatic, Left Neck
	Lymphatic, Right Neck
Cervicothoracic facet joint	Cervicothoracic Vertebral Joint
Choana	Nasopharynx
Chondroglossus muscle	Tongue, Palate, Pharynx Muscle
Chorda tympani	Facial Nerve
Choroid plexus	Cerebral Ventricle
Ciliary body	Eye, Left
	Eye, Right
Ciliary ganglion	Head and Neck Sympathetic Nerve
Circle of Willis	Intracranial Artery
Circumflex illiac artery	Femoral Artery, Right
	Femoral Artery, Left
Claustrum	Basal Ganglia
Coccygeal body	Coccygeal Glomus
Coccygeus muscle	Trunk Muscle, Left
Cochlea	Inner Ear, Left
	Inner Ear, Right
Cochlear nerve	Acoustic Nerve
Columella	Nose
Common digital vein	Foot Vein, Left
	Foot Vein, Right
Common facial vein	Face Vein, Left
	Face Vein, Right
Common fibular nerve	Peroneal Nerve
Common hepatic artery	Hepatic Artery
Common iliac (subaortic) lymph node	Lymphatic, Pelvis
Common interosseous artery	Ulnar Artery, Right
	Ulnar Artery, Left
Common peroneal nerve	Peroneal Nerve
Condyloid process	Mandible, Left
	Mandible, Right
Conus arteriosus	Ventricle, Right
Conus medullaris	Lumbar Spinal Cord
Coracoacromial ligament	Shoulder Bursa and Ligament, Right
	Shoulder Bursa and Ligament, Left
Coracobrachialis muscle	Upper Arm Muscle, Right
	Upper Arm Muscle, Left
Coracoclavicular ligament	Shoulder Bursa and Ligament, Right
	Shoulder Bursa and Ligament, Left
Coracohumeral ligament	Shoulder Bursa and Ligament, Right
	Shoulder Bursa and Ligament, Left
Coracoid process	Scapula, Left
	Scapula, Right
Corniculate cartilage	Larynx
Corpus callosum	Brain
Corpus cavernosum	Penis
Corpus spongiosum	Penis
Corpus striatum	Basal Ganglia
Corrugator supercilii muscle	Facial Muscle
Costocervical trunk	Subclavian Artery, Right
	Subclavian Artery, Left
Costoclavicular ligament	Shoulder Bursa and Ligament, Right
	Shoulder Bursa and Ligament, Left
Costotransverse joint	Thoracic Vertebral Joint
Costotransverse ligament	Thorax Bursa and Ligament, Right
	Thorax Bursa and Ligament, Left
Costovertebral joint	Thoracic Vertebral Joint
Costoxiphoid ligament	Thorax Bursa and Ligament, Right
	Thorax Bursa and Ligament, Left
Cowper's (bulbourethral) gland	Urethra
Cranial dura mater	Dura Mater
Cranial epidural space	Epidural Space
Cranial subarachnoid space	Subarachnoid Space
Cranial subdural space	Subdural Space
Cremaster muscle	Perineum Muscle
Cribriform plate	Ethmoid Bone, Right
	Ethmoid Bone, Left
Cricoid cartilage	Larynx
Cricothyroid artery	Thyroid Artery, Right
	Thyroid Artery, Left
Cricothyroid muscle	Neck Muscle, Right
	Neck Muscle, Left
Crural fascia	Subcutaneous Tissue and Fascia, Right Upper Leg
	Subcutaneous Tissue and Fascia, Left Upper Leg

Anatomical Term	PCS Description
Cubital lymph node	Lymphatic, Left Upper Extremity
	Lymphatic, Right Upper Extremity
Cubital nerve	Ulnar Nerve
Cuboid bone	Tarsal, Left
	Tarsal, Right
Cuboideonavicular joint	Tarsal Joint, Right
	Tarsal Joint, Left
Culmen	Cerebellum
Cuneiform cartilage	Larynx
Cuneonavicular ligament	Foot Bursa and Ligament, Right
	Foot Bursa and Ligament, Left
Cuneonavicular joint	Tarsal Joint, Right
	Tarsal Joint, Left
Cutaneous (transverse) cervical nerve	Cervical Plexus
Deep cervical fascia	Subcutaneous Tissue and Fascia, Anterior Neck
Deep cervical vein	Vertebral Vein, Right
	Vertebral Vein, Left
Deep circumflex iliac artery	External Iliac Artery, Right
	External Iliac Artery, Left
Deep facial vein	Face Vein, Left
	Face Vein, Right
Deep femoral artery	Femoral Artery, Right
	Femoral Artery, Left
Deep femoral (profunda femoris) vein	Femoral Vein, Right
	Femoral Vein, Left
Deep palmar arch	Hand Artery, Right
	Hand Artery, Left
Deep transverse perineal muscle	Perineum Muscle
Deferential artery	Internal Iliac Artery, Right
	Internal Iliac Artery, Left
Deltoid fascia	Subcutaneous Tissue and Fascia, Right Upper Arm
	Subcutaneous Tissue and Fascia, Left Upper Arm
Deltoid ligament	Ankle Bursa and Ligament, Right
	Ankle Bursa and Ligament, Left
Deltoid muscle	Shoulder Muscle, Right
	Shoulder Muscle, Left
Deltopectoral (infraclavicular) lymph node	Lymphatic, Left Upper Extremity
	Lymphatic, Right Upper Extremity
Dentate ligament	Dura Mater
Denticulate ligament	Spinal Meninges
Depressor anguli oris muscle	Facial Muscle
Depressor labii inferioris muscle	Facial Muscle
Depressor septi nasi muscle	Facial Muscle
Depressor supercilii muscle	Facial Muscle

Anatomical Term	PCS Description
Dermis	Skin
Descending genicular artery	Femoral Artery, Right
	Femoral Artery, Left
Diaphragma sellae	Dura Mater
Distal radioulnar joint	Wrist Joint, Right
	Wrist Joint, Left
Dorsal digital nerve	Radial Nerve
Dorsal metacarpal vein	Hand Vein, Left
	Hand Vein, Right
Dorsal metatarsal artery	Foot Artery, Right
	Foot Artery, Left
Dorsal metatarsal vein	Foot Vein, Left
	Foot Vein, Right
Dorsal scapular artery	Subclavian Artery, Right
	Subclavian Artery, Left
Dorsal scapular nerve	Brachial Plexus
Dorsal venous arch	Foot Vein, Left
	Foot Vein, Right
Dorsalis pedis artery	Anterior Tibial Artery, Right
	Anterior Tibial Artery, Left
Duct of Santorini	Pancreatic Duct, Accessory
Duct of Wirsung	Pancreatic Duct
Ductus deferens	Vas Deferens, Right
	Vas Deferens, Left
	Vas Deferens, Bilateral
	Vas Deferens
Duodenal ampulla	Ampulla of Vater
Duodenojejunal flexure	Jejunum
Dural venous sinus	Intracranial Vein
Earlobe	External Ear, Right
	External Ear, Left
	External Ear, Bilateral
Eighth cranial nerve	Acoustic Nerve
Ejaculatory duct	Vas Deferens, Right
	Vas Deferens, Left
	Vas Deferens, Bilateral
	Vas Deferens
Eleventh cranial nerve	Accessory Nerve
Encephalon	Brain
Ependyma	Cerebral Ventricle
Epidermis	Skin
Epiploic foramen	Peritoneum
Epithalamus	Thalamus
Epitroclear lymph node	Lymphatic, Left Upper Extremity
	Lymphatic, Right Upper Extremity
Erector spinae muscle	Trunk Muscle, Right
	Trunk Muscle, Left
Esophageal artery	Thoracic Aorta
Esophageal plexus	Thoracic Sympathetic Nerve
Ethmoidal air cell	Ethmoid Sinus, Right
	Ethmoid Sinus, Left

Anatomical Term	PCS Description
Extensor carpi radialis muscle	Lower Arm and Wrist Muscle, Right
Extensor carpi ulnaris muscle	Lower Arm and Wrist Muscle, Right
Extensor digitorum brevis muscle	Foot Muscle, Right
	Foot Muscle, Left
Extensor digitorum longus muscle	Lower Leg Muscle, Right
	Lower Leg Muscle, Left
Extensor hallucis brevis muscle	Foot Muscle, Right
	Foot Muscle, Left
Extensor hallucis longus muscle	Lower Leg Muscle, Right
	Lower Leg Muscle, Left
External anal sphincter	Anal Sphincter
External auditory meatus	External Auditory Canal, Right
	External Auditory Canal, Left
External maxillary artery	Face Artery
External naris	Nose
External oblique aponeurosis	Subcutaneous Tissue and Fascia, Trunk
External oblique muscle	Abdomen Muscle, Right
	Abdomen Muscle, Left
External popliteal nerve	Peroneal Nerve
External pudendal artery	Femoral Artery, Right
	Femoral Artery, Left
External pudendal vein	Greater Saphenous Vein, Right
	Greater Saphenous Vein, Left
External urethral sphincter	Urethra
Extradural space	Epidural Space
Facial artery	Face Artery
False vocal cord	Larynx
Falx cerebri	Dura Mater
Fascia lata	Subcutaneous Tissue and Fascia, Right Upper Leg
	Subcutaneous Tissue and Fascia, Left Upper Leg
Femoral head	Upper Femur, Right
	Upper Femur, Left
Femoral lymph node	Lymphatic, Left Lower Extremity
	Lymphatic, Right Lower Extremity
Femoropatellar joint	Knee Joint, Right
	Knee Joint, Left
	Knee Joint, Femoral Surface, Right
	Knee Joint, Femoral Surface, Left
Femorotibial joint	Knee Joint, Right
	Knee Joint, Left
	Knee Joint, Tibial Surface, Right
	Knee Joint, Tibial Surface, Left
Fibular artery	Peroneal Artery, Right
	Peroneal Artery, Left
Fibularis brevis muscle	Lower Leg Muscle, Right
	Lower Leg Muscle, Left

Anatomical Term	PCS Description
Fibularis longus muscle	Lower Leg Muscle, Right
	Lower Leg Muscle, Left
Fifth cranial nerve	Trigeminal Nerve
First cranial nerve	Olfactory Nerve
First intercostal nerve	Brachial Plexus
Flexor carpi ulnaris muscle	Lower Arm and Wrist Muscle, Left
	Lower Arm and Wrist Muscle, Right
Flexor digitorum brevis muscle	Foot Muscle, Right
	Foot Muscle, Left
Flexor digitorum longus muscle	Lower Leg Muscle, Right
	Lower Leg Muscle, Left
Flexor hallucis brevis muscle	Foot Muscle, Right
	Foot Muscle, Left
Flexor hallucis longus muscle	Lower Leg Muscle, Right
	Lower Leg Muscle, Left
Flexor pollicis longus muscle	Lower Arm and Wrist Muscle, Right
	Lower Arm and Wrist Muscle, Left
Foramen magnum	Occipital Bone, Right
	Occipital Bone, Left
Foramen of Monro (intraventricular)	Cerebral Ventricle
Foreskin	Prepuce
Fossa of Rosenmuller	Nasopharynx
Fourth cranial nerve	Trochlear Nerve
Fourth ventricle	Cerebral Ventricle
Fovea	Retina, Left
	Retina, Right
Frenulum labii inferioris	Lower Lip
Frenulum labii superioris	Upper Lip
Frenulum linguae	Tongue
Frontal lobe	Cerebral Hemisphere
Frontal vein	Face Vein, Left
	Face Vein, Right
Fundus uteri	Uterus
Galea aponeurotica	Subcutaneous Tissue and Fascia, Scalp
Ganglion impar (ganglion of Walther)	Sacral Sympathetic Nerve
Gasserian ganglion	Trigeminal Nerve
Gastric lymph node	Lymphatic, Aortic
Gastric plexus	Abdominal Sympathetic Nerve
Gastrocnemius muscle	Lower Leg Muscle, Right
	Lower Leg Muscle, Left
Gastrocolic ligament	Greater Omentum
Gastrocolic omentum	Greater Omentum
Gastroduodenal artery	Hepatic Artery
Gastroesophageal (GE) junction	Esophagogastric Junction
Gastrohepatic omentum	Lesser Omentum
Gastrophrenic ligament	Greater Omentum
Gastrosplenic ligament	Greater Omentum

Anatomical Term	PCS Description
Gemellus muscle	Hip Muscle, Right
	Hip Muscle, Left
Geniculate ganglion	Facial Nerve
Geniculate nucleus	Thalamus
Genioglossus muscle	Tongue, Palate, Pharynx Muscle
Genitofemoral nerve	Lumbar Plexus
Glans penis	Prepuce
Glenohumeral joint	Shoulder Joint, Right
	Shoulder Joint, Left
Glenohumeral ligament	Shoulder Bursa and Ligament, Right
	Shoulder Bursa and Ligament, Left
Glenoid fossa (of scapula)	Glenoid Cavity, Right
	Glenoid Cavity, Left
Glenoid ligament (labrum)	Shoulder Bursa and Ligament, Right
	Shoulder Bursa and Ligament, Left
Globus pallidus	Basal Ganglia
Glossoepiglottic fold	Epiglottis
Glottis	Larynx
Gluteal lymph node	Lymphatic, Pelvis
Gluteal vein	Hypogastric Vein, Right
	Hypogastric Vein, Left
Gluteus maximus muscle	Hip Muscle, Right
	Hip Muscle, Left
Gluteus medius muscle	Hip Muscle, Right
	Hip Muscle, Left
Gluteus minimus muscle	Hip Muscle, Right
	Hip Muscle, Left
Gracilis muscle	Upper Leg Muscle, Right
	Upper Leg Muscle, Left
Great auricular nerve	Cervical Plexus
Great cerebral vein	Intracranial Vein
Great saphenous vein	Greater Saphenous Vein, Right
	Greater Saphenous Vein, Left
Greater alar cartilage	Nose
Greater occipital nerve	Cervical Nerve
Greater splanchnic nerve	Thoracic Sympathetic Nerve
Greater superficial petrosal nerve	Facial Nerve
Greater trochanter	Upper Femur, Right
	Upper Femur, Left
Greater tuberosity	Humeral Head, Right
	Humeral Head, Left
Greater vestibular (Bartholin's) gland	Vestibular Gland
Greater wing	Sphenoid Bone, Right
	Sphenoid Bone, Left
Hallux	1st Toe, Left
	1st Toe, Right
Hamate bone	Carpal, Left
	Carpal, Right
Head of fibula	Fibula, Left
	Fibula, Right

Anatomical Term	PCS Description
Helix	External Ear, Right
	External Ear, Left
	External Ear, Bilateral
Hepatic artery proper	Hepatic Artery
Hepatic flexure	Ascending Colon
Hepatic lymph node	Lymphatic, Aortic
Hepatic plexus	Abdominal Sympathetic Nerve
Hepatic portal vein	Portal Vein
Hepatogastric ligament	Lesser Omentum
Hepatopancreatic ampulla	Ampulla of Vater
Humeroradial joint	Elbow Joint, Right
	Elbow Joint, Left
Humeroulnar joint	Elbow Joint, Right
	Elbow Joint, Left
Humerus, distal	Humeral Shaft
Humerus, distal involving joint	Joint, Elbow
Hyoglossus muscle	Tongue, Palate, Pharynx Muscle
Hyoid artery	Thyroid Artery, Right
	Thyroid Artery, Left
Hypogastric artery	Internal Iliac Artery, Right
	Internal Iliac Artery, Left
Hypopharynx	Pharynx
Hypophysis	Pituitary Gland
Hypothenar muscle	Hand Muscle, Right
	Hand Muscle, Left
Ileal artery	Superior Mesenteric Artery
Ileocolic artery	Superior Mesenteric Artery
Ileocolic vein	Colic Vein
Iliac crest	Pelvic Bone, Right
	Pelvic Bone, Left
Iliac fascia	Subcutaneous Tissue and Fascia, Right Upper Leg
	Subcutaneous Tissue and Fascia, Left Upper Leg
Iliac lymph node	Lymphatic, Pelvis
Iliacus muscle	Hip Muscle, Right
	Hip Muscle, Left
Iliofemoral ligament	Hip Bursa and Ligament, Right
	Hip Bursa and Ligament, Left
Iliohypogastric nerve	Lumbar Plexus
Ilioinguinal nerve	Lumbar Plexus
Iliolumbar artery	Internal Iliac Artery, Right
	Internal Iliac Artery, Left
Iliolumbar ligament	Trunk Bursa and Ligament, Right
	Trunk Bursa and Ligament, Left
Iliotibial tract (band)	Subcutaneous Tissue and Fascia, Right Upper Leg
	Subcutaneous Tissue and Fascia, Left Upper Leg
Ilium	Pelvic Bone, Right
	Pelvic Bone, Left

Anatomical Term	PCS Description
Incus	Auditory Ossicle, Right
	Auditory Ossicle, Left
Inferior cardiac nerve	Thoracic Sympathetic Nerve
Inferior cerebellar vein	Intracranial Vein
Inferior cerebral vein	Intracranial Vein
Inferior epigastric artery	External Iliac Artery, Right
	External Iliac Artery, Left
Inferior epigastric lymph node	Lymphatic, Pelvis
Inferior genicular artery	Popliteal Artery, Right
	Popliteal Artery, Left
Inferior gluteal artery	Internal Iliac Artery, Right
	Internal Iliac Artery, Left
Inferior gluteal nerve	Sacral Plexus
Inferior hypogastric plexus	Abdominal Sympathetic Nerve
Inferior labial artery	Face Artery
Inferior longitudinal muscle	Tongue, Palate, Pharynx Muscle
Inferior mesenteric ganglion	Abdominal Sympathetic Nerve
Inferior mesenteric lymph node	Lymphatic, Mesenteric
Inferior mesenteric plexus	Abdominal Sympathetic Nerve
Inferior oblique muscle	Extraocular Muscle, Right
	Extraocular Muscle, Left
Inferior pancreaticoduodenal artery	Superior Mesenteric Artery
Inferior phrenic artery	Abdominal Aorta
Inferior rectus muscle	Extraocular Muscle, Right
	Extraocular Muscle, Left
Inferior suprarenal artery	Renal Artery, Right
	Renal Artery, Left
Inferior tarsal plate	Lower Eyelid, Right
	Lower Eyelid, Left
Inferior thyroid vein	Innominate Vein, Right
	Innominate Vein, Left
Inferior tibiofibular joint	Ankle Joint, Right
	Ankle Joint, Left
Inferior turbinate	Nasal Turbinate
Inferior ulnar collateral artery	Brachial Artery, Right
	Brachial Artery, Left
Inferior vesical artery	Internal Iliac Artery, Right
	Internal Iliac Artery, Left
Infraauricular lymph node	Lymphatic, Head
Infraclavicular (deltopectoral) lymph node	Lymphatic, Left Upper Extremity
	Lymphatic, Right Upper Extremity
Infrahyoid muscle	Neck Muscle, Right
	Neck Muscle, Left
Infraparotid lymph node	Lymphatic, Head

Anatomical Term	PCS Description
Infraspinatus fascia	Subcutaneous Tissue and Fascia, Right Upper Arm
	Subcutaneous Tissue and Fascia, Left Upper Arm
Infraspinatus muscle	Shoulder Muscle, Right
	Shoulder Muscle, Left
Infundibulopelvic ligament	Uterine Supporting Structure
Inguinal canal	Inguinal Region, Right
	Inguinal Region, Left
	Inguinal Region, Bilateral
Inguinal triangle	Inguinal Region, Right
	Inguinal Region, Left
	Inguinal Region, Bilateral
Interatrial septum	Atrial Septum
Intercarpal joint	Carpal Joint, Right
	Carpal Joint, Left
Intercarpal ligament	Hand Bursa and Ligament, Right
	Hand Bursa and Ligament, Left
Interclavicular ligament	Shoulder Bursa and Ligament, Right
	Shoulder Bursa and Ligament, Left
Intercostal lymph node	Lymphatic, Thorax
Intercostal nerve	Thoracic Nerve
Intercostal muscle	Thorax Muscle, Right
	Thorax Muscle, Left
Intercostobrachial nerve	Thoracic Nerve
Intercuneiform joint	Tarsal Joint, Right
	Tarsal Joint, Left
Intermediate cuneiform bone	Tarsal, Left
	Tarsal, Right
Internal (basal) cerebral vein	Intracranial Vein
Internal anal sphincter	Anal Sphincter
Internal carotid plexus	Head and Neck Sympathetic Nerve
Internal iliac vein	Hypogastric Vein, Right
	Hypogastric Vein, Left
Internal maxillary artery	External Carotid Artery, Right
	External Carotid Artery, Left
Internal naris	Nose
Internal oblique muscle	Abdomen Muscle, Right
	Abdomen Muscle, Left
Internal pudendal artery	Internal Iliac Artery, Left
	Internal Iliac Artery, Right
Internal pudendal vein	Hypogastric Vein, Right
	Hypogastric Vein, Left
Internal thoracic artery	Internal Mammary Artery, Right
	Internal Mammary Artery, Left
	Subclavian Artery, Right
	Subclavian Artery, Left
Internal urethral sphincter	Urethra

Anatomical Term	PCS Description
Interphalangeal (IP) joint	Finger Phalangeal Joint, Right
	Finger Phalangeal Joint, Left
	Toe Phalangeal Joint, Right
	Toe Phalangeal Joint, Left
Interphalangeal ligament	Foot Bursa and Ligament, Right
	Foot Bursa and Ligament, Left
	Hand Bursa and Ligament, Right
	Hand Bursa and Ligament, Left
Interspinalis muscle	Trunk Muscle, Right
	Trunk Muscle, Left
Interspinous ligament	Trunk Bursa and Ligament, Right
	Trunk Bursa and Ligament, Left
Intertransverse ligament	Trunk Bursa and Ligament, Right
	Trunk Bursa and Ligament, Left
Intertransversarius muscle	Trunk Muscle, Right
	Trunk Muscle, Left
Interventricular foramen (Monro)	Cerebral Ventricle
Interventricular septum	Ventricular Septum
Intestinal lymphatic trunk	Cisterna Chyli
Ischiatic nerve	Sciatic Nerve
Ischiocavernosus muscle	Perineum Muscle
Ischiofemoral ligament	Hip Bursa and Ligament, Right
	Hip Bursa and Ligament, Left
Ischium	Pelvic Bone, Right
	Pelvic Bone, Left
Jejunal artery	Superior Mesenteric Artery
Jugular body	Glomus Jugulare
Jugular lymph node	Lymphatic, Left Neck
	Lymphatic, Right Neck
Labia majora	Vulva
Labia minora	Vulva
Labial gland	Upper Lip
	Lower Lip
Lacrimal canaliculus	Lacrimal Duct, Right
	Lacrimal Duct, Left
Lacrimal punctum	Lacrimal Duct, Right
	Lacrimal Duct, Left
Lacrimal sac	Lacrimal Duct, Right
	Lacrimal Duct, Left
Laryngopharynx	Pharynx
Lateral (brachial) lymph node	Lymphatic, Left Axillary
	Lymphatic, Right Axillary
Lateral canthus	Upper Eyelid, Right
	Upper Eyelid, Left
Lateral collateral ligament (LCL)	Knee Bursa and Ligament, Right
	Knee Bursa and Ligament, Left
Lateral condyle of femur	Lower Femur, Right
	Lower Femur, Left
Lateral condyle of tibia	Tibia, Left
	Tibia, Right

Anatomical Term	PCS Description
Lateral cuneiform bone	Tarsal, Left
	Tarsal, Right
Lateral epicondyle of femur	Lower Femur, Right
	Lower Femur, Left
Lateral epicondyle of humerus	Humeral Shaft, Right
	Humeral Shaft, Left
Lateral femoral cutaneous nerve	Lumbar Plexus
Lateral malleolus	Fibula, Left
	Fibula, Right
Lateral meniscus	Knee Joint, Right
	Knee Joint, Left
Lateral nasal cartilage	Nose
Lateral plantar artery	Foot Artery, Right
	Foot Artery, Left
Lateral plantar nerve	Tibial Nerve
Lateral rectus muscle	Extraocular Muscle, Right
	Extraocular Muscle, Left
Lateral sacral artery	Internal Iliac Artery, Right
	Internal Iliac Artery, Left
Lateral sacral vein	Hypogastric Vein, Right
	Hypogastric Vein, Left
Lateral sural cutaneous nerve	Peroneal Nerve
Lateral tarsal artery	Foot Artery, Right
	Foot Artery, Left
Lateral temporo-mandibular ligament	Head and Neck Bursa and Ligament
Lateral thoracic artery	Axillary Artery, Right
	Axillary Artery, Left
Latissimus dorsi muscle	Trunk Muscle, Right
	Trunk Muscle, Left
Least splanchnic nerve	Thoracic Sympathetic Nerve
Left ascending lumbar vein	Hemiazygos Vein
Left atrioventricular valve	Mitral Valve
Left auricular appendix	Atrium, Left
Left colic vein	Colic Vein
Left coronary sulcus	Heart, Left
Left gastric artery	Gastric Artery
Left gastroepiploic artery	Splenic Artery
Left gastroepiploic vein	Splenic Vein
Left inferior phrenic vein	Renal Vein, Left
Left inferior pulmonary vein	Pulmonary Vein, Left
Left jugular trunk	Thoracic Duct
Left lateral ventricle	Cerebral Ventricle
Left ovarian vein	Renal Vein, Left
Left second lumbar vein	Renal Vein, Left
Left subclavian trunk	Thoracic Duct
Left subcostal vein	Hemiazygos Vein

Anatomical Term	PCS Description
Left superior pulmonary vein	Pulmonary Vein, Left
Left suprarenal vein	Renal Vein, Left
Left testicular vein	Renal Vein, Left
Leptomeninges	Cerebral Meninges
	Spinal Meninges
Lesser alar cartilage	Nose
Lesser occipital nerve	Cervical Plexus
Lesser splanchnic nerve	Thoracic Sympathetic Nerve
Lesser trochanter	Upper Femur, Right
	Upper Femur, Left
Lesser tuberosity	Humeral Head, Right
	Humeral Head, Left
Lesser wing	Sphenoid Bone, Right
	Sphenoid Bone, Left
Levator anguli oris muscle	Facial Muscle
Levator ani muscle	Trunk Muscle, Left
Levator labii superioris alaeque nasi muscle	Facial Muscle
Levator labii superioris muscle	Facial Muscle
Levator palpebrae superioris muscle	Upper Eyelid, Right
	Upper Eyelid, Left
Levator scapulae muscle	Neck Muscle, Right
	Neck Muscle, Left
Levator veli palatini muscle	Tongue, Palate, Pharynx Muscle
Levatores costarum muscle	Thorax Muscle, Right
	Thorax Muscle, Left
Ligament of head of fibula	Knee Bursa and Ligament, Right
	Knee Bursa and Ligament, Left
Ligament of the lateral malleolus	Ankle Bursa and Ligament, Right
	Ankle Bursa and Ligament, Left
Ligamentum flavum	Trunk Bursa and Ligament, Right
	Trunk Bursa and Ligament, Left
Lingual artery	External Carotid Artery, Right
	External Carotid Artery, Left
Lingual tonsil	Tongue
Locus ceruleus	Pons
Long thoracic nerve	Brachial Plexus
Lumbar artery	Abdominal Aorta
Lumbar facet joint	Lumbar Vertebral Joint
Lumbar ganglion	Lumbar Sympathetic Nerve
Lumbar lymph node	Lymphatic, Aortic
Lumbar lymphatic trunk	Cisterna Chyli
Lumbar splanchnic nerve	Lumbar Sympathetic Nerve
Lumbosacral facet joint	Lumbosacral Joint
Lumbosacral trunk	Lumbar Nerve
Lunate bone	Carpal, Left
	Carpal, Right
Lunotriquetral ligament	Hand Bursa and Ligament, Right
	Hand Bursa and Ligament, Left

Anatomical Term	PCS Description
Macula	Retina, Left
	Retina, Right
Malleus	Auditory Ossicle, Right
	Auditory Ossicle, Left
Mammary duct	Breast, Bilateral
	Breast, Left
	Breast, Right
Mammary gland	Breast, Bilateral
	Breast, Left
	Breast, Right
Mammillary body	Hypothalamus
Mandibular nerve	Trigeminal Nerve
Mandibular notch	Mandible, Left
	Mandible, Right
Manubrium	Sternum
Masseter muscle	Head Muscle
Masseteric fascia	Subcutaneous Tissue and Fascia, Face
Mastoid (postauricular) lymph node	Lymphatic, Left Neck
	Lymphatic, Right Neck
Mastoid air cells	Mastoid Sinus, Right
	Mastoid Sinus, Left
Mastoid process	Temporal Bone, Right
	Temporal Bone, Left
Maxillary artery	External Carotid Artery, Right
	External Carotid Artery, Left
Maxillary nerve	Trigeminal Nerve
Medial canthus	Lower Eyelid, Right
	Lower Eyelid, Left
Medial collateral ligament (MCL)	Knee Bursa and Ligament, Right
	Knee Bursa and Ligament, Left
Medial condyle of femur	Lower Femur, Right
	Lower Femur, Left
Medial condyle of tibia	Tibia, Left
	Tibia, Right
Medial cuneiform bone	Tarsal, Left
	Tarsal, Right
Medial epicondyle of femur	Lower Femur, Right
	Lower Femur, Left
Medial epicondyle of humerus	Humeral Shaft, Right
	Humeral Shaft, Left
Medial malleolus	Tibia, Left
	Tibia, Right
Medial meniscus	Knee Joint, Right
	Knee Joint, Left
Medial plantar artery	Foot Artery, Right
	Foot Artery, Left
Medial plantar nerve	Tibial Nerve
Medial popliteal nerve	Tibial Nerve
Medial rectus muscle	Extraocular Muscle, Right
	Extraocular Muscle, Left
Medial sural cutaneous nerve	Tibial Nerve

Anatomical Term	PCS Description
Median antebrachial vein	Basilic Vein, Right
	Basilic Vein, Left
Median cubital vein	Basilic Vein, Right
	Basilic Vein, Left
Median sacral artery	Abdominal Aorta
Mediastinal lymph node	Lymphatic, Thorax
Meissner's (submucous) plexus	Abdominal Sympathetic Nerve
Membranous urethra	Urethra
Mental foramen	Mandible, Left
	Mandible, Right
Mentalis muscle	Facial Muscle
Mesoappendix	Mesentery
Mesocolon	Mesentery
Metacarpal ligament	Hand Bursa and Ligament, Right
	Hand Bursa and Ligament, Left
Metacarpophalangeal ligament	Hand Bursa and Ligament, Right
	Hand Bursa and Ligament, Left
Metatarsal ligament	Foot Bursa and Ligament, Right
	Foot Bursa and Ligament, Left
Metatarsophalangeal ligament	Foot Bursa and Ligament, Right
	Foot Bursa and Ligament, Left
Metatarsophalangeal (MTP) joint	Metatarsal-Phalangeal Joint, Right
	Metatarsal-Phalangeal Joint, Left
Metathalamus	Thalamus
Midcarpal joint	Carpal Joint, Right
	Carpal Joint, Left
Middle cardiac nerve	Thoracic Sympathetic Nerve
Middle cerebral artery	Intracranial Artery
Middle cerebral vein	Intracranial Vein
Middle colic vein	Colic Vein
Middle genicular artery	Popliteal Artery, Right
	Popliteal Artery, Left
Middle hemorrhoidal vein	Hypogastric Vein, Right
	Hypogastric Vein, Left
Middle rectal artery	Internal Iliac Artery, Right
	Internal Iliac Artery, Left
Middle suprarenal artery	Abdominal Aorta
Middle temporal artery	Temporal Artery, Right
	Temporal Artery, Left
Middle turbinate	Nasal Turbinate
Mitral annulus	Mitral Valve
Molar gland	Buccal Mucosa
Musculocutaneous nerve	Brachial Plexus
Musculophrenic artery	Internal Mammary Artery, Right
	Internal Mammary Artery, Left
Musculospiral nerve	Radial Nerve
Myelencephalon	Medulla Oblongata
Myenteric (Auerbach's) plexus	Abdominal Sympathetic Nerve
Myometrium	Uterus

Anatomical Term	PCS Description
Nail bed	Finger Nail
	Toe Nail
Nail plate	Finger Nail
	Toe Nail
Nasal cavity	Nose
Nasal concha	Nasal Turbinate
Nasalis muscle	Facial Muscle
Nasolacrimal duct	Lacrimal Duct, Right
	Lacrimal Duct, Left
Navicular bone	Tarsal, Left
	Tarsal, Right
Neck of femur	Upper Femur, Right
	Upper Femur, Left
Neck of humerus (anatomical) (surgical)	Humeral Head, Right
	Humeral Head, Left
Nerve to the stapedius	Facial Nerve
Neurohypophysis	Pituitary Gland
Ninth cranial nerve	Glossopharyngeal Nerve
Nostril	Nose
Obturator artery	Internal Iliac Artery, Right
	Internal Iliac Artery, Left
Obturator lymph node	Lymphatic, Pelvis
Obturator muscle	Hip Muscle, Right
	Hip Muscle, Left
Obturator nerve	Lumbar Plexus
Obturator vein	Hypogastric Vein, Right
	Hypogastric Vein, Left
Obtuse margin	Heart, Left
Occipital artery	External Carotid Artery, Right
	External Carotid Artery, Left
Occipital lobe	Cerebral Hemisphere
Occipital lymph node	Lymphatic, Left Neck
	Lymphatic, Right Neck
Occipitofrontalis muscle	Facial Muscle
Olecranon bursa	Elbow Bursa and Ligament, Right
	Elbow Bursa and Ligament, Left
Olecranon process	Ulna, Left
	Ulna, Right
Olfactory bulb	Olfactory Nerve
Ophthalmic artery	Internal Carotid Artery, Right
	Internal Carotid Artery, Left
Ophthalmic nerve	Trigeminal Nerve
Ophthalmic vein	Intracranial Vein
Optic chiasma	Optic Nerve
Optic disc	Retina, Left
	Retina, Right
Optic foramen	Sphenoid Bone, Right
	Sphenoid Bone, Left
Orbicularis oculi muscle	Upper Eyelid, Right
	Upper Eyelid, Left
Orbicularis oris muscle	Facial Muscle

Anatomical Term	PCS Description
Orbital fascia	Subcutaneous Tissue and Fascia, Face
Orbital portion of ethmoid bone	Orbit, Left
	Orbit, Right
Orbital portion of frontal bone	Orbit, Left
	Orbit, Right
Orbital portion of lacrimal bone	Orbit, Left
	Orbit, Right
Orbital portion of maxilla	Orbit, Left
	Orbit, Right
Orbital portion of palatine bone	Orbit, Left
	Orbit, Right
Orbital portion of sphenoid bone	Orbit, Left
	Orbit, Right
Orbital portion of zygomatic bone	Orbit, Left
	Orbit, Right
Oropharynx	Pharynx
Ossicular chain	Auditory Ossicle, Right
	Auditory Ossicle, Left
Otic ganglion	Head and Neck Sympathetic Nerve
Oval window	Middle Ear, Left
	Middle Ear, Right
Ovarian artery	Abdominal Aorta
Ovarian ligament	Uterine Supporting Structure
Oviduct	Fallopian Tube, Right
	Fallopian Tube, Left
Palatine gland	Buccal Mucosa
Palatine tonsil	Tonsils
Palatine uvula	Uvula
Palatoglossal muscle	Tongue, Palate, Pharynx Muscle
Palatopharyngeal muscle	Tongue, Palate, Pharynx Muscle
Palmar (volar) metacarpal vein	Hand Vein, Right
	Hand Vein, Left
Palmar (volar) digital vein	Hand Vein, Left
	Hand Vein, Right
Palmar cutaneous nerve	Median Nerve
	Radial Nerve
Palmar fascia (aponeurosis)	Subcutaneous Tissue and Fascia, Right Hand
	Subcutaneous Tissue and Fascia, Left Hand
Palmar interosseous muscle	Hand Muscle, Right
	Hand Muscle, Left
Palmar ulnocarpal ligament	Wrist Bursa and Ligament, Right
	Wrist Bursa and Ligament, Left
Palmaris longus muscle	Lower Arm and Wrist Muscle, Right
	Lower Arm and Wrist Muscle, Left
Pancreatic artery	Splenic Artery
Pancreatic plexus	Abdominal Sympathetic Nerve
Pancreatic vein	Splenic Vein
Pancreaticosplenic lymph node	Lymphatic, Aortic
Paraaortic lymph node	Lymphatic, Aortic
Pararectal lymph node	Lymphatic, Mesenteric
Parasternal lymph node	Lymphatic, Thorax
Paratracheal lymph node	Lymphatic, Thorax
Paraurethral (Skene's) gland	Vestibular Gland
Parietal lobe	Cerebral Hemisphere
Parotid lymph node	Lymphatic, Head
Parotid plexus	Facial Nerve
Pars flaccida	Tympanic Membrane, Right
	Tympanic Membrane, Left
Patellar ligament	Knee Bursa and Ligament, Right
	Knee Bursa and Ligament, Left
Patellar tendon	Knee Tendon, Right
	Knee Tendon, Left
Patellofemoral joint	Knee Joint, Right
	Knee Joint, Left
	Knee Joint, Femoral Surface, Right
	Knee Joint, Femoral Surface, Left
Pectineus muscle	Upper Leg Muscle, Right
	Upper Leg Muscle, Left
Pectoral (anterior) lymph node	Lymphatic, Left Axillary
	Lymphatic, Right Axillary
Pectoral fascia	Subcutaneous Tissue and Fascia, Chest
Pectoralis major muscle	Thorax Muscle, Left
	Thorax Muscle, Right
Pectoralis minor muscle	Thorax Muscle, Left
	Thorax Muscle, Right
Pelvic fascia	Subcutaneous Tissue and Fascia, Trunk
Pelvic splanchnic nerve	Abdominal Sympathetic Nerve
	Sacral Sympathetic Nerve
Penile urethra	Urethra
Pericardiophrenic artery	Internal Mammary Artery, Right
	Internal Mammary Artery, Left
Perimetrium	Uterus
Peroneus brevis muscle	Lower Leg Muscle, Right
	Lower Leg Muscle, Left
Peroneus longus muscle	Lower Leg Muscle, Right
	Lower Leg Muscle, Left
Petrous part of temporal bone	Temporal Bone, Right
	Temporal Bone, Left
Pharyngeal constrictor muscle	Tongue, Palate, Pharynx Muscle
Pharyngeal plexus	Vagus Nerve
Pharyngeal recess	Nasopharynx
Pharyngeal tonsil	Adenoids
Pharyngotympanic tube	Eustachian Tube, Right
	Eustachian Tube, Left
Pia mater	Cerebral Meninges
	Spinal Meninges
Pinna	External Ear, Right
	External Ear, Left
	External Ear, Bilateral

Anatomical Term	PCS Description
Piriform recess (sinus)	Pharynx
Piriformis muscle	Hip Muscle, Right
	Hip Muscle, Left
Pisiform bone	Carpal, Left
	Carpal, Right
Pisohamate ligament	Hand Bursa and Ligament, Right
	Hand Bursa and Ligament, Left
Pisometacarpal ligament	Hand Bursa and Ligament, Right
	Hand Bursa and Ligament, Left
Plantar digital vein	Foot Vein, Left
	Foot Vein, Right
Plantar fascia (aponeurosis)	Subcutaneous Tissue and Fascia, Right Foot
	Subcutaneous Tissue and Fascia, Left Foot
Plantar metatarsal vein	Foot Vein, Left
	Foot Vein, Right
Plantar venous arch	Foot Vein, Left
	Foot Vein, Right
Platysma muscle	Neck Muscle, Right
	Neck Muscle, Left
Plica semilunaris	Conjunctiva, Right
	Conjunctiva, Left
Pneumogastric nerve	Vagus Nerve
Pneumotaxic center	Pons
Pontine tegmentum	Pons
Popliteal lymph node	Lymphatic, Left Lower Extremity
	Lymphatic, Right Lower Extremity
Popliteal ligament	Knee Bursa and Ligament, Right
	Knee Bursa and Ligament, Left
Popliteal vein	Femoral Vein, Right
	Femoral Vein, Left
Popliteus muscle	Lower Leg Muscle, Right
	Lower Leg Muscle, Left
Postauricular (mastoid) lymph node	Lymphatic, Left Neck
	Lymphatic, Right Neck
Postcava	Inferior Vena Cava
Posterior (subscapular) lymph node	Lymphatic, Left Axillary
	Lymphatic, Right Axillary
Posterior auricular artery	External Carotid Artery, Right
	External Carotid Artery, Left
Posterior auricular nerve	Facial Nerve
Posterior auricular vein	External Jugular Vein, Right
	External Jugular Vein, Left
Posterior cerebral artery	Intracranial Artery
Posterior chamber	Eye, Left
	Eye, Right
Posterior circumflex humeral artery	Axillary Artery, Right
	Axillary Artery, Left
Posterior communicating artery	Intracranial Artery

Anatomical Term	PCS Description
Posterior cruciate ligament (PCL)	Knee Bursa and Ligament, Right
	Knee Bursa and Ligament, Left
Posterior facial (retromandibular) vein	Face Vein, Left
	Face Vein, Right
Posterior femoral cutaneous nerve	Sacral Plexus
Posterior inferior cerebellar artery (PICA)	Intracranial Artery
Posterior interosseous nerve	Radial Nerve
Posterior labial nerve	Pudendal Nerve
Posterior scrotal nerve	Pudendal Nerve
Posterior spinal artery	Vertebral Artery, Right
	Vertebral Artery, Left
Posterior tibial recurrent artery	Anterior Tibial Artery, Right
	Anterior Tibial Artery, Left
Posterior ulnar recurrent artery	Ulnar Artery, Right
	Ulnar Artery, Left
Posterior vagal trunk	Vagus Nerve
Preauricular lymph node	Lymphatic, Head
Precava	Superior Vena Cava
Prepatellar bursa	Knee Bursa and Ligament, Right
	Knee Bursa and Ligament, Left
Pretracheal fascia	Subcutaneous Tissue and Fascia, Anterior Neck
Prevertebral fascia	Subcutaneous Tissue and Fascia, Posterior Neck
Princeps pollicis artery	Hand Artery, Right
	Hand Artery, Left
Procerus muscle	Facial Muscle
Profunda brachii	Brachial Artery, Right
	Brachial Artery, Left
Profunda femoris (deep femoral) vein	Femoral Vein, Right
	Femoral Vein, Left
Pronator quadratus muscle	Lower Arm and Wrist Muscle, Right
	Lower Arm and Wrist Muscle, Left
Pronator teres muscle	Lower Arm and Wrist Muscle, Right
	Lower Arm and Wrist Muscle, Left
Prostatic urethra	Urethra
Proximal radioulnar joint	Elbow Joint, Right
	Elbow Joint, Left
Psoas muscle	Hip Muscle, Right
	Hip Muscle, Left
Pterygoid muscle	Head Muscle
Pterygoid process	Sphenoid Bone, Right
	Sphenoid Bone, Left
Pterygopalatine (sphenopalatine) ganglion	Head and Neck Sympathetic Nerve
Pubic ligament	Trunk Bursa and Ligament, Right
	Trunk Bursa and Ligament, Left

Anatomical Term	PCS Description
Pubis	Pelvic Bone, Right
	Pelvic Bone, Left
Pubofemoral ligament	Hip Bursa and Ligament, Right
	Hip Bursa and Ligament, Left
Pudendal nerve	Sacral Plexus
Pulmoaortic canal	Pulmonary Artery, Left
Pulmonary annulus	Pulmonary Valve
Pulmonary plexus	Thoracic Sympathetic Nerve
	Vagus Nerve
Pulmonic valve	Pulmonary Valve
Pulvinar	Thalamus
Pyloric antrum	Stomach, Pylorus
Pyloric canal	Stomach, Pylorus
Pyloric sphincter	Stomach, Pylorus
Pyramidalis muscle	Abdomen Muscle, Right
	Abdomen Muscle, Left
Quadrangular cartilage	Nasal Septum
Quadrate lobe	Liver
Quadratus femoris muscle	Hip Muscle, Right
	Hip Muscle, Left
Quadratus lumborum muscle	Trunk Muscle, Right
	Trunk Muscle, Left
Quadratus plantae muscle	Foot Muscle, Right
	Foot Muscle, Left
Quadriceps (femoris)	Upper Leg Muscle, Right
	Upper Leg Muscle, Left
	Upper Leg Tendon, Right
	Upper Leg Tendon, Left
Radial collateral ligament	Elbow Bursa and Ligament, Right
	Elbow Bursa and Ligament, Left
Radial collateral carpal ligament	Wrist Bursa and Ligament, Right
	Wrist Bursa and Ligament, Left
Radial notch	Ulna, Left
	Ulna, Right
Radial recurrent artery	Radial Artery, Right
	Radial Artery, Left
Radial vein	Brachial Vein, Right
	Brachial Vein, Left
Radialis indicis	Hand Artery, Right
	Hand Artery, Left
Radiocarpal joint	Wrist Joint, Right
	Wrist Joint, Left
Radiocarpal ligament	Wrist Bursa and Ligament, Right
	Wrist Bursa and Ligament, Left
Rectosigmoid junction	Sigmoid Colon
Radioulnar ligament	Wrist Bursa and Ligament, Right
	Wrist Bursa and Ligament, Left
Rectus abdominis muscle	Abdomen Muscle, Right
	Abdomen Muscle, Left
Rectus femoris muscle	Upper Leg Muscle, Right
	Upper Leg Muscle, Left

Anatomical Term	PCS Description
Recurrent laryngeal nerve	Vagus Nerve
Renal calyx	Kidney
	Kidney, Left
	Kidney, Right
	Kidneys, Bilateral
Renal capsule	Kidney
	Kidney, Left
	Kidney, Right
	Kidneys, Bilateral
Renal cortex	Kidney
	Kidney, Left
	Kidney, Right
	Kidneys, Bilateral
Renal plexus	Abdominal Sympathetic Nerve
Renal segment	Kidney
	Kidney, Left
	Kidney, Right
	Kidneys, Bilateral
Renal segmental artery	Renal Artery, Right
	Renal Artery, Left
Retroperitoneal lymph node	Lymphatic, Aortic
Retroperitoneal space	Retroperitoneum
Retropharyngeal lymph node	Lymphatic, Left Neck
	Lymphatic, Right Neck
Retropubic space	Pelvic Cavity
Rhinopharynx	Nasopharynx
Rhomboid major muscle	Trunk Muscle, Right
	Trunk Muscle, Left
Rhomboid minor muscle	Trunk Muscle, Right
	Trunk Muscle, Left
Right ascending lumbar vein	Azygos Vein
Right atrioventricular valve	Tricuspid Valve
Right auricular appendix	Atrium, Right
Right colic vein	Colic Vein
Right coronary sulcus	Heart, Right
Right gastric artery	Gastric Artery
Right gastroepiploic vein	Superior Mesenteric Vein
Right inferior phrenic vein	Inferior Vena Cava
Right inferior pulmonary vein	Pulmonary Vein, Right
Right jugular trunk	Lymphatic, Right Neck
Right lateral ventricle	Cerebral Ventricle
Right lymphatic duct	Lymphatic, Right Neck
Right ovarian vein	Inferior Vena Cava
Right second lumbar vein	Inferior Vena Cava
Right subclavian trunk	Lymphatic, Right Neck
Right subcostal vein	Azygos Vein

Anatomical Term	PCS Description
Right superior pulmonary vein	Pulmonary Vein, Right
Right suprarenal vein	Inferior Vena Cava
Right testicular vein	Inferior Vena Cava
Rima glottidis	Larynx
Risorius muscle	Facial Muscle
Round ligament of uterus	Uterine Supporting Structure
Round window	Inner Ear, Left
	Inner Ear, Right
Sacral ganglion	Sacral Sympathetic Nerve
Sacral lymph node	Lymphatic, Pelvis
Sacral splanchnic nerve	Sacral Sympathetic Nerve
Sacrococcygeal ligament	Trunk Bursa and Ligament, Right
	Trunk Bursa and Ligament, Left
Sacrococcygeal symphysis	Sacrococcygeal Joint
Sacroiliac ligament	Trunk Bursa and Ligament, Right
	Trunk Bursa and Ligament, Left
Sacrospinous ligament	Trunk Bursa and Ligament, Right
	Trunk Bursa and Ligament, Left
Sacrotuberous ligament	Trunk Bursa and Ligament, Right
	Trunk Bursa and Ligament, Left
Salpingopharyngeus muscle	Tongue, Palate, Pharynx Muscle
Salpinx	Fallopian Tube, Left
	Fallopian Tube, Right
Saphenous nerve	Femoral Nerve
Sartorius muscle	Upper Leg Muscle, Right
	Upper Leg Muscle, Left
Scalene muscle	Neck Muscle, Right
	Neck Muscle, Left
Scaphoid bone	Carpal, Left
	Carpal, Right
Scapholunate ligament	Hand Bursa and Ligament, Right
	Hand Bursa and Ligament, Left
Scaphotrapezium ligament	Hand Bursa and Ligament, Right
	Hand Bursa and Ligament, Left
Scarpa's (vestibular) ganglion	Acoustic Nerve
Sebaceous gland	Skin
Second cranial nerve	Optic Nerve
Sella turcica	Sphenoid Bone, Right
	Sphenoid Bone, Left
Semicircular canal	Inner Ear, Left
	Inner Ear, Right
Semimembranosus muscle	Upper Leg Muscle, Right
	Upper Leg Muscle, Left
Semitendinosus muscle	Upper Leg Muscle, Right
	Upper Leg Muscle, Left
Septal cartilage	Nasal Septum
Serratus anterior muscle	Thorax Muscle, Right
	Thorax Muscle, Left

Anatomical Term	PCS Description
Serratus posterior muscle	Trunk Muscle, Right
	Trunk Muscle, Left
Seventh cranial nerve	Facial Nerve
Short gastric artery	Splenic Artery
Sigmoid artery	Inferior Mesenteric Artery
Sigmoid flexure	Sigmoid Colon
Sigmoid vein	Inferior Mesenteric Vein
Sinoatrial node	Conduction Mechanism
Sinus venosus	Atrium, Right
Sixth cranial nerve	Abducens Nerve
Skene's (paraurethral) gland	Vestibular Gland
Small saphenous vein	Lesser Saphenous Vein, Right
	Lesser Saphenous Vein, Left
Solar (celiac) plexus	Abdominal Sympathetic Nerve
Soleus muscle	Lower Leg Muscle, Right
	Lower Leg Muscle, Left
Sphenomandibular ligament	Head and Neck Bursa and Ligament
Sphenopalatine (pterygopalatine) ganglion	Head and Neck Sympathetic Nerve
Spinal dura mater	Dura Mater
Spinal epidural space	Epidural Space
Spinal nerve, cervical	Cervical Nerve
Spinal nerve, lumbar	Lumbar Nerve
Spinal nerve, sacral	Sacral Nerve
Spinal nerve, thoracic	Thoracic Nerve
Spinal subarachnoid space	Subarachnoid Space
Spinal subdural space	Subdural Space
Spinous process	Cervical Vertebra
	Lumbar Vertebra
	Thoracic Vertebra
Spiral ganglion	Acoustic Nerve
Splenic flexure	Transverse Colon
Splenic plexus	Abdominal Sympathetic Nerve
Splenius capitis muscle	Head Muscle
Splenius cervicis muscle	Neck Muscle, Right
	Neck Muscle, Left
Stapes	Auditory Ossicle, Right
	Auditory Ossicle, Left
Stellate ganglion	Head and Neck Sympathetic Nerve
Stensen's duct	Parotid Duct, Right
	Parotid Duct, Left
Sternoclavicular ligament	Shoulder Bursa and Ligament, Right
	Shoulder Bursa and Ligament, Left
Sternocleidomastoid artery	Thyroid Artery, Right
	Thyroid Artery, Left
Sternocleidomastoid muscle	Neck Muscle, Right
	Neck Muscle, Left
Sternocostal ligament	Thorax Bursa and Ligament, Right
	Thorax Bursa and Ligament, Left

Anatomical Term	PCS Description
Styloglossus muscle	Tongue, Palate, Pharynx Muscle
Stylomandibular ligament	Head and Neck Bursa and Ligament
Stylopharyngeus muscle	Tongue, Palate, Pharynx Muscle
Subacromial bursa	Shoulder Bursa and Ligament, Right
	Shoulder Bursa and Ligament, Left
Subaortic (common iliac) lymph node	Lymphatic, Pelvis
Subclavicular (apical) lymph node	Lymphatic, Left Axillary
	Lymphatic, Right Axillary
Subclavius muscle	Thorax Muscle, Right
	Thorax Muscle, Left
Subclavius nerve	Brachial Plexus
Subcostal artery	Thoracic Aorta
Subcostal muscle	Thorax Muscle, Right
	Thorax Muscle, Left
Subcostal nerve	Thoracic Nerve
Submandibular ganglion	Facial Nerve
	Head and Neck Sympathetic Nerve
Submandibular gland	Submaxillary Gland, Right
	Submaxillary Gland, Left
Submandibular lymph node	Lymphatic, Head
Submaxillary ganglion	Head and Neck Sympathetic Nerve
Submaxillary lymph node	Lymphatic, Head
Submental artery	Face Artery
Submental lymph node	Lymphatic, Head
Submucous (Meissner's) plexus	Abdominal Sympathetic Nerve
Suboccipital nerve	Cervical Nerve
Suboccipital venous plexus	Vertebral Vein, Right
	Vertebral Vein, Left
Subparotid lymph node	Lymphatic, Head
Subscapular aponeurosis	Subcutaneous Tissue and Fascia, Right Upper Arm
	Subcutaneous Tissue and Fascia, Left Upper Arm
Subscapular artery	Axillary Artery, Right
	Axillary Artery, Left
Subscapular (posterior) lymph node	Lymphatic, Left Axillary
	Lymphatic, Right Axillary
Subscapularis muscle	Shoulder Muscle, Right
	Shoulder Muscle, Left
Substantia nigra	Basal Ganglia
Subtalar (talocalcaneal) joint	Tarsal Joint, Right
	Tarsal Joint, Left
Subtalar ligament	Foot Bursa and Ligament, Right
	Foot Bursa and Ligament, Left
Subthalamic nucleus	Basal Ganglia
Superficial epigastric artery	Femoral Artery, Left
	Femoral Artery, Right
Superficial epigastric vein	Greater Saphenous Vein, Left
	Greater Saphenous Vein, Right
Superficial circumflex iliac vein	Greater Saphenous Vein, Left
	Greater Saphenous Vein, Right
Superficial palmar arch	Hand Artery, Right
	Hand Artery, Left
Superficial palmar venous arch	Hand Vein, Left
	Hand Vein, Right
Superficial transverse perineal muscle	Perineum Muscle
Superficial temporal artery	Temporal Artery, Right
	Temporal Artery, Left
Superior cardiac nerve	Thoracic Sympathetic Nerve
Superior cerebellar vein	Intracranial Vein
Superior cerebral vein	Intracranial Vein
Superior clunic (cluneal) nerve	Lumbar Nerve
Superior epigastric artery	Internal Mammary Artery, Right
	Internal Mammary Artery, Left
Superior genicular artery	Popliteal Artery, Right
	Popliteal Artery, Left
Superior gluteal artery	Internal Iliac Artery, Right
	Internal Iliac Artery, Left
Superior gluteal nerve	Lumbar Plexus
Superior hypogastric plexus	Abdominal Sympathetic Nerve
Superior labial artery	Face Artery
Superior laryngeal artery	Thyroid Artery, Right
	Thyroid Artery, Left
Superior laryngeal nerve	Vagus Nerve
Superior longitudinal muscle	Tongue, Palate, Pharynx Muscle
Superior mesenteric ganglion	Abdominal Sympathetic Nerve
Superior mesenteric lymph node	Lymphatic, Mesenteric
Superior mesenteric plexus	Abdominal Sympathetic Nerve
Superior oblique muscle	Extraocular Muscle, Right
	Extraocular Muscle, Left
Superior olivary nucleus	Pons
Superior rectal artery	Inferior Mesenteric Artery
Superior rectal muscle	Extraocular Muscle, Right
	Extraocular Muscle, Left
Superior rectal vein	Inferior Mesenteric Vein
Superior tarsal plate	Upper Eyelid, Right
	Upper Eyelid, Left
Superior thoracic artery	Axillary Artery, Right
	Axillary Artery, Left
Superior thyroid artery	External Carotid Artery, Right
	External Carotid Artery, Left
	Thyroid Artery, Right
	Thyroid Artery, Left
Superior turbinate	Nasal Turbinate

Anatomical Term	PCS Description
Superior ulnar collateral artery	Brachial Artery, Right
	Brachial Artery, Left
Supraclavicular nerve	Cervical Plexus
Supraclavicular (Virchow's) lymph node	Lymphatic, Left Neck
	Lymphatic, Right Neck
Suprahyoid lymph node	Lymphatic, Head
Suprahyoid muscle	Neck Muscle, Right
	Neck Muscle, Left
Suprainguinal lymph node	Lymphatic, Pelvis
Supraorbital vein	Face Vein, Left
	Face Vein, Right
Suprarenal gland	Adrenal Glands, Bilateral
	Adrenal Gland, Right
	Adrenal Gland, Left
	Adrenal Gland
Suprarenal plexus	Abdominal Sympathetic Nerve
Suprascapular nerve	Brachial Plexus
Supraspinatus fascia	Subcutaneous Tissue and Fascia, Right Upper Arm
	Subcutaneous Tissue and Fascia, Left Upper Arm
Supraspinatus muscle	Shoulder Muscle, Right
	Shoulder Muscle, Left
Supraspinous ligament	Trunk Bursa and Ligament, Right
	Trunk Bursa and Ligament, Left
Suprasternal notch	Sternum
Supratrochlear lymph node	Lymphatic, Left Upper Extremity
	Lymphatic, Right Upper Extremity
Sural artery	Popliteal Artery, Right
	Popliteal Artery, Left
Sweat gland	Skin
Talocalcaneal ligament	Foot Bursa and Ligament, Right
	Foot Bursa and Ligament, Left
Talocalcaneal (subtalar) joint	Tarsal Joint, Right
	Tarsal Joint, Left
Talocalcaneonavicular joint	Tarsal Joint, Right
	Tarsal Joint, Left
Talocalcaneonavicular ligament	Foot Bursa and Ligament, Right
	Foot Bursa and Ligament, Left
Talocrural joint	Ankle Joint, Right
	Ankle Joint, Left
Talofibular ligament	Ankle Bursa and Ligament, Right
	Ankle Bursa and Ligament, Left
Talus bone	Tarsal, Left
	Tarsal, Right
Tarsometatarsal joint	Metatarsal-Tarsal Joint, Right
	Metatarsal-Tarsal Joint, Left
Tarsometatarsal ligament	Foot Bursa and Ligament, Right
	Foot Bursa and Ligament, Left
Temporal lobe	Cerebral Hemisphere
Temporalis muscle	Head Muscle
Temporoparietalis muscle	Head Muscle
Tensor fasciae latae muscle	Hip Muscle, Right
	Hip Muscle, Left
Tensor veli palatini muscle	Tongue, Palate, Pharynx Muscle
Tenth cranial nerve	Vagus Nerve
Tentorium cerebelli	Dura Mater
Teres major muscle	Shoulder Muscle, Right
	Shoulder Muscle, Left
Teres minor muscle	Shoulder Muscle, Right
	Shoulder Muscle, Left
Testicular artery	Abdominal Aorta
Thenar muscle	Hand Muscle, Right
	Hand Muscle, Left
Third cranial nerve	Oculomotor Nerve
Third occipital nerve	Cervical Nerve
Third ventricle	Cerebral Ventricle
Thoracic aortic plexus	Thoracic Sympathetic Nerve
Thoracic esophagus	Esophagus, Middle
Thoracic facet joint	Thoracic Vertebral Joint
Thoracic ganglion	Thoracic Sympathetic Nerve
Thoracoacromial artery	Axillary Artery, Right
	Axillary Artery, Left
Thoracolumbar facet joint	Thoracolumbar Vertebral Joint
Thymus gland	Thymus
Thyroarytenoid muscle	Neck Muscle, Right
	Neck Muscle, Left
Thyrocervical trunk	Thyroid Artery, Right
	Thyroid Artery, Left
Thyroid cartilage	Larynx
Tibialis anterior muscle	Lower Leg Muscle, Right
	Lower Leg Muscle, Left
Tibialis posterior muscle	Lower Leg Muscle, Right
	Lower Leg Muscle, Left
Tibiofemoral joint	Knee Joint, Right
	Knee Joint, Left
	Knee Joint, Tibial Surface, Right
	Knee Joint, Tibial Surface, Left
Tracheobronchial lymph node	Lymphatic, Thorax
Tragus	External Ear, Right
	External Ear, Left
	External Ear, Bilateral
Transversalis fascia	Subcutaneous Tissue and Fascia, Trunk
Transverse acetabular ligament	Hip Bursa and Ligament, Left
	Hip Bursa and Ligament, Right
Transverse (cutaneous) cervical nerve	Cervical Plexus
Transverse facial artery	Temporal Artery, Right
	Temporal Artery, Left

Anatomical Term	PCS Description
Transverse humeral ligament	Shoulder Bursa and Ligament, Right
	Shoulder Bursa and Ligament, Left
Transverse ligament of atlas	Head and Neck Bursa and Ligament
Transverse scapular ligament	Shoulder Bursa and Ligament, Right
	Shoulder Bursa and Ligament, Left
Transverse thoracis muscle	Thorax Muscle, Right
	Thorax Muscle, Left
Transversospinalis muscle	Trunk Muscle, Right
	Trunk Muscle, Left
Transversus abdominis muscle	Abdomen Muscle, Right
	Abdomen Muscle, Left
Trapezium bone	Carpal, Left
	Carpal, Right
Trapezius muscle	Trunk Muscle, Right
	Trunk Muscle, Left
Trapezoid bone	Carpal, Left
	Carpal, Right
Triceps brachii muscle	Upper Arm Muscle, Right
	Upper Arm Muscle, Left
Tricuspid annulus	Tricuspid Valve
Trifacial nerve	Trigeminal Nerve
Trigone of bladder	Bladder
Triquetral bone	Carpal, Left
	Carpal, Right
Trochanteric bursa	Hip Bursa and Ligament, Right
	Hip Bursa and Ligament, Left
Twelfth cranial nerve	Hypoglossal Nerve
Tympanic cavity	Middle Ear, Right
	Middle Ear, Left
Tympanic nerve	Glossopharyngeal Nerve
Tympanic part of temoporal bone	Temporal Bone, Right
	Temporal Bone, Left
Ulnar collateral ligament	Elbow Bursa and Ligament, Right
	Elbow Bursa and Ligament, Left
Ulnar collateral carpal ligament	Wrist Bursa and Ligament, Right
	Wrist Bursa and Ligament, Left
Ulnar notch	Radius, Left
	Radius, Right
Ulnar vein	Brachial Vein, Right
	Brachial Vein, Left
Umbilical artery	Internal Iliac Artery, Right
	Internal Iliac Artery, Left
Ureteral orifice	Ureter
	Ureter, Left
	Ureter, Right
	Ureters, Bilateral
Ureteropelvic junction (UPJ)	Kidney Pelvis, Right
	Kidney Pelvis, Left
Ureterovesical orifice	Ureter, Left
	Ureter, Right
Uterine artery	Internal Iliac Artery, Right
	Internal Iliac Artery, Left
Uterine cornu	Uterus
Uterine tube	Fallopian Tube, Right
	Fallopian Tube, Left
Uterine vein	Hypogastric Vein, Right
	Hypogastric Vein, Left
Vaginal artery	Internal Iliac Artery, Right
	Internal Iliac Artery, Left
Vaginal vein	Hypogastric Vein, Right
	Hypogastric Vein, Left
Vastus intermedius muscle	Upper Leg Muscle, Right
	Upper Leg Muscle, Left
Vastus lateralis muscle	Upper Leg Muscle, Right
	Upper Leg Muscle, Left
Vastus medialis muscle	Upper Leg Muscle, Right
	Upper Leg Muscle, Left
Ventricular fold	Larynx
Vermiform appendix	Appendix
Vermilion border	Lower Lip
	Upper Lip
Vertebral arch	Cervical Vertebra
	Lumbar Vertebra
	Thoracic Vertebra
Vertebral canal	Spinal Canal
Vertebral foramen	Cervical Vertebra
	Lumbar Vertebra
	Thoracic Vertebra
Vertebral lamina	Cervical Vertebra
	Lumbar Vertebra
	Thoracic Vertebra
Vertebral pedicle	Cervical Vertebra
	Lumbar Vertebra
	Thoracic Vertebra
Vesical vein	Hypogastric Vein, Right
	Hypogastric Vein, Left
Vestibular (Scarpa's) ganglion	Acoustic Nerve
Vestibular nerve	Acoustic Nerve
Vestibulocochlear nerve	Acoustic Nerve
Virchow's (supraclavicular) lymph node	Lymphatic, Left Neck
	Lymphatic, Right Neck
Vitreous body	Vitreous, Left
	Vitreous, Right
Vocal fold	Vocal Cord, Right
	Vocal Cord, Left
Volar (palmar) digital vein	Hand Vein, Left
	Hand Vein, Right
Volar (palmar) metacarpal vein	Hand Vein, Left
	Hand Vein, Right
Vomer bone	Nasal Septum (bone)

Anatomical Term	PCS Description
Xiphoid process	Sternum
Zonule of Zinn	Lens, Left
	Lens, Right
Zygomatic process of frontal bone	Frontal Bone, Right
	Frontal Bone, Left
Zygomatic process of temporal bone	Temporal Bone, Right
	Temporal Bone, Left
Zygomaticus muscle	Facial Muscle

Appendix D: Device Key and Aggregation Table

Device Key

Device Term	PCS Description
3f (Aortic) Bioprosthesis valve	Zooplastic Tissue in Heart and Great Vessels
AbioCor® Total Replacement Heart	Synthetic Substitute
Absolute Pro Vascular (OTW) Self-Expanding Stent System	Intraluminal Device
Acculink (RX) Carotid Stent System	Intraluminal Device
Acellular Hydrated Dermis	Nonautologous Tissue Substitute
Activa PC neurostimulator	Stimulator Generator, Multiple Array for Insertion in Subcutaneous Tissue and Fascia
Activa RC neurostimulator	Stimulator Generator, Multiple Array Rechargeable for Insertion in Subcutaneous Tissue and Fascia
Activa SC neurostimulator	Stimulator Generator, Single Array for Insertion in Subcutaneous Tissue and Fascia
ACUITY™ Steerable Lead	Cardiac Lead, Pacemaker for Insertion in Heart and Great Vessels Cardiac Lead, Defibrillator for Insertion in Heart and Great Vessels
Advisa (MRI)	Pacemaker, Dual Chamber for Insertion in Subcutaneous Tissue and Fascia
AMPLATZER® Muscular VSD Occluder	Synthetic Substitute
AMS 800® Urinary Control System	Artificial Sphincter in Urinary System
AneuRx® AAA Advantage®	Intraluminal Device
Annuloplasty ring	Synthetic Substitute
Artificial anal sphincter (AAS)	Artificial Sphincter in Gastrointestinal System
Artificial bowel sphincter (neosphincter)	Artificial Sphincter in Gastrointestinal System
Artificial urinary sphincter (AUS)	Artificial Sphincter in Urinary System
Ascenda Intrathecal Catheter	Infusion Device
Assurant (Cobalt) stent	Intraluminal Device
Attain Ability® Lead	Cardiac Lead, Pacemaker for Insertion in Heart and Great Vessels Cardiac Lead, Defibrillator for Insertion in Heart and Great Vessels
Attain StarFix® (OTW) Lead	Cardiac Lead, Pacemaker for Insertion in Heart and Great Vessels Cardiac Lead, Defibrillator for Insertion in Heart and Great Vessels
Autograft	Autologous Tissue Substitute

Device Term	PCS Description
Autologous artery graft	Autologous Arterial Tissue in Heart and Great Vessels Autologous Arterial Tissue in Upper Arteries Autologous Arterial Tissue in Lower Arteries Autologous Arterial Tissue in Upper Veins Autologous Arterial Tissue in Lower Veins
Autologous vein graft	Autologous Venous Tissue in Heart and Great Vessels Autologous Venous Tissue in Upper Arteries Autologous Venous Tissue in Lower Arteries Autologous Venous Tissue in Upper Veins Autologous Venous Tissue in Lower Veins
Axial Lumbar Interbody Fusion System	Interbody Fusion Device in Lower Joints
AxiaLIF® System	Interbody Fusion Device in Lower Joints
BAK/C® Interbody Cervical Fusion System	Interbody Fusion Device in Upper Joints
Bard® Composix® (E/X)(LP) mesh	Synthetic Substitute
Bard® Composix® Kugel® patch	Synthetic Substitute
Bard® Dulex™ mesh	Synthetic Substitute
Bard® Ventralex™ Hernia Patch	Synthetic Substitute
Baroreflex Activation Therapy® (BAT®)	Stimulator Lead in Upper Arteries Stimulator Generator in Subcutaneous Tissue and Fascia
Berlin Heart Ventricular Assist Device	Implantable Heart Assist System in Heart and Great Vessels
Bioactive embolization coil(s)	Intraluminal Device, Bioactive in Upper Arteries
Biventricular external heart assist system	External Heart Assist System in Heart and Great Vessels
Blood glucose monitoring system	Monitoring Device
Bone anchored hearing device	Hearing Device, Bone Conduction for Insertion in Ear, Nose, Sinus Hearing Device, in Head and Facial Bones
Bone bank bone graft	Nonautologous Tissue Substitute
Bone screw (interlocking)(lag)(pedicle)(recessed)	Internal Fixation Device in Head and Facial Bones Internal Fixation Device in Upper Bones Internal Fixation Device in Lower Bones

Device Term	PCS Description
Bovine pericardial valve	Zooplastic Tissue in Heart and Great Vessels
Bovine pericardium graft	Zooplastic Tissue in Heart and Great Vessels
Brachytherapy seeds	Radioactive Element
BRYAN® Cervical Disc System	Synthetic Substitute
BVS 5000 Ventricular Assist Device	External Heart Assist System in Heart and Great Vessels
Cardiac contractility modulation lead	Cardiac Lead in Heart and Great Vessels
Cardiac event recorder	Monitoring Device
Cardiac resynchronization therapy (CRT) lead	Cardiac Lead, Pacemaker for Insertion in Heart and Great Vessels Cardiac Lead, Defibrillator for Insertion in Heart and Great Vessels
CardioMEMS® pressure sensor	Monitoring Device, Pressure Sensor for Insertion in Heart and Great Vessels
Carotid (artery) sinus (baroreceptor) lead	Stimulator Lead in Upper Arteries
Carotid WALLSTENT® Monorail® Endoprosthesis	Intraluminal Device
Centrimag® Blood Pump	External Heart Assist System in Heart and Great Vessels
Clamp and rod internal fixation system (CRIF)	Internal Fixation Device in Upper Bones Internal Fixation Device in Lower Bones
CoAxia NeuroFlo catheter	Intraluminal Device
Cobalt/chromium head and polyethylene socket	Synthetic Substitute, Metal on Polyethylene for Replacement in Lower Joints
Cobalt/chromium head and socket	Synthetic Substitute, Metal for Replacement in Lower Joints
Cochlear implant (CI), multiple channel (electrode)	Hearing Device, Multiple Channel Cochlear Prosthesis for Insertion in Ear, Nose, Sinus
Cochlear implant (CI), single channel (electrode)	Hearing Device, Single Channel Cochlear Prosthesis for Insertion in Ear, Nose, Sinus
COGNIS® CRT-D	Cardiac Resynchronization Defibrillator Pulse Generator for Insertion in Subcutaneous Tissue and Fascia
Colonic Z-Stent®	Intraluminal Device
Complete (SE) stent	Intraluminal Device
Concerto II CRT-D	Cardiac Resynchronization Defibrillator Pulse Generator for Insertion in Subcutaneous Tissue and Fascia
CONSERVE® PLUS Total Resurfacing Hip System	Resurfacing Device in Lower Joints
Consulta CRT-D	Cardiac Resynchronization Defibrillator Pulse Generator for Insertion in Subcutaneous Tissue and Fascia
Consulta CRT-P	Cardiac Resynchronization Pacemaker Pulse Generator for Insertion in Subcutaneous Tissue and Fascia
CONTAK RENEWAL® 3 RF (HE) CRT-D	Cardiac Resynchronization Defibrillator Pulse Generator for Insertion in Subcutaneous Tissue and Fascia
Contegra Pulmonary Valved Conduit	Zooplastic Tissue in Heart and Great Vessels
Continuous Glucose Monitoring (CGM) device	Monitoring Device
CoreValve transcatheter aortic valve	Zooplastic Tissue in Heart and Great Vessels
Cormet Hip Resurfacing System	Resurfacing Device in Lower Joints
CoRoent® XL	Interbody Fusion Device in Lower Joints
Corox (OTW) Bipolar Lead	Cardiac Lead, Pacemaker for Insertion in Heart and Great Vessels Cardiac Lead, Defibrillator for Insertion in Heart and Great Vessels
Cortical strip neurostimulator lead	Neurostimulator Lead in Central Nervous System
Cultured epidermal cell autograft	Autologous Tissue Substitute
CYPHER® Stent	Intraluminal Device, Drug-eluting in Heart and Great Vessels
Cystostomy tube	Drainage Device
DBS lead	Neurostimulator Lead in Central Nervous System
DeBakey Left Ventricular Assist Device	Implantable Heart Assist System in Heart and Great Vessels
Deep brain neurostimulator lead	Neurostimulator Lead in Central Nervous System
Delta frame external fixator	External Fixation Device, Hybrid for Insertion in Upper Bones External Fixation Device, Hybrid for Reposition in Upper Bones External Fixation Device, Hybrid for Insertion in Lower Bones External Fixation Device, Hybrid for Reposition in Lower Bones
Delta III Reverse shoulder prosthesis	Synthetic Substitute, Reverse Ball and Socket for Replacement in Upper Joints
Diaphragmatic pacemaker generator	Stimulator Generator in Subcutaneous Tissue and Fascia
Direct Lateral Interbody Fusion (DLIF) device	Interbody Fusion Device in Lower Joints
Driver stent (RX) (OTW)	Intraluminal Device
DuraHeart Left Ventricular Assist System	Implantable Heart Assist System in Heart and Great Vessels
Durata® Defibrillation Lead	Cardiac Lead, Defibrillator for Insertion in Heart and Great Vessels

Device Term	PCS Description
Dynesys® Dynamic Stabilization System	Spinal Stabilization Device, Pedicle-Based for Insertion in Upper Joints Spinal Stabilization Device, Pedicle-Based for Insertion in Lower Joints
E-Luminexx™ (Biliary)(Vascular) Stent	Intraluminal Device
Electrical bone growth stimulator (EBGS)	Bone Growth Stimulator in Head and Facial Bones Bone Growth Stimulator in Upper Bones Bone Growth Stimulator in Lower Bones
Electrical muscle stimulation (EMS) lead	Stimulator Lead in Muscles
Electronic muscle stimulator lead	Stimulator Lead in Muscles
Embolization coil(s)	Intraluminal Device
Endeavor® (III)(IV) (Sprint) Zotarolimus-eluting Coronary Stent System	Intraluminal Device, Drug-eluting in Heart and Great Vessels
EndoSure® sensor	Monitoring Device, Pressure Sensor for Insertion in Heart and Great Vessels
ENDOTAK RELIANCE® (G) Defibrillation Lead	Cardiac Lead, Defibrillator for Insertion in Heart and Great Vessels
Endotracheal tube (cuffed)(double-lumen)	Intraluminal Device, Endotracheal Airway in Respiratory System
Endurant® Endovascular Stent Graft	Intraluminal Device
EnRhythm	Pacemaker, Dual Chamber for Insertion in Subcutaneous Tissue and Fascia
Enterra gastric neurostimulator	Stimulator Generator, Multiple Array for Insertion in Subcutaneous Tissue and Fascia
Epicel® cultured epidermal autograft	Autologous Tissue Substitute
Epic™ Stented Tissue Valve (aortic)	Zooplastic Tissue in Heart and Great Vessels
Epiretinal visual prosthesis	Epiretinal Visual Prosthesis in Eye
Esophageal obturator airway (EOA)	Intraluminal Device, Airway in Gastrointestinal System
Esteem® implantable hearing system	Hearing Device in Ear, Nose, Sinus
Evera (XT)(S)(DR/VR)	Defibrillator Generator for Insertion in Subcutaneous Tissue and Fascia
Everolimus-eluting coronary stent	Intraluminal Device, Drug-eluting in Heart and Great Vessels
Ex-PRESS™ mini glaucoma shunt	Synthetic Substitute
Express® (LD) Premounted Stent System	Intraluminal Device
Express® Biliary SD Monorail® Premounted Stent System	Intraluminal Device
Express® SD Renal Monorail® Premounted Stent System	Intraluminal Device

Device Term	PCS Description
External fixator	External Fixation Device in Head and Facial Bones External Fixation Device in Upper Bones External Fixation Device in Lower Bones External Fixation Device in Upper Joints External Fixation Device in Lower Joints
EXtreme Lateral Interbody Fusion (XLIF) device	Interbody Fusion Device in Lower Joints
Facet replacement spinal stabilization device	Spinal Stabilization Device, Facet Replacement for Insertion in Upper Joints Spinal Stabilization Device, Facet Replacement for Insertion in Lower Joints
FLAIR® Endovascular Stent Graft	Intraluminal Device
Flexible Composite Mesh	Synthetic Substitute
Foley catheter	Drainage Device
Formula™ Balloon-Expandable Renal Stent System	Intraluminal Device
Freestyle (Stentless) Aortic Root Bioprosthesis	Zooplastic Tissue in Heart and Great Vessels
Fusion screw (compression)(lag)(locking)	Internal Fixation Device in Upper Joints Internal Fixation Device in Lower Joints
Gastric electrical stimulation (GES) lead	Stimulator Lead in Gastrointestinal System
Gastric pacemaker lead	Stimulator Lead in Gastrointestinal System
GORE® DUALMESH®	Synthetic Substitute
Guedel airway	Intraluminal Device, Airway in Mouth and Throat
Hancock Bioprosthesis (aortic)(mitral) valve	Zooplastic Tissue
Hancock Bioprosthetic Valved Conduit	Zooplastic Tissue in Heart and Great Vessels
HeartMate II® Left Ventricular Assist Device (LVAD)	Implantable Heart Assist System in Heart and Great Vessels
HeartMate XVE® Left Ventricular Assist Device (LVAD)	Implantable Heart Assist System in Heart and Great Vessels
Herculink (RX) Elite Renal Stent System	Intraluminal Device
Hip (joint) liner	Liner in Lower Joints
Holter valve ventricular shunt	Synthetic Substitute
Ilizarov external fixator	External Fixation Device, Ring for Insertion in Upper Bones External Fixation Device, Ring for Reposition in Upper Bones External Fixation Device, Ring for Insertion in Lower Bones External Fixation Device, Ring for Reposition in Lower Bones

Device Term	PCS Description
Ilizarov-Vecklich device	External Fixation Device, Limb Lengthening for Insertion in Upper Bones External Fixation Device, Limb Lengthening for Insertion in Lower Bones
Implantable cardioverter-defibrillator (ICD)	Defibrillator Generator for Insertion in Subcutaneous Tissue and Fascia
Implantable drug infusion pump (anti-spasmodic)(chemotherapy)(pain)	Infusion Device, Pump in Subcutaneous Tissue and Fascia
Implantable gastric pacemaker generator	Stimulator Generator in Subcutaneous Tissue and Fascia
Implantable glucose monitoring device	Monitoring Device
Implantable hemodynamic monitor (IHM)	Monitoring Device, Hemodynamic for Insertion in Subcutaneous Tissue and Fascia
Implantable hemodynamic monitoring system (IHMS)	Monitoring Device, Hemodynamic for Insertion in Subcutaneous Tissue and Fascia
Implantable Miniature Telescope™ (IMT)	Synthetic Substitute, Intraocular Telescope for Replacement in Eye
Implanted (venous)(access) port	Vascular Access Device, Reservoir in Subcutaneous Tissue and Fascia
InDura, intrathecal catheter (1P) (spinal)	Infusion Device
Injection reservoir, port	Vascular Access Device, Reservoir in Subcutaneous Tissue and Fascia
Injection reservoir, pump	Infusion Device, Pump in Subcutaneous Tissue and Fascia
Interbody fusion (spine) cage	Interbody Fusion Device in Upper Joints Interbody Fusion Device in Lower Joints
Interspinous process spinal stabilization device	Spinal Stabilization Device, Interspinous Process for Insertion in Upper Joints Spinal Stabilization Device, Interspinous Process for Insertion in Lower Joints
InterStim® Therapy lead	Neurostimulator Lead in Peripheral Nervous System
InterStim® Therapy neurostimulator	Stimulator Generator Single Array for Insertion in Subcutaneous Tissue and Fascia
Intramedullary (IM) rod (nail)	Internal Fixation Device, Intramedullary in Upper Bones Internal Fixation Device, Intramedullary in Lower Bones
Intramedullary skeletal kinetic distractor (ISKD)	Internal Fixation Device, Intramedullary in Upper Bones Internal Fixation Device, Intramedullary in Lower Bones
Intrauterine Device (IUD)	Contraceptive Device in Female Reproductive System
Itrel (3)(4) neurostimulator	Stimulator Generator, Single Array for Insertion in Subcutaneous Tissue and Fascia
Joint fixation plate	Internal Fixation Device in Upper Joints Internal Fixation Device in Lower Joints
Joint liner (insert)	Liner in Lower Joints
Joint spacer (antibiotic)	Spacer in Upper Joints Spacer in Lower Joints
Kappa	Pacemaker, Dual Chamber for Insertion in Subcutaneous Tissue and Fascia
Kirschner wire (K-wire)	Internal Fixation Device in Head and Facial Bones Internal Fixation Device in Upper Bones Internal Fixation Device in Lower Bones Internal Fixation Device in Upper Joints Internal Fixation Device in Lower Joints
Knee (implant) insert	Liner in Lower Joints
Kuntscher nail	Internal Fixation Device, Intramedullary in Upper Bones Internal Fixation Device, Intramedullary in Lower Bones
LAP-BAND® Adjustable Gastric Banding System	Extraluminal Device
LifeStent® (Flexstar)(XL) Vascular Stent System	Intraluminal Device
LIVIAN™ CRT-D	Cardiac Resynchronization Defibrillator Pulse Generator for Insertion in Subcutaneous Tissue and Fascia
Loop recorder, implantable	Monitoring Device
Mark IV Breathing Pacemaker System	Stimulator Generator in Subcutaneous Tissue and Fascia
Maximo II DR (VR)	Defibrillator Generator for Insertion in Subcutaneous Tissue and Fascia
Maximo II DR CRT-D	Cardiac Resynchronization Defibrillator Pulse Generator for Insertion in Subcutaneous Tissue and Fascia
Melody® transcatheter pulmonary valve	Zooplastic Tissue in Heart and Great Vessels
Micro-Driver stent (RX) (OTW)	Intraluminal Device
MicroMed HeartAssist	Implantable Heart Assist System in Heart and Great Vessels
Micrus CERECYTE Microcoil	Intraluminal Device, Bioactive in Upper Arteries
MitraClip valve repair system	Synthetic Substitute
Mitroflow® Aortic Pericardial Heart Valve	Zooplastic Tissue in Heart and Great Vessels
Mosaic Bioprosthesis (aortic) (mitral) valve	Zooplastic Tissue in Heart and Great Vessels
MULTI-LINK (VISION)(MINI-VISION)(ULTRA) Coronary Stent System	Intraluminal Device

Device Term	PCS Description
Nasopharyngeal airway (NPA)	Intraluminal Device, Airway in Ear, Nose, Sinus
Neuromuscular electrical stimulation (NEMS) lead	Stimulator Lead in Muscles
Neurostimulator generator, multiple channel	Stimulator Generator, Multiple Array for Insertion in Subcutaneous Tissue and Fascia
Neurostimulator generator, multiple channel rechargeable	Stimulator Generator, Multiple Array Rechargeable for Insertion in Subcutaneous Tissue and Fascia
Neurostimulator generator, single channel	Stimulator Generator, Single Array for Insertion in Subcutaneous Tissue and Fascia
Neurostimulator generator, single channel rechargeable	Stimulator Generator, Single Array Rechargeable for Insertion in Subcutaneous Tissue and Fascia
Neutralization plate	Internal Fixation Device in Head and Facial Bones Internal Fixation Device in Upper Bones Internal Fixation Device in Lower Bones
Nitinol framed polymer mesh	Synthetic Substitute
Non-tunneled central venous catheter	Infusion Device
Novacor Left Ventricular Assist Device	Implantable Heart Assist System in Heart and Great Vessels
Novation® Ceramic AHS® (articulation hip system)	Synthetic Substitute, Ceramic for Replacement in Lower Joints
Omnilink Elite Vascular Balloon Expandable Stent System	Intraluminal Device
Open Pivot Aortic Valve Graft (AVG)	Synthetic Substitute
Open Pivot (mechanical) Valve	Synthetic Substitute
Optimizer™ III implantable pulse generator	Contractility Modulation Device for Insertion in Subcutaneous Tissue and Fascia
Oropharyngeal airway (OPA)	Intraluminal Device, Airway in Mouth and Throat
Ovatio™ CRT-D	Cardiac Resynchronization Defibrillator Pulse Generator for Insertion in Subcutaneous Tissue and Fascia
Oxidized zirconium ceramic hip bearing surface	Synthetic Substitute, Ceramic on Polyethylene for Replacement in Lower Joints
Paclitaxel-eluting coronary stent	Intraluminal Device, Drug-eluting in Heart and Great Vessels
Paclitaxel-eluting peripheral stent	Intraluminal Device, Drug-eluting in Upper Arteries Intraluminal Device, Drug-eluting in Lower Arteries
Partially absorbable mesh	Synthetic Substitute
Pedicle-based dynamic stabilization device	Spinal Stabilization Device, Pedicle-Based for Insertion in Upper Joints Spinal Stabilization Device, Pedicle-Based for Insertion in Lower Joints
Percutaneous endoscopic gastrojejunostomy (PEG/J) tube	Feeding Device in Gastrointestinal System
Percutaneous endoscopic gastrostomy (PEG) tube	Feeding Device in Gastrointestinal System
Percutaneous nephrostomy catheter	Drainage Device
Peripherally inserted central catheter (PICC)	Infusion Device
Pessary ring	Intraluminal Device, Pessary in Female Reproductive System
Phrenic nerve stimulator generator	Stimulator Generator in Subcutaneous Tissue and Fascia
Phrenic nerve stimulator lead	Diaphragmatic Pacemaker Lead in Respiratory System
PHYSIOMESH™ Flexible Composite Mesh	Synthetic Substitute
Pipeline™ Embolization device (PED)	Intraluminal Device
Polyethylene socket	Synthetic Substitute, Polyethylene for Replacement in Lower Joints
Polymethylmethacrylate (PMMA)	Synthetic Substitute
Polypropylene mesh	Synthetic Substitute
Porcine (bioprosthetic) valve	Zooplastic Tissue in Heart and Great Vessels
PRESTIGE® Cervical Disc	Synthetic Substitute
PrimeAdvanced neurostimulator (SureScan)(MRI Safe)	Stimulator Generator, Multiple Array for Insertion in Subcutaneous Tissue and Fascia
PROCEED™ Ventral Patch	Synthetic Substitute
Prodisc-C	Synthetic Substitute
Prodisc-L	Synthetic Substitute
PROLENE Polypropylene Hernia System (PHS)	Synthetic Substitute
Protecta XT CRT-D	Cardiac Resynchronization Defibrillator Pulse Generator for Insertion in Subcutaneous Tissue and Fascia
Protecta XT DR (XT VR)	Defibrillator Generator for Insertion in Subcutaneous Tissue and Fascia
Protégé® RX Carotid Stent System	Intraluminal Device
Pump reservoir	Infusion Device, Pump in Subcutaneous Tissue and Fascia
REALIZE® Adjustable Gastric Band	Extraluminal Device
Rebound HRD® (Hernia Repair Device)	Synthetic Substitute

Device Term	PCS Description
RestoreAdvanced neurostimulator (SureScan)(MRI Safe)	Stimulator Generator, Multiple Array Rechargeable for Insertion in Subcutaneous Tissue and Fascia
RestoreSensor neurostimulator (SureScan)(MRI Safe)	Stimulator Generator, Multiple Array Rechargeable for Insertion in Subcutaneous Tissue and Fascia
RestoreUltra neurostimulator (SureScan)(MRI Safe)	Stimulator Generator, Multiple Array Rechargeable for Insertion in Subcutaneous Tissue and Fascia
Reveal (DX)(XT)	Monitoring Device
Reverse® Shoulder Prosthesis	Synthetic Substitute, Reverse Ball and Socket for Replacement in Upper Joints
Revo MRI™ SureScan® pacemaker	Pacemaker, Dual Chamber for Insertion in Subcutaneous Tissue and Fascia
Rheos® System device	Stimulator Generator in Subcutaneous Tissue and Fascia
Rheos® System lead	Stimulator Lead in Upper Arteries
RNS System lead	Neurostimulator Lead in Central Nervous System
RNS system neurostimulator generator	Neurostimulator Generator in Head and Facial Bones
Sacral nerve modulation (SNM) lead	Stimulator Lead in Urinary System
Sacral neuromodulation lead	Stimulator Lead in Urinary System
SAPIEN transcatheter aortic valve	Zooplastic Tissue in Heart and Great Vessels
Secura (DR) (VR)	Defibrillator Generator for Insertion in Subcutaneous Tissue and Fascia
Sheffield hybrid external fixator	External Fixation Device, Hybrid for Insertion in Upper Bones External Fixation Device, Hybrid for Reposition in Upper Bones External Fixation Device, Hybrid for Insertion in Lower Bones External Fixation Device, Hybrid for Reposition in Lower Bones
Sheffield ring external fixator	External Fixation Device, Ring for Insertion in Upper Bones External Fixation Device, Ring for Reposition in Upper Bones External Fixation Device, Ring for Insertion in Lower Bones External Fixation Device, Ring for Reposition in Lower Bones
Single lead pacemaker (atrium)(ventricle)	Pacemaker, Single Chamber for Insertion in Subcutaneous Tissue and Fascia
Single lead rate responsive pacemaker (atrium)(ventricle)	Pacemaker, Single Chamber Rate Responsive for Insertion in Subcutaneous Tissue and Fascia
Sirolimus-eluting coronary stent	Intraluminal Device, Drug-eluting in Heart and Great Vessels
SJM Biocor® Stented Valve System	Zooplastic Tissue in Heart and Great Vessels
Spinal cord neurostimulator lead	Neurostimulator Lead in Central Nervous System

Device Term	PCS Description
Spiration IBV™ Valve System	Intraluminal Device, Endobronchial Valve in Respiratory System
Stent, Intraluminal (cardiovascular)(gastrointestinal)(hepatobiliary)(urinary)	Intraluminal Device
Stented tissue valve	Zooplastic Tissue in Heart and Great Vessels
Stratos LV	Cardiac Resynchronization Pacemaker Pulse Generator for Insertion in Subcutaneous Tissue and Fascia
Subcutaneous injection reservoir, port	Vascular Access Device, Reservoir in Subcutaneous Tissue and Fascia
Subcutaneous injection reservoir, pump	Infusion Device, Pump in Subcutaneous Tissue and Fascia
Subdermal progesterone implant	Contraceptive Device in Subcutaneous Tissue and Fascia
SynCardia Total Artificial Heart	Synthetic Substitute
Synchra CRT-P	Cardiac Resynchronization Pacemaker Pulse Generator for Insertion in Subcutaneous Tissue and Fascia
SyncroMed Pump	Infusion Device, Pump in Subcutaneous Tissue and Fascia
Talent® Converter	Intraluminal Device
Talent® Occluder	Intraluminal Device
Talent® Stent Graft (abdominal)(thoracic)	Intraluminal Device
TandemHeart® System	External Heart Assist System in Heart and Great Vessels
TAXUS® Liberté® Paclitaxel-eluting Coronary Stent System	Intraluminal Device, Drug-eluting in Heart and Great Vessels
Therapeutic occlusion coil(s)	Intraluminal Device
Thoracostomy tube	Drainage Device
Thoratec IVAD (implantable ventricular assist device)	Implantable Heart Assist System in Heart and Great Vessels
Thoratec Paracorporeal Ventricular Assist Device	External Heart Assist System in Heart and Great Vessels
TigerPaw® system for closure of left atrial appendage	Extraluminal Device
Tissue bank graft	Nonautologous Tissue Substitute
Tissue expander (inflatable)(injectable)	Tissue Expander in Skin and Breast Tissue Expander in Subcutaneous Tissue and Fascia
Titanium Sternal Fixation System (TSFS)	Internal Fixation Device, Rigid Plate for Insertion in Upper Bones Internal Fixation Device, Rigid Plate for Reposition in Upper Bones
Total artificial (replacement) heart	Synthetic Substitute
Tracheostomy tube	Tracheostomy Device in Respiratory System
Trifecta™ Valve (aortic)	Zooplastic Tissue in Heart and Great Vessels

Device Term	PCS Description
Tunneled central venous catheter	Vascular Access Device in Subcutaneous Tissue and Fascia
Tunneled spinal (intrathecal) catheter	Infusion Device
Two lead pacemaker	Pacemaker, Dual Chamber for Insertion in Subcutaneous Tissue and Fascia
Ultraflex™ Precision Colonic Stent System	Intraluminal Device
ULTRAPRO Hernia System (UHS)	Synthetic Substitute
ULTRAPRO Partially Absorbable Lightweight Mesh	Synthetic Substitute
ULTRAPRO Plug	Synthetic Substitute
Ultrasonic osteogenic stimulator	Bone Growth Stimulator in Head and Facial Bones Bone Growth Stimulator in Upper Bones Bone Growth Stimulator in Lower Bones
Ultrasound bone healing system	Bone Growth Stimulator in Head and Facial Bones Bone Growth Stimulator in Upper Bones Bone Growth Stimulator in Lower Bones
Uniplanar external fixator	External Fixation Device, Monoplanar for Insertion in Upper Bones External Fixation Device, Monoplanar for Reposition in Upper Bones External Fixation Device, Monoplanar for Insertion in Lower Bones External Fixation Device, Monoplanar for Reposition in Lower Bones
Urinary incontinence stimulator lead	Stimulator Lead in Urinary System
Vaginal pessary	Intraluminal Device, Pessary in Female Reproductive System
Valiant Thoracic Stent Graft	Synthetic Substitute
Vectra® Vascular Access Graft	Vascular Access Device in Subcutaneous Tissue and Fascia
Ventrio™ Hernia Patch	Synthetic Substitute
Versa	Pacemaker, Dual Chamber
Virtuoso (II) (DR) (VR)	Defibrillator Generator for Insertion in Subcutaneous Tissue and Fascia
Viva(XT)(S)	Cardiac Resynchronization Defibrillator Pulse Generator for Insertion in Subcutaneous Tissue and Fascia
WALLSTENT® Endoprosthesis	Intraluminal Device
Xact Carotid Stent System	Intraluminal Device
X-STOP® Spacer	Spinal Stabilization Device, Interspinous Process for Insertion in Upper Joints Spinal Stabilization Device, Interspinous Process for Insertion in Lower Joints
Xenograft	Zooplastic Tissue in Heart and Great Vessels
XIENCE Everolimus Eluting Coronary Stent System	Intraluminal Device, Drug-eluting in Heart and Great Vessels
XLIF® System	Interbody Fusion Device in Lower Joints
Zenith Flex® AAA Endovascular Graft	Intraluminal Device
Zenith TX2® TAA Endovascular Graft	Intraluminal Device
Zenith® Renu™ AAA Ancillary Graft	Intraluminal Device
Zilver® PTX® (paclitaxel) Drug-Eluting Peripheral Stent	Intraluminal Device, Drug-eluting in Upper Arteries Intraluminal Device, Drug-eluting in Lower Arteries
Zimmer® NexGen® LPS Mobile Bearing Knee	Synthetic Substitute
Zimmer® NexGen® LPS-Flex Mobile Knee	Synthetic Substitute
Zotarolimus-eluting coronary stent	Intraluminal Device, Drug-eluting in Heart and Great Vessels

Device Aggregation Table

This table crosswalks specific device character value definitions for specific root operations in a specific body system to the more general device character value to be used when the root operation covers a wide range of body parts and the device character represents an entire family of devices.

Specific Device	for Operation	in Body System	General Device
Autologous Arterial Tissue (A)	All applicable	Heart and Great Vessels Lower Arteries Lower Veins Upper Arteries Upper Veins	**7** Autologous Tissue Substitute
Autologous Venous Tissue (9)	All applicable	Heart and Great Vessels Lower Arteries Lower Veins Upper Arteries Upper Veins	**7** Autologous Tissue Substitute

Specific Device	for Operation	in Body System	General Device
Cardiac Lead, Defibrillator (K)	Insertion	Heart and Great Vessels	**M** Cardiac Lead
Cardiac Lead, Pacemaker (J)	Insertion	Heart and Great Vessels	**M** Cardiac Lead
Cardiac Resynchronization Defibrillator Pulse Generator (9)	Insertion	Subcutaneous Tissue and Fascia	**P** Cardiac Rhythm Related Device
Cardiac Resynchronization Pacemaker Pulse Generator (7)	Insertion	Subcutaneous Tissue and Fascia	**P** Cardiac Rhythm Related Device
Contractility Modulation Device (A)	Insertion	Subcutaneous Tissue and Fascia	**P** Cardiac Rhythm Related Device
Defibrillator Generator (8)	Insertion	Subcutaneous Tissue and Fascia	**P** Cardiac Rhythm Related Device
Epiretinal Visual Prosthesis	All applicable	Eye	**J** Synthetic Substitute
External Fixation Device, Hybrid (D)	Insertion	Lower Bones Upper Bones	**5** External Fixation Device
External Fixation Device, Hybrid (D)	Reposition	Lower Bones Upper Bones	**5** External Fixation Device
External Fixation Device, Limb Lengthening (8)	Insertion	Lower Bones Upper Bones	**5** External Fixation Device
External Fixation Device, Monoplanar (B)	Insertion	Lower Bones Upper Bones	**5** External Fixation Device
External Fixation Device, Monoplanar (B)	Reposition	Lower Bones Upper Bones	**5** External Fixation Device
External Fixation Device, Ring (C)	Insertion	Lower Bones Upper Bones	**5** External Fixation Device
External Fixation Device, Ring (C)	Reposition	Lower Bones Upper Bones	**5** External Fixation Device
Hearing Device, Bone Conduction (S)	All applicable	Head and Facial Bones	**S** Hearing Device, Bone Conduction
Hearing Device, Bone Conduction (4)	Insertion	Ear, Nose, Sinus	**S** Hearing Device
Hearing Device, Multiple Channel Cochlear Prosthesis (6)	Insertion	Ear, Nose, Sinus	**S** Hearing Device
Hearing Device, Single Channel Cochlear Prosthesis (5)	Insertion	Ear, Nose, Sinus	**S** Hearing Device
Internal Fixation Device, Intramedullary (6)	All applicable	Lower Bones Upper Bones	**4** Internal Fixation Device
Internal Fixation Device, Rigid Plate (Ø)	Insertion	Upper Bones	**4** Internal Fixation Device
Internal Fixation Device, Rigid Plate (Ø)	Reposition	Upper Bones	**4** Internal Fixation Device
Intraluminal Device, Pessary (G)	All applicable	Female Reproductive System	**D** Intraluminal Device
Intraluminal Device, Airway (B)	All applicable	Ear, Nose, Sinus Gastrointestinal System Mouth and Throat	**D** Intraluminal Device
Intraluminal Device, Bioactive (B)	All applicable	Upper Arteries	**D** Intraluminal Device
Intraluminal Device, Drug-eluting (4)	All applicable	Heart and Great Vessels Lower Arteries Upper Arteries	**D** Intraluminal Device
Intraluminal Device, Endobronchial Valve (G)	All applicable	Respiratory System	**D** Intraluminal Device
Intraluminal Device, Endotracheal Airway (E)	All applicable	Respiratory System	**D** Intraluminal Device
Intraluminal Device, Radioactive (T)	All applicable	Heart and Great Vessels	**D** Intraluminal Device
Monitoring Device, Hemodynamic (Ø)	Insertion	Subcutaneous Tissue and Fascia	**2** Monitoring Device
Monitoring Device, Pressure Sensor (Ø)	Insertion	Heart and Great Vessels	**2** Monitoring Device
Pacemaker, Dual Chamber (6)	Insertion	Subcutaneous Tissue and Fascia	**P** Cardiac Rhythm Related Device
Pacemaker, Single Chamber (4)	Insertion	Subcutaneous Tissue and Fascia	**P** Cardiac Rhythm Related Device
Pacemaker, Single Chamber Rate Responsive (5)	Insertion	Subcutaneous Tissue and Fascia	**P** Cardiac Rhythm Related Device
Spinal Stabilization Device, Facet Replacement (D)	Insertion	Lower Joints Upper Joints	**4** Internal Fixation Device
Spinal Stabilization Device, Interspinous Process (B)	Insertion	Lower Joints Upper Joints	**4** Internal Fixation Device
Spinal Stabilization Device, Pedicle-Based (C)	Insertion	Lower Joints Upper Joints	**4** Internal Fixation Device
Stimulator Generator, Multiple Array (D)	Insertion	Subcutaneous Tissue and Fascia	**M** Stimulator Generator

Specific Device	for Operation	in Body System	General Device
Stimulator Generator, Multiple Array Rechargeable (E)	Insertion	Subcutaneous Tissue and Fascia	**M** Stimulator Generator
Stimulator Generator, Single Array (B)	Insertion	Subcutaneous Tissue and Fascia	**M** Stimulator Generator
Stimulator Generator, Single Array Rechargeable (C)	Insertion	Subcutaneous Tissue and Fascia	**M** Stimulator Generator
Synthetic Substitute, Ceramic (3)	Replacement	Lower Joints	**J** Synthetic Substitute
Synthetic Substitute, Ceramic on Polyethylene (4)	Replacement	Lower Joints	**J** Synthetic Substitute
Synthetic Substitute, Intraocular Telescope (Ø)	Replacement	Eye	**J** Synthetic Substitute
Synthetic Substitute, Metal (1)	Replacement	Lower Joints	**J** Synthetic Substitute
Synthetic Substitute, Metal on Polyethylene (2)	Replacement	Lower Joints	**J** Synthetic Substitute
Synthetic Substitute, Polyethylene (Ø)	Replacement	Lower Joints	**J** Synthetic Substitute
Synthetic Substitute, Reverse Ball and Socket (Ø)	Replacement	Upper Joints	**J** Synthetic Substitute

Appendix E: Type and Type Qualifier Definitions Sections B–H

Section B–Imaging

Type (Character 3)	Definition
Computerized Tomography (CT Scan) (2)	Computer reformatted digital display of multiplanar images developed from the capture of multiple exposures of external ionizing radiation
Fluoroscopy (1)	Single plane or bi-plane real time display of an image developed from the capture of external ionizing radiation on a fluorescent screen. The image may also be stored by either digital or analog means
Magnetic Resonance Imaging (MRI) (3)	Computer reformatted digital display of multiplanar images developed from the capture of radiofrequency signals emitted by nuclei in a body site excited within a magnetic field
Plain Radiography (Ø)	Planar display of an image developed from the capture of external ionizing radiation on photographic or photoconductive plate
Ultrasonography (4)	Real time display of images of anatomy or flow information developed from the capture of reflected and attenuated high frequency sound waves

Section C–Nuclear Medicine

Type (Character 3)	Definition
Nonimaging Nuclear Medicine Assay (6)	Introduction of radioactive materials into the body for the study of body fluids and blood elements, by the detection of radioactive emissions
Nonimaging Nuclear Medicine Probe (5)	Introduction of radioactive materials into the body for the study of distribution and fate of certain substances by the detection of radioactive emissions; or, alternatively, measurement of absorption of radioactive emissions from an external source
Nonimaging Nuclear Medicine Uptake (4)	Introduction of radioactive materials into the body for measurements of organ function, from the detection of radioactive emissions
Planar Nuclear Medicine Imaging (1)	Introduction of radioactive materials into the body for single plane display of images developed from the capture of radioactive emissions
Positron Emission Tomographic (PET) Imaging (3)	Introduction of radioactive materials into the body for three dimensional display of images developed from the simultaneous capture, 18Ø degrees apart, of radioactive emissions
Systemic Nuclear Medicine Therapy (7)	Introduction of unsealed radioactive materials into the body for treatment
Tomographic (Tomo) Nuclear Medicine Imaging (2)	Introduction of radioactive materials into the body for three dimensional display of images developed from the capture of radioactive emissions

Section F–Physical Rehabilitation and Diagnostic Audiology

Type (Character 3)	Definition
Activities of Daily Living Assessment (2)	Measurement of functional level for activities of daily living
Activities of Daily Living Treatment (8)	Exercise or activities to facilitate functional competence for activities of daily living
Caregiver Training (F)	Training in activities to support patient's optimal level of function
Cochlear Implant Treatment (B)	Application of techniques to improve the communication abilities of individuals with cochlear implant
Device Fitting (D)	Fitting of a device designed to facilitate or support achievement of a higher level of function
Hearing Aid Assessment (4)	Measurement of the appropriateness and/or effectiveness of a hearing device
Hearing Assessment (3)	Measurement of hearing and related functions

Continued on next page

Section F–Physical Rehabilitation and Diagnostic Audiology

Continued from previous page

Type (Character 3)	Definition
Hearing Treatment (9)	Application of techniques to improve, augment, or compensate for hearing and related functional impairment
Motor Function Assessment/Nerve Function Assessment (1)	Measurement of motor, nerve, and related functions
Motor Treatment (7)	Exercise or activities to increase or facilitate motor function
Speech Assessment (Ø)	Measurement of speech and related functions
Speech Treatment (6)	Application of techniques to improve, augment, or compensate for speech and related functional impairment
Vestibular Assessment (5)	Measurement of the vestibular system and related functions
Vestibular Treatment (C)	Application of techniques to improve, augment, or compensate for vestibular and related functional impairment

Section F–Physical Rehabilitation and Diagnostic Audiology

Type Qualifier (Character 5)	Definition
Acoustic Reflex Decay (J)	Measures reduction in size/strength of acoustic reflex over time Includes/Examples: Includes site of lesion test
Acoustic Reflex Patterns (G)	Defines site of lesion based upon presence/absence of acoustic reflexes with ipsilateral vs. contralateral stimulation
Acoustic Reflex Threshold (H)	Determines minimal intensity that acoustic reflex occurs with ipsilateral and/or contralateral stimulation
Aerobic Capacity and Endurance (7)	Measures autonomic responses to positional changes; perceived exertion, dyspnea or angina during activity; performance during exercise protocols; standard vital signs; and blood gas analysis or oxygen consumption
Alternate Binaural or Monaural Loudness Balance (7)	Determines auditory stimulus parameter that yields the same objective sensation Includes/Examples: Sound intensities that yield same loudness perception
Anthropometric Characteristics (B)	Measures edema, body fat composition, height, weight, length and girth
Aphasia (Assessment) (C)	Measures expressive and receptive speech and language function including reading and writing
Aphasia (Treatment) (3)	Applying techniques to improve, augment, or compensate for receptive/ expressive language impairments
Articulation/Phonology (Assessment) (9)	Measures speech production
Articulation/Phonology (Treatment) (4)	Applying techniques to correct, improve, or compensate for speech productive impairment
Assistive Listening Device (5)	Assists in use of effective and appropriate assistive listening device/system
Assistive Listening System Device Selection (4)	Measures the effectiveness and appropriateness of assistive listening systems/devices
Assistive, Adaptive,Supportive or Protective Devices (9)	Explanation: Devices to facilitate or support achievement of a higher level of function in wheelchair mobility; bed mobility; transfer or ambulation ability; bath and showering ability; dressing; grooming; personal hygiene; play or leisure
Auditory Evoked Potentials (L)	Measures electric responses produced by the VIIIth cranial nerve and brainstem following auditory stimulation
Auditory Processing (Assessment) (Q)	Evaluates ability to receive and process auditory information and comprehension of spoken language
Auditory Processing (Treatment) (2)	Applying techniques to improve the receiving and processing of auditory information and comprehension of spoken language

Continued on next page

Section F–Physical Rehabilitation and Diagnostic Audiology

Continued from previous page

Type Qualifier (Character 5)	Definition
Augmentative/Alternative Communication System (Assessment) (L)	Determines the appropriateness of aids, techniques, symbols, and/or strategies to augment or replace speech and enhance communication Includes/Examples: Includes the use of telephones, writing equipment, emergency equipment, and TDD
Augmentative/Alternative Communication System (Treatment) (3)	Includes/Examples: Includes augmentative communication devices and aids
Aural Rehabilitation (5)	Applying techniques to improve the communication abilities associated with hearing loss
Aural Rehabilitation Status (P)	Measures impact of a hearing loss including evaluation of receptive and expressive communication skills
Bathing/Showering (Ø)	Includes/Examples: Includes obtaining and using supplies; soaping, rinsing, and drying body parts; maintaining bathing position; and transferring to and from bathing positions
Bathing/Showering Techniques (Ø)	Activities to facilitate obtaining and using supplies, soaping, rinsing and drying body parts, maintaining bathing position, and transferring to and from bathing positions
Bed Mobility (Assessment) (B)	Transitional movement within bed
Bed Mobility (Treatment) (5)	Exercise or activities to facilitate transitional movements within bed
Bedside Swallowing and Oral Function (H)	Includes/Examples: Bedside swallowing includes assessment of sucking, masticating, coughing, and swallowing. Oral function includes assessment of musculature for controlled movements, structures, and functions to determine coordination and phonation
Bekesy Audiometry (3)	Uses an instrument that provides a choice of discrete or continuously varying pure tones; choice of pulsed or continuous signal
Binaural Electroacoustic Hearing Aid Check (6)	Determines mechanical and electroacoustic function of bilateral hearing aids using hearing aid test box
Binaural Hearing Aid (Assessment) (3)	Measures the candidacy, effectiveness, and appropriateness of a hearing aid Explanation: Measures bilateral fit
Binaural Hearing Aid (Treatment) (2)	Explanation: Assists in achieving maximum understanding and performance
Bithermal, Binaural Caloric Irrigation (Ø)	Measures the rhythmic eye movements stimulated by changing the temperature of the vestibular system
Bithermal, Monaural Caloric Irrigation (1)	Measures the rhythmic eye movements stimulated by changing the temperature of the vestibular system in one ear
Brief Tone Stimuli (R)	Measures specific central auditory process
Cerumen Management (3)	Includes examination of external auditory canal and tympanic membrane and removal of cerumen from external ear canal
Cochlear Implant (Ø)	Measures candidacy for cochlear implant
Cochlear Implant Rehabilitation (Ø)	Applying techniques to improve the communication abilities of individuals with cochlear implant; includes programming the device, providing patients/families with information
Communicative/Cognitive Integration Skills (Assessment) (G)	Measures ability to use higher cortical functions Includes/Examples: Includes orientation, recognition, attention span, initiation and termination of activity, memory, sequencing, categorizing, concept formation, spatial operations, judgment, problem solving, generalization and pragmatic communication
Communicative/Cognitive Integration Skills (Treatment) (6)	Activities to facilitate the use of higher cortical functions Includes/Examples: Includes level of arousal, orientation, recognition, attention span, initiation and termination of activity, memory sequencing, judgment and problem solving, learning and generalization, and pragmatic communication
Computerized Dynamic Posturography (6)	Measures the status of the peripheral and central vestibular system and the sensory/motor component of balance; evaluates the efficacy of vestibular rehabilitation
Conditioned Play Audiometry (4)	Behavioral measures using nonspeech and speech stimuli to obtain frequency-specific and ear-specific information on auditory status from the patient Explanation: Obtains speech reception threshold by having patient point to pictures of spondaic words

Continued on next page

Section F–Physical Rehabilitation and Diagnostic Audiology

Continued from previous page

Type Qualifier (Character 5)	Definition
Coordination/Dexterity (Assessment) (3)	Measures large and small muscle groups for controlled goal- directed movements Explanation: Dexterity includes object manipulation
Coordination/Dexterity (Treatment) (2)	Exercise or activities to facilitate gross coordination and fine coordination
Cranial Nerve Integrity (9)	Measures cranial nerve sensory and motor functions, including tastes, smell and facial expression
Dichotic Stimuli (T)	Measures specific central auditory process
Distorted Speech (S)	Measures specific central auditory process
Dix-Hallpike Dynamic (5)	Measures nystagmus following Dix-Hallpike maneuver
Dressing (1)	Includes/Examples: Includes selecting clothing and accessories, obtaining clothing from storage, dressing, fastening and adjusting clothing and shoes, and applying and removing personal devices, prosthesis or orthosis
Dressing Techniques (1)	Activities to facilitate selecting clothing and accessories, dressing and undressing, adjusting clothing and shoes, applying and removing devices, prostheses or orthoses
Dynamic Orthosis (6)	Includes/Examples: Includes customized and prefabricated splints, inhibitory casts, spinal and other braces, and protective devices; allows motion through transfer of movement from other body parts or by use of outside forces
Ear Canal Probe Microphone (1)	Real ear measures
Ear Protector Attentuation (7)	Measures ear protector fit and effectiveness
Electrocochleography (K)	Measures the VIIIth cranial nerve action potential
Environmental, Home, Work Barriers (B)	Measures current and potential barriers to optimal function, including safety hazards, access problems and home or office design
Ergonomics and Body Mechanics (C)	Ergonomic measurement of job tasks, work hardening or work conditioning needs; functional capacity; and body mechanics
Eustachian Tube Function (F)	Measures eustachian tube function and patency of eustachian tube
Evoked Otoacoustic Emissions, Diagnostic (N)	Measures auditory evoked potentials in a diagnostic format
Evoked Otoacoustic Emissions, Screening (M)	Measures auditory evoked potentials in a screening format
Facial Nerve Function (7)	Measures electrical activity of the VIIth cranial nerve (facial nerve)
Feeding/Eating (Assessment) (2)	Includes/Examples: Includes setting up food, selecting and using utensils and tableware, bringing food or drink to mouth, cleaning face, hands, and clothing, and management of alternative methods of nourishment
Feeding/Eating (Treatment) (3)	Exercise or activities to facilitate setting up food, selecting and using utensils and tableware, bringing food or drink to mouth, cleaning face, hands, and clothing, and management of alternative methods of nourishment
Filtered Speech (Ø)	Uses high or low pass filtered speech stimuli to assess central auditory processing disorders, site of lesion testing
Fluency (Assessment) (D)	Measures speech fluency or stuttering
Fluency (Treatment) (7)	Applying techniques to improve and augment fluent speech
Gait Training/Functional Ambulation (9)	Exercise or activities to facilitate ambulation on a variety of surfaces and in a variety of environments
Gait/Balance (D)	Measures biomechanical, arthrokinematic and other spatial and temporal characteristics of gait and balance

Continued on next page

Section F–Physical Rehabilitation and Diagnostic Audiology

Continued from previous page

Type Qualifier (Character 5)	Definition
Grooming/Personal Hygiene (Assessment) (3)	Includes/Examples: Includes ability to obtain and use supplies in a sequential fashion, general grooming, oral hygiene, toilet hygiene, personal care devices, including care for artificial airways
Grooming/Personal Hygiene (Treatment) (2)	Activities to facilitate obtaining and using supplies in a sequential fashion: general grooming, oral hygiene, toilet hygiene, cleaning body, and personal care devices, including artificial airways
Hearing and Related Disorders Counseling (Ø)	Provides patients/families/caregivers with information, support, referrals to facilitate recovery from a communication disorder Includes/Examples: Includes strategies for psychosocial adjustment to hearing loss for clients and families/caregivers
Hearing and Related Disorders Prevention (1)	Provides patients/families/caregivers with information and support to prevent communication disorders
Hearing Screening (Ø)	Pass/refer measures designed to identify need for further audiologic assessment
Home Management (Assessment) (4)	Obtaining and maintaining personal and household possessions and environment Includes/Examples: Includes clothing care, cleaning, meal preparation and cleanup, shopping, money management, household maintenance, safety procedures, and childcare/parenting
Home Management (Treatment) (4)	Activities to facilitate obtaining and maintaining personal household possessions and environment Includes/Examples: Includes clothing care, cleaning, meal preparation and clean-up, shopping, money management, household maintenance, safety procedures, childcare/parenting
Instrumental Swallowing and Oral Function (J)	Definition: Measures swallowing function using instrumental diagnostic procedures Explanation: Methods include videofluoroscopy, ultrasound, manometry, endoscopy
Integumentary Integrity (1)	Includes/Examples: Includes burns, skin conditions, ecchymosis, bleeding, blisters, scar tissue, wounds and other traumas, tissue mobility, turgor and texture
Manual Therapy Techniques (7)	Techniques in which the therapist uses his/her hands to administer skilled movements Includes/Examples: Includes connective tissue massage, joint mobilization and manipulation, manual lymph drainage, manual traction, soft tissue mobilization and manipulation
Masking Patterns (W)	Measures central auditory processing status
Monaural Electroacoustic Hearing Aid Check (8)	Determines mechanical and electroacoustic function of one hearing aid using hearing aid test box
Monaural Hearing Aid (Assessment) (2)	Measures the candidacy, effectiveness, and appropriateness of a hearing aid Explanation: Measures unilateral fit
Monaural Hearing Aid (Treatment) (1)	Explanation: Assists in achieving maximum understanding and performance
Motor Function (Assessment) (4)	Measures the body's functional and versatile movement patterns Includes/Examples: Includes motor assessment scales, analysis of head, trunk and limb movement, and assessment of motor learning
Motor Function (Treatment) (3)	Exercise or activities to facilitate crossing midline, laterality, bilateral integration, praxis, neuromuscular relaxation, inhibition, facilitation, motor function and motor learning
Motor Speech (Assessment) (B)	Measures neurological motor aspects of speech production
Motor Speech (Treatment) (B)	Applying techniques to improve and augment the impaired neurological motor aspects of speech production
Muscle Performance (Assessment) (Ø)	Measures muscle strength, power and endurance using manual testing, dynamometry or computer-assisted electromechanical muscle test; functional muscle strength, power and endurance; muscle pain, tone, or soreness; or pelvic-floor musculature Explanation: Muscle endurance refers to the ability to contract a muscle repeatedly over time
Muscle Performance (Treatment) (1)	Exercise or activities to increase the capacity of a muscle to do work in terms of strength, power, and/or endurance Explanation: Muscle strength is the force exerted to overcome resistance in one maximal effort. Muscle power is work produced per unit of time, or the product of strength and speed. Muscle endurance is the ability to contract a muscle repeatedly over time

Continued on next page

Section F–Physical Rehabilitation and Diagnostic Audiology

Continued from previous page

Type Qualifier (Character 5)	Definition
Neuromotor Development (D)	Measures motor development, righting and equilibrium reactions, and reflex and equilibrium reactions
Neurophysiologic Intraoperative (8)	Monitors neural status during surgery
Non-invasive Instrumental Status (N)	Instrumental measures of oral, nasal, vocal, and velopharyngeal functions as they pertain to speech production
Nonspoken Language (Assessment) (7)	Measures nonspoken language (print, sign, symbols) for communication
Nonspoken Language (Treatment) (Ø)	Applying techniques that improve, augment, or compensate spoken communication
Oral Peripheral Mechanism (P)	Structural measures of face, jaw, lips, tongue, teeth, hard and soft palate, pharynx as related to speech production
Orofacial Myofunctional (Assessment) (K)	Measures orofacial myofunctional patterns for speech and related functions
Orofacial Myofunctional (Treatment) (9)	Applying techniques to improve, alter, or augment impaired orofacial myofunctional patterns and related speech production errors
Oscillating Tracking (3)	Measures ability to visually track
Pain (F)	Measures muscle soreness, pain and soreness with joint movement, and pain perception Includes/Examples: Includes questionnaires, graphs, symptom magnification scales or visual analog scales
Perceptual Processing (Assessment) (5)	Measures stereognosis, kinesthesia, body schema, right-left discrimination, form constancy, position in space, visual closure, figure-ground, depth perception, spatial relations and topographical orientation
Perceptual Processing (Treatment) (1)	Exercise and activities to facilitate perceptual processing Explanation: Includes stereognosis, kinesthesia, body schema, right-left discrimination, form constancy, position in space, visual closure, figure-ground, depth perception, spatial relations, and topographical orientation Includes/Examples: Includes stereognosis, kinesthesia, body schema, right-left discrimination, form constancy, position in space, visual closure, figure-ground, depth perception, spatial relations, and topographical orientation
Performance Intensity Phonetically Balanced Speech Discrimination (Q)	Measures word recognition over varying intensity levels
Postural Control (3)	Exercise or activities to increase postural alignment and control
Prosthesis (8)	Explanation: Artificial substitutes for missing body parts that augment performance or function
Psychosocial Skills (Assessment) (6)	The ability to interact in society and to process emotions Includes/Examples: Includes psychological (values, interests, self-concept); social (role performance, social conduct, interpersonal skills, self expression); self-management (coping skills, time management, self-control)
Psychosocial Skills (Treatment) (6)	The ability to interact in society and to process emotions Includes/Examples: Includes psychological (values, interests, self-concept); social (role performance, social conduct, interpersonal skills, self expression); self-management (coping skills, time management, self-control)
Pure Tone Audiometry, Air (1)	Air-conduction pure tone threshold measures with appropriate masking
Pure Tone Audiometry, Air and Bone (2)	Air-conduction and bone-conduction pure tone threshold measures with appropriate masking
Pure Tone Stenger (C)	Measures unilateral nonorganic hearing loss based on simultaneous presentation of pure tones of differing volume
Range of Motion and Joint Integrity (5)	Measures quantity, quality, grade, and classification of joint movement and/or mobility Explanation: Range of Motion is the space, distance or angle through which movement occurs at a joint or series of joints. Joint integrity is the conformance of joints to expected anatomic, biomechanical and kinematic norms

Continued on next page

Section F–Physical Rehabilitation and Diagnostic Audiology

Continued from previous page

Type Qualifier (Character 5)	Definition
Range of Motion and Joint Mobility (Ø)	Exercise or activities to increase muscle length and joint mobility
Receptive/Expressive Language (Assessment) (8)	Measures receptive and expressive language
Receptive/Expressive Language (Treatment) (B)	Applying techniques to improve and augment receptive/expressive language
Reflex Integrity (G)	Measures the presence, absence, or exaggeration of developmentally appropriate, pathologic or normal reflexes
Select Picture Audiometry (5)	Establishes hearing threshold levels for speech using pictures
Sensorineural Acuity Level (4)	Measures sensorineural acuity masking presented via bone conduction
Sensory Aids (5)	Determines the appropriateness of a sensory prosthetic device, other than a hearing aid or assistive listening system/device
Sensory Awareness/ Processing/ Integrity (6)	Includes/Examples: Includes light touch, pressure, temperature, pain, sharp/dull, proprioception, vestibular, visual, auditory, gustatory, and olfactory
Short Increment Sensitivity Index (9)	Measures the ear's ability to detect small intensity changes; site of lesion test requiring a behavioral response
Sinusoidal Vertical Axis Rotational (4)	Measures nystagmus following rotation
Somatosensory Evoked Potentials (9)	Measures neural activity from sites throughout the body
Speech/Language Screening (6)	Identifies need for further speech and/or language evaluation
Speech Threshold (1)	Measures minimal intensity needed to repeat spondaic words
Speech/Word Recognition (2)	Measures ability to repeat/identify single syllable words; scores given as a percentage; includes word recognition/speech discrimination
Speech-Language Pathology and Related Disorders Counseling (1)	Provides patients/families with information, support, referrals to facilitate recovery from a communication disorder
Speech-Language Pathology and Related Disorders Prevention (2)	Applying techniques to avoid or minimize onset and/or development of a communication disorder
Staggered Spondaic Word (3)	Measures central auditory processing site of lesion based upon dichotic presentation of spondaic words
Static Orthosis (7)	Includes/Examples: Includes customized and prefabricated splints, inhibitory casts, spinal and other braces, and protective devices; has no moving parts, maintains joint(s) in desired position
Stenger (B)	Measures unilateral nonorganic hearing loss based on simultaneous presentation of signals of differing volume
Swallowing Dysfunction (D)	Activities to improve swallowing function in coordination with respiratory function Includes/Examples: Includes function and coordination of sucking, mastication, coughing, swallowing
Synthetic Sentence Identification (5)	Measures central auditory dysfunction using identification of third order approximations of sentences and competing messages
Temporal Ordering of Stimuli (V)	Measures specific central auditory process
Therapeutic Exercise (7)	Exercise or activities to facilitate sensory awareness, sensory processing, sensory integration, balance training, conditioning, reconditioning Includes/Examples: Includes developmental activities, breathing exercises, aerobic endurance activities, aquatic exercises, stretching and ventilatory muscle training
Tinnitus Masker (Assessment) (7)	Determines candidacy for tinnitus masker
Tinnitus Masker (Treatment) (Ø)	Explanation: Used to verify physical fit, acoustic appropriateness, and benefit; assists in achieving maximum benefit

Continued on next page

Section F–Physical Rehabilitation and Diagnostic Audiology

Continued from previous page

Type Qualifier (Character 5)	Definition
Tone Decay (B)	Measures decrease in hearing sensitivity to a tone; site of lesion test requiring a behavioral response
Transfer (5)	Transitional movement from one surface to another
Transfer Training (8)	Exercise or activities to facilitate movement from one surface to another
Tympanometry (D)	Measures the integrity of the middle ear; measures ease at which sound flows through the tympanic membrane while air pressure against the membrane is varied
Unithermal Binaural Screen (2)	Measures the rhythmic eye movements stimulated by changing the temperature of the vestibular system in both ears using warm water, screening format
Ventilation/Respiration/Circulation (G)	Measures ventilatory muscle strength, power and endurance, pulmonary function and ventilatory mechanics Includes/Examples: Includes ability to clear airway, activities that aggravate or relieve edema, pain, dyspnea or other symptoms, chest wall mobility, cardiopulmonary response to performance of ADL and IAD, cough and sputum, standard vital signs
Vestibular (Ø)	Applying techniques to compensate for balance disorders; includes habituation, exercise therapy, and balance retraining
Visual Motor Integration (Assessment) (2)	Coordinating the interaction of information from the eyes with body movement during activity
Visual Motor Integration (Treatment) (2)	Exercise or activities to facilitate coordinating the interaction of information from eyes with body movement during activity
Visual Reinforcement Audiometry (6)	Behavioral measures using nonspeech and speech stimuli to obtain frequency/ear-specific information on auditory status Includes/Examples: Includes a conditioned response of looking toward a visual reinforcer (e.g., lights, animated toy) every time auditory stimuli are heard
Vocational Activities and Functional Community or Work Reintegration Skills (Assessment) (H)	Measures environmental, home, work (job/school/play) barriers that keep patients from functioning optimally in their environment Includes/Examples: Includes assessment of vocational skills and interests, environment of work (job/school/play), injury potential and injury prevention or reduction, ergonomic stressors, transportation skills, and ability to access and use community resources
Vocational Activities/Functional Community Skills/Work Reintegration Skills (Treatment) (7)	Activities to facilitate vocational exploration, body mechanics training, job acquisition, and environmental or work (job/school/play) task adaptation Includes/Examples: Includes injury prevention and reduction, ergonomic stressor reduction, job coaching and simulation, work hardening and conditioning, driving training, transportation skills, and use of community resources
Voice (Assessment) (F)	Measures vocal structure, function and production
Voice (Treatment) (C)	Applying techniques to improve voice and vocal function
Voice Prosthetic (Assessment) (M)	Determines the appropriateness of voice prosthetic/adaptive device to enhance or facilitate communication
Voice Prosthetic (Treatment) (4)	Includes/Examples: Includes electrolarynx, and other assistive, adaptive, supportive devices
Wheelchair Mobility (Assessment) (F)	Measures fit and functional abilities within wheelchair in a variety of environments
Wheelchair Mobility (Treatment) (4)	Management, maintenance and controlled operation of a wheelchair, scooter or other device, in and on a variety of surfaces and environments
Wound Management (5)	Includes/Examples: Includes non-selective and selective debridement (enzymes, autolysis, sharp debridement), dressings (wound coverings, hydrogel, vacuum-assisted closure), topical agents, etc.

Section G–Mental Health

Type (Character 3)	Definition
Biofeedback (C)	Provision of information from the monitoring and regulating of physiological processes in conjunction with cognitive-behavioral techniques to improve patient functioning or well-being Includes/Examples: Includes EEG, blood pressure, skin temperature or peripheral blood flow, ECG, electrooculogram, EMG, respirometry or capnometry, GSR/EDR, perineometry to monitor/regulate bowel/bladder activity, electrogastrogram to monitor/regulate gastric motility
Counseling (6)	The application of psychological methods to treat an individual with normal developmental issues and psychological problems in order to increase function, improve well-being, alleviate distress, maladjustment or resolve crises
Crisis Intervention (2)	Treatment of a traumatized, acutely disturbed or distressed individual for the purpose of short-term stabilization Includes/Examples: Includes defusing, debriefing, counseling, psychotherapy and/or coordination of care with other providers or agencies
Electroconvulsive Therapy (B)	The application of controlled electrical voltages to treat a mental health disorder Includes/Examples: Includes appropriate sedation and other preparation of the individual
Family Psychotherapy (7)	Treatment that includes one or more family members of an individual with a mental health disorder by behavioral, cognitive, psychoanalytic, psychodynamic or psychophysiological means to improve functioning or well-being Explanation: Remediation of emotional or behavioral problems presented by one or more family members in cases where psychotherapy with more than one family member is indicated
Group Psychotherapy (H)	Treatment of two or more individuals with a mental health disorder by behavioral, cognitive, psychoanalytic, psychodynamic or psychophysiological means to improve functioning or well-being
Hypnosis (F)	Induction of a state of heightened suggestibility by auditory, visual and tactile techniques to elicit an emotional or behavioral response
Individual Psychotherapy (5)	Treatment of an individual with a mental health disorder by behavioral, cognitive, psychoanalytic, psychodynamic or psychophysiological means to improve functioning or well-being
Light Therapy (J)	Application of specialized light treatments to improve functioning or well-being
Medication Management (3)	Monitoring and adjusting the use of medications for the treatment of a mental health disorder
Narcosynthesis (G)	Administration of intravenous barbiturates in order to release suppressed or repressed thoughts
Psychological Tests (1)	The administration and interpretation of standardized psychological tests and measurement instruments for the assessment of psychological function

Section G–Mental Health

Type Qualifier (Character 4)	Definition
Behavioral (1)	Primarily to modify behavior Includes/Examples: Includes modeling and role playing, positive reinforcement of target behaviors, response cost, and training of self-management skills
Cognitive (2)	Primarily to correct cognitive distortions and errors
Cognitive-Behavioral (8)	Combining cognitive and behavioral treatment strategies to improve functioning Explanation: Maladaptive responses are examined to determine how cognitions relate to behavior patterns in response to an event. Uses learning principles and information-processing models
Developmental (Ø)	Age-normed developmental status of cognitive, social and adaptive behavior skills
Intellectual and Psychoeducational (2)	Intellectual abilities, academic achievement and learning capabilities (including behaviors and emotional factors affecting learning)

Continued on next page

Section G–Mental Health

Continued from previous page

Type Qualifier (Character 4)	Definition
Interactive (0)	Uses primarily physical aids and other forms of non-oral interaction with a patient who is physically, psychologically or developmentally unable to use ordinary language for communication Includes/Examples: Includes the use of toys in symbolic play
Interpersonal (3)	Helps an individual make changes in interpersonal behaviors to reduce psychological dysfunction Includes/Examples: Includes exploratory techniques, encouragement of affective expression, clarification of patient statements, analysis of communication patterns, use of therapy relationship and behavior change techniques
Neurobehavioral Status/Cognitive Status (4)	Includes neurobehavioral status exam, interview(s), and observation for the clinical assessment of thinking, reasoning and judgment, acquired knowledge, attention, memory, visual spatial abilities, language functions, and planning
Neuropsychological (3)	Thinking, reasoning and judgment, acquired knowledge, attention, memory, visual spatial abilities, language functions, planning
Personality and Behavioral (1)	Mood, emotion, behavior, social functioning, psychopathological conditions, personality traits and characteristics
Psychoanalysis (4)	Methods of obtaining a detailed account of past and present mental and emotional experiences to determine the source and eliminate or diminish the undesirable effects of unconscious conflicts Explanation: Accomplished by making the individual aware of their existence, origin, and inappropriate expression in emotions and behavior
Psychodynamic (5)	Exploration of past and present emotional experiences to understand motives and drives using insight-oriented techniques to reduce the undesirable effects of internal conflicts on emotions and behavior Explanation: Techniques include empathetic listening, clarifying self-defeating behavior patterns, and exploring adaptive alternatives
Psychophysiological (9)	Monitoring and alteration of physiological processes to help the individual associate physiological reactions combined with cognitive and behavioral strategies to gain improved control of these processes to help the individual cope more effectively
Supportive (6)	Formation of therapeutic relationship primarily for providing emotional support to prevent further deterioration in functioning during periods of particular stress Explanation: Often used in conjunction with other therapeutic approaches
Vocational (1)	Exploration of vocational interests, aptitudes and required adaptive behavior skills to develop and carry out a plan for achieving a successful vocational placement Includes/Examples: Includes enhancing work related adjustment and/or pursuing viable options in training education or preparation

Section H - Substance Abuse Treatment

Type (Character 3)	Definition
Detoxification Services (2)	Detoxification from alcohol and/or drugs Explanation: Not a treatment modality, but helps the patient stabilize physically and psychologically until the body becomes free of drugs and the effects of alcohol
Family Counseling (6)	The application of psychological methods that includes one or more family members to treat an individual with addictive behavior Explanation: Provides support and education for family members of addicted individuals. Family member participation is seen as a critical area of substance abuse treatment
Group Counseling (4)	The application of psychological methods to treat two or more individuals with addictive behavior Explanation: Provides structured group counseling sessions and healing power through the connection with others
Individual Counseling (3)	The application of psychological methods to treat an individual with addictive behavior Explanation: Comprised of several different techniques, which apply various strategies to address drug addiction
Individual Psychotherapy (5)	Treatment of an individual with addictive behavior by behavioral, cognitive, psychoanalytic, psychodynamic or psychophysiological means
Medication Management (8)	Monitoring and adjusting the use of replacement medications for the treatment of addiction
Pharmacotherapy (9)	The use of replacement medications for the treatment of addiction

Appendix F: Components of the Medical and Surgical Approach Definitions

Approach	Definition	Access Location	Method	Type of Instrumentation	Example
Open (Ø)	Cutting through the skin or mucous membrane and any other body layers necessary to expose the site of the procedure.	Skin or mucous membraneany other body layers	Cutting	None	Abdominal hysterectomy
Percutaneous (3)	Entry, by puncture or minor incision, of instrumentation through the skin or mucous membrane and/or any other body layers necessary to reach the site of the procedure	Skin or mucous membrane, any other body layers	Puncture or minor incision	Without visualization	Needle biopsy of liver, Liposuction
Percutaneous endoscopic (4)	Entry, by puncture or minor incision, of instrumentation through the skin or mucous membrane and/or any other body layers necessary to reach and visualize the site of the procedure	Skin or mucous membrane, any other body layers	Puncture or minor incision	With visualization	Arthroscopy, Laparoscopic cholecystectomy
Via natural or artificial opening (7)	Entry of instrumentation through a natural or artificial external opening to reach the site of the procedure	Natural or artificial external opening	Direct entry	Without visualization	Endotracheal tube insertion, Foley catheter placement
Via natural or artificial opening endoscopic (8)	Entry of instrumentation through a natural or artificial external opening to reach and visualize the site of the procedure	Natural or artificial external opening	Direct entry with puncture or minor incision for instrumentation only	With visualization	Sigmoidoscopy, EGD, ERCP
Via natural or artificial opening with percutaneous endoscopic assistance (F)	Entry of instrumentation through a natural or artificial external opening and entry, by puncture or minor incision, of instrumentation through the skin or mucous membrane and any other body layers necessary to aid in the performance of the procedure	Skin or mucous membrane, any other body layers	Cutting	With visualization	Laparoscopic-assisted vaginal hysterectomy
External (X)	Procedures performed directly on the skin or mucous membrane and procedures performed indirectly by the application of external force through the skin or mucous membrane	Skin or mucous membrane	Direct or indirect application	None	Closed fracture reduction, Resection of tonsils

Appendix F: Components of the Medical and Surgical [illegible]

[illegible]

Appendix G: Character Meanings

Ø: Medical and Surgical

Ø: Central Nervous System

Operation–Character 3	Body Part–Character 4	Approach–Character 5	Device–Character 6	Qualifier–Character 7
1 Bypass	Ø Brain	Ø Open	Ø Drainage Device	Ø Nasopharynx
2 Change	1 Cerebral Meninges	3 Percutaneous	2 Monitoring Device	1 Mastoid Sinus
5 Destruction	2 Dura Mater	4 Percutaneous Endoscopic	3 Infusion Device	2 Atrium
8 Division	3 Epidural Space	X External	7 Autologous Tissue Substitute	3 Blood Vessel
9 Drainage	4 Subdural Space		J Synthetic Substitute	4 Pleural Cavity
B Excision	5 Subarachnoid Space		K Nonautologous Tissue Substitute	5 Intestine
C Extirpation	6 Cerebral Ventricle		M Electrode	6 Peritoneal Cavity
D Extraction	7 Cerebral Hemisphere		Y Other Device	7 Urinary Tract
F Fragmentation	8 Basal Ganglia		Z No Device	8 Bone Marrow
H Insertion	9 Thalamus			9 Fallopian Tube
J Inspection	A Hypothalamus			B Cerebral Cisterns
K Map	B Pons			F Olfactory Nerve
N Release	C Cerebellum			G Optic Nerve
P Removal	D Medulla Oblongata			H Oculomotor Nerve
Q Repair	E Cranial Nerve			J Trochlear Nerve
S Reposition	F Olfactory Nerve			K Trigeminal Nerve
T Resection	G Optic Nerve			L Abducens Nerve
U Supplement	H Oculomotor Nerve			M Facial Nerve
W Revision	J Trochlear Nerve			N Acoustic Nerve
X Transfer	K Trigeminal Nerve			P Glossopharyngeal Nerve
	L Abducens Nerve			Q Vagus Nerve
	M Facial Nerve			R Accessory Nerve
	N Acoustic Nerve			S Hypoglossal Nerve
	P Glossopharyngeal Nerve			X Diagnostic
	Q Vagus Nerve			Z No Qualifier
	R Accessory Nerve			
	S Hypoglossal Nerve			
	T Spinal Meninges			
	U Spinal Canal			
	V Spinal Cord			
	W Cervical Spinal Cord			
	X Thoracic Spinal Cord			
	Y Lumbar Spinal Cord			

Ø: Medical and Surgical

1: Peripheral Nervous System

Operation–Character 3	Body Part–Character 4	Approach–Character 5	Device–Character 6	Qualifier–Character 7
2 Change	Ø Cervical Plexus	Ø Open	Ø Drainage Device	1 Cervical Nerve
5 Destruction	1 Cervical Nerve	3 Percutaneous	2 Monitoring Device	2 Phrenic Nerve
8 Division	2 Phrenic Nerve	4 Percutaneous Endoscopic	7 Autologous Tissue Substitute	4 Ulnar Nerve
9 Drainage	3 Brachial Plexus	X External	M Neurostimulator Lead	5 Median Nerve
B Excision	4 Ulnar Nerve		Y Other Device	6 Radial Nerve
C Extirpation	5 Median Nerve		Z No Device	8 Thoracic Nerve
D Extraction	6 Radial Nerve			B Lumbar Nerve
H Insertion	8 Thoracic Nerve			C Perineal Nerve
J Inspection	9 Lumbar Plexus			D Femoral Nerve
N Release	A Lumbosacral Plexus			F Sciatic Nerve
P Removal	B Lumbar Nerve			G Tibial Nerve
Q Repair	C Pudendal Nerve			H Peroneal Nerve
S Reposition	D Femoral Nerve			X Diagnostic
U Supplement	F Sciatic Nerve			Z No Qualifier
W Revision	G Tibial Nerve			
X Transfer	H Peroneal Nerve			
	K Head and Neck Sympathetic Nerve			
	L Thoracic Sympathetic Nerve			
	M Abdominal Sympathetic Nerve			
	N Lumbar Sympathetic Nerve			
	P Sacral Sympathetic Nerve			
	Q Sacral Plexus			
	R Sacral Nerve			
	Y Peripheral Nerve			

Ø: Medical and Surgical

2: Heart and Great Vessels

Operation–Character 3	Body Part–Character 4	Approach–Character 5	Device–Character 6	Qualifier–Character 7
1 Bypass	Ø Coronary Artery, One Site	Ø Open	Ø Monitoring Device, Pressure Sensor	Ø Allogeneic
5 Destruction	1 Coronary Artery, Two Sites	3 Percutaneous	2 Monitoring Device	1 Syngeneic
7 Dilation	2 Coronary Artery, Three Sites	4 Percutaneous Endoscopic	3 Infusion Device	2 Zooplastic
8 Division	3 Coronary Artery, Four or More Sites	X External	4 Intraluminal Device, Drug-eluting	3 Coronary Artery
B Excision	4 Coronary Vein		7 Autologous Tissue Substitute	4 Coronary Vein
C Extirpation	5 Atrial Septum		8 Zooplastic Tissue	5 Coronary Circulation
F Fragmentation	6 Atrium, Right		9 Autologous Venous Tissue	6 Bifurcation
H Insertion	7 Atrium, Left		A Autologous Arterial Tissue	7 Atrium, Left
J Inspection	8 Conduction Mechanism		C Extraluminal Device	8 Internal Mammary, Right
K Map	9 Chordae Tendineae		D Intraluminal Device	9 Internal Mammary, Left
L Occlusion	A Heart		J Synthetic Substitute OR Cardiac Lead, Pacemaker (for root operation INSERTION only)	A Pacemaker Lead
N Release	B Heart, Right		K Nonautologous Tissue Substitute OR Cardiac Lead, Defibrillator (for root operation INSERTION only)	B Subclavian
P Removal	C Heart, Left		M Cardiac Lead	C Thoracic Artery
Q Repair	D Papillary Muscle		Q Implantable Heart Assist System	D Carotid
R Replacement	F Aortic Valve		R External Heart Assist System	E Defibrillator Lead
S Reposition	G Mitral Valve		T Intraluminal Device, Radioactive	F Abdominal Artery
T Resection	H Pulmonary Valve		Z No Device	G Pressure Sensor
U Supplement	J Tricuspid Valve			H Transapical
V Restriction	K Ventricle, Right			J Temporary
W Revision	L Ventricle, Left			K Left Atrial Appendage
Y Transplantation	M Ventricular Septum			P Pulmonary Trunk
	N Pericardium			Q Pulmonary Artery, Right
	P Pulmonary Trunk			R Pulmonary Artery, Left
	Q Pulmonary Artery, Right			S Biventricular
	R Pulmonary Artery, Left			T Ductus Arteriosus
	S Pulmonary Vein, Right			W Aorta
	T Pulmonary Vein, Left			X Diagnostic
	V Superior Vena Cava			Z No Qualifier
	W Thoracic Aorta			
	Y Great Vessel			

Ø: Medical and Surgical

3: Upper Arteries

Operation–Character 3	Body Part–Character 4	Approach–Character 5	Device–Character 6	Qualifier–Character 7
1 Bypass	Ø Internal Mammary Artery, Right	Ø Open	Ø Drainage Device	Ø Upper Arm Artery, Right
5 Destruction	1 Internal Mammary Artery, Left	3 Percutaneous	2 Monitoring Device	1 Upper Arm Artery, Left
7 Dilation	2 Innominate Artery	4 Percutaneous Endoscopic	3 Infusion Device	2 Upper Arm Artery, Bilateral
9 Drainage	3 Subclavian Artery, Right	X External	4 Intraluminal Device, Drug-eluting	3 Lower Arm Artery, Right
B Excision	4 Subclavian Artery, Left		7 Autologous Tissue Substitute	4 Lower Arm Artery, Left
C Extirpation	5 Axillary Artery, Right		9 Autologous Venous Tissue	5 Lower Arm Artery, Bilateral
H Insertion	6 Axillary Artery, Left		A Autologous Arterial Tissue	6 Upper Leg Artery, Right
J Inspection	7 Brachial Artery, Right		B Intraluminal Device, Bioactive	7 Upper Leg Artery, Left
L Occlusion	8 Brachial Artery, Left		C Extraluminal Device	8 Upper Leg Artery, Bilateral
N Release	9 Ulnar Artery, Right		D Intraluminal Device	9 Lower Leg Artery, Right
P Removal	A Ulnar Artery, Left		J Synthetic Substitute	B Lower Leg Artery, Left
Q Repair	B Radial Artery, Right		K Nonautologous Tissue Substitute	C Lower Leg Artery, Bilateral
R Replacement	C Radial Artery, Left		M Stimulator Lead	D Upper Arm Vein
S Reposition	D Hand Artery, Right		Z No Device	F Lower Arm Vein
U Supplement	F Hand Artery, Left			G Intracranial Artery
V Restriction	G Intracranial Artery			J Extracranial Artery, Right
W Revision	H Common Carotid Artery, Right			K Extracranial Artery, Left
	J Common Carotid Artery, Left			M Pulmonary Artery, Right
	K Internal Carotid Artery, Right			N Pulmonary Artery, Left
	L Internal Carotid Artery, Left			X Diagnostic
	M External Carotid Artery, Right			Z No Qualifier
	N External Carotid Artery, Left			
	P Vertebral Artery, Right			
	Q Vertebral Artery, Left			
	R Face Artery			
	S Temporal Artery, Right			
	T Temporal Artery, Left			
	U Thyroid Artery, Right			
	V Thyroid Artery, Left			
	Y Upper Artery			

0: Medical and Surgical

4: Lower Arteries

Operation–Character 3	Body Part–Character 4	Approach–Character 5	Device–Character 6	Qualifier–Character 7
1 Bypass	0 Abdominal Aorta	0 Open	0 Drainage Device	0 Abdominal Aorta
5 Destruction	1 Celiac Artery	3 Percutaneous	1 Radioactive Element	1 Celiac Artery
7 Dilation	2 Gastric Artery	4 Percutaneous Endoscopic	2 Monitoring Device	2 Mesenteric Artery
9 Drainage	3 Hepatic Artery	X External	3 Infusion Device	3 Renal Artery, Right
B Excision	4 Splenic Artery		4 Intraluminal Device, Drug-eluting	4 Renal Artery, Left
C Extirpation	5 Superior Mesenteric Artery		7 Autologous Tissue Substitute	5 Renal Artery, Bilateral
H Insertion	6 Colic Artery, Right		9 Autologous Venous Tissue	6 Common Iliac Artery, Right
J Inspection	7 Colic Artery, Left		A Autologous Arterial Tissue	7 Common Iliac Artery, Left
L Occlusion	8 Colic Artery, Middle		C Extraluminal Device	8 Common Iliac Arteries, Bilateral
N Release	9 Renal Artery, Right		D Intraluminal Device	9 Internal Iliac Artery, Right
P Removal	A Renal Artery, Left		J Synthetic Substitute	B Internal Iliac Artery, Left
Q Repair	B Inferior Mesenteric Artery		K Nonautologous Tissue Substitute	C Internal Iliac Arteries, Bilateral
R Replacement	C Common Iliac Artery, Right		Z No Device	D External Iliac Artery, Right
S Reposition	D Common Iliac Artery, Left			F External Iliac Artery, Left
U Supplement	E Internal Iliac Artery, Right			G External Iliac Arteries, Bilateral
V Restriction	F Internal Iliac Artery, Left			H Femoral Artery, Right
W Revision	H External Iliac Artery, Right			J Femoral Artery, Left OR Temporary (for root operation Restriction only)
	J External Iliac Artery, Left			K Femoral Arteries, Bilateral
	K Femoral Artery, Right			L Popliteal Artery
	L Femoral Artery, Left			M Peroneal Artery
	M Popliteal Artery, Right			N Posterior Tibial Artery
	N Popliteal Artery, Left			P Foot Artery
	P Anterior Tibial Artery, Right			Q Lower Extremity Artery
	Q Anterior Tibial Artery, Left			R Lower Artery
	R Posterior Tibial Artery, Right			S Lower Extremity Vein
	S Posterior Tibial Artery, Left			T Uterine Artery, Right
	T Peroneal Artery, Right			U Uterine Artery, Left
	U Peroneal Artery, Left			X Diagnostic
	V Foot Artery, Right			Z No Qualifier
	W Foot Artery, Left			
	Y Lower Artery			

Ø: Medical and Surgical

5: Upper Veins

Operation–Character 3	Body Part–Character 4	Approach–Character 5	Device–Character 6	Qualifier–Character 7
1 Bypass	Ø Azygos Vein	Ø Open	Ø Drainage Device	X Diagnostic
5 Destruction	1 Hemiazygos Vein	3 Percutaneous	2 Monitoring Device	Y Upper Vein
7 Dilation	3 Innominate Vein, Right	4 Percutaneous Endoscopic	3 Infusion Device	Z No Qualifier
9 Drainage	4 Innominate Vein, Left	X External	7 Autologous Tissue Substitute	
B Excision	5 Subclavian Vein, Right		9 Autologous Venous Tissue	
C Extirpation	6 Subclavian Vein, Left		A Autologous Arterial Tissue	
D Extraction	7 Axillary Vein, Right		C Extraluminal Device	
H Insertion	8 Axillary Vein, Left		D Intraluminal Device	
J Inspection	9 Brachial Vein, Right		J Synthetic Substitute	
L Occlusion	A Brachial Vein, Left		K Nonautologous Tissue Substitute	
N Release	B Basilic Vein, Right		Z No Device	
P Removal	C Basilic Vein, Left			
Q Repair	D Cephalic Vein, Right			
R Replacement	F Cephalic Vein, Left			
S Reposition	G Hand Vein, Right			
U Supplement	H Hand Vein, Left			
V Restriction	L Intracranial Vein			
W Revision	M Internal Jugular Vein, Right			
	N Internal Jugular Vein, Left			
	P External Jugular Vein, Right			
	Q External Jugular Vein, Left			
	R Vertebral Vein, Right			
	S Vertebral Vein, Left			
	T Face Vein, Right			
	V Face Vein, Left			
	Y Upper Vein			

Ø: Medical and Surgical

6: Lower Veins

Operation–Character 3	Body Part–Character 4	Approach–Character 5	Device–Character 6	Qualifier–Character 7
1 Bypass	Ø Inferior Vena Cava	Ø Open	Ø Drainage Device	5 Superior Mesenteric Vein
5 Destruction	1 Splenic Vein	3 Percutaneous	2 Monitoring Device	6 Inferior Mesenteric Vein
7 Dilation	2 Gastric Vein	4 Percutaneous Endoscopic	3 Infusion Device	9 Renal Vein, Right
9 Drainage	3 Esophageal Vein	X External	7 Autologous Tissue Substitute	B Renal Vein, Left
B Excision	4 Hepatic Vein		9 Autologous Venous Tissue	C Hemorrhoidal Plexus
C Extirpation	5 Superior Mesenteric Vein		A Autologous Arterial Tissue	T Via Umbilical Vein
D Extraction	6 Inferior Mesenteric Vein		C Extraluminal Device	X Diagnostic
H Insertion	7 Colic Vein		D Intraluminal Device	Y Lower Vein
J Inspection	8 Portal Vein		J Synthetic Substitute	Z No Qualifier
L Occlusion	9 Renal Vein, Right		K Nonautologous Tissue Substitute	
N Release	B Renal Vein, Left		Z No Device	
P Removal	C Common Iliac Vein, Right			
Q Repair	D Common Iliac Vein, Left			
R Replacement	F External Iliac Vein, Right			
S Reposition	G External Iliac Vein, Left			
U Supplement	H Hypogastric Vein, Right			
V Restriction	J Hypogastric Vein, Left			
W Revision	M Femoral Vein, Right			
	N Femoral Vein, Left			
	P Greater Saphenous Vein, Right			
	Q Greater Saphenous Vein, Left			
	R Lesser Saphenous Vein, Right			
	S Lesser Saphenous Vein, Left			
	T Foot Vein, Right			
	V Foot Vein, Left			
	Y Lower Vein			

Ø: Medical and Surgical

7: Lymphatic and Hemic Systems*

Operation–Character 3	Body Part–Character 4	Approach–Character 5	Device–Character 6	Qualifier–Character 7
2 Change	Ø Lymphatic, Head	Ø Open	Ø Drainage Device	Ø Allogeneic
5 Destruction	1 Lymphatic, Right Neck	3 Percutaneous	3 Infusion Device	1 Syngeneic
9 Drainage	2 Lymphatic, Left Neck	4 Percutaneous Endoscopic	7 Autologous Tissue Substitute	2 Zooplastic
B Excision	3 Lymphatic, Right Upper Extremity	X External	C Extraluminal Device	X Diagnostic
C Extirpation	4 Lymphatic, Left Upper Extremity		D Intraluminal Device	Z No Qualifier
D Extraction	5 Lymphatic, Right Axillary		J Synthetic Substitute	
H Insertion	6 Lymphatic, Left Axillary		K Nonautologous Tissue Substitute	
J Inspection	7 Lymphatic, Thorax		Y Other Device	
L Occlusion	8 Lymphatic, Internal Mammary, Right		Z No Device	
N Release	9 Lymphatic, Internal Mammary, Left			
P Removal	B Lymphatic, Mesenteric			
Q Repair	C Lymphatic, Pelvis			
S Reposition	D Lymphatic, Aortic			
T Resection	F Lymphatic, Right Lower Extremity			
U Supplement	G Lymphatic, Left Lower Extremity			
V Restriction	H Lymphatic, Right Inguinal			
W Revision	J Lymphatic, Left Inguinal			
Y Transplantation	K Thoracic Duct			
	L Cisterna Chyli			
	M Thymus			
	N Lymphatic			
	P Spleen			
	Q Bone Marrow, Sternum			
	R Bone Marrow, Iliac			
	S Bone Marrow, Vertebral			
	T Bone Marrow			

* Includes lymph vessels and lymph nodes.

Ø: Medical and Surgical

8: Eye

Operation–Character 3	Body Part–Character 4	Approach–Character 5	Device–Character 6	Qualifier–Character 7
Ø Alteration	Ø Eye, Right	Ø Open	Ø Drainage Device OR Synthetic Substitute, Intraocular Telescope (for root operation REPLACEMENT only)	3 Nasal Cavity
1 Bypass	1 Eye, Left	3 Percutaneous	1 Radioactive Element	4 Sclera
2 Change	2 Anterior Chamber, Right	7 Via Natural or Artificial Opening	3 Infusion Device	X Diagnostic
5 Destruction	3 Anterior Chamber, Left	8 Via Natural or Artificial Opening Endoscopic	5 Epiretinal Visual Prosthesis	Z No Qualifier
7 Dilation	4 Vitreous, Right	X External	7 Autologous Tissue Substitute	
9 Drainage	5 Vitreous, Left		C Extraluminal Device	
B Excision	6 Sclera, Right		D Intraluminal Device	
C Extirpation	7 Sclera, Left		J Synthetic Substitute	
D Extraction	8 Cornea, Right		K Nonautologous Tissue Substitute	
F Fragmentation	9 Cornea, Left		Y Other Device	
H Insertion	A Choroid, Right		Z No Device	
J Inspection	B Choroid, Left			
L Occlusion	C Iris, Right			
M Reattachment	D Iris, Left			
N Release	E Retina, Right			
P Removal	F Retina, Left			
Q Repair	G Retinal Vessel, Right			
R Replacement	H Retinal Vessel, Left			
S Reposition	J Lens, Right			
T Resection	K Lens, Left			
U Supplement	L Extraocular Muscle, Right			
V Restriction	M Extraocular Muscle, Left			
W Revision	N Upper Eyelid, Right			
X Transfer	P Upper Eyelid, Left			
	Q Lower Eyelid, Right			
	R Lower Eyelid, Left			
	S Conjunctiva, Right			
	T Conjunctiva, Left			
	V Lacrimal Gland, Right			
	W Lacrimal Gland, Left			
	X Lacrimal Duct, Right			
	Y Lacrimal Duct, Left			

Ø: Medical and Surgical

9: Ear, Nose, Sinus*

Operation–Character 3	Body Part–Character 4	Approach–Character 5	Device–Character 6	Qualifier–Character 7
Ø Alteration	Ø External Ear, Right	Ø Open	Ø Drainage Device	Ø Endolymphatic
1 Bypass	1 External Ear, Left	3 Percutaneous	4 Hearing Device, Bone Conduction	X Diagnostic
2 Change	2 External Ear, Bilateral	4 Percutaneous Endoscopic	5 Hearing Device, Single Channel Cochlear Prosthesis	Z No Qualifier
5 Destruction	3 External Auditory Canal, Right	7 Via Natural or Artificial Opening	6 Hearing Device, Multiple Channel Cochlear Prosthesis	
7 Dilation	4 External Auditory Canal, Left	8 Via Natural or Artificial Opening Endoscopic	7 Autologous Tissue Substitute	
8 Division	5 Middle Ear, Right	X External	B Intraluminal Device, Airway	
9 Drainage	6 Middle Ear, Left		D Intraluminal Device	
B Excision	7 Tympanic Membrane, Right		J Synthetic Substitute	
C Extirpation	8 Tympanic Membrane, Left		K Nonautologous Tissue Substitute	
D Extraction	9 Auditory Ossicle, Right		S Hearing Device	
H Insertion	A Auditory Ossicle, Left		Y Other Device	
J Inspection	B Mastoid Sinus, Right		Z No Device	
M Reattachment	C Mastoid Sinus, Left			
N Release	D Inner Ear, Right			
P Removal	E Inner Ear, Left			
Q Repair	F Eustachian Tube, Right			
R Replacement	G Eustachian Tube, Left			
S Reposition	H Ear, Right			
T Resection	J Ear, Left			
U Supplement	K Nose			
W Revision	L Nasal Turbinate			
	M Nasal Septum			
	N Nasopharynx			
	P Accessory Sinus			
	Q Maxillary Sinus, Right			
	R Maxillary Sinus, Left			
	S Frontal Sinus, Right			
	T Frontal Sinus, Left			
	U Ethmoid Sinus, Right			
	V Ethmoid Sinus, Left			
	W Sphenoid Sinus, Right			
	X Sphenoid Sinus, Left			
	Y Sinus			

* Includes sinus ducts.

Ø: Medical and Surgical

B: Respiratory System

Operation–Character 3	Body Part–Character 4	Approach–Character 5	Device–Character 6	Qualifier–Character 7
1 Bypass	Ø Tracheobronchial Tree	Ø Open	Ø Drainage Device	Ø Allogeneic
2 Change	1 Trachea	3 Percutaneous	1 Radioactive Element	1 Syngeneic
5 Destruction	2 Carina	4 Percutaneous Endoscopic	2 Monitoring Device	2 Zooplastic
7 Dilation	3 Main Bronchus, Right	7 Via Natural or Artificial Opening	3 Infusion Device	4 Cutaneous
9 Drainage	4 Upper Lobe Bronchus, Right	8 Via Natural or Artificial Opening Endoscopic	7 Autologous Tissue Substitute	6 Esophagus
B Excision	5 Middle Lobe Bronchus, Right	X External	C Extraluminal Device	X Diagnostic
C Extirpation	6 Lower Lobe Bronchus, Right		D Intraluminal Device	Z No Qualifier
D Extraction	7 Main Bronchus, Left		E Intraluminal Device, Endotracheal Airway	
F Fragmentation	8 Upper Lobe Bronchus, Left		F Tracheostomy Device	
H Insertion	9 Lingula Bronchus		G Intraluminal Endobronchial Valve	
J Inspection	B Lower Lobe Bronchus, Left		J Synthetic Substitute	
L Occlusion	C Upper Lung Lobe, Right		K Nonautologous Tissue Substitute	
M Reattachment	D Middle Lung Lobe, Right		M Diaphragmatic Pacemaker Lead	
N Release	F Lower Lung Lobe, Right		Y Other Device	
P Removal	G Upper Lung Lobe, Left		Z No Device	
Q Repair	H Lung Lingula			
S Reposition	J Lower Lung Lobe, Left			
T Resection	K Lung, Right			
U Supplement	L Lung, Left			
V Restriction	M Lungs, Bilateral			
W Revision	N Pleura, Right			
Y Transplantation	P Pleura, Left			
	Q Pleura			
	R Diaphragm, Right			
	S Diaphragm, Left			
	T Diaphragm			

0: Medical and Surgical

C: Mouth and Throat

Operation–Character 3	Body Part–Character 4	Approach–Character 5	Device–Character 6	Qualifier–Character 7
0 Alteration	0 Upper Lip	0 Open	0 Drainage Device	0 Single
2 Change	1 Lower Lip	3 Percutaneous	1 Radioactive Element	1 Multiple
5 Destruction	2 Hard Palate	4 Percutaneous Endoscopic	5 External Fixation Device	2 All
7 Dilation	3 Soft Palate	7 Via Natural or Artificial Opening	7 Autologous Tissue Substitute	X Diagnostic
9 Drainage	4 Buccal Mucosa	8 Via Natural or Artificial Opening Endoscopic	B Intraluminal Device, Airway	Z No Qualifier
B Excision	5 Upper Gingiva	X External	C Extraluminal Device	
C Extirpation	6 Lower Gingiva		D Intraluminal Device	
D Extraction	7 Tongue		J Synthetic Substitute	
F Fragmentation	8 Parotid Gland, Right		K Nonautologous Tissue Substitute	
H Insertion	9 Parotid Gland, Left		Y Other Device	
J Inspection	A Salivary Gland		Z No Device	
L Occlusion	B Parotid Duct, Right			
M Reattachment	C Parotid Duct, Left			
N Release	D Sublingual Gland, Right			
P Removal	F Sublingual Gland, Left			
Q Repair	G Submaxillary Gland, Right			
R Replacement	H Submaxillary Gland, Left			
S Reposition	J Minor Salivary Gland			
T Resection	M Pharynx			
U Supplement	N Uvula			
V Restriction	P Tonsils			
W Revision	Q Adenoids			
X Transfer	R Epiglottis			
	S Larynx			
	T Vocal Cord, Right			
	V Vocal Cord, Left			
	W Upper Tooth			
	X Lower Tooth			
	Y Mouth and Throat			

0: Medical and Surgical

D: Gastrointestinal System

Operation–Character 3	Body Part–Character 4	Approach–Character 5	Device–Character 6	Qualifier–Character 7
1 Bypass	0 Upper Intestinal Tract	0 Open	0 Drainage Device	0 Allogeneic
2 Change	1 Esophagus, Upper	3 Percutaneous	1 Radioactive Element	1 Syngeneic
5 Destruction	2 Esophagus, Middle	4 Percutaneous Endoscopic	2 Monitoring Device	2 Zooplastic
7 Dilation	3 Esophagus, Lower	7 Via Natural or Artificial Opening	3 Infusion Device	3 Vertical
8 Division	4 Esophagogastric Junction	8 Via Natural or Artificial Opening Endoscopic	7 Autologous Tissue Substitute	4 Cutaneous
9 Drainage	5 Esophagus	X External	B Intraluminal Device, Airway	5 Esophagus
B Excision	6 Stomach		C Extraluminal Device	6 Stomach
C Extirpation	7 Stomach, Pylorus		D Intraluminal Device	9 Duodenum
F Fragmentation	8 Small Intestine		J Synthetic Substitute	A Jejunum
H Insertion	9 Duodenum		K Nonautologous Tissue Substitute	B Ileum
J Inspection	A Jejunum		L Artificial Sphincter	H Cecum
L Occlusion	B Ileum		M Stimulator Lead	K Ascending Colon
M Reattachment	C Ileocecal Valve		U Feeding Device	L Transverse Colon
N Release	D Lower Intestinal Tract		Y Other Device	M Descending Colon
P Removal	E Large Intestine		Z No Device	N Sigmoid Colon
Q Repair	F Large Intestine, Right			P Rectum
R Replacement	G Large Intestine, Left			Q Anus
S Reposition	H Cecum			X Diagnostic
T Resection	J Appendix			Z No Qualifier
U Supplement	K Ascending Colon			
V Restriction	L Transverse Colon			
W Revision	M Descending Colon			
X Transfer	N Sigmoid Colon			
Y Transplantation	P Rectum			
	Q Anus			
	R Anal Sphincter			
	S Greater Omentum			
	T Lesser Omentum			
	U Omentum			
	V Mesentery			
	W Peritoneum			

Ø: Medical and Surgical

F: Hepatobiliary System and Pancreas

Operation–Character 3	Body Part–Character 4	Approach–Character 5	Device–Character 6	Qualifier–Character 7
1 Bypass	Ø Liver	Ø Open	Ø Drainage Device	Ø Allogeneic
2 Change	1 Liver, Right Lobe	3 Percutaneous	1 Radioactive Element	1 Syngeneic
5 Destruction	2 Liver, Left Lobe	4 Percutaneous Endoscopic	2 Monitoring Device	2 Zooplastic
7 Dilation	4 Gallbladder	7 Via Natural or Artificial Opening	3 Infusion Device	3 Duodenum
8 Division	5 Hepatic Duct, Right	8 Via Natural or Artificial Opening Endoscopic	7 Autologous Tissue Substitute	4 Stomach
9 Drainage	6 Hepatic Duct, Left	X External	C Extraluminal Device	5 Hepatic Duct, Right
B Excision	8 Cystic Duct		D Intraluminal Device	6 Hepatic Duct, Left
C Extirpation	9 Common Bile Duct		J Synthetic Substitute	7 Hepatic Duct, Caudate
F Fragmentation	B Hepatobiliary Duct		K Nonautologous Tissue Substitute	8 Cystic Duct
H Insertion	C Ampulla of Vater		Y Other Device	9 Common Bile Duct
J Inspection	D Pancreatic Duct		Z No Device	B Small Intestine
L Occlusion	F Pancreatic Duct, Accessory			C Large Intestine
M Reattachment	G Pancreas			X Diagnostic
N Release				Z No Qualifier
P Removal				
Q Repair				
R Replacement				
S Reposition				
T Resection				
U Supplement				
V Restriction				
W Revision				
Y Transplantation				

Ø: Medical and Surgical

G: Endocrine System

Operation–Character 3	Body Part–Character 4	Approach–Character 5	Device–Character 6	Qualifier–Character 7
2 Change	Ø Pituitary Gland	Ø Open	Ø Drainage Device	X Diagnostic
5 Destruction	1 Pineal Body	3 Percutaneous	2 Monitoring Device	Z No Qualifier
8 Division	2 Adrenal Gland, Left	4 Percutaneous Endoscopic	3 Infusion Device	
9 Drainage	3 Adrenal Gland, Right	X External	Y Other Device	
B Excision	4 Adrenal Glands, Bilateral		Z No Device	
C Extirpation	5 Adrenal Gland			
H Insertion	6 Carotid Body, Left			
J Inspection	7 Carotid Body, Right			
M Reattachment	8 Carotid Bodies, Bilateral			
N Release	9 Para-aortic Body			
P Removal	B Coccygeal Glomus			
Q Repair	C Glomus Jugulare			
S Reposition	D Aortic Body			
T Resection	F Paraganglion Extremity			
W Revision	G Thyroid Gland Lobe, Left			
	H Thyroid Gland Lobe, Right			
	J Thyroid Gland Isthmus			
	K Thyroid Gland			
	L Superior Parathyroid Gland, Right			
	M Superior Parathyroid Gland, Left			
	N Inferior Parathyroid Gland, Right			
	P Inferior Parathyroid Gland, Left			
	Q Parathyroid Glands, Multiple			
	R Parathyroid Gland			
	S Endocrine Gland			

Ø: Medical and Surgical

H: Skin and Breast*

Operation–Character 3	Body Part–Character 4	Approach–Character 5	Device–Character 6	Qualifier–Character 7
Ø Alteration	Ø Skin, Scalp	Ø Open	Ø Drainage Device	3 Full Thickness
2 Change	1 Skin, Face	3 Percutaneous	1 Radioactive Element	4 Partial Thickness
5 Destruction	2 Skin, Right Ear	7 Via Natural or Artificial Opening	7 Autologous Tissue Substitute	5 Latissimus Dorsi Myocutaneous Flap
8 Division	3 Skin, Left Ear	8 Via Natural or Artificial Opening Endoscopic	J Synthetic Substitute	6 Transverse Rectus Abdominis Myocutaneous Flap
9 Drainage	4 Skin, Neck	X External	K Nonautologous Tissue Substitute	7 Deep Inferior Epigastric Artery Perforator Flap
B Excision	5 Skin, Chest		N Tissue Expander	8 Superficial Inferior Epigastric Artery Flap
C Extirpation	6 Skin, Back		Y Other Device	9 Gluteal Artery Perforator Flap
D Extraction	7 Skin, Abdomen		Z No Device	D Multiple
H Insertion	8 Skin, Buttock			X Diagnostic
J Inspection	9 Skin, Perineum			Z No Qualifier
M Reattachment	A Skin, Genitalia			
N Release	B Skin, Right Upper Arm			
P Removal	C Skin, Left Upper Arm			
Q Repair	D Skin, Right Lower Arm			
R Replacement	E Skin, Left Lower Arm			
S Reposition	F Skin, Right Hand			
T Resection	G Skin, Left Hand			
U Supplement	H Skin, Right Upper Leg			
W Revision	J Skin, Left Upper Leg			
X Transfer	K Skin, Right Lower Leg			
	L Skin, Left Lower Leg			
	M Skin, Right Foot			
	N Skin, Left Foot			
	P Skin			
	Q Finger Nail			
	R Toe Nail			
	S Hair			
	T Breast, Right			
	U Breast, Left			
	V Breast, Bilateral			
	W Nipple, Right			
	X Nipple, Left			
	Y Supernumerary Breast			

* Includes skin and breast glands and ducts.

Ø: Medical and Surgical

J: Subcutaneous Tissue and Fascia

Operation–Character 3	Body Part–Character 4	Approach–Character 5	Device–Character 6	Qualifier–Character 7
Ø Alteration	Ø Subcutaneous Tissue and Fascia, Scalp	Ø Open	Ø Monitoring Device, Hemodynamic	B Skin and Subcutaneous Tissue
2 Change	1 Subcutaneous Tissue and Fascia, Face	3 Percutaneous	1 Radioactive Element	C Skin, Subcutaneous Tissue and Fascia
5 Destruction	4 Subcutaneous Tissue and Fascia, Anterior Neck	X External	2 Monitoring Device	X Diagnostic
8 Division	5 Subcutaneous Tissue and Fascia, Posterior Neck		3 Infusion Device	Z No Qualifier
9 Drainage	6 Subcutaneous Tissue and Fascia, Chest		4 Pacemaker, Single Chamber	
B Excision	7 Subcutaneous Tissue and Fascia, Back		5 Pacemaker, Single Chamber Rate Responsive	
C Extirpation	8 Subcutaneous Tissue and Fascia, Abdomen		6 Pacemaker, Dual Chamber	
D Extraction	9 Subcutaneous Tissue and Fascia, Buttock		7 Autologous Tissue Substitute OR Cardiac Resynchronization Pacemaker Pulse Generator (for root operation INSERTION only)	
H Insertion	B Subcutaneous Tissue and Fascia, Perineum		8 Defibrillator Generator	
J Inspection	C Subcutaneous Tissue and Fascia, Pelvic Region		9 Cardiac Resynchronization Defibrillator Pulse Generator	
N Release	D Subcutaneous Tissue and Fascia, Right Upper Arm		A Contractility Modulation Device	
P Removal	F Subcutaneous Tissue and Fascia, Left Upper Arm		B Stimulator Generator, Single Array	
Q Repair	G Subcutaneous Tissue and Fascia, Right Lower Arm		C Stimulator Generator, Single Array Rechargeable	
R Replacement	H Subcutaneous Tissue and Fascia, Left Lower Arm		D Stimulator Generator, Multiple Array	
U Supplement	J Subcutaneous Tissue and Fascia, Right Hand		E Stimulator Generator, Multiple Array Rechargea	
W Revision	K Subcutaneous Tissue and Fascia, Left Hand		H Contraceptive Device	
X Transfer	L Subcutaneous Tissue and Fascia, Right Upper Leg		J Synthetic Substitute	
	M Subcutaneous Tissue and Fascia, Left Upper Leg		K Nonautologous Tissue Substitute	
	N Subcutaneous Tissue and Fascia, Right Lower Leg		M Stimulator Generator	
	P Subcutaneous Tissue and Fascia, Left Lower Leg		N Tissue Expander	
	Q Subcutaneous Tissue and Fascia, Right Foot		P Cardiac Rhythm Related Device	
	R Subcutaneous Tissue and Fascia, Left Foot		V Infusion Pump	
	S Subcutaneous Tissue and Fascia, Head and Neck		W Reservoir	
	T Subcutaneous Tissue and Fascia, Trunk		X Vascular Access Device	
	V Subcutaneous Tissue and Fascia, Upper Extremity		Y Other Device	
	W Subcutaneous Tissue and Fascia, Lower Extremity		Z No Device	

Ø: Medical and Surgical

K: Muscles

Operation–Character 3	Body Part–Character 4	Approach–Character 5	Device–Character 6	Qualifier–Character 7
2 Change	Ø Head Muscle	Ø Open	Ø Drainage Device	Ø Skin
5 Destruction	1 Facial Muscle	3 Percutaneous	7 Autologous Tissue Substitute	1 Subcutaneous Tissue
8 Division	2 Neck Muscle, Right	4 Percutaneous Endoscopic	J Synthetic Substitute	2 Skin and Subcutaneous Tissue
9 Drainage	3 Neck Muscle, Left	X External	K Nonautologous Tissue Substitute	6 Transverse Rectus Abdominis Myocutaneous Flap
B Excision	4 Tongue, Palate, Pharynx Muscle		M Stimulator Lead	X Diagnostic
C Extirpation	5 Shoulder Muscle, Right		Y Other Device	Z No Qualifier
H Insertion	6 Shoulder Muscle, Left		Z No Device	
J Inspection	7 Upper Arm Muscle, Right			
M Reattachment	8 Upper Arm Muscle, Left			
N Release	9 Lower Arm and Wrist Muscle, Right			
P Removal	B Lower Arm and Wrist Muscle, Left			
Q Repair	C Hand Muscle, Right			
S Reposition	D Hand Muscle, Left			
T Resection	F Trunk Muscle, Right			
U Supplement	G Trunk Muscle, Left			
W Revision	H Thorax Muscle, Right			
X Transfer	J Thorax Muscle, Left			
	K Abdomen Muscle, Right			
	L Abdomen Muscle, Left			
	M Perineum Muscle			
	N Hip Muscle, Right			
	P Hip Muscle, Left			
	Q Upper Leg Muscle, Right			
	R Upper Leg Muscle, Left			
	S Lower Leg Muscle, Right			
	T Lower Leg Muscle, Left			
	V Foot Muscle, Right			
	W Foot Muscle, Left			
	X Upper Muscle			
	Y Lower Muscle			

Ø: Medical and Surgical

L: Tendons*

Operation–Character 3	Body Part–Character 4	Approach–Character 5	Device–Character 6	Qualifier–Character 7
2 Change	Ø Head and Neck Tendon	Ø Open	Ø Drainage Device	X Diagnostic
5 Destruction	1 Shoulder Tendon, Right	3 Percutaneous	7 Autologous Tissue Substitute	Z No Qualifier
8 Division	2 Shoulder Tendon, Left	4 Percutaneous Endoscopic	J Synthetic Substitute	
9 Drainage	3 Upper Arm Tendon, Right	X External	K Nonautologous Tissue Substitute	
B Excision	4 Upper Arm Tendon, Left		Y Other Device	
C Extirpation	5 Lower Arm and Wrist Tendon, Right		Z No Device	
J Inspection	6 Lower Arm and Wrist Tendon, Left			
M Reattachment	7 Hand Tendon, Right			
N Release	8 Hand Tendon, Left			
P Removal	9 Trunk Tendon, Right			
Q Repair	B Trunk Tendon, Left			
R Replacement	C Thorax Tendon, Right			
S Reposition	D Thorax Tendon, Left			
T Resection	F Abdomen Tendon, Right			
U Supplement	G Abdomen Tendon, Left			
W Revision	H Perineum Tendon			
X Transfer	J Hip Tendon, Right			
	K Hip Tendon, Left			
	L Upper Leg Tendon, Right			
	M Upper Leg Tendon, Left			
	N Lower Leg Tendon, Right			
	P Lower Leg Tendon, Left			
	Q Knee Tendon, Right			
	R Knee Tendon, Left			
	S Ankle Tendon, Right			
	T Ankle Tendon, Left			
	V Foot Tendon, Right			
	W Foot Tendon, Left			
	X Upper Tendon			
	Y Lower Tendon			

* Includes synovial membrane.

Ø: Medical and Surgical

M: Bursae and Ligaments*

Operation–Character 3	Body Part–Character 4	Approach–Character 5	Device–Character 6	Qualifier–Character 7
2 Change	Ø Head and Neck Bursa and Ligament	Ø Open	Ø Drainage Device	X Diagnostic
5 Destruction	1 Shoulder Bursa and Ligament, Right	3 Percutaneous	7 Autologous Tissue Substitute	Z No Qualifier
8 Division	2 Shoulder Bursa and Ligament, Left	4 Percutaneous Endoscopic	J Synthetic Substitute	
9 Drainage	3 Elbow Bursa and Ligament, Right	X External	K Nonautologous Tissue Substitute	
B Excision	4 Elbow Bursa and Ligament, Left		Y Other Device	
C Extirpation	5 Wrist Bursa and Ligament, Right		Z No Device	
D Extraction	6 Wrist Bursa and Ligament, Left			
J Inspection	7 Hand Bursa and Ligament, Right			
M Reattachment	8 Hand Bursa and Ligament, Left			
N Release	9 Upper Extremity Bursa and Ligament, Right			
P Removal	B Upper Extremity Bursa and Ligament, Left			
Q Repair	C Trunk Bursa and Ligament, Right			
S Reposition	D Trunk Bursa and Ligament, Left			
T Resection	F Thorax Bursa and Ligament, Right			
U Supplement	G Thorax Bursa and Ligament, Left			
W Revision	H Abdomen Bursa and Ligament, Right			
X Transfer	J Abdomen Bursa and Ligament, Left			
	K Perineum Bursa and Ligament			
	L Hip Bursa and Ligament, Right			
	M Hip Bursa and Ligament, Left			
	N Knee Bursa and Ligament, Right			
	P Knee Bursa and Ligament, Left			
	Q Ankle Bursa and Ligament, Right			
	R Ankle Bursa and Ligament, Left			
	S Foot Bursa and Ligament, Right			
	T Foot Bursa and Ligament, Left			
	V Lower Extremity Bursa and Ligament, Right			
	W Lower Extremity Bursa and Ligament, Left			
	X Upper Bursa and Ligament			
	Y Lower Bursa and Ligament			

* Includes synovial membrane.

0: Medical and Surgical

N: Head and Facial Bones

Operation–Character 3	Body Part–Character 4	Approach–Character 5	Device–Character 6	Qualifier–Character 7
2 Change	0 Skull	0 Open	0 Drainage Device	X Diagnostic
5 Destruction	1 Frontal Bone, Right	3 Percutaneous	4 Internal Fixation Device	Z No Qualifier
8 Division	2 Frontal Bone, Left	4 Percutaneous Endoscopic	5 External Fixation Device	
9 Drainage	3 Parietal Bone, Right	X External	7 Autologous Tissue Substitute	
B Excision	4 Parietal Bone, Left		J Synthetic Substitute	
C Extirpation	5 Temporal Bone, Right		K Nonautologous Tissue Substitute	
H Insertion	6 Temporal Bone, Left		M Bone Growth Stimulator	
J Inspection	7 Occipital Bone, Right		N Neurostimulator Generator	
N Release	8 Occipital Bone, Left		S Hearing Device	
P Removal	B Nasal Bone		Y Other Device	
Q Repair	C Sphenoid Bone, Right		Z No Device	
R Replacement	D Sphenoid Bone, Left			
S Reposition	F Ethmoid Bone, Right			
T Resection	G Ethmoid Bone, Left			
U Supplement	H Lacrimal Bone, Right			
W Revision	J Lacrimal Bone, Left			
	K Palatine Bone, Right			
	L Palatine Bone, Left			
	M Zygomatic Bone, Right			
	N Zygomatic Bone, Left			
	P Orbit, Right			
	Q Orbit, Left			
	R Maxilla, Right			
	S Maxilla, Left			
	T Mandible, Right			
	V Mandible, Left			
	W Facial Bone			
	X Hyoid Bone			

Ø: Medical and Surgical

P: Upper Bones

Operation–Character 3	Body Part–Character 4	Approach–Character 5	Device–Character 6	Qualifier–Character 7
2 Change	Ø Sternum	Ø Open	Ø Drainage Device OR Internal Fixation Device, Rigid Plate (for root operation INSERTION only)	X Diagnostic
5 Destruction	1 Rib, Right	3 Percutaneous	4 Internal Fixation Device	Z No Qualifier
8 Division	2 Rib, Left	4 Percutaneous Endoscopic	5 External Fixation Device	
9 Drainage	3 Cervical Vertebra	X External	6 Internal Fixation Device, Intramedullary	
B Excision	4 Thoracic Vertebra		7 Autologous Tissue Substitute	
C Extirpation	5 Scapula, Right		8 External Fixation Device, Limb Lengthening	
H Insertion	6 Scapula, Left		B External Fixation Device, Monoplanar	
J Inspection	7 Glenoid Cavity, Right		C External Fixation Device, Ring	
N Release	8 Glenoid Cavity, Left		D External Fixation Device, Hybrid	
P Removal	9 Clavicle, Right		J Synthetic Substitute	
Q Repair	B Clavicle, Left		K Nonautologous Tissue Substitute	
R Replacement	C Humeral Head, Right		M Bone Growth Stimulator	
S Reposition	D Humeral Head, Left		Y Other Device	
T Resection	F Humeral Shaft, Right		Z No Device	
U Supplement	G Humeral Shaft, Left			
W Revision	H Radius, Right			
	J Radius, Left			
	K Ulna, Right			
	L Ulna, Left			
	M Carpal, Right			
	N Carpal, Left			
	P Metacarpal, Right			
	Q Metacarpal, Left			
	R Thumb Phalanx, Right			
	S Thumb Phalanx, Left			
	T Finger Phalanx, Right			
	V Finger Phalanx, Left			
	Y Upper Bone			

Ø: Medical and Surgical

Q: Lower Bones

Operation–Character 3	Body Part–Character 4	Approach–Character 5	Device–Character 6	Qualifier–Character 7
2 Change	Ø Lumbar Vertebra	Ø Open	Ø Drainage Device	X Diagnostic
5 Destruction	1 Sacrum	3 Percutaneous	4 Internal Fixation Device	Z No Qualifier
8 Division	2 Pelvic Bone, Right	4 Percutaneous Endoscopic	5 External Fixation Device	
9 Drainage	3 Pelvic Bone, Left	X External	6 Internal Fixation Device, Intramedullary	
B Excision	4 Acetabulum, Right		7 Autologous Tissue Substitute	
C Extirpation	5 Acetabulum, Left		8 External Fixation Device, Limb Lengthening	
H Insertion	6 Upper Femur, Right		B External Fixation Device, Monoplanar	
J Inspection	7 Upper Femur, Left		C External Fixation Device, Ring	
N Release	8 Femoral Shaft, Right		D External Fixation Device, Hybrid	
P Removal	9 Femoral Shaft, Left		J Synthetic Substitute	
Q Repair	B Lower Femur, Right		K Nonautologous Tissue Substitute	
R Replacement	C Lower Femur, Left		M Bone Growth Stimulator	
S Reposition	D Patella, Right		Y Other Device	
T Resection	F Patella, Left		Z No Device	
U Supplement	G Tibia, Right			
W Revision	H Tibia, Left			
	J Fibula, Right			
	K Fibula, Left			
	L Tarsal, Right			
	M Tarsal, Left			
	N Metatarsal, Right			
	P Metatarsal, Left			
	Q Toe Phalanx, Right			
	R Toe Phalanx, Left			
	S Coccyx			
	Y Lower Bone			

Ø: Medical and Surgical

R: Upper Joints*

Operation–Character 3	Body Part–Character 4	Approach–Character 5	Device–Character 6	Qualifier–Character 7
2 Change	Ø Occipital-cervical Joint	Ø Open	Ø Drainage Device OR Synthetic Substitute, Reverse Ball and Socket (for root operation REPLACEMENT only)	Ø Anterior Approach, Anterior Column
5 Destruction	1 Cervical Vertebral Joint	3 Percutaneous	3 Infusion Device	1 Posterior Approach, Posterior Column
9 Drainage	2 Cervical Vertebral Joint, 2 or more	4 Percutaneous Endoscopic	4 Internal Fixation Device	6 Humeral Surface
B Excision	3 Cervical Vertebral Disc	X External	5 External Fixation Device	7 Glenoid Surface
C Extirpation	4 Cervicothoracic Vertebral Joint		7 Autologous Tissue Substitute	J Posterior Approach, Anterior Column
G Fusion	5 Cervicothoracic Vertebral Disc		8 Spacer	X Diagnostic
H Insertion	6 Thoracic Vertebral Joint		A Interbody Fusion Device	Z No Qualifier
J Inspection	7 Thoracic Vertebral Joint, 2 to 7		B Spinal Stabilization Device, Interspinous Process	
N Release	8 Thoracic Vertebral Joint, 8 or more		C Spinal Stabilization Device, Pedicle-Based	
P Removal	9 Thoracic Vertebral Disc		D Spinal Stabilization Device, Facet Replacement	
Q Repair	A Thoracolumbar Vertebral Joint		J Synthetic Substitute	
R Replacement	B Thoracolumbar Vertebral Disc		K Nonautologous Tissue Substitute	
S Reposition	C Temporomandibular Joint, Right		Y Other Device	
T Resection	D Temporomandibular Joint, Left		Z No Device	
U Supplement	E Sternoclavicular Joint, Right			
W Revision	F Sternoclavicular Joint, Left			
	G Acromioclavicular Joint, Right			
	H Acromioclavicular Joint, Left			
	J Shoulder Joint, Right			
	K Shoulder Joint, Left			
	L Elbow Joint, Right			
	M Elbow Joint, Left			
	N Wrist Joint, Right			
	P Wrist Joint, Left			
	Q Carpal Joint, Right			
	R Carpal Joint, Left			
	S Metacarpocarpal Joint, Right			
	T Metacarpocarpal Joint, Left			
	U Metacarpophalangeal Joint, Right			
	V Metacarpophalangeal Joint, Left			
	W Finger Phalangeal Joint, Right			
	X Finger Phalangeal Joint, Left			
	Y Upper Joint			

* Includes synovial membrane.

Ø: Medical and Surgical

S: Lower Joints*

Operation–Character 3	Body Part–Character 4	Approach–Character 5	Device–Character 6	Qualifier–Character 7
2 Change	Ø Lumbar Vertebral Joint	Ø Open	Ø Drainage Device OR Synthetic Substitute, Polyethylene (for root operation REPLACEMENT only)	Ø Anterior Approach, Anterior Column
5 Destruction	1 Lumbar Vertebral Joint, 2 or more	3 Percutaneous	1 Synthetic Substitute, Metal	1 Approach, Posterior Posterior Column
9 Drainage	2 Lumbar Vertebral Disc	4 Percutaneous Endoscopic	2 Synthetic Substitute, Metal on Polyethylene	9 Cemented
B Excision	3 Lumbosacral Joint	X External	3 Infusion Device OR Synthetic Substitute, Ceramic (for root operation REPLACEMENT only)	A Uncemented
C Extirpation	4 Lumbosacral Disc		4 Internal Fixation Device OR Synthetic Substitute, Ceramic on Polyethylene (for root operation REPLACEMENT only)	C Patellar Surface
G Fusion	5 Sacrococcygeal Joint		5 External Fixation Device	J Posterior Approach, Anterior Column
H Insertion	6 Coccygeal Joint		7 Autologous Tissue Substitute	X Diagnostic
J Inspection	7 Sacroiliac Joint, Right		8 Spacer	Z No Qualifier
N Release	8 Sacroiliac Joint, Left		9 Liner	
P Removal	9 Hip Joint, Right		A Interbody Fusion Device	
Q Repair	B Hip Joint, Left		B Resurfacing Device OR Spinal Stabilization Device, Interspinous Process (for root operation INSERTION only)	
R Replacement	C Knee Joint, Right		C Spinal Stabilization Device, Pedicle-Based	
S Reposition	D Knee Joint, Left		D Spinal Stabilization Device, Facet Replacement	
T Resection	F Ankle Joint, Right		J Synthetic Substitute	
U Supplement	G Ankle Joint, Left		K Nonautologous Tissue Substitute	

* Includes synovial membrane.

Continued on next page

Ø: Medical and Surgical

S: Lower Joints*

(continued from previous page)

Operation–Character 3	Body Part–Character 4	Approach–Character 5	Device–Character 6	Qualifier–Character 7
W Revision	H Tarsal Joint, Right		Y Other Device	
	J Tarsal Joint, Left		Z No Device	
	K Metatarsal-Tarsal Joint, Right			
	L Metatarsal-Tarsal Joint, Left			
	M Metatarsal-Phalangeal Joint, Right			
	N Metatarsal-Phalangeal Joint, Left			
	P Toe Phalangeal Joint, Right			
	Q Toe Phalangeal Joint, Left			
	Y Lower Joint			

Ø: Medical and Surgical

T: Urinary System

Operation–Character 3	Body Part–Character 4	Approach–Character 5	Device–Character 6	Qualifier–Character 7
1 Bypass	Ø Kidney, Right	Ø Open	Ø Drainage Device	Ø Allogeneic
2 Change	1 Kidney, Left	3 Percutaneous	2 Monitoring Device	1 Syngeneic
5 Destruction	2 Kidneys, Bilateral	4 Percutaneous Endoscopic	3 Infusion Device	2 Zooplastic
7 Dilation	3 Kidney Pelvis, Right	7 Via Natural or Artificial Opening	7 Autologous Tissue Substitute	3 Kidney Pelvis, Right
8 Division	4 Kidney Pelvis, Left	8 Via Natural or Artificial Opening Endoscopic	C Extraluminal Device	4 Kidney Pelvis, Left
9 Drainage	5 Kidney	X External	D Intraluminal Device	6 Ureter, Right
B Excision	6 Ureter, Right		J Synthetic Substitute	7 Ureter, Left
C Extirpation	7 Ureter, Left		K Nonautologous Tissue Substitute	8 Colon
D Extraction	8 Ureters, Bilateral		L Artificial Sphincter	9 Colocutaneous
F Fragmentation	9 Ureter		M Stimulator Lead	A Ileum
H Insertion	B Bladder		Y Other Device	B Bladder
J Inspection	C Bladder Neck		Z No Device	C Ileocutaneous
L Occlusion	D Urethra			D Cutaneous
M Reattachment				X Diagnostic
N Release				Z No Qualifier
P Removal				
Q Repair				
R Replacement				
S Reposition				
T Resection				
U Supplement				
V Restriction				
W Revision				
X Transfer				
Y Transplantation				

Ø: Medical and Surgical

U: Female Reproductive System

Operation–Character 3	Body Part–Character 4	Approach–Character 5	Device–Character 6	Qualifier–Character 7
1 Bypass	Ø Ovary, Right	Ø Open	Ø Drainage Device	Ø Allogeneic
2 Change	1 Ovary, Left	3 Percutaneous	1 Radioactive Element	1 Syngeneic
5 Destruction	2 Ovaries, Bilateral	4 Percutaneous Endoscopic	3 Infusion Device	2 Zooplastic
7 Dilation	3 Ovary	7 Via Natural or Artificial Opening	7 Autologous Tissue Substitute	5 Fallopian Tube, Right
8 Division	4 Uterine Supporting Structure	8 Via Natural or Artificial Opening Endoscopic	C Extraluminal Device	6 Fallopian Tube, Left
9 Drainage	5 Fallopian Tube, Right	F Via Natural or Artificial Opening With Percutaneous Endoscopic Assistance	D Intraluminal Device	9 Uterus
B Excision	6 Fallopian Tube, Left	X External	G Intraluminal Device, Pessary	X Diagnostic
C Extirpation	7 Fallopian Tubes, Bilateral		H Contraceptive Device	Z No Qualifier
D Extraction	8 Fallopian Tube		J Synthetic Substitute	
F Fragmentation	9 Uterus		K Nonautologous Tissue Substitute	
H Insertion	B Endometrium		Y Other Device	
J Inspection	C Cervix		Z No Device	
L Occlusion	D Uterus and Cervix			
M Reattachment	F Cul-de-sac			
N Release	G Vagina			
P Removal	H Vagina and Cul-de-sac			
Q Repair	J Clitoris			
S Reposition	K Hymen			
T Resection	L Vestibular Gland			
U Supplement	M Vulva			
V Restriction	N Ova			
W Revision				
X Transfer				
Y Transplantation				

Ø: Medical and Surgical

V: Male Reproductive System

Operation–Character 3	Body Part–Character 4	Approach–Character 5	Device–Character 6	Qualifier–Character 7
1 Bypass	Ø Prostate	Ø Open	Ø Drainage Device	J Epididymis, Right
2 Change	1 Seminal Vesicle, Right	3 Percutaneous	1 Radioactive Element	K Epididymis, Left
5 Destruction	2 Seminal Vesicle, Left	4 Percutaneous Endoscopic	3 Infusion Device	N Vas Deferens, Right
7 Dilation	3 Seminal Vesicles, Bilateral	7 Via Natural or Artificial Opening	7 Autologous Tissue Substitute	P Vas Deferens, Left
9 Drainage	4 Prostate and Seminal Vesicles	8 Via Natural or Artificial Opening Endoscopic	C Extraluminal Device	X Diagnostic
B Excision	5 Scrotum	X External	D Intraluminal Device	Z No Qualifier
C Extirpation	6 Tunica Vaginalis, Right		J Synthetic Substitute	
H Insertion	7 Tunica Vaginalis, Left		K Nonautologous Tissue Substitute	
J Inspection	8 Scrotum and Tunica Vaginalis		Y Other Device	
L Occlusion	9 Testis, Right		Z No Device	
M Reattachment	B Testis, Left			
N Release	C Testes, Bilateral			
P Removal	D Testis			
Q Repair	F Spermatic Cord, Right			
R Replacement	G Spermatic Cord, Left			
S Reposition	H Spermatic Cords, Bilateral			
T Resection	J Epididymis, Right			
U Supplement	K Epididymis, Left			
W Revision	L Epididymis, Bilateral			
	M Epididymis and Spermatic Cord			
	N Vas Deferens, Right			
	P Vas Deferens, Left			
	Q Vas Deferens, Bilateral			
	R Vas Deferens			
	S Penis			
	T Prepuce			
	V Male External Genitalia			

Ø: Medical and Surgical

W: Anatomical Regions, General

Operation–Character 3	Body Region–Character 4	Approach–Character 5	Device–Character 6	Qualifier–Character 7
Ø Alteration	Ø Head	Ø Open	Ø Drainage Device	Ø Vagina
1 Bypass	1 Cranial Cavity	3 Percutaneous	1 Radioactive Element	1 Penis
2 Change	2 Face	4 Percutaneous Endoscopic	3 Infusion Device	2 Stoma
3 Control	3 Oral Cavity and Throat	7 Via Natural or Artificial Opening	7 Autologous Tissue Substitute	4 Cutaneous
4 Creation	4 Upper Jaw	8 Via Natural or Artificial Opening Endoscopic	J Synthetic Substitute	9 Pleural Cavity, Right
8 Division	5 Lower Jaw	X External	K Nonautologous Tissue Substitute	B Pleural Cavity, Left
9 Drainage	6 Neck		Y Other Device	G Peritoneal Cavity
B Excision	8 Chest Wall		Z No Device	J Pelvic Cavity
C Extirpation	9 Pleural Cavity, Right			X Diagnostic
F Fragmentation	B Pleural Cavity, Left			Y Lower Vein
H Insertion	C Mediastinum			Z No Qualifier
J Inspection	D Pericardial Cavity			
M Reattachment	F Abdominal Wall			
P Removal	G Peritoneal Cavity			
Q Repair	H Retroperitoneum			
U Supplement	J Pelvic Cavity			
W Revision	K Upper Back			
	L Lower Back			
	M Perineum, Male			
	N Perineum, Female			
	P Gastrointestinal Tract			
	Q Respiratory Tract			
	R Genitourinary Tract			

0: Medical and Surgical

X: Anatomical Regions, Upper Extremities

Operation–Character 3	Body Part–Character 4	Approach–Character 5	Device–Character 6	Qualifier–Character 7
0 Alteration	0 Forequarter, Right	0 Open	0 Drainage Device	0 Complete
2 Change	1 Forequarter, Left	3 Percutaneous	1 Radioactive Element	1 High
3 Control	2 Shoulder Region, Right	4 Percutaneous Endoscopic	3 Infusion Device	2 Mid
6 Detachment	3 Shoulder Region, Left	X External	7 Autologous Tissue Substitute	3 Low
9 Drainage	4 Axilla, Right		J Synthetic Substitute	4 Complete 1st Ray
B Excision	5 Axilla, Left		K Nonautologous Tissue Substitute	5 Complete 2nd Ray
H Insertion	6 Upper Extremity, Right		Y Other Device	6 Complete 3rd Ray
J Inspection	7 Upper Extremity, Left		Z No Device	7 Complete 4th Ray
M Reattachment	8 Upper Arm, Right			8 Complete 5th Ray
P Removal	9 Upper Arm, Left			9 Partial 1st Ray
Q Repair	B Elbow Region, Right			B Partial 2nd Ray
R Replacement	C Elbow Region, Left			C Partial 3rd Ray
U Supplement	D Lower Arm, Right			D Partial 4th Ray
W Revision	F Lower Arm, Left			F Partial 5th Ray
X Transfer	G Wrist Region, Right			L Thumb, Right
	H Wrist Region, Left			M Thumb, Left
	J Hand, Right			N Toe, Right
	K Hand, Left			P Toe, Left
	L Thumb, Right			X Diagnostic
	M Thumb, Left			Z No Qualifier
	N Index Finger, Right			
	P Index Finger, Left			
	Q Middle Finger, Right			
	R Middle Finger, Left			
	S Ring Finger, Right			
	T Ring Finger, Left			
	V Little Finger, Right			
	W Little Finger, Left			

Ø: Medical and Surgical

Y: Anatomical Regions, Lower Extremities

Operation–Character 3	Body Part–Character 4	Approach–Character 5	Device–Character 6	Qualifier–Character 7
Ø Alteration	Ø Buttock, Right	Ø Open	Ø Drainage Device	Ø Complete
2 Change	1 Buttock, Left	3 Percutaneous	1 Radioactive Element	1 High
3 Control	2 Hindquarter, Right	4 Percutaneous Endoscopic	3 Infusion Device	2 Mid
6 Detachment	3 Hindquarter, Left	X External	7 Autologous Tissue Substitute	3 Low
9 Drainage	4 Hindquarter, Bilateral		J Synthetic Substitute	4 Complete 1st Ray
B Excision	5 Inguinal Region, Right		K Nonautologous Tissue Substitute	5 Complete 2nd Ray
H Insertion	6 Inguinal Region, Left		Y Other Device	6 Complete 3rd Ray
J Inspection	7 Femoral Region, Right		Z No Device	7 Complete 4th Ray
M Reattachment	8 Femoral Region, Left			8 Complete 5th Ray
P Removal	9 Lower Extremity, Right			9 Partial 1st Ray
Q Repair	A Inguinal Region, Bilateral			B Partial 2nd Ray
U Supplement	B Lower Extremity, Left			C Partial 3rd Ray
W Revision	C Upper Leg, Right			D Partial 4th Ray
	D Upper Leg, Left			F Partial 5th Ray
	E Femoral Region, Bilateral			X Diagnostic
	F Knee Region, Right			Z No Qualifier
	G Knee Region, Left			
	H Lower Leg, Right			
	J Lower Leg, Left			
	K Ankle Region, Right			
	L Ankle Region, Left			
	M Foot, Right			
	N Foot, Left			
	P 1st Toe, Right			
	Q 1st Toe, Left			
	R 2nd Toe, Right			
	S 2nd Toe, Left			
	T 3rd Toe, Right			
	U 3rd Toe, Left			
	V 4th Toe, Right			
	W 4th Toe, Left			
	X 5th Toe, Right			
	Y 5th Toe, Left			

1: Obstetrics

Ø: Pregnancy

Operation–Character 3	Body Part–Character 4	Approach–Character 5	Device–Character 6	Qualifier–Character 7
2 Change	Ø Products of Conception	Ø Open	3 Monitoring Electrode	Ø Classical
9 Drainage	1 Products of Conception, Retained	3 Percutaneous	Y Other Device	1 Low Cervical
A Abortion	2 Products of Conception, Ectopic	4 Percutaneous Endoscopic	Z No Device	2 Extraperitoneal
D Extraction		7 Via Natural or Artificial Opening		3 Low Forceps
E Delivery		8 Via Natural or Artificial Opening Endoscopic		4 Mid Forceps
H Insertion		X External		5 High Forceps
J Inspection				6 Vacuum
P Removal				7 Internal Version
Q Repair				8 Other
S Reposition				9 Fetal Blood
T Resection				A Fetal Cerebrospinal Fluid
Y Transplantation				B Fetal Fluid, Other
				C Amniotic Fluid, Therapeutic
				D Fluid, Other
				E Nervous System
				F Cardiovascular System
				G Lymphatics & Hemic
				H Eye
				J Ear, Nose & Sinus
				K Respiratory System
				L Mouth & Throat
				M Gastrointestinal System
				N Hepatobiliary & Pancreas
				P Endocrine System
				Q Skin
				R Musculoskeletal System
				S Urinary System
				T Female Reproductive System
				U Amniotic Fluid, Diagnostic
				V Male Reproductive System
				W Laminaria
				X Abortifacient
				Y Other Body Systems
				Z No Qualifier

2: Placement

W: Anatomical Regions

Operation–Character 3	Body Region Character 4	Approach–Character 5	Device–Character 6	Qualifier–Character 7
0 Change	0 Head	X External	0 Traction Apparatus	Z No Qualifier
1 Compression	1 Face		1 Splint	
2 Dressing	2 Neck		2 Cast	
3 Immobilization	3 Abdominal Wall		3 Brace	
4 Packing	4 Chest Wall		4 Bandage	
5 Removal	5 Back		5 Packing Material	
6 Traction	6 Inguinal Region, Right		6 Pressure Dressing	
	7 Inguinal Region, Left		7 Intermittent Pressure Device	
	8 Upper Extremity, Right		8 Stereotatic Apparatus	
	9 Upper Extremity, Left		9 Wire	
	A Upper Arm, Right		Y Other Device	
	B Upper Arm, Left		Z No Device	
	C Lower Arm, Right			
	D Lower Arm, Left			
	E Hand, Right			
	F Hand, Left			
	G Thumb, Right			
	H Thumb, Left			
	J Finger, Right			
	K Finger, Left			
	L Lower Extremity, Right			
	M Lower Extremity, Left			
	N Upper Leg, Right			
	P Upper Leg, Left			
	Q Lower Leg, Right			
	R Lower Leg, Left			
	S Foot, Right			
	T Foot, Left			
	U Toe, Right			
	V Toe, Left			

2: Placement

Y: Anatomical Orifices

Operation–Character 3	Body Orifice–Character 4	Approach Character–5	Device Character–6	Qualifier Character–7
0 Change	0 Mouth and Pharynx	X External	5 Packing Material	Z No Qualifier
4 Packing	1 Nasal			
5 Removal	2 Ear			
	3 Anorectal			
	4 Female Genital Tract			
	5 Urethra			

3: Administration
Ø: Circulatory

Operation–Character 3	Body System/Region Character 4	Approach–Character 5	Substance–Character 6	Qualifier–Character 7
2 Transfusion	3 Peripheral Vein	Ø Open	A Stem Cells, Embryonic	Ø Autologous
	4 Central Vein	3 Percutaneous	B 4-Factor Prothrombin Complex Concentrate	1 Nonautologous
	5 Peripheral Artery	7 Via Natural or Artificial Opening	G Bone Marrow	Z No Qualifier
	6 Central Artery		H Whole Blood	
	7 Products of Conception, Circulatory		J Serum Albumin	
			K Frozen Plasma	
			L Fresh Plasma	
			M Plasma Cryoprecipitate	
			N Red Blood Cells	
			P Frozen Red Cells	
			Q White Cells	
			R Platelets	
			S Globulin	
			T Fibrinogen	
			V Antihemophilic Factors	
			W Factor IX	
			X Stem Cells, Cord Blood	
			Y Stem Cells, Hematopoietic	

3: Administration
C: Indwelling Device

Operation–Character 3	Body System/Region Character 4	Approach–Character 5	Substance–Character 6	Qualifier–Character 7
1 Irrigation	Z None	X External	8 Irrigating Substance	Z No Qualifier

3: Administration

E: Physiological Systems and Anatomical Regions

Operation–Character 3	Body System/Region–Character 4	Approach–Character 5	Substance–Character 6	Qualifier–Character 7
Ø Introduction	Ø Skin and Mucous Membranes	Ø Open	Ø Antineoplastic	Ø Autologous
1 Irrigation	1 Subcutaneous Tissue	3 Percutaneous	1 Thrombolytic	1 Nonautologous
	2 Muscle	7 Via Natural or Artificial Opening	2 Anti-infective	2 High-dose Interleukin-2
	3 Peripheral Vein	8 Via Natural or Artificial Opening Endoscopic	3 Anti-inflammatory	3 Low-dose Interleukin-2
	4 Central Vein	X External	4 Serum, Toxoid and Vaccine	4 Liquid Brachytherapy Radioisotope
	5 Peripheral Artery		5 Adhesion Barrier	5 Other Antineoplastic
	6 Central Artery		6 Nutritional Substance	6 Recombinant Human-activated Protein C
	7 Coronary Artery		7 Electrolytic and Water Balance Substance	7 Other Thrombolytic
	8 Heart		8 Irrigating Substance	8 Oxazolidinones
	9 Nose		9 Dialysate	9 Other Anti-infective
	A Bone Marrow		A Stem Cells, Embryonic	A Anti-infective Envelope
	B Ear		B Local Anesthetic	B Recombinant Bone Morphogenetic Protein
	C Eye		C Regional Anesthetic	C Other Substance
	D Mouth and Pharynx		D Inhalation Anesthetic	D Nitric Oxide
	E Products of Conception		E Stem Cells, Somatic	F Other Gas
	F Respiratory Tract		F Intracirculatory Anesthetic	G Insulin
	G Upper GI		G Other Therapeutic Substance	H Human B-type Natriuretic Peptide
	H Lower GI		H Radioactive Substance	J Other Hormone
	J Biliary and Pancreatic Tract		K Other Diagnostic Substance	K Immunostimulator
	K Genitourinary Tract		L Sperm	L Immunosuppressive
	L Pleural Cavity		M Pigment	M Monoclonal Antibody
	M Peritoneal Cavity		N Analgesics, Hypnotics, Sedatives	N Blood Brain Barrier Disruption
	N Male Reproductive		P Platelet Inhibitor	P Clofarabine
	P Female Reproductive		Q Fertilized Ovum	X Diagnostic
	Q Cranial Cavity and Brain		R Antiarrhythmic	Z No Qualifier
	R Spinal Canal		S Gas	
	S Epidural Space		T Destructive Agent	
	T Peripheral Nerves and Plexi		U Pancreatic Islet Cells	
	U Joints		V Hormone	
	V Bones		W Immunotherapeutic	
	W Lymphatics		X Vasopressor	
	X Cranial Nerves			
	Y Pericardial Cavity			

4: Measurement and Monitoring

A: Physiological Systems

Operation–Character 3	Body System–Character 4	Approach–Character 5	Function/Device–Character 6	Qualifier–Character 7
Ø Measurement	Ø Central Nervous	Ø Open	Ø Acuity	Ø Central
1 Monitoring	1 Peripheral Nervous	3 Percutaneous	1 Capacity	1 Peripheral
	2 Cardiac	4 Percutaneous Endoscopic	2 Conductivity	2 Portal
	3 Arterial	7 Via Natural or Artificial Opening	3 Contractility	3 Pulmonary
	4 Venous	8 Via Natural or Artificial Opening Endoscopic	4 Electrical Activity	4 Stress
	5 Circulatory	X External	5 Flow	5 Ambulatory
	6 Lymphatic		6 Metabolism	6 Right Heart
	7 Visual		7 Mobility	7 Left Heart
	8 Olfactory		8 Motility	8 Bilateral
	9 Respiratory		9 Output	9 Sensory
	B Gastrointestinal		B Pressure	A Guidance
	C Biliary		C Rate	B Motor
	D Urinary		D Resistance	C Coronary
	F Musculoskeletal		F Rhythm	D Intracranial
	H Products of Conception, Cardiac		G Secretion	F Other Thoracic
	J Products of Conception, Nervous		H Sound	G Intraoperative
	Z None		J Pulse	Z No Qualifier
			K Temperature	
			L Volume	
			M Total Activity	
			N Sampling and Pressure	
			P Action Currents	
			Q Sleep	
			R Saturation	

4: Measurement and Monitoring

B: Physiological Devices

Operation–Character 3	Body System–Character 4	Approach–Character 5	Function/Device–Character 6	Qualifier–Character 7
Ø Measurement	Ø Central Nervous	X External	S Pacemaker	Z No Qualifier
	1 Peripheral Nervous		T Defibrillator	
	2 Cardiac		V Stimulator	
	9 Respiratory			
	F Musculoskeletal			

5: Extracorporeal Assistance and Performance

A: Physiological Systems

Operation–Character 3	Body System–Character 4	Duration–Character 5	Function–Character 6	Qualifier–Character 7
0 Assistance	2 Cardiac	0 Single	0 Filtration	0 Balloon Pump
1 Performance	5 Circulatory	1 Intermittent	1 Output	1 Hyperbaric
2 Restoration	9 Respiratory	2 Continuous	2 Oxygenation	2 Manual
	C Biliary	3 Less than 24 Consecutive Hours	3 Pacing	3 Membrane
	D Urinary	4 24-96 Consecutive Hours	4 Rhythm	4 Nonmechanical
		5 Greater than 96 Consecutive Hours	5 Ventilation	5 Pulsatile Compression
		6 Multiple		6 Other Pump
				7 Continuous Positive Airway Pressure
				8 Intermittent Positive Airway Pressure
				9 Continuous Negative Airway Pressure
				B Intermittent Negative Airway Pressure
				C Supersaturated
				D Impeller Pump
				Z No Qualifier

6: Extracorporeal Therapies

A: Physiological Systems

Operation–Character 3	Body System–Character 4	Duration–Character 5	Qualifier–Character 6	Qualifier–Character 7
0 Atmospheric Control	0 Skin	0 Single	Z No Qualifier	0 Erythrocytes
1 Decompression	1 Urinary	1 Multiple		1 Leukocytes
2 Electromagnetic Therapy	2 Central Nervous			2 Platelets
3 Hyperthermia	3 Musculoskeletal			3 Plasma
4 Hypothermia	5 Circulatory			4 Head and Neck Vessels
5 Pheresis	Z None			5 Heart
6 Phototherapy				6 Peripheral Vessels
7 Ultrasound Therapy				7 Other Vessels
8 Ultraviolet Light Therapy				T Stem Cells, Cord Blood
9 Shock Wave Therapy				V Stem Cells, Hematopoietic
				Z No Qualifier

7: Osteopathic

W: Anatomical Regions

Operation–Character 3	Body Region–Character 4	Approach–Character 5	Method–Character 6	Qualifier–Character 7
0 Treatment	0 Head	X External	0 Articulatory-Raising	Z None
	1 Cervical		1 Fascial Release	
	2 Thoracic		2 General Mobilization	
	3 Lumbar		3 High Velocity-Low Amplitude	
	4 Sacrum		4 Indirect	
	5 Pelvis		5 Low Velocity-High Amplitude	
	6 Lower Extremities		6 Lymphatic Pump	
	7 Upper Extremities		7 Muscle Energy-Isometric	
	8 Rib Cage		8 Muscle Energy-Isotonic	
	9 Abdomen		9 Other Method	

8: Other Procedures

C: Indwelling Devices

Operation–Character 3	Body Region–Character 4	Approach–Character 5	Method–Character 6	Qualifier–Character 7
0 Other procedures	1 Nervous System	X External	6 Collection	J Cerebrospinal Fluid
	2 Circulatory System			K Blood
				L Other Fluid

8: Other Procedures

E: Physiological Systems and Anatomical Regions

Operation–Character 3	Body Region–Character 4	Approach–Character 5	Method–Character 6	Qualifier–Character 7
0 Other Procedures	1 Nervous System	0 Open	0 Acupuncture	0 Anesthesia
	2 Circulatory System	3 Percutaneous	1 Therapeutic Massage	1 In Vitro Fertilization
	9 Head and Neck Region	4 Percutaneous Endoscopic	6 Collection	2 Breast Milk
	H Integumentary System and Breast	7 Via Natural or Artificial Opening	B Computer Assisted Procedure	3 Sperm
	K Musculoskeletal System	8 Via Natural or Artificial Opening Endoscopic	C Robotic Assisted Procedure	4 Yoga Therapy
	U Female Reproductive System	X External	D Near Infrared Spectroscopy	5 Meditation
	V Male Reproductive System		Y Other Method	6 Isolation
	W Trunk Region			7 Examination
	X Upper Extremity			8 Suture Removal
	Y Lower Extremity			9 Piercing
	Z None			C Prostate
				D Rectum
				F With Fluoroscopy
				G With Computerized Tomography
				H With Magnetic Resonance Imaging
				Z No Qualifier

9: Chiropractic

W: Anatomical Regions

Operation–Character 3	Body Region–Character 4	Approach–Character 5	Method–Character 6	Qualifier–Character 7
B Manipulation	Ø Head	X External	B Non-Manual	Z None
	1 Cervical		C Indirect Visceral	
	2 Thoracic		D Extra-Articular	
	3 Lumbar		F Direct Visceral	
	4 Sacrum		G Long Lever Specific Contact	
	5 Pelvis		H Short Lever Specific Contact	
	6 Lower Extremities		J Long and Short Lever Specific Contact	
	7 Upper Extremities		K Mechanically Assisted	
	8 Rib Cage		L Other Method	
	9 Abdomen			

B: Imaging

Body System–Character 2	Type–Character 3	Meanings–Character 4	Contrast–Character 5	Qualifier–Character 6	Qualifier–Character 7
Ø Central Nervous System	Ø Plain Radiography	See next page	Ø High Osmolar	Ø Unenhanced and Enhanced	Ø Intraoperative
2 Heart	1 Fluoroscopy		1 Low Osmolar	1 Laser	1 Densitometry
3 Upper Arteries	2 Computerized Tomography (CT Scan)		Y Other Contrast	2 Intravascular Optical Coherence	3 Intravascular
4 Lower Arteries	3 Magnetic Resonance Imaging (MRI)		Z None	Z None	4 Transesophageal
5 Veins	4 Ultrasonography				A Guidance
7 Lymphatic System					Z None
8 Eye					
9 Ear, Nose, Mouth and Throat					
B Respiratory System					
D Gastrointestinal System					
F Hepatobiliary System and Pancreas					
G Endocrine System					
H Skin, Subcutaneous Tissue and Breast					
L Connective Tissue					
N Skull and Facial Bones					
P Non-Axial Upper Bones					
Q Non-Axial Lower Bones					
R Axial Skeleton, Except Skull and Facial Bones					
T Urinary System					
U Female Reproductive System					
V Male Reproductive System					
W Anatomical Regions					
Y Fetus and Obstetrical					

B: Imaging

Body Part—Character 4 Meanings

Body System–Character 2		Body Part–Character 4	
Ø	Central Nervous System	Ø	Brain
		7	Cisterna
		8	Cerebral Ventricle(s)
		9	Sella Turcica/Pituitary Gland
		B	Spinal Cord
		C	Acoustic Nerves
2	Heart	Ø	Coronary Artery, Single
		1	Coronary Arteries, Multiple
		2	Coronary Artery Bypass Graft, Single
		3	Coronary Artery Bypass Grafts, Multiple
		4	Heart, Right
		5	Heart, Left
		6	Heart, Right and Left
		7	Internal Mammary Bypass Graft, Right
		8	Internal Mammary Bypass Graft, Left
		B	Heart with Aorta
		C	Pericardium
		D	Pediatric Heart
		F	Bypass Graft, Other
3	Upper Arteries	Ø	Thoracic Aorta
		1	Brachiocephalic-Subclavian Artery, Right
		2	Subclavian Artery, Left
		3	Common Carotid Artery, Right
		4	Common Carotid Artery, Left
		5	Common Carotid Arteries, Bilateral
		6	Internal Carotid Artery, Right
		7	Internal Carotid Artery, Left
		8	Internal Carotid Arteries, Bilateral
		9	External Carotid Artery, Right
		B	External Carotid Artery, Left
		C	External Carotid Arteries, Bilateral
		D	Vertebral Artery, Right
		F	Vertebral Artery, Left
		G	Vertebral Arteries, Bilateral
		H	Upper Extremity Arteries, Right
		J	Upper Extremity Arteries, Left
		K	Upper Extremity Arteries, Bilateral
		L	Intercostal and Bronchial Arteries
		M	Spinal Arteries
		N	Upper Arteries, Other
		P	Thoraco-Abdominal Aorta
		Q	Cervico-Cerebral Arch
		R	Intracranial Arteries
		S	Pulmonary Artery, Right
		T	Pulmonary Artery, Left
		V	Ophthalmic Arteries

Continued on next page

B: Imaging

Body Part—Character 4 Meanings

Continued from previous page

Body System–Character 2		Body Part–Character 4	
4	Lower Arteries	Ø	Abdominal Aorta
		1	Celiac Artery
		2	Hepatic Artery
		3	Splenic Arteries
		4	Superior Mesenteric Artery
		5	Inferior Mesenteric Artery
		6	Renal Artery, Right
		7	Renal Artery, Left
		8	Renal Arteries, Bilateral
		9	Lumbar Arteries
		B	Intra-Abdominal Arteries, Other
		C	Pelvic Arteries
		D	Aorta and Bilateral Lower Extremity Arteries
		F	Lower Extremity Arteries, Right
		G	Lower Extremity Arteries, Left
		H	Lower Extremity Arteries, Bilateral
		J	Lower Arteries, Other
		K	Celiac and Mesenteric Arteries
		L	Femoral Artery
		M	Renal Artery Transplant
		N	Penile Arteries
5	Veins	Ø	Epidural Veins
		1	Cerebral and Cerebellar Veins
		2	Intracranial Sinuses
		3	Jugular Veins, Right
		4	Jugular Veins, Left
		5	Jugular Veins, Bilateral
		6	Subclavian Vein, Right
		7	Subclavian Vein, Left
		8	Superior Vena Cava
		9	Inferior Vena Cava
		B	Lower Extremity Veins, Right
		C	Lower Extremity Veins, Left
		D	Lower Extremity Veins, Bilateral
		F	Pelvic (Iliac) Veins, Right
		G	Pelvic (Iliac) Veins, Left
		H	Pelvic (Iliac) Veins, Bilateral
		J	Renal Vein, Right
		K	Renal Vein, Left
		L	Renal Veins, Bilateral
		M	Upper Extremity Veins, Right
		N	Upper Extremity Veins, Left
		P	Upper Extremity Veins, Bilateral
		Q	Pulmonary Vein, Right
		R	Pulmonary Vein, Left
		S	Pulmonary Veins, Bilateral
		T	Portal and Splanchnic Veins
		V	Veins, Other
		W	Dialysis Shunt/Fistula
7	Lymphatic System	Ø	Abdominal/Retroperitoneal Lymphatics, Unilateral
		1	Abdominal/Retroperitoneal Lymphatics, Bilateral
		4	Lymphatics, Head and Neck
		5	Upper Extremity Lymphatics, Right
		6	Upper Extremity Lymphatics, Left
		7	Upper Extremity Lymphatics, Bilateral
		8	Lower Extremity Lymphatics, Right
		9	Lower Extremity Lymphatics, Left
		B	Lower Extremity Lymphatics, Bilateral
		C	Lymphatics, Pelvic

Continued on next page

B: Imaging

Body Part—Character 4 Meanings

Continued from previous page

Body System–Character 2		Body Part–Character 4	
8	Eye	0	Lacrimal Duct, Right
		1	Lacrimal Duct, Left
		2	Lacrimal Ducts, Bilateral
		3	Optic Foramina, Right
		4	Optic Foramina, Left
		5	Eye, Right
		6	Eye, Left
		7	Eyes, Bilateral
9	Ear, Nose, Mouth and Throat	0	Ear
		2	Paranasal Sinuses
		4	Parotid Gland, Right
		5	Parotid Gland, Left
		6	Parotid Glands, Bilateral
		7	Submandibular Gland, Right
		8	Submandibular Gland, Left
		9	Submandibular Glands, Bilateral
		B	Salivary Gland, Right
		C	Salivary Gland, Left
		D	Salivary Glands, Bilateral
		F	Nasopharynx/Oropharynx
		G	Pharynx and Epiglottis
		H	Mastoids
		J	Larynx
B	Respiratory System	2	Lung, Right
		3	Lung, Left
		4	Lungs, Bilateral
		6	Diaphragm
		7	Tracheobronchial Tree, Right
		8	Tracheobronchial Tree, Left
		9	Tracheobronchial Trees, Bilateral
		B	Pleura
		C	Mediastinum
		D	Upper Airways
		F	Trachea/Airways
		G	Lung Apices
D	Gastrointestinal System	1	Esophagus
		2	Stomach
		3	Small Bowel
		4	Colon
		5	Upper GI
		6	Upper GI and Small Bowel
		7	Gastrointestinal Tract
		8	Appendix
		9	Duodenum
		B	Mouth/Oropharynx
		C	Rectum
F	Hepatobiliary System and Pancreas	0	Bile Ducts
		1	Biliary and Pancreatic Ducts
		2	Gallbladder
		3	Gallbladder and Bile Ducts
		4	Gallbladder, Bile Ducts and Pancreatic Ducts
		5	Liver
		6	Liver and Spleen
		7	Pancreas
		8	Pancreatic Ducts
		C	Hepatobiliary System, All
G	Endocrine System	0	Adrenal Gland, Right
		1	Adrenal Gland, Left
		2	Adrenal Glands, Bilateral
		3	Parathyroid Glands
		4	Thyroid Gland

Continued on next page

B: Imaging

Body Part—Character 4 Meanings

Continued from previous page

Body System–Character 2		Body Part–Character 4	
H	Skin, Subcutaneous Tissue and Breast	Ø	Breast, Right
		1	Breast, Left
		2	Breasts, Bilateral
		3	Single Mammary Duct, Right
		4	Single Mammary Duct, Left
		5	Multiple Mammary Ducts, Right
		6	Multiple Mammary Ducts, Left
		7	Extremity, Upper
		8	Extremity, Lower
		9	Abdominal Wall
		B	Chest Wall
		C	Head and Neck
		D	Subcutaneous Tissue, Head/Neck
		F	Subcutaneous Tissue, Upper Extremity
		G	Subcutaneous Tissue, Thorax
		H	Subcutaneous Tissue, Abdomen and Pelvis
		J	Subcutaneous Tissue, Lower Extremity
L	Connective Tissue	Ø	Connective Tissue, Upper Extremity
		1	Connective Tissue, Lower Extremity
		2	Tendons, Upper Extremity
		3	Tendons, Lower Extremity
N	Skull and Facial Bones	Ø	Skull
		1	Orbit, Right
		2	Orbit, Left
		3	Orbits, Bilateral
		4	Nasal Bones
		5	Facial Bones
		6	Mandible
		7	Temporomandibular Joint, Right
		8	Temporomandibular Joint, Left
		9	Temporomandibular Joints, Bilateral
		B	Zygomatic Arch, Right
		C	Zygomatic Arch, Left
		D	Zygomatic Arches, Bilateral
		F	Temporal Bones
		G	Tooth, Single
		H	Teeth, Multiple
		J	Teeth, All
P	Non-Axial Upper Bones	Ø	Sternoclavicular Joint, Right
		1	Sternoclavicular Joint, Left
		2	Sternoclavicular Joints, Bilateral
		3	Acromioclavicular Joints, Bilateral
		4	Clavicle, Right
		5	Clavicle, Left
		6	Scapula, Right
		7	Scapula, Left
		8	Shoulder, Right
		9	Shoulder, Left
		A	Humerus, Right
		B	Humerus, Left
		C	Hand/Finger Joint, Right
		D	Hand/Finger Joint, Left
		E	Upper Arm, Right
		F	Upper Arm, Left
		G	Elbow, Right
		H	Elbow, Left
		J	Forearm, Right
		K	Forearm, Left

Continued on next page

B: Imaging

Body Part—Character 4 Meanings

Continued from previous page

Body System–Character 2		Body Part–Character 4	
P	Non-Axial Upper Bones	L	Wrist, Right
		M	Wrist, Left
		N	Hand, Right
		P	Hand, Left
		Q	Hands and Wrists, Bilateral
		R	Finger(s), Right
		S	Finger(s), Left
		T	Upper Extremity, Right
		U	Upper Extremity, Left
		V	Upper Extremities, Bilateral
		W	Thorax
		X	Ribs, Right
		Y	Ribs, Left
Q	Non-Axial Lower Bones	Ø	Hip, Right
		1	Hip, Left
		2	Hips, Bilateral
		3	Femur, Right
		4	Femur, Left
		7	Knee, Right
		8	Knee, Left
		9	Knees, Bilateral
		B	Tibia/Fibula, Right
		C	Tibia/Fibula, Left
		D	Lower Leg, Right
		F	Lower Leg, Left
		G	Ankle, Right
		H	Ankle, Left
		J	Calcaneus, Right
		K	Calcaneus, Left
		L	Foot, Right
		M	Foot, Left
		P	Toe(s), Right
		Q	Toe(s), Left
		R	Lower Extremity, Right
		S	Lower Extremity, Left
		V	Patella, Right
		W	Patella, Left
		X	Foot/Toe Joint, Right
		Y	Foot/Toe Joint, Left

Continued on next page

B: Imaging

Body Part—Character 4 Meanings

Continued from previous page

Body System–Character 2		Body Part–Character 4	
R	Axial Skeleton, Except Skull and Facial Bones	0	Cervical Spine
		1	Cervical Disc(s)
		2	Thoracic Disc(s)
		3	Lumbar Disc(s)
		4	Cervical Facet Joint(s)
		5	Thoracic Facet Joint(s)
		6	Lumbar Facet Joint(s)
		7	Thoracic Spine
		8	Thoracolumbar Joint
		9	Lumbar Spine
		B	Lumbosacral Joint
		C	Pelvis
		D	Sacroiliac Joints
		F	Sacrum and Coccyx
		G	Whole Spine
		H	Sternum
T	Urinary System	0	Bladder
		1	Kidney, Right
		2	Kidney, Left
		3	Kidneys, Bilateral
		4	Kidneys, Ureters and Bladder
		5	Urethra
		6	Ureter, Right
		7	Ureter, Left
		8	Ureters, Bilateral
		9	Kidney Transplant
		B	Bladder and Urethra
		C	Ileal Diversion Loop
		D	Kidney, Ureter and Bladder, Right
		F	Kidney, Ureter and Bladder, Left
		G	Ileal Loop, Ureters and Kidneys
		J	Kidneys and Bladder
U	Female Reproductive System	0	Fallopian Tube, Right
		1	Fallopian Tube, Left
		2	Fallopian Tubes, Bilateral
		3	Ovary, Right
		4	Ovary, Left
		5	Ovaries, Bilateral
		6	Uterus
		8	Uterus and Fallopian Tubes
		9	Vagina
		B	Pregnant Uterus
		C	Uterus and Ovaries
V	Male Reproductive System	0	Corpora Cavernosa
		1	Epididymis, Right
		2	Epididymis, Left
		3	Prostate
		4	Scrotum
		5	Testicle, Right
		6	Testicle, Left
		7	Testicles, Bilateral
		8	Vasa Vasorum
		9	Prostate and Seminal Vesicles
		B	Penis

Continued on next page

B: Imaging

Body Part—Character 4 Meanings

Continued from previous page

Body System–Character 2		Body Part–Character 4	
W	Anatomical Regions	Ø	Abdomen
		1	Abdomen and Pelvis
		3	Chest
		4	Chest and Abdomen
		5	Chest, Abdomen and Pelvis
		8	Head
		9	Head and Neck
		B	Long Bones, All
		C	Lower Extremity
		F	Neck
		G	Pelvic Region
		H	Retroperitoneum
		J	Upper Extremity
		K	Whole Body
		L	Whole Skeleton
		M	Whole Body, Infant
		P	Brachial Plexus
Y	Fetus and Obstetrical	Ø	Fetal Head
		1	Fetal Heart
		2	Fetal Thorax
		3	Fetal Abdomen
		4	Fetal Spine
		5	Fetal Extremities
		6	Whole Fetus
		7	Fetal Umbilical Cord
		8	Placenta
		9	First Trimester, Single Fetus
		B	First Trimester, Multiple Gestation
		C	Second Trimester, Single Fetus
		D	Second Trimester, Multiple Gestation
		F	Third Trimester, Single Fetus
		G	Third Trimester, Multiple Gestation

C: Nuclear Medicine

Body System–Character 2	Type–Character 3	Meanings–Character 4	Radionuclide–Character 5	Qualifier–Character 6	Qualifier–Character 7
Ø Central Nervous System	1 Planar Nuclear Medicine Imaging	See next Page	1 Technetium 99m (Tc-99m)	Z None	Z None
2 Heart	2 Tomographic (Tomo) Nuclear Medicine Imaging		7 Cobalt 58 (Co-58)		
5 Veins	3 Positron Emission Tomographic (PET) Imaging		8 Samarium 153 (Sm-153)		
7 Lymphatic and Hematologic System	4 Nonimaging Nuclear Medicine Uptake		9 Krypton (Kr-81m)		
8 Eye	5 Nonimaging Nuclear Medicine Probe		B Carbon 11 (C-11)		
9 Ear, Nose, Mouth and Throat	6 Nonimaging Nuclear Medicine Assay		C Cobalt 57 (Co-57)		
B Respiratory System	7 Systemic Nuclear Medicine Therapy		D Indium 111 (In-111)		
D Gastrointestinal System			F Iodine 123 (I-123)		
F Hepatobiliary System and Pancreas			G Iodine 131 (I-131)		
G Endocrine System			H Iodine 125 (I-125)		
H Skin, Subcutaneous Tissue and Breast			K Fluorine 18 (F-18)		
P Musculoskeletal System			L Gallium 67 (Ga-67)		
T Urinary System			M Oxygen 15 (O-15)		
V Male Reproductive System			N Phosphorus 32 (P-32)		
W Anatomical Regions			P Strontium 89 (Sr-89)		
			Q Rubidium 82 (Rb-82)		
			R Nitrogen 13 (N-13)		
			S Thallium 2Ø1 (Tl-2Ø1)		
			T Xenon 127 (Xe-127)		
			V Xenon 133 (Xe-133)		
			W Chromium (Cr-51)		
			Y Other Radionuclide		
			Z None		

C: Nuclear Medicine

Body Part—Character 4 Meanings

Body System–Character 2	Body Part–Character 4
Ø Central Nervous System	Ø Brain 5 Cerebrospinal Fluid Y Central Nervous System
2 Heart	6 Heart, Right and Left G Myocardium Y Heart
5 Veins	B Lower Extremity Veins, Right C Lower Extremity Veins, Left D Lower Extremity Veins, Bilateral N Upper Extremity Veins, Right P Upper Extremity Veins, Left Q Upper Extremity Veins, Bilateral R Central Veins Y Veins
7 Lymphatic and Hematologic System	Ø Bone Marrow 2 Spleen 3 Blood 5 Lymphatics, Head and Neck D Lymphatics, Pelvic J Lymphatics, Head K Lymphatics, Neck L Lymphatics, Upper Chest M Lymphatics, Trunk N Lymphatics, Upper Extremity P Lymphatics, Lower Extremity Y Lymphatic and Hematologic System
8 Eye	9 Lacrimal Ducts, Bilateral Y Eye
9 Ear, Nose, Mouth and Throat	B Salivary Glands, Bilateral Y Ear, Nose, Mouth and Throat
B Respiratory System	2 Lungs and Bronchi Y Respiratory System
D Gastrointestinal System	5 Upper Gastrointestinal Tract 7 Gastrointestinal Tract Y Digestive System
F Hepatobiliary System and Pancreas	4 Gallbladder 5 Liver 6 Liver and Spleen C Hepatobiliary System, All Y Hepatobiliary System and Pancreas
G Endocrine System	1 Parathyroid Glands 2 Thyroid Gland 4 Adrenal Glands, Bilateral Y Endocrine System
H Skin, Subcutaneous Tissue and Breast	Ø Breast, Right 1 Breast, Left 2 Breasts, Bilateral Y Skin, Subcutaneous Tissue and Breast

Continued on next page

C: Nuclear Medicine

Body Part—Character 4 Meanings

Continued from previous page

Body System–Character 2		Body Part–Character 4	
P	Musculoskeletal System	1	Skull
		2	Cervical Spine
		3	Skull and Cervical Spine
		4	Thorax
		5	Spine
		6	Pelvis
		7	Spine and Pelvis
		8	Upper Extremity, Right
		9	Upper Extremity, Left
		B	Upper Extremities, Bilateral
		C	Lower Extremity, Right
		D	Lower Extremity, Left
		F	Lower Extremities, Bilateral
		G	Thoracic Spine
		H	Lumbar Spine
		J	Thoracolumbar Spine
		N	Upper Extremities
		P	Lower Extremities
		Y	Musculoskeletal System, Other
		Z	Musculoskeletal System, All
T	Urinary System	3	Kidneys, Ureters and Bladder
		H	Bladder and Ureters
		Y	Urinary System
V	Male Reproductive System	9	Testicles, Bilateral
		Y	Male Reproductive System
W	Anatomical Regions	Ø	Abdomen
		1	Abdomen and Pelvis
		3	Chest
		4	Chest and Abdomen
		6	Chest and Neck
		B	Head and Neck
		D	Lower Extremity
		G	Thyroid
		J	Pelvic Region
		M	Upper Extremity
		N	Whole Body
		Y	Anatomical Regions, Multiple
		Z	Anatomical Region, Other

D: Radiation Therapy

Body System–Character 2	Modality–Character 3	Meanings–Character 4	Modality-Qualifier Character 5	Isotope–Character 6	Qualifier–Character 7
0 Central and Peripheral Nervous System	0 Beam Radiation	See next Page	0 Photons <1 MeV	7 Cesium 137 (Cs-137)	0 Intraoperative
7 Lymphatic and Hematologic System	1 Brachytherapy		1 Photons 1 - 10 MeV	8 Iridium 192 (Ir-192)	Z None
8 Eye	2 Stereotactic Radiosurgery		2 Photons >10 MeV	9 Iodine 125 (I-125)	
9 Ear, Nose, Mouth and Throat	Y Other Radiation		3 Electrons	B Palladium 103 (Pd-103)	
B Respiratory System			4 Heavy Particles (Protons, Ions)	C Californium 252 (Cf-252)	
D Gastrointestinal System			5 Neutrons	D Iodine 131 (I-131)	
F Hepatobiliary System and Pancreas			6 Neutron Capture	F Phosphorus 32 (P-32)	
G Endocrine System			7 Contact Radiation	G Strontium 89 (Sr-89)	
H Skin			8 Hyperthermia	H Strontium 90 (Sr-90)	
M Breast			9 High Dose Rate (HDR)	Y Other Isotope	
P Musculoskeletal System			B Low Dose Rate (LDR)	Z None	
T Urinary System			C Intraoperative Radiation Therapy (IORT)		
U Female Reproductive System			D Stereotactic Other Photon Radiosurgery		
V Male Reproductive System			F Plaque Radiation		
W Anatomical Regions			G Isotope Administration		
			H Stereotactic Particulate Radiosurgery		
			J Stereotactic Gamma Beam Radiosurgery		
			K Laser Interstitial Thermal Therapy		

D. Radiation Therapy

Treatment Site—Character 4 Meanings

Body System–Character 2		Treatment Site–Character 4	
Ø	Central and Peripheral Nervous System	Ø	Brain
		1	Brain Stem
		6	Spinal Cord
		7	Peripheral Nerve
7	Lymphatic and Hematologic System	Ø	Bone Marrow
		1	Thymus
		2	Spleen
		3	Lymphatics, Neck
		4	Lymphatics, Axillary
		5	Lymphatics, Thorax
		6	Lymphatics, Abdomen
		7	Lymphatics, Pelvis
		8	Lymphatics, Inguinal
8	Eye	Ø	Eye
9	Ear, Nose, Mouth and Throat	Ø	Ear
		1	Nose
		3	Hypopharynx
		4	Mouth
		5	Tongue
		6	Salivary Glands
		7	Sinuses
		8	Hard Palate
		9	Soft Palate
		B	Larynx
		C	Pharynx
		D	Nasopharynx
		F	Oropharynx
B	Respiratory System	Ø	Trachea
		1	Bronchus
		2	Lung
		5	Pleura
		6	Mediastinum
		7	Chest Wall
		8	Diaphragm
D	Gastrointestinal System	Ø	Esophagus
		1	Stomach
		2	Duodenum
		3	Jejunum
		4	Ileum
		5	Colon
		7	Rectum
		8	Anus
F	Hepatobiliary System and Pancreas	Ø	Liver
		1	Gallbladder
		2	Bile Ducts
		3	Pancreas
G	Endocrine System	Ø	Pituitary Gland
		1	Pineal Body
		2	Adrenal Glands
		4	Parathyroid Glands
		5	Thyroid

Continued on next page

D. Radiation Therapy

Treatment Site—Character 4 Meanings

Continued from previous page

Body System–Character 2		Treatment Site–Character 4	
H	Skin	2	Skin, Face
		3	Skin, Neck
		4	Skin, Arm
		5	Skin, Hand
		6	Skin, Chest
		7	Skin, Back
		8	Skin, Abdomen
		9	Skin, Buttock
		B	Skin, Leg
		C	Skin, Foot
M	Breast	Ø	Breast, Left
		1	Breast, Right
P	Musculoskeletal System	Ø	Skull
		2	Maxilla
		3	Mandible
		4	Sternum
		5	Rib(s)
		6	Humerus
		7	Radius/Ulna
		8	Pelvic Bones
		9	Femur
		B	Tibia/Fibula
		C	Other Bone
T	Urinary System	Ø	Kidney
		1	Ureter
		2	Bladder
		3	Urethra
U	Female Reproductive System	Ø	Ovary
		1	Cervix
		2	Uterus
V	Male Reproductive System	Ø	Prostate
		1	Testis
W	Anatomical Regions	1	Head and Neck
		2	Chest
		3	Abdomen
		4	Hemibody
		5	Whole Body
		6	Pelvic Region

F: Physical Rehabilitation and Diagnostic Audiology

Ø: Rehabilitation

See next page for Character 5 Meanings

Type–Character 3	Body System–Body Region–Character 4	Equipment – Character 6	Qualifier–Character 7
Ø Speech Assessment	Ø Neurological System - Head and Neck	1 Audiometer	Z None
1 Motor and/or Nerve Function Assessment	1 Neurological System - Upper Back / Upper Extremity	2 Sound Field / Booth	
2 Activities of Daily Living Assessment	2 Neurological System - Lower Back / Lower Extremity	4 Electroacoustic Immitance / Acoustic Reflex	
6 Speech Treatment	3 Neurological System - Whole Body	5 Hearing Aid Selection / Fitting / Test	
7 Motor Treatment	4 Circulatory System - Head and Neck	7 Electrophysiologic	
8 Activities of Daily Living Treatment	5 Circulatory System - Upper Back / Upper Extremity	8 Vestibular / Balance	
9 Hearing Treatment	6 Circulatory System - Lower Back / Lower Extremity	9 Cochlear Implant	
B Cochlear Implant Treatment	7 Circulatory System - Whole Body	B Physical Agents	
C Vestibular Treatment	8 Respiratory System - Head and Neck	C Mechanical	
D Device Fitting	9 Respiratory System - Upper Back / Upper Extremity	D Electrotherapeutic	
F Caregiver Training	B Respiratory System - Lower Back / Lower Extremity	E Orthosis	
	C Respiratory System - Whole Body	F Assistive, Adaptive, Supportive or Protective	
	D Integumentary System - Head and Neck	G Aerobic Endurance and Conditioning	
	F Integumentary System - Upper Back / Upper Extremity	H Mechanical or Electromechanical	
	G Integumentary System - Lower Back / Lower Extremity	J Somatosensory	
	H Integumentary System - Whole Body	K Audiovisual	
	J Musculoskeletal System - Head and Neck	L Assistive Listening	
	K Musculoskeletal System - Upper Back / Upper Extremity	M Augmentative / Alternative Communication	
	L Musculoskeletal System - Lower Back / Lower Extremity	N Biosensory Feedback	
	M Musculoskeletal System - Whole Body	P Computer	
	N Genitourinary System	Q Speech Analysis	
	Z None	S Voice Analysis	
		T Aerodynamic Function	
		U Prosthesis	
		V Speech Prosthesis	
		W Swallowing	
		X Cerumen Management	
		Y Other Equipment	
		Z None	

F: Physical Rehabilitation and Diagnostic Audiology

0: Rehabilitation

Type Qualifier—Character 5 Meanings

Type–Character 3		Type Qualifier–Character 5	
Ø	Speech Assessment	Ø	Filtered Speech
		1	Speech Threshold
		2	Speech/Word Recognition
		3	Staggered Spondaic Word
		4	Sensorineural Acuity Level
		5	Synthetic Sentence Identification
		6	Speech and/or Language Screening
		7	Nonspoken Language
		8	Receptive/Expressive Language
		9	Articulation/Phonology
		B	Motor Speech
		C	Aphasia
		D	Fluency
		F	Voice
		G	Communicative/Cognitive Integration Skills
		H	Bedside Swallowing and Oral Function
		J	Instrumental Swallowing and Oral Function
		K	Orofacial Myofunctional
		L	Augmentative/Alternative Communication System
		M	Voice Prosthetic
		N	Non-invasive Instrumental Status
		P	Oral Peripheral Mechanism
		Q	Performance Intensity Phonetically Balanced Speech Discrimination
		R	Brief Tone Stimuli
		S	Distorted Speech
		T	Dichotic Stimuli
		V	Temporal Ordering of Stimuli
		W	Masking Patterns
		X	Other Specified Central Auditory Processing
1	Motor and/or Nerve Function Assessment	Ø	Muscle Performance
		1	Integumentary Integrity
		2	Visual Motor Integration
		3	Coordination/Dexterity
		4	Motor Function
		5	Range of Motion and Joint Integrity
		6	Sensory Awareness/Processing/Integrity
		7	Facial Nerve Function
		9	Somatosensory Evoked Potentials
		B	Bed Mobility
		C	Transfer
		D	Gait and/or Balance
		F	Wheelchair Mobility
		G	Reflex Integrity
2	Activities of Daily Living Assessment	Ø	Bathing/Showering
		1	Dressing
		2	Feeding/Eating
		3	Grooming/Personal Hygiene
		4	Home Management
		5	Perceptual Processing
		6	Psychosocial Skills
		7	Aerobic Capacity and Endurance
		8	Anthropometric Characteristics
		9	Cranial Nerve Integrity
		B	Environmental, Home and Work Barriers
		C	Ergonomics and Body Mechanics
		D	Neuromotor Development
		F	Pain
		G	Ventilation, Respiration and Circulation
		H	Vocational Activities and Functional Community or Work Reintegration Skills

Continued on next page

F: Physical Rehabilitation and Diagnostic Audiology

0: Rehabilitation

Type Qualifier—Character 5 Meanings

Continued from previous page

Type–Character 3		Type Qualifier–Character 5	
6	Speech Treatment	Ø	Nonspoken Language
		1	Speech-Language Pathology and Related Disorders Counseling
		2	Speech-Language Pathology and Related Disorders Prevention
		3	Aphasia
		4	Articulation/Phonology
		5	Aural Rehabilitation
		6	Communicative/Cognitive Integration Skills
		7	Fluency
		8	Motor Speech
		9	Orofacial Myofunctional
		B	Receptive/Expressive Language
		C	Voice
		D	Swallowing Dysfunction
7	Motor Treatment	Ø	Range of Motion and Joint Mobility
		1	Muscle Performance
		2	Coordination/Dexterity
		3	Motor Function
		4	Wheelchair Mobility
		5	Bed Mobility
		6	Therapeutic Exercise
		7	Manual Therapy Techniques
		8	Transfer Training
		9	Gait Training/Functional Ambulation
8	Activities of Daily Living Treatment	Ø	Bathing/Showering Techniques
		1	Dressing Techniques
		2	Grooming/Personal Hygiene
		3	Feeding/Eating
		4	Home Management
		5	Wound Management
		6	Psychosocial Skills
		7	Vocational Activities and Functional Community or Work Reintegration Skills
9	Hearing Treatment	Ø	Hearing and Related Disorders Counseling
		1	Hearing and Related Disorders Prevention
		2	Auditory Processing
		3	Cerumen Management
B	Cochlear Implant Treatment	Ø	Cochlear Implant Rehabilitation
C	Vestibular Treatment	Ø	Vestibular
		1	Perceptual Processing
		2	Visual Motor Integration
		3	Postural Control
D	Device Fitting	Ø	Tinnitus Masker
		1	Monaural Hearing Aid
		2	Binaural Hearing Aid
		3	Augmentative/Alternative Communication System
		4	Voice Prosthetic
		5	Assistive Listening Device
		6	Dynamic Orthosis
		7	Static Orthosis
		8	Prosthesis
		9	Assistive, Adaptive, Supportive or Protective Devices

Continued on next page

F: Physical Rehabilitation and Diagnostic Audiology

0: Rehabilitation

Type Qualifier—Character 5 Meanings

Continued from previous page

Type–Character 3	Type Qualifier–Character 5
F Caregiver Training	Ø Bathing/Showering Technique
	1 Dressing
	2 Feeding and Eating
	3 Grooming/Personal Hygiene
	4 Bed Mobility
	5 Transfer
	6 Wheelchair Mobility
	7 Therapeutic Exercise
	8 Airway Clearance Techniques
	9 Wound Management
	B Vocational Activities and Functional Community or Work Reintegration Skills
	C Gait Training/Functional Ambulation
	D Application, Proper Use and Care of Assistive, Adaptive, Supportive or Protective Devices
	F Application, Proper Use and Care of Orthoses
	G Application, Proper Use and Care of Prosthesis
	H Home Management
	J Communication Skills

F: Physical Rehabilitation and Diagnostic Audiology

1: Diagnostic Audiology

Type–Character 3	Body System–Body Region–Character 4	Meanings–Character 5	Equipment–Character 6	Qualifer–Character 7
3 Hearing Assessment	Z None	See next page	Ø Occupational Hearing	Z None
4 Hearing Aid Assessment			1 Audiometer	
5 Vestibular Assessment			2 Sound Field / Booth	
			3 Tympanometer	
			4 Electroacoustic Immitance / Acoustic Reflex	
			5 Hearing Aid Selection / Fitting / Test	
			6 Otoacoustic Emission (OAE)	
			7 Electrophysiologic	
			8 Vestibular / Balance	
			9 Cochlear Implant	
			K Audiovisual	
			L Assistive Listening	
			P Computer	
			Y Other Equipment	
			Z None	

F: Physical Rehabilitation and Diagnostic Audiology

1: Diagnostic Audiology

Type Qualifier—Character 5 Meanings

Type–Character 3		Type Qualifier–Character 5	
3	Hearing Assessment	Ø	Hearing Screening
		1	Pure Tone Audiometry, Air
		2	Pure Tone Audiometry, Air and Bone
		3	Bekesy Audiometry
		4	Conditioned Play Audiometry
		5	Select Picture Audiometry
		6	Visual Reinforcement Audiometry
		7	Alternate Binaural or Monaural Loudness Balance
		8	Tone Decay
		9	Short Increment Sensitivity Index
		B	Stenger
		C	Pure Tone Stenger
		D	Tympanometry
		F	Eustachian Tube Function
		G	Acoustic Reflex Patterns
		H	Acoustic Reflex Threshold
		J	Acoustic Reflex Decay
		K	Electrocochleography
		L	Auditory Evoked Potentials
		M	Evoked Otoacoustic Emissions, Screening
		N	Evoked Otoacoustic Emissions, Diagnostic
		P	Aural Rehabilitation Status
		Q	Auditory Processing
4	Hearing Aid Assessment	Ø	Cochlear Implant
		1	Ear Canal Probe Microphone
		2	Monaural Hearing Aid
		3	Binaural Hearing Aid
		4	Assistive Listening System/Device Selection
		5	Sensory Aids
		6	Binaural Electroacoustic Hearing Aid Check
		7	Ear Protector Attentuation
		8	Monaural Electroacoustic Hearing Aid Check
5	Vestibular Assessment	Ø	Bithermal, Binaural Caloric Irrigation
		1	Bithermal, Monaural Caloric Irrigation
		2	Unithermal Binaural Screen
		3	Oscillating Tracking
		4	Sinusoidal Vertical Axis Rotational
		5	Dix-Hallpike Dynamic
		6	Computerized Dynamic Posturography
		7	Tinnitus Masker

G: Mental Health

Z: Body System—None

Type–Character 3	Type Qualifier –Character 4	Qualifier–Character 5	Qualifier–Character 6	Qualifier–Character 7
1 Psychological Tests	Ø Developmental 1 Personality and Behavioral 2 Intellectual and Psychoeducational 3 Neuropsychological 4 Neurobehavioral and Cognitive Status	Z None	Z None	Z None
2 Crisis Intervention	Z None			
3 Medication Management	Z None			
5 Individual Psychotherapy	Ø Interactive 1 Behavioral 2 Cognitive 3 Interpersonal 4 Psychoanalysis 5 Psychodynamic 6 Supportive 8 Cognitive-Behavioral 9 Psychophysiological			
6 Counseling	Ø Educational 1 Vocational 3 Other Counseling			
7 Family Psychotherapy	2 Other Family Psychotherapy			
B Electroconvulsive Therapy	Ø Unilateral-Single Seizure 1 Unilateral-Multiple Seizure 2 Bilateral-Single Seizure 3 Bilateral-Multiple Seizure 4 Other Electroconvulsive Therapy			
C Biofeedback	9 Other Biofeedback			
F Hypnosis	Z None			
G Narcosynthesis	Z None			
H Group Psychotherapy	Z None			
J Light Therapy	Z None			

H: Substance Abuse Treatment

Z: Body System—None

Type–Character 3	Type Qualifier–Character 4	Qualifier–Character 5	Qualifier–Character 6	Qualifier–Character 7
2 Detoxification Services	Z None	Z None	Z None	Z None
3 Individual Counseling	Ø Cognitive			
	1 Behavioral			
	2 Cognitive-Behavioral			
	3 12-Step			
	4 Interpersonal			
	5 Vocational			
	6 Psychoeducation			
	7 Motivational Enhancement			
	8 Confrontational			
	9 Continuing Care			
	B Spiritual			
	C Pre/Post-Test Infectious Disease			
4 Group Counseling	Ø Cognitive			
	1 Behavioral			
	2 Cognitive-Behavioral			
	3 12-Step			
	4 Interpersonal			
	5 Vocational			
	6 Psychoeducation			
	7 Motivational Enhancement			
	8 Confrontational			
	9 Continuing Care			
	B Spiritual			
	C Pre/Post-Test Infectious Disease			
5 Individual Psychotherapy	Ø Cognitive			
	1 Behavioral			
	2 Cognitive-Behavioral			
	3 12-Step			
	4 Interpersonal			
	5 Interactive			
	6 Psychoeducation			
	7 Motivational Enhancement			
	8 Confrontational			
	9 Supportive			
	B Psychoanalysis			
	C Psychodynamic			
	D Psychophysiological			
6 Family Counseling	3 Other Family Counseling			
8 Medication Management	Ø Nicotine Replacement			
	1 Methadone Maintenance			
	2 Levo-alpha-acetyl-methadol (LAAM)			
	3 Antabuse			
	4 Naltrexone			
	5 Naloxone			
	6 Clonidine			
	7 Bupropion			
	8 Psychiatric Medication			
	9 Other Replacement Medication			
9 Pharmacotherapy	Ø Nicotine Replacement			
	1 Methadone Maintenance			
	2 Levo-alpha-acetyl-methadol (LAAM)			
	3 Antabuse			
	4 Naltrexone			
	5 Naloxone			
	6 Clonidine			
	7 Bupropion			
	8 Psychiatric Medication			
	9 Other Replacement Medication			

Appendix H: Answers to Coding Exercises

Medical Surgical Section

Procedure	Code
Excision of malignant melanoma from skin of right ear	ØHB2XZZ
Laparoscopy with excision of endometrial implant from left ovary	ØUB14ZZ
Percutaneous needle core biopsy of right kidney	ØTBØ3ZX
EGD with gastric biopsy	ØDB68ZX
Open endarterectomy of left common carotid artery	Ø3CJØZZ
Excision of basal cell carcinoma of lower lip	ØCB1XZZ
Open excision of tail of pancreas	ØFBGØZZ
Percutaneous biopsy of right gastrocnemius muscle	ØKBS3ZX
Sigmoidoscopy with sigmoid polypectomy	ØDBN8ZZ
Open excision of lesion from right Achilles tendon	ØLBNØZZ
Open resection of cecum	ØDTHØZZ
Total excision of pituitary gland, open	ØGTØØZZ
Explantation of left failed kidney, open	ØTT1ØZZ
Open left axillary total lymphadenectomy	Ø7T6ØZZ (RESECTION is coded for cutting out a chain of lymph nodes.)
Laparoscopic-assisted total vaginal hysterectomy	ØUT9FZZ
Right total mastectomy, open	ØHTTØZZ
Open resection of papillary muscle	Ø2TDØZZ (The papillary muscle refers to the heart and is found in the *Heart and Great Vessels* body system.)
Radical retropubic prostatectomy, open	ØVTØØZZ
Laparoscopic cholecystectomy	ØFT44ZZ
Endoscopic bilateral total maxillary sinusectomy	Ø9TQ4ZZ, Ø9TR4ZZ
Amputation at right elbow level	ØX6BØZZ
Right below-knee amputation, proximal tibia/fibula	ØY6HØZ1 (The qualifier *High* here means the portion of the tib/fib closest to the knee.)
Fifth ray carpometacarpal joint amputation, left hand	ØX6KØZ8 (A *complete* ray amputation is through the carpometacarpal joint.)
Right leg and hip amputation through ischium	ØY62ØZZ (The *Hindquarter* body part includes amputation along any part of the hip bone.)

Procedure	Code
DIP joint amputation of right thumb	ØX6LØZ3 (The qualifier *low* here means through the distal interphalangeal joint.)
Right wrist joint amputation	ØX6JØZØ (Amputation at the wrist joint is actually complete amputation of the hand.)
Trans-metatarsal amputation of foot at left big toe	ØY6NØZ9 (A *partial* amputation is through the shaft of the metatarsal bone.)
Mid-shaft amputation, right humerus	ØX68ØZ2
Left fourth toe amputation, mid-proximal phalanx	ØY6WØZ1 (The qualifier *High* here means anywhere along the proximal phalanx.)
Right above-knee amputation, distal femur	ØY6CØZ3
Cryotherapy of wart on left hand	ØH5GXZZ
Percutaneous radiofrequency ablation of right vocal cord lesion	ØC5T3ZZ
Left heart catheterization with laser destruction of arrhythmogenic focus, A-V node	Ø2583ZZ
Cautery of nosebleed	Ø95KXZZ
Transurethral endoscopic laser ablation of prostate	ØV5Ø8ZZ
Cautery of oozing varicose vein, left calf	Ø65Y3ZZ (The approach is coded *Percutaneous* because that is the normal route to a vein. No mention is made of approach, because likely the skin has eroded at that spot.)
Laparoscopy with destruction of endometriosis, bilateral ovaries	ØU524ZZ
Laser coagulation of right retinal vessel hemorrhage, percutaneous	Ø85G3ZZ (The *Retinal Vessel* body-part values are in the *Eye* body system.)
Thoracoscopic pleurodesis, left side	ØB5P4ZZ
Percutaneous insertion of Greenfield IVC filter	Ø6HØ3DZ
Forceps total mouth extraction, upper and lower teeth	ØCDWXZ2, ØCDXXZ2
Removal of left thumbnail	ØHDQXZZ (No separate body-part value is given for thumbnail, so this is coded to *Fingernail*.)
Extraction of right intraocular lens without replacement, percutaneous	Ø8DJ3ZZ

Procedure	Code
Laparoscopy with needle aspiration of ova for in vitro fertilization	ØUDN4ZZ
Nonexcisional debridement of skin ulcer, right foot	ØHDMXZZ
Open stripping of abdominal fascia, right side	ØJD8ØZZ
Hysteroscopy with D&C, diagnostic	ØUDB8ZX
Liposuction for medical purposes, left upper arm	ØJDF3ZZ (The *Percutaneous* approach is inherent in the liposuction technique.)
Removal of tattered right ear drum fragments with tweezers	Ø9D77ZZ
Microincisional phlebectomy of spider veins, right lower leg	Ø6DY3ZZ
Routine Foley catheter placement	ØT9B7ØZ
Incision and drainage of external perianal abscess	ØD9QXZZ
Percutaneous drainage of ascites	ØW9G3ZZ (This is drainage of the cavity and not the peritoneal membrane itself.)
Laparoscopy with left ovarian cystotomy and drainage	ØU914ZZ
Laparotomy and drain placement for liver abscess, right lobe	ØF91ØØZ
Right knee arthrotomy with drain placement	ØS9CØØZ
Thoracentesis of left pleural effusion	ØW9B3ZZ (This is drainage of the pleural cavity)
Phlebotomy of left median cubital vein for polycythemia vera	Ø59C3ZZ (The median cubital vein is a branch of the basilic vein)
Percutaneous chest tube placement for right pneumothorax	ØW993ØZ
Endoscopic drainage of left ethmoid sinus	Ø99V4ZZ
External ventricular CSF drainage catheter placement via burr hole	ØØ963ØZ
Removal of foreign body, right cornea	Ø8C8XZZ
Percutaneous mechanical thrombectomy, left brachial artery	Ø3C83ZZ
Esophagogastroscopy with removal of bezoar from stomach	ØDC68ZZ
Foreign body removal, skin of left thumb	ØHCGXZZ (There is no specific value for thumb skin, so the procedure is coded to *Hand*.)
Transurethral cystoscopy with removal of bladder stone	ØTCB8ZZ
Forceps removal of foreign body in right nostril	Ø9CKXZZ (Nostril is coded to the *Nose* body-part value.)
Laparoscopy with excision of old suture from mesentery	ØDCV4ZZ
Incision and removal of right lacrimal duct stone	Ø8CXØZZ

Procedure	Code
Nonincisional removal of intraluminal foreign body from vagina	ØUCG7ZZ (The approach *External* is also a possibility. It is assumed here that since the patient went to the doctor to have the object removed, that it was not in the vaginal orifice.)
Right common carotid endarterectomy, open	Ø3CHØZZ
Open excision of retained sliver, subcutaneous tissue of left foot	ØJCRØZZ
Extracorporeal shockwave lithotripsy (ESWL), bilateral ureters	ØTF6XZZ, ØTF7XZZ (The *Bilateral Ureter* body-part value is not available for the root operation FRAGMENTATION, so the procedures are coded separately.)
Endoscopic retrograde cholangiopancreatography (ERCP) with lithotripsy of common bile duct stone	ØFF98ZZ (ERCP is performed through the mouth to the biliary system via the duodenum, so the approach value is *Via Natural or Artificial Opening Endoscopic*.)
Thoracotomy with crushing of pericardial calcifications	Ø2FNØZZ
Transurethral cystoscopy with fragmentation of bladder calculus	ØTFB8ZZ
Hysteroscopy with intraluminal lithotripsy of left fallopian tube calcification	ØUF68ZZ
Division of right foot tendon, percutaneous	ØL8V3ZZ
Left heart catheterization with division of bundle of HIS	Ø2883ZZ
Open osteotomy of capitate, left hand	ØP8NØZZ (The capitate is one of the carpal bones of the hand.)
EGD with esophagotomy of esophagogastric junction	ØD848ZZ
Sacral rhizotomy for pain control, percutaneous	Ø18R3ZZ
Laparotomy with exploration and adhesiolysis of right ureter	ØTN6ØZZ
Incision of scar contracture, right elbow	ØHNDXZZ (The skin of the elbow region is coded to *Lower Arm*.)
Frenulotomy for treatment of tongue-tie syndrome	ØCN7XZZ (The frenulum is coded to the body-part value *Tongue*.)
Right shoulder arthroscopy with coracoacromial ligament release	ØMN14ZZ
Mitral valvulotomy for release of fused leaflets, open approach	Ø2NGØZZ
Percutaneous left Achilles tendon release	ØLNP3ZZ
Laparoscopy with lysis of peritoneal adhesions	ØDNW4ZZ

Procedure	Code
Manual rupture of right shoulder joint adhesions under general anesthesia	ØRNJXZZ
Open posterior tarsal tunnel release	Ø1NGØZZ (The nerve released in the posterior tarsal tunnel is the tibial nerve.)
Laparoscopy with freeing of left ovary and fallopian tube	ØUN14ZZ, ØUN64ZZ
Liver transplant with donor matched liver	ØFYØØZØ
Orthotopic heart transplant using porcine heart	Ø2YAØZ2 (The donor heart comes from an animal [pig], so the qualifier value is *Zooplastic.*)
Right lung transplant, open, using organ donor match	ØBYKØZØ
Transplant of large intestine, organ donor match	ØDYEØZØ
Left kidney/pancreas organ bank transplant	ØFYGØZØ, ØTY1ØZØ
Replantation of avulsed scalp	ØHMØXZZ
Reattachment of severed right ear	Ø9MØXZZ
Reattachment of traumatic left gastrocnemius avulsion, open	ØKMTØZZ
Closed replantation of three avulsed teeth, lower jaw	ØCMXXZ1
Reattachment of severed left hand	ØXMKØZZ
Right open palmaris longus tendon transfer	ØLX5ØZZ
Endoscopic radial to median nerve transfer	Ø1X64Z5
Fasciocutaneous flap closure of left thigh, open	ØJXMØZC (The qualifier identifies the body layers in addition to fascia included in the procedure.)
Transfer left index finger to left thumb position, open	ØXXPØZM
Percutaneous fascia transfer to fill defect, anterior neck	ØJX43ZZ
Trigeminal to facial nerve transfer, percutaneous endoscopic	ØØXK4ZM
Endoscopic left leg flexor hallucis longus tendon transfer	ØLXP4ZZ
Right scalp advancement flap to right temple	ØHXØXZZ
Bilateral TRAM pedicle flap reconstruction status post mastectomy, muscle only, open	ØKXKØZ6, ØKXLØZ6 (The transverse rectus abdominus muscle (TRAM) flap is coded for each flap developed.)
Skin transfer flap closure of complex open wound, left lower back	ØHX6XZZ
Open fracture reduction, right tibia	ØQSGØZZ
Laparoscopy with gastropexy for malrotation	ØDS64ZZ
Left knee arthroscopy with reposition of anterior cruciate ligament	ØMSP4ZZ
Open transposition of ulnar nerve	Ø1S4ØZZ
Closed reduction with percutaneous internal fixation of right femoral neck fracture	ØQS634Z
Trans-vaginal intraluminal cervical cerclage	ØUVC7DZ

Procedure	Code
Cervical cerclage using Shirodkar technique	ØUVC7ZZ
Thoracotomy with banding of left pulmonary artery using extraluminal device	Ø2VRØCZ
Restriction of thoracic duct with intraluminal stent, percutaneous	Ø7VK3DZ
Craniotomy with clipping of cerebral aneurysm	Ø3VGØCZ (The clip is placed lengthwise on the outside wall of the widened portion of the vessel.)
Nonincisional, trans-nasal placement of restrictive stent in right lacrimal duct	Ø8VX7DZ
Catheter-based temporary restriction of blood flow in abdominal aorta for treatment of cerebral ischemia	Ø4VØ3DJ
Percutaneous ligation of esophageal vein	Ø6L33ZZ
Percutaneous embolization of left internal carotid-cavernous fistula	Ø3LL3DZ
Laparoscopy with bilateral occlusion of fallopian tubes using Hulka extraluminal clips	ØUL74CZ
Open suture ligation of failed AV graft, left brachial artery	Ø3L8ØZZ
Percutaneous embolization of vascular supply, intracranial meningioma	Ø3LG3DZ
Percutaneous embolization of right uterine artery, using coils	Ø4LE3DT
Open occlusion of left atrial appendage, using extraluminal pressure clips	Ø2L7ØCK
Percutaneous suture exclusion of left atrial appendage, via femoral artery access	Ø2L73ZK
ERCP with balloon dilation of common bile duct	ØF798ZZ
PTCA of two coronary arteries, LAD with stent placement, RCA with no stent	Ø27Ø3DZ, Ø27Ø3ZZ (A separate procedure is coded for each artery dilated, since the device value differs for each artery.)
Cystoscopy with intraluminal dilation of bladder neck stricture	ØT7C8ZZ
Open dilation of old anastomosis, left femoral artery	Ø47LØZZ
Dilation of upper esophageal stricture, direct visualization, with Bougie sound	ØD717ZZ
PTA of right brachial artery stenosis	Ø3773ZZ
Transnasal dilation and stent placement in right lacrimal duct	Ø87X7DZ
Hysteroscopy with balloon dilation of bilateral fallopian tubes	ØU778ZZ
Tracheoscopy with intraluminal dilation of tracheal stenosis	ØB718ZZ
Cystoscopy with dilation of left ureteral stricture, with stent placement	ØT778DZ
Open gastric bypass with Roux-en-Y limb to jejunum	ØD16ØZA
Right temporal artery to intracranial artery bypass using Gore-Tex graft, open	Ø31SØJG
Tracheostomy formation with tracheostomy tube placement, percutaneous	ØB113F4

Procedure	Code
PICVA (percutaneous in situ coronary venous arterialization) of single coronary artery	Ø21Ø3D4
Open left femoral-popliteal artery bypass using cadaver vein graft	Ø41LØKL
Shunting of intrathecal cerebrospinal fluid to peritoneal cavity using synthetic shunt	ØØ16ØJ6
Colostomy formation, open, transverse colon to abdominal wall	ØD1LØZ4
Open urinary diversion, left ureter, using ileal conduit to skin	ØT17ØZC
CABG of LAD using left internal mammary artery, open off-bypass	Ø21ØØZ9
Open pleuroperitoneal shunt, right pleural cavity, using synthetic device	ØW19ØJG
Percutaneous placement of ventriculoperitoneal shunt for treatment of hydrocephalus	ØØ163J6
End-of-life replacement of spinal neurostimulator generator, multiple array, in lower abdomen	ØJH8ØDZ (Taking out of the old generator is coded separately to the root operation *Removal*)
Percutaneous insertion of spinal neurostimulator lead, lumbar spinal cord	ØØHV3MZ
Percutaneous placement of broken pacemaker lead in left atrium	Ø2H73MZ (Taking out the broken pacemaker lead is coded separately to the root operation *Removal*.)
Open placement of dual chamber pacemaker generator in chest wall	ØJH6Ø6Z
Percutaneous placement of venous central line in right internal jugular	Ø5HM33Z
Open insertion of multiple channel cochlear implant, left ear	Ø9HEØ6Z
Percutaneous placement of Swan-Ganz catheter in superior vena cava	Ø2HV32Z (The Swan-Ganz catheter is coded to the device value *Monitoring Device* because it monitors pulmonary artery output.)
Bronchoscopy with insertion of brachytherapy seeds, right main bronchus	ØBHØ81Z
Placement of intrathecal infusion pump for pain management, percutaneous	ØJH73VZ (The device resides principally in the subcutaneous tissue of the back, so it is coded to body system *Subcutaneous Tissue and Fascia*.)
Open insertion of interspinous process device into lumbar vertebral joint	ØQHØØ4Z
Open placement of bone growth stimulator, left femoral shaft	ØQHYØMZ
Cystoscopy with placement of brachytherapy seeds in prostate gland	ØVHØ81Z
Percutaneous insertion of Greenfield IVC filter	Ø6HØ3DZ

Procedure	Code
Full-thickness skin graft to right lower arm, autograft (do not code graft harvest for this exercise)	ØHRDX73
Excision of necrosed left femoral head with bone bank bone graft to fill the defect, open	ØQR7ØKZ
Penetrating keratoplasty of right cornea with donor matched cornea, percutaneous approach	Ø8R83KZ
Bilateral mastectomy with concomitant saline breast implants, open	ØHRVØJZ
Excision of abdominal aorta with Gore-Tex graft replacement, open	Ø4RØØJZ
Total right knee arthroplasty with insertion of total knee prosthesis	ØSRCØJZ
Bilateral mastectomy with free TRAM flap reconstruction	ØHRVØ76
Tenonectomy with graft to right ankle using cadaver graft, open	ØLRSØKZ
Mitral valve replacement using porcine valve, open	Ø2RGØ8Z
Percutaneous phacoemulsification of right eye cataract with prosthetic lens insertion	Ø8RJ3JZ
Transcatheter replacement of pulmonary valve using of bovine jugular vein valve	Ø2RH38Z
Total left hip replacement using ceramic on ceramic prosthesis, without bone cement	ØSRBØ3A
Aortic valve annuloplasty using ring, open	Ø2UFØJZ
Laparoscopic repair of left inguinal hernia with marlex plug	ØYU64JZ
Autograft nerve graft to right median nerve, percutaneous endoscopic (do not code graft harvest for this exercise)	Ø1U547Z
Exchange of liner in femoral component of previous left hip replacement, open approach	ØSUSØ9Z (Taking out of the old liner is coded separately to the root operation *Removal*)
Anterior colporrhaphy with polypropylene mesh reinforcement, open approach	ØUUGØJZ
Implantation of CorCap cardiac support device, open approach	Ø2UAØJZ
Abdominal wall herniorrhaphy, open, using synthetic mesh	ØWUFØJZ
Tendon graft to strengthen injured left shoulder using autograft, open (do not code graft harvest for this exercise)	ØLU2Ø7Z
Onlay lamellar keratoplasty of left cornea using autograft, external approach	Ø8U9X7Z
Resurfacing procedure on right femoral head, open approach	ØSURØBZ
Exchange of drainage tube from right hip joint	ØS2YXØZ
Tracheostomy tube exchange	ØB21XFZ
Change chest tube for left pneumothorax	ØW2BXØZ
Exchange of cerebral ventriculostomy drainage tube	ØØ2ØXØZ

Procedure	Code
Foley urinary catheter exchange	ØT2BXØZ (This is coded to *Drainage Device* because urine is being drained.)
Open removal of lumbar sympathetic neurostimulator lead	Ø1PYØMZ
Nonincisional removal of Swan-Ganz catheter from right pulmonary artery	Ø2PYX2Z
Laparotomy with removal of pancreatic drain	ØFPGØØZ
Extubation, endotracheal tube	ØBP1XDZ
Nonincisional PEG tube removal	ØDP6XUZ
Transvaginal removal of brachytherapy seeds	ØUPH71Z
Transvaginal removal of extraluminal cervical cerclage	ØUPD7CZ
Incision with removal of K-wire fixation, right first metatarsal	ØQPNØ4Z
Cystoscopy with retrieval of left ureteral stent	ØTP98DZ
Removal of nasogastric drainage tube for decompression	ØDP6XØZ
Removal of external fixator, left radial fracture	ØPPJX5Z
Reposition of Swan-Ganz catheter insertion in superior vena cava	Ø2WYX2Z
Open revision of right hip replacement, with readjustment of prosthesis	ØSW9ØJZ
Adjustment of position, pacemaker lead in left ventricle, percutaneous	Ø2WA3MZ
External repositioning of Foley catheter to bladder	ØTWBXØZ
Taking out loose screw and putting larger screw in fracture repair plate, left tibia	ØQWHØ4Z
Revision of VAD reservoir placement in chest wall, causing patient discomfort, open	ØJWTØWZ
Thoracotomy with exploration of right pleural cavity	ØWJ9ØZZ
Diagnostic laryngoscopy	ØCJS8ZZ
Exploratory arthrotomy of left knee	ØSJDØZZ
Colposcopy with diagnostic hysteroscopy	ØUJD8ZZ
Digital rectal exam	ØDJD7ZZ
Diagnostic arthroscopy of right shoulder	ØRJJ4ZZ
Endoscopy of maxillary sinus	Ø9JY4ZZ
Laparotomy with palpation of liver	ØFJØØZZ
Transurethral diagnostic cystoscopy	ØTJB8ZZ
Colonoscopy, discontinued at sigmoid colon	ØDJD8ZZ
Percutaneous mapping of basal ganglia	ØØK83ZZ
Heart catheterization with cardiac mapping	Ø2K83ZZ
Intraoperative whole brain mapping via craniotomy	ØØKØØZZ
Mapping of left cerebral hemisphere, percutaneous endoscopic	ØØK74ZZ
Intraoperative cardiac mapping during open heart surgery	Ø2K8ØZZ
Hysteroscopy with cautery of post-hysterectomy oozing and evacuation of clot	ØW3R8ZZ
Open exploration and ligation of post-op arterial bleeder, left forearm	ØX3FØZZ

Procedure	Code
Control of post-operative retroperitoneal bleeding via laparotomy	ØW3HØZZ
Reopening of thoracotomy site with drainage and control of post-op hemopericardium	ØW3DØZZ
Arthroscopy with drainage of hemarthrosis at previous operative site, right knee	ØY3F4ZZ
Radiocarpal fusion of left hand with internal fixation, open	ØRGPØ4Z
Posterior spinal fusion at L1-L3 level with BAK cage interbody fusion device, open	ØSG1ØAJ
Intercarpal fusion of right hand with bone bank bone graft, open	ØRGQØKZ
Sacrococcygeal fusion with bone graft from same operative site, open	ØSG5Ø7Z
Interphalangeal fusion of left great toe, percutaneous pin fixation	ØSGQ34Z
Suture repair of left radial nerve laceration	Ø1Q6ØZZ (The approach value is *Open*, though the surgical exposure may have been created by the wound itself.)
Laparotomy with suture repair of blunt force duodenal laceration	ØDQ9ØZZ
Perineoplasty with repair of old obstetric laceration, open	ØWQNØZZ
Suture repair of right biceps tendon laceration, open	ØLQ3ØZZ
Closure of abdominal wall stab wound	ØWQFØZZ
Cosmetic face lift, open, no other information available	ØWØ2ØZZ
Bilateral breast augmentation with silicone implants, open	ØHØVØJZ
Cosmetic rhinoplasty with septal reduction and tip elevation using local tissue graft, open	Ø9ØKØ7Z
Abdominoplasty (tummy tuck), open	ØWØFØZZ
Liposuction of bilateral thighs	ØJØL3ZZ, ØJØM3ZZ
Creation of penis in female patient using tissue bank donor graft	ØW4NØK1
Creation of vagina in male patient using synthetic material	ØW4MØJØ
Laparoscopic vertical (sleeve) gastrectomy	ØDB64Z3
Left uterine artery embolization with intraluminal biosphere injection	Ø4LF3DU

Obstetrics

Procedure	Code
Abortion by dilation and evacuation following laminaria insertion	10A07ZW
Manually assisted spontaneous abortion	10E0XZZ (Since the pregnancy was not artificially terminated, this is coded to *Delivery* because it captures the procedure objective. The fact that it was an abortion will be identified in the diagnosis code.)
Abortion by abortifacient insertion	10A07ZX
Bimanual pregnancy examination	10J07ZZ
Extraperitoneal C-section, low transverse incision	10D00Z2
Fetal spinal tap, percutaneous	10903ZA
Fetal kidney transplant, laparoscopic	10Y04ZS
Open in utero repair of congenital diaphragmatic hernia	10Q00ZK (Diaphragm is classified to the *Respiratory* body system in the *Medical and Surgical* section.)
Laparoscopy with total excision of tubal pregnancy	10T24ZZ
Transvaginal removal of fetal monitoring electrode	10P073Z

Placement

Procedure	Code
Placement of packing material, right ear	2Y42X5Z
Mechanical traction of entire left leg	2W6MX0Z
Removal of splint, right shoulder	2W5AX1Z
Placement of neck brace	2W32X3Z
Change of vaginal packing	2Y04X5Z
Packing of wound, chest wall	2W44X5Z
Sterile dressing placement to left groin region	2W27X4Z
Removal of packing material from pharynx	2Y50X5Z
Placement of intermittent pneumatic compression device, covering entire right arm	2W18X7Z
Exchange of pressure dressing to left thigh	2W0PX6Z

Administration

Procedure	Code
Peritoneal dialysis via indwelling catheter	3E1M39Z
Transvaginal artificial insemination	3E0P7LZ
Infusion of total parenteral nutrition via central venous catheter	3E0436Z
Esophagogastroscopy with Botox injection into esophageal sphincter	3E0G8GC (Botulinum toxin is a paralyzing agent with temporary effects; it does not sclerose or destroy the nerve.)
Percutaneous irrigation of knee joint	3E1U38Z
Epidural injection of mixed steroid and local anesthetic for pain control	3E0S33Z and 3E0U3NZ (This is coded to the substance value *Anti-inflammatory*.)
Transfusion of antihemophilic factor, (nonautologous) via arterial central line	30263V1
Transabdominal in vitro fertilization, implantation of donor ovum	3E0P3Q1
Autologous bone marrow transplant via central venous line	30243G0
Implantation of anti-microbial envelope with cardiac defibrillator placement, open	3E0102A
Sclerotherapy of brachial plexus lesion, alcohol injection	3E0T3TZ
Percutaneous peripheral vein injection, glucarpidase	3E033GQ
Introduction of anti-infective envelope into subcutaneous tissue, open	3E0102A

Measurement and Monitoring

Procedure	Code
Cardiac stress test, single measurement	4A02XM4
EGD with biliary flow measurement	4A0C85Z
Right and left heart cardiac catheterization with bilateral sampling and pressure measurements	4A023N8
Temperature monitoring, rectal	4A1Z7KZ
Peripheral venous pulse, external, single measurement	4A04XJ1
Holter monitoring	4A12X45
Respiratory rate, external, single measurement	4A09XCZ
Fetal heart rate monitoring, transvaginal	4A1H7CZ
Visual mobility test, single measurement	4A07X7Z
Left ventricular cardiac output monitoring from pulmonary artery wedge (Swan-Ganz) catheter	4A1239Z
Olfactory acuity test, single measurement	4A08X0Z

Extracorporeal Assistance and Performance

Procedure	Code
Intermittent mechanical ventilation, 16 hours	5A1935Z
Liver dialysis, single encounter	5A1CØØZ
Cardiac countershock with successful conversion to sinus rhythm	5A22Ø4Z
IPPB (intermittent positive pressure breathing) for mobilization of secretions, 22 hours	5AØ9358
Renal dialysis, series of encounters	5A1D6ØZ
IABP (intra-aortic balloon pump) continuous	5AØ221Ø
Intra-operative cardiac pacing, continuous	5A1223Z
ECMO (extracorporeal membrane oxygenation), continuous	5A15223
Controlled mechanical ventilation (CMV), 45 hours	5A1945Z (The endotracheal tube associated with the mechanical ventilation procedure is considered a component of the equipment used in performing the procedure and is not coded separately.)
Pulsatile compression boot with intermittent inflation	5AØ2115 (This is coded to the function value *Cardiac Output*, because the purpose of such compression devices is to return blood to the heart faster.)

Extracorporeal Therapies

Procedure	Code
Donor thrombocytapheresis, single encounter	6A55ØZ2
Bili-lite phototherapy, series treatment	6A651ZZ
Whole body hypothermia, single treatment	6A4ZØZZ
Circulatory phototherapy, single encounter	6A65ØZZ
Shock wave therapy of plantar fascia, single treatment	6A93ØZZ
Antigen-free air conditioning, series treatment	6AØZ1ZZ
TMS (transcranial magnetic stimulation), series treatment	6A221ZZ
Therapeutic ultrasound of peripheral vessels, single treatment	6A75ØZ6
Plasmapheresis, series treatment	6A551Z3
Extracorporeal electromagnetic stimulation (EMS) for urinary incontinence, single treatment	6A21ØZZ

Osteopathic

Procedures	Code
Isotonic muscle energy treatment of right leg	7WØ6X8Z
Low velocity-high amplitude osteopathic treatment of head	7WØØX5Z
Lymphatic pump osteopathic treatment of left axilla	7WØ7X6Z
Indirect osteopathic treatment of sacrum	7WØ4X4Z
Articulatory osteopathic treatment of cervical region	7WØ1XØZ

Other Procedures

Procedure	Code
Near infrared spectroscopy of leg vessels	8EØ23DZ
CT computer assisted sinus surgery	8EØ9XBG (The primary procedure is coded separately.)
Suture removal, abdominal wall	8EØWXY8
Isolation after infectious disease exposure	8EØZXY6
Robotic assisted open prostatectomy	8EØWØCZ (The primary procedure is coded separately.)
In vitro fertilization	8EØZXY1

Chiropractic

Procedure	Code
Chiropractic treatment of lumbar region using long lever specific contact	9WB3XGZ
Chiropractic manipulation of abdominal region, indirect visceral	9WB9XCZ
Chiropractic extra-articular treatment of hip region	9WB6XDZ
Chiropractic treatment of sacrum using long and short lever specific contact	9WB4XJZ
Mechanically-assisted chiropractic manipulation of head	9WBØXKZ

Imaging

Procedure	Code
Noncontrast CT of abdomen and pelvis	BW21ZZZ
Intravascular ultrasound, left subclavian artery	B342ZZ3
Fluoroscopic guidance for insertion of central venous catheter in SVC, low osmolar contrast	B5181ZA
Chest x-ray, AP/PA and lateral views	BW03ZZZ
Endoluminal ultrasound of gallbladder and bile ducts	BF43ZZZ
MRI of thyroid gland, contrast unspecified	BG34YZZ
Esophageal videofluoroscopy study with oral barium contrast	BD11YZZ
Portable x-ray study of right radius/ulna shaft, standard series	BP0JZZZ
Routine fetal ultrasound, second trimester twin gestation	BY4DZZZ
CT scan of bilateral lungs, high osmolar contrast with densitometry	BB240ZZ
Fluoroscopic guidance for percutaneous transluminal angioplasty (PTA) of left common femoral artery, low osmolar contrast	B41G1ZZ

Nuclear Medicine

Procedure	Code
Tomo scan of right and left heart, unspecified radiopharmaceutical, qualitative gated rest	C226YZZ
Technetium pentetate assay of kidneys, ureters, and bladder	CT631ZZ
Uniplanar scan of spine using technetium oxidronate, with first-pass study	CP151ZZ
Thallous chloride tomographic scan of bilateral breasts	CH22SZZ
PET scan of myocardium using rubidium	C23GQZZ
Gallium citrate scan of head and neck, single plane imaging	CW1BLZZ
Xenon gas nonimaging probe of brain	C050VZZ
Upper GI scan, radiopharmaceutical unspecified, for gastric emptying	CD15YZZ
Carbon 11 PET scan of brain with quantification	C030BZZ
Iodinated albumin nuclear medicine assay, blood plasma volume study	C763HZZ

Radiation Therapy

Procedure	Code
Plaque radiation of left eye, single port	D8Y0FZZ
8 MeV photon beam radiation to brain	D0011ZZ
IORT of colon, 3 ports	DDY5CZZ
HDR brachytherapy of prostate using palladium-103	DV109BZ
Electron radiation treatment of right breast, with custom device	DM013ZZ
Hyperthermia oncology treatment of pelvic region	DWY68ZZ
Contact radiation of tongue	D9Y57ZZ
Heavy particle radiation treatment of pancreas, four risk sites	DF034ZZ
LDR brachytherapy to spinal cord using iodine	D016B9Z
Whole body Phosphorus 32 administration with risk to hematopoetic system	DWY5GFZ

Physical Rehabilitation and Diagnostic Audiology

Procedure	Code
Bekesy assessment using audiometer	F13Z31Z
Individual fitting of left eye prosthesis	F0DZ8UZ
Physical therapy for range of motion and mobility, patient right hip, no special equipment	F07L0ZZ
Bedside swallow assessment using assessment kit	F00ZHYZ
Caregiver training in airway clearance techniques	F0FZ8ZZ
Application of short arm cast in rehabilitation setting	F0DZ7EZ (Inhibitory cast is listed in the equipment reference table under E, *Orthosis*.)
Verbal assessment of patient's pain level	F02ZFZZ
Caregiver training in communication skills using manual communication board	F0FZJMZ (Manual communication board is listed in the equipment reference table under M, *Augmentative/ Alternative Communication*.)
Group musculoskeletal balance training exercises, whole body, no special equipment	F07M6ZZ (Balance training is included in the motor treatment reference table under *Therapeutic Exercise*.)
Individual therapy for auditory processing using tape recorder	F09Z2KZ (Tape recorder is listed in the equipment reference table under *Audiovisual Equipment*.)

Mental Health

Procedure	Code
Cognitive-behavioral psychotherapy, individual	GZ58ZZZ
Narcosynthesis	GZGZZZZ
Light therapy	GZJZZZZ
ECT (electroconvulsive therapy), unilateral, multiple seizure	GZB1ZZZ
Crisis intervention	GZ2ZZZZ
Neuropsychological testing	GZ13ZZZ
Hypnosis	GZFZZZZ
Developmental testing	GZ1ØZZZ
Vocational counseling	GZ61ZZZ
Family psychotherapy	GZ72ZZZ

Substance Abuse Treatment

Procedure	Code
Naltrexone treatment for drug dependency	HZ94ZZZ
Substance abuse treatment family counseling	HZ63ZZZ
Medication monitoring of patient on methadone maintenance	HZ81ZZZ
Individual interpersonal psychotherapy for drug abuse	HZ54ZZZ
Patient in for alcohol detoxification treatment	HZ2ZZZZ
Group motivational counseling	HZ47ZZZ
Individual 12-step psychotherapy for substance abuse	HZ53ZZZ
Post-test infectious disease counseling for IV drug abuser	HZ3CZZZ
Psychodynamic psychotherapy for drug dependent patient	HZ5CZZZ
Group cognitive-behavioral counseling for substance abuse	HZ42ZZZ

Appendix I: Procedure Combination Tables

The tables below were developed to help simplify the relationship between ICD-1Ø-PCS coding and MS-DRG assignment. The Centers for Medicare & Medicaid Services (CMS) has identified in the MS-DRG v31R Definitions Manual certain procedure combinations that must occur in order to assign a specific MS-DRG. There are many factors influencing MS-DRG assignment, including principal and secondary diagnoses, MCC or CC use, sex of the patient, and discharge status. These tables should be used only as a guide.

Note: In some cases the Combination Only and Combination Member codes are not identified as having any other procedures that, when coded together, would influence the MS-DRG assignment. These codes are listed under a footnote titled "No Procedure Combinations Specified" directly under the table in which the code is found.

DRG ØØ1-ØØ2 Heart Transplant or Implant of Heart Assist System

Insertion With Removal of Heart Assist System

Type of Heart Assist System	Code as appropriate Insertion by approach	Code also as appropriate Removal of Heart Assist System by approach
External	Ø2HA[Ø,4]R[S,Z] or Ø2HA3RS	Ø2PA[Ø,3,4]RZ

Revision With Removal of Heart Assist System

Type of Heart Assist System	Code as appropriate Revision by approach	Code also as appropriate Removal of Heart Assist System by approach
Implantable	Ø2WA[Ø,3,4]QZ	Ø2PA[Ø,3,4]RZ
External	Ø2WA[Ø,3,4]RZ	Ø2PA[Ø,3,4]RZ

DRG ØØ8 Simultaneous Pancreas/Kidney Transplant

Transplanted Body Part Laterality	Code Transplant as appropriate by tissue type			Code also Pancreas Transplant as appropriate by tissue type		
	Allogeneic	Syngeneic	Zooplastic	Allogeneic	Syngeneic	Zooplastic
Kidney, Right	ØTYØØZØ	ØTYØØZ1	ØTYØØZ2	ØFYGØZØ	ØFYGØZ1	ØFYGØZ2
Kidney, Left	ØTY1ØZØ	ØTY1ØZ1	ØTY1ØZ2	ØFYGØZØ	ØFYGØZ1	ØFYGØZ2

DRG Ø23-Ø27 Craniotomy

Site of Neurostimulator Lead	Code as appropriate Insertion of Lead by approach	Code also as appropriate Insertion of Device by type and subcutaneous site						
		Neuro-stimulator Generator	Stimulator Multiple Array Code as appropriate by approach			Stimulator Multiple Array, Rechargeable Code as appropriate by approach		
		Skull	Chest	Back	Abdomen	Chest	Back	Abdomen
Brain	ØØHØ[Ø,3,4]MZ	ØNHØØNZ	ØJH6[Ø,3]DZ	ØJH7[Ø,3]DZ	ØJH8[Ø,3]DZ	ØJH6[Ø,3]EZ	ØJH7[Ø,3]EZ	ØJH8[Ø,3]EZ
Cerebral Ventricle	ØØH6[Ø,3,4]MZ	ØNHØØNZ	ØJH6[Ø,3]DZ	ØJH7[Ø,3]DZ	ØJH8[Ø,3]DZ	ØJH6[Ø,3]EZ	ØJH7[Ø,3]EZ	ØJH8[Ø,3]EZ

DRG Ø28-Ø3Ø Spinal Procedures

Generator Type	Insertion of Generator by Site			Code also as appropriate Insertion of Neurostimulator Lead by approach	
	Chest	Abdomen	Back	Spinal Canal	Spinal Cord
Single Array	ØJH6[Ø,3]BZ	ØJH8[Ø,3]BZ	ØJH7[Ø,3]BZ	ØØHU[Ø,3,4]MZ	ØØHV[Ø,3,4]MZ
Single Array, Rechargeable	ØJH6[Ø,3]CZ	ØJH8[Ø,3]CZ	ØJH7[Ø,3]CZ	ØØHU[Ø,3,4]MZ	ØØHV[Ø,3,4]MZ
Multiple Array	ØJH6[Ø,3]DZ	ØJH8[Ø,3]DZ	ØJH7[Ø,3]DZ	ØØHU[Ø,3,4]MZ	ØØHV[Ø,3,4]MZ
Multiple Array, Rechargeable	ØJH6[Ø,3]EZ	ØJH8[Ø,3]EZ	ØJH7[Ø,3]EZ	ØØHU[Ø,3,4]MZ	ØØHV[Ø,3,4]MZ

DRG Ø4Ø-Ø42 Peripheral and Cranial Nerve and Other Nervous System Procedures

Insertion of Neurostimulator Lead With Device

Site of Neurostimulator Lead	Code as appropriate Insertion by approach	Code also as appropriate Insertion of Device by type and subcutaneous site					
		Stimulator Single Array Code as appropriate by approach			Stimulator Single Array, Rechargeable Code as appropriate by approach		
		Chest	Back	Abdomen	Chest	Back	Abdomen
Cranial Nerve	ØØHE[Ø,3,4]MZ	ØJH6[Ø,3]BZ	ØJH7[Ø,3]BZ	ØJH8[Ø,3]BZ	ØJH6[Ø,3]CZ	ØJH7[Ø,3]CZ	ØJH8[Ø,3]CZ
Peripheral Nerve	Ø1HY[Ø,3,4]MZ	ØJH6[Ø,3]BZ	ØJH7[Ø,3]BZ	ØJH8[Ø,3]BZ	ØJH6[Ø,3]CZ	ØJH7[Ø,3]CZ	ØJH8[Ø,3]CZ
Stomach	ØDH6[Ø,3,4]MZ	ØJH6[Ø,3]BZ	ØJH7[Ø,3]BZ	ØJH8[Ø,3]BZ	ØJH6[Ø,3]CZ	ØJH7[Ø,3]CZ	ØJH8[Ø,3]CZ
		Stimulator Multiple Array Code as appropriate by approach			Stimulator Multiple Array, Rechargeable Code as appropriate by approach		
		Chest	Back	Abdomen	Chest	Back	Abdomen
Cranial Nerve	ØØHE[Ø,3,4]MZ	ØJH6[Ø,3]DZ	ØJH7[Ø,3]DZ	ØJH8[Ø,3]DZ	ØJH6[Ø,3]EZ	ØJH7[Ø,3]EZ	ØJH8[Ø,3]EZ
Peripheral Nerve	Ø1HY[Ø,3,4]MZ	ØJH6[Ø,3]DZ	ØJH7[Ø,3]DZ	ØJH8[Ø,3]DZ	ØJH6[Ø,3]EZ	ØJH7[Ø,3]EZ	ØJH8[Ø,3]EZ
Stomach	ØDH6[Ø,3,4]MZ	ØJH6[Ø,3]DZ	ØJH7[Ø,3]DZ	ØJH8[Ø,3]DZ	ØJH6[Ø,3]EZ	ØJH7[Ø,3]EZ	ØJH8[Ø,3]EZ

Insertion of Generator and Lead(s) Only

Generator Type	Insertion of Generator by Site		Code also as appropriate Insertion of Cardiac Leads by Site		
	Chest	Abdomen	Coronary Vein	Atrium	Ventricle
Single Chamber	ØJH6[Ø,3]4Z	ØJH8[Ø,3]4Z	Ø2H4[Ø,4][J,M]Z	Ø2H[6,7][Ø,4][J,M]Z or Ø2H[6,7]3JZ	Ø2H[K,L][Ø,3,4][J,M]Z
Single Chamber RR	ØJH6[Ø,3]5Z	ØJH8[Ø,3]5Z	Ø2H4[Ø,4][J,M]Z	Ø2H[6,7][Ø,4][J,M]Z or Ø2H[6,7]3JZ	Ø2H[K,L][Ø,3,4][J,M]Z
Dual Chamber	ØJH6[Ø,3]6Z	ØJH8[Ø,3]6Z	—	—	Ø2H[K,L]3JZ
Cardiac Resynch Pacemaker Pulse Generator	ØJH6[Ø,3]7Z	ØJH8[Ø,3]7Z	Ø2H4[Ø,3,4][J,M]Z or Ø2H43KZ	Ø2H[6,7][Ø,3,4][J,M]Z	Ø2H[K,L][Ø,3,4][J,M]Z
Cardiac Rhythm Related	ØJH6[Ø,3]PZ	ØJH8[Ø,3]PZ	Ø2H4[Ø,4][J,M]Z	Ø2H[6,7][Ø,3,4][J,M]Z	Ø2H[K,L][Ø,3,4][J,M]Z

DRG Ø4Ø-Ø42 Peripheral and Cranial Nerve and Other Nervous System Procedures

(Continued)

Insertion of Generator and Lead(s) into the Coronary Vein, Atrium or Ventricle With Removal of Cardiac Rhythm Device

Generator Type	Insertion of Generator by Site		Code also as appropriate Insertion of Leads by Site			Code also
	Chest	Abdomen	Coronary Vein	Atrium	Ventricle	Removal Cardiac Rhythm Device
Single Chamber	ØJH6[Ø,3]4Z	ØJH8[Ø,3]4Z	Ø2H4[Ø,4][J,M]Z	Ø2H[6,7][Ø,3,4][J,M]Z	Ø2H[K,L][Ø,3,4][J,M]Z	ØJPT[Ø,3]PZ
Single Chamber RR	ØJH6[Ø,3]5Z	ØJH8[Ø,3]5Z	Ø2H4[Ø,4][J,M]Z	Ø2H[6,7][Ø,3,4][J,M]Z	Ø2H[K,L][Ø,3,4][J,M]Z	ØJPT[Ø,3]PZ
Dual Chamber	ØJH6[Ø,3]6Z	ØJH8[Ø,3]6Z	Ø2H4[Ø,4][J,M]Z	Ø2H[6,7][Ø,3,4][J,M]Z	Ø2H[K,L][Ø,3,4][J,M]Z	ØJPT[Ø,3]PZ

Insertion of Generator and Leads into the Pericardium With or Without Removal of Cardiac Rhythm Device

Generator Type	Insertion of Generator by Site		Code also as appropriate Insertion of Cardiac Leads by Type		If Performed – Code also
	Chest	Abdomen	Pericardium		Removal Cardiac Rhythm Device
			Pacemaker	Cardiac	
Single Chamber	ØJH6[Ø,3]4Z	ØJH8[Ø,3]4Z	Ø2HN[Ø,3,4]JZ	Ø2HN[Ø,3,4]MZ	ØJPT[Ø,3]PZ
Single Chamber RR	ØJH6[Ø,3]5Z	ØJH8[Ø,3]5Z	Ø2HN[Ø,3,4]JZ	Ø2HN[Ø,3,4]MZ	ØJPT[Ø,3]PZ
Dual Chamber	ØJH6[Ø,3]6Z	ØJH8[Ø,3]6Z	Ø2HN[Ø,3,4]JZ	Ø2HN[Ø,3,4]MZ	ØJPT[Ø,3]PZ
Cardiac Resynch Pacemaker Pulse Generator	ØJH6[Ø,3]7Z	ØJH8[Ø,3]7Z	Ø2HN[Ø,3,4]JZ	Ø2HN[Ø,3,4]MZ	—
Cardiac Rhythm Related	ØJH6[Ø,3]PZ	ØJH8[Ø,3]PZ	Ø2HN[Ø,3,4]JZ	Ø2HN[Ø,3,4]MZ	—

Insertion of Generator and Lead(s) With Removal of Cardiac Rhythm Device and Leads

Generator Type	Insertion of Generator by Site		Code also as appropriate Insertion of Cardiac Leads by Site		Code also	
	Chest	Abdomen	Atrium	Ventricle	Removal of Cardiac Rhythm Device	Removal of Heart Lead
Single Chamber	ØJH6[Ø,3]4Z	ØJH8[Ø,3]4Z	Ø2H[6,7]3JZ	Ø2H[K,L]3JZ	ØJPT[Ø,3]PZ	Ø2PA[Ø,3,4,X]MZ
Single Chamber RR	ØJH6[Ø,3]5Z	ØJH8[Ø,3]5Z	Ø2H[6,7]3JZ	Ø2H[K,L]3JZ	ØJPT[Ø,3]PZ	Ø2PA[Ø,3,4,X]MZ
Dual Chamber	ØJH6[Ø,3]6Z	ØJH8[Ø,3]6Z	Ø2H[6,7]3JZ	Ø2H[K,L]3JZ	ØJPT[Ø,3]PZ	Ø2PA[Ø,3,4,X]MZ
Cardiac Resynch Pacemaker Pulse Generator	ØJH6[Ø,3]7Z	ØJH8[Ø,3]7Z	Ø2H[6,7]3JZ	Ø2H[K,L]3JZ	—	Ø2PA[Ø,3,4,X]MZ
Cardiac Rhythm Related	ØJH6[Ø,3]PZ	ØJH8[Ø,3]PZ	Ø2H[6,7]3JZ	Ø2H[K,L]3JZ	—	Ø2PA[Ø,3,4,X]MZ

DRG 222-227 Cardiac Defibrillator Implant

Insertion of Generator With Insertion of Lead(s) into Coronary Vein, Atrium or Ventricle

Generator Type	Insertion of Generator by Site		Code also as appropriate Insertion of Leads by site					
	Chest	Abdomen	Coronary Vein	Atrium		Ventricle		
				Right	Left	Right	Left	
Defibrillator	ØJH6[Ø,3]8Z	ØJH8[Ø,3]8Z	Ø2H4[Ø,3,4]KZ	Ø2H6[Ø,3,4]KZ	Ø2H7[Ø,3,4]KZ	Ø2HK[Ø,3,4]KZ	Ø2HL[Ø,3,4]KZ	
Cardiac Resynch Defibrillator Pulse Generator	ØJH6[Ø,3]9Z	ØJH8[Ø,3]9Z	Ø2H4[Ø,3,4]KZ or Ø2H43[J,M]Z	Ø2H6[Ø,3,4]KZ	Ø2H7[Ø,3,4]KZ	Ø2HK[Ø,3,4]KZ	Ø2HL[Ø,3,4]KZ	
Contractility Modulation Device	ØJH6[Ø,3]AZ	ØJH8[Ø,3]AZ	—	—	—	—	Ø2HL[Ø,3,4]MZ	

Insertion of Generator with Insertion of Lead(s) into Pericardium

Generator Type	Insertion of Generator by Site		Code also as appropriate Insertion of Leads by Type		
	Chest	Abdomen	Pericardium		
			Pacemaker	Defibrillator	Cardiac
Defibrillator	ØJH6[Ø,3]8Z	ØJH8[Ø,3]8Z	Ø2HN[Ø,3,4]JZ	Ø2HN[Ø,3,4]KZ	Ø2HN[Ø,3,4]MZ
Cardiac Resynch Defibrillator Pulse Generator	ØJH6[Ø,3]9Z	ØJH8[Ø,3]9Z	Ø2HN[Ø,3,4]JZ	Ø2HN[Ø,3,4]KZ	Ø2HN[Ø,3,4]MZ

DRG 242-244 Permanent Cardiac Pacemaker Implant

Insertion of Generator and Lead(s) Only

Generator Type	Insertion of Generator by Site		Code also as appropriate Insertion of Cardiac Leads by Site		
	Chest	Abdomen	Coronary Vein	Atrium	Ventricle
Single Chamber	ØJH6[Ø,3]4Z	ØJH8[Ø,3]4Z	Ø2H4[Ø,4][J,M]Z	Ø2H[6,7][Ø,4][J,M]Z or Ø2H[6,7]3JZ	Ø2H[K,L][Ø,3,4][J,M]Z
Single Chamber RR	ØJH6[Ø,3]5Z	ØJH8[Ø,3]5Z	Ø2H4[Ø,4][J,M]Z	Ø2H[6,7][Ø,4][J,M]Z or Ø2H[6,7]3JZ	Ø2H[K,L][Ø,3,4][J,M]Z
Dual Chamber	ØJH6[Ø,3]6Z	ØJH8[Ø,3]6Z	—	—	Ø2H[K,L]3JZ
Cardiac Resynch Pacemaker Pulse Generator	ØJH6[Ø,3]7Z	ØJH8[Ø,3]7Z	Ø2H4[Ø,3,4][J,M]Z or Ø2H43KZ	Ø2H[6,7][Ø,3,4][J,M]Z	Ø2H[K,L][Ø,3,4][J,M]Z
Cardiac Rhythm Related	ØJH6[Ø,3]PZ	ØJH8[Ø,3]PZ	Ø2H4[Ø,4][J,M]Z	Ø2H[6,7][Ø,3,4][J,M]Z	Ø2H[K,L][Ø,3,4][J,M]Z

Insertion of Generator and Lead(s) into the Coronary Vein, Atrium or Ventricle With Removal of Cardiac Rhythm Device

Generator Type	Insertion of Generator by Site		Code also as appropriate Insertion of Cardiac Leads by site			Code also
	Chest	Abdomen	Coronary Vein	Atrium	Ventricle	Removal Cardiac Rhythm Device
Single Chamber	ØJH6[Ø,3]4Z	ØJH8[Ø,3]4Z	Ø2H4[Ø,4][J,M]Z	Ø2H[6,7][Ø,3,4][J,M]Z	Ø2H[K,L][Ø,3,4][J,M]Z	ØJPT[Ø,3]PZ
Single Chamber RR	ØJH6[Ø,3]5Z	ØJH8[Ø,3]5Z	Ø2H4[Ø,4][J,M]Z	Ø2H[6,7][Ø,3,4][J,M]Z	Ø2H[K,L][Ø,3,4][J,M]Z	ØJPT[Ø,3]PZ
Dual Chamber	ØJH6[Ø,3]6Z	ØJH8[Ø,3]6Z	Ø2H4[Ø,4][J,M]Z	Ø2H[6,7][Ø,3,4][J,M]Z	Ø2H[K,L][Ø,3,4][J,M]Z	ØJPT[Ø,3]PZ

DRG 242-244 Permanent Cardiac Pacemaker Implant *(Continued)*

Insertion of Generator and Lead(s) into the Pericardium With or Without Removal of Cardiac Rhythm Device

Generator Type	Insertion of Generator by Site		Code also as appropriate Insertion of Leads by type		If Performed–Code also
	Chest	Abdomen	Pericardium		Removal Cardiac Rhythm Device
			Pacemaker	Cardiac	
Single Chamber	ØJH6[Ø,3]4Z	ØJH8[Ø,3]4Z	Ø2HN[Ø,3,4]JZ	Ø2HN[Ø,3,4]MZ	ØJPT[Ø,3]PZ
Single Chamber RR	ØJH6[Ø,3]5Z	ØJH8[Ø,3]5Z	Ø2HN[Ø,3,4]JZ	Ø2HN[Ø,3,4]MZ	ØJPT[Ø,3]PZ
Dual Chamber	ØJH6[Ø,3]6Z	ØJH8[Ø,3]6Z	Ø2HN[Ø,3,4]JZ	Ø2HN[Ø,3,4]MZ	ØJPT[Ø,3]PZ
Cardiac Resynch Pacemaker Pulse Generator	ØJH6[Ø,3]7Z	ØJH8[Ø,3]7Z	Ø2HN[Ø,3,4]JZ	Ø2HN[Ø,3,4]MZ	—
Cardiac Rhythm Related	ØJH6[Ø,3]PZ	ØJH8[Ø,3]PZ	Ø2HN[Ø,3,4]JZ	Ø2HN[Ø,3,4]MZ	—

Insertion of Generator and Lead(s) With Removal of Cardiac Rhythm Device and Leads

Generator Type	Insertion of Generator by Site		Code also as appropriate Insertion of Cardiac Leads by Site		Code also	
	Chest	Abdomen	Atrium	Ventricle	Removal of Cardiac Rhythm Device	Removal of Heart Lead
Single Chamber	ØJH6[Ø,3]4Z	ØJH8[Ø,3]4Z	Ø2H[6,7]3JZ	Ø2H[K,L]3JZ	ØJPT[Ø,3]PZ	Ø2PA[Ø,3,4,X]MZ
Single Chamber RR	ØJH6[Ø,3]5Z	ØJH8[Ø,3]5Z	Ø2H[6,7]3JZ	Ø2H[K,L]3JZ	ØJPT[Ø,3]PZ	Ø2PA[Ø,3,4,X]MZ
Dual Chamber	ØJH6[Ø,3]6Z	ØJH8[Ø,3]6Z	Ø2H[6,7]3JZ	Ø2H[K,L]3JZ	ØJPT[Ø,3]PZ	Ø2PA[Ø,3,4,X]MZ
Cardiac Resynch Pacemaker Pulse Generator	ØJH6[Ø,3]7Z	ØJH8[Ø,3]7Z	Ø2H[6,7]3JZ	Ø2H[K,L]3JZ	—	Ø2PA[Ø,3,4,X]MZ
Cardiac Rhythm Related	ØJH6[Ø,3]PZ	ØJH8[Ø,3]PZ	Ø2H[6,7]3JZ	Ø2H[K,L]3JZ	—	Ø2PA[Ø,3,4,X]MZ

DRG 258-259 Cardiac Pacemaker Device Replacement

Generator Type	Insertion of Generator by Site		Code also as appropriate Insertion Cardiac Rhythm Device by approach	
	Chest	Abdomen	Open	Percutaneous
Pacemaker, Single Chamber	ØJH6[Ø,3]4Z	ØJH8[Ø,3]4Z	ØJPTØPZ	ØJPT3PZ
Pacemaker, Single Chamber Rate Responsive	ØJH6[Ø,3]5Z	ØJH8[Ø,3]5Z	ØJPTØPZ	ØJPT3PZ
Pacemaker, Dual Chamber	ØJH6[Ø,3]6Z	ØJH8[Ø,3]6Z	ØJPTØPZ	ØJPT3PZ

DRG 26Ø-262 Cardiac Pacemaker Revision Except Device Replacement

Site	Removal of Lead by approach	Code also as appropriate Insertion by percutaneous approach of Cardiac Leads by site			
		Atrium		Ventricle	
		Right	Left	Right	Left
Heart	Ø2PA[Ø,3,4,X]MZ	Ø2H63JZ	Ø2H73JZ	Ø2HK3JZ	Ø2HL3JZ

DRG 264 Other Circulatory Procedures

Device Type	Insertion of Device by approach	Code also as appropriate insertion of Hemodynamic Monitoring Device by Subcutaneous Site	
		Chest	Abdomen
Monitoring Device, Pressure Sensor	Ø2HK[Ø,3,4]ØZ	ØJH6[Ø,3]ØZ	ØJH8[Ø,3]ØZ
Monitoring Device	Ø2HK[Ø,3,4]2Z	ØJH6[Ø,3]ØZ	ØJH8[Ø,3]ØZ

DRG 326-328 Stomach, Esophageal and Duodenal Procedures

Site	Resection by Open Approach	Code also as appropriate Resection of Pancreas by Open Approach
Duodenum	ØDT9ØZZ	ØFTGØZZ

DRG 344-346 Minor Small and Large Bowel Procedures

Site	Repair by Open Approach	Code also as appropriate Repair by external approach of Abdominal Wall Stoma
Small Intestine	ØDQ8ØZZ	ØWQFXZ2
Duodenum	ØDQ9ØZZ	ØWQFXZ2
Jejunum	ØDQAØZZ	ØWQFXZ2
Ileum	ØDQBØZZ	ØWQFXZ2
Large Intestine	ØDQEØZZ	ØWQFXZ2
Large Intestine, Right	ØDQFØZZ	ØWQFXZ2
Large Intestine, Left	ØDQGØZZ	ØWQFXZ2
Cecum	ØDQHØZZ	ØWQFXZ2
Ascending Colon	ØDQKØZZ	ØWQFXZ2
Transverse Colon	ØDQLØZZ	ØWQFXZ2
Descending Colon	ØDQMØZZ	ØWQFXZ2
Sigmoid Colon	ØDQNØZZ	ØWQFXZ2

DRG 485-489 Knee Procedures

Joint	Removal of Liner by open approach	Code also as appropriate Supplement of Tibial Surface by site
Knee, RT	ØSPCØ9Z	ØSUVØ9Z
Knee, LT	ØSPDØ9Z	ØSUWØ9Z

DRG 461-462 Bilateral or Multiple Major Joint Procedures of Lower Extremity

Joint	Removal of Device by approach	Code also as appropriate Replacement of Device with Synthetic Substitute by Device Type			
		Metal	Metal on Poly	Ceramic	Synth Subst
Hip, Right	ØSP9ØJZ	ØSR9Ø1[9,A,Z]	ØSR9Ø2[9,A,Z]	ØSR9Ø3[9,A,Z]	ØSR9ØJ[9,A,Z]
Hip, Left	ØSPBØJZ	ØSRBØ1[9,A,Z]	ØSRBØ2[9,A,Z]	ØSRBØ3[9,A,Z]	ØSRBØJ[9,A,Z]
Knee, Right	ØSPC[Ø,4]JZ	—	—	—	ØSRCØJ[9,A,Z]
Knee, Left	ØSPD[Ø,4]JZ	—	—	—	ØSRDØJ[9,A,Z]

DRG 466-468 Revision of Hip or Knee Replacement

Removal of Hip Joint Liner With Supplement of Liner

Joint	Removal of Liner by open approach	Code also as appropriate Supplement of Liner by Site		
		Joint	Acetabular Surface	Femoral Surface
Hip, RT	ØSP9Ø9Z	ØSU9Ø9Z	ØSUAØ9Z	ØSURØ9Z
Hip, LT	ØSPBØ9Z	ØSUBØ9Z	ØSUEØ9Z	ØSUSØ9Z

Removal of Hip Joint Device With Replacement

Hip Joint/Surface	Removal by Open approach of Synthetic Substitute	Code also as appropriate Replacement by Open approach With Synthetic Substitute by Device Type				
		Polyethylene	Metal	Metal on Poly	Ceramic	Synth Subst
Joint, Right	ØSP9ØJZ	—	ØSR9Ø1[9,A,Z]	ØSR9Ø2[9,A,Z]	ØSR9Ø3[9,A,Z]	ØSR9ØJ[9,A,Z]
Joint, Left	ØSPBØJZ	—	ØSRBØ1[9,A,Z]	ØSRBØ2[9,A,Z]	ØSRBØ3[9,A,Z]	ØSRBØJ[9,A,Z]
Acetabular Surface, Right	ØSP9ØJZ	ØSRAØØ[9,A,Z]	ØSRAØ1[9,A,Z]	—	ØSRAØ3[9,A,Z]	ØSRAØJ[9,A,Z]
Acetabular Surface, Left	ØSPBØJZ	ØSREØØ[9,A,Z]	ØSREØ1[9,A,Z]	—	ØSREØ3[9,A,Z]	ØSREØJ[9,A,Z]
Femoral Surface, Right	ØSP9ØJZ	—	ØSRRØ1[9,A,Z]	—	ØSRRØ3[9,A,Z]	ØSRRØJ[9,A,Z]
Femoral Surface, Left	ØSPBØJZ	—	ØSRSØ1[9,A,Z]	—	ØSRSØ3[9,A,Z]	ØSRSØJ[9,A,Z]

Removal of Knee Joint Device With Replacement

Site	Removal of Device by approach		Code also as appropriate Replacement of Device by Site		
	Open	Percutaneous Endoscopic	Joint	Femoral Surface	Tibial Surface
Knee Joint, RT	ØSPCØJZ	—	ØSRCØJ[9,A,Z]	ØSRTØJZ	ØSRVØJZ
Knee Joint, RT	—	ØSPC4JZ	ØSRCØJ[9,A,Z]	—	—
Knee Joint, LT	ØSPDØJZ	—	ØSRDØJ[9,A,Z]	ØSRUØJZ	ØSRWØJZ
Knee Joint, LT	—	ØSPD4JZ	ØSRDØJ[9,A,Z]	—	—

DRG 49Ø-491 Back and Neck Procedures, Except Spinal Fusion

Generator Type	Insertion of Generator by Site			Code also as appropriate Insertion Neurostimulator Lead by approach and Site	
	Chest	Abdomen	Back	Spinal Canal	Spinal Cord
Single Array	ØJH6[Ø,3]BZ	ØJH8[Ø,3]BZ	ØJH7[Ø,3]BZ	ØØHU[Ø,3,4]MZ	ØØHV[Ø,3,4]MZ
Single Array, Rechargeable	ØJH6[Ø,3]CZ	ØJH8[Ø,3]CZ	ØJH7[Ø,3]CZ	ØØHU[Ø,3,4]MZ	ØØHV[Ø,3,4]MZ
Multiple Array	ØJH6[Ø,3]DZ	ØJH8[Ø,3]DZ	ØJH7[Ø,3]DZ	ØØHU[Ø,3,4]MZ	ØØHV[Ø,3,4]MZ
Multiple Array, Rechargeable	ØJH6[Ø,3]EZ	ØJH8[Ø,3]EZ	ØJH7[Ø,3]EZ	ØØHU[Ø,3,4]MZ	ØØHV[Ø,3,4]MZ

DRG 515-517 Other Musculoskeletal System and Connective Tissue Procedures

Site	Reposition of Vertebra by percutaneous approach	Code also as appropriate Supplement With Synthetic Substitute by Percutaneous Approach at site of Repositioned Vertebra
Cervical	ØPS33ZZ	ØPU33JZ
Coccyx	ØQSS3ZZ	ØQUS3JZ
Lumbar	ØQSØ3ZZ	ØQUØ3JZ
Sacrum	ØQS13ZZ	ØQU13JZ
Thoracic	ØPS43ZZ	ØPU43JZ

DRG 582-583 Mastectomy for Malignancy

Site	Resection by Open approach	Code also as appropriate Resection of Lymph Nodes by Open approach by site			Code also as appropriate Resection of Thorax Muscle by Open approach	
		Axillary	Internal Mammary	Thorax	Right	Left
Breast, Right	ØHTTØZZ	Ø7T5ØZZ	Ø7T8ØZZ	Ø7T7ØZZ	ØKTHØZZ	—
Breast, Left	ØHTUØZZ	Ø7T6ØZZ	Ø7T9ØZZ	Ø7T7ØZZ	—	ØKTJØZZ
Breast, Bilateral	ØHTVØZZ	Ø7T5ØZZ and Ø7T6ØZZ	Ø7T8ØZZ and Ø7T9ØZZ	Ø7T7ØZZ	ØKTHØZZ	ØKTJØZZ

DRG 584-585 Breast Biopsy, Local Excision and Other Breast procedures

Resection of Breast With Resection of Lymph Nodes and Thorax Muscle

Site	Resection by Open approach	Code also as appropriate Resection of Lymph Nodes by Open approach by site			Code also as appropriate Resection of Thorax Muscle by Open approach	
		Axillary	Internal Mammary	Thorax	Right	Left
Breast, Right	ØHTTØZZ	Ø7T5ØZZ	Ø7T8ØZZ	Ø7T7ØZZ	ØKTHØZZ	—
Breast, Left	ØHTUØZZ	Ø7T6ØZZ	Ø7T9ØZZ	Ø7T7ØZZ	—	ØKTJØZZ
Breast, Bilateral	ØHTVØZZ	Ø7T5ØZZ and Ø7T6ØZZ	Ø7T8ØZZ and Ø7T9ØZZ	Ø7T7ØZZ	ØKTHØZZ	ØKTJØZZ

Replacement of Breast Tissue

Site	Replacement by Percutaneous approach with Autologous Tissue	Code also as appropriate Extraction of Subcutaneous Tissue by Percutaneous approach					
		Abdomen	Back	Buttock	Chest	Leg, Upper, Right	Leg, Upper, Left
Breast, Right	ØHRT37Z	ØJD83ZZ	ØJD73ZZ	ØJD93ZZ	ØJD63ZZ	ØJDL3ZZ	ØJDM3ZZ
Breast, Left	ØHRU37Z	ØJD83ZZ	ØJD73ZZ	ØJD93ZZ	ØJD63ZZ	ØJDL3ZZ	ØJDM3ZZ
Breast, Bilateral	ØHRV37Z	ØJD83ZZ	ØJD73ZZ	ØJD93ZZ	ØJD63ZZ	ØJDL3ZZ	ØJDM3ZZ

DRG 628-630 Other Endocrine, Nutritional and Metabolic Procedures

Hip Joint/Surface	Removal by Open approach	Code also as appropriate Replacement by Open approach With Synthetic Substitute by Device Type				
		Polyethylene	Metal	Metal on Poly	Ceramic	Synth Subst
Joint, Right	ØSP9ØJZ	—	ØSR901[9,A,Z]	ØSR902[9,A,Z]	ØSR903[9,A,Z]	ØSR9ØJ[9,A,Z]
Joint, Left	ØSPBØJZ	—	ØSRBØ1[9,A,Z]	ØSRBØ2[9,A,Z]	ØSRBØ3[9,A,Z]	ØSRBØJ[9,A,Z]
Acetabular Surface, Right	ØSP9ØJZ	ØSRAØØ[9,A,Z]	ØSRAØ1[9,A,Z]	—	ØSRAØ3[9,A,Z]	ØSRAØJ[9,A,Z]
Acetabular Surface, Left	ØSPBØJZ	ØSREØØ[9,A,Z]	ØSREØ1[9,A,Z]	—	ØSREØ3[9,A,Z]	ØSREØJ[9,A,Z]
Femoral Surface, Right	ØSP9ØJZ	—	ØSRRØ1[9,A,Z]	—	ØSRRØ3[9,A,Z]	ØSRRØJ[9,A,Z]
Femoral Surface, Left	ØSPBØJZ	—	ØSRSØ1[9,A,Z]	—	ØSRSØ3[9,A,Z]	ØSRSØJ[9,A,Z]

DRG 665-667 Prostatectomy

Site	Resection by approach				Code also as appropriate Resection of Seminal Vesicles, Bilateral by approach	
	Open	Percutaneous Endoscopic	Via Natural or Artificial Opening	Via Natural or Artificial Opening Endoscopic	Open	Percutaneous Endoscopic
Prostate	ØVTØØZZ	ØVTØ4ZZ	ØVTØ7ZZ	ØVTØ8ZZ	ØVT3ØZZ	ØVT34ZZ

DRG 7Ø7-7Ø8 Major Male Pelvic Procedures

Site	Resection by approach				Code also as appropriate Resection of Seminal Vesicles, Bilateral by approach	
	Open	Percutaneous Endoscopic	Via Natural or Artificial Opening	Via Natural or Artificial Opening Endoscopic	Open	Percutaneous Endoscopic
Prostate	ØVTØØZZ	ØVTØ4ZZ	ØVTØ7ZZ	ØVTØ8ZZ	ØVT3ØZZ	ØVT34ZZ

DRG 734-735 Pelvic Evisceration, Radical Hysterectomy and Radical Vulvectomy

Code as appropriate the procedures performed

Procedure	Resection by Site								Code also as appropriate Excision of Inguinal Lymph Nodes by approach	
	Bladder	Cervix	Fallopian Tubes, Bilateral	Ovaries, Bilateral	Urethra	Uterus	Vagina	Vulva	Right	Left
Radical Vulvectomy	—	—	—	—	—	—	—	ØUTM[Ø,X]ZZ	Ø7BH[Ø,4]ZZ	Ø7BJ[Ø,4]ZZ
Pelvic Evisceration	ØTTBØZZ	ØUTCØZZ	ØUT7ØZZ	ØUT2ØZZ	ØTTDØZZ	ØUT9ØZZ	ØUTGØZZ	—	—	—

Radical Hysterectomy	Resection by Site		
	Cervix	Uterus	Uterine Support Structure
Vaginal	ØUTC[7,8]ZZ	ØUT9[7,8]ZZ	ØUT4[7,8]ZZ
Abdominal, Endoscopic	ØUTC4ZZ	ØUT9[4,F]ZZ	ØUT44ZZ
Abdominal, Open	ØUTCØZZ	ØUT9ØZZ	ØUT4ØZZ

DRG 895-897 Alcohol/Drug Abuse or Dependence

	Substance Abuse Treatment	Code also as appropriate Counseling by type	
		Individual	Group
Detoxification from alcohol and/or drugs	HZ2ZZZZ	HZ3[Ø,1,2,3,4,5,6,7,8,9,B]ZZZ	HZ4[Ø,1,2,3,4,5,6,7,8,9,B]ZZZ

DRG 9Ø7-9Ø9 Other Procedures for Injuries

Insertion of Generator and Lead(s) Only

Generator Type	Insertion of Generator by Site		Code also as appropriate Insertion of Cardiac Leads by Site		
	Chest	Abdomen	Coronary Vein	Atrium	Ventricle
Single Chamber	ØJH6[Ø,3]4Z	ØJH8[Ø,3]4Z	Ø2H4[Ø,4][J,M]Z	Ø2H[6,7][Ø,4][J,M]Z or Ø2H[6,7]3JZ	Ø2H[K,L][Ø,3,4][J,M]Z
Single Chamber RR	ØJH6[Ø,3]5Z	ØJH8[Ø,3]5Z	Ø2H4[Ø,4][J,M]Z	Ø2H[6,7][Ø,4][J,M]Z or Ø2H[6,7]3JZ	Ø2H[K,L][Ø,3,4][J,M]Z
Dual Chamber	ØJH6[Ø,3]6Z	ØJH8[Ø,3]6Z	—	—	Ø2H[K,L]3JZ
Cardiac Resynch Pacemaker Pulse Generator	ØJH6[Ø,3]7Z	ØJH8[Ø,3]7Z	Ø2H4[Ø,3,4][J,M]Z or Ø2H43KZ	Ø2H[6,7][Ø,3,4][J,M]Z	Ø2H[K,L][Ø,3,4][J,M]Z
Cardiac Rhythm Related	ØJH6[Ø,3]PZ	ØJH8[Ø,3]PZ	Ø2H4[Ø,4][J,M]Z	Ø2H[6,7][Ø,3,4][J,M]Z	Ø2H[K,L][Ø,3,4][J,M]Z

DRG 907-909 Other Procedures for Injuries *(Continued)*

Insertion of Generator and Lead(s) into the Coronary Vein, Atrium or Ventricle With Removal of Cardiac Rhythm Device

Generator Type	Insertion of Generator by Site		Code also as appropriate Insertion of Cardiac Leads by site			Code also
	Chest	Abdomen	Coronary Vein	Atrium	Ventricle	Removal Cardiac Rhythm Device
Single Chamber	ØJH6[Ø,3]4Z	ØJH8[Ø,3]4Z	Ø2H4[Ø,4][J,M]Z	Ø2H[6,7][Ø,3,4][J,M]Z	Ø2H[K,L][Ø,3,4][J,M]Z	ØJPT[Ø,3]PZ
Single Chamber RR	ØJH6[Ø,3]5Z	ØJH8[Ø,3]5Z	Ø2H4[Ø,4][J,M]Z	Ø2H[6,7][Ø,3,4][J,M]Z	Ø2H[K,L][Ø,3,4][J,M]Z	ØJPT[Ø,3]PZ
Dual Chamber	ØJH6[Ø,3]6Z	ØJH8[Ø,3]6Z	Ø2H4[Ø,4][J,M]Z	Ø2H[6,7][Ø,3,4][J,M]Z	Ø2H[K,L][Ø,3,4][J,M]Z	ØJPT[Ø,3]PZ

Insertion of Generator and Lead(s) into the Pericardium With or Without Removal of Cardiac Rhythm Device

Generator Type	Insertion of Generator by Site		Code also as appropriate Insertion of Leads by type		If Performed –Code also
			Pericardium		
	Chest	Abdomen	Pacemaker	Cardiac	Removal Cardiac Rhythm Device
Single Chamber	ØJH6[Ø,3]4Z	ØJH8[Ø,3]4Z	Ø2HN[Ø,3,4]JZ	Ø2HN[Ø,3,4]MZ	ØJPT[Ø,3]PZ
Single Chamber RR	ØJH6[Ø,3]5Z	ØJH8[Ø,3]5Z	Ø2HN[Ø,3,4]JZ	Ø2HN[Ø,3,4]MZ	ØJPT[Ø,3]PZ
Dual Chamber	ØJH6[Ø,3]6Z	ØJH8[Ø,3]6Z	Ø2HN[Ø,3,4]JZ	Ø2HN[Ø,3,4]MZ	ØJPT[Ø,3]PZ
Cardiac Resynch Pacemaker Pulse Generator	ØJH6[Ø,3]7Z	ØJH8[Ø,3]7Z	Ø2HN[Ø,3,4]JZ	Ø2HN[Ø,3,4]MZ	—
Cardiac Rhythm Related	ØJH6[Ø,3]PZ	ØJH8[Ø,3]PZ	Ø2HN[Ø,3,4]JZ	Ø2HN[Ø,3,4]MZ	—

Insertion of Generator and Lead(s) With Removal of Cardiac Rhythm Device and Leads

Generator Type	Insertion of Generator by Site		Code also as appropriate Insertion of Cardiac Leads by Site		Code also	
	Chest	Abdomen	Atrium	Ventricle	Removal of Cardiac Rhythm Device	Removal of Heart Lead
Single Chamber	ØJH6[Ø,3]4Z	ØJH8[Ø,3]4Z	Ø2H[6,7]3JZ	Ø2H[K,L]3JZ	ØJPT[Ø,3]PZ	Ø2PA[Ø,3,4,X]MZ
Single Chamber RR	ØJH6[Ø,3]5Z	ØJH8[Ø,3]5Z	Ø2H[6,7]3JZ	Ø2H[K,L]3JZ	ØJPT[Ø,3]PZ	Ø2PA[Ø,3,4,X]MZ
Dual Chamber	ØJH6[Ø,3]6Z	ØJH8[Ø,3]6Z	Ø2H[6,7]3JZ	Ø2H[K,L]3JZ	ØJPT[Ø,3]PZ	Ø2PA[Ø,3,4,X]MZ
Cardiac Resynch Pacemaker Pulse Generator	ØJH6[Ø,3]7Z	ØJH8[Ø,3]7Z	Ø2H[6,7]3JZ	Ø2H[K,L]3JZ	—	Ø2PA[Ø,3,4,X]MZ
Cardiac Rhythm Related	ØJH6[Ø,3]PZ	ØJH8[Ø,3]PZ	Ø2H[6,7]3JZ	Ø2H[K,L]3JZ	—	Ø2PA[Ø,3,4,X]MZ

Non-OR procedure combinations

Note: The following table identifies procedure combinations that are considered Non-OR even though one or more procedures of the combination are considered valid DRG OR procedures

Dilation With Removal of Intraluminal Device.

Approach	Code as appropriate Dilation by Site					Code also as appropriate Removal of Intraluminal Device by Site	
	Hepatic Duct, Right	Hepatic Duct, Left	Cystic Duct	Common Bile Duct	Pancreatic Duct	Hepatobiliary Duct	Pancreatic Duct
Via Natural or Artificial Opening	ØF757DZ	ØF767DZ	ØF787DZ	ØF797DZ	ØF7D7DZ	ØFPB7DZ	ØFPD7DZ
Via Natural or Artificial Opening Endoscopic	ØF758DZ	ØF768DZ	ØF788DZ	ØF798DZ	ØF7D8DZ	ØFPB8DZ	ØFPD8DZ

Insertion With Removal of Intraluminal Device

Approach	Code as appropriate Insertion of Intraluminal Device into Hepatobiliary Duct	Code also as appropriate Removal of Intraluminal Device by Site	
		Hepatobiliary Duct	Pancreatic Duct
Via Natural or Artificial Opening	ØFHB7DZ	ØFPB7DZ	ØFPD7DZ
Via Natural or Artificial Opening Endoscopic	ØFHB8DZ	ØFPB8DZ	ØFPD8DZ

Insertion With Removal of Intraluminal Device

Approach	Code as appropriate Insertion of Intraluminal Device into Hepatobiliary Duct	Code also as appropriate Removal of Intraluminal Device by Site	
		Hepatobiliary Duct	Pancreatic Duct
Via Natural or Artificial Opening	ØFHB7DZ	—	—
External	—	ØFPBXDZ	ØFPDXDZ

Appendix J: Administration/Substance Key

This key classifies substances listed by trade name or synonym to a PCS character in the Administration section indicated in the sixth-character Substance or seventh-character Qualifier column.

Trade Name or Synonym	PCS Substance Category
AIGISRx Antibacterial Envelope	Anti-Infective Envelope
Antimicrobial envelope	Anti-Infective Envelope
Bone morphogenetic protein 2 (BMP 2)	Recombinant Bone Morphogenetic Protein
Clolar	Clofarabine
Kcentra	4-Factor Prothrombin Complex Concentrate
Nesiritide	Human B-type Natriutretic Peptide
rhBMP-2	Recombinant Bone Morphogenetic Protein
Seprafilm	Adhesion Barrier
Tissue Plasminogen Activator (tPA)(r-tPA)	Other Thrombolytic
Voraxaze	Glucarpidase
Zyvox	Oxazolidinones

Appendix K: Illustrations

Peripheral Nervous System

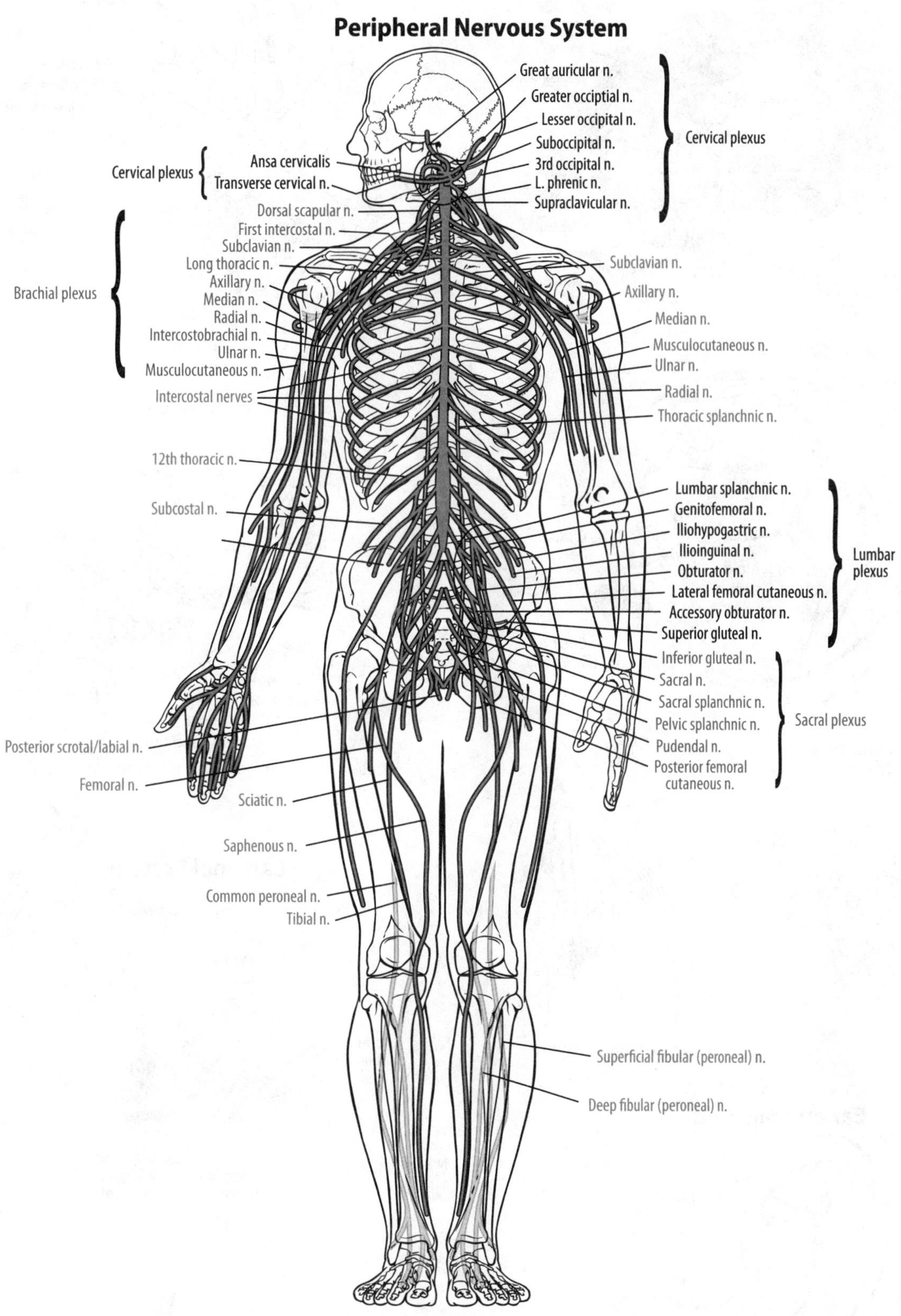

Brain

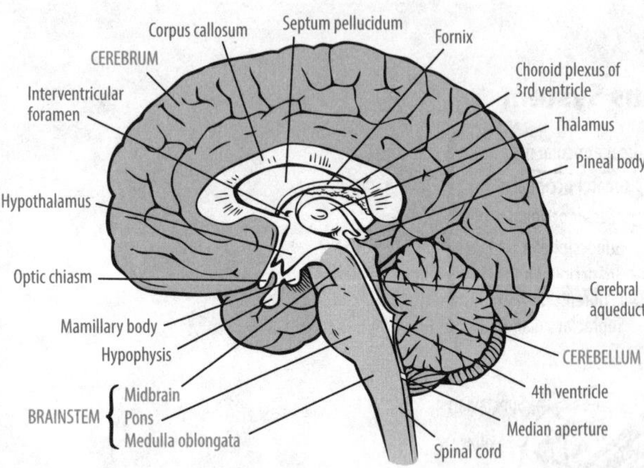

Cranial Nerves

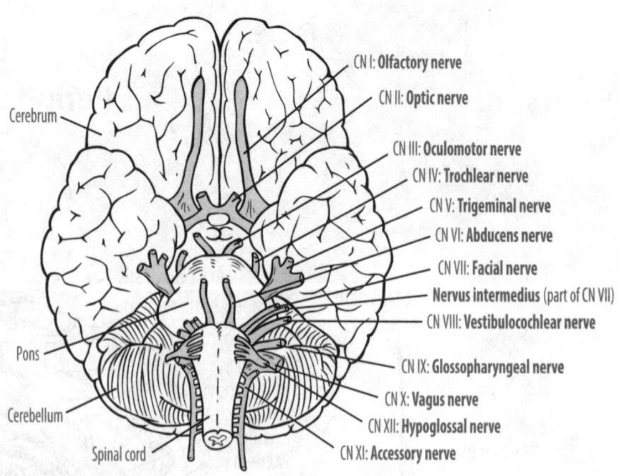

Eye

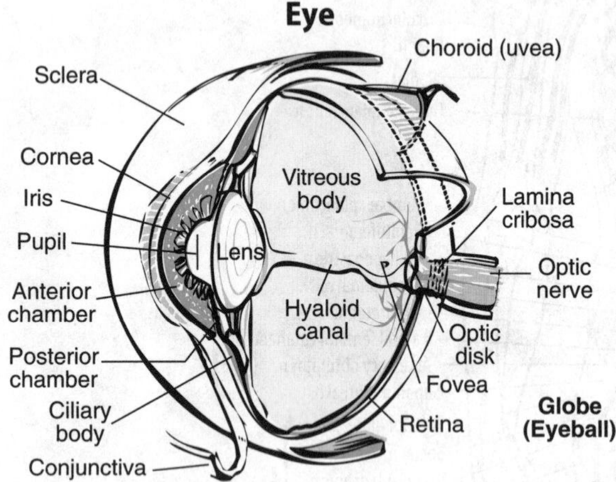

Middle Ear

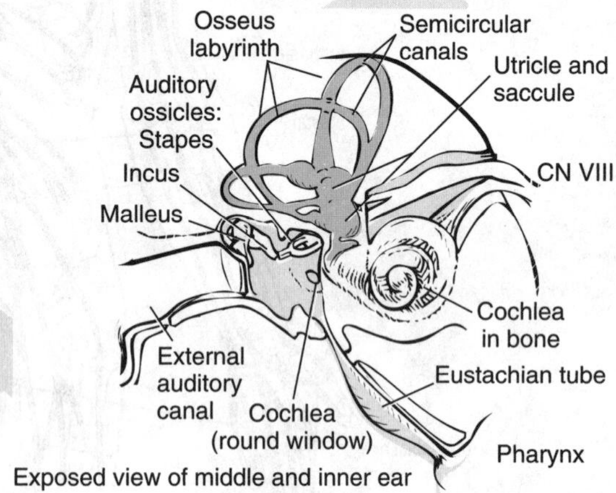

Exposed view of middle and inner ear

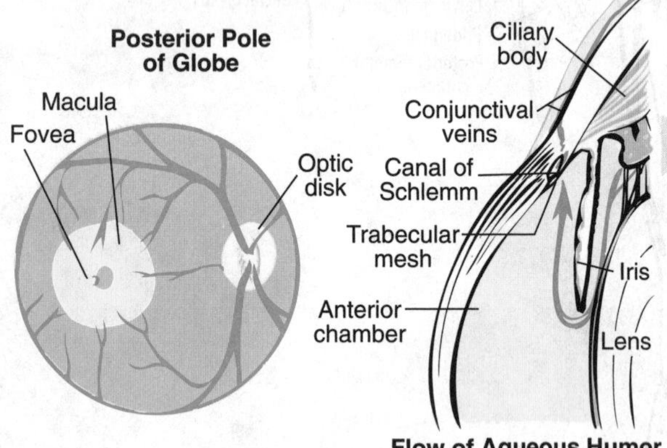

Flow of Aqueous Humor

Lacrimal System

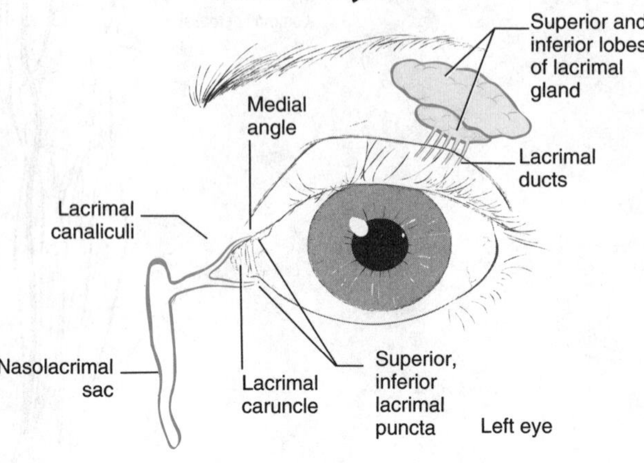

Ear and Mastoid

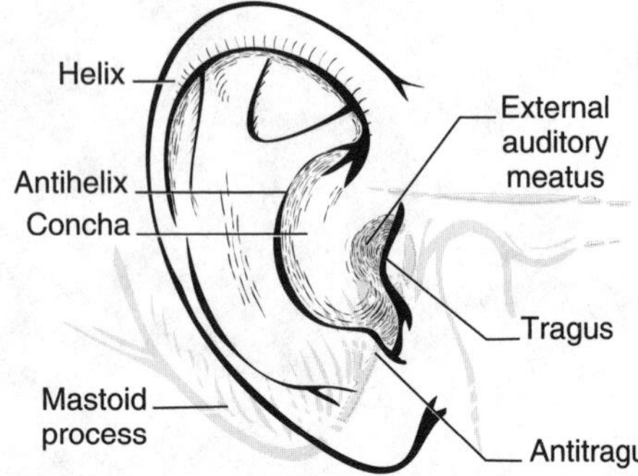

Arteries

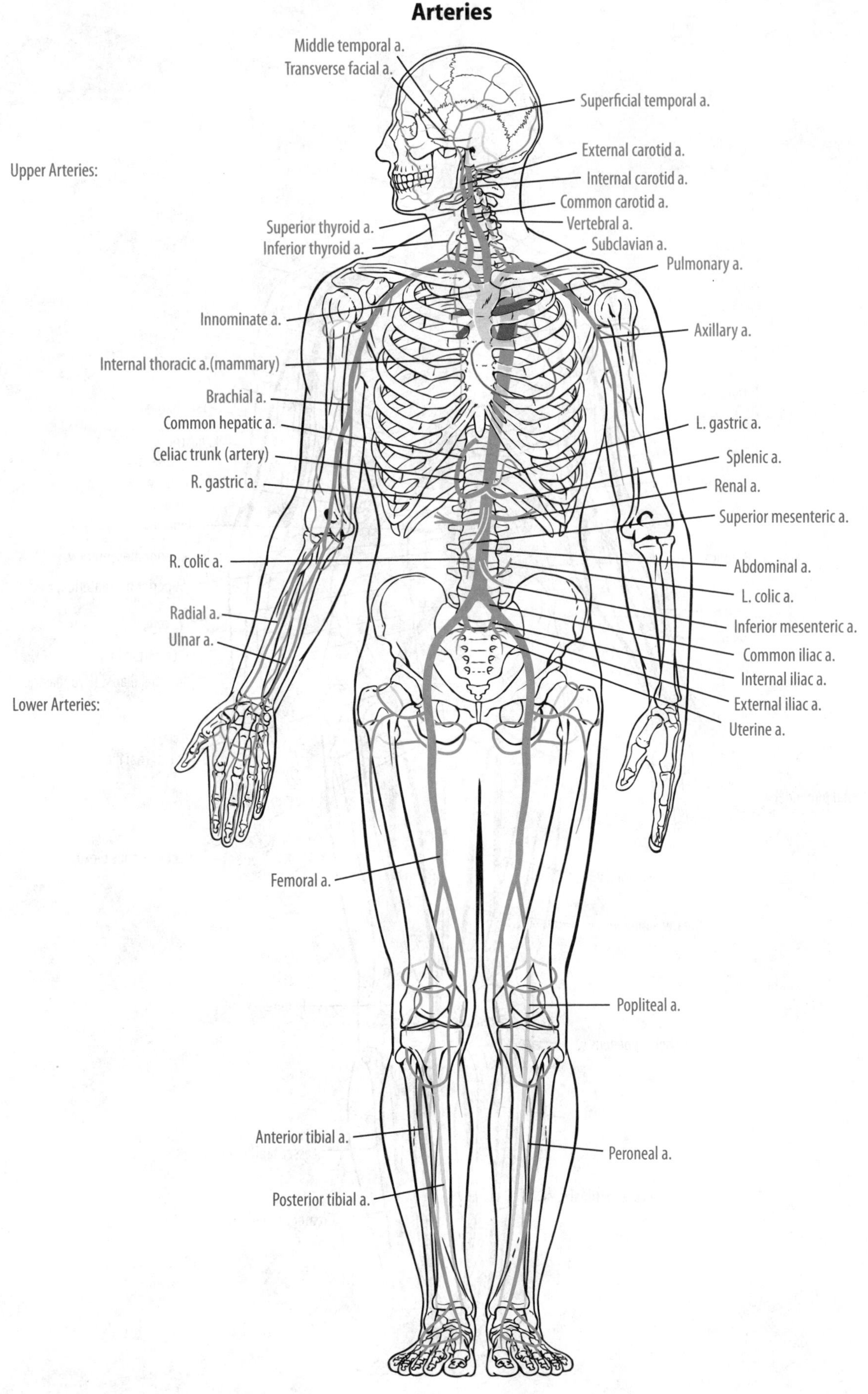

Middle temporal a.
Transverse facial a.
Superficial temporal a.
Upper Arteries:
External carotid a.
Internal carotid a.
Common carotid a.
Superior thyroid a.
Vertebral a.
Inferior thyroid a.
Subclavian a.
Pulmonary a.
Innominate a.
Axillary a.
Internal thoracic a.(mammary)
Brachial a.
Common hepatic a.
L. gastric a.
Celiac trunk (artery)
Splenic a.
R. gastric a.
Renal a.
Superior mesenteric a.
R. colic a.
Abdominal a.
L. colic a.
Radial a.
Inferior mesenteric a.
Ulnar a.
Common iliac a.
Internal iliac a.
Lower Arteries:
External iliac a.
Uterine a.
Femoral a.
Popliteal a.
Anterior tibial a.
Peroneal a.
Posterior tibial a.

Veins

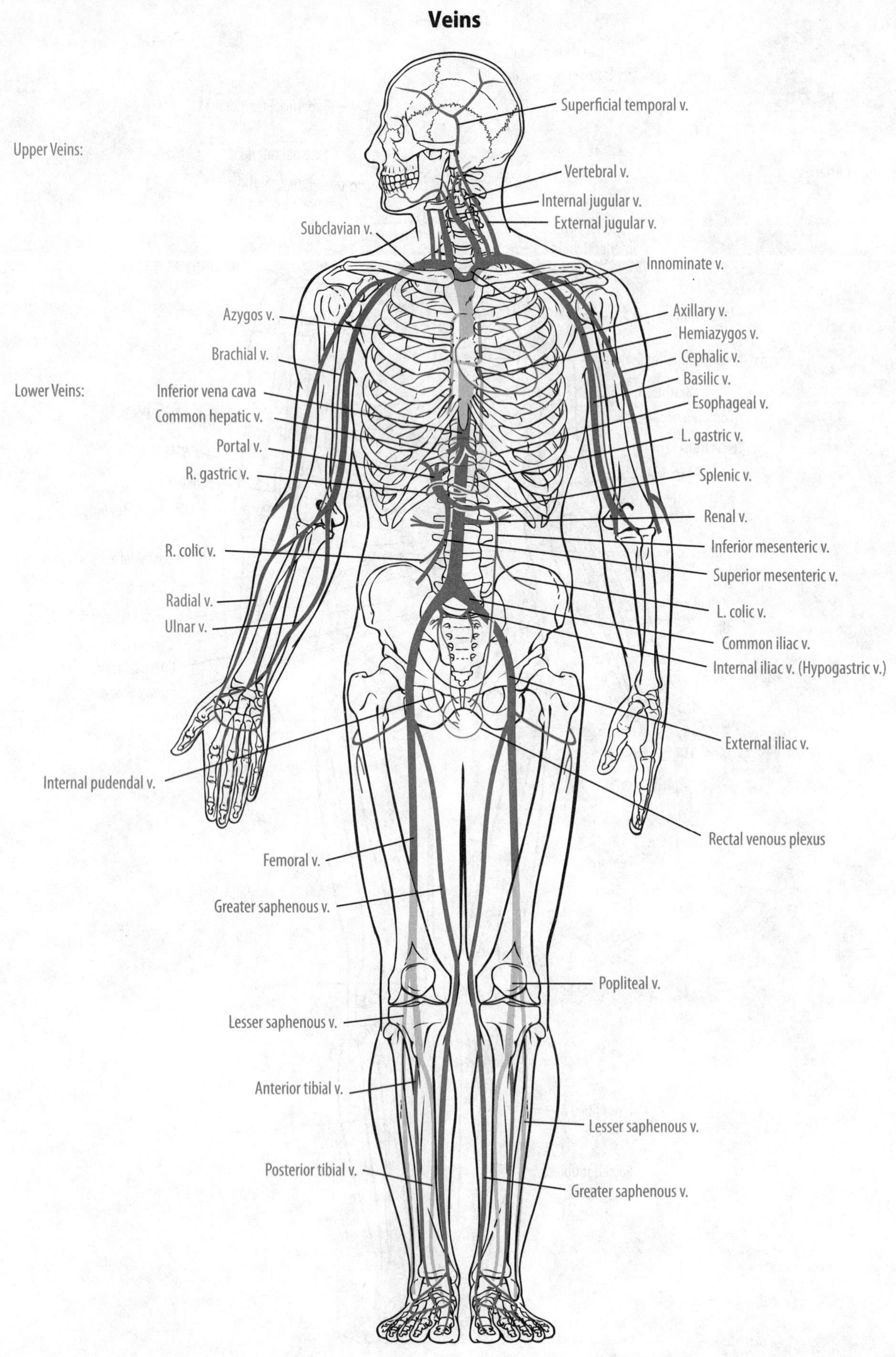
Upper Veins:
Lower Veins:
Superficial temporal v.
Vertebral v.
Internal jugular v.
External jugular v.
Subclavian v.
Innominate v.
Azygos v.
Axillary v.
Hemiazygos v.
Brachial v.
Cephalic v.
Basilic v.
Inferior vena cava
Esophageal v.
Common hepatic v.
L. gastric v.
Portal v.
R. gastric v.
Splenic v.
Renal v.
R. colic v.
Inferior mesenteric v.
Superior mesenteric v.
Radial v.
L. colic v.
Ulnar v.
Common iliac v.
Internal iliac v. (Hypogastric v.)
External iliac v.
Internal pudendal v.
Rectal venous plexus
Femoral v.
Greater saphenous v.
Popliteal v.
Lesser saphenous v.
Anterior tibial v.
Lesser saphenous v.
Posterior tibial v.
Greater saphenous v.

Anatomy of Heart

Superior vena cava
Aorta
Pulmonary artery
Pulmonary vein
Aortic valve
Pulmonary valve
Right atrium
Left atrium
Tricuspid valve
Mitral valve
Right ventricle
Chorda tendinae
Inferior vena cava
Left ventricle

Arteries of Heart

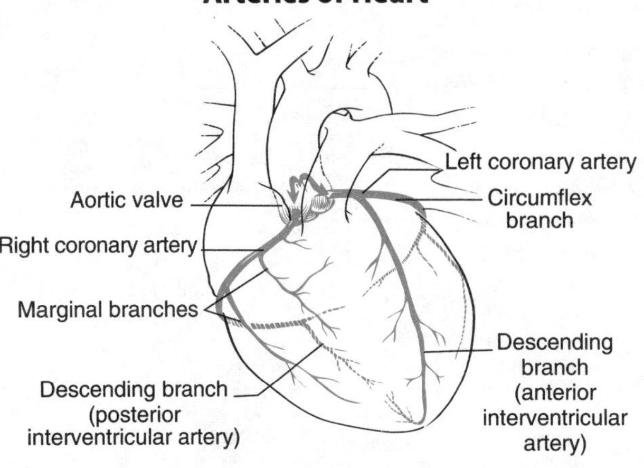

Cerebrovascular Arteries

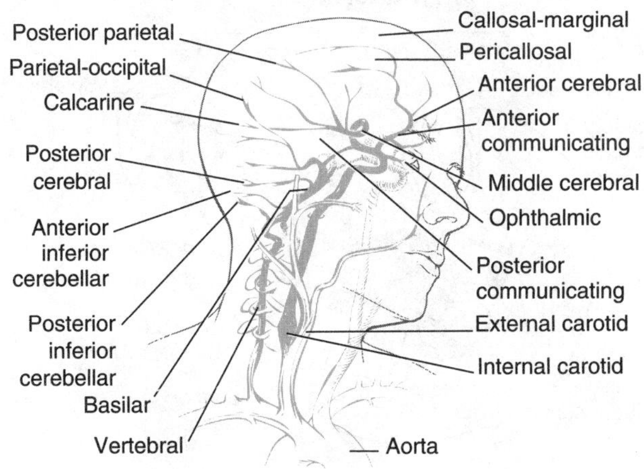

Veins of Head and Neck

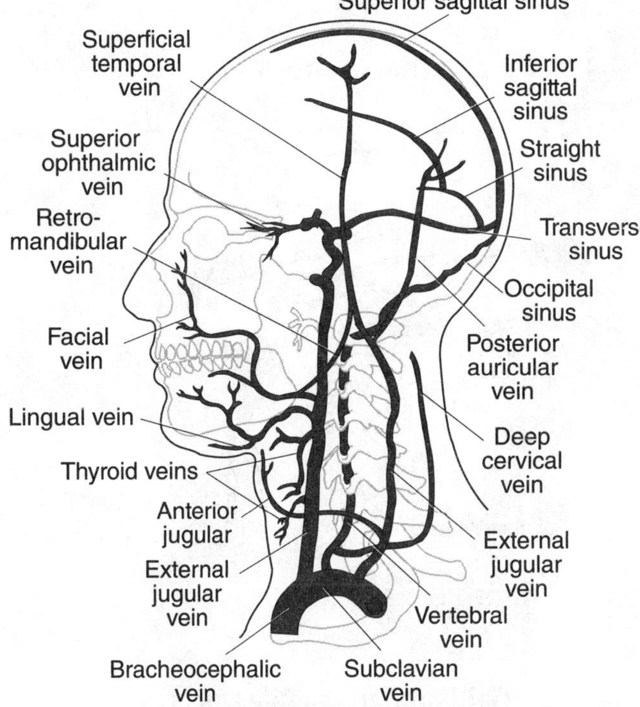

Lymphatic System of Head and Neck

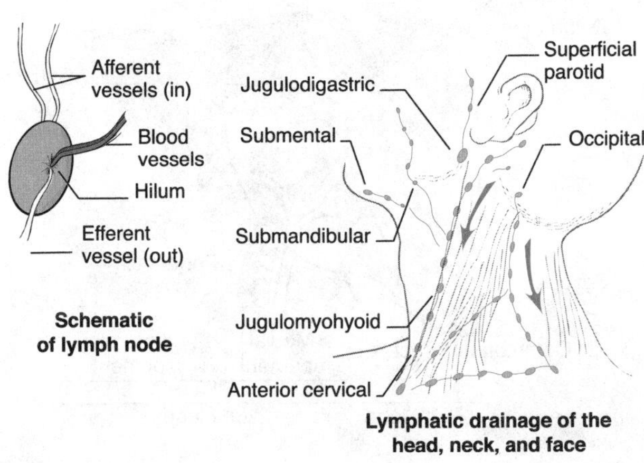

Lymph Nodes

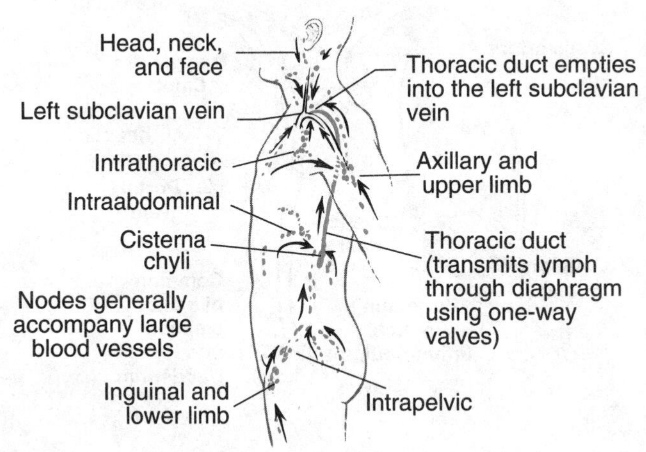

Respiratory System

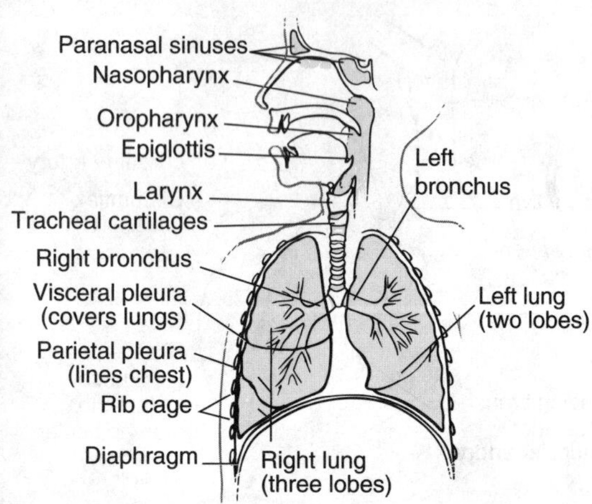

Paranasal Sinuses

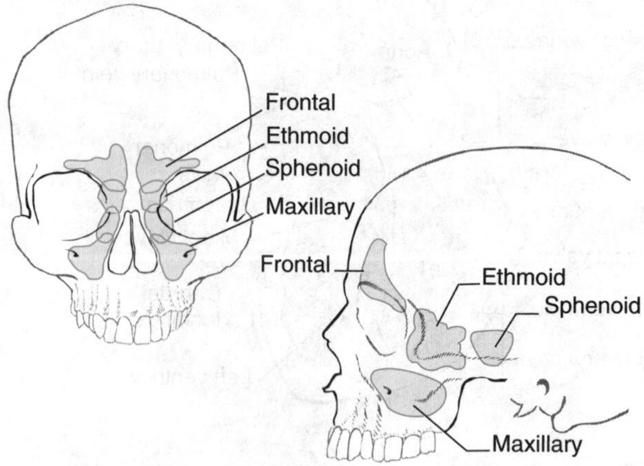

Oral Cavity

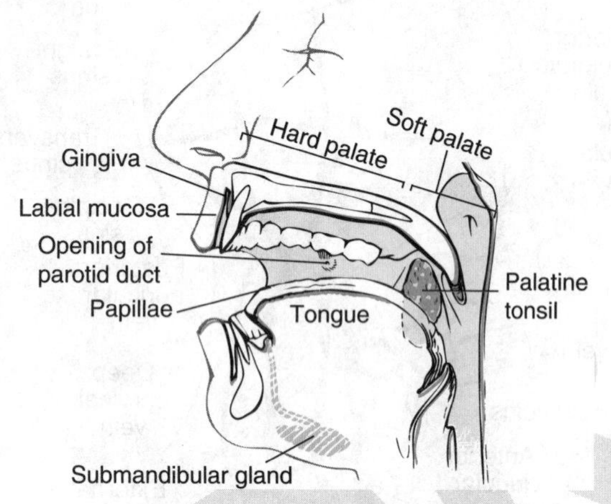

Pancreas

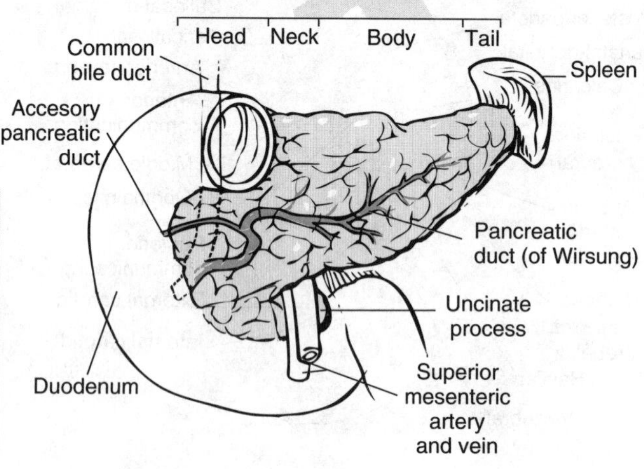

Gallbladder and Bile Ducts

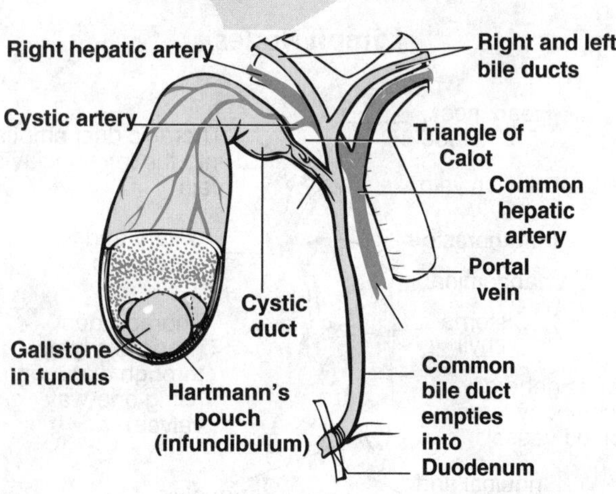

Liver

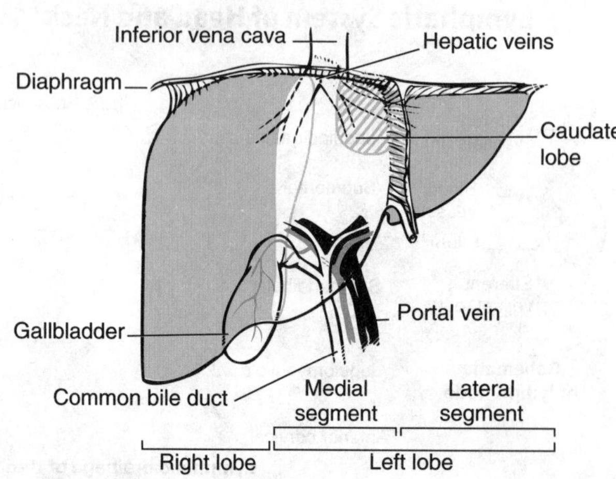

Gastrointestinal System

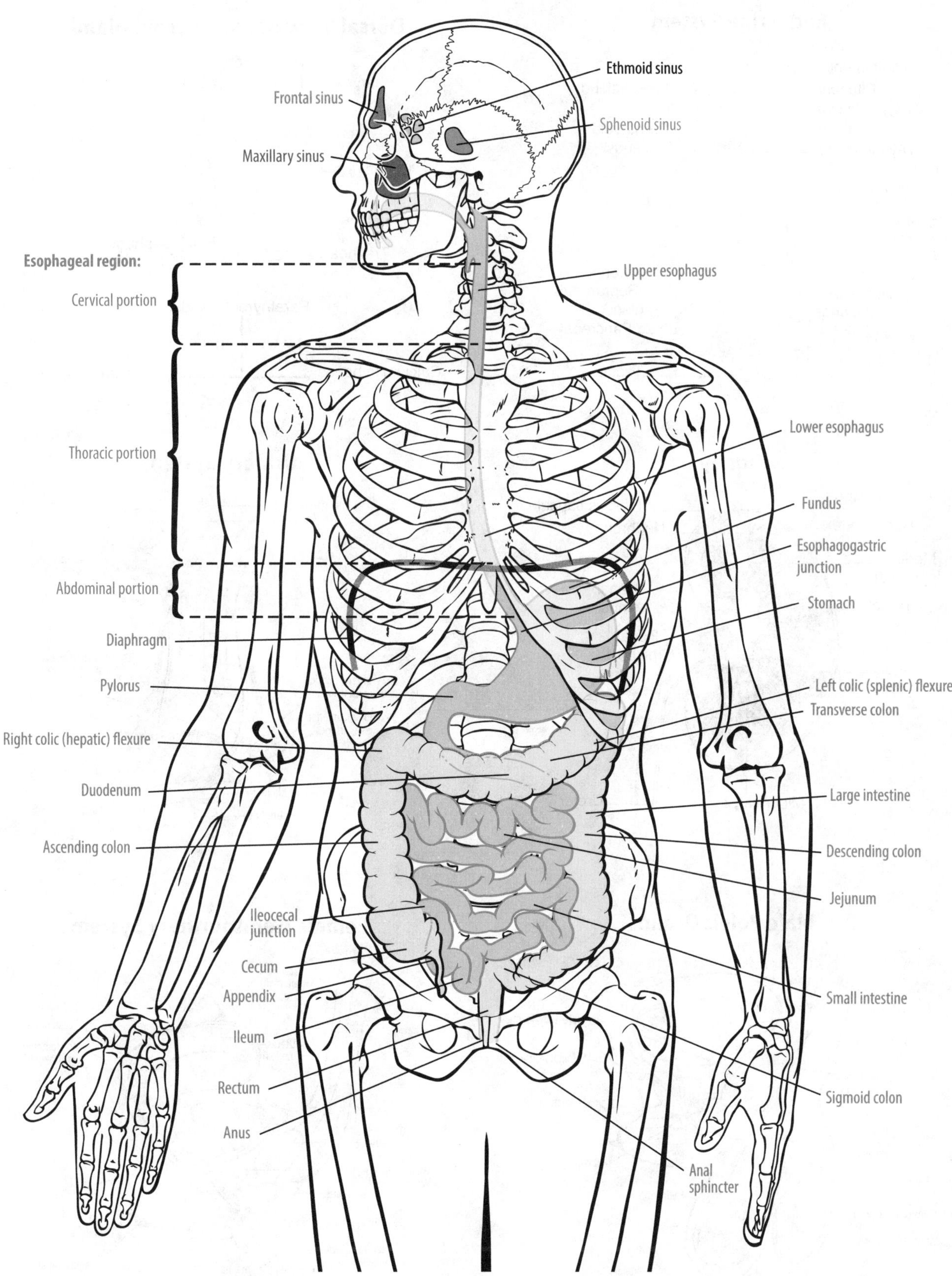

Endocrine System

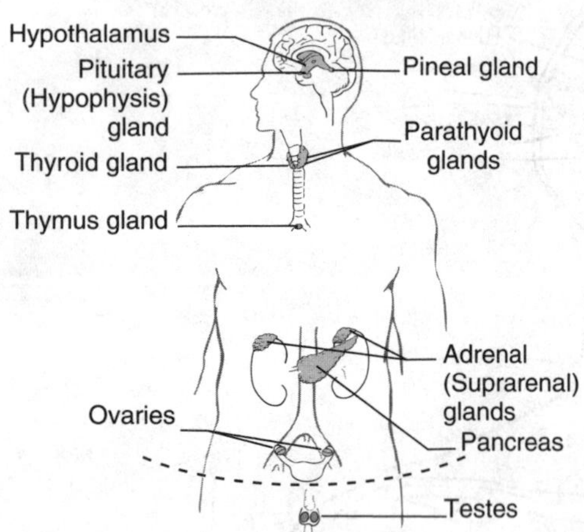

Dorsal View of Parathyroid Gland

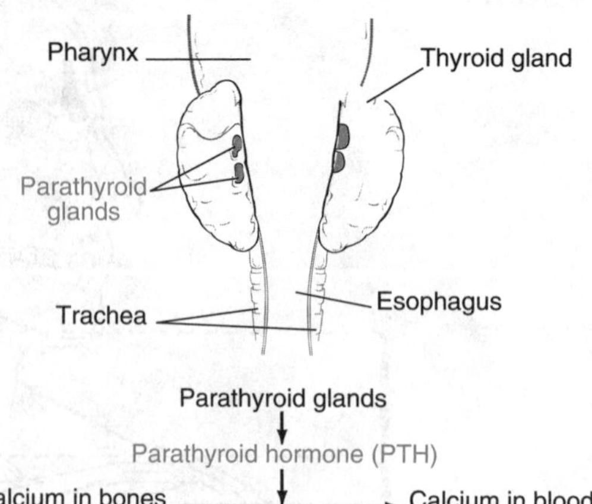

Kidney

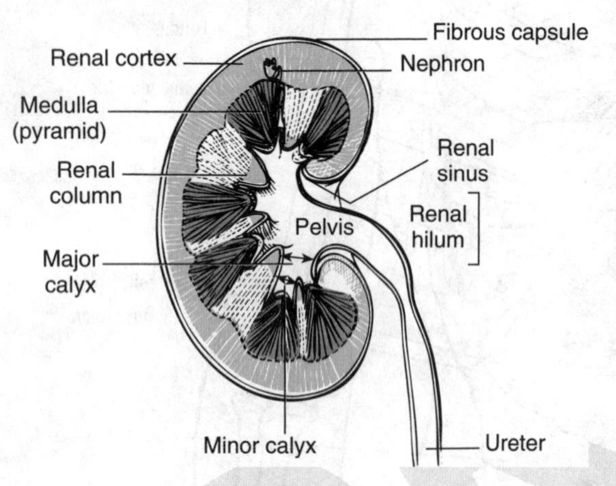

Urinary System

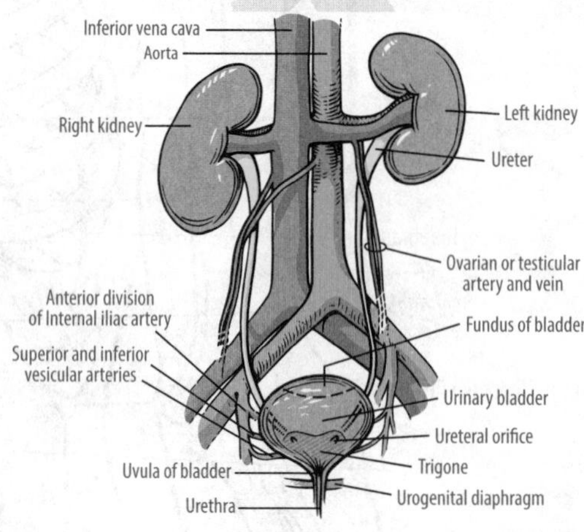

Male Pelvic Organs

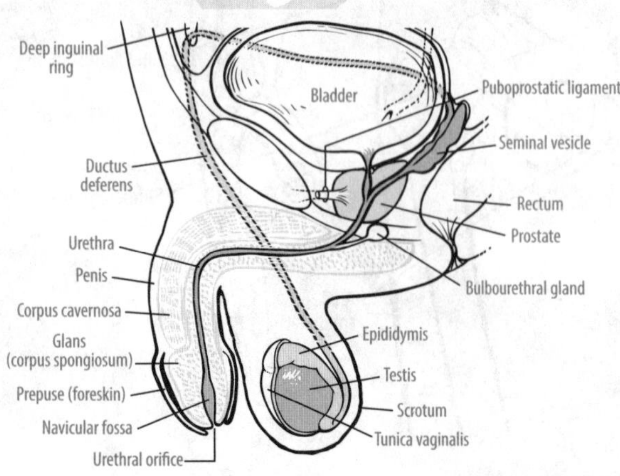

Female Genitourinary System

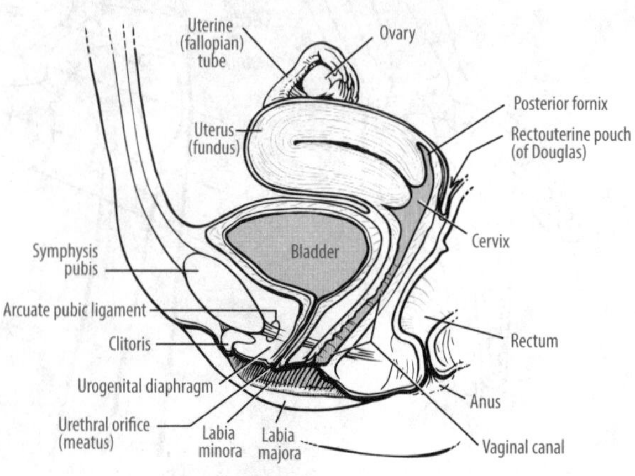

Joints

Shoulder (Anterior View)

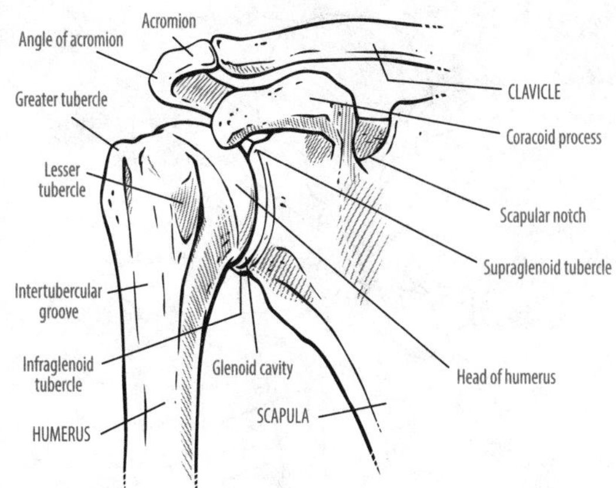

Shoulder (Posterior View)

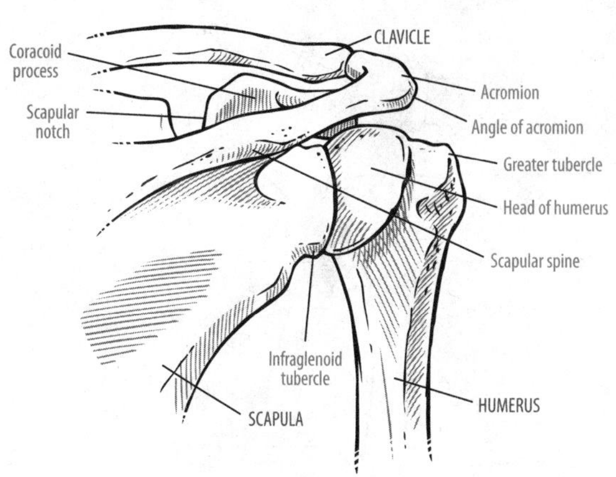

Elbow (Anterior View)

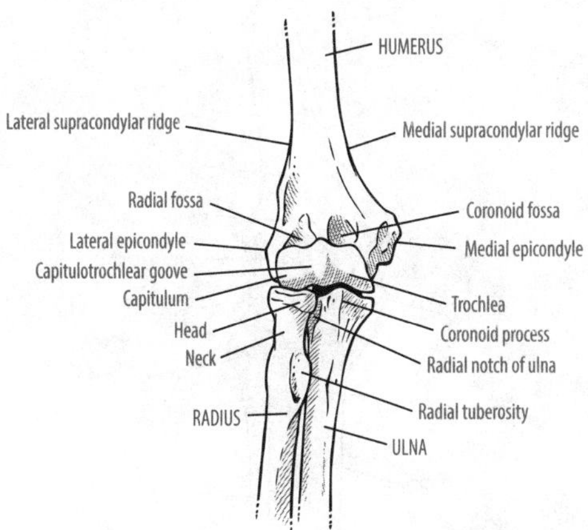

Elbow (Posterior View)

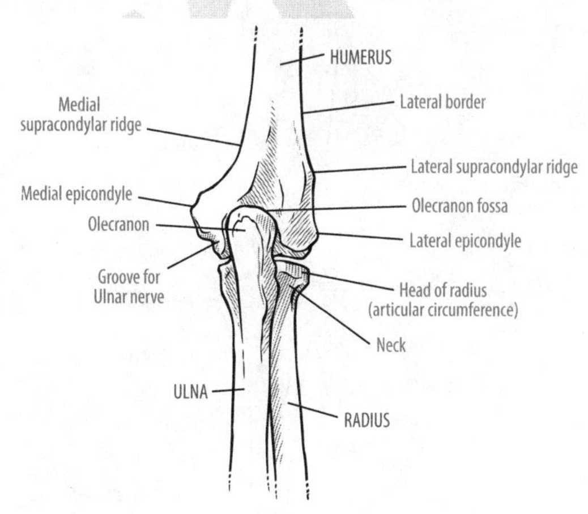

Hand

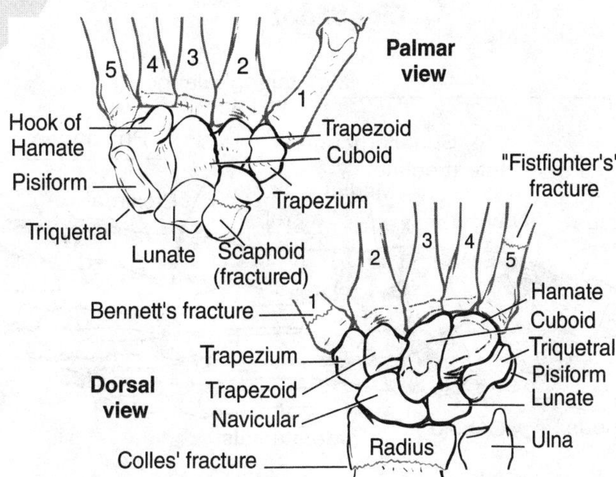

Joints

Hip (Anterior View)

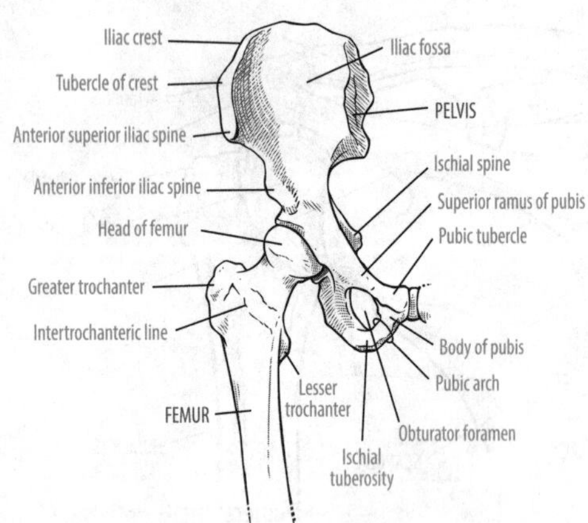

Hip (Posterior View)

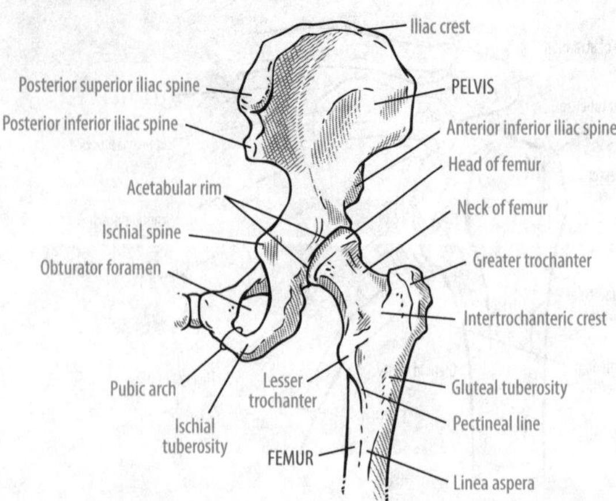

Knee (Anterior View)

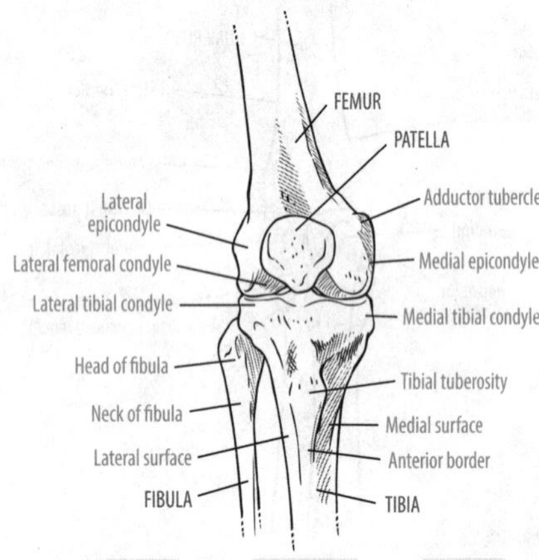

Knee (Posterior View)

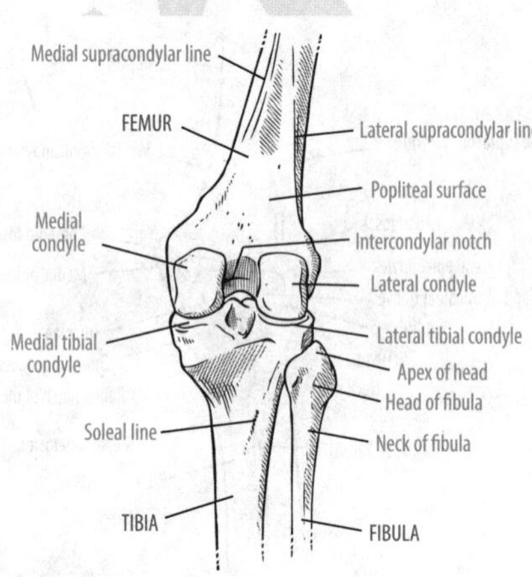

Right Foot

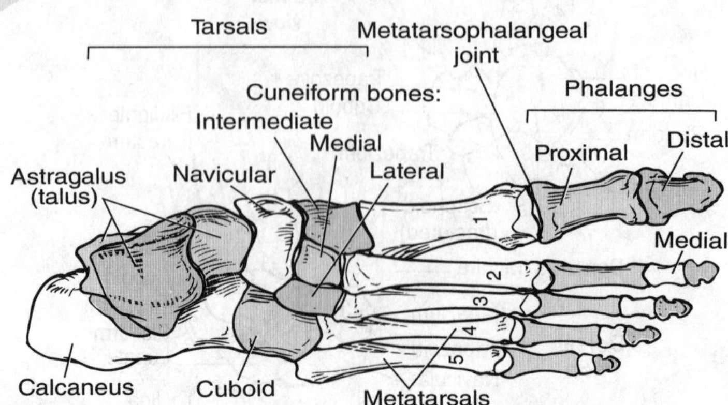

Bones/Joints

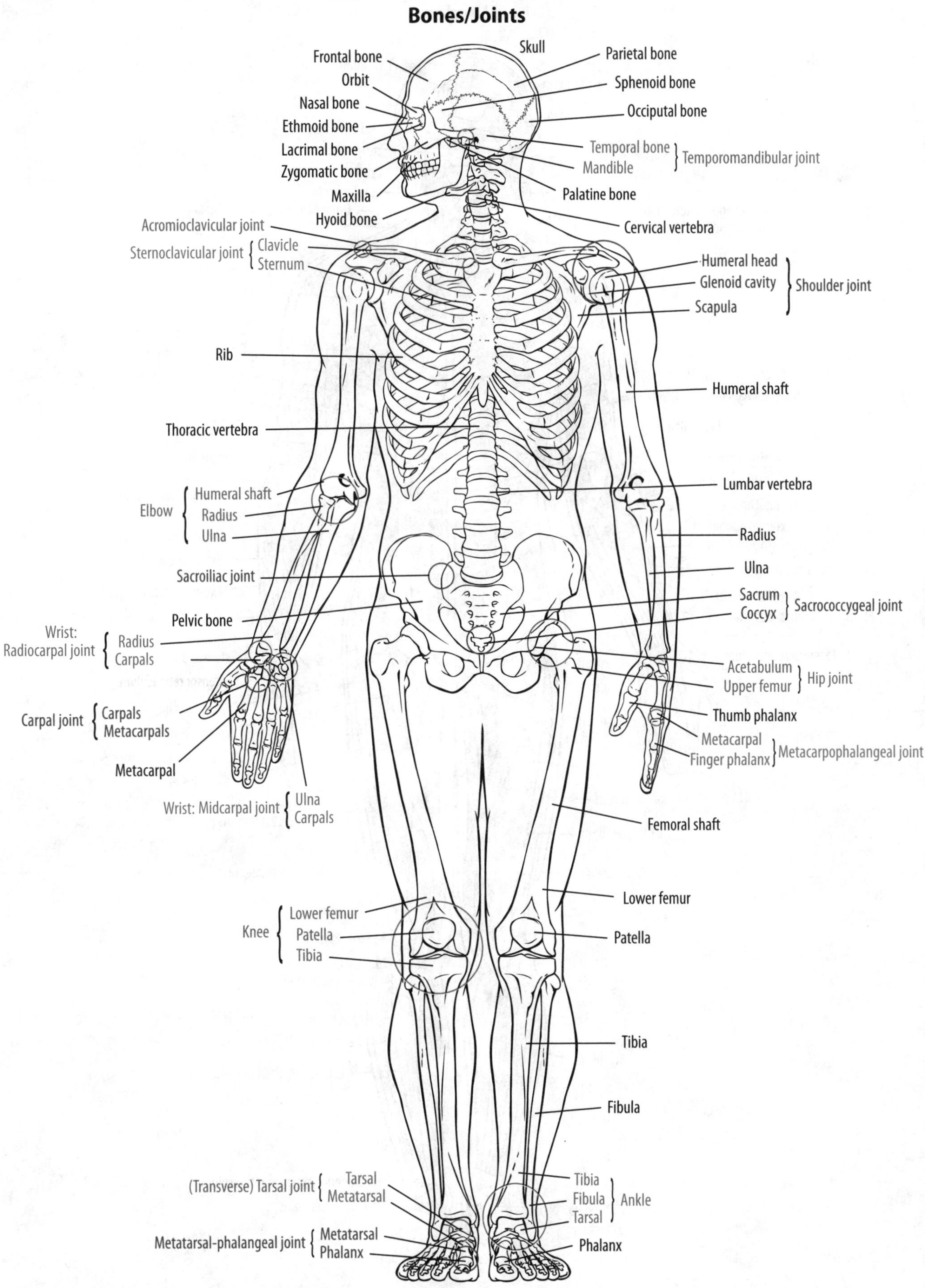

Muscles

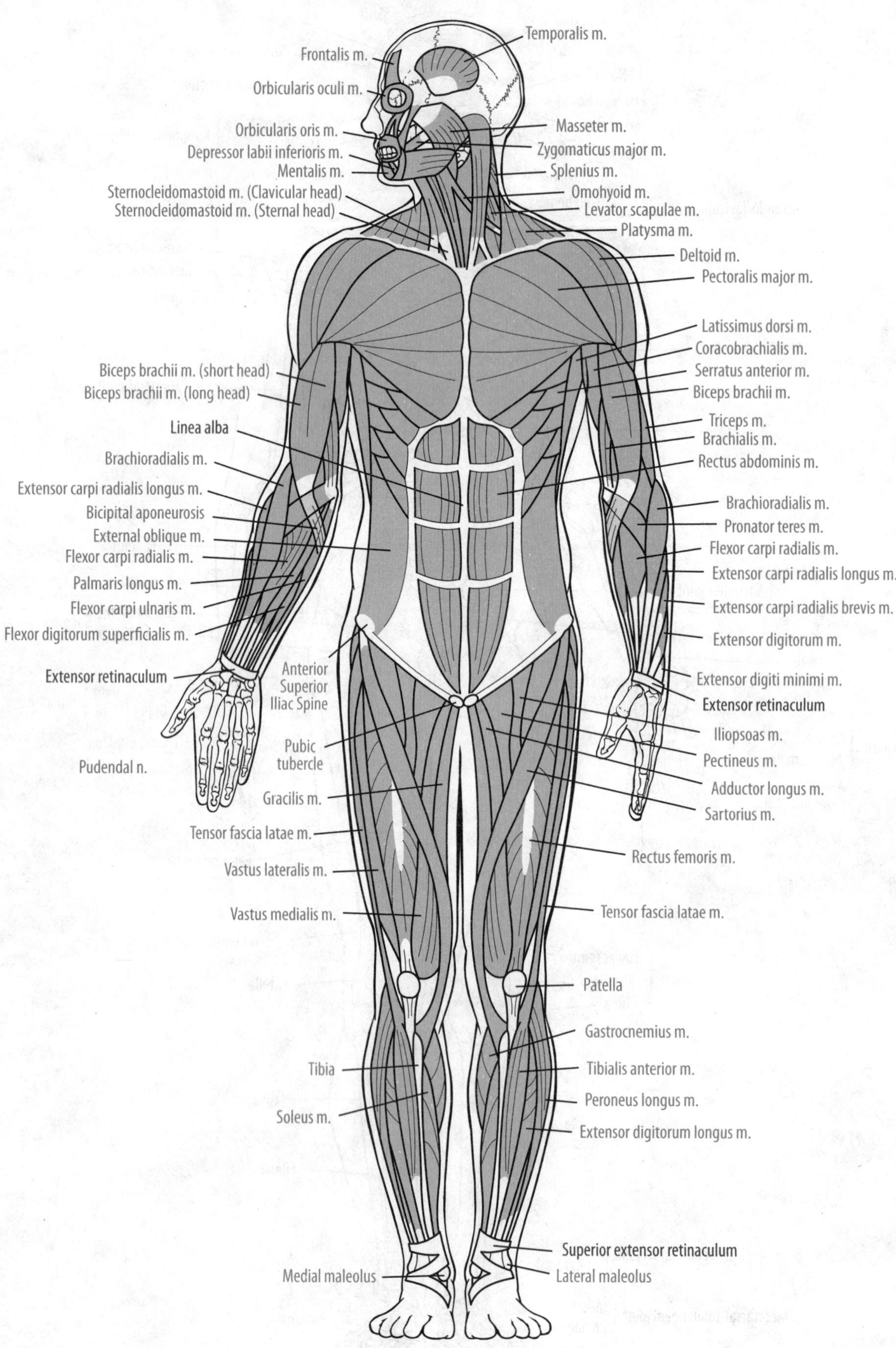
Temporalis m.
Frontalis m.
Orbicularis oculi m.
Masseter m.
Orbicularis oris m.
Zygomaticus major m.
Depressor labii inferioris m.
Mentalis m.
Splenius m.
Sternocleidomastoid m. (Clavicular head)
Omohyoid m.
Sternocleidomastoid m. (Sternal head)
Levator scapulae m.
Platysma m.
Deltoid m.
Pectoralis major m.
Latissimus dorsi m.
Coracobrachialis m.
Biceps brachii m. (short head)
Serratus anterior m.
Biceps brachii m. (long head)
Biceps brachii m.
Triceps m.
Linea alba
Brachialis m.
Brachioradialis m.
Rectus abdominis m.
Extensor carpi radialis longus m.
Brachioradialis m.
Bicipital aponeurosis
Pronator teres m.
External oblique m.
Flexor carpi radialis m.
Flexor carpi radialis m.
Extensor carpi radialis longus m.
Palmaris longus m.
Flexor carpi ulnaris m.
Extensor carpi radialis brevis m.
Flexor digitorum superficialis m.
Extensor digitorum m.
Anterior Superior Iliac Spine
Extensor retinaculum
Extensor digiti minimi m.
Extensor retinaculum
Iliopsoas m.
Pubic tubercle
Pectineus m.
Pudendal n.
Adductor longus m.
Gracilis m.
Sartorius m.
Tensor fascia latae m.
Rectus femoris m.
Vastus lateralis m.
Vastus medialis m.
Tensor fascia latae m.
Patella
Gastrocnemius m.
Tibia
Tibialis anterior m.
Peroneus longus m.
Soleus m.
Extensor digitorum longus m.
Superior extensor retinaculum
Medial maleolus
Lateral maleolus